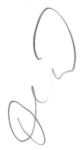

Comprehensive Management of Skull Base Tumors

Second Edition

Ehab Y. Hanna, MD, FACS
Professor, Vice Chairman, and Director of
    Skull Base Surgery
Department of Head and Neck Surgery
Medical Director, Head and Neck Center
University of Texas MD Anderson Cancer
    Center
Houston, Texas

Franco DeMonte, MD, FRCSC, FACS
Mary Beth Pawelek Chair in Neurosurgery
Professor of Neurosurgery and Head and
    Neck Surgery
Director, David C. Nicholson Microsurgical
    and Endoscopic Center for Clinical
    Applications Laboratory
Director, Skull Base Program
Department of Neurosurgery
University of Texas MD Anderson Cancer
    Center
Houston, Texas

LIBRARY OF
CONGRESS
SURPLUS
DUPLICATE

1688 illustrations

Thieme
New York • Stuttgart • Delhi • Rio de Janeiro

Library of Congress Cataloging-in-Publication Data is available with the publisher.

Thieme Medical Publishers, Inc.
333 Seventh Avenue, New York, NY 10001 USA
+1 800 782 3488, customerservice@thieme.com

Cover design: Thieme Publishing Group
Cover illustration by Ian Suk © Franco DeMonte,
    Department of Neurosurgery, University of Texas,
    MD Anderson Cancer Center
Typesetting by TNQ Technologies, India

Printed in USA by King Printing Company, Inc.

ISBN 978-1-62623-532-8

Also available as an e-book:
eISBN 978-1-62623-533-5

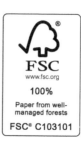

This book is dedicated to
My Wife, Sylvie,
For her grace, sacrifice, and support;
Our daughters, Gabrielle Grace "Gigi" Hanna and Camille Lauren Hanna,
For the joy and blessing they bring to our lives;
My parents
Who encouraged me to follow my dreams;
My Mentors
Who inspired me to pursue excellence;
My fellows, residents, and students,
Who continue to teach me;
And my patients,
Whose endurance, resilience, and faith continue to amaze me.

– Ehab Y. Hanna, MD, FACS

Dedicated to Paula, with love and thanks!

– Franco DeMonte, MD, FRCSC, FACS

Contents

Section I: General Principles

Carolina Martins, Georgios A. Zenonos, Ezequiel Goldschmidt, Juan C. Fernandez-Miranda, and Albert L. Rhoton Jr.[†]

Diana Bell, Gregory N. Fuller, and Adel K. El-Naggar

[†]Deceased

Contents

†Deceased

Contents

13   Cerebrovascular Management in Skull Base Tumors 220

Anoop P. Patel, Sabareesh K. Natarajan, Basavaraj Ghodke, and Laligam N. Sekhar

14   Quality of Life and Measures of Outcome for Patients with Skull Base Tumors 242

John R. De Almeida and Dan M. Fliss

15   Pediatric Skull Base Surgery 251

Nidal Muhanna, Alon Pener Tesler, and Dan M. Fliss

Contents

Contents

Contents

40 Craniopharyngiomas

Alan Siu, Sanjeet Rangarajan, Christopher J. Farrell, Marc Rosen, and James J. Evans

41 Epidermoids, Dermoids, and Other Cysts of the Skull Base 606

Samuel P. Gubbels, Bruce J. Gantz, Paul W. Gidley, and Franco DeMonte

Contents

Videos

Video **5.1:** Baseline facial nerve electromyography (EMG) activity.

Video **5.2:** Facial nerve electromyography (EMG) activity during tumor dissection.

Video **5.3:** Stimulated facial nerve electromyography (EMG) activity.

Video **11.1:** Normal modified barium swallow study.

Video **11.2:** Normal fiberoptic endoscopic evaluation of swallowing.

Video **11.3:** Flaccid ataxic dysarthria.

Video **11.4:** Silent aspiration on modified barium swallow (MBS).

Video **11.5:** Videostroboscopy right vocal fold paralysis.

Video **11.6:** Right pharyngeal weakness on modified barium swallow (MBS).

Video **11.7:** Videostroboscopy following thyroplasty.

Video **16.1:** Endoscopic view of normal nasal anatomy.

Video **16.2:** Esthesioneuroblastoma of the left nasal cavity.

Video **16.3:** Robotic trans-antral approach to sinonasal region and the central skull base.

Video **22.1:** Endoscopic endonasal transsphenoidal resection of pituitary macroadenoma.

Video **30.1:** Surgical management of patient with intestinal-type adenocarcinoma (ITAC).

Video **30.2:** Multidisciplinary management of sinonasal undifferentiated carcinoma (SNUC).

Preface

Over a decade has passed since the publication of the successful first edition of *Comprehensive Management of Skull Base Tumors*, and much has happened in the intervening years. Major advances have been made in the surgical, radiotherapeutic, and chemotherapeutic management of skull base neoplasms. Coincident has been the rapidly advancing understanding of the biology and molecular underpinnings of such tumors. The latter has opened new doors to individualized therapeutics and holds tremendous promise for continued advances.

This revised and updated second edition is again intended as a comprehensive guide to navigate the complexity of contemporary multidisciplinary management of patients with tumors affecting the skull base. Tumor-specific chapters are expanded to emphasize the significant advances in molecular characterization of these tumors and discuss potential novel treatments based on this data.

We have organized this book into the following three sections: general principles, site-specific chapters, and tumor-specific chapters. Section one covers general topics pertinent to all patients with neoplasms of the skull base, regardless of specific location or tumor type. Of note is the expanded coverage of endonasal skull base anatomy and surgical principles. Radiotherapeutic principles and management are covered over two chapters in order to emphasize the significant advances in this area over the past decade, such as proton therapy and stereotactic radiation. Other topics covered include pathology, genetics, clinical evaluation, diagnostic imaging, anesthesia, surgical reconstruction, prosthetic rehabilitation, chemotherapy and targeted therapy, evaluation and rehabilitation of speech and swallowing, functional outcomes and quality of life issues, neurocognitive assessment, and cerebrovascular management.

Section two covers site-specific information regarding the various anatomic regions of the cranial base, including surgical anatomy, regional pathology, differential diagnosis, clinical assessment, diagnostic imaging, and surgical approaches.

Section three covers tumor-specific topics such as tumor incidence and epidemiology, pathology, staging, multidisciplinary treatment, outcome, and prognosis. The chapters comprehensively cover the varied sinonasal malignancies, sarcomas of the skull base, vascular skull base tumors, chordomas and chondrosarcomas, meningiomas, schwannomas, paragangliomas, pituitary tumors, craniopharyngiomas, epidermoids, and other cysts of the skull base, and fibro-osseous disease.

The organizational structure, by design, incorporates some redundancy of topics, although discussed from a variety of perspectives by differing authors. Rather than being detrimental, we see this as an expression of the reality of the diversity of opinion evident in the management of these rare and difficult tumors, where many nonmutually exclusive points of view exist.

We have gathered a group of contributors with incredible expertise. These authors truly represent the world's experts on their specific topics, and we are deeply grateful for their contribution.

Ehab Y. Hanna, MD, FACS
Franco DeMonte, MD, FRCSC, FACS

Acknowledgments

We sincerely thank all the contributors to this second edition for their work. Special thoughts go out to Albert L. Rhoton Jr. and Walter S. Jellish, great physicians and great friends who, sadly, are no longer with us to see the publication of this book to which they are important contributors.

Ehab Y. Hanna, MD, FACS
Franco DeMonte, MD, FRCSC, FACS

Contributors

Remo Accorona, MD
Division of Otorhinolaryngology
"San Maurizio" Hospital
Bolzano, Italy

Badih Adada, MD, FACS
John and Margaret Kruppa Chair in Neurosciences
Chairman, Department of Neurosurgery
Director, Neuroscience Center
Cleveland Clinic Florida
Weston, Florida

Siviero Agazzi, MD, MBA, FACS
Professor and Vice Chairman
Director, Division of Cranial Surgery
Department of Neurosurgery
University of South Florida
Tampa, Florida

Ossama Al-Mefty, MD, FACS
Director of Skull Base Surgery
Brigham and Women's Hospital
Harvard Medical School
Boston, Massachusetts

Joao Paulo Almeida, MD
Clinical Fellow
Division of Neurosurgery
Toronto Western Hospital
University of Toronto
Toronto, Ontario, Canada

Jaimie Payne Anderson, MS, CCC, SLP
Speech-Language Pathologist
Cleveland Clinic Florida
Weston, Florida

Ramsey Ashour, MD
Assistant Professor
Department of Neurosurgery
Dell Medical School
University of Texas
Austin, Texas

Karolyn H. Au, MD, MSc, FRCS(C)
Assistant Professor
Division of Neurosurgery
University of Alberta
Edmonton, Alberta, Canada

Samer Ayoubi, MD
Consultant Neurosurgeon
Department of Neurosurgery
Abbassi Medical Centre
Damascus, Syria

Denise Barringer, MS, CCC-SLP, BCS-S
Manager, Speech Pathology and Audiology
Head and Neck Center
University of Texas MD Anderson Cancer Center
Houston, Texas

Paolo Battaglia, MD
Assistant Professor
Department of Otorhinolaryngology–Head and Neck
  Surgery
Head and Neck Surgery & Forensic Dissection
  Research Center
University of Insubria, ASST Sette Laghi
Varese, Italy

Erasmo Barros da Silva Jr., MD, MSc
Department of Neurosurgery
Neuro-Oncology Division
Instituto de Neurologia de Curitiba
Curitiba, Brazil

Diana Bell, MD
Associate Professor
Head and Neck Section
Departments of Pathology and Head and Neck Surgery
University of Texas MD Anderson Cancer Center
Houston, Texas

Robert S. Benjamin, MD
Clinical Professor
Department of Sarcoma Medical Oncology
University of Texas MD Anderson Cancer Center
Houston, Texas

Jurij R. Bilyk, MD, FACS
Attending Surgeon, Oculoplastic and Orbital Surgery
  Service
Wills Eye Hospital
Professor of Ophthalmology
Thomas Jefferson University Hospital
Philadelphia, Pennsylvania

Luis A. B. Borba, MD, PhD, IFAANS
Professor and Chairman
Department of Neurosurgery
Federal University of Parana
Mackenzie Medical School
Curitiba, Brazil

Mariana E. Bradshaw, PhD, ABPP
Associate Professor
Section of Neuropsychology
Department of Neuro-Oncology
University of Texas MD Anderson Cancer Center
Houston, Texas

Paul D. Brown, MD
Professor
Co-Section Chief, CNS/Pediatrics
Co-Chair, CNS Disease Group
Department of Radiation Oncology
Mayo Clinic
Rochester, Minnesota

Gregory G. Capra, MD
Assistant Professor of Surgery
Uniformed Services University of the Health Sciences
Department of Otolaryngology
Naval Medical Center Portsmouth
Portsmouth, Virginia

Ricardo L. Carrau, MD
Professor and Lynne Shepard Jones Chair in Head and
   Neck Oncology
Director, Comprehensive Skull Base Surgery Program
Departments of Otolaryngology–Head and Neck Surgery,
   Neurological Surgery, and Speech and Hearing Sciences
The Ohio State University
Columbus, Ohio

Paolo Castelnuovo, MD, FACS, FRCS(Ed)
Professor and Chairman
Department of Otorhinolaryngology–Head and Neck
   Surgery
Head and Neck Surgery & Forensic Dissection Research
   Center
University of Insubria, ASST Sette Laghi
Varese, Italy

Marc C. Chamberlain, MD
Professor
Department of Neurology and Neurological Surgery
University of Washington
Fred Hutchinson Cancer Research Center
Seattle, Washington

Jimmy Yu Wai Chan, MD, MS, PhD
Division of Head and Neck Surgery
Department of Surgery
Queen Mary Hospital
University of Hong Kong
Hong Kong

Maurício Coelho Neto, MD
Director of Skull Base Surgery
Neurological Institute of Curitiba
Curitiba, Brazil

William T. Couldwell, MD, PhD, FACS
Professor and Chair
Department of Neurosurgery
University of Utah
Salt Lake City, Utah

John R. De Almeida, MD, MSc, FRCSC
Assistant Professor
Department of Otolaryngology–Head and Neck Surgery
Princess Margaret Cancer Center/University Health
   Network
University of Toronto
Toronto, Ontario, Canada

Franco DeMonte, MD, FRCSC, FACS
Mary Beth Pawelek Chair in Neurosurgery
Professor of Neurosurgery and Head and Neck Surgery
Director, David C. Nicholson Microsurgical and Endoscopic
   Center for Clinical Applications Laboratory
Director, Skull Base Program
Department of Neurosurgery
University of Texas MD Anderson Cancer Center
Houston, Texas

Colin L. W. Driscoll, MD
Professor and Chair
Department of Otorhinolaryngology–Head and Neck
   Surgery
Mayo Clinic
Rochester, Minnesota

Charles S. Ebert Jr., MD, MPH, FACS, FARS, FAAOA
Director, NeuroRhinology: Advanced Rhinology and
   Endoscopic Skull Base Surgery Fellowship
Medical Director, Otolaryngic Allergy Services
Associate Director, Residency Program
Associate Professor
Department of Otolaryngology–Head and Neck Surgery
University of North Carolina
Chapel Hill, North Carolina

Steven B. Edelstein, MD, FASA
Professor and Interim Chairman
Department of Anesthesiology and Perioperative
  Medicine
Loyola University Medical Center
Maywood, Illinois

Adel K. El-Naggar, MD, PhD
Head & Neck Pathology
University of Texas MD Anderson Cancer Center
Houston, Texas

James J. Evans, MD, FACS, FAANS
Professor of Neurological Surgery and Otolaryngology
Chief, Brain Tumor and Stereotactic Radiosurgery
  Division
Director, Cranial Base and Pituitary Surgery
Director, Cranial Base and Endoscopic Surgery Fellowship
Thomas Jefferson University
Philadelphia, Pennsylvania

Christopher J. Farrell, MD
Assistant Professor
Department of Neurosurgery
Sidney Kimmel Medical College at Thomas Jefferson
  University
Philadelphia, Pennsylvania

Juan C. Fernandez-Miranda, MD, FACS
Professor of Neurosurgery, Medicine and, by courtesy,
  ENT-Head and Neck Surgery
Surgical Director of Brain Tumor, Skull Base, and
  Pituitary Centers
Stanford University Medical Center
Palo Alto, California

Dan M. Fliss, MD
Professor and Chairman
Department of Otolaryngology Head & Neck Surgery
  and Maxillofacial Surgery
Director, Interdisciplinary Center for Head & Neck Surgical
  Oncology
Tel Aviv Sourasky Medical Center
Sackler School of Medicine Tel Aviv University
Tel Aviv, Israel

Mathieu Forgues, MD
Chief Resident
Department of Otolaryngology–Head and Neck Surgery
Louisiana State University Health Sciences Center
New Orleans, Louisiana

Steven J. Frank, MD, FACR
The Bessie McGoldrick Professor of Clinical Cancer
  Research
Executive Director, Particle Therapy Institute
Professor and Deputy Head, Department of Radiation
  Oncology
University of Texas MD Anderson Cancer Center
Houston, Texas

Jacob Freeman, MD
Ocala Neurosurgical Center
Ocala, Florida

Rick A. Friedman, MD, PhD
Professor of Otolaryngology and Neurosurgery
Director of Otology and Neurotology and the UCSD
  Acoustic Neuroma Center
University of California San Diego
San Diego, California

Gregory N. Fuller, MD, PhD
Professor and Deputy Chair
Chief Neuropathologist
Department of Anatomical Pathology
University of Texas MD Anderson Cancer Center
Houston, Texas

Bruce J. Gantz, MD
Professor and Head
Department of Otolaryngology–Head and Neck Surgery
University of Iowa Hospitals and Clinics
Iowa City, Iowa

Paul A. Gardner, MD
Associate Professor
Departments of Neurological Surgery and Otolaryngology
Co-Director, UPMC Center for Cranial Base Surgery
University of Pittsburgh School of Medicine
Pittsburgh, Pennsylvania

Basavaraj Ghodke, MD, DNB
Professor of Radiology and Neurological Surgery
University of Washington
Seattle, Washington

Steven L. Giannotta, MD
Professor and Chair
Program Director
Martin H. Weiss Chair in Neurological Surgery
Department of Neurological Surgery
Keck School of Medicine
University of Southern California
Los Angeles, California

Paul W. Gidley, MD, FACS
Professor
Otology-Neurotology
Department of Head and Neck Surgery
University of Texas MD Anderson Cancer Center
Houston, Texas

Lawrence E. Ginsberg, MD
Professor of Radiology and Head and Neck Surgery
Deputy Chair and Vice Chair for Clinical Operations
Department of Neuroradiology
University of Texas MD Anderson Cancer Center
Houston, Texas

Michael Gleeson, MD, FRCS, FRACS, FDS
Emeritus Professor of Otolaryngology and Skull Base
 Surgery
The National Hospital for Neurology & Neurosurgery
Guy's, King's & St Thomas' Hospitals
The Great Ormond Street Hospital for Sick Children
London, England, United Kingdom

Ezequiel Goldschmidt, MD, PhD
Chief Resident
Department of Neurosurgery
University of Pittsburgh
Pittsburgh, Pennsylvania

Samuel P. Gubbels, MD, FACS
Director, University of Colorado Health Hearing and
 Balance Clinics
Associate Professor, Department of Otolaryngology
University of Colorado School of Medicine
Aurora, Colorado

**Patrick J. Gullane, CM, OOnt, MB, FRCSC, FACS, Hon
FRACS, Hon FRCS, Hon FRCSI**
Wharton Chair in Head and Neck Surgery
Professor, Department of Otolaryngology–Head and Neck
 Surgery
Professor of Surgery
University of Toronto
Toronto, Ontario, Canada

Ehab Y. Hanna, MD, FACS
Professor, Vice Chairman, and Director of
 Skull Base Surgery
Department of Head and Neck Surgery
Medical Director, Head and Neck Center
University of Texas MD Anderson Cancer Center
Houston, Texas

David J. Howard, FRCS, FRCSEd
Professor of Head and Neck Oncology
Imperial College London
Honorary Consultant ENT and Head and Neck Surgeon
Imperial NHS Trust & the Royal National Throat, Nose and
 Ear Hospital
University College London Hospitals NHS Trust
London, England, United Kingdom

John A. Jane Jr., MD
The W. Gayle Crutchfield Professor of Neurosurgery
Professor of Pediatrics
Neurosurgery Residency Program Director
Department of Neurosurgery
University of Virginia
Charlottesville, Virginia

Walter S. Jellish†, PhD
Professor and Chairman
Department of Anesthesiology
Loyola University Medical Center
Maywood, Illinois

Alexandra Kammen, MD
Resident Physician
Department of Neurosurgery
University of Southern California
Los Angeles, California

Panagiotis Kerezoudis, MD, MS
Resident
Department of Neurologic Surgery
Mayo Clinic
Rochester, Minnesota

Cristine N. Klatt-Cromwell, MD
Assistant Professor
Otolaryngology Head and Neck Surgery, Rhinology, and
 Anterior Skull Base Surgery
Washington University in St. Louis
St. Louis, Missouri

Dennis H. Kraus, MD, FACS
Vice Chairman, Department of Otolaryngology–Head and
 Neck Surgery
Lenox Hill Hospital
Director, Center for Head & Neck Oncology
New York Head & Neck Institute
New York, New York
Northwell Health Cancer Institute
Greenlawn, New York
Professor, Department of Otolaryngology
Zucker School of Medicine at Hofstra/Northwell
Hempstead, New York

---

†Deceased

Michael E. Kupferman, MD, MBA
Senior Vice President, Clinical and Academic Network
  Development
Professor
Department of Head and Neck Surgery
University of Texas MD Anderson Cancer Center
Houston, Texas

Jan S. Lewin, PhD, BCS-S
Professor
Department of Head and Neck Surgery
Chief, Section of Speech Pathology and Audiology
Director, Voice Center
University of Texas MD Anderson Cancer Center
Houston, Texas

Michael J. Link, MD
Professor of Neurosurgery and Otolaryngology
Program Director, Neurosurgical Skull Base Fellowship
Department of Neurologic Surgery
Mayo Clinic
Rochester, Minnesota

Joshua W. Lucas, MD
Neurosurgeon
Mercy Medical Group
Dignity Health Neurological Institute
Sacramento, California

Valerie J. Lund, MS, FRCS, FRCSEd, FACSHon, CBE
Professor Emeritus in Rhinology
University College London
Honorary Consultant ENT and Anterior Skull Base
  Surgeon,
Royal National Throat, Nose and Ear Hospital
University College London Hospitals NHS Trust
London, England, United Kingdom

Ashley Kay Maglione, OD, FAAO
Assistant Professor
Department of Neuro-Ophthalmic Disease
Salus University: The Eye Institute of the Pennsylvania
  College of Optometry
Philadelphia, Pennsylvania

Carolina Martins, MD, PhD
Neurosurgeon
Director of Research and Education
Hospital Metropolitano Oeste Pelópidas
  Silveira—IMIP/SES/SUS
Professor, Department of Neuropsychiatry
Federal University of Pernambuco - UFPE
Recife, Brazil

Davide Mattavelli, MD
Assistant Professor
Unit of Otorhinolaryngology–Head and Neck Surgery
Department of Medical and Surgical Specialties,
  Radiological Sciences, and Public Health
University of Brescia
Brescia, Italy

Daniel P. McCormick, MBBS(Hons), FRACS OHNS
ENT, Head & Neck Surgeon
Department of Surgery
St Vincent's Hospital
Melbourne, Australia

Rahul Mehta, MD, MS, FRCS(Edin)
Associate Professor
Department of Otolaryngology–Head Neck Surgery
Louisiana State University Health Sciences Center
New Orleans, Louisiana

Matthew Mifsud, MD
Assistant Professor
Department of Otolaryngology–Head and Neck Surgery
University of South Florida College of Medicine
Tampa, Florida

Kelsey Moody, OD, FAAO
Assistant Professor of Ophthalmology
Section of Optometry
Emory Eye Center
Atlanta, Georgia

Eric J. Moore, MD
Professor
Department of Otorhinolaryngology–Head and Neck
  Surgery
Mayo Clinic
Rochester, Minnesota

Jacques J. Morcos, MD, FRCS(Eng), FRCS(Ed), FAANS
Professor and Co-Chairman, Department of Neurological
  Surgery
Professor of Clinical Neurosurgery and Otolaryngology
Division Chief, Cranial Neurosurgery, Jackson Memorial
  Hospital
Director, Cerebrovascular and Skull Base Fellowship
  Program
University of Miami
Miami, Florida

Nidal Muhanna MD, PhD
Director of the Head and Neck Surgery Unit
Department of Otolaryngology, Head and Neck and
  Maxillofacial Surgery
Tel Aviv Sourasky Medical Center
Tel Aviv, Israel

Marc-Elie Nader, MD, CM, MSc, FRCSC
Assistant Professor of Otology, Neurotology, and Skull
  Base Surgery
Department of Head and Neck Surgery
University of Texas MD Anderson Cancer Center
Houston, Texas

Sabareesh K. Natarajan, MD
Assistant Professor of Neurological Surgery and Radiology
Division Director, Open Vascular & Endovascular
  Neurosurgery Program
Division Director, Skull Base & Cranial Microsurgery
  Program
Department of Neurological Surgery
University of Massachusetts Medical School
Worcester, Massachusetts

Piero Nicolai, MD
Professor and Chairman
Department of Otorhinolaryngology–Head and Neck
  Surgery
University of Brescia
Brescia, Italy

Gustavo Fabiano Nogueira, MD
Chairman of the ENT Department
Co-Director of the Center for Cranial Base Surgery
Neurological Institute of Curitiba
Head of the ENT Department
Hospital Universitário Evangelico Mackenzie de Curitiba
Curitiba, Brazil

Daniel W. Nuss, MD, FACS
George D. Lyons Professor and Chairman
Skull Base Surgery, Complex Head and Neck Oncology
Department of Otolaryngology-Head and Neck Surgery
Louisiana State University School of Medicine, LSU Health
Sciences Center
New Orleans, Louisiana

Kerry D. Olsen, MD
Joseph I. and Barbara Ashkins Professor of Surgery
Mayo Clinic
Rochester, Minnesota

Michael Paci, MD, FRCSC
Neurosurgeon
Northern Light Eastern Maine Medical Center
Bangor, Maine

Anoop P. Patel, MD
Assistant Professor of Neurosurgery
University of Washington
Seattle, Washington

Alon Pener-Tessler, MD
Department of Otolaryngology Head and Neck and
  Maxillofacial Surgery
Tel Aviv Sourasky Medical Center
Sackler School of Medicine, Tel Aviv University
Tel Aviv, Israel

Kyle D. Perry, MD
Senior Pathologist
Pathology and Laboratory Medicine Product Line
Henry Ford Health System
Detroit, Michigan

Jack Phan, MD, PhD
Associated Professor
Director of Head and Neck Stereotactic Radiation
  Therapy Program
Director of Clinical Research, Head and Neck Section
Department of Radiation Oncology
University of Texas MD Anderson Cancer Center
Houston, Texas

Daniel L. Price, MD
Department of Otorhinolaryngology–Head and Neck
  Surgery
Mayo Clinic
Rochester, Minnesota

Amol Raheja, MBBS, MCH
Assistant Professor
Department of Neurosurgery
All India Institute of Medical Sciences
New Delhi, India

Ricardo Ramina, MD, PhD
Chairman, Neurosurgical Department
Neurological Institute of Curitiba
Curitiba, Brazil

Sanjeet Rangarajan, MD, M.Eng
Director of Rhinology and Endoscopic Skull Base Surgery
Assistant Professor
Department of Otolaryngology–Head and Neck Surgery
University of Tennessee Health Science Center
Memphis, Tennessee

Marcio S. Rassi, MD
Department of Neurosurgery
Brigham and Women's Hospital
Harvard Medical School
Boston, Massachusetts

Ravin Ratan, MD
Assistant Professor
Department of Sarcoma Medical Oncology
University of Texas MD Anderson Cancer Center
Houston, Texas

Shaan M. Raza, MD, FAANS
Associate Professor of Neurosurgery and Head and Neck
    Surgery
Vice Chairman–Education
Skull Base Program
Department of Neurosurgery
University of Texas MD Anderson Cancer Center
Houston, Texas

Albert L. Rhoton Jr†., MD
R. D. Keene Family Professor and Chairman Emeritus
Department of Neurosurgery
University of Florida College of Medicine
Gainesville, Florida

Marc R. Rosen, MD
Professor of Otolaryngology-Head and Neck Surgery and
    Neurological Surgery
Co-Director, Jefferson Center for Minimally Invasive
    Cranial Base Surgery
Department of Otolaryngology–Head and Neck Surgery
Thomas Jefferson University
Philadelphia, Pennsylvania

Laligam N. Sekhar, MD, FACS, FAANS
Professor and Vice Chairman
Director of Cranial Base and Cerebrovascular Surgery
Department of Neurological Surgery
University of Washington
Harborview Medical Center
Seattle, Washington

Komal Shah, MD
University of Texas MD Anderson Cancer Center
Houston, Texas

Parth V. Shah, MD
Department of Otolaryngology–Head and Neck Surgery
University of North Carolina
Chapel Hill, North Carolina

Alan Siu, MD
Department of Neurosurgery
Thomas Jefferson University
Philadelphia, Pennsylvania

Carl H. Snyderman, MD, MBA
Professor
Departments of Otolaryngology and Neurological Surgery
Co-Director, UPMC Center for Cranial Base Surgery
University of Pittsburgh School of Medicine
Pittsburgh, Pennsylvania

Shirley Y. Su, MBBS, FRACS
Associate Professor
Skull Base Tumor Program
Departments of Head and Neck Surgery and Neurosurgery
University of Texas MD Anderson Cancer Center
Houston, Texas

**Somasundaram Subramaniam, MBBCH, MMED, DOHNS,
    FRCS-ORL Eng**
Consultant and Clinical Director
Department of Otolaryngology–Head and Neck Surgery
Ng Teng Fong General Hospital Singapore
National University Health Services
Adjunct Assistant Professor
Department of Otolaryngology
National University of Singapore
Singapore

Sophie Taillibert, MD
Department of Neurology
Pitié-Salpétrière Hospital
Paris, France

Brian D. Thorp, MD, FACS, FARS
Assistant Professor
Departments of Otolaryngology–Head and Neck Surgery
    and Neurosurgery
University of North Carolina
Chapel Hill, North Carolina

Mario Turri-Zanoni, MD
Consultant in Skull Base Surgery
Department of Otorhinolaryngology–Head and Neck
    Surgery
Head and Neck Surgery & Forensic Dissection Research
    Center
University of Insubria, ASST Sette Laghi
Varese, Italy

Harry R. Van Loveren, MD
David W. Cahill Professor and Chair
Department of Neurosurgery and Brain Repair
Vice-Dean of Clinical Affairs
CEO, Byrd Alzheimer's Center and Research Institute
Director, USF Health Neuroscience Institute
University of South Florida Morsani College of Medicine
Tampa, Florida

†Deceased

Ashwin Viswanathan, MD
Clinical Associate Professor
Department of Neurosurgery
University of Texas MD Anderson Cancer Center
Houston, Texas

Michael Y. Wang, MD, FACS
Professor, Neurological Surgery & Rehab Medicine
Spine Fellowship Director
Chief of Neurosurgery, University of Miami Hospital
University of Miami Miller School of Medicine
Miami, Florida

Tony R. Wang, MD
Resident Physician
Department of Neurosurgery
University of Virginia Health System
Charlottesville, Virginia

Adam M. Zanation, MD, FACS
Harold C. Pillsbury Distinguished Professor
Departments of Otolaryngology–Head and Neck Surgery
  and Neurosurgery
University of North Carolina
Chapel Hill, North Carolina

Georgios A. Zenonos, MD
Assistant Professor of Neurological Surgery
Associate Director, Center for Skull Base Surgery
University of Pittsburgh Medical Center
Pittsburgh, Pennsylvania

I

1 Surgical Anatomy of the Cranial Base: Transcranial and Endonasal Approaches

Carolina Martins, Georgios A. Zenonos, Ezequiel Goldschmidt, Juan C. Fernandez-Miranda, and Albert L. Rhoton Jr.[†]

Summary

In this chapter, we focus on surgically relevant anatomy, specifically as it pertains to approaches designed to manage skull base pathology. In view of the significant expansion of endoscopic endonasal approaches' role in the treatment of skull base lesions, the modern skull base surgeon should be facile with both transcranial and endonasal approaches. Following this principle, we will briefly review some of the traditional skull base anatomy, with which most skull base surgeons are familiar, and will then discuss some basic principles of endonasal skull base anatomy.

Keywords: skull base anatomy, endoscopic anatomy, endoscopic approaches, surgical anatomy

1.1 Cranial Base Anatomy from the Transcranial Perspective

1.1.1 Anterior Cranial Base

The anterior cranial base is formed by three different bones: frontal, ethmoid, and sphenoid (▶ Fig. 1.1). The lateral aspect of the floor of the anterior cranial fossa comprises the orbital process of the frontal bone, whereas the deepened central anterior skull base is formed by the ethmoid bone. The cribriform plate lies in the center and is perforated by multiple small dural invaginations containing the olfactory filia, whereas the crista galli protrudes along the midline as the main anterior bony attachment of the falx. The horizontal cribriform plate is bounded laterally by the vertical lateral lamella of the ethmoid bone. The lateral lamella joins the cribriform plate to the fovea ethmoidalis of the frontal bone, which covers the roof of the ethmoid sinus.[1]

The sphenoid bone forms the posterior part of the anterior cranial base (▶ Fig. 1.2). Posterior to the cribriform plate is the planum sphenoidale, which forms the roof of the sphenoid sinus on the exocranial side of the skull base. It is bordered laterally by the lesser wings of the sphenoid bone, which medially and posteriorly form the anterior clinoid processes, which are landmarks for the clinoidal internal carotid artery (ICA) as well as the optic nerves. Above the cribriform plate and the planum sphenoidale lie the olfactory bulb and tract, respectively, which run in the olfactory sulcus of the frontal lobe. Posteriorly, the planum is separated from the prechiasmatic sulcus by the limbus of the sphenoid, a surgical landmark for localization of the optic canal and falciform ligament.[2]

The anterior skull base is intimately related to the paranasal sinuses as well as the orbit. The ethmoid sinuses lie in between the orbits. Directly posterior we find the sphenoid sinus. The frontal sinus lies anteriorly between the thin posterior plate and thicker anterior plate of the frontal bone. The orbit is roughly pyramidal and is related superiorly to the frontal sinus,

medially to the ethmoid sinus, and inferiorly to the maxillary sinus. The medial wall is formed from anterior to posterior by the orbital process of the frontal bone and the lacrimal, ethmoid, and sphenoid bones. The floor of the orbit is formed by the maxilla and by the zygoma anterolaterally. The infraorbital groove transmitting the infraorbital nerve is found on the orbital floor. The lateral wall is formed by the frontal and zygomatic bones anteriorly and by the greater and lesser wings of the sphenoid bone posteriorly, separated by the superior orbital fissure. It is essential to realize that although the anterior lateral wall is related to the temporalis muscle, the posterior lateral wall is related to the middle fossa and the temporal lobe. The orbital roof is formed mainly by the orbital process of the frontal bone, although the lesser wing of the sphenoid contributes to some extent posteriorly. The orbital apex comprises three main portals: the superior and inferior orbital fissures and the optic canal. The annulus of Zinn, the common tendinous attachment of the orbital muscles, separates the orbital apex into lateral and medial compartments. The lateral superior orbital fissure transmits the lacrimal, frontal, and trochlear nerves as well as the superior ophthalmic vein. The superior and inferior divisions of the oculomotor nerve as well as the nasociliary and abducens nerves are transmitted within the annulus of Zinn in the medial compartment of the superior orbital fissure. Superomedially within the annulus of Zinn, we find the optic canal transmitting the optic nerve and ophthalmic artery. The ophthalmic artery arises from the supraclinoidal ICA just medial to the anterior clinoid process. After running inferiorly and laterally to the optic nerve, the ophthalmic artery within the orbital apex crosses superiorly and gives off the supratrochlear and frontal arteries (important for vascularized pericranial flaps) as well as the anterior and posterior ethmoidal arteries. Notably, in 7 to 13% of cases, the optic canal can be completely encompassed within posterior ethmoidal cells (Onodi cells), and if this is not acknowledged on review of preoperative imaging, the optic nerves can be injured during endonasal approaches.[3] The inferior ophthalmic vein joins the superior ophthalmic vein at the orbital apex to drain into the cavernous sinus.

1.1.2 Middle Cranial Base

A detailed understanding of the anatomy of the sphenoid bone is crucial for both open and endoscopic endonasal approaches. The body of the sphenoid bone forms the central portion of the middle skull base. The sphenoidal body is cuboidal in shape and houses the sphenoidal sinus, which is the portal for most endoscopic approaches. The sides of the sphenoid body are grooved by the ICA as it transitions from the petrous segment over the foramen lacerum to the cavernous segment. The lateral aspect of the middle skull base is roughly triangular, limited by the sphenoid ridge anteriorly and by the petrous ridge posteriorly. The floor consists of the greater wing of the sphenoid anteriorly, the petrous apex of the temporal bone medially, and the squamous temporal bone laterally.

[†]Deceased

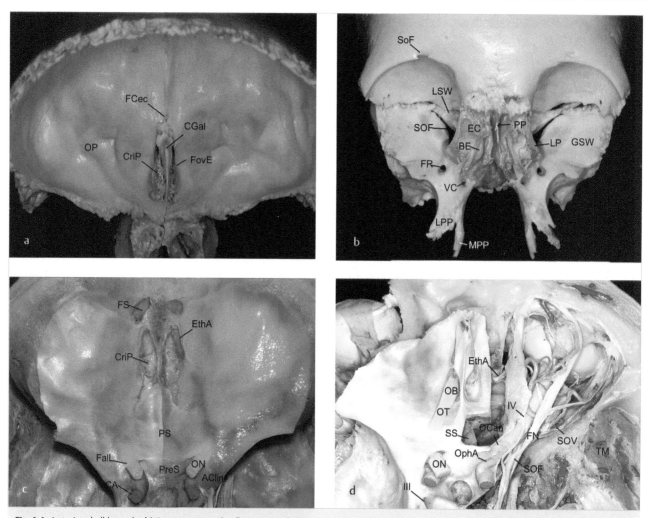

Fig. 1.1 Anterior skull base. **(a, b)** Bony anatomy. **(c, d)** Nerves and vascular content. AClin, anterior clinoid process; BE, bulla ethmoidalis; CA, carotid artery; CGal, crista galli; CriP, cribriform plate; EC, ethmoidal cells; EthA, ethmoidal artery; FalL, falciform ligament; F Cec, foramen cecum; FN, frontal nerve; FovE, fovea ethmoidalis; FR, foramen rotundum; FS, frontal sinus; GSW, greater sphenoid wing; III, third cranial nerve; IV, fourth cranial nerve; LP, lamina papyracea; LPP, lateral pterygoid plate; LSW, lesser sphenoid wing; MPP, medial pterygoid plate; OB, olfactory bulb; OCan, optic canal; OphA, ophthalmic artery; OP, orbital plate; OT, olfactory tract; PP, perpendicular plate; PreS, prechiasmatic sulcus; ON, optic nerve; PS, planum sphenoidale; SOF, superior orbital fissure; SoF, supraorbital foramen; SOV, superior ophthalmic vein; SS, sphenoid sinus; TM, temporalis muscle; VC, vidian canal.

The medial and lateral pterygoid plates project down from the pterygoid body on either side of the sphenoid sinus and articulate with the palatine bone anteriorly. The greater wings extending from the inferior sphenoid body and the lesser wings extending from the superolateral aspect of the body have been described as resembling bat's wings from a superior view. The anterior clinoid process has two attachments to the sphenoid bone: the superior one forms the roof of the optic canal as it joins the planum, whereas the inferior one, the optic strut, forms the floor of the optic canal. The optic strut, when it is well pneumatized, forms a recess that corresponds to the lateral opticocarotid recess endoscopically. The prechiasmatic sulcus is a groove that extends between the two optic canals. This sulcus is bound posteriorly by the tuberculum sella and anteriorly by the limbus of the sphenoid bone. Between the tuberculum sellae anteriorly, the dorsum sellae and posterior clinoids posteriorly, and the cavernous sinuses

and cavernous carotids on either side lies the sella turcica with the pituitary gland (▶ Fig. 1.3).

Occasionally a middle clinoid process, a bony prominence that extends from the superolateral aspect of the sella toward the tip of the anterior clinoid process, can be developed enough to connect to the anterior clinoid process, completely encasing the clinoidal ICA in a caroticoclinoidal ligament.[4] Usually, however, the anterior genu of the parasellar carotid is only partially encased. The middle clinoid is an endonasal landmark, for it marks the roof of the cavernous sinus as well as the transition between the cavernous and paraclinoidal segments of the ICA.[4] The diaphragma is a dural fold that extends from the tuberculum to the dorsum sellae, forming the roof of the sellar turcica. The pituitary stalk traverses the plane of the diaphragma through a central aperture—the pituitary aperture. Notably, the arachnoid does not usually follow the stalk inferiorly through the aperture, and thus the contents of the pituitary fossa are

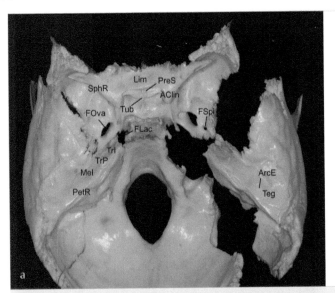 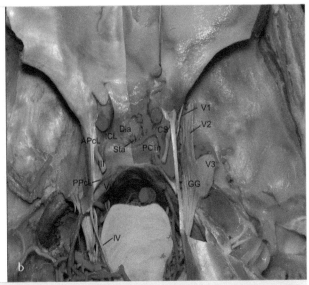

Fig. 1.2 **(a)** Bony anatomy. **(b)** Vascular content and nerves. AClin, anterior clinoid; APCl, anterior petroclinoidal ligament; ArcE, arcuate eminence; Dia, diaphragm sellae; FLac, foramen lacerum; FSpi, foramen spinosum; GG, gasserian ganglion; ICL, interclinoidal ligament; IV, fourth cranial nerve; Lim, limbus sphenoidale; PreS, prechiasmatic sulcus; PClin, posterior clinoid; PetR, petrous ridge; PPcl, posterior petroclinoidal ligament; SphR, sphenoid ridge; Sta, pituitary stalk; Teg, tegmen; Trl, trigeminal impression; TrP, trigeminal prominence; Tub, tuberculum sella; V1 first trigeminal division; V2, second trigeminal division; V3, third trigeminal division.

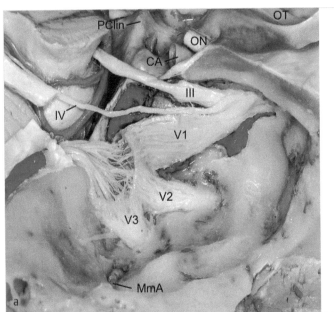 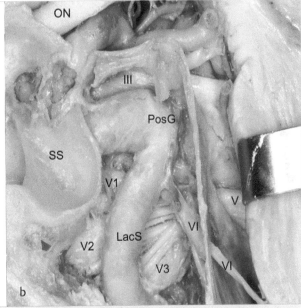

Fig. 1.3 Cavernous sinus from **(a)** an open and **(b)** an endoscopic perspective. CA, carotid artery; III, third cranial nerve; IV, fourth cranial nerve; LacS, lacerum segment; MmA, middle meningeal artery; ON, optic nerve; OT, olfactory tract; PClin, posterior clinoid; PosG, posterior genu; SS, sphenoid sinus; V, trigeminal root; V1, first trigeminal division; V2, second trigeminal division; V3, third trigeminal division; VI, sixth cranial nerve.

normally not bathed in cerebrospinal fluid.[5] Laterally the diaphragma is continuous with the dura of the cavernous sinus.

Several important foramina are found in the middle cranial fossa. The superior orbital fissure connects the middle fossa and the cavernous sinus to the orbit and its contents. The foramen rotundum lies inferior to the superior orbital fissure and transmits the maxillary division of the trigeminal nerve. The two are separated by a bony island—the maxillary strut of the sphenoid

bone. The foramen rotundum has an average length of approximately 4 mm and actually presents as more of a canal than a foramen.[6] Posterolateral to the foramen rotundum, the foramen ovale transmits the mandibular division of the trigeminal nerve and may also serve as the conduit for an accessory meningeal artery, the lesser superficial petrosal nerve (LSPN), and emissary veins to the pterygoid plexus. These neurovascular structures may also exit or enter the skull base using their own independent foramina. Immediately posterolateral to the foramen ovale we find the foramen spinosum transmitting the middle meningeal artery. The foramen lacerum lies medial to the foramen ovale and is formed by the confluence of the petrous, sphenoid, and occipital bones. Its inferior compartment comprises fibrocartilage, whereas the superior compartment contains the lacerum segment of the ICA. The foramen lacerum is actually the continuation of the petrous carotid canal. The inconstant foramen of Vesalius is seen within an island of bone bridging the foramen ovale and foramen lacerum, which we call the "mandibular strut." It transmits an emissary vein from the pterygoid plexus to the cavernous sinus. Immediately posterolateral to the foramen spinosum, the innominate foramen transmits the LSPN, which courses toward the foramen ovale. Medial and parallel to the LSPN, the greater superficial petrosal nerve (GSPN) exits through its homonymous foramen and courses parallel to the petrous ridge toward the foramen lacerum, where the GSPN joins the deep petrosal nerve and enters the vidian canal to become the nerve of the vidian canal. The GSPN can be traced posteriorly to the geniculate ganglion of the facial nerve. The course of the GSPN is an important landmark for the horizontal segment of the petrous carotid, which lies just inferior and medial to this nerve.[7]

Other anatomical landmarks of the middle skull base, from medial to lateral, include the trigeminal impression on the petrous ridge, which accommodates cranial nerve (CN) V in its course from the posterior cranial fossa to Meckel's cave. The ICA runs in its bony canal just under this area, which may be dehiscent. The trigeminal impression is followed posterolaterally by the trigeminal prominence and then by the meatal impression, which corresponds to the underlying internal acoustic canal. Proceeding more laterally, we find the arcuate eminence, which corresponds to an elevation created by the underlying superior semicircular canal, and then the flattened paper-thin roof of the tympanic cavity and mastoid air cells—the tegmen tympani and tegmen mastoideum, respectively.

An essential component of the middle skull base is the cavernous sinus, a large venous compartment encased within two layers of dura, which surrounds the sella turcica and is continuous anteriorly with the superior orbital fissure. It is surrounded by five walls of dura. The anterior wall is formed by the periosteal layer of dura overlying the sella anteriorly as it separates from its meningeal layer laterally. The meningeal layer continues posteriorly to form the medial wall as it surrounds the pituitary gland. The posterior wall faces the posterior cranial fossa and is formed by an extension of the periosteal layer between petrous apex and dorsum sella. The roof is continuous with the diaphragma and lateral wall and is formed by the oculomotor triangle posteriorly and the clinoidal triangle anteriorly. The lateral and medial walls meet at the inferior limit or floor of the cavernous sinus, which corresponds to the maxillary division of the trigeminal nerve and Meckel's cave posteriorly. The lateral wall is essentially a continuation of the outer or periosteal dural layer of the middle fossa. The meningeal layer of the middle fossa and the periosteal layers come together at the anterior petroclinoidal fold, which corresponds to the transition of the lateral wall to the roof.[2] Multiple venous structures drain into the cavernous sinus, such as the basilar plexus, ophthalmic veins, foramen rotundum, foramen ovale, foramen of Vesalius, and sphenoparietal sinus. The cavernous sinus then drains into the superior and inferior petrosal sinuses, which then drain into the transverse and sigmoid sinuses, respectively. The cavernous carotid has a short ascending segment, a posterior genu, a horizontal segment, and an anterior genu that continues as the paraclinoidal carotid. Two major branches come off the cavernous carotid: (1) the meningohypophyseal trunk, which arises from the posterior genu and gives off the inferior hypophyseal arteries, the tentorial artery of Bernasconi and Cassinary, and the dorsal meningeal artery, and (2) the inferolateral trunk, which arises from the horizontal segment and supplies the lateral wall and the first two divisions of the trigeminal nerve. These branches may also arise independently from the ICA. The inferolateral trunk courses between the abducens medially and V1 laterally to the lateral wall of the cavernous sinus. An inconstant third branch is McConnell's capsular artery, which has inferior and superior branches; the inferior branch arises medially from the horizontal segment, just anterior to the inferolateral trunk, to supply the anterior and inferior sellar dura, whereas the superior branch supplies the dura of the tuberculum sella and prechiasmatic sulcus.[2]

There are multiple important anatomical relationships within the cavernous sinus. The abducens nerve and the carotid sympathetic plexus are the only nerves that course within the sinus itself; all others are related to the lateral cavernous sinus wall. The abducens nerve enters the cavernous sinus just behind the posterior ascending cavernous carotid, then courses inferior and laterally to the horizontal segment of the carotid, lying just medial to V1 on its way to the superior orbital fissure. The oculomotor nerve, coursing from the interpeduncular fossa, enters the roof of the cavernous sinus within the oculomotor triangle, which is formed by the anterior petroclinoidal ligament laterally (extending from petrous apex to anterior clinoid), the posterior petroclinoidal ligament posteromedially (extending from petrous apex to posterior clinoid), and the interclinoidal ligament anteromedially (extending between the anterior and posterior clinoids). The dural membrane between these three dural folds forms the posterior roof of the cavernous sinus. The oculomotor nerve courses just lateral and parallel to the interclinoidal ligament and is surrounded by a thin invagination of the oculomotor triangle dura containing arachnoid and CSF (also known as the oculomotor cistern or interdural segment of the oculomotor nerve) before being incorporated into the lateral wall of the cavernous sinus under the clinoidal triangle, which forms the anterior roof of the cavernous sinus. The trochlear nerve enters the cavernous sinus in the posterolateral corner of the oculomotor triangle, just posterior to the junction of the anterior and posterior petroclinoidal ligaments. Here it lies posterior and lateral to CN III. It is then incorporated into the lateral wall of the cavernous sinus between the oculomotor nerve superiorly and V1 inferiorly, with which it forms the supra- and infratrochlear triangles, respectively.

1.1.3 Posterior Skull Base

The anterior wall of the posterior fossa is formed by the posterior surface of the petrous bone laterally and the clivus in the midline. The posterior and lateral confines are formed by the occipital bone, whereas the roof is formed by the tentorium cerebelli. The floor ends at the level of the foramen magnum.

The posterior surface of the petrous bone has two important foramina: (1) the internal auditory canal transmitting the seventh and eighth nerve complexes, as well as the labyrinthine branches of the anteroinferior cerebellar artery, to the inner ear and (2) the vestibular aqueduct, which transmits the endolymphatic duct, located lateral to the internal auditory canal. The jugular foramen is found below these two foramina and is formed by the junction of the jugular process of the petrous bone with the occipital bone. The jugular foramen has a posterolateral compartment (the pars venosa, which contains the jugular bulb and CNs X and XI) and an anteromedial compartment (the pars nervosa, which contains the glossopharyngeal nerve, the inferior petrosal sinus as it courses toward the jugular bulb, and usually a posterior meningeal branch from the ascending pharyngeal artery). Inferior and medial to the jugular foramen lies the hypoglossal canal with the hypoglossal nerve.

The vertebral arteries give off the posterior inferior cerebellar arteries ventral to the lower CNs before joining to form the basilar artery at the pontomedullary junction. The basilar artery gives off the anteroinferior cerebellar artery (AICA) just distal to the vertebrobasilar junction (▶ Fig. 1.4). The AICAs loop close to the internal acoustic canal and are intimately related to the VII–VIII complex. The superior cerebellar arteries arise from the distal basilar artery just before it bifurcates into the two posterior cerebral arteries.

From the external surface, such as that encountered when performing a far lateral craniotomy, the posterior skull base is protected by the mastoid tip and the suboccipital musculature. The sternocleidomastoid muscle arises from the mastoid tip, whereas the digastric muscle arises just medial, from the mastoid groove. The occipital artery usually courses medial to the mastoid tip. Deep to the sternocleidomastoid lie the splenius

capitis and longissimus capitis muscles, whereas posteriorly in the midline lays the trapezius, with the semispinalis capitis arising deep to it. A very important anatomical landmark is the suboccipital triangle containing the vertebral artery with its venous plexus. The suboccipital triangle is exposed when the muscles superficial to it are reflected off the superior nuchal line and occipital squama. The muscles forming this triangle are the superior and inferior oblique and the rectus capitis posterior major. The superior oblique and the rectus major attach at the inferior nuchal line, a landmark for identifying the suboccipital triangle. The C1 lateral process, the site of attachment for both oblique muscles, serves as a key landmark for identifying the location of the transverse foramen and of the vertebral artery as it exits the foramen and grooves the C1 arch. Identification of the vertebral artery within this triangle is needed to safely access the occipital condyle and C1 mass, which can be drilled to provide ventral access to the foramen magnum, lower clivus, and craniocervical junction (▶ Fig. 1.5; ▶ Fig. 1.6).

1.2 Cranial Base Anatomy from the Endonasal Perspective

1.2.1 The Sphenoid Sinus

Central to almost all endoscopic endonasal approaches to the skull base is the anatomy of the sphenoid sinus. The sphenoid sinus can range in pneumatization from the conchal type, in which there is almost no pneumatization, to the sellar type (most common), in which pneumatization is sufficient to expose variable amounts of the sellar floor. The presellar pneumatization pattern has some pneumatization but does not extend posteriorly beyond the plane of the tuberculum sellae. Pneumatization of the sinus increases after birth and is more or less finalized by late adolescence.[8] In the center of the sinus, a round bulge corresponds to the anterior surface of the sella turcica. Below the sella, pneumatization of the clivus creates a depression called the clival recess in between the paraclival segments of the ICA.[9] The paraclival carotids superiorly enter the cavernous sinus to turn anteriorly in a horizontal plane before looping again posteriorly, with the apex of the anterior loop corresponding to the middle clinoid process.[4] Notably, the middle clinoid forms a small depression just medial to the carotid and lateral to the sella. This anterior loop borders the sella on either side and is endoscopically referred to as the "parasellar carotid." This anterior loop or anterior genu of the parasellar carotid is prominent on either side of the sella and corresponds to the carotid prominence. One to multiple septations usually exist within the sphenoid sinus; their anatomy is extremely variable and almost never corresponds to the midline. Notably, in approximately 80% of cases, the septations lead to the carotid prominences posteriorly.[10] Above the carotid prominence on either side is another prominence that corresponds to the precanalicular segment of the optic nerve and then the optic canal as it courses from posterior and medial to anterior and lateral toward the orbit. The optic and carotid prominences are separated laterally by a very important endoscopic landmark, the lateral opticocarotid recess, which is the endoscopic correlate of the optic strut. The depth of this recess essentially corresponds to the degree of pneumatization of the optic strut.[9] Medially,

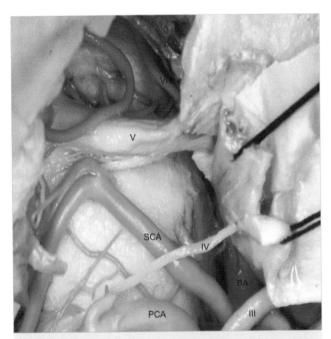

Fig. 1.4 Left posterior petrosectomy view. BA, basilar artery; III, third cranial nerve; IV, fourth cranial nerve; PCA, posterior cerebral artery; SCA, superior cerebellar artery; V, fifth cranial nerve.

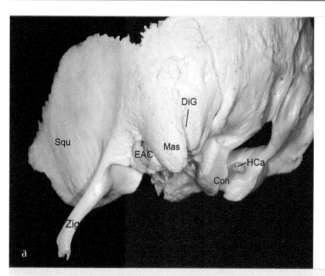
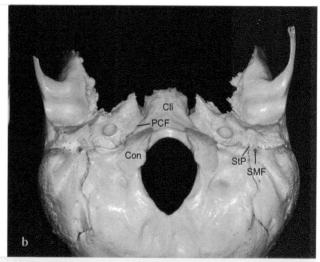

Fig. 1.5 Posterior fossa, bony anatomy, **(a)** lateral and **(b)** inferior views. Cli, clivus; Con, condyle; DiG, digastric groove; EAC, external acoustic canal; HCa, hypoglossal canal; Mas, mastoid process; PCF, petroclinoid fissure; SMF, styloid mastoid foramen; Squ, squamous plate; StP, styloid process; Zig, zygomatic arch.

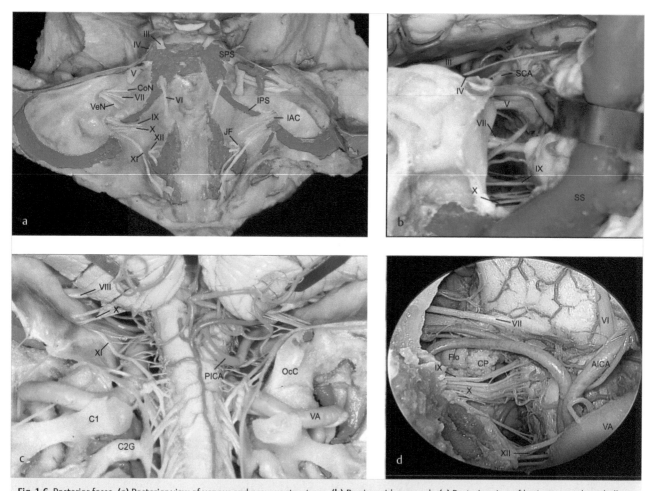

Fig. 1.6 Posterior fossa. **(a)** Posterior view of venous and nervous structures. **(b)** Presigmoid approach. **(c)** Posterior view of brainstem and cerebellum. **(d)** Endoscopic view of the pontomedullary sulcus. AICA, anteroinferior cerebellar artery; C2G, C2 ganglion; Con, cochlear nerve; CP, choroid plexus; Flo, flocculus; IAC, internal auditory canal; III, third cranial nerve; IPS, inferior petrosal sinus; IV, fourth cranial nerve; IX, ninth cranial nerve; JF, jugular foramen; OcC, occipital condyle; PICA, posterior inferior cerebellar artery; SCA, superior cerebellar artery; SPS, superior petrosal sinus; SS, sigmoid sinus; VA, vertebral artery; VeN, vestibular nerve; V, fifth cranial nerve; VI, sixth cranial nerve; VII, seventh cranial nerve; X, tenth cranial nerve; XI, eleventh cranial nerve; XII, twelfth cranial nerve.

the medial opticocarotid recess is another variable depression bordering the carotid and optic prominences as well as the superolateral aspect of the sellar prominence. The two medial opticocarotid recesses are the lateral extensions of the tubercular recess, a depression that borders the superior aspect of the sellar prominence and that corresponds to the tuberculum intracranially.[9] The depressions corresponding to the middle clinoids are slightly inferior to the medial opticocarotid recesses.

1.2.2 The Pituitary Gland and Suprasellar Space

The pituitary gland comprises an anterior lobe, or adenohypophysis, and a smaller posterior lobe, or neurohypophysis. Embryologically, the posterior lobe derives from the diencephalon, is slightly lighter in color, and produces oxytocin and vasopressin, whereas the anterior lobe is derived from an invagination of the oral ectoderm and produces all the remaining pituitary hormones. The superior hypophyseal arteries, which arise from the inferomedial aspect of the supraclinoidal or paraclinoidal ICA, provide blood supply to the anterior gland and pituitary stalk.[11,12,13] Each of these arteries may give off three branches: (1) a recurrent branch to the optic nerve; (2) an anastomotic branch to the undersurface of the chiasm and upper infundibulum, which anastomoses with the homonymous contralateral branch; and (3) a descending branch to the lower infundibulum and the diaphragma.[13] The capillary plexus of the superior hypophyseal arteries drains into the anterior gland by a portal venous system, facilitating the delivery of the hypothalamic hormone–releasing factors to the adenohypophysis.[11,12,13] The blood supply to the posterior gland, by contrast, comes from the inferior hypophyseal arteries, which are branches of the meningohypophyseal trunk of the cavernous carotid.[11,12] Notably, however, extensive collateralization exists between the superior and inferior hypophyseal systems, and recent clinical evidence suggests that bilateral sacrifice of inferior hypophyseal arteries does not cause permanent posterior pituitary dysfunction.[14] The majority of the pituitary gland is covered by an outer periosteal layer of dura as well as an inner meningeal layer. Laterally, these separate to form part of the cavernous sinus. The meningeal layer remains attached to the pituitary forming the medial wall of the cavernous sinus, whereas the periosteal layer continues laterally to form the sphenoidal (or anterior) wall of the cavernous sinus. Between these two layers are multiple intercavernous venous connections having great variability. The venous outflow of the gland is to the cavernous sinus through the gland's meningeal dural layer.[11,12]

Removing the tuberculum sella and prechiasmatic sulcus up to the level of the limbus of the sphenoid provides access to the suprasellar space and its infrachiasmatic, suprachiasmatic, and retrochiasmatic areas (▶ Fig. 1.7). The infundibulum in the infrachiasmatic space is covered by the arachnoid of the suprasellar cistern and, posteriorly, the membrane of Lillequist. Important structures in this space are the ophthalmic arteries, arising from the ICAs just above the distal dural ring and coursing ventral to the optic nerves initially. These arteries subsequently loop lateral and superior to the optic nerves once within the orbit.

1.2.3 Anterior Cranial Base

Removal of bone anterior to the limbus provides access to the base of the frontal lobe. After a complete ethmoidectomy and frontal sinusotomy, the surgical corridor can be widened to include all the area encompassed by the two midorbits laterally, the anterior table of the frontal sinus anteriorly, and the suprachiasmatic space posteriorly. Two major arteries can be seen coursing across the ethmoid roof. The posterior ethmoid artery

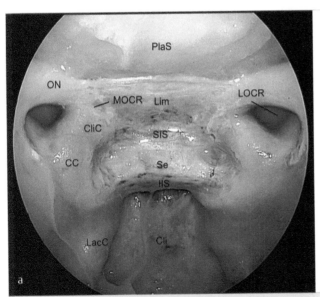
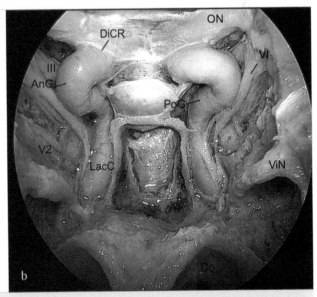

Fig. 1.7 Endoscopic view of **(a)** the sella and the parasellar region and **(b)** cavernous sinus. AnG, anterior genu; CC, cavernous carotid; Cli, clivus; CliC, clinoidal carotid; DiCR, distal carotid ring; III, third cranial nerve; IIS, inferior intercavernous sinus; LacC, lacerum carotid; Lim, limbus; LOCR, lateral opticocarotid recess; MOCR, medial opticocarotid recess; ON, optic nerve; PlaS, planum sphenoidale; PoG, posterior genu; Se, sella; SIS, superior intercavernous sinus; V2, second trigeminal division; VI, sixth cranial nerve; ViN, vidian nerve.

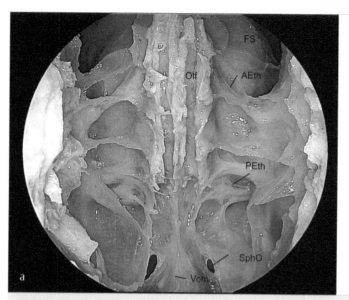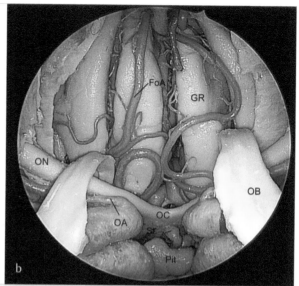

Fig. 1.8 Endoscopic view of **(a)** the anterior skull base bony and **(b)** brain anatomy. AEth, anterior ethmoidal artery; FoA, fronto-orbital artery; GR, gyrus rectus; OA, ophthalmic artery; OB, olfactory bulb; OC, optic chiasm; Olf, olfactory fibers; ON, optic nerve; PEth, posterior ethmoidal artery; Pit, pituitary gland; SphO, sphenoid ostium; St, stalk; Vom, vomer.

is found at the junction of the planum sphenoidale and the cribriform plate; it usually runs directly from lateral to medial, completely encased in bone (▶ Fig. 1.8). The anterior ethmoid artery, however, is more variable and is sometimes found in a bony mesentery as a result of pneumatization of the ethmoid roof around it. It also tends to run obliquely across the skull base from posterolateral to anteromedial. It is important to identify these vessels and avoid transecting them too close to the orbit lest they retract into the orbit, resulting in a retrobulbar hemorrhage.[15] Just anterior to the crista, at the frontoethmoidal junction, lies the foramen cecum, which occasionally may transmit an anterior nasal emissary vein. This can serve as a portal of spread for tumors or infections but can also serve as an anatomical landmark.

1.2.4 The Cavernous Sinus

From an endonasal route, because the cavernous carotid is encountered first when operating within the cavernous sinus, the cavernous sinus can be helpfully divided into venous compartments based on their relationship to the carotid: a superior, an inferior, a posterior, and a lateral compartment. The superior compartment lies between the horizontal cavernous segment of the carotid and the roof of the cavernous sinus. Within this compartment, the paraclinoidal carotid is found anteromedially as it courses superiorly and posteriorly, the dura of the oculomotor triangle is found posterolaterally, and the interclinoidal ligament is found superomedially. Conversely, below the horizontal carotid and between the posterior genu and the anterior or sphenoidal wall of the cavernous sinus lies the inferior compartment, which houses the sympathetic plexus as well as the abducens nerve coursing inferolaterally to the horizontal segment of the carotid. The abducens is also found just posterior to the short ascending segment of the cavernous carotid as it enters the posterior compartment of the cavernous sinus, which is defined as the area behind the posterior genu (▶ Fig. 1.3). The

lateral compartment is located lateral to the horizontal segment of the cavernous carotid and contains the abducens nerve coursing within the sinus, as well as CNs III, IV, and V1, contained within the lateral wall of the cavernous sinus as they course toward the superior orbital fissure. Notably, CN V2 abuts the cavernous sinus floor but is not contained within its wall.

1.2.5 The Clival and Petroclival Regions

An understanding of the anatomy of the clivus is essential for any transclival endoscopic approach. The clivus (Latin for "slope") forms the central part of the skull base and is formed by the synostosis of the sphenoid and occipital bones. It is wedge-shaped in a midsagittal section and is separated from the petrous bone on either side by the petroclival fissure.[16] This fissure contains a groove that accommodates the inferior petrosal sinus in its most cranial end. The cranial surface of the clivus is covered by two layers of dura, the periosteal and the meningeal. Prominent venous channels between these two layers of dura form the "basilar venous plexus," which is continuous with the cavernous sinus rostrally and with the internal and external vertebral plexus inferiorly. The two layers of dura are subsequently penetrated by the abducens nerve in the lateralmost part of the clivus; this dural envelope or interdural segment of the abducens nerve forms Dorello's canal, which is surrounded by trabeculated venous channels and lies immediately rostral to the inferior petrosal sinus.[17] The petrosphenoidal ligament, coursing between the superior border of the pyramid of the petrous bone and the lateral margin of the dorsum sellae (a.k.a. Gruber's ligament), forms the roof of Dorello's canal. Occasionally this ligament can be calcified at the superior crest of the petrous pyramid, forming a posterior sphenoidal process, or at the lateral margin of the dorsum sellae, forming a posterior-inferior clinoid process.[16] In an endonasal approach to Dorello's canal, the petrosphenoidal ligament is actually located behind the abducens nerve, not above it.

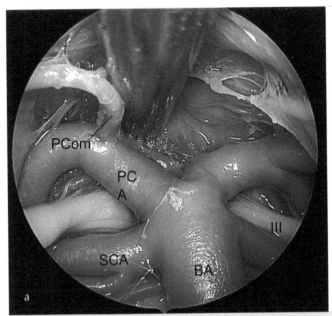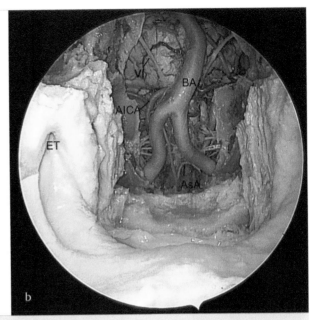

Fig. 1.9 (a, b) Endoscopic view of the posterior fossa. AICA, anteroinferior cerebellar artery; AsA, anterior spinal artery; BA, basilar artery; ET, Eustachian tube; III, third cranial nerve; PCA, posterior cerebral artery; Pcom, posterior communicating artery; SCA, superior cerebellar artery; VI, sixth cranial nerve.

Ventrally, the clivus forms the floor of the sphenoid sinus, which is bordered by the vomer with its alae. Its outer surface is covered by thick fibrous tissue, which is continuous laterally with the fibrocartilage of the foramen lacerum. Approximately 1 cm anterior and superior to the foramen magnum, the pharyngeal tubercle corresponds to the fixation point of the pharyngeal raphe and the anterior longitudinal ligament and is conceptually the posterior extension of the roof of the pharynx. Lateral to the pharyngeal tubercle we find two lines: the superior and inferior clival lines, which correspond to the attachment of the longus capitis major and the rectus capitis anterior. The muscular layer is covered by a fascial layer, the nasopharyngeal fascia. The resection of these layers and the anterior atlanto-occipital membrane exposes the lower clivus, occipital condyle, atlanto-occipital joint, and apical and alar ligaments. In addition to the pharyngeal tubercle, the supracondylar groove is a landmark on the clivus for localizing the hypoglossal canal, which is located just deep at the same craniocaudal level.[18,19,20]

1.2.6 Subdivision of the Ventral Clivus

Based on the "rule of three" classification for the posterior fossa originally proposed by Rhoton,[21] the clivus can be divided into three regions—upper, middle, and lower—based on the relationship of the three clival regions with the three cerebellar arteries (superior cerebellar, anteroinferior cerebellar, posterior inferior cerebellar), the related CNs (III, VI, XII), the subdivisions of the brainstem (midbrain, pons, medulla), and the cerebellum (superior, middle, and inferior cerebellar peduncle; ▶ Fig. 1.9).

We have since built on this concept to provide an endonasal surgical classification that may help in better understanding and predicting the anatomical relationships encountered during endoscopic endonasal transclival surgery.[22] The subdivisions of the clivus based on this approach are analyzed in

▶ Table 1.1. The surgically relevant anatomy of each of the three subdivisions of the clivus is presented hereafter.

Upper Clivus

The upper clivus is contained within the anatomical boundaries of the sellar and parasellar regions and is thus known as the "sellar clivus." It is formed by the posterior clinoids and the dorsum sellae and is the smallest of the three clival segments. Laterally, it is limited by the upper extension of the petroclival fissure, whereas inferiorly it is bound by the sellar floor. The sellar floor lies a few millimeters above the level at which Dorello's canal transmits the abducens nerve to the posterior compartment of the cavernous sinus, which also constitutes the transition point between the upper and middle clival segments of the transcranial classification.[23] An endoscopic superior transclival approach provides midline access to the interpeduncular cistern, the basilar apex, the mammillary bodies, and the floor of the third ventricle. The oculomotor nerves and the posterior communicating arteries limit the exposure laterally, whereas the superior limits of the exposure are the suprasellar cistern and the infrachiasmatic and tuberoinfundibular regions. Further lateral exposure allows access to the tentorial edge, the uncus, the trochlear nerve, and the posterior root of the trigeminal nerve. Anterior access to the upper clivus requires transposition of the pituitary, which can be achieved in one of three ways: (1) The *extradural pituitary transposition* involves upward mobilization of the gland with both its meningeal and periosteal dura.[24,25,26] Although this is the least disruptive to the arterial supply and venous outflow of the gland, it also provides the least exposure, which most of the time is inadequate for performing a complete posterior clinoidectomy or accessing the interpeduncular cistern. (2) The *interdural pituitary transposition* is essentially a transcavernous approach between the meningeal (medial) and periosteal (lateral) layers of the

Table 1.1 Endoscopic surgical subdivision of the clivus

Clival segment	Bone removed	ICA segment	Arachnoid cistern	Arteries	Nerves	Lateral extension
Upper clivus	Sellar floor Dorsum sella Posterior clinoids	Parasellar (paraclinoidal and intracavernous)	Interpeduncular	Basilar apex (SCA, PCA)	III	Cavernous sinus (parasellar) Suprasellar
Middle clivus	Clival recess of sphenoid bone Sphenoid floor Paraclival carotid canal	Paraclival Lacerum	Prepontine	Basilar trunk (AICA)	VI (IV–V–VII–VIII)	Medial petrous apex Meckel's cave
Lower clivus	Basilar part occipital bone Foramen magnum Jugular tubercle Medial condyle	Lacerum Petrosal Parapharyngeal	Premedullary	Vertebral arteries (PICA)	XII (IX–X–XI)	Transjugular tubule Transcondylar Infrapetrous Parapharyngeal

Abbreviations: AICA, anteroinferior cerebellar artery; ICA, internal carotid artery; PCA, posterior cerebral artery; PICA, posterior inferior cerebellar artery; SCA, superior cerebellar artery.

cavernous sinus.[14] This approach allows preservation of the venous outflow of the pituitary, because the meningeal layer of the gland is preserved, while providing excellent mobilization of the gland. Although the inferior hypophyseal arteries must be carefully identified, coagulated, and divided, there has been no report of pituitary dysfunction as a result, suggesting adequate collateral supply from the superior hypophyseal arteries.[14] (3) The *intradural transposition* of the pituitary provides the highest degree of mobilization, but the necessary detachment of the gland from its meningeal layer of dura also carries the highest risk for pituitary dysfunction.[25]

Middle Clivus

The middle clivus is also known as the "sphenoidal clivus," and it extends from the floor of the sella to the roof of the choana. It is the tallest of the three segments. A middle transclival approach provides access to the ventral pons and prepontine cistern, to the basilar trunk and AICA, and to the cisternal segment of the abducens nerve. The sphenoidal clivus is limited laterally by the paraclival ICA and the petroclival fissure. The foramen lacerum lies inferolaterally, roughly at the level of the floor of the sphenoid body. An important endoscopic anatomical relationship is that of the vidian nerve within the vidian canal at the medial base of the pterygoid body, coursing toward the lateral portion of the foramen lacerum, which is an excellent landmark for localizing the lacerum segment of the carotid when other landmarks are distorted by pathology. Laterally, the middle transclival exposure is limited by the interdural segment of CN VI.

Lower Clivus

The inferior clivus, also known as the "nasopharyngeal clivus," extends from the roof of the choana to the foramen magnum and is shorter, but wider, than the middle clivus. The inferior transclival approach through this segment exposes the premedullary cistern and ventral medullary surface, the vertebral arteries, the vertebrobasilar junction, and the posterior inferior cerebellar arteries, as well as CNs IX–X–XI–XII. Through this ventral exposure, the hypoglossal nerves are found anteroinferiorly, whereas the lower CNs are situated posterosuperiorly. Exposure of the lower clivus requires detachment of the nasopharyngeal

fascia and the underlying longus capitis and rectus capitis muscles from the ventral surface of clivus. This exposure also provides access to critical structures of the craniocervical junction: the anterior atlanto-occipital membrane, the ring of C1, the capsule of the atlanto-occipital joint, the apical ligament, and the tectorial membrane. Laterally, the lower clivus is limited by the Eustachian tubes, which are attached to the medial pterygoid plate laterally and superiorly to the fibrocartilage filling the lower segment of the foramen lacerum. Transection or mobilization of the Eustachian tube provides further exposure to the inferoventral petroclival fissure, which extends from the foramen lacerum to the jugular foramen. The lower clival segment is divided by the hypoglossal canal into two compartments[20]: (1) the tubercular or superior compartment, corresponding to the ventral aspect of the jugular tubercle, the drilling of which provides access to the cisternal segment of CNs IX–X–XI in their course toward the jugular foramen,[19] and (2) the inferior or condylar compartment, which corresponds to the ventral occipital condyle. Drilling of the medial condyle provides access to the vertebral artery as it enters the dura of the posterior fossa. In our experience, drilling of less than 20% of the condyle is required to obtain enough lateral access in the foramen magnum, an amount that does not significantly affect craniocervical stability if the remainder of the condyle is structurally intact.[18,27]

1.2.7 Petroclival Region and Jugular Foramen

Lateral expansion of the lower transclival approach to access tumors extending lateral to the petroclival junction can be achieved with a transpterygoid infravidian approach followed by a sublacerum or infrapetrous approach,[28,29] so that after removal of the posterior wall of the maxillary sinus, the pterygopalatine fossa is exposed and its contents mobilized laterally to expose the vidian nerve. The pterygopalatine and palatosphenoidal arteries need to be sacrificed in this process.[30] The palatosphenoidal artery is located behind the sphenoid process of the palatine bone and represents a key landmark for proper identification of the vidian nerve entering the vidian canal. Subsequently, by drilling the base of the pterygoid, the surgeon can skeletonize the vidian nerve in the vidian canal and follow it posteriorly to the foramen lacerum. The soft tissue of the inferior compartment of the foramen lacerum (sublacerum) can then be resected, achieving detachment and mobilization of the Eustachian tube. The bone between the horizontal petrous carotid and the Eustachian tube in the inferior surface of the petrous bone can be drilled (infrapetrous). Transection of the Eustachian tube and drilling of the carotid canal inferiorly can expand the surgical corridor even more laterally to the ventral aspect of the jugular foramen. Furthermore, transection of the Eustachian tube allows wide access to the parapharyngeal space and any pathology that may extend here. Unfortunately, no bony landmarks exist for the parapharyngeal ICA in this area, so image guidance and/or Doppler ultrasound become integral.

1.3 Conclusion

Mastery of the surgically relevant anatomy is an essential component of a good skull base surgeon. The current chapter provides an introductory overview of key anatomical details. The interested reader should further expand on specific anatomical topics as contained in the listed references.

References

[1] Fernandez-Miranda JC. Intracranial region. In: Standring S, ed. Gray's Anatomy: Philadelphia, PA: Elsevier Health Sciences; 2015:429–442

[2] Patel CR, Fernandez-Miranda JC, Wang WH, Wang EW. Skull base anatomy. Otolaryngol Clin North Am. 2016; 49(1):9–20

[3] Tomovic S, Esmaeili A, Chan NJ, et al. High-resolution computed tomography analysis of the prevalence of Onodi cells. Laryngoscope. 2012; 122(7): 1470–1473

[4] Fernandez-Miranda JC, Tormenti M, Latorre F, Gardner P, Snyderman C. Endoscopic endonasal middle clinoidectomy: anatomic, radiological, and technical note. Neurosurgery. 2012; 71(2) Suppl Operative:ons233–ons239

[5] Campero A, Martins C, Yasuda A, Rhoton AL, Jr. Microsurgical anatomy of the diaphragma sellae and its role in directing the pattern of growth of pituitary adenomas. Neurosurgery. 2008; 62(3):717–723

[6] Grewal SS, Kurbanov A, Anaizi A, Keller JT, Theodosopoulos PV, Zimmer LA. Endoscopic endonasal approach to the maxillary strut: anatomical review and case series. Laryngoscope. 2014; 124(8):1739–1743

[7] Shao YX, Xie X, Liang HS, Zhou J, Jing M, Liu EZ. Microsurgical anatomy of the greater superficial petrosal nerve. World Neurosurg. 2012; 77(1): 172–182

[8] Hamid O, El Fiky L, Hassan O, Kotb A, El Fiky S. Anatomic variations of the sphenoid sinus and their impact on trans-sphenoid pituitary surgery. Skull Base. 2008; 18(1):9–15

[9] Peris-Celda M, Kucukyuruk B, Monroy-Sosa A, Funaki T, Valentine R, Rhoton AL, Jr. The recesses of the sellar wall of the sphenoid sinus and their intracranial relationships. Neurosurgery. 2013; 73(2) Suppl Operative: ons117–ons131

[10] Fernandez-Miranda JC, Prevedello DM, Madhok R, et al. Sphenoid septations and their relationship with internal carotid arteries: anatomical and radiological study. Laryngoscope. 2009; 119(10):1893–1896

[11] Daniel PM. Anatomy of the hypothalamus and pituitary gland. J Clin Pathol Suppl (Assoc Clin Pathol). 1976; 7:1–7

[12] Lechan RM, Toni R. Functional anatomy of the hypothalamus and pituitary. In: De Groot LJ, Beck-Peccoz P, Chrousos G, et al., eds. Endotext. South Dartmouth, MA: MDText.com, Inc.; 2000–2016

[13] Krisht AF, Barrow DL, Barnett DW, Bonner GD, Shengalaia G. The microsurgical anatomy of the superior hypophyseal artery. Neurosurgery. 1994; 35 (5):899–903

[14] Fernandez-Miranda JC, Gardner PA, Rastelli MM, Jr, et al. Endoscopic endonasal transcavernous posterior clinoidectomy with interdural pituitary transposition. J Neurosurg. 2014; 121(1):91–99

[15] Cecchini G. Anterior and posterior ethmoidal artery ligation in anterior skull base meningiomas: a review on microsurgical approaches. World Neurosurg. 2015; 84(4):1161–1165

[16] Hofmann E, Prescher A. The clivus: anatomy, normal variants and imaging pathology. Clin Neuroradiol. 2012; 22(2):123–139

[17] Ono K, Arai H, Endo T, et al. Detailed MR imaging anatomy of the abducent nerve: evagination of CSF into Dorello canal. AJNR Am J Neuroradiol. 2004; 25(4):623–626

[18] Wang WH, Abhinav K, Wang E, Snyderman C, Gardner PA, Fernandez-Miranda JC. Endoscopic endonasal transclival transcondylar approach for foramen magnum meningiomas: surgical anatomy and technical note. Oper Neurosurg (Hagerstown). 2016; 12(2):153–162

[19] Fernandez-Miranda JC, Morera VA, Snyderman CH, Gardner P. Endoscopic endonasal transclival approach to the jugular tubercle. Neurosurgery. 2012; 71(1) Suppl Operative:146–158, discussion 158–159

[20] Morera VA, Fernandez-Miranda JC, Prevedello DM, et al. "Far-medial" expanded endonasal approach to the inferior third of the clivus: the transcondylar and transjugular tubercle approaches. Neurosurgery. 2010; 66(6) Suppl Operative:211–219, discussion 219–220

[21] Rhoton AL, Jr. The cerebellar arteries. Neurosurgery. 2000; 47(3) Suppl:S29–S68

[22] Fernandez-Miranda JC, Gardner PA, Snyderman CH, et al. Clival chordomas: a pathological, surgical, and radiotherapeutic review. Head Neck. 2014; 36(6): 892–906

[23] Sekhar LN, Jannetta PJ, Burkhart LE, Janosky JE. Meningiomas involving the clivus: a six-year experience with 41 patients. Neurosurgery. 1990; 27(5):764–781

[24] Kassam A, Snyderman CH, Mintz A, Gardner P, Carrau RL. Expanded endonasal approach: the rostrocaudal axis. Part II. Posterior clinoids to the foramen magnum. Neurosurg Focus. 2005; 19(1):E4

[25] Kassam AB, Prevedello DM, Thomas A, et al. Endoscopic endonasal pituitary transposition for a transdorsum sellae approach to the interpeduncular cistern. Neurosurgery. 2008; 62(3) Suppl 1:57–72, discussion 72–74

[26] Silva D, Attia M, Schwartz TH. Endoscopic endonasal posterior clinoidectomy. J Neurosurg. 2015; 122(2):478–479

[27] Kooshkabadi A, Choi PA, Koutourousiou M, et al. Atlanto-occipital instability following endoscopic endonasal approach for lower clival lesions: experience with 212 cases. Neurosurgery. 2015; 77(6):888–897

[28] Scopel TF, Fernandez-Miranda JC, Pinheiro-Neto CD, et al. Petrous apex cholesterol granulomas: endonasal versus infracochlear approach. Laryngoscope. 2012; 122(4):751–761

[29] Paluzzi A, Gardner P, Fernandez-Miranda JC, et al. Endoscopic endonasal approach to cholesterol granulomas of the petrous apex: a series of 17 patients: clinical article. J Neurosurg. 2012; 116(4):792–798

[30] Pinheiro-Neto CD, Fernandez-Miranda JC, Rivera-Serrano CM, et al. Endoscopic anatomy of the palatovaginal canal (palatosphenoidal canal): a landmark for dissection of the vidian nerve during endonasal transpterygoid approaches. Laryngoscope. 2012; 122(1):6–12

2 The Pathology of Tumors and Tumorlike Lesions of the Skull Base

Diana Bell, Gregory N. Fuller, and Adel K. El-Naggar

Summary

The skull base is the location for a wide variety of benign and malignant tumors of ectodermal, endodermal, and mesodermal origins. The majority of tumors at these locations are malignant, and, over the last decade, such tumors have shown dramatic improvement in patient survival, partly due to the development and use of endoscopy and improvements in pathology. Novel diagnostic markers for skull base tumors, along with a growing body of evidence, show the importance of immunophenotyping and genotyping for differentiating among these neoplasms. The identification of molecular abnormalities underlying sinonasal neoplasms, as well as those responsible for carcinogenesis, is critical to the development of specific targeted therapies and design of clinical trials.

Keywords: skull base neoplasms, histogenesis, immunophenotype, molecular genotype, biomarkers

2.1 Introduction

The skull base is the location for a wide variety of benign and malignant tumors. Per cubic centimeter, the sinonasal tract gives rise to a greater diversity of neoplasms than any other site in the human body. The diversity of these histogenetically and biologically heterogeneous neoplasms of ectodermal, endodermal, and mesodermal origins partly arises from the anatomic complexity and highly varied tissues of this compact area. The vast majority of tumors at these locations are malignant, with only a small percentage being benign or tumorlike lesions.

Malignant sinonasal tract tumors comprise < 1% of all neoplasms, including about 3% of those of the upper aerodigestive tract. Paranasal disease and malignancies have showed dramatic improvements in patient survival, from 20% in the 1950s to 60 to 80% in the current decade's literature. This advancement has been closely tied to the development and use of endoscopy and to improvements in pathology. In the past 5 years, several studies have identified novel diagnostic markers for skull base tumors, and a growing body of evidence shows the importance of immunophenotyping and genotyping for differentiating among these neoplasms. Differentiating these tumor types may have a clinical impact, as advances in therapeutic intervention could increase survival rates, improve quality of life, and occasionally result in a cure. Conventional treatment continues to include surgical resection, often followed by chemoradiotherapy. The identification of molecular abnormalities underlying sinonasal neoplasms and those responsible for carcinogenesis is critical to the development of specific targeted therapies and design of clinical trials.

Although the majority of tumors at this location are of primary origin, metastasis can be encountered and thus will be discussed. Nonmetastatic tumors are either primary or an extension from neighboring structures.

2.2 Biopsies and Frozen Sections

The evaluation of sinonasal pathology typically requires a tissue biopsy, the tissue may be limited by the accessibility of the target region. Obtaining adequate and representative materials is essential for accurate diagnosis and better planning of patient management. The initial assessment of these tumors is commonly conducted intraoperatively for either provisional or definitive diagnosis and/or to verify adequacy for representative tissue. Communication with the pathologist at the time of frozen section is key to coordinating patient care. At this stage, nonneoplastic processes, lymphoma, and metastatic neoplasms can be determined. For primary tumors, the frozen tissue biopsy may be adequate for diagnosis and for planning of ancillary tests, but efforts to secure additional tissue for permanent processing are strongly recommended for optimal morphologic assessment and biomarker characterization.

2.3 Nonneoplastic and Congenital Lesions

2.3.1 Encephalocele

Depending on the age of the patient and the location of the lesion, diagnosis of an encephalocele may be made by imaging prior to submitting histology. Frequently, encephaloceles extending into the nasal cavity or sinus include meninges and glial tissue associated with fibrosis.[1,2]

2.3.2 Nasal Glial Heterotopia

This is a congenital malformation in which ectopic glial tissue is found without connection to intracranial structures.[3] Nasal glial heterotopia may present as an extranasal, intranasal, or mixed intranasal and subcutaneous mass. Patients may also present with symptoms and findings of nasal polyp, chronic sinusitis, and otitis media. Radiological confirmation of the lack of intracranial communication is stressed so as to avoid complications such as cerebrospinal fluid leak. Generally these lesions present as smooth, homogenous tan soft tissue–mimicking brain parenchyma. Histologically, they are typically composed of neural tissue with fibrosis and astrocytic proliferation (▶ Fig. 2.1).

Differential Diagnosis

This entity can be differentiated from encephalocele, which frequently shows meninges.

2.3.3 Respiratory Epithelial Adenomatoid Hamartoma

Respiratory epithelial adenomatoid hamartoma (REAH), a benign proliferation of minor seromucinous glands of the sinonasal

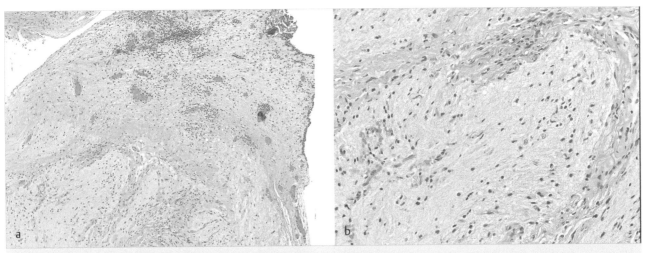

Fig. 2.1 (a, b) Nasal glial heterotopia, typically composed of neural tissue with fibrosis.

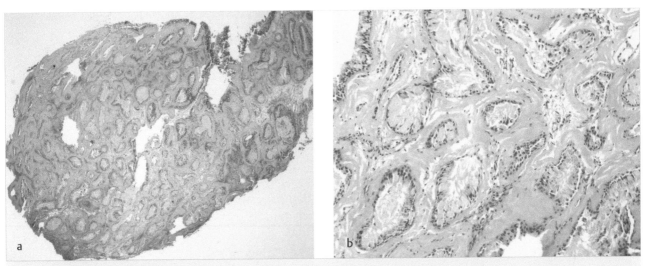

Fig. 2.2 (a, b) Adenomatoid hamartoma composed of respiratory epithelial-lined spaces and glandular structures.

tract, occurs more commonly in men than women during the sixth decade of life. Major symptoms include nasal obstruction, epistaxis, and recurrent sinusitis. These lesions appear normally as polypoid tan to reddish brown, rubbery tissue nodules.[4,5,6] Histologically, they are formed of numerous glandular structures lined by ciliated respiratory epithelium with thickened basement membrane and intervening fibrotic and/or edematous stroma (▶ Fig. 2.2).

Differential Diagnosis

These lesions may be confused with Schneiderian inverted papilloma and sinonasal adenocarcinomas. The benign glandular structures lined by columnar cells that form these lesions are key to differentiating REAH from both these entities. Another important consideration in the differential diagnosis is chondromesenchymal hamartoma. These lesions, which have a REAH-like glandular proliferation associated with small islands of chondroid material within the stroma, typically occur in children; they may be a manifestation of a

germline DICER1 mutation and may be associated with pleuropulmonary blastomas. Complete excision is curative for REAH, with no recurrences reported to date.[6]

2.3.4 Seromucinous Hamartomas

In seromucinous hamartomas the underlying glandular component consists predominantly of seromucinous glands, in contrast to REAH. Smaller tubules, ducts, and glands are present in a lobular arrangement; the glands may be surrounded by stromal hyalinization, and a chronic lymphoplasmacellular infiltrate is typically present. By analogy, these resemble the microglandular adenosis of the breast.[5,6]

Differential Diagnosis

REAH with florid seromucinous glandular proliferation and low-grade nonintestinal adenocarcinomas may be challenging for the diagnosis of seromucinous hamartomas.

2.3.5 Ectopic Pituitary Adenoma

Pituitary adenomas may occur in the sphenoid bone and sinuses, either as a separate lesion or as an extension from a primary adenoma arising in the sella.[7,8] Embryonic residue along the Rathke's pouch formation is the presumed derivation. Females are more affected than males (2:1). Patients may present with nasal obstruction, headache, or epistaxis. Approximately half of patients exhibit hormonal abnormalities. Histologically, an ectopic pituitary adenoma is identical to that of a conventional pituitary adenoma with monotonous round cells (▶ Fig. 2.3).

Differential Diagnosis

This lesion should be differentiated from carcinoid tumor, olfactory neuroblastoma (ONB), and other small undifferentiated tumors at these locations. Immunohistochemical staining for hormonal receptors, especially for adrenocorticotropic hormone and prolactin, is helpful.

2.3.6 Inflammatory Pseudotumor

This is a benign reactive process in which a spindle cell tumor–like proliferation with inflammatory component is the cardinal feature.[9,10,11] They may arise at any site in the skull base regions.

Histopathology

These tumors are composed of spindle cell proliferation admixed with chronic inflammatory and plasma cells. Immunohistochemically, the spindle cells express weak smooth muscle actin characteristic of myofibroblast.

Differential Diagnosis

These lesions may be confused with some benign and malignant mesenchymal tumors and fibromatosis. The inflammatory cells and the myofibroblastic nature are keys to their proper identification.

2.3.7 Sinonasal Polyps

These polypoid growths originate from the Schneiderian epithelial lining of the sinonasal cavities. They evolve as a result of fluid accumulation of the mucosa, most commonly as a result of nasal allergy and repeated sinusitis. Frequently, maxillary polyps may extend via the sinus openings into nasal or nasopharyngeal locations. The majority of polyps occurring in children are associated with asthma or cystic fibrosis (20–30%). In adult patients, they are often secondary to chronic sinusitis and allergy.[12,13,14] Generally, sinonasal polyps grossly appear smooth, glistening, and translucent or opaque.

Histologically, the epithelium of nasal polyps is commonly respiratory, with or without mild hyperplasia or squamous metaplasia. The core is edematous, with numerous vessels and scattered inflammatory cells. In allergic polyps, the dominant cells are eosinophils, whereas inflammatory polyps feature chronic and a few acute inflammatory cells. Scattered minor salivary gland structures are also seen. Commonly, secondary changes due to infarction and organization are observed.

Differential Diagnosis

These lesions should be differentiated from angiofibroma and from small cell tumors forming a polypoid mass. Angiofibroma is a specific benign entity that features proliferation of vascular spaces with satellite bland stromal cells in young male patients. Rhabdomyosarcoma, lymphoma, and melanoma are more cellular and can be readily excluded using respective markers.

2.3.8 Sinonasal (Schneiderian) Papilloma

There are three histologic subtypes of this entity: (1) the exophytic, which is typically squamous in histology and almost always affects the nasal septum; (2) cylindrical cells, which are characterized by stratified columnar epithelial lining; and (3) the inverted papilloma, of which a transitional-like squamous proliferation in an inward growth is the cardinal feature.[15,16,17,18,19,20]

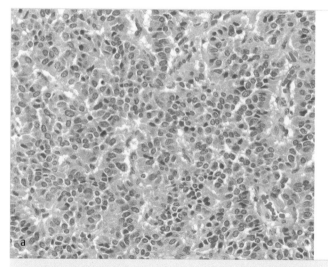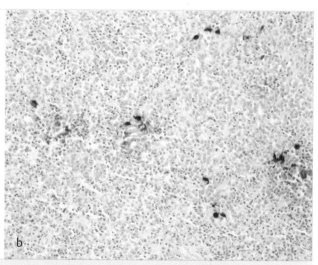

Fig. 2.3 Pituitary adenoma with (a) uniform endocrine cells and (b) sparse adrenocorticotropic hormone.

The latter types originate from the lateral nasal wall, middle meatus, and paranasal sinuses. Both cylindrical and inverted papillomas affect one side of the nasal and paranasal sinuses, with fewer than 5% occurring bilaterally.

2.3.9 Human Papillomavirus

Low- and high-risk human papillomavirus (HPV) subtypes have been identified in inverted and exophytic papillomas by in situ hybridizations and polymerase chain reactions. No clear association between HPV status and malignant transformation has been established.

2.3.10 Exophytic Sinonasal (Schneiderian) Papilloma

Generally, exophytic Schneiderian papilloma is a lobular mass composed histologically of bland squamous epithelium around fibrovascular cores.

2.3.11 Cylindrical Cell Papilloma

A generally exophytic papillomatous proliferation, histologically lined by multilayered columnar epithelium with and without oncocytic features. Microcysts with neutrophils within the epithelium are common (▶ Fig. 2.4).

2.3.12 Inverted Sinonasal (Schneiderian) Papilloma

Grossly, inverted papillomas are typically tan to gray polypoid soft tissue having a mulberry appearance. These lesions affect more males than females and occur in older age. Keratinization may be present in some lesions, potentially indicating progression. Characteristic features of this lesion are inward invagination and presence of cellular structures formed of transitional-like epithelium having intraepithelial microcysts filled with macrophages, cellular debris, and mucinlike materials. Malignant transformation may occur in 10% of these lesions. Identifying dysplasia and carcinoma in situ in these lesions is critical for predicting the malignant progression of these lesions (▶ Fig. 2.4).

Differential Diagnosis

All three types of Schneiderian papilloma must be differentiated from carcinomas: the exophytic type from papillary squamous carcinomas, cylindrical cell papilloma from sinonasal adenocarcinomas, and the inverted type primarily from squamous carcinoma, which will show dyskeratosis, dysplasia, and stromal desmoplasia in response to invasion.

2.4 Inflammatory and Granulomatous Conditions

2.4.1 Allergic Fungal Sinusitis

This entity results from an allergic reaction to persistent fungal organisms leading to mass formation.[21,22,23] It may occur at any age, without gender predominance. The main symptoms are nasal discharge and rhinorrhea over a protracted period. The overall appearance of tissues from these lesions is that of tan butterlike material with debris.

The cardinal microscopic features include characteristic alternating layers of mucin and degenerating cells with eosinophilic materials and cells. Numerous intact and degenerating eosinophils and granules are present. Occasionally crystalloid eosinophilic deposition (Charcot–Leyden) crystals are found. Tissue invasion by hyphae is not identified in this disorder.

Ancillary Markers

Fungal stains may reveal degenerated noninvasive fungal forms in allergic mucin secretion. Culture is necessary for speciation of the fungal organism; the most common is *Aspergillus* sp.

Differential Diagnosis

The most common differential diagnoses of this entity are invasive fungal infection, mycetoma (fungal ball), or inflammatory polyp. Invasive fungal infections are characterized by vascular invasion by fungal organism, tissue necrosis, and a lack of layered secretions. Mycetoma shows sheets of fungal hyphae without tissue invasion. Inflammatory polyp can be excluded based on the lack of alternating layers and eosinophilic materials and cells.

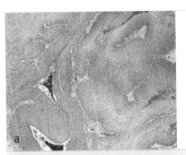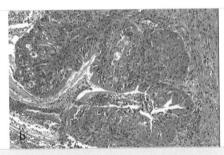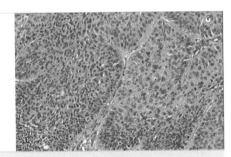

Fig. 2.4 (a) Inverted Schneiderian papilloma composed of an epithelial proliferation within submucosa. **(b)** Cylindrical cell papilloma with characteristic bland columnar epithelial-lined papillae and microcystic formation. **(c)** Squamous carcinoma arising from inverted papilloma, with nuclear pleomorphism and atypical mitoses.

2.4.2 Invasive Fungal Sinusitis

Invasive fungal sinusitis is a potentially life-threatening condition characterized by fungal organisms that invade tissue and blood vessels, leading to massive tissue necrosis.[24,25] Most commonly it is seen in immunocompromised patients and in patients who have poorly controlled diabetes mellitus. Infections spread rapidly to involve the central nervous system, which may lead to the patient's death. Normally, tissue fragments are tan-gray, soft, and necrotic.

Histologically, fungal hyphae are identified with invading tissues and specifically with the blood vessels leading to massive necrosis (▶ Fig. 2.5). Zygomycoses (*Rhizopus/Rhizomucor*) and *Aspergillus* are the most common organisms. Cultures should be taken for definitive species identification.

Differential Diagnosis

The most common differential diagnoses of this entity are allergic fungal sinusitis and infectious agents. Invasive fungal infections are characterized by vascular invasion by fungal organism, tissue necrosis, a lack of layered secretions. Inflammatory polyp can be excluded based on the lack of alternating layers and eosinophilic materials and cells.

2.4.3 Rhinoscleroma

Rhinoscleroma is a chronic progressive granulomatous inflammation caused by *Klebsiella rhinoscleromatis*, a gram-negative bacterium.[26,27] The disease is rare in the United States but is endemic in developing counties. Females are slightly affected more than males in the second to third decades of life. The natural history of the disease includes exudative, proliferative, and fibrotic phases. The exudative stage is characterized by purulent discharge, acute and chronic inflammation, and mucosal edema and congestion. The proliferative phase is characterized by granulomatous formation and multiple nodular inflammatory and ulcerating masses. The terminal phase is fibrotic, leading to stenosis.

The overall appearance of this lesion is that of polypoid and friable soft tissue in the proliferative phase. The histologic features are those of chronic inflammatory conditions, with extensive histiocytic cells that have vacuolation containing *Klebsiella* microorganisms (Mikulicz cells; ▶ Fig. 2.6). The fibrotic stage is nondiagnostic of the condition.

Differential Diagnosis

Other infectious agents, including mycobacterial infections and syphilis, should also be considered.

2.4.4 Granulomatosis with Polyangiitis

Formally known as Wegener's granulomatosis, this destructive granulomatous condition is of unknown etiology. The disease, although systemic in nature, most commonly affects the upper respiratory tract, and it affects all ages and both genders. Common complaints are nasal stuffiness, rhinitis, and pain. Nasal septal destruction is common in young patients.[28,29,30,31]

Generally, tissues obtained from these lesions comprise fragments of necrotic-appearing materials. Histologically, the characteristic features include small vessel inflammation with granulomatous features, geographic necrosis, and basophilic debris as a result of cellular degeneration.

Ancillary Markers

Up to 85% of patients who have granulomatosis with polyangiitis are positive for serologic testing with antineutrophil cytoplasmic antibodies (c-ANCA).

Differential Diagnosis

All infections associated with granulomatous inflammation would be included in the differential diagnosis and should be excluded by negative cultures. NK/T-cell lymphoma might show necrosis and may be included.

2.4.5 Histiocytosis-X (Eosinophilic Granuloma)

Histiocytosis-X (eosinophilic granuloma) is the most prevalent of these rare conditions, which also include two related

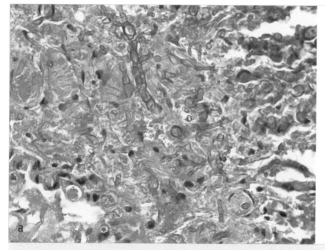
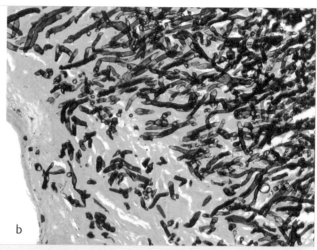

Fig. 2.5 (a) Invasive fungal sinusitis with fungal hyphae invading vasculature. **(b)** A silver stain highlights the fungal hyphae.

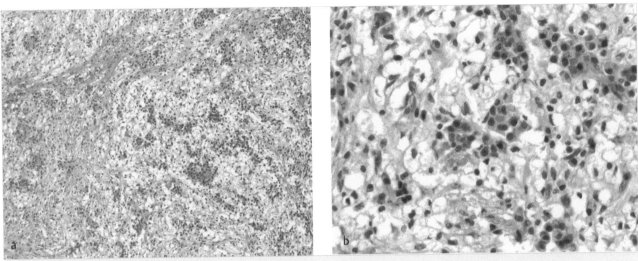

Fig. 2.6 (a, b) Rhinoscleroma; inflammatory infiltrate including the characteristic vacuolated histiocytes (Mikulicz cells).

conditions, Hand-Schüller-Christian syndrome and Lettere-Siwe disease. This disease can be localized or systemic and frequently involves head and neck sites, including the flat bones of the skull and sinonasal tract. Although age at presentation varies widely, this condition is most common in younger groups (< 20 years). Symptoms are nonspecific and include middle ear infections and destructive bony structures.[32,33,34,35,36]

The cardinal histologic features are proliferation of large histiocytes with cytoplasmic vacuolation and marked eosinophilic infiltrate. The characteristic electron-dense Birbeck granules are often seen on electron-optic examinations.

Differential Diagnosis

The conditions most frequently confused with this entity are Hodgkin's disease and lymphoma NK/T-cell type.

2.4.6 Myospherulosis

This is an iatrogenically induced lesion caused by reaction to petroleum, lanolin-based products, and fat necrosis.[37] Typically patients present having undergone surgery with petroleum-based nasal packing. Symptoms include sinusitis, pain, and swelling.

The main histologic findings are pseudocystic formations containing nonrefractile small spherules and fibrosis.

Differential Diagnosis

Coccidioidomycosis fungal infection.

2.5 Malignant Epithelial Neoplasms

Sinonasal malignancy most commonly affects the maxillary sinus (60%), nasal cavity (22%), ethmoid sinus (15%), and, less frequently, frontal and sphenoid sinuses (3%; ▶ Table 2.1).

A wide variety of malignant neoplasms of different cellular lineages arises in this location. The most common malignancies are

Table 2.1 Incidence of malignant sinonasal tumors

- < 1% of all neoplasm tumors
- 3% of head and neck malignancy

Sites

• Maxillary	60%
• Nasal cavity	22%
• Ethmoid	15%
• Frontal and sphenoid	3%

Histology

• Epithelial	55%
• Mesenchymal	30%
• Neuroectodermal	15%
• Other	5%

carcinomas (55%), followed by nonepithelial tumors (30%), neuroectodermal tumors (15%), and miscellaneous entities (5%).[38,39]

2.5.1 Squamous Carcinoma

Squamous carcinoma typically occurs in elderly individuals who are in their sixth and seventh decades; it is more common in males (2:1). The most common sites are maxillary sinus, nasal cavity, ethmoid, frontal, and sphenoid sinus.[40,41,42,43] Usually these carcinomas are typical ulcerated and indurate with exophytic features; sinus tumors are bulky and composed of friable light tan tumor tissues.

Histologically, squamous features should be identified and the extent of differentiation graded (well, moderately, or poorly). Tumors originating from the nasal cavity are generally keratinizing and well differentiated. Tumors of the paranasal sinuses and skull base are nonkeratinizing carcinomas with intermediate to poor differentiation (▶ Fig. 2.7). The poorly differentiated carcinomas, also called Schneiderian carcinomas, most likely originate from preexisting inverted papillomas (▶ Fig. 2.4c).

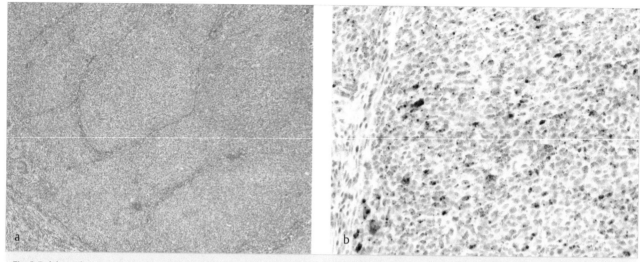

Fig. 2.7 **(a)** Nonkeratinizing squamous carcinoma with **(b)** nuclear human papillomavirus high-risk signals (RNA-scope in situ hybridization).

Differential Diagnosis

Squamous carcinoma may occasionally pose a diagnostic challenge on small biopsy specimens with sialometaplasia, pseudoepitheliomatous hyperplasia, and Schneiderian papilloma and should be differentiated from sinonasal undifferentiated carcinoma (SNUC).

2.5.2 Sinonasal Undifferentiated Carcinoma

SNUC was originally defined by Frierson et al[44] as a "high-grade epithelial neoplasm of the nasal cavity and paranasal sinuses of uncertain histogenesis with or without neuroendocrine differentiation but without evidence of squamous or glandular differentiation." The World Health Organization (WHO) redefined SNUC as a highly aggressive and clinicopathologically distinct carcinoma of uncertain histogenesis that typically presents with locally extensive disease. SNUC is reputed to be refractory to even the most radical therapy and to carry a poor prognosis, particularly when the tumor transgresses the cranial base.

It seems likely that SNUC arises from Schneiderian epithelium and thus is of ectodermal derivation. In light of the overlapping clinical, anatomical, microscopic, and ultrastructural findings in olfactory neuroblastoma (ON) and neuroendocrine carcinoma (NEC), their origins may share both cells of Schneiderian mucosa and cells of olfactory neuroepithelium.[45,46] It has also been proposed that SNUC would be best categorized as a large-cell NEC.[45]

SNUC is a high-grade, undifferentiated carcinoma characterized by primitive malignant epithelial cells with high mitotic figures and cellular necrosis.[44,45,46,47,48,49] Patients are typically elderly males who present in a late stage of disease (▶ Table 2.2). Tumors originate most commonly from the nasal cavity, ethmoid sinus, and maxillary sinus, but site of origin may be difficult to ascertain at presentation. These tumors are typically large, involving multiple adjacent structures that have ill-defined borders. They present as light tan soft tissue fragments.

Table 2.2 Clinicopathologic features of undifferentiated carcinoma of the skull base

Feature	SNUC	NEC	NPC type
Grade	High	High	High
Incidence	Rare	Rare	<0.5%
M/F	3:1	–	3:1
LN mets	30%	–	Common
Mortality	80%	50–60%	50–60%
Risk factor	–	–	EBV
Site	Nasal cavity and sinus	Maxillary sinus	Nasopharynx

Abbreviations: EBV, Epstein-Barr virus; LN mets, lymph node metastasis; M/F, male/female; NEC, neuroendocrine carcinoma; NPC, nasopharyngeal carcinoma; SNUC, sinonasal undifferentiated cancer.

Histologically, SNUC comprises sheets of undifferentiated cells having a low nuclear–cytoplasmic ratio, prominent nucleoli, and reticular and clear nuclei with high mitotic rate and necrotic features (▶ Fig. 2.8). No squamous or glandular differentiation should be present.

Differential Diagnosis

The diagnosis and etiology of this entity is a subject of controversy that frequently arises as a result of management issues. Because of poor differentiation, they are most often confused with poorly differentiated sinonasal carcinomas (Schneiderian/squamous), as already described; NEC; and the solid form of adenoid cystic carcinoma (ACC). Immunohistochemical markers are crucial to the diagnosis of this entity. Positive epithelial lineage markers and absence of focal neuroendocrine marker exclude neuroblastoma, NEC, lymphoma, melanoma, and primitive neuroectodermal tumor (PNET). Lack of lymphoid infiltrate, along with accurate localization, is crucial for the exclusion of nasopharyngeal-type carcinoma (▶ Table 2.2).

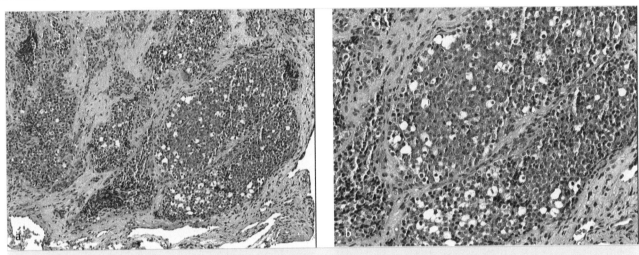

Fig. 2.8 **(a)** Sinonasal undifferentiated carcinoma forms nests, lobules, trabeculae, and sheets in the absence of squamous or glandular differentiation. **(b)** Nuclei are medium to large and are surrounded by small amounts of eosinophilic cytoplasm that lacks a syncytial quality; nucleoli are single and prominent.

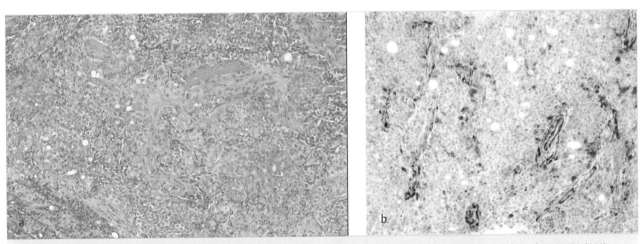

Fig. 2.9 **(a)** SMARCB1 (INI1)-deficient carcinomas grow as epithelioid nests in the sinonasal submucosa. **(b)** Complete loss of SMARCB1 (INI1) immunohistochemical expression (positive staining highlights vessels as internal control).

2.5.3 SMARCB1 (INI1)-Deficient Sinonasal Carcinoma

Recently, a unique subset of sinonasal carcinomas was identified that is characterized by basaloid/rhabdoid tumor morphology and loss of expression of SMARCB1 (INI1). These tumors appear to be restricted to the sinonasal tract, and their unique clinical, morphological, and immunohistochemical features seem to warrant their inclusion as a separate new entity among the existing high-grade sinonasal neoplasms.[50,51,52] Separation from the other types of sinonasal malignancies is important, for identification of SMARCB1 (INI1) deficiency may provide a new target for novel treatment approaches and could ultimately lead to improved patient survival. At the moment, these tumors are viewed as a subset of SNUCs.[52]

Morphologically these carcinomas are characterized by rounded or anastomosing nests of tumor cells set in a fibrous stroma. In some cases a prominent exophytic component with papillary fronds can be noted, but generally the tumors show a cohesive pattern of growth. Further characteristics include peripheral palisading as well as radial growth around blood vessels that impart a pseudorosette-like pattern. The tumors are highly infiltrative and often show invasion of the underlying bone. Cytologically, the cells have large round nuclei and prominent nucleoli (▶ Fig. 2.9). The cytoplasm can vary and ranges from scant (basaloid) to more abundant with prominent eccentric eosinophilic cytoplasm (rhabdoid). Necrosis and a high mitotic rate are common findings. Isolated cases contained scattered ductlike spaces, but squamous or glandular differentiation is not a feature of reported SMARCB1-deficient sinonasal carcinomas.

SMARCB1 (INI1) is a tumor suppressor gene located on chromosome 22q11.2. Its gene product, SMARCB1 (INI1), is ubiquitously expressed in nuclei of all normal tissues. *SMARCB1* gene inactivation has been implicated in the pathogenesis of a diverse group of malignant neoplasms that tend to share rhabdoid cytomorphology.

2.5.4 Nasopharyngeal Carcinoma

These tumors are classified into keratinizing and nonkeratinizing phenotypes and correspond to WHO type I and II/III grades.[48,53,54,55,56,57,58] Pathogenesis is strongly linked to Epstein-Barr virus (EBV) infection and a diet high in nitrosamines, including salted fish and fermented food (▶ Table 2.2).

The histopathologic characteristics of these tumors vary by WHO classification. The keratinizing type (WHO-I) is composed of tumor nests with squamous features, including keratinization and intercellular bridges. The nonkeratinizing type (WHO-II/III) is composed of sheets of undifferentiated malignant epithelial cells intimately intermingled with chronic inflammatory infiltrate, which is often EBV-positive (▶ Fig. 2.10).

Ancillary Markers

On histologic examination, EBV can be identified by in situ hybridization for EBV-encoded RNA. Most commonly, EBV is identified in nonkeratinizing types (WHO-II/III). Serology for EBV-encoded RNA is also available.

Differential Diagnosis

The nonkeratinizing phenotype must be differentiated primarily from the SNUC and from NEC. The presence of lymphocytic infiltrate and the lack of neuroendocrine markers helps confirm the diagnosis.

2.5.5 Nuclear Protein in Testis Carcinoma

Nuclear protein in testis (NUT) carcinomas are rare, clinically aggressive carcinomas. They are characterized by a translocation involving the *NUT* gene on chromosome 15q14 and, in most cases, the bromodomain-containing 4 (*BRD4*) gene on chromosome 19p13.1, resulting in a *BRD4-NUT* fusion gene.[59,60,61]

NUT carcinomas are composed of undifferentiated basaloid cells with focal, often abrupt, squamous differentiation (▶ Fig. 2.11). NUT carcinomas can mimic other undifferentiated neoplasms, such as pediatric small blue cell tumors, germ cell tumors, Ewing's sarcoma, lymphoma, and SNUC.[57,58,59,60,61,62] NUT carcinomas have an epithelial immunophenotype and focally express keratin, p63, CK7, CK20, and CK34, which reflect varying degrees of squamous differentiation. An extensive panel of immunostains (e.g., desmin, myoglobin, smooth muscle actin, muscle actin, chromogranin, synaptophysin, leukocyte common antigen, placental alkaline phosphatase, S-100 protein, alpha fetoprotein, neuron-specific enolase, CD57, CD99, HMB45) are not expressed in NUT carcinomas. Oncoviruses, such as EBV and HPV, have

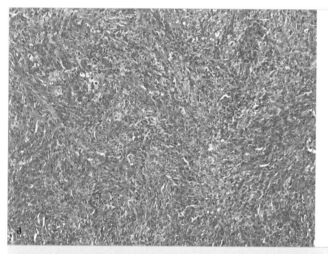
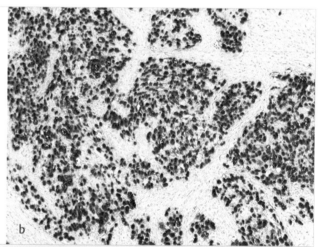

Fig. 2.10 (a) Nasopharyngeal carcinoma, undifferentiated type (WHO-III) showing undifferentiated neoplastic cells with cleared nuclei in a prominent lymphoid background. (b) The tumor is positive for Epstein-Barr virus (EBER in situ hybridization).

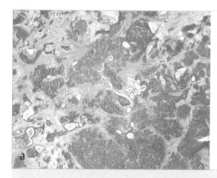
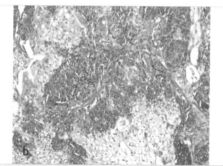
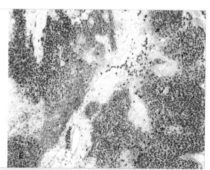

Fig. 2.11 (a, b) Nuclear protein in testis (NUT) carcinomas are composed of undifferentiated basaloid cells with focal, often abrupt, squamous differentiation. (c) An anti-NUT monoclonal antibody is strongly positive within the tumor, aiding diagnosis.

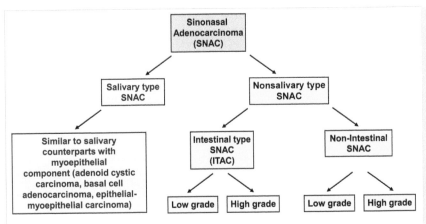

Fig. 2.12 World Health Organization classification of sinonasal adenocarcinomas.

never been identified in NUT carcinomas; their presence would likely exclude this diagnosis. Demonstration of the NUT translocation is required for the diagnosis of NUT carcinomas; this can be achieved by karyotyping, reverse transcription polymerase chain reaction, or fluorescence in situ hybridization.

A monoclonal antibody to NUT was developed for use in immunohistochemistry (IHC) and has a sensitivity of 87%, a specificity of 100%, a negative predictive value of 99%, and a positive predictive value of 100% when tested in a large panel of carcinoma tissues.[63] The use of this antibody helps distinguish NUT carcinomas from other poorly differentiated sinonasal carcinomas, thereby contributing to their clinicopathological characterization.[63] In view of the anecdotal favorable responses of NMCs to certain treatment regimens, including chemotherapy according to Ewing's sarcoma protocols or docetaxel and radiotherapy,[64,65] the distinction of NUT carcinomas from other sinonasal carcinomas appears to be of clinical relevance. Any poorly differentiated midline carcinoma or head and neck tumor lacking lineage-specific differentiation markers should be considered for immunostaining for NUT or rearrangement testing.

2.5.6 Sinonasal Adenocarcinoma

These tumors originate from either the respiratory epithelium or the underlying seromucinous glands (▶ Fig. 2.12; ▶ Table 2.3). Tumors of respiratory epithelial derivation are frequently located in the nasal cavity and the ethmoid sinus, whereas those arising from the subepithelial glands frequently affect the nasal cavity and the maxillary sinus.[6] Salivary-type tumors appear as large, nodular, light tan soft masses, whereas intestinal-type adenocarcinomas tend to be bulky, friable, and soft with ulcerated surface.

2.5.7 Salivary-Type Adenocarcinomas

The most frequent phenotype affecting the minor salivary gland of the skull base is ACC. Less frequent subtypes are mucoepidermoid, acinic cell, and low-grade papillary adenocarcinoma.[6] The histopathologic features are those of their primary salivary counterparts.

Table 2.3 Sinonasal adenocarcinomas

Factor	Salivary	Nonsalivary	
		Intestinal	Seromucinous type
Origin	Minor salivary gland	Respiratory mucosa	Minor salivary gland
Age (years)	30–70	60–70	30–70
Gender	Equal	More in males	Equal
Prognosis	• Depends on stage • 50%	• Depends on differentiation • Stage	• Depends on stage • 50%
Recurrence	High (60%)	High	Yes
Risk factor	–	• Wood worker • Leather worker	–
Markers	S-100, keratins, SMA	K-ras, keratins 7 and 20	S-100, keratins, SMA

Differential Diagnosis

The differential diagnosis is mainly of the solid form of ACC, which should not be confused with basaloid squamous or NECs. The lack of squamous differentiation, neuroendocrine markers, and anaplastic features favors ACC.

2.5.8 Human Papillomavirus–Related Carcinoma with Adenoid Cystic–Like Features

As in conventional ACC, HPV-related carcinoma with ACC-like features demonstrates a dual population of ductal and basal cells with solid and cribriform growth (▶ Fig. 2.13). Squamous dysplasia may be seen in the overlying surface epithelium but without infiltrating squamous carcinoma.[64,65] The biphasic phenotype mirrors ACC, with CK7 and c-kit in epithelial cells, whereas p63 and p40 SMA decorate the abluminal cells. These tumors strongly express p16 and HPV types 31 and 33.[6,66,67,68]

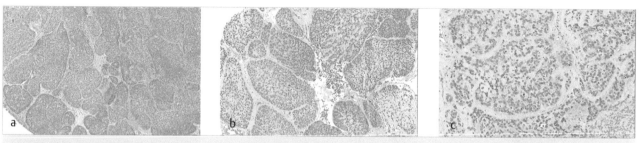

Fig. 2.13 (a–c) Human papillomavirus–related carcinoma with adenoid cystic carcinoma–like features demonstrates a dual population of ductal and basal cells with solid and cribriform growth.

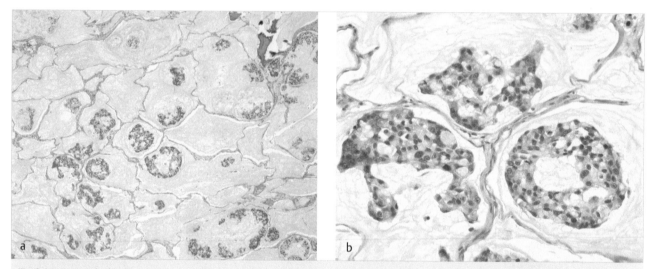

Fig. 2.14 Sinonasal adenocarcinoma, nonsalivary, intestinal type. **(a)** In the mucinous (colloidal) variant, the neoplastic cells are floating in pools of mucin. **(b)** Goblet and signet ring cells are present on higher magnification.

2.5.9 Nonsalivary Gland Adenocarcinoma

Tumors in this category are divided into intestinal and nonintestinal (seromucinous) adenocarcinomas. The intestinal adenocarcinoma is identical to those arising in the intestinal tract. These tumors arise in patients who have a history of exposure to hardwoods, leather, and certain chemical manufacturing processes. They tend to occur in the ethmoid sinus and nasal cavity. The nonintestinal adenocarcinomas are typically seromucinous adenocarcinoma and affect the ethmoid and maxillary sinuses.[6,69,70,71,72,73,74]

Histologically, the intestinal type is typically that of the colonic adenocarcinoma phenotype but may show mucinous and signet ring features (▸ Fig. 2.14). The seromucinous type is usually low-grade, with back-to-back cuboidal-lined glands and cords (▸ Fig. 2.15a). Some cases may be composed of clear cells and resemble renal cell carcinoma (RCC; ▸ Fig. 2.15b), staining with antibodies to CA-IX but less reliably with antibodies to CD10 and RCC.[75]

Differential Diagnosis

The intestinal form should be differentiated from metastasis from salivary and intestinal primaries to the skull base areas, which should be clinically excluded (▸ Table 2.3).

2.6 Mesenchymal Tumors

2.6.1 Benign Tumors

Various benign tumors similar to those originating in other soft tissues may arise in the skull base region.

2.6.2 Lobular Capillary Hemangioma (Pyogenic Granuloma)

This relatively common benign vascular lesion represents approximately 25% of the nonepithelial neoplasms of the sinonasal tract and skull base region. This entity is frequently found in the nasal septum (60%) and is most commonly identified in adolescent boys and young women. Local trauma and hormonal factors may play an etiologic role in the development of this entity. Intermittent painless epistaxis is the most common symptom.[76,77]

Usually a polypoid red to purple nodular growth is identified with mucosal ulceration. Histologically, lobular capillary hemangiomas are composed of fairly organized vascular proliferations with lobular formation (▸ Fig. 2.16). An inflammatory infiltrate may be present.

Differential Diagnosis

The differential diagnoses of these lesions are mainly vascular polyp, nasopharyngeal angiofibroma, hemangiopericytoma, and

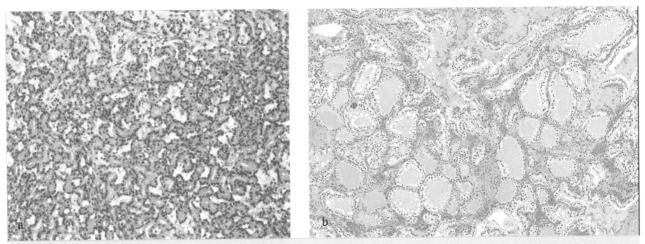

Fig. 2.15 (a) Sinonasal adenocarcinoma, nonsalivary, nonintestinal (sero-mucinous) type, formed by bland cuboidal back-to-back glands filling the stroma. **(b)** The clear cell variant mirrors renal clear cell carcinoma morphology.

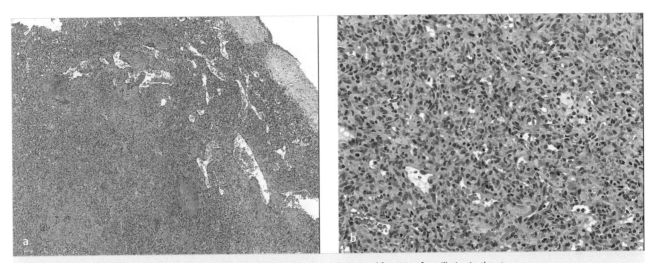

Fig. 2.16 (a, b) Lobular hemangioma (a.k.a. pyogenic granuloma) with a lobular proliferation of capillaries in the stroma.

low-grade angiosarcoma. The lobular architecture is the key finding of capillary hemangioma, which lacks the stellate stroma of an angiofibroma and the highly cellular spindled cells of a hemangiopericytoma.

2.6.3 Glomangiopericytoma (Sinonasal Hemangiopericytoma)

An uncommon nonepithelial neoplasm is composed of spindle cell proliferation of hybrid pericyte and myxoid differentiation. The tumor can present at any age, and patients most commonly complain of nasal obstruction epistaxis and pain. The nasal cavity and the paranasal sinuses are typically affected.[67,68,69,70]

In general, these tumors appear typically as a polypoid gray to red soft, fleshy tissue mass. Histologically, these lesions manifest as subepithelial spindled to round, markedly compacted cell proliferation with complex vascularity (▶ Fig. 2.17). The cells may form a variety of patterns, including fascicular, storiform, and palisading morphology with interspersed vascular

spaces in different size and forms; mitosis and mild cellular pleomorphism may also be seen.

Ancillary Markers

On IHC, the spindled cells are positive for smooth muscle actin and beta-catenin and are negative for CD34, which will highlight the vessels.

Differential Diagnosis

This tumor should be readily differentiated from reactive pyogenic granuloma, cellular hemangioma and nasopharyngeal angiofibroma, benign and low-grade smooth muscle tumors, solitary fibrous tumor, and spindle cell sarcomas (synovial sarcoma and fibrosarcoma). Immunohistochemical markers may be used to exclude some of these entities. In solitary fibrosis tumors, there is lower cellularity and positivity for STAT6, CD34, and bcl-2 in the spindled cells, which can help differentiate these entities.[71,72,73]

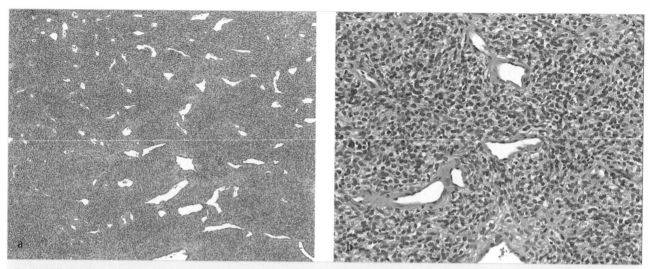

Fig. 2.17 (a, b) Glomangiopericytoma (sinonasal hemangiopericytoma) showing proliferation of spindled cells with intervening hyalinized staghorn vascular spaces.

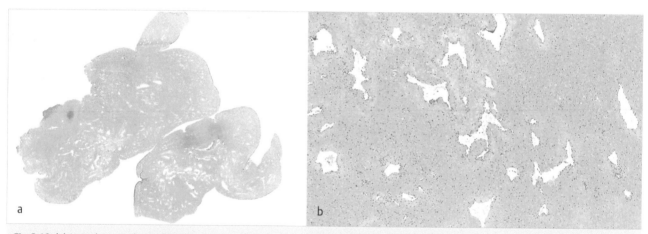

Fig. 2.18 (a) Nasopharyngeal angiofibroma may be confused with vascular and inflammatory polyps (low-power), but (b) fibrous stroma with prominent vessels is a cardinal morphological feature.

2.6.4 Nasopharyngeal Angiofibroma

This benign, highly vascular mesenchymal neoplasm arises predominantly in young males. Lesions arise in the roof of the nasopharynx, and patients' symptoms typically include nasal obstruction, epistaxis and drainage, and, less commonly, facial deformities, proptosis, deafness, sinusitis, and palliative swelling.[73,74,75]

Usually angiofibroma presents as rounded, nonencapsulated, gray-white soft tissue masses covered with smooth mucosa and spongy cut surface appearance. The cardinal histologic features of these lesions are richly thin-walled vascular formations in fibrotic connective background with stromal cell proliferation (▶ Fig. 2.18).

Differential Diagnosis

Angiofibromas may be confused with vascular and inflammatory polyp, hemangiopericytomas, vascular proliferations, hemangiomas, and pyogenic granulomas.[73,74,75]

2.6.5 Myxoma

These intraosseous, ill-defined lesions comprise mucomyxoid stroma with scattered stellate cells. If a fibrous component is visible, they are called myxofibroma. Although they most commonly present in the jaw, the maxilla may be affected. These lesions affect females more than they do males.[76,77] Usually they appear as unencapsulated, well-circumscribed, nodular, tan to white gelatinous lesions. Histologically, they are characterized by sparsely scattered, stellate-shaped mesenchymal cells in a myxoid background.

2.6.6 PEComa (Perivascular Epithelioid Cell Tumor)

The perivascular epithelioid cell tumors (PEComa) family includes mesenchymal tumors that consist of perivascular epithelioid cells. The most common tumors in the PEComa family are renal angiomyolipoma and pulmonary lymphangioleiomyomatosis

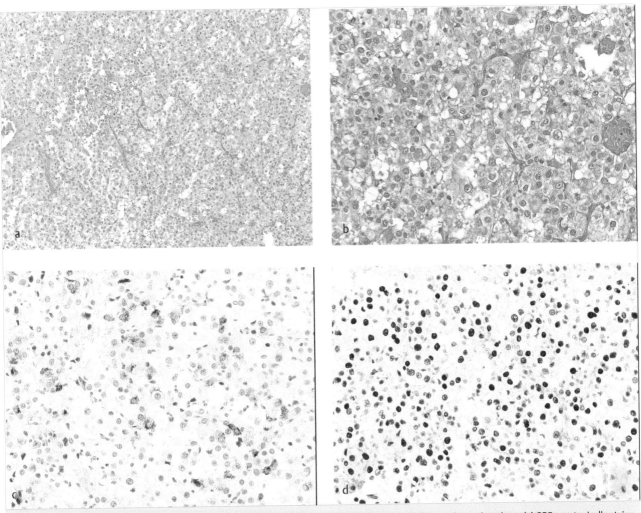

Fig. 2.19 (a, b) PEComa consists of perivascular epithelioid cells with clear/granular cytoplasm and central round nucleus. (c) PEComa typically stains for melanocytic markers (HMB45), and (d) a subset will stain for TFE3.

(both of which are more common in patients who have tuberous sclerosis).[78,79,80]

Histologically, the tumor shows a trabecular and nested architecture, composed of epithelioid cells having clear to granular eosinophilic cytoplasm (▶ Fig. 2.19). Some PEComas are dominated by spindle cells and show a sheetlike grown pattern. Marked nuclear atypia, prominent nucleoli, high mitotic activity, and necrosis are features of malignant transformation. On IHC, the tumor cells are positive for smooth muscle actin and desmin, as well as for the melanocytic markers HMB-45 and microphthalmia transcription factor.

The majority of PEComas harbor *TSC1/TSC2* (tuberous sclerosis complex) mutations. Inactivation of *TSC2* releases the inhibition of Rheb, resulting in mTOR activation—hence the use of mTOR inhibitors (sirolimus, temsirolimus) for this class of tumors, with demonstrated clinical efficacy. A large subset of PEComas lack the TSC2 mutations and instead harbor TFE3 gene rearrangements. TFE3 gene rearrangements also define alveolar soft part sarcomas as a consequence of the translocation t(X; 17).[78,79,80] Differential diagnosis includes leiomyosarcoma, melanoma, and alveolar soft part sarcoma.

Table 2.4 Clinical features of rhabdomyosarcoma subtypes

Feature	Embryonal	Alveolar
Site	Nasopharynx more than sinonasal tract	
Age	Children/young adults	Adults
Outcome	Young: 60% Adults: 10%	Poor
Incidence	80%	20%

2.7 Malignant Neoplasms

2.7.1 Rhabdomyosarcoma

Though a relatively uncommon mesenchymal malignancy of the skull base region, rhabdomyosarcoma is the most common sarcoma of the head and neck and is the most frequent childhood sarcoma. The sinonasal tract and the nasopharynx are the most commonly affected sites. The embryonal type is the most common type in children, whereas the alveolar subtype predominates in an older age group. Patients present with swelling, bleeding, visual symptoms, and sinusitis (▶ Table 2.4).[73,81,82,83]

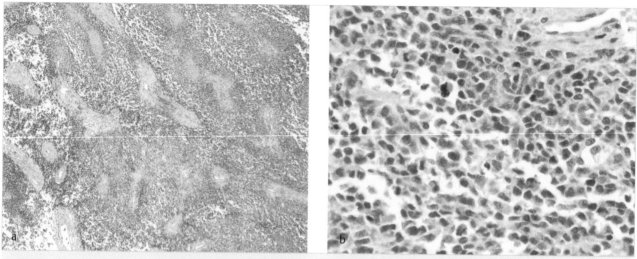

Fig. 2.20 (a) Rhabdomyosarcoma, alveolar pattern. (b) Rhabdoid cells with eccentric nuclei and pink cytoplasm are a tipoff toward establishing a diagnosis for this small round cell malignancy.

Normally the tumor may be either small gray/red or large, polypoid, and fleshy. The botryoid variant exhibits grapelike features.

Histologically, these tumors are classified into the embryonal phenotype for the vast majority of skull base rhabdomyosarcomas and are composed of primitive small round to spindled monotonous cell proliferation in sheets. A myxoid stroma may be present, giving rise to the botryoid variant. The alveolar phenotype is less common and is composed of tumor cells with eosinophilic cytoplasm in clusters separated by fibrous septa (▶ Fig. 2.20). Rhabdomyoblasts and multinucleated giant cells may be seen.

Ancillary Markers

Immunohistochemical markers, including desmin, myo-D, and myogenin, are necessary for diagnosis, especially of the embryonal form.

Differential Diagnosis

Tumors that may be confused with embryonal rhabdomyosarcoma include lymphoma, neuroblastoma, Ewing's sarcoma/PNET, and melanoma. Immunophenotyping is critical for diagnosis (▶ Fig. 2.21; ▶ Table 2.5).

2.7.2 Fibrosarcoma

This is the most frequent mesenchymal malignancy of the sinonasal tract, affecting the maxillary sinus, nasal cavity, and ethmoid region most frequently.[73,84,85] Normally the tumor presents as light tan and fleshy with a smooth surface having soft to firm consistency. Histologically, the tumor typically forms sweeping spindle cell interlacing bundles extending to surrounding tissue cells with moderate to low mitotic activity.

Differential Diagnosis

A variety of spindle cell benign and malignant tumors must be differentiated from this lesion, including neurofibroma, rhabdomyo- and synovial sarcomas, hemangiopericytoma, spindle cell carcinoma, and spindle cell melanoma. Reactive myofibroblastic

tumors and fibromatosis should also be included. Immunohistochemical markers will exclude neural, skeletal muscle, and spindle cell carcinoma if keratin is positive, but spindle cell carcinoma is phenotypically more pleomorphic and may contain an epithelial component. Synovial sarcoma may exhibit a mixed pattern, but testing for the t(X;18) fusion gene is helpful for differentiating a purely spindle cell form.

2.7.3 Synovial Sarcoma

Synovial sarcoma may involve the skull base region as extension from oropharynx or adjacent structures. The tumor affects the young age groups, having a median of 25 years and exhibiting male predominance.[73,86,87,88,89,90,91]

Histologically, synovial sarcoma may present as a pure spindle cell variant (monophasic) or in a biphasic form in which both spindle and epithelial components are present (▶ Fig. 2.22). The epithelioid component is typically composed of cuboidal or columnar epithelial cells forming cords, nests, and pseudoglandular spaces intermingled with a spindle cell proliferation.

Ancillary Markers

Cytokeratins of low and high molecular weight and epithelial membrane antigen (EMA) are positive in epithelial tumor cells. Transducin-like enhancer of split 1 (TLE1) expression is a highly specific biomarker for synovial sarcoma in the setting of differential diagnosis of unclassified high-grade sarcomas.[88,89] In cases of monomorphic spindle cells, in situ hybridization or polymerase chain reactions for the t(X;18) (p11.2; q11;2) translocation is complementary (▶ Fig. 2.21; ▶ Table 2.5).

Differential Diagnosis

This entity should be differentiated from spindle-forming tumors, including spindle cell carcinoma, fibrosarcoma, melanoma, and metastatic carcinoma to the base of skull. The combined features of clinicopathologic and immunohistochemical markers should be integrated in the diagnosis of this entity.

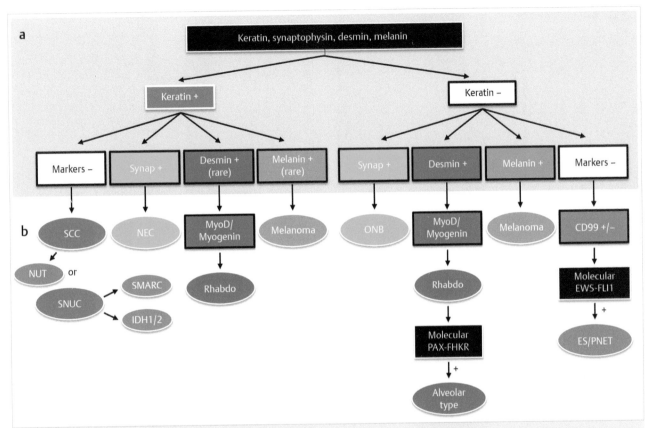

Fig. 2.21 Work-up algorithm for undifferentiated skull base tumors. **(a)** Initial panel of immunohistochemical markers. **(b)** Ancillary immunohistochemical and molecular markers and diagnoses. ES/PNET, Ewing sarcoma/peripheral neuroectodermal tumor; NEC, neuroendocrine carcinoma; ONB, olfactory neuroblastoma; Rhabdo, rhabdomyosarcoma; SCC, squamous cell carcinoma; SNUC, sinonasal undifferentiated carcinoma; Synap, synaptophysin.

2.7.4 Hemangioendothelioma/Epithelioid Hemangioendothelioma

Epithelioid hemangioendothelioma (EHE) is a rare low- to intermediate-grade mesenchymal neoplasm characterized by short cords and nests of epithelioid tumor cells with endothelial differentiation set in a myxohyaline matrix (▶ Fig. 2.13b,c; ▶ Fig. 2.23).[92,93,94] Primary sites include skin, superficial and deep soft tissues, visceral organs, and bone. Anecdotal cases of primary hemangioendothelioma of the skull base have been described.[92,93] Although the majority behave in an indolent fashion, there is an approximately 20% risk of widespread metastasis and death from disease.[94] The diagnosis of EHE may be challenging, particularly on limited biopsy, with mimickers including metastatic carcinoma, myoepithelial, and chondroid neoplasms. EHE of the bone and extraskeletal sites has a highly specific recurrent translocation, t(1;3)(p36.3; q23–25), resulting in a *WWTR1-CAMTA1* fusion transcript.[94]

2.7.5 Angiosarcoma

Angiosarcoma of the skull base region is rare, and diagnosis is based on the identification of abnormal vascular features and the use of immunohistochemical markers to support lineage (▶ Fig. 2.24).[95,96]

2.7.6 Chordoma

Chordoma is a low- to intermediate-grade malignant neoplasm originating from the notochord. The skull base accounts for approximately 32% of the cases and the cervical spine for approximately 5%. Rarely, chordoma has been reported in extra-axial locations such as nasopharynx, paranasal sinuses, oropharynx, and the soft tissue of the neck. Lesions affecting the head and neck region frequently occur in middle-aged patients and in those who are in their sixties. Patients typically present with neurological symptoms, headache, and progressive pain.[97,98,99,100]

Chordoma is a characteristically lobulated myxoid, expansive mass with mucus and a slippery appearance. Histologically, it is divided into classic, chondroid, and dedifferentiated phenotypes. The classic type is marked by a lobulated growth pattern with cords and islands of polygonal and vacuolated cells in myxomucoid background (▶ Fig. 2.25). The characteristic vacuolated and eosinophilic cell is called a physaliphorous cell. The chondroid type exhibits the same features along with areas of hyaline cartilaginous tissue. Dedifferentiated signifying transformation to a high-grade sarcoma shows marked cytologic atypia and high cellularity.

Table 2.5 Clinicohistopathologic and genetic features of small round cell tumors of the sinonasal area

Diagnosis	Age (y)/location	Histopathology/architecture	Mitotic activity/necrosis	Cytomorphology	Anaplasia or marked atypia	Cytogenetic/molecular	Immunohistochemistry
Malignant epithelial sinonasal small round blue cell tumors							
Small cell carcinoma, neuroendocrine type	26–77/superior or posterior nasal cavity, maxillary, ethmoid sinuses	Sheets, ribbons, or nests of closely packed cells with nuclear molding	Frequent/common	Monotonous small cells with hyperchromatic nuclei, inconspicuous or absent nucleoli, and minimal cytoplasm	Variable		CD56, Cytokeratin (punctate perinuclear), Chromogranin (variable), NSE (variable), Synaptophysin (variable), TTF-1 (variable)
Sinonasal undifferentiated carcinoma	20–80/nasal cavity, maxillary antrum, ethmoid sinuses, often with extension into adjacent sites	Tumor cells may be arranged in nests, lobules, trabeculae, or sheets	Frequent/common	Medium-sized nuclei with prominent nucleoli surrounded by scant eosinophilic cytoplasm	Common	No recurrent cytogenetic change; No c-kit activating mutations or gene amplification	Pankeratin, CK7, CK8, CK19, Ki-67 (most cells, variable intensity), NSE (occasional), EMA (occasional), CD99 (rare), Synaptophysin (rare), S-100 protein (rare), Chromogranin (rare)
Squamous cell carcinoma (nonkeratinizing)	55–65/maxillary sinus, nasal cavity, ethmoid sinus, sphenoid, and frontal sinuses	Ribbons, nests, or strands; underlying tissue invasion often features well-delineated border	Variable/limited	Poorly differentiated form most difficult to distinguish from other undifferentiated small round cell tumors, such as neuroendocrine carcinoma and olfactory neuroblastoma	Common		Pankeratin, EMA, CK5/6, CK8, CK13, CK14, CK19
Neuroectodermal sinonasal small round blue cell tumors							
Ewing's sarcoma/primitive neuroectodermal tumor	<30/maxillary sinus, nasal fossa	Sheets, lobules (less commonly cords or trabeculae may cause dx difficulty with carcinoid or undifferentiated carcinoma) of uniformly round cells; ± Homer-Wright rosettes	Variable/common	Small to intermediate-sized cells with poorly defined, scant, or vacuolated cytoplasm and round nuclei with fine chromatin	Infrequent	t(11;22)(q24;q12) EWSR1-FLI1 (~95%), t(21;22)(q22;q12) EWSR1-ERG (~5%), Other EWSR1 or FUS variants (<5%)	CD99 (membranous pattern), Vimentin, FLI1, NSE (variable), Synaptophysin (variable), AE1/AE3 and CAM5.2 (occasional)

Table 2.5 (*Continued*) Clinicohistopathologic and genetic features of small round cell tumors of the sinonasal area

Diagnosis	Age (y)/location	Histopathology/architecture	Mitotic activity/necrosis	Cytomorphology	Anaplasia or marked atypia	Cytogenetic/molecular	Immunohistochemistry
Mucosal malignant melanoma	40–70/nasal septum, paranasal sinuses (particularly maxillary).	Commonly deeply infiltrative with ulceration and frequent pseudopapillary architecture.	Frequent/common	Amelanotic small round cell or larger melanotic epithelioid or spindle-shaped cells; nuclear molding and/or prominent eosinophilic nucleoli possibly present	Common	CDKN2A/p16 (9p21) PTEN (10q23) 1q+,6p+,8q+	S-100 protein; Vimentin; HMB45 (usually); Melan-A (usually); Microphthalmia transcription factor (variable); Tyrosinase (variable)
Olfactory neuroblastoma	Broad age range (<10 to >80)/roof of nasal cavity, cribriform plate	Localized to submucosa; lobular to solid growth pattern in higher-grade neoplasms; rosettes (Homer-Wright and Flexner-Wintersteiner) may be present	Variable/variable	Uniformly, small cells having scant cytoplasm and round nuclei with fine to coarse granular chromatin and occasional small nucleoli (grade-dependent)	Variable (more common in high-grade tumors)	Complex with aCGH studies demonstrating gain of 13q, 20q, and loss of Xp as most frequent in high-stage tumors	Neuron-specific enolase; CD56; Synaptophysin (usually); S-100 protein (supporting sustentacular cells); CD57 (Leu7) (variable); Chromogranin (variable); GFAP (variable); Keratin (occasional)
Mesenchymal sinonasal small round blue cell tumors							
Desmoplastic small round blue cell	15–35/sinonasal case report 1	Nests of undifferentiated cells embedded in a prominent desmoplastic stroma	Frequent/common	Small, round–oval cells with scant-moderate cytoplasm and hyperchromatic nuclei with inconspicuous nucleoli; intracytoplasmic inclusions or vacuoles may be seen	Infrequent	t(11;22)(p13;q12) EWSR1-WT1	Desmin (perinuclear dot-like pattern); Pankeratin, EMA, AE1/AE3, CAM5.2; Vimentin; WT1; NSE (usually); CD57 (usually); Synaptophysin (occasional); CD99 (occasional)
Rhabdomyosarcoma	<20 y/nasopharynx[sinonasal tract	Embryonal subtype (ERMS): alternating hyper- and hypocellular areas with myxoid or sparsely collagenized stroma. Alveolar subtype (ARMS): collagenous fibrous septa separate nests of tumor cells with loss of central cohesion. Solid ARMS: sheets of tumor cells without fibrous septa	Variable/limited	Small round cells with scant cytoplasm ± scattered cells with eosinophilic cytoplasm and cross-striations	Common	ERMS: gain of all or portions of chromosomes 2, 7, 8, 11, 12, 13, and/or 20 with or without loss of 22. 11p15 LOH. ARMS: t(2;13)(q35;q14) PAX3-FOXO1 (50–60%) t(1;13)(p36;q14) PAX7-FOXO1 (*20%) Other PAX3 variants (1%) Fusion neg. (20–30%)	Desmin; Myogenin (nuclear); myo-D1 (nuclear); Myoglobin (cytoplasmic); Vimentin (usually); CD56 (usually); Myosin (variable)

Table 2.5 (*Continued*) Clinicohistopathologic and genetic features of small round cell tumors of the sinonasal area

Diagnosis	Age (y)/location	Histopathology/architecture	Mitotic activity/necrosis	Cytomorphology	Anaplasia or marked atypia	Cytogenetic/molecular	Immunohistochemistry
Synovial sarcoma (poorly differentiated)	<50/maxillary, sphenoid, ethmoid, and frontal sinuses	Often solidly packed small round cells with richly vascular hemangiopericytoma-like pattern; may be focal within a typical biphasic or monophasic synovial sarcoma or may represent the predominant pattern; other poorly differentiated forms include large (epithelioid) cell and high-grade spindle cell	Variable/variable	Poorly differentiated small cell pattern composed of small cells with high nuclear-to-cytoplasmic ratios may be exceedingly difficult to distinguish from other small round cell tumors	Infrequent	t(X;18)(p11.2;q11.2) SYT-SSX1 or SYT-SSX2 (>99%)	EMA BCL2 TLE1 Vimentin Cytokeratin (variable) CD99 (variable) S-100 (occasional)
Hematolymphoid sinonasal small round blue cell tumors							
Extramedullary plasmacytoma	35–75/nasal cavity, paranasal sinuses, nasal cavity	Diffuse infiltrate of uniform (well-differentiated) to pleomorphic (anaplastic) neoplastic plasma cells Amyloid deposits (11–38%)	Variable/uncommon	Small to large (well to poorly differentiated) cells with fine to coarse nuclear chromatin and prominent nucleoli; intracytoplasmic crystals, Dutcher bodies, and perinuclear hof may be present	Occasional	14q32 (IGH) [although unlike multiple myeloma lacks t(11;14)] -13 or 13q-	Light chain restriction CD138 CD38 CD45 VS38 EMA (variable) CD79a (variable) CD31 (occasional) CD56 (occasional)
Extranodal NK/T cell lymphoma, nasal	50–75/nasal cavity, paranasal sinuses, nasopharynx	Diffuse neoplastic lymphoid proliferation with angiocentric/angiodestructive growth pattern, mucosal ulceration, pseudoepitheliomatous hyperplasia, and frequent associated inflammatory infiltrate	Frequent/common	Small or medium-sized cells to large transformed cells with round, oval, or irregular nuclei and azurophilic cytoplasmic granules	Common	del(6)(q21–25) i(6)(p10) EBV (ISH) 10% with T cell receptor gene rearrangement, no immunoglobulin light or heavy chain rearrangements	CD2 CD3e (cytoplasmic) Granzyme B Perforin CD45 CD56 (cytoplasmic) (usually) TIA-1 (usually)

Abbreviations: TLE1, Transducer-like enhancer of split 1; TIA-1, T cell intracellular antigen 1

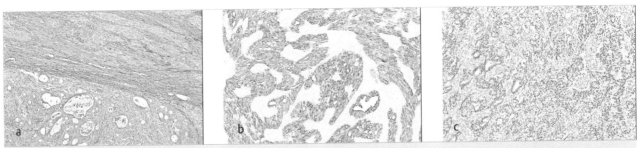

Fig. 2.22 (a) Biphasic synovial sarcoma with glandular and spindle cell component; immunoreactivity with (b) antikeratin and (c) TLE1.

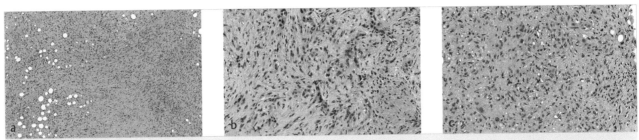

Fig. 2.23 (a–c) Epithelioid hemangioendothelioma is a low- to intermediate-grade mesenchymal neoplasm characterized by short cords and nests of epithelioid tumor cells with endothelial differentiation set in a myxohyaline matrix.

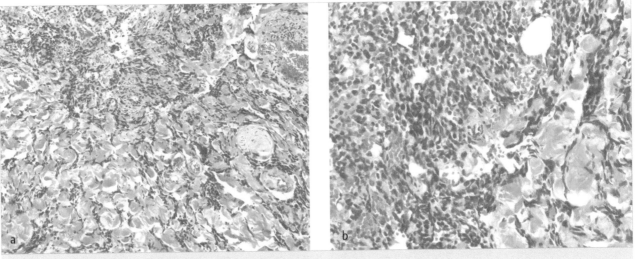

Fig. 2.24 (a, b) Angiosarcoma with atypical neoplastic cells forming vascular spaces.

Ancillary Markers

Chordoma is characteristically immunoreactive to cytokeratin, S-100, and EMA markers. Brachyury and its nuclear expression (a marker of notochordal differentiation) is highly specific for chordoma.[73,101,102]

Differential Diagnosis

Chordoma should be differentiated from mucinous adenocarcinoma, myxoma, and cartilaginous neoplasms. Immunohistochemical stains typically aid in the diagnosis. In particular, reactivity to brachyury and keratin helps exclude chondrosarcoma.

2.7.7 Chondrosarcoma

Chondrosarcomas may present as an extension from a maxillary primary. They present in a wide range of age groups, with the mesenchymal phenotype affecting mainly patients who are in the second and third decades of life. The most common presenting symptoms are craniofacial bone expansion and pain.[73,103,104] Typically these tumors manifest as translucent, cartilaginous, and scattered calcifications. Myxomatous areas with lobulation are commonly seen.

The histologic spectrum seen in these tumors ranges from benign-appearing hyaline cartilaginous lesions to highly cellular malignant spindle cell sarcoma. The characteristic malignant chondrocytic cells must be identified. The tumor can manifest

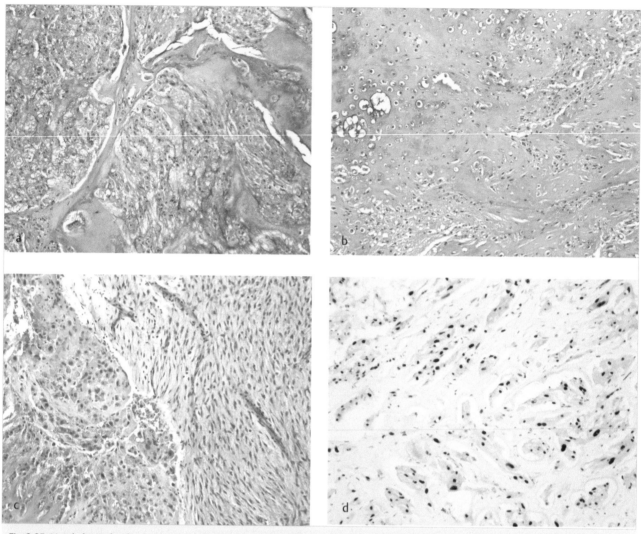

Fig. 2.25 Morphologic chordoma subtypes: **(a)** conventional; **(b)** chondroid; **(c)** spindle type/dedifferentiated. **(d)** Expression of T brachyuri is characteristic for chordoma.

as myxoid, clear cell, dedifferentiated, and mesenchymal phenotypes. Mesenchymal chondrosarcoma is rare and may cause differential diagnostic difficulties. These tumors are composed of highly cellular spindle cell proliferations in interlacing short fascicles with focal cartilaginous formations.

Differential Diagnosis

The main differential diagnosis includes enchondroma, osteochondroma, and chondroblastic osteosarcoma and chordoma. Mesenchymal chondrosarcoma should be differentiated from spindle cell malignant tumors and primitive sinonasal tumors. CD99 and SOX9 markers are typically positive in mesenchymal chondrosarcoma and could be of use in the diagnosis of this entity.

2.7.8 Osteosarcoma

Osteosarcoma is a rare tumor in the skull base region. The tumor most commonly represents an extension from maxillary origin.[73,100,105,106] Usually osteosarcoma manifests as an ill-defined, irregular, tan-yellow tissue mass with gritty (bone) sensation.

Histologically, these tumors exhibit malignant cellular proliferation with osteoid bone formation. The degree of cellularity and anaplastic cellular features reflects the grade of these tumors. The most common type of osteosarcoma is the osteogenic phenotype.

Differential Diagnosis

This tumor should be differentiated from other bone-forming lesions, including osteoblastoma, chondrosarcoma with osteoid formation, dedifferentiated chondrosarcoma, and chondroblastic osteosarcoma. Radiologic and histopathologic correlation are important.

2.8 Neurogenic Neoplasms

The tumors are derived from neuroglial origin and manifest as a primitive small cell growth, morphologic similarities that may lead to misclassification. The most frequently encountered entities at the skull base are ONB and the primitive neuroectodermal group of tumors.

2.8.1 Olfactory Neuroblastoma

This entity arises from neuroepithelium in the upper aspect of the nasal cavity and in the roof of the nose and the cribriform plate of the ethmoid sinus. They comprise approximately 5% sinonasal tract malignancies. ONB affects both genders equally, with bimodal age clustering at the first and second and the fourth and fifth decades of life. These tumors typically present as a unilateral nasal mass with obstruction and bleeding symptoms.[107,108,109,110] Comparison with other primitive sinonasal tumors is made in ▶ Table 2.5.

Grossly, ONBs are light tan soft tissue masses. Histologically, tumors are composed of small uniform sheets and nests of primitive basal cells featuring minimal cytoplasm with neurofibrillary background and occasionally with neuroepithelial pseudorosetting features (Homer-Wright structure; ▶ Fig. 2.26). True rosette formation with ductlike spaces (Flexner-Wintersteiner rosette) is rare. High-grade tumors are characterized by large pleomorphic cells and necrosis. The Hyams grading system, proposed in the late 1980s by the American Forces Institute of Pathology,[109] captures the spectrum of ONB maturation, from indolent disease to more aggressive behavior. A score from 1 to 4 is given based on the degree of expression of key adverse features: mitotic activity, nuclear pleomorphism, rosette formations, necrosis, disorganized architecture, sparse fibrillary matrix (▶ Fig. 2.27).

In the last decade, histopathologic Hyams grading has been proven to accurately characterize the tumor's biology and to be an independent predictor of locoregionally aggressive disease and worse disease-free survival (DFS).[111,112] The Hyams grading system remains a valuable asset when dealing with clinically advanced ONB and contemplating adjuvant therapy. The histopathologic grade of ONB offers added value to the clinical stage and should thus complement it in decision making.

Ancillary Markers

Negative staining for keratin, synaptophysin, and other neuroendocrine and muscle markers establishes the diagnosis of ONB. Amplification of c-Myc oncogene and loss of chromosome 1p have been considered poor prognostic markers.

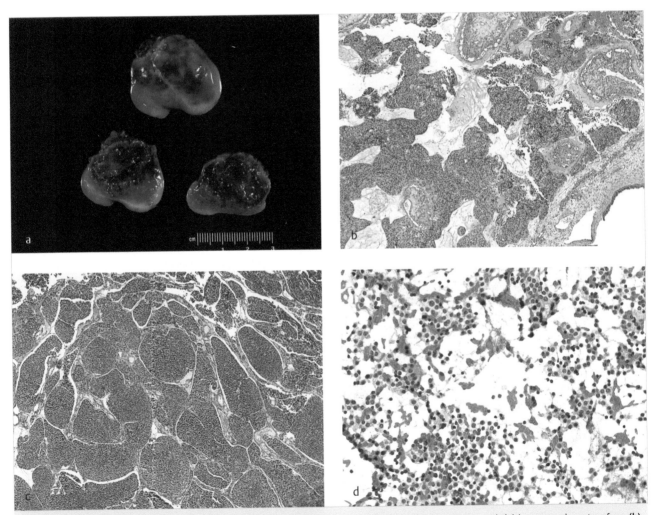

Fig. 2.26 Olfactory neuroblastoma (ONB) classical case scenario: gross appearance of polypoid red-gray mass, with (a) hypervascular cut surface, (b) frozen section diagnosis, and (d) touch preparation of nasal cavity mass. (c) Hematoxylin and eosin at low power with lobulated architectural pattern (ONB low grade).

HYAM's	Grade I	Grade II	Grade III	Grade IV
Architecture	Lobular	Lobular	Lobular	Lobular
Mitotic activity	Absent	Present	Prominent	Marked
Nuclear pleomorphism	Absent	Moderate	Prominent	Marked
Fibrillary matrix	Prominent	Present	Minimal	Absent
Rosettes	HW	HW	FW	FW
Necrosis	Absent	Absent	+/- Present	Common
Hematoxylin and Eosin		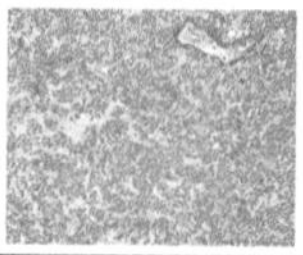	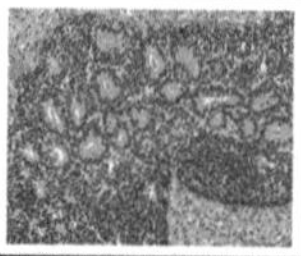	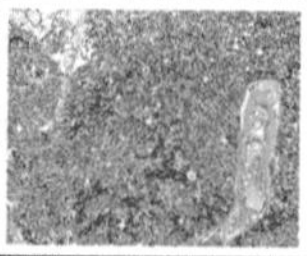

Fig. 2.27 Key features and criteria for Hyams grades I, II, III, and IV, with their corresponding histopathologic hematoxilin and eosin (H&E) slides.

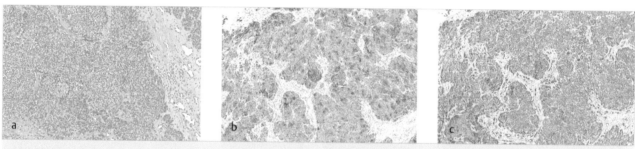

Fig. 2.28 (a) Ewing's sarcoma/primitive neuroectodermal tumor growing in sheets of monotonous small cells. Tumor cells are diffusely positive for (b) CD99 and (c) Fli1.

Differential Diagnosis

Tumors to be differentiated from ONB include lymphoma, melanoma, small round cell (Ewing's sarcoma/PNET) tumor, rhabdomyosarcoma, and ACC (solid form). Immunohistochemical profiles, including a spectrum of different cell lineage, are crucial to the diagnosis (▶ Fig. 2.21; ▶ Table 2.5).

2.8.2 Ewing Family Tumors

Ewing family tumors (EFTs), previously known as Ewing's sarcoma and PNET, are interrelated primitive round cell malignancies of neuroectodermal derivation. They represent a spectrum of morphologic entities that share common molecular genetic features. These uncommon childhood and young adult tumors affect the skull base and the sinonasal tract regions in approximately 5% of patients. The maxillary sinus and the nasal fossa are the most commonly affected sites.[73,113,114,115,116] Generally these tumors present as light tan, soft, and fleshy tissues with hemorrhage and mucosal ulceration. Histologically, the tumor presents in sheets and nests of densely uniform small cell proliferation (▶ Fig. 2.28).

2.8.3 Adamantinoma-Like Ewing Family Tumors

These sarcomas have divergent epithelial differentiation and are characterized by the same *EWSR1* alteration seen in conventional Ewing family tumors (EFT).[117,118] Morphologically, they display nested epithelial architecture with peripheral nuclear palisading, basement-membrane material and occasional keratinization (▶ Fig. 2.29).

Ancillary Markers

CD99 (MIC2) is generally diffusely positive; nuclear expression of Fli-1 and NKX2.2 also supports the diagnosis. Chromogranin, synaptophysin, and low molecular weight cytokeratin are often expressed in a subset of EFT. The adamantinoma-like variant is strongly positive for high molecular weight cytokeratin, p40 and p63. Polymerase chain reaction (PCR)-based methods for detecting the EWS/FLI gene fusion transcript and in situ hybridization of chromosomes t(11;22) or t(21;22) are helpful in confirming the diagnosis (▶ Fig. 2.21; ▶ Table 2.5).

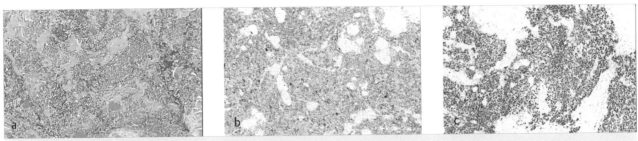

Fig. 2.29 **(a)** Adamantinoma-like Ewing's sarcoma displays a nested epithelial architecture with peripheral nuclear palisading, basement-membrane material and occasional keratinization, positive for **(b)** high molecular weight cytokeratin and **(c)** p40.

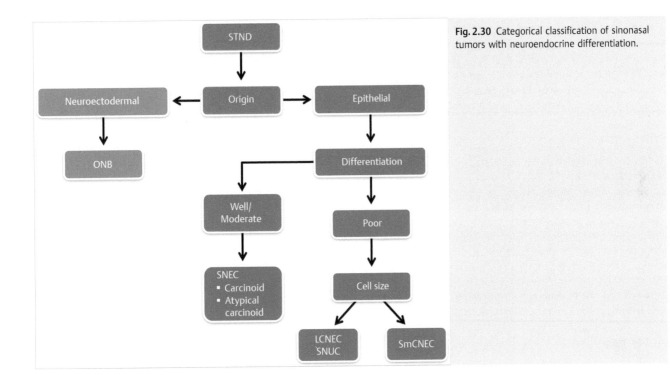

Fig. 2.30 Categorical classification of sinonasal tumors with neuroendocrine differentiation.

Differential Diagnosis

The differential diagnosis includes all small round cell tumors, lymphoma, melanoma, rhabdomyosarcoma, small cell carcinoma, and pituitary adenoma. A combined cytomorphologic and immunohistochemical markers panel is sufficient for establishing the diagnosis.

2.9 Neuroendocrine Neoplasms

2.9.1 Neuroendocrine Carcinoma

This malignancy has divergent differentiation along both the epithelial and neuroendocrine lineages. The classical scheme divides these tumors into three types: carcinoid, atypical carcinoid, and small cell carcinoma.[45,119,120] Grading uses a classification scheme that includes well-differentiated NEC (i.e., carcinoid), moderately differentiated NEC (i.e., atypical carcinoid), and poorly differentiated NEC (i.e., small "oat"-cell NEC; ▶ Fig. 2.30). These are uncommon tumors at the sinonasal and skull base sites but frequently lead to differential diagnostic difficulties.[45,119,120]

2.9.2 Carcinoid and Atypical Carcinoid Tumors

Histologically, carcinoid tumors are composed of organoid structures, including cell nests, glandular structures, and cords of monotonous basaloid cells with clear or granular cytoplasm. Atypical carcinoid lesions exhibit these organized features as well but also have evidence of mitotic activity, cellular pleomorphism, and necrosis.

2.9.3 Large Cell Neuroendocrine Carcinoma

In the respiratory tract, large cell neuroendocrine carcinoma (LCNEC) is composed of organoid nests, trabeculae, and rosettes, with peripheral palisading of nuclei. The cells are large, having low nuclear/cytoplasmic ratio, nucleoli or vesicular chromatin, and more than 11 mitoses per 10 high-power fields (HPF)/ 2 mm², Ki-67 > 20%. Neuroendocrine features are seen on IHC or electron microscopy.[121,122]

2.9.4 Small Cell Neuroendocrine Carcinoma

Irrespective of the site of occurrence, small cell neuroendocrine carcinoma (SCNEC) is hypercellular and exhibits variegated growth patterns, including ribbons, cords, and sheets. The cells are small and have hyperchromasia, no nucleoli, minimal cytoplasm, and abundant necrosis. Crush artifact of the neoplastic cells is characteristically seen; the Azzopardi effect (i.e., smudged hematoxylinic deposits in blood vessel walls) may be noted. Neural-like rosettes can be seen in SCNEC, although this is uncommon. Reactivity with the following antibodies may be present: keratin cocktail (may show punctate perinuclear positivity), chromogranin, and synaptophysin.[45,119,120] Glandular (with mucin production) or squamous differentiation can be seen in neuroendocrine neoplasms.[45] Small cell carcinoma is generally composed of undifferentiated small cell proliferations, lacking organization, with high levels of mitotic activities and necrosis (▶ Fig. 2.31). The differential diagnosis of these tumors depends on the state of differentiations for carcinoid and atypical carcinoid.[120]

Differential Diagnosis

The differential diagnosis may include adenocarcinoma and pituitary adenoma. For SCNEC, a host of small undifferentiated tumors of different lineages should be included in the diagnosis. Immunohistochemical, molecular, and histomorphologic characteristics should be integrated.

Achaete-scute homologue 1 (*ASH1*) is a key player in modulating neuroendocrine differentiation in tumor cells and may provide a useful marker for cancers that have neuroendocrine features. ASH1 expression levels are inversely associated with the degree of tumor differentiation (high-grade tumors show increased expression of this protein), which correlates well with studies indicating that expression of ASH1 appears to be restricted to immature cells.[123]

2.9.5 Paraganglioma

Sinonasal and skull base paraganglioma are extremely rare.[45,124] They are likely to be derived from dispersed neuroendocrine cells with the sinonasal mucosal covering. Tumors at this location may behave aggressively.[124] The histologic characteristics of these tumors are typical of those at traditional sites, with classical Zellballen organization and vascularization (▶ Fig. 2.32).

Ancillary Markers

Immunohistochemically, cells comprising these tumors are positive for neuroendocrine markers and negative for keratin. A helpful feature is the positivity for S-100 protein in sustentacular cells bordering the Zellballen.

2.9.6 Melanoma

Primary melanoma in the sinonasal tract accounts for less than 1% of all melanomas. These tumors afflict patients in their fifth and sixth decades of life with equal gender distribution. The most frequently affected sites are the anterior nasal septum and the maxillary antrum. Symptoms are nasal obstruction, epistaxis, and nasal mass or polyp (▶ Table 2.6).[125,126,127]

Melanomas usually appear as a small to large polypoid light tan, brown, or black mass. Histologically, the cytomorphologic features are identical to those of melanoma of the skin, in which spindle, rounded, and epithelioid cells forming nests, sheets and fascicles may be found (▶ Fig. 2.33). These phenotypes may or may not exhibit melanin pigmentation. Mucosal involvement and epidermoid migration of melanocytic cells is a helpful diagnostic feature when present.

Ancillary Markers

This tumor is negative for keratin and reactive to melanocytic markers, including HMB-45, Melan-A, MART-1, tyrosinase, and S-100. Mutations in KIT are frequently found, whereas BRAF and NRAS mutations are rarely found except in conjunctival melanomas that carry BRAF mutations. Mutations in the TERT promoter region are also found in mucosal melanomas.[128]

Differential Diagnosis

Melanoma at these locations should be differentiated from metastatic melanoma and primary undifferentiated skull base

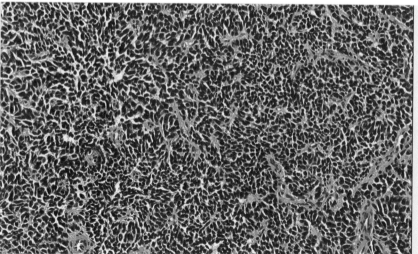

Fig. 2.31 Small cell carcinoma with an organoid pattern of growth (ribbons, rosettes) of small to medium-sized cells exhibiting minimal cytoplasm, hyperchromatic, indistinct nucleoli, and nuclear molding. Mitoses are frequent.

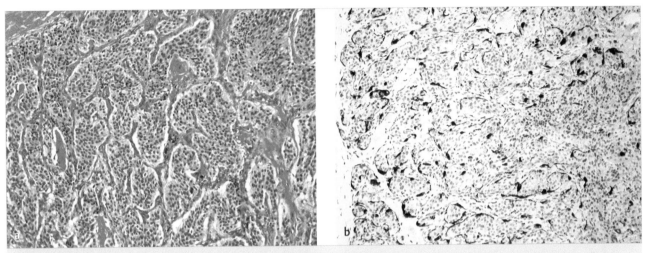

Fig. 2.32 (a) Paraganglioma with nested neuroendocrine cells (Zellballen) surrounded by thin vasculature. **(b)** Peripheral sustentacular cells are highlighted by S-100.

Table 2.6 Characteristics of mucosal melanoma

- <1% of all melanomas
- <5% of sinonasal tumors
- M/F: 1:1
- Age: Fifth to eighth decades
- Race: Japanese
- Site:
  - Anterior septum
  - Maxillary antrum
- Poor prognosis
- Adverse features:
  - >3.0 cm size
  - Advanced age
  - Vascular invasion

Abbreviation: M/F, male/female.

neoplasms, including undifferentiated carcinoma, neuroendocrine tumor, neuroblastoma, lymphoma, and small peripheral neuroectodermal tumors and rhabdomyosarcoma. Immunohistochemical markers are fundamental in differentiating these tumors (► Fig. 2.21; ► Table 2.5).

2.9.7 Melanotic Neuroectodermal Tumor of Infancy

Melanotic neuroectodermal tumor of infancy are extremely rare tumors that have a predilection for the head and neck region and that exhibit evidence of neural, epithelial, mesenchymal and neuroectodermal differentiation.[45,129] Histological characteristic features consist of a biphasic population of large and small cells forming alveolar or tubular-like structures in a dense fibrotic stroma (► Fig. 2.34).

Ancillary Studies

Immunohistochemically, the larger cells are positive for cytokeratin, vimentin, and HMB-45, with variable immunoreactivity for EMA. Both small and large cells are usually positive for

neuroendocrine markers. Surgical excision with free margins is curative in almost all cases.[45,129]

2.9.8 Biphenotypic Sinonasal Sarcoma

Biphenotypic sinonasal sarcoma (BSNS) is a low-grade sarcoma with neural and myogenic differentiation that arises exclusively in the sinonasal tract, predominantly in the superior nasal cavity and ethmoid sinuses, with rare extension into the cribriform plate, cranial vault, or orbit. It has been described as more frequent in women, and symptoms include difficulty breathing, facial pain and pressure, and nasal congestion.[73]

BSNSs are poorly circumscribed, infiltrative hypercellular lesions composed of uniform spindle cells arranged in medium to long fascicles; classic herringbone areas are noted in most cases (► Fig. 2.35). Collagen wisps are frequently present between tumor cells; a hemangiopericytoma-like vascular pattern is also identified.[73,114]

Ancillary Studies

Phenotypically, BSNSs typically coexpress smooth muscle actins (SMA, MSA) and S100 > nuclear beta-catenin has been reported. Most reported cases demonstrate rearrangements of *PAX3*: *PAX3-MAML3* fusion is specific for this entity, but *PAX3-NCOA1* and *PAX3-FOXO1* (previously described under alveolar rhabdomyosarcoma) are described in a subset of BSNSs.[130]

Differential Diagnosis

The differential diagnosis of BSNSs includes benign and malignant spindle cell neoplasms: low-grade fibrosarcoma, cellular schwannoma, malignant peripheral nerve sheath tumor, leiomyosarcoma, monophasic synovial sarcoma, spindle cell melanoma, solitary fibrous tumor, and glomangiopericytoma. Most patients are treated with surgical resection with or without adjuvant radiotherapy. Local recurrence has been reported in up to 40% of the cases, with no reported metastases or tumor-related deaths thus far (2019).

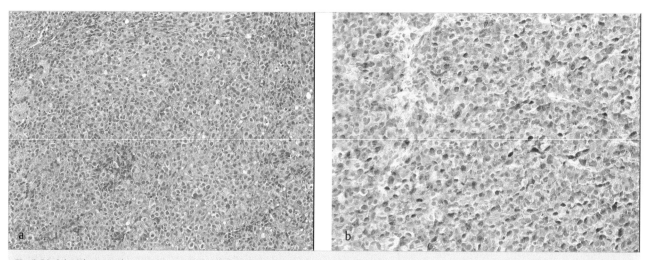

Fig. 2.33 (a) Melanoma showing prominent nucleoli and growing in sheets, (b) diffusely reactive with anti-S100 (nuclear and cytoplasmic pattern).

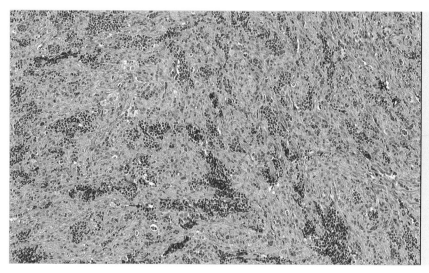

Fig. 2.34 Melanotic neuroectodermal tumor of infancy showing biphasic pattern with small neuroblastic cells and large epithelioid cells.

Fig. 2.35 (a–c) Biphenotypic sinonasal sarcoma: a low-grade sarcoma that exhibits both neural and myogenic differentiation. On histologic sections it displays hypercellular fascicles of bland spindle cells. Of note in (a) are entrapped respiratory seromucinous glands.

2.9.9 Desmoplastic Small Round Cell Tumor

Desmoplastic small round cell tumor (DSRCT) is an uncommon and aggressive malignancy that occurs on serosal surfaces, primarily in adolescent males. Generally it presents as an abdominal or pelvic mass, although cases have been described in various locations, such as pleura, lung, pericardium, femur, hypothenar area, and brachial plexus. In the head and neck region, it is relatively rare.[128,129] Although there are aggressive treatment modalities, such as a combination of radiotherapy, CT, and surgery, the overall progression-free 5-year survival rate of patients is 18%.[131,132]

Ancillary Studies

Diagnosis is based mainly on pathologic evaluation, including IHC and cytogenetic analysis. Morphologically, the tumor shows an alveolar and nested arrangement of small monotonous round cells (▶ Fig. 2.36). Immunoreactivity with desmin, WT1 is usually strong, with variable positivity for neuroendocrine markers (NSE, chromogranin, synaptophysin) and keratins (CAM 5.2). This tumor has an unique translocation t(11:22)(p:13, q:12), resulting in EWS/WT1 gene fusion that is diagnostic for DSRCT.

2.10 Lymphoproliferative Disorders

2.10.1 Sinus Histiocytosis with Massive Lymphadenopathy (Rosai-Dorfman Disease)

This rare idiopathic, histiocytic, proliferative disorder is typically found in young black women. It affects the paranasal sinuses, the nasal cavity, and the eyes; patients present with nasal obstruction, proptosis, cranial nerve deficits, mass, and fever.[133] Usually lymphoreticular tumors appear as polypoid gray to yellow soft tissue masses. Histologically, they show marked sinus expansion with lymphoplasmacytic proliferation. The sinuses are also filled with histiocytic cells and have lymphocytes and red cells in their cytoplasm (lymphophagocytosis/emperipolesis; ▶ Fig. 2.37).

Ancillary Markers

Diagnosis may be aided by staining histiocytic markers, including S-100 protein and CD68.

Differential Diagnosis

Rosai-Dorfman disease must be differentiated from infectious entities, such as rhinoscleroma, lepromatous leprosy, and malignant, and histiocytic lymphoma.

2.10.2 Lymphoma

Although rare, most lymphoproliferative lesion that arise from the skull base region[134,135] are B-cell lineage lymphomas and sinonasal NK/T-cell lymphomas. These tumors may affect the nasal cavity and paranasal sinuses and may extend to involve any adjacent structures. Patients present with nasal obstruction, epistaxis, proptosis, or mass lesion. NK/T-cell lymphoma is seen in adults, with a male predominance. Lymphoproliferative tumors appear grossly as soft and tan-gray and are often described as "fish-flesh" soft tissue masses.

Histology will vary depending on the underlying entity, but most will show sheets of atypical lymphoid cells with a diffuse growth pattern infiltrating the stroma (▶ Fig. 2.38). The tumor cells are frequently angiocentric around blood vessels in the NK/T-cell type. Prominent necrosis is also common in this specific entity, leading to a midline facial destructive process.

Ancillary Markers

Diagnosis is aided by staining lymphoid markers, including CD45 and lineage markers (such as, B-cell CD20; T-cell CD3, CD4, and CD8) among a multitude of other markers, such as CD56. On histologic samples, EBV can be identified by in situ hybridization for EBV-encoded RNA, which is almost universally positive in the NK/T-cell type lymphoma and may be associated with some diffuse B-cell lymphomas. When lymphoma is

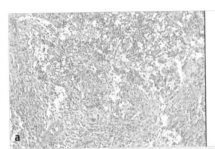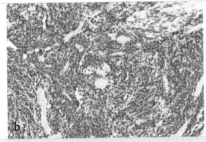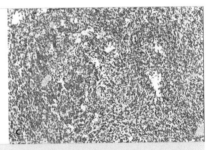

Fig. 2.36 (a) Desmoplastic small round cell tumor showing alveolar and nested arrangement of small monotonous round cells. Immunophenotype with (b) antidesmin (membranous pattern of distribution) and (c) WT1 (nuclear, as part of the *EWSR1-WT1* fusion gene signature).

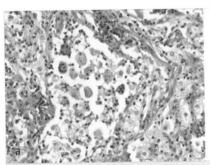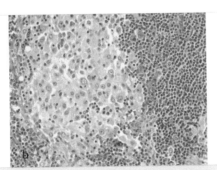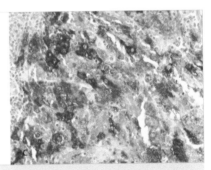

Fig. 2.37 Rosai-Dorfman disease. (a, b) The sinuses are also filled with histiocytic cell with lymphocytes and red cells in their cytoplasm (lymphophagocytosis/emperipolesis); (c) S100 aids by staining the histiocytes.

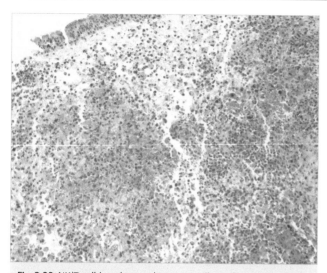

Fig. 2.38 NK/T-cell lymphoma: the tumor cells are frequently angio-centric around blood vessels; prominent necrosis is also common in this specific entity.

suspected, fresh tissue should be sent for flow cytometric analysis along with tissue for permanent histologic examination.

Differential Diagnosis

This lesion may mimic small, round, blue cell tumors (▶ Fig. 2.21; Table 2-5) and undifferentiated carcinomas (sinonasal and nasopharyngeal). If prominent necrosis is present, then granulomatosis with polyangiitis (Wegener's) and other chronic lesions may be considered. IHC for carcinoma and small round cell tumor and fungal stains excludes these entities.

2.11 Miscellaneous

2.11.1 Teratocarcinosarcoma

This rare skull base and sinonasal tract malignant tumor is composed of carcinomatous, sarcomatous, and immature neural elements. The most frequent sites are the ethmoid and maxillary sinuses, as well as the nasal cavity in elderly male patients.

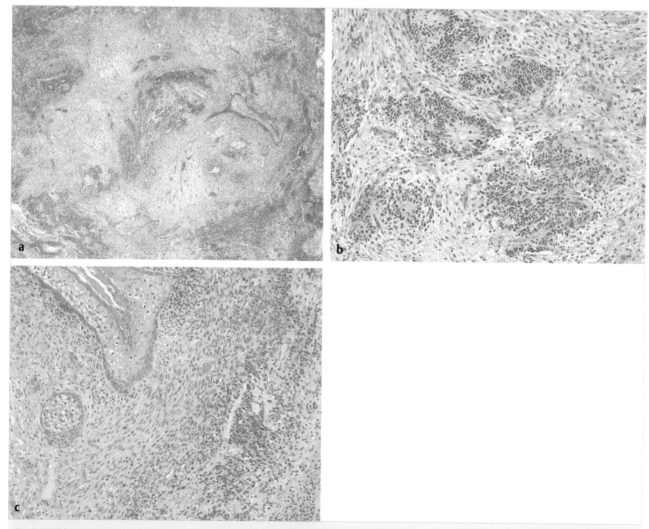

Fig. 2.39 (a) Heterogeneous morphology of teratocarcinosarcoma with varying proportions of benign and malignant epithelial, mesenchymal, and neuroepithelial elements; **(b)** true neuroepithelial rosettes. **(c)** Primitive small round cells adjacent to spindled stroma and fetal-type (glycogenated) squamous mucosa (*left side*).

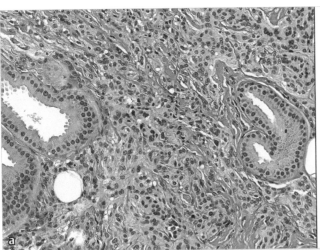
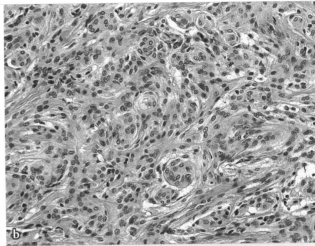

Fig. 2.40 Meningioma. (a) Ceruminous glands, recognized by cytoplasmic lipofuscin pigment and apocrine secretions, are embedded within meningothelial sheets. (b) Meningothelial-type meningioma with characteristic whirling.

Grossly, these rare tumors appear as a bulky, polypoid, and friable light tan to red mass.

Histologically, the tumor is characteristically composed of a high-grade carcinomatous component admixed with sarcomatous and immature neural elements (▶ Fig. 2.39). Benign and malignant germ cell elements may also be present. The carcinoma can be either squamous or adeno- or neuroendocrine, and the sarcoma can be cartilaginous, bony, or skeletal muscle in nature. The neural elements may contain primitive rosettes with neurofibrillary features.[136,137,138,139]

Differential Diagnosis

This tumor causes a differential diagnostic dilemma if a dominant component is present on small biopsy samples. The diagnosis may depend on the available tissue component.

2.11.2 Meningioma

Histologically, skull base meningiomas are identical morphologically to their primary meningeal origin but tend to be locally invasive, frequently showing characteristic whirling (▶ Fig. 2.40). They are typically meningothelial or fibroblastic, but other types may also be found.[140,141,142]

2.11.3 Ameloblastoma

Ameloblastoma is a tumor of intermediate malignancy and odontogenic origin that arises from enamel organ, residual dental lamina, the epithelial lining of dentigerous or follicular cysts, or, rarely, heterotopic embryonal enamel in the sinonasal tract. Ameloblastoma at the base of skull are typically an extension from tumors originating in the molar region of the maxillary antrum. They can frequently cause presentation with nasal symptoms without a history of dental complaints.[143]

Histologically, the solid form manifests as cellular, follicular structures with palisading basal cells that have branding cords and cellular islets (▶ Fig. 2.41). The cystic form manifests as varied spaces lined by palisading basal cells with squamous

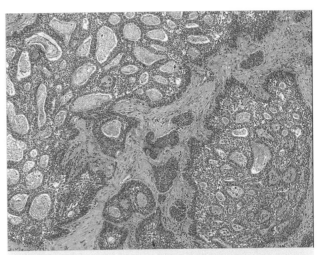

Fig. 2.41 Palisading basaloid epithelium with central stellate reticulum mimicking dental elements are key morphological features of ameloblastoma.

metaplasia that has central satellite appearing cells. Extraosseous ameloblastoma may histologically mimic basal cell carcinoma, and efforts must be made to exclude this possibility.

2.12 Metastatic Neoplasms

Isolated metastatic tumors in this region are very rare, but tumors may occur in metastasis to multiple other sites. RCC is by far the most common source. Others include breast, lung, melanoma, and testicular tumors, in descending order of frequency. Isolated incidences of metastasis from various other tumors have also been reported.

Metastatic tumors affect both genders equally, notwithstanding gender-specific influence. In female patients, breast, gynecologic, and thyroid tumors, in descending order, are the most frequent primary origins. In male patients, lung, prostate, kidney and bone, in descending order, are the most common

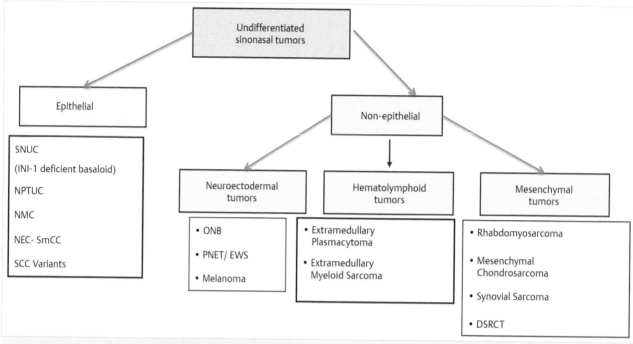

Fig. 2.42 Practical diagnostic algorithm for sinonasal undifferentiated neoplasms.

sites.[144,145,146] ▶ Fig. 2.42 summarizes a practical diagnostic algorithm for sinonasal undifferentiated neoplasms.

References

[1] Lai SY, Kennedy DW, Bolger WE. Sphenoid encephaloceles: disease management and identification of lesions within the lateral recess of the sphenoid sinus. Laryngoscope. 2002; 112(10):1800–1805

[2] Jabre A, Tabaddor R, Samaraweera R. Transsphenoidal meningoencephalocele in adults. Surg Neurol. 2000; 54(2):183–187, discussion 187–188

[3] Penner CR, Thompson L. Nasal glial heterotopia: a clinicopathologic and immunophenotypic analysis of 10 cases with a review of the literature. Ann Diagn Pathol. 2003; 7(6):354–359

[4] Khan RA, Chernock RD, Lewis JS, Jr. Seromucinous hamartoma of the nasal cavity: a report of two cases and review of the literature. Head Neck Pathol. 2011; 5(3):241–247

[5] Bullock MJ. Low-grade epithelial proliferations of the sinonasal tract. Head Neck Pathol. 2016; 10(1):47–59

[6] Stelow EB. Glandular neoplasia of the sinonasal tract. Surg Pathol Clin. 2017; 10(1):89–102

[7] Thompson LD, Seethala RR, Müller S. Ectopic sphenoid sinus pituitary adenoma (ESSPA) with normal anterior pituitary gland: a clinicopathologic and immunophenotypic study of 32 cases with a comprehensive review of the english literature. Head Neck Pathol. 2012; 6(1):75–100

[8] Hyrcza MD, Ezzat S, Mete O, et al. Pituitary adenomas presenting as sinonasal or nasopharyngeal masses: a case series illustrating potential diagnostic pitfalls. Am J Surg Path. 2016:Dec 22. PMID: 28009611 2017;41(4);525–534

[9] Alyono JC, Shi Y, Berry GJ, et al. Inflammatory pseudotumors of the skull base: a meta-analysis. Otol Neurotol. 2015; 36(8):1432–1438

[10] Newlin HE, Werning JW, Mendenhall WM. Plasma cell granuloma of the maxillary sinus: a case report and literature review. Head Neck. 2005; 27 (8):722–728

[11] Maruya S, Kurotaki H, Hashimoto T, Ohta S, Shinkawa H, Yagihashi S. Inflammatory pseudotumour (plasma cell granuloma) arising in the maxillary sinus. Acta Otolaryngol. 2005; 125(3):322–327

[12] Polzehl D, Moeller P, Riechelmann H, Perner S. Distinct features of chronic rhinosinusitis with and without nasal polyps. Allergy. 2006; 61(11): 1275–1279

[13] Garavello W, Gaini RM. Histopathology of routine nasal polypectomy specimens: a review of 2,147 cases. Laryngoscope. 2005; 115(10):1866–1868

[14] Kizil Y, Aydil U, Ceylan A, Uslu S, Baştürk V, İleri F. Analysis of choanal polyps. J Craniofac Surg. 2014; 25(3):1082–1084

[15] Lawson W, Kaufman MR, Biller HF. Treatment outcomes in the management of inverted papilloma: an analysis of 160 cases. Laryngoscope. 2003; 113(9): 1548–1556

[16] Udager AM, McHugh JB. Human papillomavirus-associated neoplasms of the head and neck. Surg Pathol Clin. 2017; 10(1):35–55

[17] Chan JK. Virus-associated neoplasms of the nasopharynx and sinonasal tract: diagnostic problems. Mod Pathol. 2017; 30 s1:S68–S83

[18] Lisan Q, Laccourreye O, Bonfils P. Sinonasal inverted papilloma: from diagnosis to treatment. Eur Ann Otorhinolaryngol Head Neck Dis. 2016; 133(5):337–341

[19] Lewis JS, Jr. Sinonasal squamous cell carcinoma: a review with emphasis on emerging histologic subtypes and the role of human papillomavirus. Head Neck Pathol. 2016; 10(1):60–67

[20] Adriaensen GF, Lim KH, Georgalas C, Reinartz SM, Fokkens WJ. Challenges in management of inverted papilloma: a review of 72 revision cases. Laryngoscope. 2016; 126(2):322–328

[21] Hartwick RW, Batsakis JG. Sinus aspergillosis and allergic fungal sinusitis. Ann Otol Rhinol Laryngol. 1991; 100(5 Pt 1) 5pt1:427–430

[22] Granville L, Chirala M, Cernoch P, Ostrowski M, Truong LD. Fungal sinusitis: histologic spectrum and correlation with culture. Hum Pathol. 2004; 35(4): 474–481

[23] Taxy JB. Paranasal fungal sinusitis: contributions of histopathology to diagnosis: a report of 60 cases and literature review. Am J Surg Pathol. 2006; 30 (6):713–720

[24] Kontoyiannis DP, Lionakis MS, Lewis RE, et al. Zygomycosis in a tertiary-care cancer center in the era of Aspergillus-active antifungal therapy: a case-control observational study of 27 recent cases. J Infect Dis. 2005; 191 (8):1350–1360

[25] Parikh SL, Venkatraman G, DelGaudio JM. Invasive fungal sinusitis: a 15-year review from a single institution. Am J Rhinol. 2004; 18(2):75–81

[26] Botelho-Nevers E, Gouriet F, Lepidi H, et al. Chronic nasal infection caused by Klebsiella rhinoscleromatis or Klebsiella ozaenae: two forgotten infectious diseases. Int J Infect Dis. 2007; 11(5):423–429

[27] Quevedo J. Scleroma in Guatemala, with a study of the disease based on the experience of 108 cases. Ann Otol Rhinol Laryngol. 1949; 58(3):613–645, illust

[28] Keni SP, Wiley EL, Dutra JC, Mellott AL, Barr WG, Altman KW. Skull base Wegener's granulomatosis resulting in multiple cranial neuropathies. Am J Otolaryngol. 2005; 26(2):146–149

[29] Heffner DK. Wegener's granulomatosis is not a granulomatous disease. Ann Diagn Pathol. 2002; 6(5):329–333

[30] Bajema IM, Hagen EC, van der Woude FJ, Bruijn JA. Wegener's granulomatosis: a meta-analysis of 349 literary case reports. J Lab Clin Med. 1997; 129 (1):17–22

[31] Montone KT, LiVolsi VA. LiVolsi VA. Inflammatory and infectious lesions of the sinonasal tract. Surg Pathol Clin. 2017; 10(1):125–154

[32] Buchmann L, Emami A, Wei JL. Primary head and neck Langerhans cell histiocytosis in children. Otolaryngol Head Neck Surg. 2006; 135(2):312–317

[33] Krishna H, Behari S, Pal L, et al. Solitary Langerhans-cell histiocytosis of the clivus and sphenoid sinus with parasellar and petrous extensions: case report and a review of literature. Surg Neurol. 2004; 62(5):447–454

[34] Davis SE, Rice DH. Langerhans' cell histiocytosis: current trends and the role of the head and neck surgeon. Ear Nose Throat J. 2004; 83(5):340–344 passim

[35] Boston M, Derkay CS. Langerhans' cell histiocytosis of the temporal bone and skull base. Am J Otolaryngol. 2002; 23(4):246–248

[36] Brisman JL, Feldstein NA, Tarbell NJ, et al. Eosinophilic granuloma of the clivus: case report, follow-up of two previously reported cases, and review of the literature on cranial base eosinophilic granuloma. Neurosurgery. 1997; 41(1):273–278, discussion 278–279

[37] Sindwani R, Cohen JT, Pilch BZ, Metson RB. Myospherulosis following sinus surgery: pathological curiosity or important clinical entity? Laryngoscope. 2003; 113(7):1123–1127

[38] Tsai EC, Santoreneos S, Rutka JT. Tumors of the skull base in children: review of tumor types and management strategies. Neurosurg Focus. 2002; 12(5):e1

[39] Richardson MS. Pathology of skull base tumors. Otolaryngol Clin North Am. 2001; 34(6):1025–1042, vii

[40] Porceddu S, Martin J, Shanker G, et al. Paranasal sinus tumors: Peter MacCallum Cancer Institute experience. Head Neck. 2004; 26(4):322–330

[41] Dulguerov P, Jacobsen MS, Allal AS, Lehmann W, Calcaterra T. Nasal and paranasal sinus carcinoma: are we making progress? A series of 220 patients and a systematic review. Cancer. 2001; 92(12):3012–3029

[42] Wieneke JA, Thompson LD, Wenig BM. Basaloid squamous cell carcinoma of the sinonasal tract. Cancer. 1999; 85(4):841–854

[43] Robbins KT, Ferlito A, Silver CE, et al. Contemporary management of sinonasal cancer. Head Neck. 2011; 33(9):1352–1365

[44] Frierson HF, Jr, Mills SE, Fechner RE, Taxy JB, Levine PA. Sinonasal undifferentiated carcinoma. An aggressive neoplasm derived from schneiderian epithelium and distinct from olfactory neuroblastoma. Am J Surg Pathol. 1986; 10(11):771–779

[45] Mills SE. Neuroectodermal neoplasms of the head and neck with emphasis on neuroendocrine carcinomas. Mod Pathol. 2002; 15(3):264–278

[46] Jeng YM, Sung MT, Fang CL, et al. Sinonasal undifferentiated carcinoma and nasopharyngeal-type undifferentiated carcinoma: two clinically, biologically, and histopathologically distinct entities. Am J Surg Pathol. 2002; 26 (3):371–376

[47] Franchi A, Moroni M, Massi D, Paglierani M, Santucci M. Sinonasal undifferentiated carcinoma, nasopharyngeal-type undifferentiated carcinoma, and keratinizing and nonkeratinizing squamous cell carcinoma express different cytokeratin patterns. Am J Surg Pathol. 2002; 26(12):1597–1604

[48] Bell D, Hanna EY. Sinonasal undifferentiated carcinoma: morphological heterogeneity, diagnosis, management and biological markers. Expert Rev Anticancer Ther. 2013; 13(3):285–296

[49] Franchi A, Palomba A, Cardesa A. Current diagnostic strategies for undifferentiated tumours of the nasal cavities and paranasal sinuses. Histopathology. 2011; 59(6):1034–1045

[50] Bishop JA, Antonescu CR, Westra WH. SMARCB1 (INI-1)-deficient carcinomas of the sinonasal tract. Am J Surg Pathol. 2014; 38(9):1282–1289

[51] Agaimy A, Koch M, Lell M, et al. SMARCB1(INI1)-deficient sinonasal basaloid carcinoma: a novel member of the expanding family of SMARCB1-deficient neoplasms. Am J Surg Pathol. 2014; 38(9):1274–1281

[52] Bell D, Hanna EY, Agaimy A, Weissferdt A. Reappraisal of sinonasal undifferentiated carcinoma: SMARCB1 (INI1)-deficient sinonasal carcinoma: a single-institution experience. Virchows Arch. 2015; 467(6):649–656

[53] Chan JKC, Bray F, McCarron P, et al. Nasopharyngeal carcinoma. In: El-Naggar AK, Chan JKC, Grandis JR, Takata T, Slootweg P, eds. Pathology and Genetics of Head and Neck Tumours. Lyon, France: IARC Press; 2017:65–70. Chan JKC, Slootweg P, Series eds. World Health Organization Classification of Tumours

[54] Wei WI, Sham JS. Nasopharyngeal carcinoma. Lancet. 2005; 365(9476): 2041–2054

[55] Lo KW, To KF, Huang DP. Focus on nasopharyngeal carcinoma. Cancer Cell. 2004; 5(5):423–428

[56] Shi W, Pataki I, MacMillan C, et al. Molecular pathology parameters in human nasopharyngeal carcinoma. Cancer. 2002; 94(7):1997–2006

[57] Dawson CW, Port RJ, Young LS. The role of the EBV-encoded latent membrane proteins LMP1 and LMP2 in the pathogenesis of nasopharyngeal carcinoma (NPC). Semin Cancer Biol. 2012; 22(2):144–153

[58] Hsu HC, Chen CL, Hsu MM, Lynn TC, Tu SM, Huang SC. Pathology of nasopharyngeal carcinoma. Proposal of a new histologic classification correlated with prognosis. Cancer. 1987; 59(5):945–951

[59] French CA. Pathogenesis of NUT midline carcinoma. Annu Rev Pathol. 2012; 7:247–265

[60] French CA, Kutok JL, Faquin WC, et al. Midline carcinoma of children and young adults with NUT rearrangement. J Clin Oncol. 2004; 22(20):4135–4139

[61] Hsieh MS, French CA, Liang CW, Hsiao CH. NUT midline carcinoma: case report and review of the literature. Int J Surg Pathol. 2011; 19(6):808–812

[62] Stelow EB, Bellizzi AM, Taneja K, et al. NUT rearrangement in undifferentiated carcinomas of the upper aerodigestive tract. Am J Surg Pathol. 2008; 32 (6):828–834

[63] Haack H, Johnson LA, Fry CJ, et al. Diagnosis of NUT midline carcinoma using a NUT-specific monoclonal antibody. Am J Surg Pathol. 2009; 33(7):984–991

[64] Mertens F, Wiebe T, Adlercreutz C, Mandahl N, French CA. Successful treatment of a child with t(15;19)-positive tumor. Pediatr Blood Cancer. 2007; 49 (7):1015–1017

[65] Engleson J, Soller M, Panagopoulos I, Dahlén A, Dictor M, Jerkeman M. Midline carcinoma with t(15;19) and BRD4-NUT fusion oncogene in a 30-year-old female with response to docetaxel and radiotherapy. BMC Cancer. 2006; 6:69

[66] Bishop JA, Guo TW, Smith DF, et al. Human papillomavirus-related carcinomas of the sinonasal tract. Am J Surg Pathol. 2013; 37(2):185–192

[67] Bishop JA, Ogawa T, Stelow EB, et al. Human papillomavirus-related carcinoma with adenoid cystic-like features: a peculiar variant of head and neck cancer restricted to the sinonasal tract. Am J Surg Pathol. 2013; 37 (6):836–844

[68] Bishop JA. Recently described neoplasms of the sinonasal tract. Semin Diagn Pathol. 2016; 33(2):62–70

[69] Yom SS, Rashid A, Rosenthal DI, et al. Genetic analysis of sinonasal adenocarcinoma phenotypes: distinct alterations of histogenetic significance. Mod Pathol. 2005; 18(3):315–319

[70] Cathro HP, Mills SE. Immunophenotypic differences between intestinal-type and low-grade papillary sinonasal adenocarcinomas: an immunohistochemical study of 22 cases utilizing CDX2 and MUC2. Am J Surg Pathol. 2004; 28 (8):1026–1032

[71] Choi HR, Sturgis EM, Rashid A, et al. Sinonasal adenocarcinoma: evidence for histogenetic divergence of the enteric and nonenteric phenotypes. Hum Pathol. 2003; 34(11):1101–1107

[72] Neto AG, Pineda-Daboin K, Luna MA. Sinonasal tract seromucous adenocarcinomas: a report of 12 cases. Ann Diagn Pathol. 2003; 7(3):154–159

[73] Franchi A, Gallo O, Santucci M. Clinical relevance of the histological classification of sinonasal intestinal-type adenocarcinomas. Hum Pathol. 1999; 30 (10):1140–1145

[74] Franquemont DW, Fechner RE, Mills SE. Histologic classification of sinonasal intestinal-type adenocarcinoma. Am J Surg Pathol. 1991; 15(4):368–375

[75] Zur KB, Brandwein M, Wang B, Som P, Gordon R, Urken ML. Primary description of a new entity, renal cell-like carcinoma of the nasal cavity: van Meegeren in the house of Vermeer. Arch Otolaryngol Head Neck Surg. 2002; 128 (4):441–447

[76] Smith SC, Patel RM, Lucas DR, McHugh JB. Sinonasal lobular capillary hemangioma: a clinicopathologic study of 34 cases characterizing potential for local recurrence. Head Neck Pathol. 2013; 7(2):129–134

[77] Mills SE, Cooper PH, Fechner RE. Lobular capillary hemangioma: the underlying lesion of pyogenic granuloma. A study of 73 cases from the oral and nasal mucous membranes. Am J Surg Pathol. 1980; 4(5):470–479

[78] Wagner AJ, Malinowska-Kolodziej I, Morgan JA, et al. Clinical activity of mTOR inhibition with sirolimus in malignant perivascular epithelioid cell tumors: targeting the pathogenic activation of mTORC1 in tumors. J Clin Oncol. 2010; 28(5):835–840

[79] Dickson MA, Schwartz GK, Antonescu CR, Kwiatkowski DJ, Malinowska IA. Extrarenal perivascular epithelioid cell tumors (PEComas) respond to mTOR inhibition: clinical and molecular correlates. Int J Cancer. 2013; 132(7): 1711–1717

[80] Agaram NP, Sung YS, Zhang L, et al. Dichotomy of genetic abnormalities in PEComas with therapeutic implications. Am J Surg Pathol. 2015; 39(6): 813–825

[81] Iezzoni JC, Mills SE. "Undifferentiated" small round cell tumors of the sinonasal tract: differential diagnosis update. Am J Clin Pathol. 2005; 124 Suppl: S110–S121

[82] Sorensen PH, Lynch JC, Qualman SJ, et al. PAX3-FKHR and PAX7-FKHR gene fusions are prognostic indicators in alveolar rhabdomyosarcoma: a report from the children's oncology group. J Clin Oncol. 2002; 20(11): 2672–2679

[83] Parham DM. Pathologic classification of rhabdomyosarcomas and correlations with molecular studies. Mod Pathol. 2001; 14(5):506–514

[84] Heffner DK, Gnepp DR. Sinonasal fibrosarcomas, malignant schwannomas, and "Triton" tumors. A clinicopathologic study of 67 cases. Cancer. 1992; 70 (5):1089–1101

[85] Frankenthaler R, Ayala AG, Hartwick RW, Goepfert H. Fibrosarcoma of the head and neck. Laryngoscope. 1990; 100(8):799–802

[86] Potter BO, Sturgis EM. Sarcomas of the head and neck. Surg Oncol Clin N Am. 2003; 12(2):379–417

[87] Argani P, Zakowski MF, Klimstra DS, Rosai J, Ladanyi M. Detection of the SYT-SSX chimeric RNA of synovial sarcoma in paraffin-embedded tissue and its application in problematic cases. Mod Pathol. 1998; 11(1):65–71

[88] Valente AL, Tull J, Zhang S. Specificity of TLE1 expression in unclassified high-grade sarcomas for the diagnosis of synovial sarcoma. Appl Immunohistochem Mol Morphol. 2013; 21(5):408–413

[89] Chuang HC, Hsu SC, Huang CG, Hsueh S, Ng KF, Chen TC. Reappraisal of TLE-1 immunohistochemical staining and molecular detection of SS18-SSX fusion transcripts for synovial sarcoma. Pathol Int. 2013; 63(12):573–580

[90] Thway K, Fisher C. Synovial sarcoma: defining features and diagnostic evolution. Ann Diagn Pathol. 2014; 18(6):369–380

[91] Li WS, Liao IC, Wen MC, Lan HH, Yu SC, Huang HY. BCOR-CCNB3-positive soft tissue sarcoma with round-cell and spindle-cell histology: a series of four cases highlighting the pitfall of mimicking poorly differentiated synovial sarcoma. Histopathology. 2016; 69(5):792–801

[92] Ma SR, Li KC, Xu YQ, Wang YM, Ma WL, Li Q. Primary epithelioid hemangioendothelioma in the clival region: a case report and literature review. Neuropathology. 2011; 31(5):519–522

[93] Fernandes AL, Ratilal B, Mafra M, Magalhaes C. Aggressive intracranial and extra-cranial epithelioid hemangioendothelioma: a case report and review of the literature. Neuropathology. 2006; 26(3):201–205

[94] Hart JL, Edgar MA, Gardner JM. Vascular tumors of bone. Semin Diagn Pathol. 2014; 31(1):30–38

[95] Nelson BL, Thompson LD. Sinonasal tract angiosarcoma: a clinicopathologic and immunophenotypic study of 10 cases with a review of the literature. Head Neck Pathol. 2007; 1(1):1–12

[96] Heffner DK. Sinonasal angiosarcoma? Not likely (a brief description of infarcted nasal polyps). Ann Diagn Pathol. 2010; 14(4):233–234

[97] Hoch BL, Nielsen GP, Liebsch NJ, Rosenberg AE. Base of skull chordomas in children and adolescents: a clinicopathologic study of 73 cases. Am J Surg Pathol. 2006; 30(7):811–818

[98] St Martin M, Levine SC. Chordomas of the skull base: manifestations and management. Curr Opin Otolaryngol Head Neck Surg. 2003; 11(5):324–327

[99] Campbell RG, Prevedello DM, Ditzel Filho L, Otto BA, Carrau RL. Contemporary management of clival chordomas. Curr Opin Otolaryngol Head Neck Surg. 2015; 23(2):153–161

[100] George B, Bresson D, Herman P, Froelich S. Chordomas: a review. Neurosurg Clin N Am. 2015; 26(3):437–452

[101] Wang K, Tian K, Wang L, et al. Brachyury: A sensitive marker, but not a prognostic factor, for skull base chordomas. Mol Med Rep. 2015; 12(3): 4298–4304

[102] Bell D, Raza SM, Bell AH, Fuller GN, DeMonte F. Whole-transcriptome analysis of chordoma of the skull base. Virchows Arch. 2016; 469(4):439–449

[103] Kakkar A, Nambirajan A, Suri V, et al. Primary bone tumors of the skull: spectrum of 125 cases, with review of literature. J Neurol Surg B Skull Base. 2016; 77(4):319–325

[104] Awad M, Gogos AJ, Kaye AH. Skull base chondrosarcoma. J Clin Neurosci. 2016; 24:1–5

[105] Panda NK, Jain A, Eshwara Reddy CE. Osteosarcoma and chondrosarcoma of the maxilla. Br J Oral Maxillofac Surg. 2003; 41(5):329–333

[106] Padilla RJ, Murrah VA. The spectrum of gnathic osteosarcoma: caveats for the clinician and the pathologist. Head Neck Pathol. 2011; 5(1):92–99

[107] Faragalla H, Weinreb I. Olfactory neuroblastoma: a review and update. Adv Anat Pathol. 2009; 16(5):322–331

[108] Ow TJ, Bell D, Kupferman ME, Demonte F, Hanna EY. Esthesioneuroblastoma. Neurosurg Clin N Am. 2013; 24(1):51–65

[109] Hyams VJ. Olfactory neuroblastoma (case 6). In: Batsakis JG, Hyams VJ, Morales AR, eds. Special Tumors of the Head and Neck. Chicago: ASCP Press; 1982:24–29

[110] Su SY, Bell D, Hanna EY. Esthesioneuroblastoma, neuroendocrine carcinoma, and sinonasal undifferentiated carcinoma: differentiation in diagnosis and treatment. Int Arch Otorhinolaryngol. 2014; 18 Suppl 2:S149–S156

[111] Van Gompel JJ, Giannini C, Olsen KD, et al. Long-term outcome of esthesioneuroblastoma: hyams grade predicts patient survival. J Neurol Surg B Skull Base. 2012; 73(5):331–336

[112] Bell D, Saade R, Roberts D, et al. Prognostic utility of Hyams histological grading and Kadish-Morita staging systems for esthesioneuroblastoma outcomes. Head Neck Pathol. 2015; 9(1):51–59

[113] Fisher C. The diversity of soft tissue tumours with EWSR1 gene rearrangements: a review. Histopathology. 2014; 64(1):134–150

[114] Rooper LM, Bishop JA. Sinonasal small round blue cell tumors: an immunohistochemical approach. Surg Pathol Clin. 2017; 10(1):103–123

[115] Thompson LD. Small round blue cell tumors of the sinonasal tract: a differential diagnosis approach. Mod Pathol. 2017; 30(s1) S1:S1–S26

[116] Hafezi S, Seethala RR, Stelow EB, et al. Ewing's family of tumors of the sinonasal tract and maxillary bone. Head Neck Pathol. 2011; 5(1):8–16

[117] Bishop JA, Alaggio R, Zhang L, Seethala RR, Antonescu CR. Adamantinoma-like Ewing family tumors of the head and neck: a pitfall in the differential diagnosis of basaloid and myoepithelial carcinomas. Am J Surg Pathol. 2015; 39(9):1267–1274

[118] Lezcano C, Clarke MR, Zhang L, Antonescu CR, Seethala RR. Adamantinoma-like Ewing sarcoma mimicking basal cell adenocarcinoma of the parotid gland: a case report and review of the literature. Head Neck Pathol. 2015; 9 (2):280–285

[119] Fitzek MM, Thornton AF, Varvares M, et al. Neuroendocrine tumors of the sinonasal tract. Results of a prospective study incorporating chemotherapy, surgery, and combined proton-photon radiotherapy. Cancer. 2002; 94(10): 2623–2634

[120] Bell D, Hanna EY, Weber RS, et al. Neuroendocrine neoplasms of the sinonasal region. Head Neck. 2016; 38 Suppl 1:E2259–E2266

[121] Shah K, Perez-Ordóñez B. Neuroendocrine neoplasms of the sinonasal tract: neuroendocrine carcinomas and olfactory neuroblastoma. Head Neck Pathol. 2016; 10(1):85–94

[122] Thompson ED, Stelow EB, Mills SE, et al. Large cell neuroendocrine carcinoma of the head and neck: a clinicopathologic series of 10 cases with an emphasis on HPV status. Am J Surg Pathol. 2016; 40(4):471–478

[123] Taggart MW, Hanna EY, Gidley P, Weber RS, Bell D. Achaete-scute homolog 1 expression closely correlates with endocrine phenotype and degree of differentiation in sinonasal neuroendocrine tumors. Ann Diagn Pathol. 2015; 19(3):154–156

[124] Woolen S, Gemmete JJ. Paragangliomas of the head and neck. Neuroimaging Clin N Am. 2016; 26(2):259–278

[125] Thompson LD, Wieneke JA, Miettinen M. Sinonasal tract and nasopharyngeal melanomas: a clinicopathologic study of 115 cases with a proposed staging system. Am J Surg Pathol. 2003; 27(5):594–611

[126] Jarrom D, Paleri V, Kerawala C, et al. Mucosal melanoma of the upper airways tract mucosal melanoma: a systematic review with meta-analyses of treatment. Head Neck. 2017; 39(4):819–825

[127] Houette A, Gilain L, Mulliez A, Mom T, Saroul N. Prognostic value of two tumour staging classifications in patients with sinonasal mucosal melanoma. Eur Ann Otorhinolaryngol Head Neck Dis. 2016; 133(5):313–317

[128] Mikkelsen LH, Larsen AC, von Buchwald C, Drzewiecki KT, Prause JU, Heegaard S. Mucosal malignant melanoma - a clinical, oncological, pathological and genetic survey. APMIS. 2016; 124(6):475–486

[129] Rachidi S, Sood AJ, Patel KG, et al. Melanotic neuroectodermal tumor of infancy: a systematic review. J Oral Maxillofac Surg. 2015; 73(10):1946–1956

[130] Fritchie KJ, Jin L, Wang X, et al. Fusion gene profile of biphenotypic sinonasal sarcoma: an analysis of 44 cases. Histopathology. 2016; 69(6):930–936

[131] Fletcher CD. Distinctive soft tissue tumors of the head and neck. Mod Pathol. 2002; 15(3):324–330

[132] Thway K, Noujaim J, Zaidi S, et al. Desmoplastic small round cell tumor: pathology, genetics, and potential therapeutic strategies. Int J Surg Pathol. 2016; 24(8):672–684

[133] Yoon AJ, Parisien M, Feldman F, Young-In Lee F. Extranodal Rosai-Dorfman disease of bone, subcutaneous tissue and paranasal sinus mucosa with a review of its pathogenesis. Skeletal Radiol. 2005; 34(10):653–657

[134] Rodriguez J, Romaguera JE, Manning J, et al. Nasal-type T/NK lymphomas: a clinicopathologic study of 13 cases. Leuk Lymphoma. 2000; 39(1–2):139–144

[135] Abbondanzo SL, Wenig BM. Non-Hodgkin's lymphoma of the sinonasal tract. A clinicopathologic and immunophenotypic study of 120 cases. Cancer. 1995; 75(6):1281–1291

[136] Shimazaki H, Aida S, Tamai S, Miyazawa T, Nakanobou M. Sinonasal terato-carcinosarcoma: ultrastructural and immunohistochemical evidence of neuroectodermal origin. Ultrastruct Pathol. 2000; 24(2):115–122

[137] Pai SA, Naresh KN, Masih K, Ramarao C, Borges AM. Teratocarcinosarcoma of the paranasal sinuses: a clinicopathologic and immunohistochemical study. Hum Pathol. 1998; 29(7):718–722

[138] Smith SL, Hessel AC, Luna MA, Malpica A, Rosenthal DI, El-Naggar AK. Sinonasal teratocarcinosarcoma of the head and neck: a report of 10 patients treated at a single institution and comparison with reported series. Arch Otolaryngol Head Neck Surg. 2008; 134(6):592–595

[139] Misra P, Husain Q, Svider PF, Sanghvi S, Liu JK, Eloy JA. Management of sinonasal teratocarcinosarcoma: a systematic review. Am J Otolaryngol. 2014; 35 (1):5–11

[140] Ho KL. Primary meningioma of the nasal cavity and paranasal sinuses. Cancer. 1980; 46(6):1442–1447

[141] Gump WC. Meningiomas of the pediatric skull base: a review. J Neurol Surg B Skull Base. 2015; 76(1):66–73

[142] Cornelius JF, Slotty PJ, Steiger HJ, Hänggi D, Polivka M, George B. Malignant potential of skull base versus non-skull base meningiomas: clinical series of 1,663 cases. Acta Neurochir (Wien). 2013; 155(3):407–413

[143] Schafer DR, Thompson LD, Smith BC, Wenig BM. Primary ameloblastoma of the sinonasal tract: a clinicopathologic study of 24 cases. Cancer. 1998; 82 (4):667–674

[144] Flocks RH, Boatman DL. Incidence of head and neck metastases from genitourinary neoplasms. Laryngoscope. 1973; 83(9):1527–1539

[145] Deconde AS, Sanaiha Y, Suh JD, Bhuta S, Bergsneider M, Wang MB. Metastatic disease to the clivus mimicking clival chordomas. J Neurol Surg B Skull Base. 2013; 74(5):292–299

[146] Remenschneider AK, Sadow PM, Lin DT, Gray ST. Metastatic renal cell carcinoma to the sinonasal cavity: a case series. J Neurol Surg Rep. 2013; 74(2): 67–72

Suggested Readings

Andrews T, Kountakis SE, Maillard AA. Myxomas of the head and neck. Am J Otolaryngol. 2000; 21(3):184–189

Asimakopoulos P, Syed MI, Andrews T, Syed S, Williams A. Sinonasal glomangiopericytoma: Is anything new? Ear Nose Throat J. 2016; 95(2):E1–E5

Beham A, Beham-Schmid C, Regauer S, Auböck L, Stammberger H. Nasopharyngeal angiofibroma: true neoplasm or vascular malformation? Adv Anat Pathol. 2000; 7(1):36–46

Chuang IC, Liao KC, Huang HY, et al. NAB2-STAT6 gene fusion and STAT6 immunoexpression in extrathoracic solitary fibrous tumors: the association between fusion variants and locations. Pathol Int. 2016; 66(5):288–296

Kao YC, Lin PC, Yen SL, et al. Clinicopathological and genetic heterogeneity of the head and neck solitary fibrous tumours: a comparative histological, immunohistochemical and molecular study of 36 cases. Histopathology. 2016; 68(4): 492–501

López F, Triantafyllou A, Snyderman CH, et al. Nasal juvenile angiofibroma: Current perspectives with emphasis on management. Head Neck. 2017; 39(5): 1033–1045

Purgina B, Lai CK. Distinctive head and neck bone and soft tissue neoplasms. Surg Pathol Clin. 2017; 10(1):223–279

Windfuhr JP, Schwerdtfeger FP. Myxoma of the lateral skull base: clinical features and management. Laryngoscope. 2004; 114(2):249–254

3 Imaging of Skull Base Neoplasms

Komal Shah and Lawrence E. Ginsberg

Summary

The goals of this chapter are to provide an overview of the imaging appearances of the more common skull base neoplasms, provide imaging strategies, and review ways in which certain imaging features provide clues to tumor type and benign versus malignant pathology. However, this chapter does not depict every conceivable skull base tumor.

Keywords: radiology, imaging, MR, CT, skull base, tumor, head and neck cancer

3.1 Introduction

Management of skull base neoplasms requires a team whose members are dedicated and specifically experienced at dealing with these unique tumors. The radiologist is no exception, for imaging plays a vital role in the diagnosis and posttreatment evaluation of skull base tumors. Although radiologists have traditionally concerned themselves with preoperative diagnosis, such a goal is not attainable in every case. Thus the goal of imaging known or suspected skull base tumors is several-fold. First, some patients who are suspected, but not known, to have a skull base tumor (based on pain, cranial neuropathy, etc.) require imaging simply to establish or exclude such a diagnosis. For those who have known skull base tumors, the role of imaging is to establish the full extent and location of the abnormality, outline areas of possible spread and secondary effects on adjacent structures, exclude nodal disease, and, finally, suggest a possible histologic diagnosis.[1] In some cases, distinguishing tumor from benign disease entities such as skull base osteomyelitis and other inflammations is a critical role of imaging. Obviously the radiologist can suggest a diagnosis when possible, and in fact for many lesions the imaging is quite characteristic.[1,2]

3.2 Selection of Imaging Modality

For lesions of the sinonasal cavity and skull base, unlike at some anatomical sites in the head and neck, MR and CT are complementary. At the University of Texas MD Anderson Cancer Center, virtually all patients who have such lesions will be imaged using both modalities prior to therapy, and many will have both modalities following therapy, at least early on.

The advantages of CT include its ability to detect calcification and bone—important in lesions that either destroy bone or produce some characteristic bony or calcific change. The latter include the classic sunburst periosteal new bone formation in osteosarcoma, the mineralized chondroid matrix of chondrosarcoma, and the hyperostotic reaction typical of certain types of meningioma. CT may also have value, through the multiplanar reconstruction capability of multidetector-row technology, for providing very high-quality images in virtually any plane of section. Furthermore, CT angiography has value, in cases of certain hypervascular lesions, such as glomus tumors or juvenile

angiofibroma, for establishing that a lesion is indeed hypervascular and then for assisting in surgical planning.

The advantages of MR include its ability to distinguish tumor within a paranasal sinus from obstructed secretions, something not always possible with CT. MR is better able to detect small soft tissue tumor components, particularly those near bony surfaces for which the enhancement may be inconspicuous on CT, such as with intracranial spread of a sinonasal malignancy. MR is also more accurate in detecting tumor extension through neural foramina and canals, whether by direct or perineural mechanisms.

3.3 Anterior Cranial Base

The anterior cranial base comprises the orbital and ethmoid roofs and the cribriform plates. Tumors seldom primarily arise within these bony structures—most generally originate intracranially and extend inferiorly through the skull base (e.g., meningioma; ► Fig. 3.1) or by extending intracranially from an origin in the upper nasoethmoid or frontal sinus region.[3] The latter are typically sinonasal malignancies (► Fig. 3.2; ► Fig. 3.3).

Anterior cranial fossa meningiomas often arise at the olfactory groove or tuberculum sella (► Fig. 3.1).[4] These benign dural tumors may extend inferiorly, growing directly through the ethmoid roof (fovea ethmoidalis) and cribriform plate into the nasal cavity and/or ethmoid sinuses. In such cases, it is generally evident radiographically that the bulk (or so-called "epicenter") of the tumor is intracranial. In addition, characteristic imaging features of meningioma—such as relatively homogeneous isointensity on T1-weighted images; iso- or slightly hyperintense signal on T2-weighted images; and bright homogeneous enhancement following gadolinium-based IV contrast administration, often with a so-called dural tail of enhancement—make the diagnosis of meningioma straightforward in most cases (► Fig. 3.1).[4]

Sinonasal malignancies may arise in the upper nasoethmoid region. Typical histologic tumor types include olfactory neuroblastoma (esthesioneuroblastoma), sinonasal undifferentiated carcinoma, squamous cell carcinoma, and neuroendocrine carcinoma.[3] Other tumor types are less common. Although the imaging characteristics of these lesions are relatively nonspecific, imaging is important in evaluating for intracranial spread, which will often have implications for surgical therapy. CT can often make this determination, but MR is better in this regard (► Fig. 3.2; ► Fig. 3.3). On CT, sinonasal malignancies generally enhance to a mild or moderate degree. When they involve bone, the pattern is usually one of destruction; sclerosis of bone is uncommon. With MR, sinonasal malignancies are typically close to muscle or brain in signal on T1- and T2-weighted sequences and enhance to varying degrees with contrast administration. Obstructed sinonasal secretions are usually low-signal on T1 and high-signal on T2. If chronic or inspissated, sinus mucosal secretions may become hyperintense (high-signal) on T1-weighted images (► Fig. 3.3).[3] Review of all sequences generally allows determination of whether sinus is

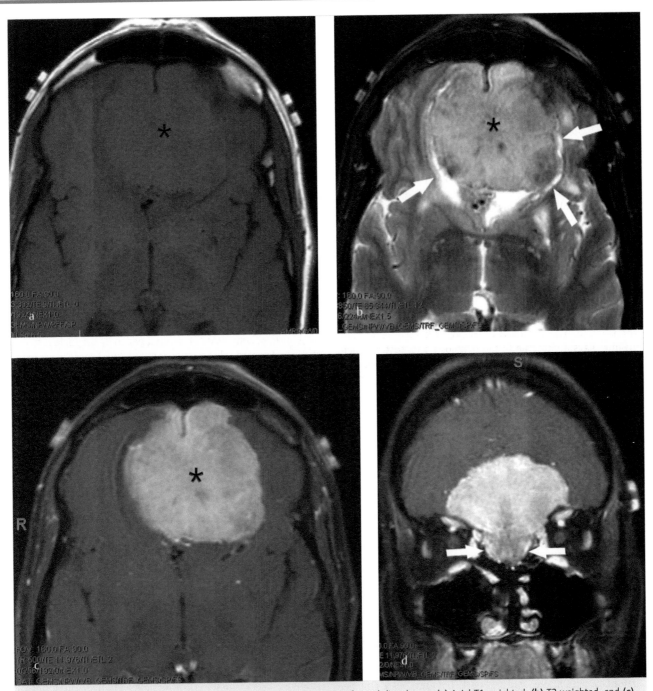

Fig. 3.1 Olfactory groove meningioma in a 53-year-old woman complaining of visual disturbance. **(a)** Axial T1-weighted, **(b)** T2-weighted, and **(c)** postcontrast T1-weighted axial MR images each demonstrate a large subfrontal mass (*asterisks*). Seen are the classic signal characteristics and bright homogenous enhancement typical of meningioma. The T2-weighted image demonstrates so-called CSF-clefts, representing pockets of cerebrospinal fluid (CSF) between the lesion and brain surface that are characteristic of an extra-axial lesion (*arrows* in **b**). **(d)** Coronal postcontrast T1-weighted image demonstrating downward, nasoethmoid tumor extension (*arrows*).

involved with tumor or merely obstructed. It is important to always image the neck in cases of sinonasal malignancy, for such lesions may present with, or recur as, nodal disease.

3.4 Central Skull Base

The central skull base (CSB) includes primarily the sphenoid bone and its various parts as well as adjacent structures such as the cavernous sinus, sella turcica, and parasellar region. A very large variety of tumors may afflict the CSB.[1,2,3] As with the anterior cranial base, lesions may arise intracranially and secondarily involve the sphenoid bone. Alternatively, lesions may arise primarily within the sphenoid bone, or arise inferiorly or anteriorly, and secondarily affect it by upward or posterior spread.

The most common intracranially arising lesion to affect the CSB is meningioma.[4] Various aspects of the CSB may be

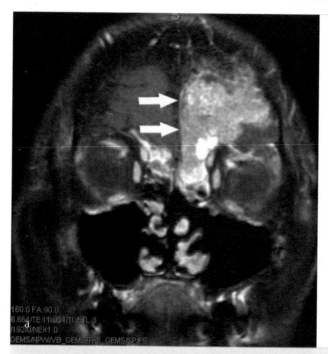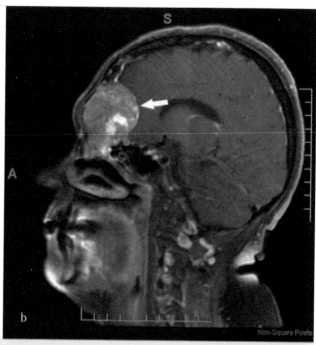

Fig. 3.2 Squamous cell carcinoma of the frontal and ethmoid sinuses in a 66-year-old woman presenting with bloody nasal and oral secretions and subsequent left eye visual changes. **(a)** Coronal and **(b)** sagittal T1-weighted postcontrast MR images demonstrate a large, somewhat heterogeneously but brightly enhancing mass lesion filling the frontal and nasoethmoid regions with obvious posterior extension into the epidural space (*arrows*).

involved, including the planum sphenoidale and tuberculum sella, the anterior clinoid, the greater sphenoid wing, the parasellar region and cavernous sinus, and the petroclival region (▶ Fig. 3.4; ▶ Fig. 3.5). In most of these locations, the lesion is merely dural in location; while there may be some reactive bony sclerosis or hyperostosis, the bone is uninvolved.[4] One exception is hyperostosing en plaque meningioma of the greater sphenoid wing, which is associated with a very striking sclerotic response, or hyperostosis, because meningioma cells actually involve the bone.[4,5] This bony involvement has a very characteristic radiographic appearance, including intraorbital extension (▶ Fig. 3.6).[1,4,5]

Although most meningiomas, other than the hyperostosing sphenoid wing type, remain confined to the dural space, some meningiomas may invade the CSB in an aggressive, almost malignant manner.[1,4] The imaging for such invasion can be dramatic, and if the diagnosis of meningioma is unknown, the radiologic diagnosis may be more difficult (▶ Fig. 3.7). Such meningiomas may achieve massive size and may extend directly through the bone, or through neural foramina, into extracranial spaces such as the pterygopalatine fossa, orbit, or masticator space. Such lesions may be grossly destructive of bone. It should be kept in mind, for any location, that dural metastases may be radiographically indistinguishable from meningioma. In a known cancer patient, a lesion that resembles a meningioma on the first imaging study may be a dural metastasis; the finding of growth on serial imaging should raise that possibility (▶ Fig. 3.8).[6,7] Finally, another lesion that can be radiographically confused with meningioma is the rare, highly vascular malignancy hemangiopericytoma. These also have the potential to be highly destructive of the cranial base (▶ Fig. 3.9).

Another common benign CSB lesion is the pituitary adenoma.[1,8,9,10,11] Some macroadenomas (those greater than 1 cm) may become giant adenomas (greater than 5 cm) and/or invade the CSB. Such cases may present a diagnostic challenge to the radiologist. There is no imaging feature with which to specifically differentiate giant pituitary adenoma from other CSB masses, except that an adenoma should encompass the pituitary gland and may demonstrate cavernous sinus invasion without perineural spread (PNS). Accordingly, the radiologist should consider pituitary adenoma when confronted with a large, destructive CSB mass and should check hormone levels, especially prolactin (▶ Fig. 3.10).

One relatively uncommon benign tumor that arises near, and that may secondarily affect, the CSB is the juvenile angiofibroma. These highly vascular tumors typically present with epistaxis in teenage males and have very characteristic imaging features.[1,12] They arise in or near the sphenopalatine foramen, the opening between the pterygopalatine fossa and the nasal cavity. Tumor components are often seen in the nasal cavity and nasopharynx. These aggressive lesions often invade the clivus and sphenoid sinus. Because of the hypervascularity, juvenile angiofibromas enhance brightly on CT. On MR, they have small foci of low signal, so-called flow voids, that represent rapidly flowing arterial supply to the tumor (▶ Fig. 3.11). Vascular studies such as catheter angiography, CT angiography, and MR angiography can provide a surgical road map or facilitate preoperative embolization (▶ Fig. 3.11e).

One final intracranial (and sometimes also extracranial) lesion affecting the CSB is peripheral nerve sheath tumor arising from the trigeminal nerve. Histologically such tumors can be schwannoma or neurofibroma, but the imaging appearance of each is similar to that of the other.[2,6] These usually benign

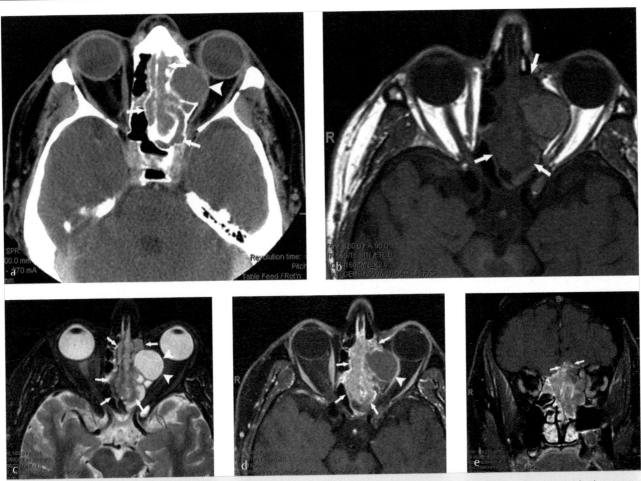

Fig. 3.3 Olfactory neuroblastoma (esthesioneuroblastoma) in the upper nasal cavity in a 47-year-old man complaining of anosmia and subsequent development epistaxis and congestion. **(a)** Axial postcontrast CT demonstrating relatively nondescript and nonenhancing soft tissue filling the left nasoethmoid region and, to a lesser extent, the right nasal cavity (*arrows*). There is an enlarged, airless left ethmoid air cell mucocele that is slightly less dense than the tumor (*arrowhead*). Notice that no overt bone destruction is evident, although there could be in this entity. **(b)** Axial T1-weighted, **(c)** T2-weighted, and **(d)** postcontrast axial T1-weighted MR images demonstrate the characteristic findings of sinonasal malignancy. The lesion is isointense to muscle and other soft tissue (*arrows* in **b**). Notice on the T2-weighted image (*arrows* in **c**) that the tumor is relatively isointense to brain and not nearly as high-signal or hyperintense as obstructed secretions in the left ethmoid mucocele (*arrowheads* in **c**). **(d)** The lesion enhances brightly, unlike obstructed secretions in the mucocele (*arrowhead*). **(e)** Coronal postcontrast T1-weighted MR image shows intracranial extension through the cribriform plate and ethmoid roof (*arrows*).

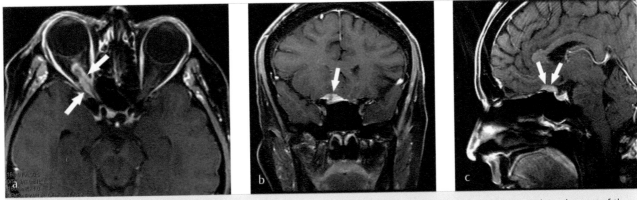

Fig. 3.4 A 53-year-old woman presenting with decreased visual acuity in the right eye. Dx: tuberculum sella meningioma with involvement of the optic sheath/canal. **(a)** Axial, **(b)** coronal, and **(c)** sagittal T1-weighted postcontrast MR images demonstrate enhancing tumor in a characteristic elongated manner along the surface of the right optic nerve (*arrows* in **a**). Tumor extends up the tuberculum sella onto the planum sphenoidale (*arrows* in **b** and **c**).

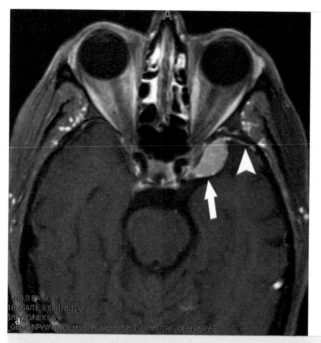
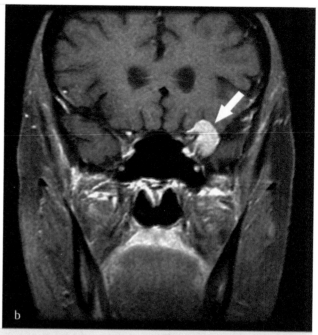

Fig. 3.5 Noninvasive greater sphenoid wing meningioma in an asymptomatic 75-year-old woman. This lesion was picked up on a routine lymphoma screening CT. **(a)** Axial and **(b)** coronal postcontrast T1-weighted MR images reveal a homogenously brightly enhancing mass lesion (*arrows*) along the left anterior clinoid process, superior orbital fissure, and greater sphenoid wing region. An obvious dural tail or enhancement of dura extends from the tumor, characteristic but not diagnostic of meningioma (*arrowhead* in **a**).

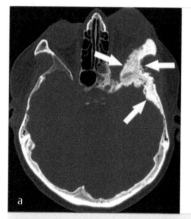
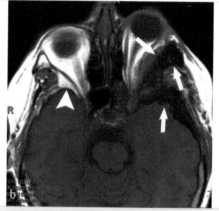
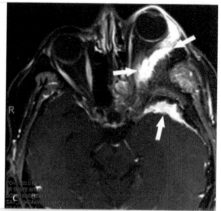

Fig. 3.6 Hyperostosing en plaque greater sphenoid wing meningioma in a 54-year-old woman presenting with left-sided headaches and progressive visual loss in the left eye. **(a)** Axial bone window CT image demonstrates left proptosis and gross bone thickening or hyperostosis of the left greater sphenoid wing and lateral orbital wall (*arrows*). **(b)** Axial precontrast and **(c)** fat-suppressed postcontrast T1-weighted MR images show that the bone marrow is markedly abnormal (*arrows* in **b**) as opposed to the normal marrow in the right sphenoid triangle, depicted by an arrowhead. Enhancing soft tissue (extraosseous) meningioma can be seen in the left orbit and behind the greater sphenoid wing (*arrows* in **c**).

lesions can arise from the main trigeminal trunk and extend along any of its branches or may arise within one of its three divisions. Such lesions often cause widening of foramina or other benign bony remodeling (as opposed to destruction) of the CSB (▶ Fig. 3.12).

Among primarily extracranial malignancies that may affect the CSB, probably the most common is nasopharyngeal carcinoma (NPC).[1,8,13,14] Owing to its location immediately inferior to the clivus, upward spread of NPC very commonly involves the CSB. If the nasopharyngeal component is relatively small (▶ Fig. 3.13), the radiologist must bear in mind the possibility of NPC. As opposed to some malignancies that tend to destroy bone—and even though NPC may do exactly this—NPC often has a tendency to infiltrate in a nondestructive manner.[15] For this reason, MR imaging is more sensitive than CT for detecting such involvement (▶ Fig. 3.14). Of course, NPC can also cause skull base destruction, which CT also plays a role in detecting.[15] Because MR is also more sensitive for detecting intracranial spread via perineural and direct mechanisms, we prefer to use MR as the main imaging modality in cases of NPC.[16]

Another type of extracranial malignancy that may secondarily affect the CSB is head and neck malignancy with PNS of

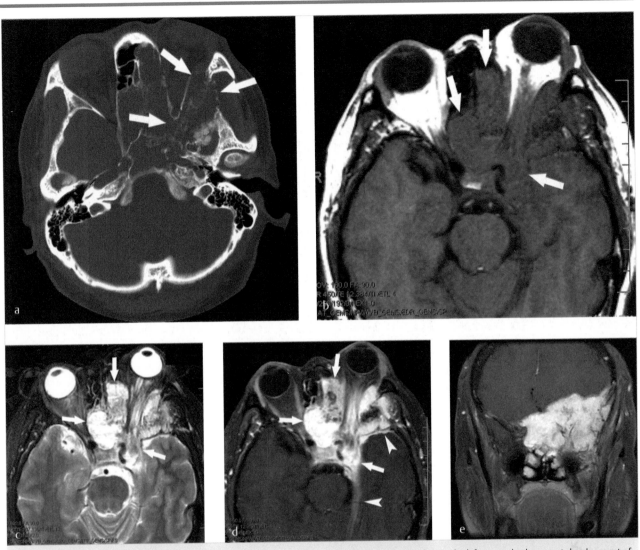

Fig. 3.7 Massive skull base meningioma in a 61-year-old woman presenting with progressive vision loss in the left eye and subsequent development of proptosis. **(a)** Axial CT bone window demonstrates a permeative type of bone destruction (*arrows*). **(b)** Axial T1-weighted, **(c)** T2-weighted, and **(d)** postcontrast axial T1-weighted MR images demonstrate extensive soft tissue tumor infiltrating the nasoethmoid region, left cavernous sinus, and left orbit (*arrows*). Note the dural tail along the incisura and sphenoid wing (*arrowheads* in **d**). **(e)** Coronal postcontrast MR image demonstrates the extensive nature of this lesion.

tumor.[17,18,19] A thorough description is beyond the scope of this chapter. The most common manner in which the CSB is affected is in a patient who has a known, or sometimes an unknown, malignancy of the face (most commonly in a V2 distribution, such as the cheek; ▶ Fig. 3.15) or a lesion of the lower lip or palate (or, less commonly, of other mucosal surfaces). Common tumor types include squamous cell carcinoma, adenoid cystic carcinoma, and desmoplastic melanoma.[18] Such lesions may spread proximally, toward the central nervous system, along the branch of the trigeminal nerve that innervates the primary site. For the cheek and palate, this would be the infraorbital (▶ Fig. 3.15) or palatine nerves (▶ Fig. 3.16), respectively, with tumor spread to the pterygopalatine fossa.

From here, tumor can spread posteriorly along the main trunk of the maxillary nerve, through foramen rotundum, and into the cavernous sinus or further posteriorly into Meckel's cave or even onto the main trigeminal trunk.[18] For lesions of

the lower lip or gingiva, tumor can access the inferior alveolar branch of V3 and then spread upward onto the main trunk of the mandibular nerve (▶ Fig. 3.17), through foramen ovale, and into Meckel's cave. Though perhaps best considered in the temporal bone section, PNS along the facial nerve may arise from primary or secondary parotid gland tumors (▶ Fig. 3.18).

Recognition of PNS is a critical function of the radiologist, because failure to recognize it—unfortunately a common occurrence—can have a very adverse effect on treatment outcome. Characteristically, PNS occurs in the form of, or at the time of, tumor recurrence (▶ Fig. 3.15), not necessarily at the time of diagnosis or initial therapy. In other cases, unfortunately, PNS is not recognized until late in the patient's course, as a progression of disease that went undiagnosed and untreated at clinical presentation.

Metastases are the most common malignancies that arise directly in the skull base.[3] Such lesions may be lytic or blastic,

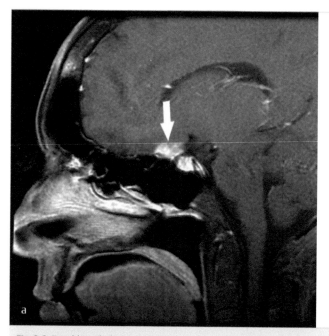
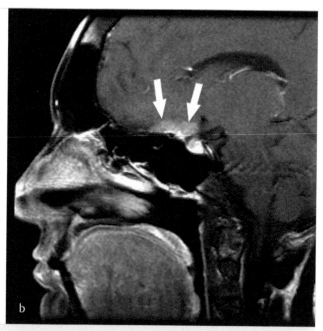

Fig. 3.8 Dural-based planum sphenoidale metastasis initially believed to be meningioma in a 47-year-old woman who has metastatic breast carcinoma. **(a)** Sagittal T1 postcontrast MR image demonstrates a small enhancing lesion along the planum sphenoidale (*arrow*). Note similarity with the meningioma shown in Fig. 3.4. **(b)** Sagittal T1-weighted postcontrast MR image 8 months later shows clear progression of this lesion (*arrows*), which prompted surgery.

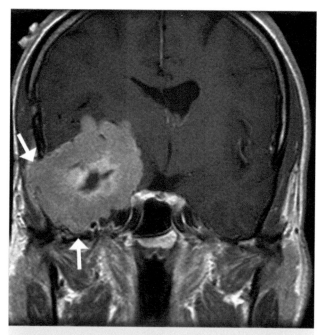

Fig. 3.9 Masticator space and middle cranial fossa/skull base hemangiopericytoma in a 45-year-old man who presented with headache, nausea, and vomiting. Coronal postcontrast T1-weighted MR image demonstrates a large, moderately enhancing mass encompassing the middle cranial fossa and obvious destruction through the calvarium (*arrows*). There is a central area of nonenhancement, representing necrosis. Though indistinguishable from an aggressive meningioma, this proved to be a hemangiopericytoma at surgery.

depending on the primary malignancy; both are common (► Fig. 3.19). Their imaging is generally straightforward, except that small lesions may be subtle.

Primary CSB malignancies include chordoma and chondrosarcoma. Chordomas are notochord-derived malignancies that occur in the sacrococcygeal region (50%), spine (15%), and clivus (35%).[1,3] They may also occasionally occur off midline. Most chordomas occur in mid- to late adulthood. Radiographically, they appear as expansile lytic lesions, with internal areas of fragmented bone that are most readily seen on CT (► Fig. 3.20). On MR they have characteristic T2 signal hyperintensity within the soft tissue mass component. Some degree of extracranial and/or intracranial extension is typical, the latter of which often results in brainstem compression.

Chondrosarcomas may also arise in the CSB.[1,3] These cartilage-derived malignancies tend to occur in proximity to the various synchondroses. Common locations include the petroclival fissure and the upper nasal septum/vomer region (► Fig. 3.21; ► Fig. 3.22; ► Fig. 3.23). Chondrosarcoma may also involve the greater sphenoid wing more laterally, often with masticator space components (► Fig. 3.23). On imaging, many, though not all, will have a mineralized chondroid matrix seen in chondroid tumors anywhere—calcifications in an "arcs and rings" pattern (► Fig. 3.21; ► Fig. 3.23). On MR, although signal intensity varies, marked heterogeneity is often seen, particularly on postcontrast T1-weighted images (► Fig. 3.22). A lesion in the appropriate location and having typical imaging features should suggest the possibility of chondrosarcoma.

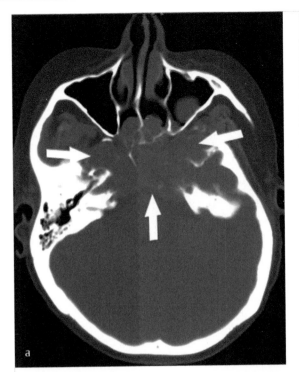
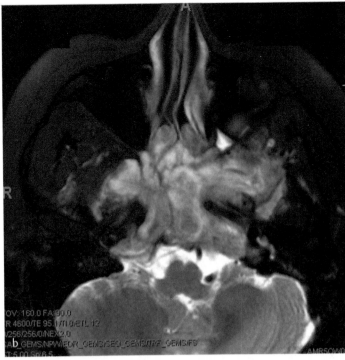
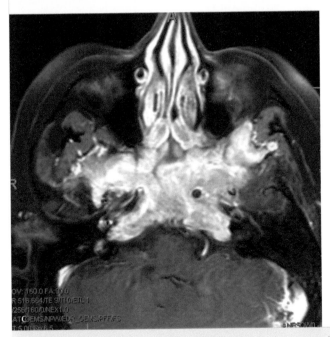
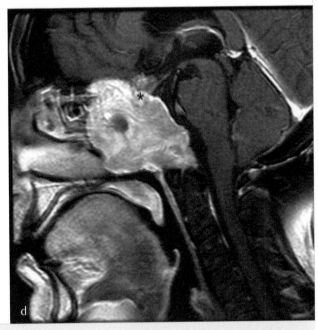

Fig. 3.10 Massive pituitary adenoma in a 48-year-old man who presented with only severe headache. **(a)** Axial CT bone window reveals a large destructive process involving the central skull base (CSB; *arrows*). **(b)** Axial T2 and **(c)** postcontrast T1-weighted MR images, respectively, reveal a large minimally and somewhat heterogeneously hyperintense and brightly enhancing mass involving virtually the entire CSB. **(d)** Sagittal image revealing complete replacement of the sphenoid sinus and clivus. Notice that although the lesion encompasses the sella (*asterisk*), there is no suprasellar extension, so the diagnosis of pituitary adenoma was less than obvious. The patient's prolactin level was 344214, indicating prolactinoma.

3.5 Posterior Cranial Base

For the purposes of this chapter, the posterior cranial base includes the temporal bone and the lower occipital structures, such as the foramen magnum, hypoglossal canal, and the jugular foramen/carotid canal. Many different tumors may affect the temporal bone. Among extracranial lesions that affect the temporal bone secondarily, lesions of the external ear are probably the most common.[20] Periauricular lesions may also grow into the temporal bone. Histologic tumor types include squamous cell, adenoid cystic carcinoma of the external canal, melanoma, and basal cell carcinoma.[20] When imaging skin lesions in and

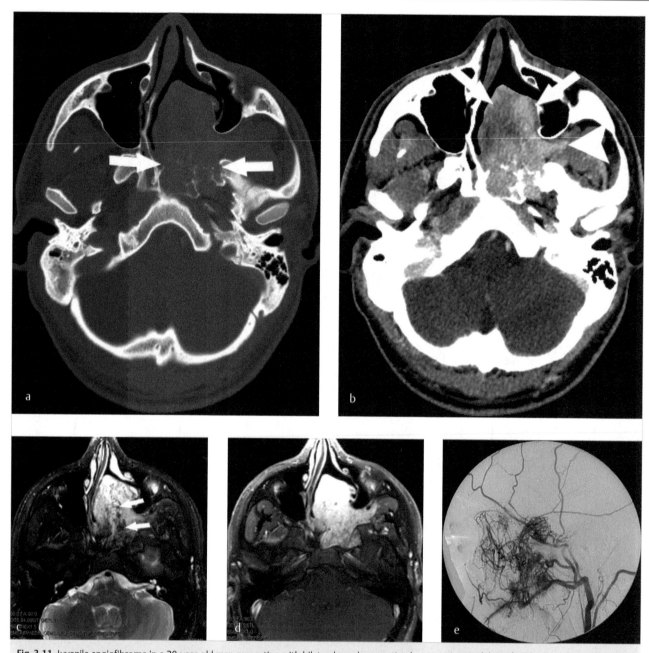

Fig. 3.11 Juvenile angiofibroma in a 20-year-old man presenting with bilateral nasal congestion but no epistaxis. **(a)** Axial CT bone window revealing a large mass with destruction of the mid and left aspects of the central skull base (*arrows*). **(b)** Contrast-enhanced CT soft tissue window reveals a moderately enhancing mass lesion corresponding to the areas of bone destruction (*arrows*). **(c)** Axial T2-weighted and **(d)** T1-weighted postcontrast MR images reveal a hyperintense, enhancing lesion. Central areas of signal void represent blood vessels and are so-called "flow voids" (*arrows in* **c**). **(e)** Lateral view of an external carotid angiogram in a different patient who has a juvenile angiofibroma reveals marked tumor hypervascularity.

around the ear, CT with high-resolution bone windows is critical for assessing the bony structures (▶ Fig. 3.24).

The temporal bone may also be infiltrated by petrous region meningiomas. While the diagnosis of meningioma is often fairly straightforward, occasionally a meningioma may be primarily infiltrative, without much dural disease; in such cases the diagnosis can be difficult, for the imaging may be quite nonspecific

(▶ Fig. 3.25). If so, then only biopsy can differentiate from infiltrative malignancies such as sarcoma or leukemic infiltration (▶ Fig. 3.26).

Intrinsic temporal bone tumors are relatively uncommon, although of course metastases can occur in the temporal bone (▶ Fig. 3.27). Vestibular schwannoma is addressed hereafter, in the discussion of cerebellopontine lesions, but it should be

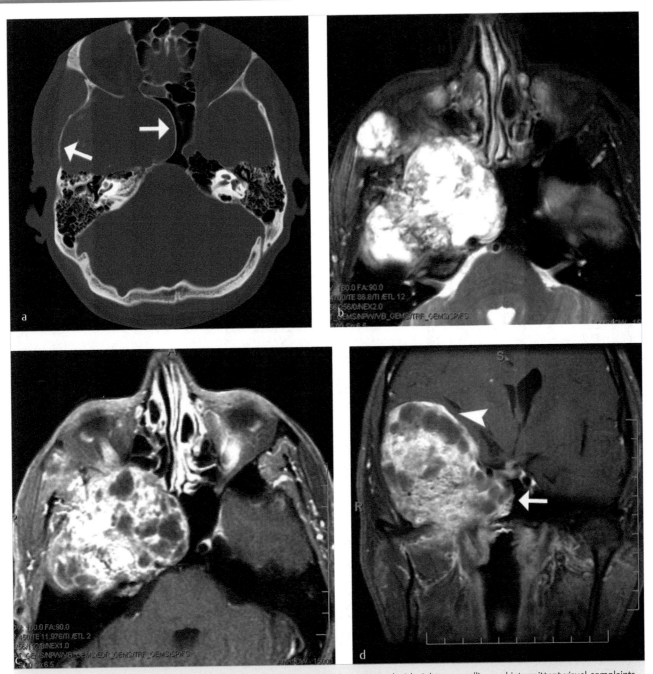

Fig. 3.12 Massive trigeminal/skull base schwannoma in a 44-year-old man who presented with right eye swelling and intermittent visual complaints. **(a)** Axial CT bone window reveals benign bony remodeling (*arrows*) with the lateral wall of the sphenoid sinus pushed medially. **(b)** Axial T2, **(c)** axial postcontrast T1, and **(d)** coronal postcontrast T1 MR images reveal a very large heterogeneously T2 hyperintense and brightly enhancing extra-axial mass lesion centered at and above the floor of the right middle cranial fossa. The coronal image shows obvious tumor extending into the sphenoid sinus (*arrow*) and elevation of the right temporal lobe (*arrowhead*). This was not a straightforward diagnosis, but the lack of bony destruction or edema in the brain argued for a slow growing process such as, in this case, schwannoma.

noted that schwannomas of the facial nerve typically present in the intratympanic portion of the facial nerve, which earns them a mention in a discussion of temporal bone tumors. These benign lesions typically present with facial neuropathy.[21] Commonly involved segments include the geniculate ganglion, the descending facial nerve, and the greater superficial petrosal nerve. This last is a branch of the facial nerve containing preganglionic parasympathetic fibers destined to innervate the lacrimal gland and vasomotor nerves of the nasal cavity and palate.[22] The nerve emerges from the geniculate ganglion and

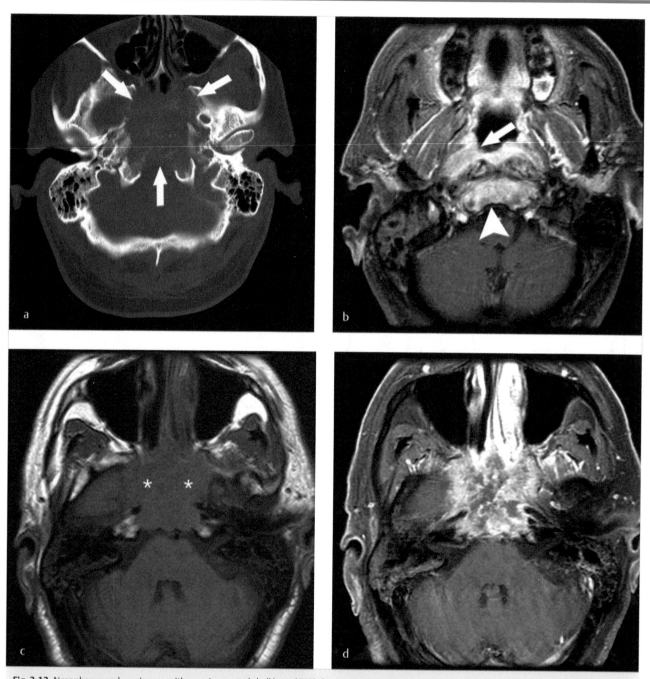

Fig. 3.13 Nasopharyngeal carcinoma with massive central skull base (CSB) destruction in a 55-year-old man presenting with headache and subsequent development of diplopia. **(a)** Axial CT bone window reveals gross destruction of the CSB (*arrows*). **(b)** Axial T1 postcontrast MR image demonstrates a small mass in the right fossa of Rosenmüller (*arrow*). There is also abnormal enhancement in the clivus, indicating tumor involvement (*arrowhead*). **(c)** Axial T1 noncontrast and **(d)** T1 postcontrast MR images show replacement of the normal T1 hyperintense bone marrow of the clivus (*asterisks* in **c**), as well as heterogeneously bright contrast enhancement. Skull base involvement in nasopharyngeal carcinoma indicates T3 staging.

exits the facial hiatus to become intracranial, along the spheno-petrosal synchondrosis in the floor of the middle cranial fossa.[22] A tumor along this portion of the facial nerve can present as an extra-axial mass along the roof or intracranial surface of the petrous bone and may be confused radiographically with a

meningioma. Recognition of the branches of the facial nerve or enlargement of the facial hiatus, along with a history of facial neuropathy, should suggest the correct diagnosis (▶ Fig. 3.28).

Intracranial lesions can involve the posterior cranial base by either growing anteroinferiorly or by arising adjacent to, say,

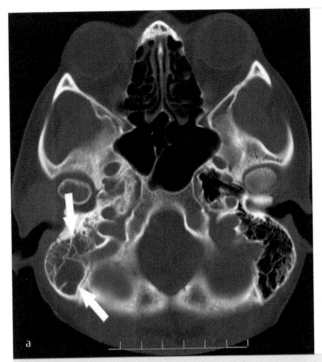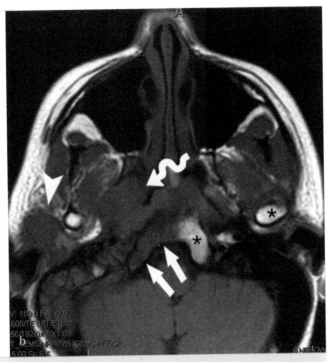

Fig. 3.14 Nasopharyngeal carcinoma. **(a)** Axial CT bone window shows no discernible abnormality in the lower clivus. **(b)** Axial T1-weighted MR image shows abnormal hypointense signal in the right side of the clivus (*arrows*), indicating tumor infiltration. The primary cancer is also visible (*squiggly arrow* in **b**). The normal marrow demonstrates T1 hyperintense fat signal, as seen in the left side of the clivus and left mandibular condyles (*asterisks* in **b**). Also, note right parotid metastasis (*arrowhead* in **b**) and right mastoid effusion, owing to Eustachian tube obstruction (*arrows* in **a**). This case demonstrates MRI's utility for evaluating for skull base infiltration in cases in which CT may be normal.

the temporal bone. Examples of anteroinferior extension include posterior fossa meningiomas, which tend to grow through neural foramina such as the jugular foramen (▶ Fig. 3.29).[4] The meningioma may or, often, may not have a bony reaction and may be difficult to distinguish from nerve sheath tumors. Nerve sheath tumors grow through neural foramina by their nature and may involve either the nerves within the jugular foramen (▶ Fig. 3.30) or, less commonly, the hypoglossal canal (▶ Fig. 3.31). These lesions cause a characteristic nondestructive widening or expansion of the neural foramina as seen on CT and exhibit other typical imaging features of peripheral nerve sheath tumor on CT and MR (▶ Fig. 3.30).

Other benign intracranial neoplasms adjacent to the temporal bone include the cerebellopontine lesions, which comprise vestibular schwannoma, meningioma, and epidermoid cyst. Vestibular schwannomas are quite variable in size and shape but generally involve the internal auditory canal (IAC) to some extent. Some are entirely intracanalicular (within the IAC), and others primarily involve the cistern but extend into the IAC (▶ Fig. 3.32; ▶ Fig. 3.33). Vestibular schwannomas typically enhance brightly but may contain areas of cystic change or necrosis, which do not enhance. Bilateral vestibular schwannomas are associated with type II neurofibromatosis (▶ Fig. 3.33), as are schwannomas of other cranial nerves and meningiomas.[6]

The most common jugular foramen neoplasm is the glomus tumor.[2] These so-called paragangliomas are hypervascular,

usually benign but aggressive tumors that arise from paraganglia cells in various locations in the body. In the head and neck, the carotid sheath (glomus caroticum or vagale) or, for this discussion, the jugular foramen (glomus jugulare) are typical locations. On CT, these characteristically cause a "moth-eaten" or permeative pattern of bone destruction (▶ Fig. 3.34).[2] They also enhance quite brightly due to their hypervascular nature. On MR, when 2.5 cm or so is exceeded, they usually have internal flow voids representing their vascularity (▶ Fig. 3.33) in what is sometimes referred to as a "salt-and-pepper" appearance. Coronal CT reconstructions are probably the best way to determine whether the lesion is extending into the hypotympanum (glomus jugulotympanicum). Angiography can play a role here, whether by catheter or using MR/CT techniques, by providing vascular road mapping preoperatively or facilitating embolization.

3.6 Marrow Space

Prior sections of this chapter illustrated how precise localization can allow specific diagnoses to be suggested. However, pathologies such as metastasis (▶ Fig. 3.27), lymphoma, and plasmacytoma can nonspecifically involve the marrow space and dura.

Lymphoma that is limited to the marrow space might not be identifiable by CT. MR typically shows low T1 signal, high T2

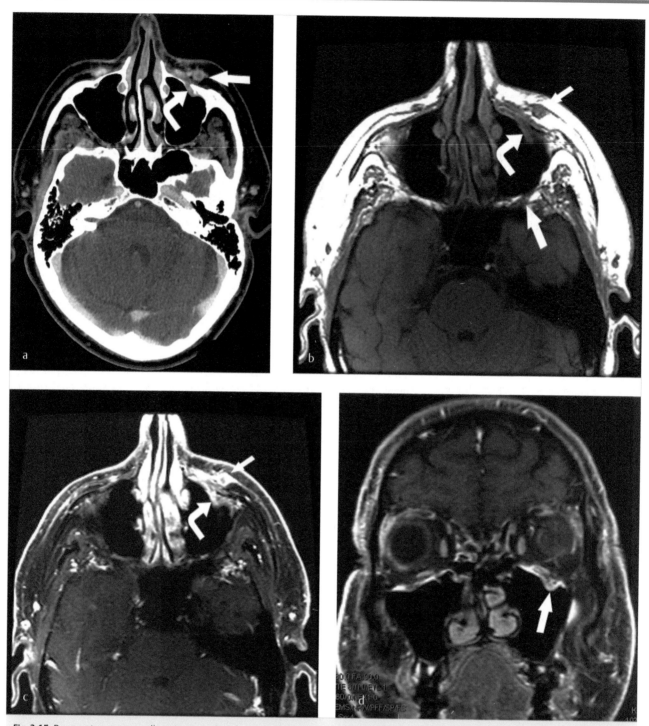

Fig. 3.15 Recurrent squamous cell carcinoma in the left premaxillary region in a 62-year-old man who had previously undergone Mohs resection, now presenting with left facial (V2) paresthesias. This case demonstrates perineural tumor spread along the infraorbital branch of the maxillary nerve. **(a)** Axial postcontrast CT image demonstrates a subcutaneous mass anterior to the left maxillary sinus (*straight arrow*). There is also abnormal density within the infraorbital foramen and anterior aspect of the left infraorbital canal (*curved arrow*). Axial **(b)** pre- and **(c)** postcontrast T1-weighted MR images reveal enhancing tumor in a premaxillary region (*small arrows*) as well as abnormal signal and enhancement along the course of the infraorbital nerve (*curved arrow*). More posteriorly, tumor can be seen actually coursing into the pterygopalatine fossa (*large arrow* in **b**). **(d)** Coronal T1 postcontrast MR with fat suppression reveals enlargement of the infraorbital nerve along the orbital floor or maxillary sinus roof (*arrow*).

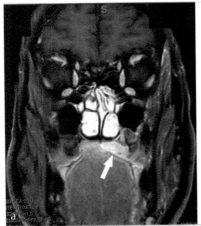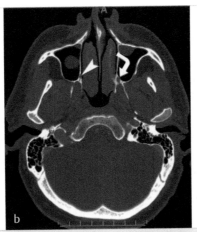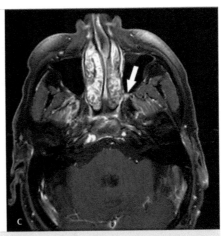

Fig. 3.16 Adenoid cystic carcinoma of the left hard palate with perineural spread along the palatine branches of the maxillary nerve in a 55-year-old whose dentist discovered a palatal mass. There was no clinical evidence of neuropathy. **(a)** Coronal T1 postcontrast MR image reveals a mass in the left side of the hard palate (*arrow*). **(b)** Axial CT bone window shows enlargement of the left greater palatine foramen (*arrow*). Note the normal right greater palatine foramen (*arrowhead*). **(c)** Axial postcontrast T1 MR image shows abnormal enhancement in the left pterygopalatine fossa (*arrow*), indicating spread of perineural tumor to at least this level. From here, tumor can spread posteriorly in a retrograde fashion, either through foramen rotundum or along the vidian nerve.

signal, short-TI inversion recovery (STIR) signal, and moderate to intense enhancement. Extramedullary lymphoma, however, shows low T2 signal. T1 signal and postcontrast T1 characteristics of extramedullary lymphoma are similar to marrow lymphoma. ▶ Fig. 3.35 shows Burkitt lymphoma involving the marrow space, nasal cavity, and dura.

Myeloma or plasmacytoma in the marrow space is typically seen as a lytic lesion on CT. MRI is more sensitive than CT, for it can detect myeloma or plasmacytoma in the marrow that is not visible on CT; both have an appearance similar to that of lymphoma on MRI. Marrow lesions are bright on T2 and STIR, and demonstrate soft tissue signal on T1, with moderate to intense enhancement.[23] Extramedullary myeloma and plasmacytoma can show low or moderate signal on T2-weighted MR images.[24] Typically, the lesions show soft tissue signal on T1 and moderate to intense enhancement (▶ Fig. 3.36).

Lymphoma and plasmacytoma do not require complete resection for treatment, because they are responsive to radiation and chemotherapy. Accordingly, suggestion of the diagnosis is an aid to preoperative planning. A specific diagnosis at frozen section may be difficult but when available can spare the patient an extensive resection.

PET/CT has an important, well-defined role in diagnosis and response assessment for lymphoma.[25,26] The use of PET/CT for diagnosis and response assessment in multiple myeloma is likely to increase in coming years.[23,27]

3.7 Conclusion

Tumors of the skull base encompass a huge variety of lesions, and imaging appearance can vary even for a given diagnosis. As a result, and because of the often nonspecific nature of imaging findings, diagnosis is not always possible prior to biopsy. It is the radiologist's job to confirm the presence of disease and to precisely define the extent of tumor. In many cases, doing so will suggest a likely diagnosis. This chapter was designed to give readers an appreciation, and a healthy respect, for the spectrum of imaging findings associated with skull base neoplasms. The skull base radiologist must accept that he or she will not always be correct—only through experience can one learn the many nuances of this field. As difficult as initial diagnosis is, posttreatment, and especially postoperative imaging, in the patient population is even more difficult. There is no substitute for experience and—to be frank—the wisdom born of error.

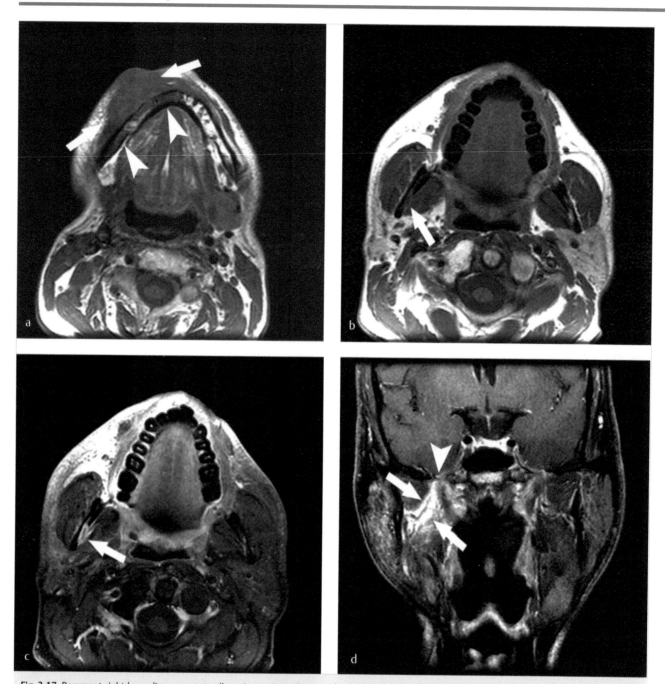

Fig. 3.17 Recurrent right lower lip squamous cell carcinoma in a 42-year-old man who had previously undergone biopsy and Mohs surgery as well as subsequent wedge resection and neck dissection for prior recurrences. (a) Axial T1-weighted MR image reveals a large recurrence in the right lower lip, very close to the mental foramen (*arrows*). Note the probable tumor infiltration of the right mandibular marrow cavity (*arrowheads*). Axial (b) pre- and (c) postcontrast T1-weighted MR images reveal abnormal signal intensity and enhancement in the mandibular foramen for the right inferior alveolar nerve (*arrows*). (d) Coronal T1-postcontrast MR image reveals tumor extending in an upward and medial direction from the mandibular foramen along the course of the main mandibular nerve trunk (*arrows*), approaching foramen ovale (*arrowhead*).

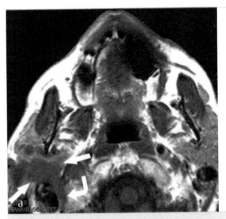
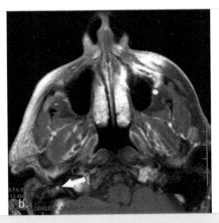
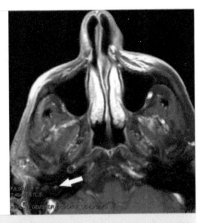

Fig. 3.18 Parotid salivary duct carcinoma associated with perineural spread along the descending segment of the right facial nerve in a 67-year-old man who presented with right-sided facial neuropathy for which an initial MR was said to be negative. **(a)** Axial noncontrast T1-weighted MR image reveals a mass in the right parotid gland (*arrows*). Note the posterior extension of disease toward the stylomastoid foramen (*curved arrow*). **(b, c)** Axial T1 postcontrast MR images at progressively cephalad positions revealing enlargement and excessive enhancement of the right descending facial nerve segment (*arrows*).

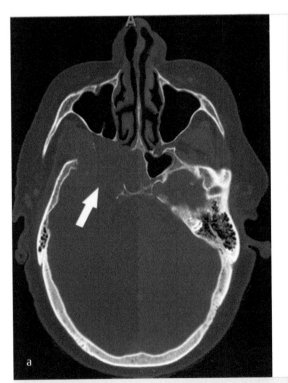
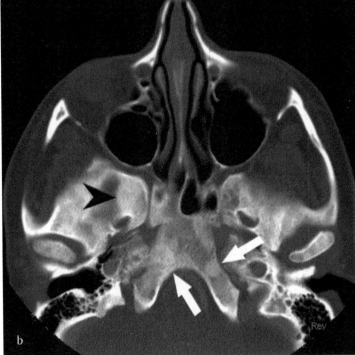

Fig. 3.19 Two patients with skull base metastasis. **(a)** Axial CT bone window demonstrating a large lytic and destructive metastasis from lung carcinoma (*arrow*). **(b)** Axial CT bone window in a patient with metastatic breast carcinoma showing blastic lesions in the clivus (*arrows*) and the right side of the central skull base lateral to the vidian canal (*arrowhead*).

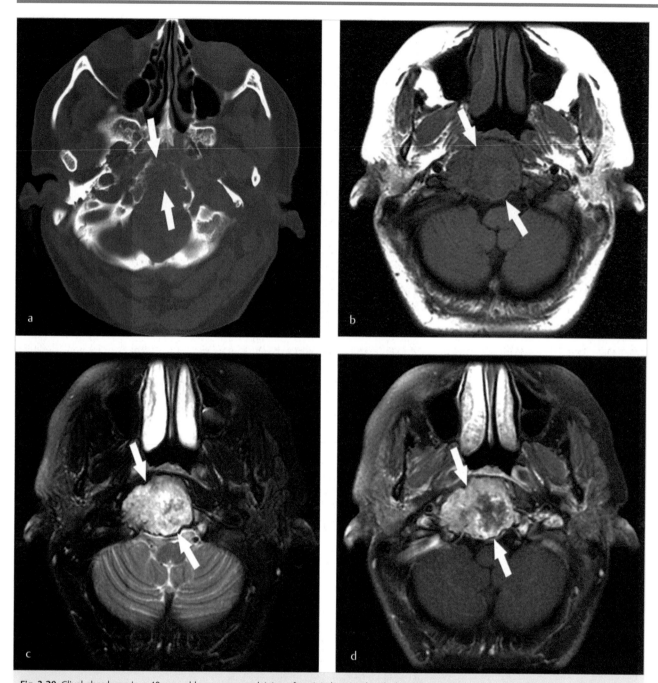

Fig. 3.20 Clival chordoma in a 40-year-old woman complaining of occipital region headache radiating to the right neck. **(a)** CT bone window demonstrates a large destructive lesion involving the clivus (*arrows*). **(b)** Axial T1, **(c)** T2, and **(d)** postcontrast T1-weighted MR images reveal a well-circumscribed mass lesion in the central skull base that is isointense on T1 and hyperintense on T2 and that enhances moderately with some heterogeneity (*arrows*). The bright signal on T2 is strongly suggestive of chordoma.

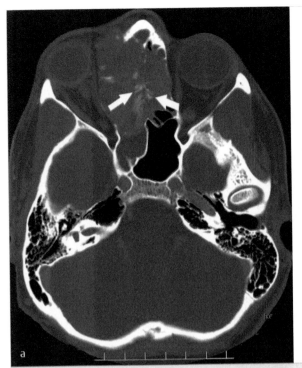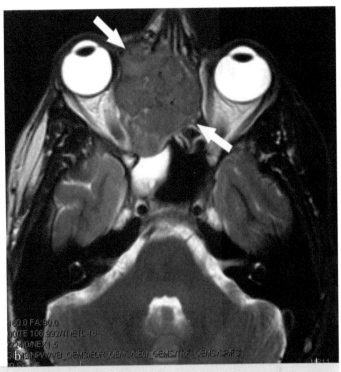

Fig. 3.21 Nasoethmoid chondrosarcoma in a 38-year-old woman presenting with progressive sinus symptoms, including congestion and epistaxis. **(a)** Axial CT bone window reveals a destructive mass with internal "arcs and rings" pattern of calcification representing the chondroid matrix (*arrows*). **(b)** Axial T2-weighted MR image revealing a relatively homogeneous isointense mass in the nasoethmoid region (*arrows*). Chondrosarcomas are often, but not always, heterogeneous on T2 and postcontrast MR images.

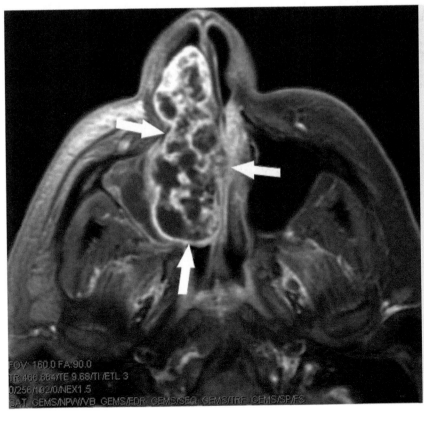

Fig. 3.22 Nasoethmoid chondrosarcoma in a different patient. Axial T1 postcontrast MR image reveals the marked heterogeneity that is characteristic of some chondrosarcomas, although the appearance can be variable.

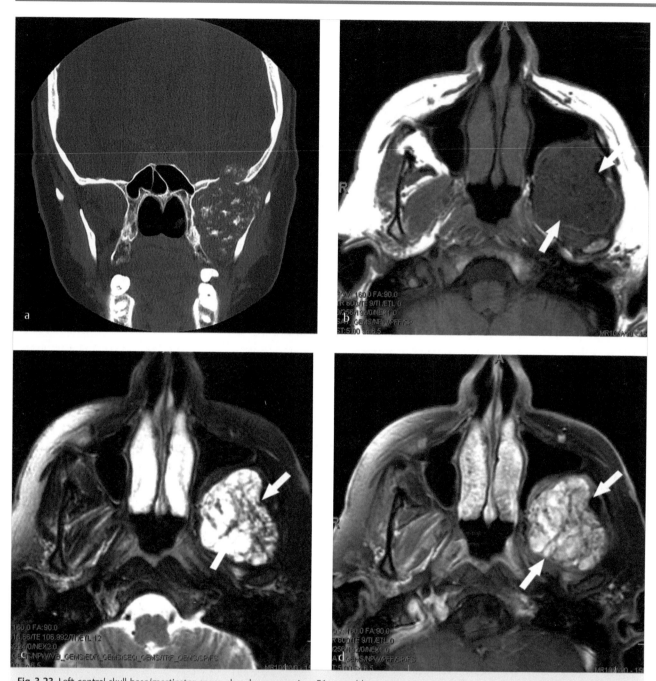

Fig. 3.23 Left central skull base/masticator space chondrosarcoma in a 51-year-old woman presenting with severe headaches. **(a)** Coronal bone window CT revealing a mass destroying the floor of the middle cranial fossa (*arrow*). Note the marked chondroid calcifications. **(b)** Axial T1, **(c)** T2, and **(d)** postcontrast T1-weighted MR images reveal a somewhat heterogeneous mass that is isointense on T1 and hyperintense on T2 and that enhances brightly following gadolinium administration. This is a fairly classic appearance for chondrosarcoma given the heterogeneity as well as chondroid calcifications.

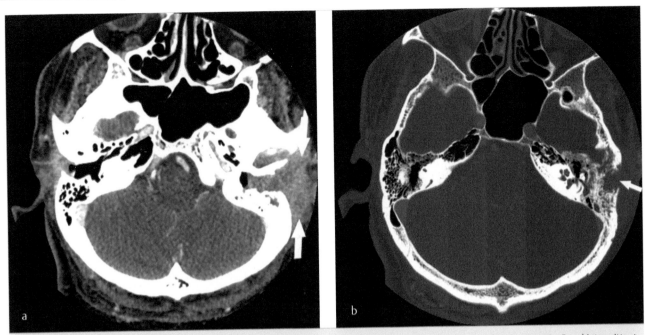

Fig. 3.24 Adenoid cystic carcinoma of the left external auditory canal in a 60-year-old man with a 2-year history of "ear congestion" and intermittent otorrhea. **(a)** Axial postcontrast CT (soft tissue window) demonstrates a large mass about the left external canal and external ear (*arrow*). **(b)** Axial CT bone window reveals gross destruction of the temporal bone (*arrow*).

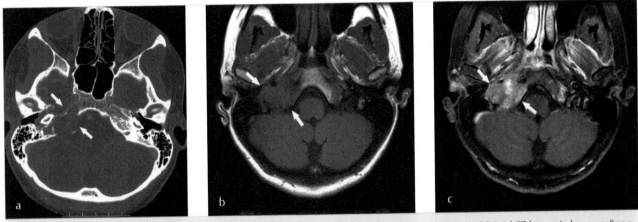

Fig. 3.25 Infiltrating neoplasm of the right temporal bone. The diagnosis ultimately proved to be meningioma. **(a)** Axial CT bone window revealing a destructive, somewhat permeative pattern of bony infiltration in the right temporal bone (*arrows*). Axial **(b)** pre- and **(c)** postcontrast T1-weighted MR images show a T1 isointense, mildly enhancing mass replacing the normal temporal bone structures and lower clivus (*arrows*). The imaging is nonspecific, and the differential diagnosis should include other entities, such as metastasis.

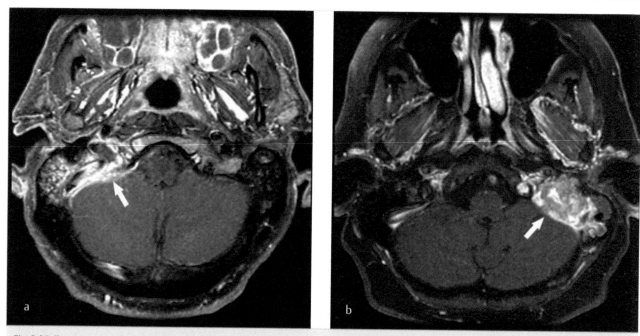

Fig. 3.26 Two patients with nonspecific infiltrative masses of the temporal bone. (a) Axial postcontrast, T1-weighted MR image reveals a patient with leukemic infiltration of the right temporal bone (*arrow*). (b) Axial postcontrast T1-weighted MR revealing a large enhancing mass in the left temporal bone (*arrow*) that proved to be a high-grade sarcoma. The imaging for these lesions, as well as that for the meningioma in ▶ Fig. 3.25, is nonspecific.

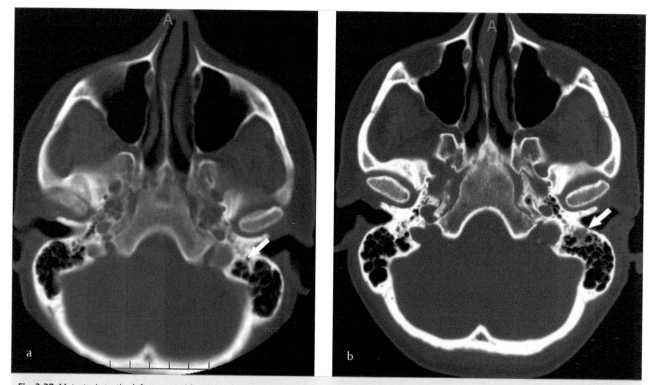

Fig. 3.27 Metastasis to the left temporal bone resulting in facial neuropathy in a patient who has metastatic carcinoma of the cervix. (a) CT bone window obtained for evaluation of cervical lymphadenopathy, but prior to the onset of facial palsy, showing normal descending left facial nerve canal (*arrow*). (b) Axial CT bone window following onset of left facial neuropathy. Note the new destructive lytic lesion corresponding to the location of the left descending facial nerve canal (*arrow*).

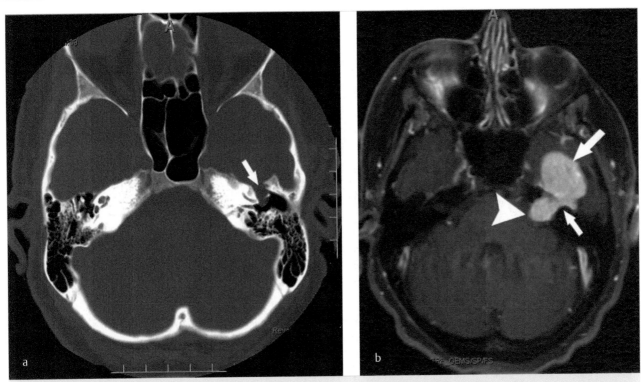

Fig. 3.28 Facial schwannoma with greater superficial petrosal nerve and middle cranial fossa involvement in a 53-year-old woman with a many-year history of facial neuropathy and progressive hearing loss. **(a)** Axial CT bone window reveals enlargement of the facial hiatus for the left greater superficial petrosal nerve (*arrow*). There is a soft tissue mass at the location for the geniculate ganglion (*arrowhead*). **(b)** Axial postcontrast T1-weighted MR image reveals a homogeneous, brightly enhancing mass lesion with a component in the middle cranial fossa (*large arrow*), the labyrinthine portion of the facial nerve (*small arrow*), and the internal auditory canal (*arrowhead*).

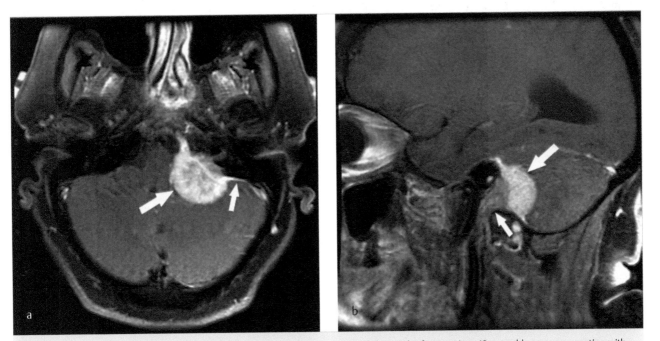

Fig. 3.29 Left-sided cerebellopontine angle (CPA) meningioma with involvement of the jugular foramen in a 43-year-old woman presenting with tinnitus and progressive left-sided hearing loss. **(a)** Axial and **(b)** sagittal postcontrast T1-weighted MR images reveal a dural-based extra axial mass lesion in the left CPA (*large arrows*). Note extension into the jugular foramen (*small arrow* in **b**). A so-called dural tail of enhancement is best seen in the axial image extending laterally from the lesion (*smaller arrow* in **a**).

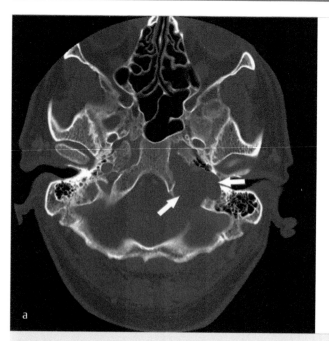
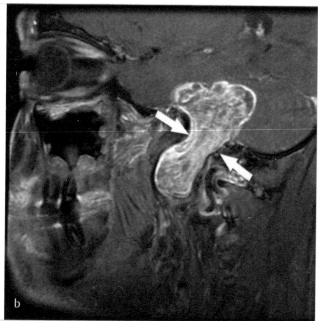

Fig. 3.30 Jugular schwannoma in a 52-year-old man presenting who has a hissing sound in the left ear and left-side sensorineural hearing loss. **(a)** Axial CT bone window reveals benign expansion and remodeling, without destruction, in the left jugular foramen (*arrow*). **(b)** Sagittal postcontrast T1-weighted MR image shows a heterogeneously but brightly enhancing mass lesion extending from the posterior fossa through a widened jugular foramen (*arrows*) and into the upper carotid space.

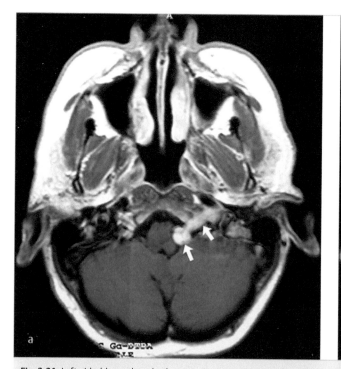
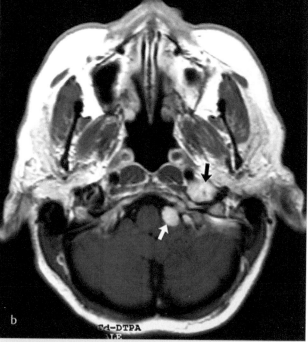

Fig. 3.31 Left-sided hypoglossal schwannoma in a patient presenting with headache and left tongue fasciculations. **(a,b)** Axial postcontrast T1-weighted MR images through the posterior fossa reveal a dumbbell-shaped enhancing tumor with a component in the cerebellomedullary angle (*white arrows*) and extending through the hypoglossal canal into the upper carotid space (*black arrow* in **b**).

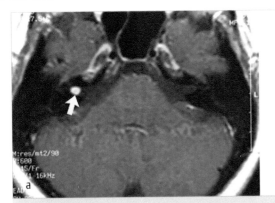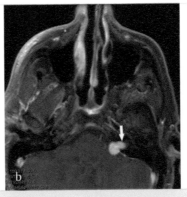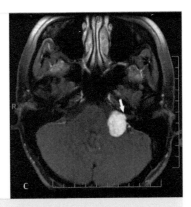

Fig. 3.32 Assortment of vestibular schwannomas. **(a)** Axial postcontrast T1-weighted MR image through the posterior fossa reveals a small intracanalicular enhancing mass representing a vestibular schwannoma in the right internal auditory canal (IAC; *arrow*). **(b)** Axial postcontrast T1-weighted MR image revealing a dumbbell-like mass extending from the cerebellopontine angle into a widened left IAC (*arrow*). A small dural tail appears to extend posterolaterally, away from the lesion; however, such a tail is not specific for meningioma but can also be seen in other lesions. **(c)** Axial postcontrast T1-weighted MR image shows a larger vestibular schwannoma that is primarily cisternal in location, with only minimal extension into the IAC (*arrow*). Acoustic vestibular schwannomas come in different sizes and shapes.

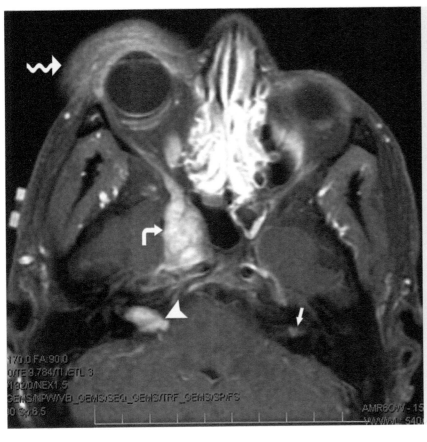

Fig. 3.33 Neurofibromatosis type II in a patient with long-standing disease and multiple manifestations. Axial T1 postcontrast MR image through the posterior fossa and skull base reveals bilateral acoustic vestibular schwannomas, with a larger right-sided lesion (*arrowhead*) and the left-sided lesion intracanalicular (*small arrow*). Incidental note is also made of an enhancing mass within the right cavernous sinus (*curved arrow*) representing a trigeminal schwannoma, as well as (only partially seen on this image) a large plexiform neurofibroma involving the upper eyelid (*squiggly arrow*).

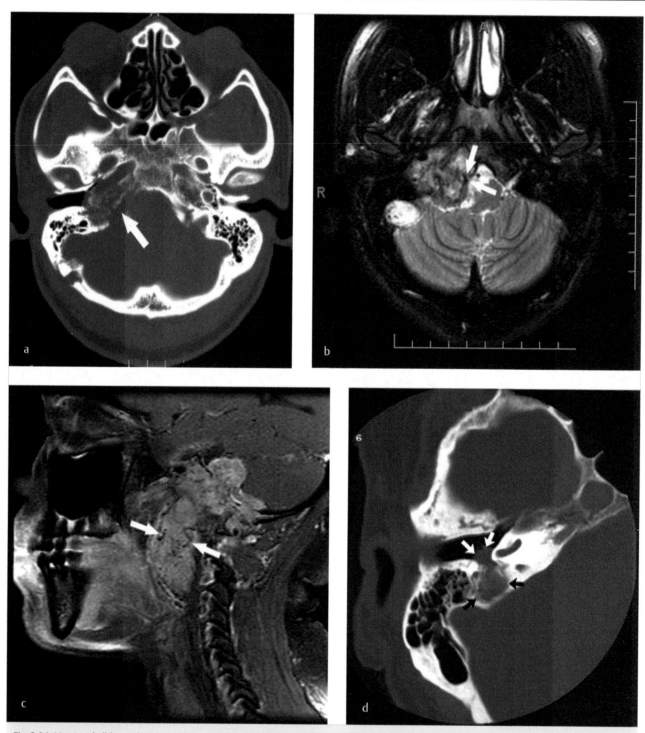

Fig. 3.34 Massive skull base glomus tumor in a 32-year-old woman with long-standing occipital region headache and progressive lower cranial neuropathies. **(a)** Axial CT bone window reveals a permeative type of bony destruction in the right temporal bone in the region of the jugular foramen (*arrow*). **(b)** Axial T2 and **(c)** sagittal T1 postcontrast MR images reveal a large mass lesion. Note internal areas of heterogeneity, some of which are dotlike and others of which are curvilinear (*arrows*), representing flow voids within this hypervascular lesion. The sagittal image amply demonstrates inferior extension into the upper carotid space. **(d)** Axial CT bone window through the temporal bone in a different patient with a jugular foramen glomus tumor (*black arrows*) with extension into the tympanic cavity (*white arrows*). Accordingly, this is properly termed a glomus jugulotympanicum.

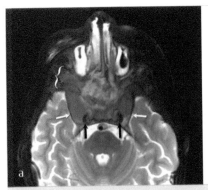
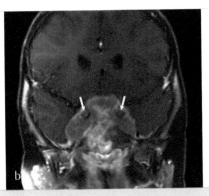
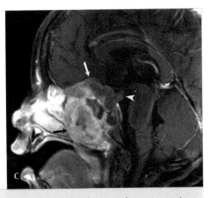

Fig. 3.35 Burkitt lymphoma in a 3-year-old boy with new onset of bilateral vision loss. **(a)** Axial fat-saturated T2-weighted image shows a massive tumor of the nasal cavity, clivus, and cavernous sinuses (*white arrows*). The lymphoma surrounds the cavernous carotid arteries (*black arrows*) and extends through the pterygopalatine fossa into the right retromaxillary space (*bracket*). **(b)** Coronal fat-saturated T1 postcontrast MR image shows moderate tumor enhancement, suprasellar extension, and complete encasement of bilateral optic nerves (*white arrows*). **(c)** Sagittal fat-saturated T1 postcontrast MR image shows lymphoma in the nasal cavity (*black arrow*) extending into the epidural space of the anterior cranial fossa (*white arrow*) and suprasellar region. The pituitary gland is displaced posteriorly (*arrowhead*).

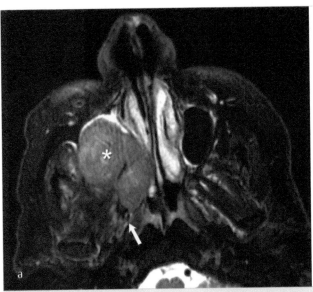
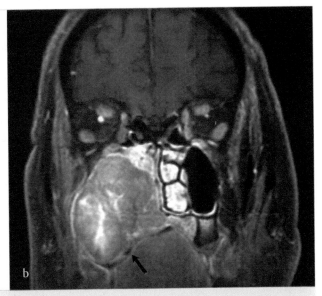

Fig. 3.36 Plasmacytoma in a 74-year-old man presenting with epistaxis, nasal obstruction and ill-fitting dentures. **(a)** Axial fat-saturated T2 MR image depicts a maxillary sinus mass (*asterisk*) with low T2 signal and destruction of the right pterygoid process (*white arrow*). **(b)** Coronal fat-saturated T1 postcontrast MR image shows heterogeneous moderate to intense enhancement and involvement of the left alveolar ridge (*black arrow*).

References

[1] Ginsberg LE. Neoplastic diseases affecting the central skull base: CT and MR imaging. AJR Am J Roentgenol. 1992; 159(3):581–589

[2] Harnsberger HR, Wiggins RH, Hudgins PA, et al. Diagnostic Imaging: Head and Neck, 1st ed. Salt Lake City, UT: Amirsys; 2004

[3] Som PM, Brandwein MS. Tumors and tumor-like conditions. In: Som PM, Curtin HD, eds. Head and Neck Imaging. St. Louis: Mosby; 2003

[4] Ginsberg LE, Moody DM. Meningiomas: imaging. In: Wilkins RH, Reangachary SS, (eds): Neurosurgery, 2nd ed. New York: McGraw-Hill, 1996, Vol 1:855–872

[5] Kim KS, Rogers LF, Goldblatt D. CT features of hyperostosing meningioma en plaque. AJR Am J Roentgenol. 1987; 149(5):1017–1023

[6] Ginsberg LE. Contrast enhancement in meningeal and extra-axial disease. Neuroimaging Clin N Am. 1994; 4(1):133–152

[7] Laidlaw JD, Kumar A, Chan A. Dural metastases mimicking meningioma. Case report and review of the literature. J Clin Neurosci. 2004; 11(7):780–783

[8] Curtin HD, Rabinov J, Som PM. Skull base: embryology, anatomy, and pathology. In: Som PM, Curtin HD, eds. Head and Neck Imaging. St. Louis: Mosby; 2003

[9] Fischbein NJ, Kaplan MJ. Magnetic resonance imaging of the central skull base. Top Magn Reson Imaging. 1999; 10(5):325–346

[10] Levy RA, Quint DJ. Giant pituitary adenoma with unusual orbital and skull base extension. AJR Am J Roentgenol. 1998; 170(1):194–196

[11] Minniti G, Jaffrain-Rea M-L, Santoro A, et al. Giant prolactinomas presenting as skull base tumors. Surg Neurol. 2002; 57(2):99–103, discussion 103–104

[12] Weinstein MA, Levine H, Duchesneau PM, Tucker HM. Diagnosis of juvenile angiofibroma by computed tomography. Radiology. 1978; 126(3):703–705

[13] Ishida H, Mohri M, Amatsu M. Invasion of the skull base by carcinomas: histopathologically evidenced findings with CT and MRI. Eur Arch Otorhinolaryngol. 2002; 259(10):535–539

[14] Chong VF, Mukherji SK, Ng SH, et al. Nasopharyngeal carcinoma: review of how imaging affects staging. J Comput Assist Tomogr. 1999; 23(6):984–993

[15] Chong VF, Fan YF. Skull base erosion in nasopharyngeal carcinoma: detection by CT and MRI. Clin Radiol. 1996; 51(9):625–631

[16] Chong VF, Fan YF, Khoo JB. Nasopharyngeal carcinoma with intracranial spread: CT and MR characteristics. J Comput Assist Tomogr. 1996; 20(4): 563–569

[17] Ginsberg LE, Demonte F. Palatal adenoid cystic carcinoma presenting as perineural spread to the cavernous sinus. Skull Base Surg. 1998; 8(1):39–43

[18] Ginsberg LE. Imaging of perineural tumor spread in head and neck cancer. In: Som PM, Curtin HD, eds. Head and Neck Imaging. St. Louis: Mosby; 2003

[19] Ginsberg LE. Imaging of perineural tumor spread in head and neck cancer. Semin Ultrasound CT MR. 1999; 20(3):175–186

[20] Dinehart SM, Jansen GT. Cancer of the skin. In: Myers EN, Suen JY, eds. Cancer of the Head and Neck. Philadelphia, PA: W.B. Saunders; 1996:143–159

[21] Ginsberg LE, DeMonte F. Diagnosis please. Case 16: facial nerve schwannoma with middle cranial fossa involvement. Radiology. 1999; 213(2):364–368

[22] Ginsberg LE, De Monte F, Gillenwater AM. Greater superficial petrosal nerve: anatomy and MR findings in perineural tumor spread. AJNR Am J Neuroradiol. 1996; 17(2):389–393

[23] Ferraro R, Agarwal A, Martin-Macintosh EL, Peller PJ, Subramaniam RM. MR imaging and PET/CT in diagnosis and management of multiple myeloma. Radiographics. 2015; 35(2):438–454

[24] Tirumani SH, Shinagare AB, Jagannathan JP, Krajewski KM, Munshi NC, Ramaiya NH. MRI features of extramedullary myeloma. AJR Am J Roentgenol. 2014; 202(4):803–810

[25] Barrington SF, Mikhaeel NG, Kostakoglu L, et al. Role of imaging in the staging and response assessment of lymphoma: consensus of the International Conference on Malignant Lymphomas Imaging Working Group. J Clin Oncol. 2014; 32(27):3048–3058

[26] Johnson SA, Kumar A, Matasar MJ, Schöder H, Rademaker J. Imaging for Staging and Response Assessment in Lymphoma. Radiology. 2015; 276(2): 323–338

[27] Agarwal A, Chirindel A, Shah BA, Subramaniam RM. Evolving role of FDG PET/CT in multiple myeloma imaging and management. AJR Am J Roentgenol. 2013; 200(4):884–890

4 Head, Neck, and Neuro-otologic Assessment of Patients with Skull Base Tumors

Paul W. Gidley

Summary

This chapter discusses the head and neck examination with particular attention to neuro-otologic diagnosis. The physical examination is conducted in a systematic fashion to avoid missing important findings. The cranial nerves are examined carefully, because pathology often produces subtle findings. Cranial nerve anatomy and syndromes are tabulated for easy reference. Special tests for assessing hearing and balance are discussed, with particular attention to findings that suggest acoustic neuroma.

Keywords: acoustic neuroma, audiogram, auditory brainstem response, cranial nerve, endolymphatic sac tumor, meningioma, otoacoustic emissions, physical examination, tuning fork test, videonystagmography

4.1 Introduction

The art of history taking, physical examination, and creation of a differential diagnosis develops through practice. Key to this art is an understanding of the subtleties of symptoms and signs, especially those associated with neurologic diseases. This chapter discusses the basics of the neuro-otologic examination. Site-specific symptoms and signs will be explored to help the physician learn the cause of these maladies. This chapter is meant to be a foundation from which to work toward a proper differential diagnosis and treatment plan for each patient.

This interaction between physician and patient, which establishes the basic rapport and tenor of the physician–patient relationship, is supplanted and not replaced by technology. The daily and long-term outcomes of treatment are readily measured and tracked by noting the symptoms and signs of disease, whether at the bedside or in the outpatient setting.

It is assumed that the reader, being either a resident or a well-seasoned practitioner, is already familiar with the basics of history and physical examination. This chapter's objectives are to discuss the physical signs associated with neuro-otologic disease and to discuss the ancillary audiometric, vestibular, and electrophysiologic tests used to discern disease processes. Special attention is paid to the cranial nerve (CN) examination. This chapter will not discuss individual disease states except to discuss the signs and symptoms that are indicative of a particular disease process.

4.2 Physical Examination

Owing to the compact and complex regional anatomy of the head and neck, the neuro-otologic examination requires practice and experience to refine. As with a general physical examination, a head-to-toe organization is systematic and simple to perform for completeness. In doing so, CNs are checked when moving from site to site, although a dedicated and rigorous CN examination requires additional techniques and observation.

On initial introduction to the patient, one might identify obvious facial paralysis or a wet, weak, or hoarse voice. Regardless,

the examining physician should avoid being sidetracked by these overt signs and should instead conduct a systematic review to look for all abnormalities. The reader probably has experienced a patient who has long-standing facial paralysis but whose presenting complaint is totally unrelated to that finding. Additionally, patients frequently present with a complaint of ear pain whose cause is discovered only after a careful history and physical examination: vocal fold malignancy.

4.2.1 Head, Scalp, and Skin Exams

Occasionally, the obvious does escape our attention. The head and neck are covered by skin, but sometimes this skin is overlooked to examine the ear canals or nasal passages instead. The posterior surface of the pinna is often overlooked but can harbor malignant disease. The sun-exposed portions need to be examined for premalignant or malignant conditions. Patients who have already had skin excisions need to be queried about the pathologic diagnosis from these sites considering melanoma's and squamous cell carcinoma's propensity for metastatic and perineural spread (▶ Fig. 4.1).

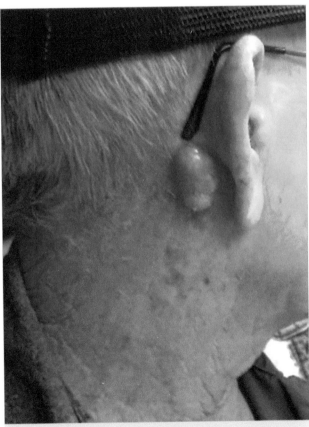

Fig. 4.1 Metastatic carcinoma to the right mastoid tip following Mohs excision of facial squamous cell carcinoma.

At times, the skin of the head and neck provides the diagnosis, as in the case of adenoma sebaceum and tuberous sclerosis or port-wine stain and Sturge-Weber syndrome. A list of neurocutaneous disorders that affect the head and neck, as well as their constituent findings and genetic causes, is given in ▶ Table 4.1.[1,2,3,4,5,6,7,8,9]

4.2.2 Eye, Orbit, and Eye Movement Exams

Patients who have primary eye complaints are typically seen first by an ophthalmologist. Certainly patients who present with skull base tumors that affect the orbit, eye movements, or visual pathways should have a rigorous ophthalmologic evaluation. A close working relationship with a neuro-ophthalmologist is necessary for any skull base team. The following description of the eye

examination is provided to highlight the important signs and symptoms to discover and note in patients who have skull base tumors.

Eye and Orbit

The symmetry of the orbits and eyes should be compared. The globes should be compared to look for proptosis. The status of the lids should be examined, not only to identify lesions but also to inspect their conformity to the globe. Ectropion is very common with facial paralysis, and corrective measures can be performed to minimize its effects. The status of the conjunctiva should be noted for inflammation or irritation: this, too, is a frequent sign accompanying facial paralysis. The size and reactivity of the pupils should be documented: this is done both with a flashlight, looking for direct and indirect responses, and with convergence. Visual fields can be estimated by testing peripheral

Table 4.1 A listing of neurocutaneous disorders that affect the head and neck, their congeners, associated findings and genetic cause

Diagnosis	Dermatologic manifestation	Associated findings	Genetic cause
Ataxia telangiectasia[a,b]	Cutaneous telangiectasia	Progressive neurologic deterioration Immunodeficiency High incidence of neoplasms (lymphoid tumors, 10–15%)	*ATM*
Neurofibromatosis type 1[b,c]	Café au lait spots	Multiple neurofibromas Lisch nodules of the iris Optic glioma	17q11.2-Neurofibromin
Neurofibromatosis type 2[d,e]		Bilateral acoustic neuromas Schwannomas of other nerves Meningiomas Ependymomas Gliomas	*NF2*-22q12.2-Merlin
PHACE syndrome[f]	Cutaneous and airway hemangiomas	Posterior fossa malformations (Dandy-Walker) Arterial anomalies Coarctation of the aorta and cardiac defects Eye abnormalities	X-linked dominance Developmental disorder
Sturge-Weber syndrome[g,h]	Port wine stain	Leptomeningeal angioma Choroidal angioma Epilepsy (80%) Learning disabilities	Sporadic Somatic mutation
Tuberous sclerosis[g]	Adenoma sebaceum (facial angiomatosis)	Epilepsy (78%) Learning disabilities Giant cell astrocytoma Cardiac rhabdomyosarcoma Lymphangiomatosis Renal angiomyolipoma	TSC1–9q34-hamartin TSC2–16p13.3-tuberin
Von-Hippel Lindau[d,i]		Cerebellar hemangioblastoma (60%) Retinal angiomas (60%) Renal, pancreatic cysts Renal cell carcinoma (40%) Pheochromocytomas Endolymphatic sac tumors	*VHL*-3q 11-"VHL protein"

Abbreviation: PHACE, posterior fossa, hemangiomas, arterial anomalies, coarctation of the aorta and cardiac defects, and eye abnormalities.
[a]Bott L, Thumerelle C, Cuvellier JC, Deschildre A, Vallée L, Sardet A. [Ataxia-telangiectasia: a review]. Arch Pediatr 2006;13(3):293–298.
[b]Taylor AM, Byrd PJ. Molecular pathology of ataxia telangiectasia. J Clin Pathol 2005;58(10):1009–1015.
[c]Kreusel KM. Ophthalmological manifestations in VHL and NF 1: pathological and diagnostic implications. Fam Cancer 2005;4(1):43–47.
[d]Patel NP, Mhatre AN, Lalwani AK. Molecular pathogenesis of skull base tumors. Otol Neurotol 2004;25(4):636–643.
[e]Xiao GH, Chernoff J, Testa JR. NF2: the wizardry of merlin. Genes Chromosomes Cancer 2003;38(4):389–399.
[f]Smith DS, Lee KK, Milczuk HA. Otolaryngologic manifestations of PHACE syndrome. Int J Pediatr Otorhinolaryngol 2004;68(11):1445–1450.
[g]Cross JH. Neurocutaneous syndromes and epilepsy-issues in diagnosis and management. Epilepsia 2005;46(Suppl 10):17–23.
[h]Comi AM. Pathophysiology of Sturge-Weber syndrome. J Child Neurol 2003;18(8):509–516.
[i]Freedman SF, Amedee RG, Molony T. Neurotologic manifestations of von Hippel Lindau disease. Ear Nose Throat J 1992;71(12):655–658.

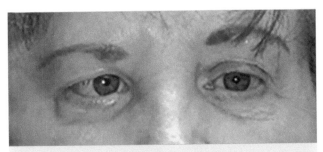

Fig. 4.2 Right abducens palsy from recurrent adenoid cystic carcinoma of the right parotid and temporal bone.

vision. Finally, an estimate of vision can be gained by testing each eye separately using a handheld Snellen eye chart held about 14 inches from the eyes.

Eye Movements

Normal eye movements depend on the equal function of CNs III, IV, and VI and their innervated muscles. A basic test of eye movements involves having the patient follow the examiner's finger. All the extraocular muscles are tested in nine different positions (straight ahead, right, left, up, down, as well as diagonally right up, right down, left up, and left down).[10] Sixth nerve palsy is common with disease in the petrous apex (▶ Fig. 4.2). The CNs, with their muscles and their actions, are listed in ▶ Table 4.2.[11]

Nystagmus

Nystagmus is an involuntary, rhythmic movement of the eyes. The term is derived from the Greek word *nystagmos*, for nodding.[12] Nystagmus can be generally divided into two broad categories: jerk nystagmus and pendular nystagmus.[13] In pendular nystagmus, the two phases of nystagmus are of equal length. Jerk nystagmus, the more relevant of the two in this discussion, has two components: a slow phase followed by a fast phase. Its direction is named for the direction of the fast component. The primary plane or axis of nystagmus is described as horizontal, vertical, rotatory, or direction-changing. Classically, horizontal nystagmus is associated with peripheral lesions. The fast component is toward the unaffected ear. Vertical and direction-changing nystagmus are generally signs of central pathology. The time of onset can be described as spontaneous (occurring without provocation), latent (some delay in onset, usually after a change in position), gaze-evoked (brought out with certain eye movements), or positional (brought out by certain positions).

Spontaneous nystagmus represents an imbalance in the vestibular–ocular reflex (VOR) and can be either central or peripheral in origin.[14] Spontaneous nystagmus is best evaluated by examining the eyes through Frenzel lenses. These 10+ diopter lenses not only magnify fine movements but also eliminate visual fixation that could overpower a vestibular nystagmus.[14] Spontaneous nystagmus that does not abate with visual fixation probably represents central pathology. Pure vertical, torsional, or linear nystagmus cannot be explained by involvement of a single canal or single labyrinth and implies a central etiology.[14]

Table 4.2 Eye movements: the cranial nerves, muscles, actions, and deficits

Cranial nerve	Muscle	Action	Deficit
III – Oculomotor	Medial rectus	Adduction	Eye is outward, downward, and dilated; upper lid ptosis
	Superior rectus	1. Elevation 2. Adduction, intorsion	
	Inferior rectus	1. Depression 2. Adduction and extorsion	
	Inferior oblique	1. Elevation 2. Extorsion and abduction	
III – Oculomotor, parasympathetics	Ciliary muscle	Constriction of the pupil	
VI – Superior oblique	Superior oblique	1. Depression 2. Intorsion and abduction	Skew deviation, head tilted toward weak side
VI – Abducens	Lateral rectus	Abduction	Cannot move eye laterally past midline

Source: Reproduced with permission from Kandell E, Schwartz J, Jessell T, eds. Principles of Neural Science. New York, NY: McGraw-Hill; 2000.

Gaze nystagmus can be elicited by having the patient follow the examiner's finger as it performs a +-type movement, thus evoking either lateral gaze or upward or downward gaze nystagmus. Gaze-evoked nystagmus most often occurs as a side effect of medications or toxins.[10] Horizontal gaze-evoked nystagmus usually indicates a lesion in the brainstem or cerebellum; vertical gaze-evoked nystagmus is found in midbrain lesions that involve the interstitial nucleus of Cajal.[15] Gaze nystagmus has been described as first-degree (occurs only with gazing in the direction of the fast component), second-degree (occurs in the direction of the fast component and straight ahead), and third-degree (occurs in all three directions of gaze). The significance of these distinctions is that first-degree nystagmus is seen with a peripheral lesion but second- and third-degree with central pathology.[16]

Congenital nystagmus generally beats horizontally at various frequencies and amplitudes and increases with fixation.[10]

Bruns's nystagmus is associated with large posterior fossa tumors. This nystagmus involves a coarse, large-amplitude horizontal gaze nystagmus toward the tumor side and a fine, high-frequency gaze nystagmus away from the tumor side,[14] thought to result from bilateral compression of the flocculus.[17]

Dynamic vestibular imbalance can be assessed by passive head movement and observation of the patient's eyes. Dynamic visual acuity is assessed by passively rotating the patient's head at or above 2 Hz while he or she reads a Snellen eye chart at the standard distance. A drop in visual acuity of more than one line indicates abnormal gain in the VOR.[18] A computerized form of this test has also been developed[19] and might be useful as a clinical tool for separating unilateral from bilateral vestibular hypofunction.

Positional nystagmus is provoked using the Dix-Hallpike maneuver.[20] In this test the patient is seated on an examining table or bed and is instructed to turn the head to the right side, then recline backward as quickly as possible. The examiner watches the patient's eyes for any nystagmus and asks the patient whether he or she feels dizzy. If nystagmus is present, then its length of latency and duration should be noted. After this nystagmus or dizziness disappears, the patient is asked to return to an upright sitting position; again the eyes are examined for nystagmus. Patients who have benign paroxysmal positional vertigo will have a latent (usually 2–5 s), geotropic (nystagmus beats toward the ground), rotatory nystagmus that reverses (reversibility) when seated upright. The duration and strength of the nystagmus lessens with each subsequent test when performed in repetition (fatigability).

Head Thrust Test

The head thrust test (HTT) is a bedside test with which to assess the VOR.[21] The test is performed by asking the patient to focus on a target. The examiner gently grasps the head, and a small-amplitude (5–10°), high-acceleration (3,000–4,000°/s/s) thrust is applied. The examiner watches the eyes at the end of the head thrust for a corrective saccade. Normal individuals do not use a corrective saccade: their eyes stay fixed on the target. Patients who have vestibular hypofunction use a corrective saccade after the head thrust, and the saccade is toward the side of the lesion. This corrective saccade returns the eye to the target and indicates a decreased gain (eye velocity/head velocity) of the VOR.[22] The specificity of HTT for identifying lateral semicircular canal pathology is very high (95–100%), and it correlates 100% with surgical vestibular nerve section.[23] In patients who have lesser degrees of unilateral hypofunction, the sensitivity is as low as 34 to 39% but the specificity remains as high as 95 to 100%.[24,25,26] The sensitivity of this test can be improved by 30° of cervical flexion (making the horizontal canal horizontal).[22]

Head-Shaking Nystagmus

Head-shaking nystagmus (HSN)[27] is used to demonstrate asymmetry in the velocity storage that can occur with either central or peripheral lesions. In this test, the patient's head is shaken either actively or passively in the horizontal plane for 10 to 15 seconds with the eyes closed. After stopping and opening the eyes, nystagmus will be seen beating away from the side of the lesion.[14] In this test, Frenzel lenses are indispensable, because the nystagmus is often fine and fleeting. HSN can also be performed with electronystagmography (ENG) and is discussed in the Electronystagmography section, following.

4.2.3 Ear Exams

Pinna and External Auditory Canal

The external ear includes the pinna, the membranous external auditory meatus, and the bony ear canal. In one's eagerness to examine the eardrum, the pinna might be overlooked. Fully 15 to 20% of head and neck skin cancers occur on the external ear, and 55% are along the helix.[28,29,30] The examination should not be limited to the protruding parts of the pinna but rather should also include the postauricular skin (▶ Fig. 4.3).

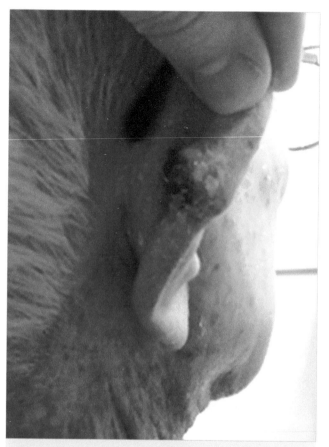

Fig. 4.3 Squamous cell carcinoma on the posterior surface of the right pinna.

A distinction is made here between the external auditory meatus, which is the cartilaginous outer third of the ear canal, and the bony ear canal, which is the bony two-thirds of the external ear canal. The membranous meatus has a thick squamous epithelium, is hair-covered, and contains the cerumen glands (▶ Fig. 4.4a), whereas the bony canal is lined by a thin squamous epithelium without any modified sweat glands or hair (▶ Fig. 4.4b).

Tympanic Membrane and Middle Ear

These structures are best evaluated with a handheld otoscope, an otomicroscope, and an otoendoscope. Each modality gives a slightly different but complementary view of the ear canal and tympanic membrane (TM). Each also allows testing of TM movement, either with a bulb attachment to the otoscope or through a Siegle otoscope viewed through the microscope. Occasionally patients have a narrowed or oddly shaped ear canal that cannot be adequately evaluated using an oval or round speculum. In such circumstances, a pediatric or adult nasal speculum can be helpful.

Ear endoscopes have been available for the past few decades and have become a part of the surgical treatment of many middle ear diseases. These endoscopes are 6 cm long and are 2.7 or 4 mm in diameter; 0 and 30° varieties are available. These endoscopes can provide an unparalleled view of middle ear structures, surpassing that available through a microscope or a

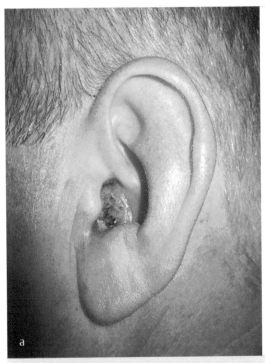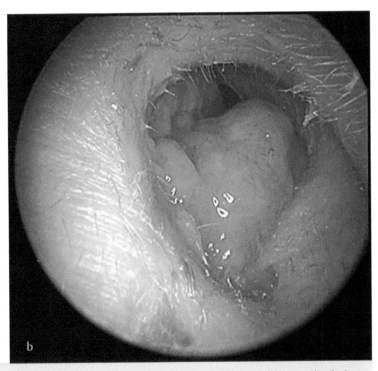

Fig. 4.4 (a) Squamous cell carcinoma of left external auditory meatus. This tumor involved only the cartilaginous canal and did not involve the bony canal; thus it did not require lateral temporal bone resection. **(b)** Squamous cell carcinoma of the right external auditory canal. This tumor requires a lateral temporal bone resection.

handheld otoscope. Additionally, high-quality photodocumentation of ear canal, eardrum, and middle ear pathology can be captured easily using an endoscope (▶ Fig. 4.5).

Tuning Fork Examination

In a bygone era, tuning fork examination represented the state of the art in audiometric assessment. With the advent of calibrated audiometers, the tuning fork examination has lost its centrality in measuring a patient's hearing. It has not lost its importance, however, in giving the attentive clinician valuable information regarding hearing. Although the history of otology and audiometry includes several tuning fork tests, only the Weber and Rinne tests are performed routinely.

The Weber test is performed by striking the tuning fork and then placing it on the patient's forehead, philtrum, or upper incisors and asking the patient where the sound is heard best: right side, left side, or midline (or equally in both ears). The sound is perceived as louder in an ear that has a conductive loss or in an ear that has better sensorineural hearing when no conductive component is present in the other ear. Interestingly, patients who have unilateral, congenital conductive hearing loss do not have lateralization to that side.

The Rinne test is performed by striking the tuning fork and then asking the patient to compare for loudness the sound produced with the fork on the mastoid versus in front of the ear canal. A normal result (also called a "positive Rinne") is that the loudness is greater in front of the ear, by air conduction (AC), than it is by bone conduction (BC; also noted as AC > BC). In a conductive loss larger than about 25 dB with a 512 Hz fork, the sound is louder on the bone than it is

through air conduction (noted as a "negative Rinne" or as BC > AC).

These tests are easy to perform in the outpatient clinic or at the bedside. They provide a quick assessment of hearing and can be used to check audiometric findings.[31,32]

4.2.4 Nose and Nasopharynx Exams

Anterior rhinoscopy demonstrates the health of the nasal mucosa, the status of the turbinates, and the anatomy of the septum. Boggy, purplish, congested turbinates with thin, clear nasal mucus are often an indicator of allergic or irritant rhinitis. Polyps and other masses are noted. Pathology in the nose should be more closely examined using rigid nasal endoscopes. Doing so allows evaluation of the paranasal sinus meati and permits an adequate measurement of the extent of the disease (▶ Fig. 4.6).

The nasopharynx can be examined indirectly using a heated mirror through the oral cavity; however, only a few patients permit an adequate examination with this approach. The nasopharynx is much better assessed using an endoscope. In this circumstance, the Eustachian tube orifice, posterior and lateral pharyngeal wall, and palate movement can be examined. Palatal myoclonus is best examined using nasopharyngeal endoscopy, because the mouth opening required for a peroral examination eliminates this tremor.

Fine Eustachian tube endoscopes are developed and are being evaluated. They could help shed light on and aid in the treatment of disorders such as patulous or obstructed Eustachian tube.[33]

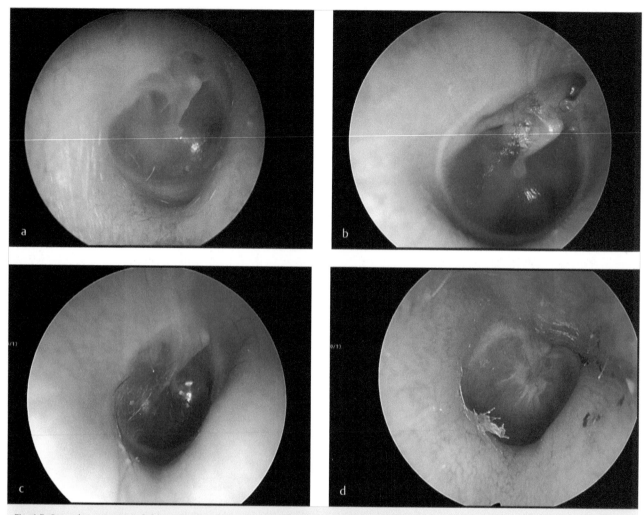

Fig. 4.5 Otoendoscopic view of the ear canal and tympanic membrane in four different patients. **(a)** Normal. **(b)** Serous otitis media following radiation treatment for oropharyngeal cancer. **(c)** Paraganglioma of middle ear (glomus tympanicum). **(d)** Giant cell tumor of temporomandibular joint involving ear canal.

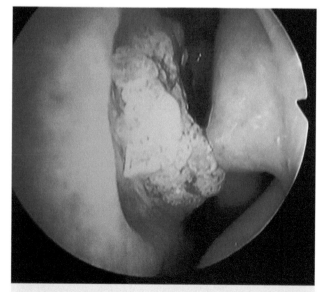

Fig. 4.6 Inverting papilloma of the left nasal septum.

4.2.5 Oral Cavity and Oropharynx Exams

Even a cursory evaluation of the oral mucosa allows examination of the state of the oral mucosa, teeth, and tongue. Pathologies in the oral cavity are a frequent cause of referred otalgia. Tongue protrusion and movement from side to side adequate denotes normal hypoglossal nerve function, whereas fasciculations and atrophy are indicators of abnormal hypoglossal function. The protruding tongue will point to the side of the lesion. The parotid and submandibular ducts are easily assessed by examining their drainage while massaging the respective gland.

The oropharynx is separated from the oral cavity by an imaginary plane through the hard–soft palate junction superiorly and the circumvallate papillae inferiorly. It contains the palatine tonsils, if still present, the lingual tonsils, the soft palate, and the mucosa of the lateral and posterior pharyngeal walls. The examiner should note the status of this mucosa. Frequently, chronic postnasal drainage will produce cobblestoning of the

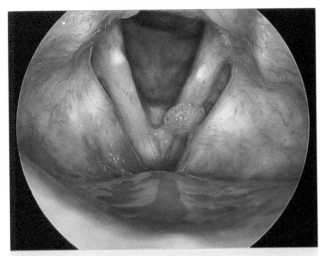

Fig. 4.7 Endoscopic laryngeal photo showing left true vocal fold papilloma. (Courtesy of Jan Lewin, MD.)

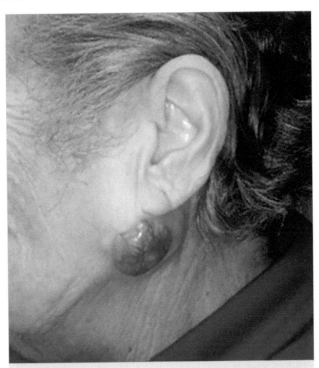

Fig. 4.8 Left parotid adenoid cystic carcinoma. This tumor is located in the tail of the parotid, and it extended up to the stylomastoid foramen. The patient's facial nerve function is normal.

posterior pharyngeal wall. The movement of the palate should be noted. Unilateral palate weakness, from a glossopharyngeal injury, will allow the uvula to be pulled toward the intact (normal) side. Gag reflex can be elicited by touching the base of the tongue or the lateral pharyngeal walls. A uvula that is bifid or that contains a thin membrana pellucida might be indicators of a submucous cleft palate. This finding warrants digital palpation of the hard palate to assess for occult cleft.

4.2.6 Exams of the Larynx

Laryngeal assessment begins with the interview, noting the patient's voice quality. Wet, weak, or breathy voices are signs of vocal fold weakness. Speech fluency, by contrast, is directed by higher cortical structures. Expressive aphasia from a lesion in Broca's area is an example of an abnormal fluency. Dysarthria, or difficult, poorly articulated speech, might result from abnormal hypoglossal or facial nerve function.

A basic examination of laryngeal function includes mirror examination, but only an exceptional patient permits an unhurried examination using this technique. Flexible fiberoptic endoscopy under topical nasal anesthetic is the preferred initial method for assessing vocal fold function. Patients who have or will have vocal fold paralysis should be evaluated by a speech pathologist. Videostroboscopy provides an excellent assessment of vocal fold anatomy and function and can discern various degrees of weakness better than flexible endoscopy can. Additionally, videographic and photographic documentation of vocal fold function and appearance is much better with videostroboscopy than through a flexible fiberoptic scope (▶ Fig. 4.7).

Laryngeal function is controlled by the vagus nerve, a mixed nerve that carries motor, sensory and parasympathetic impulses. Its first branch in the neck is the superior laryngeal nerve, which has two branches: an internal laryngeal branch that carries sensation from the mucosa above the true vocal folds and an external branch that is motor to the cricopharyngeal muscles. This muscle tilts the thyroid cartilage on the cricoid cartilage and produces the tightening of the vocal fold needed to make high-pitch phonation.

The remainder of the laryngeal muscles and the sensation of the vocal folds and mucosa of the tracheobronchial tree are innervated by the vagus and its inferior or recurrent laryngeal nerve. This nerve branch loops under the arch of the aorta on the left side of the neck and the subclavian on the right side. Nonrecurrent nerves (nerves that do not descend into the mediastinum before going to the larynx) have been well described. This situation occurs more commonly on the right side and is constantly on the minds of thyroid surgeons.

The recurrent laryngeal nerve innervates both the adductors and abductors of the vocal folds. Accordingly, recovery from laryngeal neurotmesis might be limited due to synkinesis of laryngeal innervation.

Injury or loss of vagal (and, for that matter, glossopharyngeal) function at the skull base can produce severe dysphagia and aspiration, because both the motor and sensory functions are lost, removing the protective mechanisms of the upper aerodigestive tract.

4.2.7 Neck, Parotid, and Thyroid Exams

The neck and, by extension, the parotid glands should be examined by palpation for any masses or lymphadenopathy. Cervical adenopathy should be reported based on its location and size. For malignant disease, location and size of lymphadenopathy is important for tumor staging. The parotid glands should be palpated for any masses, especially in patients who have facial paralysis (▶ Fig. 4.8; ▶ Fig. 4.9). Loss of a single branch of the facial nerve is due to malignant involvement until proven otherwise. Complete facial paralysis can occur from parotid tumors at the stylomastoid foramen. Deep lobe

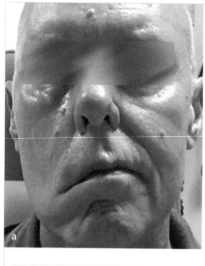
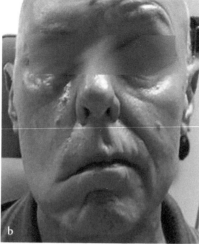
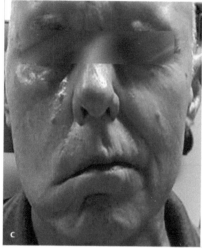
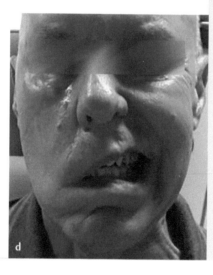

Fig. 4.9 Recurrent right parotid mucoepidermoid carcinoma causing complete facial paralysis. **(a)** Face at rest. **(b)** Eyebrows raised. **(c)** Eyes closed tightly. **(d)** Forceful smile.

tumors can also cause facial paralysis and can escape palpation; only through imaging studies can these tumors be found.

The thyroid gland sits on top of the trachea, just below the level of the cricoid cartilage and above the sternal notch. Palpating this part of the neck while asking the patient to swallow moves the gland under the examiner's fingers. A normal gland is usually not able to be palpated. A solitary tumor should be further investigated with ultrasound and fine needle aspiration. Diffuse swelling of the gland might indicate goiter. Vocal fold paralysis associated with a thyroid nodule should be attributed to malignant disease until proven otherwise.

Finally, the spinal accessory nerve (CN XI) function is tested. This nerve innervates the sternocleidomastoid (SCM) and trapezius muscles. To test the SCM muscle, the patient is asked to turn his or her head slightly to the right while the examiner applies an opposite force against the right jaw and face and palpates the strength in the left SCM. The head is turned slightly to the left to test the strength of the right SCM muscle. The patient should be asked to shrug his or her shoulders while the examiner applies resistance to measure trapezius strength.

4.2.8 Exams of the Cranial Nerves

Meyerhoff's dictum is "any symptom suggestive of cranial neuropathy must alert the clinician to the possibility of a skull base or intracranial space occupying lesion."[34] For the most part, the CN examination is performed while progressing through the head and neck physical examination. Eye, palate, tongue, vocal fold, and shoulder/head movement have been already discussed in the sections related to each organ system.

This space does not permit discussion of the complex anatomy of the CNs or their brainstem and skull base relations, but some of these details have been summarized in ▶ Table 4.3.[35,36,37] Here, the nerves that are not readily examined in a routine examination are described as part of a neuro-otologic examination.

Olfactory Nerve Exams

Although taste and smell provide excellent sensory stimulation, they are perhaps the least tested sensory functions.[38] The sense of smell occurs when odorants come into contact with olfactory receptors in olfactory receptor neurons (ORN).[39] The ORN are bipolar cells that penetrate the cribriform plate to synapse with glomeruli cells in the olfactory bulb. These glomeruli cells then

Table 4.3 Cranial nerves and their nuclei, brainstem location, and function

Cranial nerve	Brainstem nucleus	Brainstem location	Function	Deficit
I – Olfactory	None (olfactory glomerulus in olfactory bulb)	None (Olfactory tract to anterior perforated substance and pyriform lobe)	Olfaction	Anosmia
II – Optic	None (ganglion cell layer in retina, optic tracts project to lateral geniculate body)	None (diencephalon)	Vision	Blindness
III – Oculomotor	Oculomotor nucleus (lateral somatic cell column)	Midbrain (level of superior colliculus)	Extraocular muscle movement	Diplopia, outward and downward deviation of eye
III – Oculomotor (SVE)	Oculomotor nucleus (caudal central group)	Midbrain (level of superior colliculus)	Levator palpebrae	Ptosis
III – Oculomotor, parasympathetics (GVE)	Edinger-Westphal nucleus	Midbrain (level of superior colliculus)	Dilator of the pupil via NCG of V1	"Blown pupil"
III – Oculomotor, sympathetics	Superior cervical ganglion of sympathetic chain		Constrictor of pupil Mueller's muscle in upper eyelid	Horner's syndrome
IV – Trochlear, motor (GSE)	Trochlear nucleus	Midbrain (level of inferior colliculus)	Superior oblique	Vertical diplopia (trouble walking down stairs)
V – Trigeminal, motor (SVE)	Motor nucleus of V	Pontine tegmentum	Muscles of mastication, accessory muscles of mastication (tensor tympani, tensor veli palatine)	Weakness of muscles of mastication
V – Trigeminal, sensory (GSA)	Principal sensory, geniculate ganglion	Pontine tegmentum	Light touch and pressure	Loss of sensation in distribution
V – Trigeminal, sensory (GSA)	Descending, spinal tract and nucleus of V, geniculate ganglion	Pons to C2–C4	Pain and temperature	Loss of sensation in distribution
V – Trigeminal, sensory (GSA)	Mesencephalic nucleus of V (no peripheral ganglion)	Midbrain	Proprioception from the TMJ	Loss of jaw jerk reflex
VI – Abducens (GSE)	Abducens nucleus	Pons	Motor to lateral rectus mus	Diplopia, eye does not abduct
VII – Facial, motor (SVE)	Facial motor nucleus	Pons	Muscles of facial function, buccinators, platysma, stapedius mm	Facial paralysis, loss of stapedial reflex (hyperacusis)
VII – Facial, sensation (GSA)	Intermediate nerve, geniculate ganglion, spinal trigeminal tract	Pons	Sensation of ear canal	Numbness of ear canal (Hitselberger's sign)
VII – Facial, sensation (SVA)	Intermediate nerve, geniculate ganglion, nucleus solitarius ("gustatory nucleus")	Pons	Sensation of taste for anterior two-thirds of the tongue	Loss of taste, anterior two-thirds of the tongue
VII – Facial, parasympathetics (GVE)	Superior salivatory nucleus, intermediate nerve	Pons	Lacrimal gland and nasal mucosa via GSPN and PtPG (V2) Submandibular gland via chorda tympani (and lingual nerve–V3)	Dry eyes, nose, mouth
VIII – Cochlear nerve	Cochlear nuclei (dorsal and ventral)	Pons	Hearing	Deafness
VIII – Vestibular nerves	Vestibular nuclei (superior, medial, lateral, inferior)	Pons	Balance	Imbalance
IX – Glossopharyngeal, sensory (GSA)	Superior ganglion, in neck, spinal trigeminal nucleus	Medulla	Sensation to postauricular skin	Numbness
IX – Glossopharyngeal, sensory (GVA)	Inferior salivatory	Medulla	Sensory to base of tongue and upper pharynx	Loss of gag reflex
IX – Glossopharyngeal, motor (SVE)	Nucleus ambiguus	Medulla	Motor to stylopharyngeus and superior constrictor mm	Dysphagia
IX – Glossopharyngeal, special sensory (SVA)	Nucleus solitarius ("gustatory nucleus")	Medulla	Taste, base of tongue, baroreceptor	Lack of pharyngeal taste, loss or carotid sinus reflex

(Continued)

Table 4.3 *(Continued)* Cranial nerves and their nuclei, brainstem location, and function

Cranial nerve	Brainstem nucleus	Brainstem location	Function	Deficit
IX – Glossopharyngeal, parasympathetic (GVE)	Inferior salivatory nucleus	Medulla	Parotid gland via otic ganglion (lesser petrosal nerve and auriculotemporal branch of V3)	Xerostomia
X – Vagus, motor (SVE)	Nucleus ambiguus	Spinomedullary junction	Vocal fold movement, pharyngeal constrictors, cricopharyngeus	Hoarseness, dysphagia, aspiration
X – Vagus, sensation (GSA)	Superior ganglion, in neck, spinal trigeminal tract	Spinomedullary junction	Postauricular skin and ear canal	Numbness
X – Vagus, sensation (GVA)	Inferior (or nodal) ganglion in neck, nucleus solitarius	Spinomedullary junction	Hypopharynx, larynx, and tracheobronchial tree	Dysphagia, aspiration
X – Vagus, special sensation (SVA)	Inferior (or nodal) ganglion in neck, nucleus solitarius	Spinomedullary junction	Taste, tip of epiglottis	Lack of laryngeal taste
X – Vagus, parasympathetics (GVE)	Dorsal motor nucleus	Spinomedullary junction	Parasympathetic to the GI tract	
XI – Spinal accessory, cranial root (SVE)	Nucleus ambiguus	Medulla and C1–C3	Motor to SCM and trapezius	Weakness of shoulder
XI – Spinal accessory, spinal root (GSE)	Rootlets from C1 to C3			
XII – Hypoglossal (GSE)	Hypoglossal nucleus	Spinomedullary junction	Motor to the tongue	Dysarthria

Abbreviations: GI, gastrointestinal; GSA, general somatic afferent; GSE, general somatic efferent; GSPN, greater superficial petrosal nerve; GVA, general visceral afferent; GVE, general visceral efferent; NCG, nasociliary ganglion; PtPG, pterygopalatine ganglion; SCM, sternocleidomastoid; SVA, special visceral afferent; SVE, somatic visceral efferent; TMJ, temporomandibular joint.
Source: Data from Nemzek WR, The trigeminal nerve, Top Magn Reson Imaging 1996;8(3):132–154; Saper C, Brain stem, reflexive behavior, and the cranial nerves, In: Kandell E, Schwartz J, Jessell T, eds., Principles of Neural Science, New York: McGraw-Hill; 2000, Carpenter M, Core Text of Neuroanatomy, 3rd ed, Baltimore: Williams and Wilkins; 1985.

synapse with mitral cells that carry the signal into the piriform cortex. From the piriform, connections with the hippocampus, amygdala, and orbitofrontal cortex combine to give the associated sensory, memory, or hedonic reactions.[39] Tests of olfaction are becoming more important as their significance in predicting Parkinson's disease and Alzheimer's disease is recognized.[39,40]

Anosmia, or the inability to smell, can be evaluated based on conductive or sensorineural causes.[41] Olfactory epithelium is located high inside the nose, on the upper middle turbinate and roof of the nose. Odorants must be able to pass through a patent nasal airway, and the patient must be able to generate sufficient nasal airflow (by sniffing) to bring odorants into contact with the olfactory epithelium. The patient who has severe obstructive nasal polyposis represents a form of conductive anosmia, because the polyps prevent airflow through the nose. Furthermore, a laryngectomee is unable to move any air through the nasal passages, because all his or her airflow is through the tracheostoma.

Sensorineural anosmia can result from either damaged olfactory mucosa, such as might occur after a viral upper respiratory tract infection, or shearing of the olfactory nerve as a result of head trauma. Tumors in the sinonasal tract and esthesioblastomas can produce anosmia through obstruction and/or destruction along the olfactory pathway. Olfactory loss from intracerebral tumors (glioma, olfactory meningioma, esthesioneuroblastoma, and adenocarcinoma) has been described.[39] For this reason, patients who have anosmia and a normal nasal endoscopic examination should undergo MRI imaging.[39]

Olfaction can be measured in several ways. A simple test of smell might include waved household products such as coffee, cinnamon, mint, or water under the nose and closed eyes and asking the patient to respond to the question of "Do you smell this item?"[13,42] Eighty percent of the normal population can identify the odor of coffee.[34] A patient who professes not to smell anything can be further tested in a similar fashion using ammonium, which triggers response from V2, being a mucosal irritant. All normal patients sense the nasal irritation of ammonia.[34] A "no" response in this circumstance might indicate that the patient is being less than honest.

A better form of testing uses the University of Pennsylvania Smell Identification Test (UPSIT).[43] This test uses 40 scratch-and-sniff odors that patients try to identify by matching to a four-option response panel. Patients are required to answer all questions and to guess at an answer even if they smell nothing. The number of correct answers is matched in a nomogram divided by gender and age range to determine the level of olfaction: normal, hyposmia, anosmia, malingering. Because patients have a one-in-four chance of getting any question correct through guessing, a patient who has missed all 40 questions has probably intentionally avoided correct answers.[40] This test is performed with both nostrils open and thus cannot give side-specific values. Nonetheless, this method of testing has been widely verified and is valued for its accuracy in providing a qualitative measurement of smell.[41]

Trigeminal Nerve

The trigeminal nerve is perhaps the most complex nerve of the head and neck. It has origins from four different brainstem nuclei, and it carries both sensory and motor function. Its three main trunks pass through three different foramina in the skull base, and each trunk has an associated parasympathetic ganglion.

The trigeminal nerve has general somatic and general visceral afferent function. The somatic afferents are for cutaneous sensation of the skin of the head and neck. The first division, V1, supplies sensation to the cornea and conjunctiva, the upper eyelid, the eyebrow, and the scalp as far posterior as the vertex. The second division, V2, supplies sensation to the skin of the nose, cheek, and upper lip; to the maxillary teeth; and to the mucosa of the nose and the roof of the mouth. The third division, V3, provides sensation to the skin of the lower lip, chin, and lower third of the face; to the mandibular teeth; and to the mucosa of the cheeks, lower lip, and floor of mouth. The general somatic afferents of CN V are also carried on V3 to the anterior two-thirds of the tongue. Light touch, pinprick, and temperature can be tested for each division of the trigeminal nerve.

The motor function of the trigeminal nerve is carried on V3 to the masticatory muscles (masseter, temporalis, medial, and lateral pterygoid) and to the accessory muscles of mastication (mylohyoid, anterior belly of the digastric, tensor tympani, and tensor veli palatini). Motor strength is difficult to assess clinically, but the tone of the masseter and temporalis can be palpated while the patient grinds his or her teeth.

Corneal Reflex

The description of the corneal reflex rightfully belongs between the discussion of trigeminal and facial nerve function, because it involves both nerves. The corneal reflex arc is composed of afferents from corneal epithelium through the V1 into the brainstem, where it synapses through one or two interneurons and connects to the facial nuclei to produce muscular contraction of the orbicularis oculi muscles. Normally, unilateral corneal irritation produces bilateral orbicularis oculi contraction.

The test is performed by asking the patient to look slightly nasally while a wisp of cotton is placed on the temporal portion of the cornea. Care is taken to prevent the patient from seeing the cotton approach the eye. In the case of a trigeminal nerve lesion, no muscular contraction will be elicited in either eye. In the case of a facial nerve lesion, the muscular contraction will be absent on the side of the lesion but will still be present on the normal side.

Facial Nerve

Being the motor supply to the face, the facial nerve controls several wide-ranging functions. Under control of the facial nerve, the buccinator muscle aids in mastication by helping keep the food bolus on the occlusal surface of the molars and not in the gingivobuccal sulcus. The perioral muscles aid in articulation of speech (for labial and plosive sounds). The orbicularis oculi protects the eye by closing the lids and by moving a lubricating coating of tears over the cornea. Last, and perhaps most important, it allows nonverbal communication of emotion through facial muscle contractions.

Like the trigeminal nerve, the facial nerve has an intricate anatomy, including the longest bony course of any CN; conveys motor, general sensory, and special sensory functions; and is the primary pathway for two parasympathetic ganglia (sphenopalatine and submandibular). Because the facial nerve has many different branches along its course, each having a testable function, a topographic method of testing was previously used to determine the site of lesion, so that testing lacrimation (Shirmer's test), taste (electrogustometry), salivation, stapedial reflexes, and facial muscle function could provide the examiner with the location of the lesion. However, this topographic testing has largely been supplanted by modern imaging techniques and thus is no longer in wide use. Acoustic reflex testing is performed and will be discussed in the section on audiometric testing.

Facial muscle function is tested by asking the patient to "raise your eyebrows"; "close your eyes tightly," even against resistance; "wrinkle your nose"; "puff out your cheeks"; "pucker your lips"; and "show your teeth" (▶ Fig. 4.6). In cases of complete paralysis, the examiner presses his or her thumbs on the midline of the patient's face to prevent the unopposed normal side from distorting the examination of the paralyzed side.

Facial function should be reported for each area of the face, because just one branch might be paralyzed. Single-branch facial paralysis strongly suggests tumor.[44] Any individual who has progressive facial weakness should be considered to have a tumor of the facial nerve until proven otherwise.[44] The American Academy of Otolaryngology has approved the House-Brackmann scale as a measure of facial function for reporting results in its publications (▶ Table 4.4).[45]

The constellation of CN abnormalities can be grouped according to recognizable patterns. These patterns, which are often eponymous, can help in deducing the underlying pathologic process. Several such syndromes are listed in ▶ Table 4.5.[41,46,47,48,49,50,51,52]

4.2.9 Gait and Balance Testing

A general neurologic examination of upper and lower body strength and sensation and of cerebellar function should be performed, looking for light touch, vibratory sensation, fine and rapid motor skills, and finger-to-nose testing.[13]

Gait

Patients are asked to walk for 15 feet and then return, allowing assessment of gait. The observer should note the posture, head position, arm motion, and gait. Foot drop or poor posture might be indicators of imbalance. One should note how the patient turns around: does he or she use a quick method without needing to stop, or does he or her make several small steps to turn around? The latter might be an indication of a vestibular pathology.

Next the patient is asked to walk heel to toe (tandem gait) for 15 feet. The examiner should accompany the patient to guard against fall. An abnormal tandem gait is loss of balance more than three times within 15 feet.

Table 4.4 The House-Brackmann facial nerve grading system

Grade	Description	Characteristics
I	Normal	Normal facial function in all areas
II	Slight dysfunction	Gross: slight weakness noticeable on close inspection; may have very slight synkinesis
		At rest: normal symmetry and tone
		Motion
		Forehead: moderate to good function
		Eye: complete closure with minimum effort
		Mouth: slight asymmetry
III	Moderate dysfunction	Gross: obvious but not disfiguring difference between two sides; noticeable but not severe synkinesis, contracture, and/or hemifacial spasm
		At rest: normal symmetry and tone
		Motion
		Forehead: slight to moderate function
		Eye: complete closure with effort
		Mouth: slightly weak with maximum effort
IV	Moderately severe dysfunction	Gross: obvious weakness and/or disfiguring asymmetry
		At rest: normal symmetry and tone
		Motion
		Forehead: none
		Eye: incomplete closure
		Mouth: asymmetric with maximum effort
V	Severe dysfunction	Gross: only barely perceptible motion
		At rest: asymmetry
		Motion
		Forehead: none
		Eye: incomplete closure
		Mouth: slight movement
VI	Total paralysis	No movement

Source: Reproduced with permission from House JW, Brackmann DE. Facial nerve grading system. Otolaryngol Head Neck Surg, 1985;93(2):146–147.

Stance

Moritz Heinrich Romberg first published his description of tabes dorsalis in 1846.[53] Romberg test is performed with eyes closed, feet together, arms folded across the chest, and head extended.[54] A sharpened Romberg test is performed with feet tandem (heel to toe), eyes closed, arms folded across the chest, and head extended. A simplified Romberg test is performed with feet together, arms at the side, head in a neutral position, and eyes closed. The examiner looks for increased body sway and protects the patient from falling. This can be done by asking the patient to stand between two chairs with his or her back about 50 cm from the wall. Normal individuals can maintain a Romberg posture for 30 seconds with eyes closed. Romberg posture relies on normal proprioception (dorsal columns), and an abnormal Romberg often indicates disease outside of the labyrinths.[54]

Patients are then asked to stand on one leg with eyes open and then with eyes closed. Normal patients can easily stand on one leg for 15 seconds. Inability to stand on one leg indicates imbalance and highlights the need for normal muscle and joint strength and normal proprioception to maintain balance.

Fukuda Test

The Fukuda[55] (also called Unterberger[56]) stepping test is performed with eyes closed and arms outstretched while the patient marches in place. The examiner watches the patient's movement during 50 marched steps. Forward movement (> 1 meter) or turning movement (> 45°, usually toward the side of the lesion) are significant findings in the Fukuda test.[57] This is a test of vestibulospinal and proprioceptive contributions for balance control.[58] Some reports have shown good sensitivity of this test,[57] but others have discounted its usefulness.[56,59]

Clinical Test of Sensory Integration and Balance

The Clinical Test of Sensory Integration and Balance (CTSIB) series of tests uses simple objects to test static and dynamic equilibrium.[54,60] Romberg postures with eyes open and closed are used to mimic test situations 4 and 5 as found in computerized dynamic posturography (CDP).[54] Thick upholstery foam, a rigid cover, and a lampshade are used to create the "foam and dome" test modalities. These simple clinical tasks of static and dynamic equilibrium can reliably distinguish vestibular disorder patients from normal subjects.[61]

Table 4.5 Cranial nerve syndromes

Syndrome	Cranial nerves involved	Most likely cause(s)
Foster Kennedy syndrome[a]	I (ipsilateral hyposmia or anosmia) II (ipsilateral optic atrophy and central papilledema)	Tumor of olfactory grove and sphenoidal ridge
Orbital apex[b]	III, IV, VI, V1	Inflammatory (sarcoid, systemic lupus erythematosus, Wegener's, Graves's)
Cavernous sinus[b,c]	III, IV, VI, V1, V2 + sympathetics	Infectious (fungal, bacterial, viral)
Superior orbital fissure (Rochon-Duvigneaud or Foix) syndrome[b,d]	III, IV, V1, VI	Tumors (nasopharyngeal, adenoid cystic, squamous cell, lymphoma) Iatrogenic (sinonasal or orbitofacial surgery) Vascular (carotid aneurysm, carotid cavernous fistula) Mucocele Idiopathic (Tolosa-Hunt) Thrombosis Sellar tumors Trauma
Retrosphenoidal space (Jacod)[d]	II, III, IV, V, VI	Tumors of the middle fossa
Petrous apex (Gradenigo's syndrome)[d]	V, VI	Chronic otitis Cholesterol granuloma Chondrosarcoma
Miller-Fisher syndrome	VI, VII	Rhombencephalitis (herpes, Guillain-Barre)
Internal auditory canal[d]	VII, VII	Acoustic neuroma Meningioma Epidermoid tumor
Cerebellopontine angle[d,e]	V, VII, VIII, IX, X, XI	Meningioma Acoustic neuroma Epidermoid tumor
Jugular foramen (Vernet's)[d,e,f]	IX, X, XI	Neoplasm Carotid aneurysm
Schmitt's[e] or Collet-Sicard[f,g,h] syndrome	IX, X, XI, XII without Horner's syndrome	
Retropharyngeal syndrome of Villaret[g]	IX, X, XI, XII with Horner's syndrome	

[a]Wrobel BB, Leopold DA. Clinical assessment of patients with smell and taste disorders. Otolaryngol Clin North Am 2004;37(6):1127–1142.
[b]Yeh S, Foroozan R. Orbital apex syndrome. Curr Opin Ophthalmol 2004;15(6):490–498.
[c]Johnston JL. Parasellar syndromes. Curr Neurol Neurosci Rep 2002;2(5):423–431.
[d]Zaffaroni M, Baldini SM, Ghezzi A. Cranial nerve, brainstem and cerebellar syndromes in the differential diagnosis of multiple sclerosis. Neurol Sci 2001;22(Suppl 2):S74–S78.
[e]Krasnianski M, Neudecker S, Zierz S. [The Schmidt and Vernet classical syndrome. Alternating brain stem syndromes that do not exist?]. Nervenarzt 2003;74(12):1150–1154.
[f]Schweinfurth JM, Johnson JT, Weissman J. Jugular foramen syndrome as a complication of metastatic melanoma. Am J Otolaryngol 1993;14(3):168–174.
[g]Paparounas K, Gotsi A, Apostolou F, Akritidis N. Collet-Sicard syndrome disclosing glomus tumor of the skull base. Eur Neurol 2003;49(2):103–105.
[h]Chacon G, Alexandraki I, Palacio C. Collet-Sicard syndrome: an uncommon manifestation of metastatic prostate cancer. South Med J 2006;99(8):898–899.

4.3 Audiometric, Vestibular, and Electromyographic Tests

These tests provide valuable insight into the disease process and help in measuring function. The following text is not meant to describe how to perform each test; where indicated, a rudimentary description is given to familiarize the reader with how the test is performed as well as, more important, how to interpret its results and place them into the framework of the entire clinical picture.

Electrodiagnostic testing is a wide field of medical practice. Audiologists, neurologists, neuromuscular specialists, and physiatrists perform one or more of these tests as part of their regular practice and are the recognized experts in performing these

tests. Liberal use of these consultants is necessary for evaluation of patients who have skull base tumors. The allotted space does not permit this chapter to be an exhaustive resource; accordingly, certain tests are eliminated even if they might provide insight into disease processes (e.g., electrogustometry).

The bulk of medical literature relating to audiometric testing and skull base tumors concerns the diagnosis of acoustic neuroma (AN). ANs account for 5 to 10% of intracranial tumors and 80 to 90% of posterior fossa tumors.[62] Since Cushing recognized hearing loss as the presenting symptom of ANs,[63] scientists and physicians have tried to develop better audiometric tests to identify their presence. The history of neuro-otologic diagnosis for ANs has included reflex decay, alternate binaural loudness, and Bekesy audiometry,[64,65] but these modalities have been replaced by auditory brainstem response (ABR) and MRI. The following topics will primarily relate the findings of audiometry and vestibular testing to ANs. The findings of other tumors, such as meningiomas and epidermoids, will be presented where significant differences are found.

4.3.1 Basic Audiometry

The audiogram is the most fundamental element of otologic and neuro-otologic evaluation after the history and physical examination. A basic audiogram consists of pure tone audiometry, speech audiometry, immittance testing (e.g., tympanogram), and acoustic reflex testing. Only a brief description of each test is permitted in this chapter; the interested reader is directed to other reference works for an in-depth discussion of their finer points.[66,67,68,69]

Pure tone audiometry is the measurement of the lowest threshold at which a tone is heard. A calibrated audiometer delivers sound at a specific frequency (pitch) and specific intensity (loudness). The test is performed by an audiologist in a soundproof booth using either circumaural headphones or ear inserts for air conduction levels and a bone vibrator for bone conduction levels. Masking sound is given to the nontest ear via an ear canal insert and is the physiologic equivalent of covering one eye during a vision test.

The results of pure tone tests are placed on the audiogram, using conventional symbols to designate the ear, the modality (air or bone conduction), and the use of masking. The intensity levels of air conduction at 500, 1,000, and 2,000 Hz (and occasionally 3,000 or 4,000 Hz) are averaged producing a pure tone average (PTA). Hearing loss can be grouped into three different categories: conductive, sensorineural, and mixed.

Conductive hearing loss indicates that the sound-conducting mechanism of the ear is impaired. This condition can occur as a result of any process that blocks the ear canal or impairs the vibration of the TM or ossicles. TM perforations, cholesteatoma, cerumen impaction, otitis media, ear canal cancers (▶ Fig. 4.10), and otosclerosis are common causes of conductive hearing loss (▶ Fig. 4.11).

Sensorineural hearing loss indicates that the defect in hearing lies within either the cochlea or the auditory nervous pathway. Sensorineural hearing loss commonly occurs in cases of presbycusis, noise-induced hearing loss, ototoxicity (▶ Fig. 4.12), and ANs (▶ Fig. 4.13).

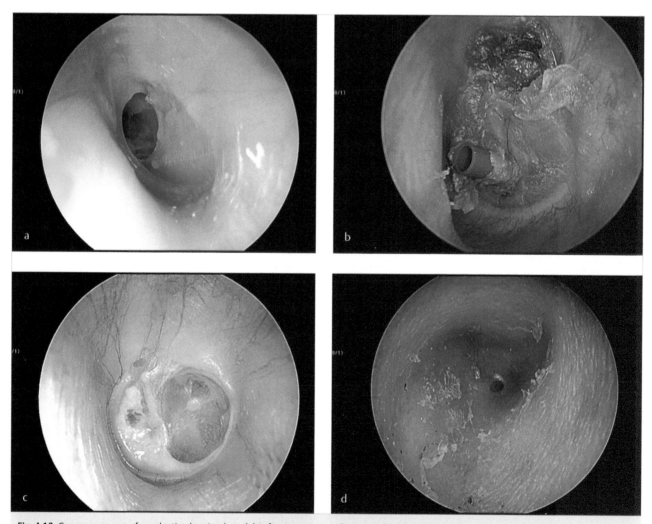

Fig. 4.10 Common causes of conductive hearing loss. **(a)** Left tympanic membrane perforation. **(b)** Pars flaccida cholesteatoma. **(c)** Myringostapediopexy and loss of incus. **(d)** Canal stenosis following radiotherapy for nasopharyngeal cancer.

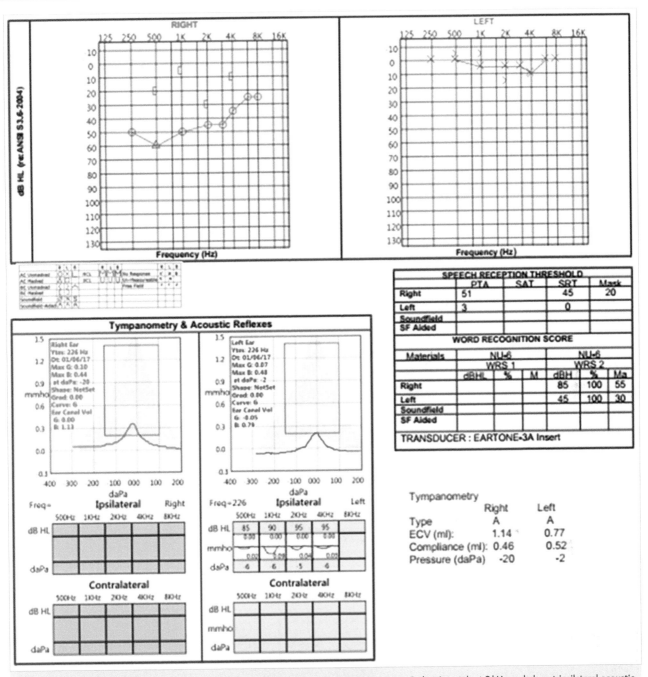

Fig. 4.11 Audiogram demonstrating right conductive hearing loss due to otosclerosis. Notice Carhart's notch at 2 kHz and absent ipsilateral acoustic reflexes in the right ear.

Mixed hearing loss means that both conductive and sensorineural hearing loss (SNHL) types are present in an ear.

A threshold for perceiving words can be achieved by using spondaic words. The lowest level, at which 50% of words are perceived, is called the speech reception threshold (SRT). The PTA and SRT should agree within 5 to 10 dB of each other.

Speech audiometry measures word understanding. Phonetically balanced (PB) words are presented via air conduction at a presentation level 40 dB over the SRT or PTA (also called 40 dB

sensation level or 40 dB normal hearing level [nHL]). The percentage of words understood is recorded as the speech discrimination score (SDS). Generally speaking, word understanding improves as intensity is increased for cochlear or sensory hearing loss. However, retrocochlear hearing loss might demonstrate a worsening of word understanding with increased intensity in what is called PB rollover. A compilation of differences between sensory or cochlear hearing loss and retrocochlear or neural hearing loss is presented in ▶ Table 4.6.[70,71,72,73,74]

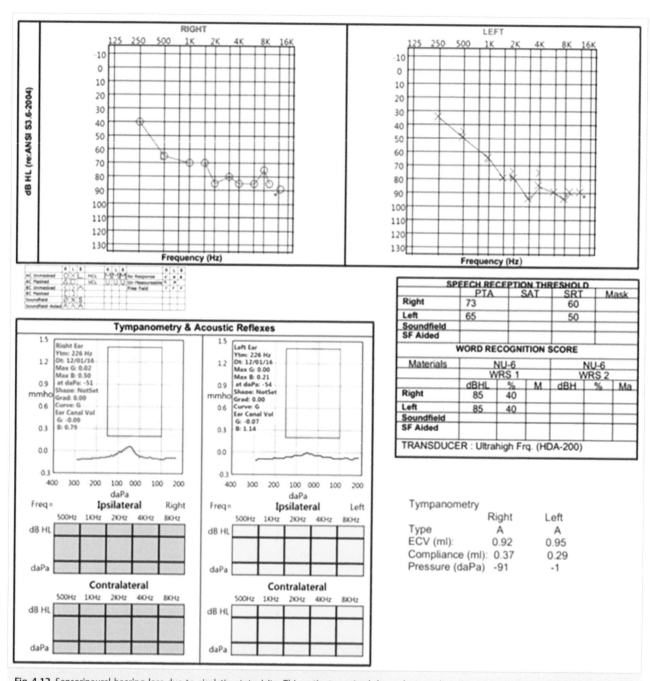

Fig. 4.12 Sensorineural hearing loss due to cisplatin ototoxicity. This patient received doxorubicin and cisplatin (total dose 480 mg/M²) as part of treatment for high-grade pleomorphic spindle cell sarcoma.

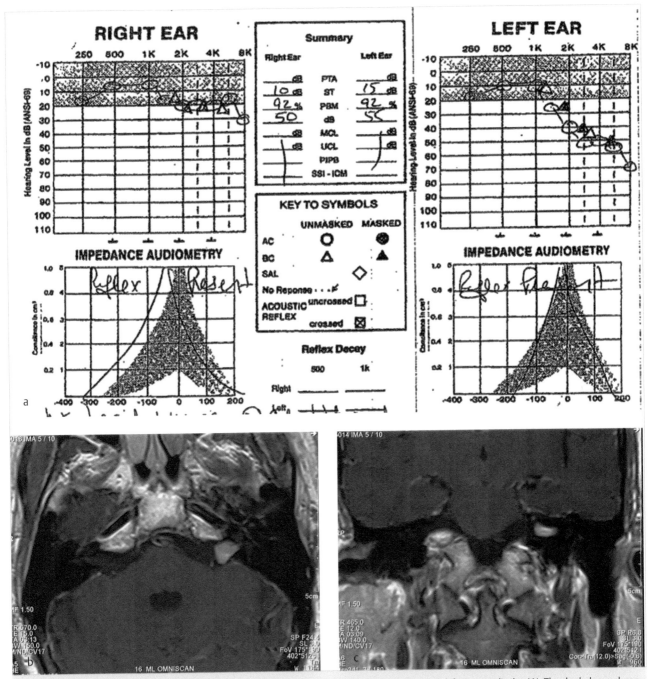

Fig. 4.13 Left sensorineural hearing loss due to acoustic neuroma (AN). Audiogram from patient with left intracanalicular AN. The shaded area shows the normal hearing range. There is left sensorineural hearing loss above 1 KHz. The right ear hearing is essentially normal. The word recognition score phonetically balanced maximum is 92% for each ear. The tympanograms are normal Type A bilaterally. The auditory reflexes are present bilaterally. **(a)** Audiogram. Contrast-enhanced **(b)** axial and **(c)** coronal.

Table 4.6 A compilation of differences between sensory (cochlear) versus neural (retrocochlear) hearing loss

	Site of pathology	Pure tone audiometry[a]	Speech discrimination[a]	Secondary findings[b,c]	Speech discrimination[a]	ABR[d]	OAE[e]
Sensory or cochlear	Hair cell	Decreased	Preserved, until widespread cochlear damage	Recruitment	Preserved, until widespread cochlear damage	Intact	Absent
Neural or retrocochlear	Auditory nerve	Relatively unaffected	Decreased	Auditory fatigue or tone decay	Decreased	Abnormal or absent	Intact

Abbreviations: ABR, auditory brainstem response; OAE, otoacoustic emissions.
[a]Walsh TE, Goodman A. Speech discrimination in central auditory lesions. Laryngoscope 1955;65(1):1–8.
[b]Dix MR, Hallpike CS. The otoneurological diagnosis of tumours of the VIII nerve. Proc R Soc Med 1958;51(11):889–896.
[c]Hirsch A, Anderson H. Audiologic test results in 96 patients with tumours affecting the eighth nerve. A clinical study with emphasis on the early audiological diagnosis. Acta Otolaryngol Suppl 1980;369:1–26.
[d]Clemis JD, Mc Gee T. Brain stem electric response audiometry in the differential diagnosis of acoustic tumors. Laryngoscope 1979;89(1):31–42.
[e]Telischi F. An objective method of analyzing cochlear versus noncochlear patterns of distortion-product otoacoustic emissions in patients with acoustic neuromas. Laryngoscope 2000;110(4):553–562.

Prior to ABR and MRI, site of lesion testing was of paramount importance in discerning patients who might have an AN. However, because up to 20% of AN patients might demonstrate a cochlear rather than a retrocochlear pattern of hearing loss, retrocochlear audiometric testing is of little benefit.[75]

The American Academy of Otolaryngology Committee on Hearing and Equilibrium[76] composed a classification system for reporting hearing results in AN surgery. This classification system uses PTA and SDS to stratify patients into four different classes of hearing level (▶ Table 4.7).

Alternatively, some authors report hearing results as "unchanged," "serviceable," "measurable," or "not measurable." In this context, *serviceable* means PTA ≤ 50 dB and SDS ≥ 50%, *unchanged* means hearing within 15 dB PTA and 15% SDS of preoperative levels, and *measurable* means any other hearing; *not measurable* is self-explanatory.[77]

Immittance testing uses an impedance bridge to measure changes in TM compliance. Compliance of the TM is affected by perforations, middle ear fluid or tumor, and the reflex contraction of middle ear muscles. Several important findings can be made using this type of testing. Immittance testing gives clues to the status of the TM (intact, perforated, or floppy) and the status of the middle ear (aerated or fluid-filled). These findings are denoted on a tympanogram, but this has little significance for the discussion of skull base tumors unless the tumor or spinal fluid invades the middle ear and produces a flat tympanogram.

Acoustic reflex testing, by contrast, has more significance for neuro-otologic diagnosis of skull base tumors. Using the impedance bridge, compliance of the TM can be measured in response to a tone burst given either ipsi- or contralaterally. In response to loud sound (85–110 dB), a reflex contraction of the stapedial muscle will occur bilaterally. A normal reflex requires an intact TM, an air-filled middle ear, normal movement of the ossicles, no worse than 35 dB hearing loss, and an intact facial nerve (stapedial muscle). A defect anywhere along this pathway can produce an absent or reduced acoustic reflex. The sensitivity of acoustic reflex testing for ANs has been quoted as anywhere between 21 and 90%.[75,78,79,80,81,82,83,84]

Acoustic reflex decay is defined as a 50% loss of middle ear contractility in response to a tone administered 10 dB above threshold. The sensitivity of reflex decay has been reported to be from 36 to 100% for ANs.[75,78,79,81,82,83,84,85]

Table 4.7 AAO-HNS hearing classification

Class	PTA	SDS
A	≤ 30 dB	≥ 70%
B	> 30 dB, ≤ 50 dB	≥ 50%
C	> 50 dB	≥ 50%
D	Any level	≤ 50%

Abbreviations: PTA, pure tone average; SDS, speech discrimination score.
Source: Reproduced with permission from Committee on Hearing and Equilibrium guidelines for the evaluation of hearing preservation in acoustic neuroma (vestibular schwannoma), American Academy of Otolaryngology–Head and Neck Surgery Foundation, Inc, Otolaryngol Head Neck Surg, 1995;113(3):179–180.

Acoustic Neuroma

Hearing loss is found in up to 95% of patients who have an AN.[75] By the same token, normal hearing is reported in 3 to 12% of AN patients.[75,81,86,87,88] The current level of clinical detection of ANs is approximately 1 in 100,000 persons per year,[89] although vastly higher numbers of tumors must be present and escaping detection considering the 1% observed rate of acoustic tumors found at autopsy.[90] Indeed, a significant number of ANs are found serendipitously on MRI performed for unrelated complaints.[91] In general, degree of hearing loss is significantly linked to tumor size, so that up to 33% of intracanalicular tumors are associated with normal hearing.[83] However, there are many reports of individual large tumors (> 2 cm) associated with normal hearing and small tumors (< 1 cm) associated with anacusis.[92]

Schuknecht calculated that 75% of nerve fibers need to be destroyed before pure tone hearing is affected, given an intact organ of Corti.[93] The distribution of high-frequency nerve fibers on the periphery and low-frequency fibers centrally in the acoustic nerve accounts for the high-frequency hearing loss found in early acoustic tumor development: Hearing deteriorates by as much as 2.4 dB per year while ANs are observed.[94] Speech discrimination also significantly deteriorates over time in observed ANs.[94] In the series of tumors described by Selesnick and Jackler,[88] high-frequency asymmetry at 4 KHz was a more sensitive indicator of an AN than difference in either SRT or SDS.

Although the classic presentation of an AN is a unilateral progressive SNHL with poor speech discrimination,[95] experts do not agree on what exactly constitutes a significant asymmetry.[75,96,97] As a rule of thumb, a significant asymmetry in hearing is described as an interaural SRT difference greater than 15 dB, an interaural SDS difference greater than 12 to 20%, or an interaural 4 kHz difference greater than 15 dB.[75]

Obholzer et al,[98] seeking to define appropriate audiometric criteria for referral for MRI, reviewed 392 MRIs performed in one year; the 36 ANs found and 92 randomly selected "normals" were included for the analysis. Audiometric data and clinical histories were evaluated to look for findings that might be indicative of AN. The researchers used the published protocols of seven different studies to analyze audiometric data. Their study supports the use of interaural asymmetry at two neighboring frequencies of > 15 dB if the mean threshold in the better ear was ≤ 30 dB (unilateral hearing loss) and an interaural difference of 20 dB if the mean threshold is greater than 30 dB in the better ear (bilateral asymmetric hearing loss). These criteria had a 97% sensitivity and 49% specificity for AN. The most sensitive individual frequency asymmetry was for 15 dB at 2 KHz, with a sensitivity of 91% and a specificity of 60%. The most sensitive criterion was a difference of 15 dB at any frequency (sensitivity 100% and specificity 29%).

Several authors have examined hearing levels as a predictor of hearing preservation in AN surgery. In a multivariate logistic analysis of preoperative hearing variables predictive of hearing preservation, Robinette et al[99] examined the audiometric tests results of 104 AN patients. Only word recognition score (WR40) was found to be a significant determinant after accounting for small tumor size (≤ 2.0 cm). Additionally, they found that patients who had hearing preserved had a higher rate of normal acoustic reflexes than those patients who did not have hearing preserved.[99]

Other Tumors

In 1997, Baguley et al[100] published a series of cerebellopontine angle (CPA) meningiomas and performed a review of the literature. In their series, 80% (20 of 25 patients) had abnormal pure tone testing, and 50% (10 of 20) had abnormal SDS (i.e. < 90%). Interestingly, the five patients who had normal audiometry had large tumors (two in the 2.5–3.4 cm range and three > 4.5 cm); similarly, 9 of 10 patients who had normal SDS were found to have large tumors (2.5 cm or larger). In combined with the other series reviewed, 37 of 61 (61%) patients had abnormal PTA and 22 of 42 (52%) had abnormal SDS.[100]

Doyle and De La Cruz[101] reported audiometric results in 13 patients who had CPA epidermoid tumors. Four patients had PTA greater than 30 dB; SDS was reduced out of proportion to pure tone hearing.

Quaranta et al[102] described the audiometric features in a report of 11 CPA epidermoid tumors. Their series consisted of tumors that measured 3.5 to 7 cm in maximum diameter. They found symmetric hearing in six patients; another four had asymmetric hearing loss that was worse on the tumor side.

In a report on 10 epidermoid tumors, Kaylie et al[103] found normal hearing in three, but the remainder had varying levels of hearing loss, from mild to anacusis.

4.3.2 Auditory Brainstem Responses

In the history of methods for diagnosing ANs, ABR represented a giant advance and promised a much less invasive test. Prior to its development, audiologists had developed many different tests with which to stress the auditory nerve so as to determine its function. As the preceding paragraphs indicate, many of these tests lacked the specificity or sensitivity necessary to identify tumors. However, after a patient was identified as possibly having an AN, he or she would have been subjected to either an air-contrast or a Pantopaque posterior fossa myelogram or to polytomograms of the internal auditory canal (IAC). These tests were not only invasive but were also extremely painful and potentially morbid. They were not recommended lightly.

In 1971, when ABR was introduced, its significance for AN screening had not yet been realized[104]; however, before the close of the decade, ABR's sensitivity in identifying ANs was well established.[105] Unfortunately for ABR, its heyday was relatively short-lived. MRI with gadolinium contrast enhancement was introduced in 1988,[96] since which time MRI has been nearly 100% sensitive for ANs as small as 4 mm.[106,107]

ABR is performed with a ground electrode on the vertex and another electrode on the earlobe or mastoid of the stimulated ear. Clicks or tone burst are given at 20/second or faster rates. Click stimulus estimates hearing in the range of 1000 to 4000 Hz. Intensity can be varied but is generally given at 70 dB; with lower intensities the amplitude response decreases and latency increases. Bandpass filters are set from 30 or 100 to 3000 Hz and are used to encompass the spectrum of response while reducing undesirable activity. ABR is influenced by age, gender, and body temperature but is not greatly affected by state of arousal or sedative medications.[108]

By convention, ABR waveforms are numbered I through V, with each numeral indicating a positive waveform. These waveforms have been correlated with structures within the auditory pathway: I for the distal eighth nerve, II for the proximal eighth nerve, III for the cochlear nucleus, IV for the olivary complex, and V for the lateral lemniscus (▸ Fig. 4.14).

Acoustic Neuroma

Auditory brainstem response's place in the diagnosis of acoustic tumors still provokes debate among neuro-otologists. Although some use ABR to screen all patients who have asymmetric hearing loss, others reserve ABR for patients who have only a low probability of tumor (▸ Table 4.8),[62,75,96] preferring to use MRI for patients who have a higher probability of tumor.[96] Certainly MRI could be used for all suspicious cases if availability and cost were not considerations, but that is not the case in today's health care environment.

These arguments are largely based on ABR's sensitivity for diagnosing AN. In large retrospective series of tumor patients, normal ABR can be seen in 2 to 18% of patients.[105,109,110] In their series of 309 CPA tumors, Marangos et al[110] found normal ABR in 50 of 261 sporadic ANs, 3 of 29 ANs due to NF-2, and 4 of 17 meningiomas. Their study further demonstrates, quite elegantly, the impact of MRI and the steady decrease in average tumor size by year of initial diagnosis. Among their study population, in 1986 the average tumor size was 36 mm (± 10 mm), whereas in 1999 the average decreased to 16 mm (± 5 mm).

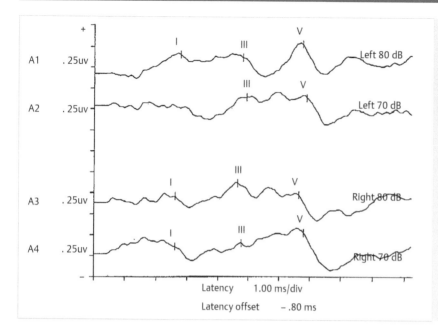

Fig. 4.14 Normal auditory brainstem response. Auditory brainstem response of patient depicted in ► Fig. 4.13. Click stimulus was performed at 70 and 80 dB for each ear. Note that latency increases with lower intensities. In this patient, the absolute latency of wave V is 5.96 for the left ear and 5.84 for the right ear (within normal limits). The interpeak latencies I to V are 4.00 for the left and 4.04 for the right (within normal limits).

Table 4.8 Probability of an acoustic neuroma based on symptoms and signs

Probability	Factors
Low (<5% chance)	Isolated vertigo Symmetrical hearing loss Historically explainable unilateral hypoacusis or tinnitus
Moderate (5–30% chance)	Sudden SNHL Unexplained tinnitus
High (>30% chance)	Combination of "classic symptoms and findings": • Unilateral SNHL • Tinnitus • Decreased speech discrimination

Abbreviations: SNHL, sensorineural hearing loss.
Source: Data from Gordon ML, Cohen NL, Efficacy of auditory brainstem response as a screening test for small acoustic neuromas, Am J Otol 1995;16(2):136–139; Selesnick SH, Jackler RK, Clinical manifestations and audiologic diagnosis of acoustic neuromas, Otolaryngol Clin North Am 1992;25(3):521–551; Welling DB, Glasscock ME III, Woods CI, Jackson CG, Acoustic neuroma: a cost-effective approach, Otolaryngol Head Neck Surg 1990;103(3):364–370.

Use of ABR as a screening tool has been examined in prospective studies. Ruckenstein et al[97] performed a prospective study of patients who had asymmetric hearing loss examined with both ABR and MRI to determine ABR's sensitivity, specificity, positive predictive value, and negative predictive value. Their small study included only 47 patients who met the inclusion criteria: 8 had significant pathology on MRI, 5 of which were ANs, but ABR was normal in 3 of these patients, and all 3 had tumors smaller than 1.5 cm; 14 patients had an abnormality in ABR testing that was not demonstrable by MRI. In this preliminary study, ABR's sensitivity for diagnosing significant retrocochlear pathology was 63%, its specificity was 64%, its positive predictive value was 26% for AN, and its negative predictive value was 89%.[97] Similar results were published by

Ferguson et al,[106] although their protocol used contrast-enhanced CT as a prerequisite for MRI imaging.

Cueva[111] published a follow-up study to that of Ruckenstein et al[97] and examined 312 adult patients who had asymmetric hearing loss using ABR and MRI prospectively. He found 31 patients who had retrocochlear pathology by MRI: 24 ANs and a collection of other pathologies (including 2 glomus jugulares and 1 petrous apex cholesterol granuloma). ABR was abnormal in 22 of these 31 patients, with 9 patients having normal ABR, 7 of whom had an AN; all 7 tumors were 16 mm or smaller. It should be noted that tumors as small as 5 mm were the cause of an abnormal ABR by these criteria. By Cueva's calculations, ABR's sensitivity was 71% and its specificity was 74%. He recommended use of MRI for patients who have asymmetric hearing loss, noting that if ABR is relied on as a screening test, 29 patients of every 1,000 screened will be missed.[111]

Overall sensitivity rates of ANs by ABR range from 88 to 95%.[62,97,109,112,113,114,115,116] There are several reasons for such a wide range of positive findings: (1) testing parameters, (2) tumor size, (3) tumor location (intracanalicular versus extracanalicular), and (4) involved nerve (superior versus inferior vestibular nerve).

Waveform latencies and waveform morphologies have been studied by various authors. The most common indicators of pathology have been (1) an interaural wave I to V latency difference (IT5 or ILD I–V) > 0.2 msec, (2) a wave I–V interpeak latency (I–V IPL) > 4.4 msec, and/or (3) poor waveform morphology, with either absent wave or no response. Absolute latencies are not as useful as interpeak latencies for diagnosis of ANs, because absolute latency is affected by many factors, such as click intensity, hearing loss, and age.[117] Some authors have not used interpeak latencies, because wave I or II is difficult to identify even in normal listeners.[112] Additionally, waveform amplitude is not used as a criterion, being highly variable.[112] A compilation of criteria used by several authors is presented in ► Table 4.9.

Table 4.9 Definitions of abnormal auditory brainstem response

Authors	Interaural wave V latency difference, msec (ILD-V) (a.k.a. IT5)	Absolute wave V latency, msec	Interaural latency difference of I–V, msec (ILD I–V)	I–V interpeak latency, msec (I–V IPL)	Waveform morphology
House JW, Brackmann DE. Brainstem audiometry in neurotologic diagnosis. Arch Otolaryngol 1979;105(6):305–309	>0.2	>6			Absence of wave V
Bauch CD, Rose DE, Harner SG. Auditory brain stem response results from 255 patients with suspected retrocochlear involvement. Ear Hear 1982;3(2):83–86	>0.2	>6.1			No response or poor overall waveform at high intensities
Josey AF, Glasscock ME III, Musiek FE. Correlation of ABR and medical imaging in patients with cerebellopontine angle tumors. Am J Otol 1988;9(Suppl):12–16	>0.4			>4.4	Absence of V despite good hearing
Weiss MH, Kisiel DL, Bhatia P. Predictive value of brainstem evoked response in the diagnosis of acoustic neuroma. Otolaryngol Head Neck Surg 1990;103(4):583–585	≥0.4	>6.03		≥4.45	
Wilson DF, Hodgson RS, Gustafson MF, Hogue S, Mills L. The sensitivity of auditory brainstem response testing in small acoustic neuromas. Laryngoscope 1992;102(9):961–964	≥0.4		≥0.4	≥4.4	Poor morphology in spite of adequate hearing
Dornhoffer JL, Helms J, Hoehmann DH. Presentation and diagnosis of small acoustic tumors. Otolaryngol Head Neck Surg 1994;111(3 Pt 1):232–235	≥0.4	>5.9			
Chandrasekhar SS, Brackmann DE, Devgan KK. Utility of auditory brainstem response audiometry in diagnosis of acoustic neuromas. Am J Otol 1995;16(1):63–67	>0.2				Abnormal ipsilateral or contralateral waveforms
Gordon ML, Cohen NL. Efficacy of auditory brainstem response as a screening test for small acoustic neuromas. Am J Otol 1995;16(2):136–139		"Abnormally prolonged"	>0.2		Abnormal or absent waveform morphology
Berrettini S, Ravecca F, Sellari-Franceschini S, Bruschini P, Casani A, Padolecchia R. Acoustic neuroma: correlations between morphology and otoneurological manifestations. J Neurol Sci 1996;144(1–2):24–33		(>2 standard deviations above normal limit for the patient's age and gender)	>0.3	>4.3	
Ferguson MA, Smith PA, Lutman ME, Mason SM, Coles RR, Gibbin KP. Efficiency of tests used to screen for cerebello-pontine angle tumours: a prospective study. Br J Audiol 1996;30(3):159–176		>6.10 (male) >5.97 (female)	>0.3	>4.58 (male) >4.34 (female)	
Ruckenstein MJ, Cueva RA, Morrison DH, Press G. A prospective study of ABR and MRI in the screening for vestibular schwannomas. Am J Otol 1996;17(2):317–320	>0.2	Abnormal absolute wave V latency			Absent or poor waveform morphology
Saleh EA, Aristegui M, Naguib MB, Cokesser Y, Landolfi M, Sanna M. Normal hearing in acoustic neuroma patients: a critical evaluation. Am J Otol 1996;17(1):127–132	>0.3	>6		≥4.4	Absent waves if adequate PTA
Zappia JJ, O'Connor CA, Wiet RJ, Dinces EA. Rethinking the use of auditory brainstem response in acoustic neuroma screening. Laryngoscope 1997;107(10):1388–1392	>0.2				Absent or abnormal waveform morphology
Godey B, Morandi X, Beust L, Brassier G, Bourdinière J. Sensitivity of auditory brainstem response in acoustic neuroma screening. Acta Otolaryngol 1998;118(4):501–504	>0.2		>0.2	>4.4	Absent or abnormal waveforms

(Continued)

Table 4.9 *(Continued)* Definitions of abnormal auditory brainstem response

Authors	Interaural wave V latency difference, msec (ILD-V) (a.k.a. IT5)	Absolute wave V latency, msec	Interaural latency difference of I–V, msec (ILD I–V)	I–V interpeak latency, msec (I–V IPL)	Waveform morphology
Noguchi Y, Komatsuzaki A, Nishida H. Cochlear microphonics for hearing preservation in vestibular schwannoma surgery. Laryngoscope 1999;109(12):1982–1987	≥0.3			≥4.4	
El-Kashlan HK, Eisenmann D, Kileny PR. Auditory brain stem response in small acoustic neuromas. Ear Hear 2000;21(3):257–262	>0.4	>7.75		>4.4	Complete absence of waves if adequate PTA or absence of waves beyond wave I
Haapaniemi JJ, Laurikainen ET, Johansson R, Rinne T, Varpula M. Audiovestibular findings and location of an acoustic neuroma. Eur Arch Otorhinolaryngol 2000;257(5):237–241	≥0.4		≥0.4	≥4.4	Abnormal or absent
Marangos N, Maier W, Merz R, Laszig R. Brainstem response in cerebellopontine angle tumors. Otol Neurotol 2001;22(1):95–99	>0.3		>0.2	>4.4	
Rupa V, Job A, George M, Rajshekhar V. Cost-effective initial screening for vestibular schwannoma: auditory brainstem response or magnetic resonance imaging? Otolaryngol Head Neck Surg 2003;128(6):823–828	≥0.3			≥4.4	Absence of one or more waves, poor waveform morphology
Cueva RA. Auditory brainstem response versus magnetic resonance imaging for the evaluation of asymmetric sensorineural hearing loss. Laryngoscope 2004;114(10):1686–1692	>0.2	Abnormal absolute wave V latency			Absent or distorted waveform morphology

Abbreviations: ILD, interaural latency difference; IPL, interpeak latency; PTA, pure tone average.

Table 4.10 Auditory brainstem response sensitivity with respect to tumor size

Study	Patients	≤10 mm	11–20 mm	>21 mm
Gordon ML, Cohen NL. Efficacy of auditory brainstem response as a screening test for small acoustic neuromas. Am J Otol 1995;16(2):136–139	105	69%	88%	100%
Chandrasekhar SS, Brackmann DE, Devgan KK. Utility of auditory brainstem response audiometry in diagnosis of acoustic neuromas. Am J Otol 1995;16(1):63–67	197	83%	97%	100%
Bauch CD, Olsen WO, Pool AF. ABR indices: sensitivity, specificity, and tumor size. Am J audiol 1996;5(1):97–104		82%		
Zappia JJ, O'Connor CA, Wiet RJ, Dinces EA. Rethinking the use of auditory brainstem response in acoustic neuroma screening. Laryngoscope 1997;107(10):1388–1392	111	89%	98%	100%

Study	Patients	<15 mm	16–25 mm	>25 mm
Marangos N, Maier W, Merz R, Laszig R. Brainstem response in cerebellopontine angle tumors. Otol Neurotol 2001;22(1):95–99	309	59.3%	82.7%	96.7%

Study	Patients	Intracanalicular	Extracanalicular
Wilson DF, Hodgson RS, Gustafson MF, Hogue S, Mills L. The sensitivity of auditory brainstem response testing in small acoustic neuromas. Laryngoscope 1992;102(9):961–964	40	66%	96%
Godey B, Morandi X, Beust L, Brassier G, Bourdinière J. Sensitivity of auditory brainstem response in acoustic neuroma screening. Acta Otolaryngol 1998;118(4):501–504	89	77%	94%

Many different studies have examined the sensitivity of ABR by tumor size (▸ Table 4.10), and a statistically significant positive correlation between tumor size and wave V latency has been reported.[92] Additionally, when ABR waveforms from the contralateral ear are abnormal (e.g., a delayed wave V or prolonged wave I–V interval), a tumor larger than 2 cm should be suspected.[118] Thus it is concluded that ABR is nearly 100% sensitive for tumors larger than 2 cm.[62,116,119] For this reason, ABR is a desirable screening test in the elderly and poor surgical risk patients, for both of whom surgery may be indicated only for a symptomatic, large tumor.[61,111]

However, to give a reasonable chance of hearing preservation, tumors should be diagnosed as early (small) as possible, where small is defined as 2 cm or smaller.[99,120] ABR sensitivity rates for tumors smaller than 1 cm range from 63 to 93%.[62,97,113,114,115,116] Healthy patients who have unilateral symptoms (hearing loss, poor discrimination, and tinnitus) should have MRI with gadolinium enhancement to find an AN.

ABR still provides excellent insight into the physiology of the acoustic nerve, which may have important implications for hearing preservation. Matthies and Samii[121] found that preoperative ABR was more important than preoperative hearing quality when estimating the chances of hearing preservation. They found that the presence of wave III correlated with better postoperative results, especially SDSs.[121]

Robinette et al[99] found similar results regarding the presence of waves I, III, and V when looking at preoperative predictors of hearing preservation. They reported that when these three waves were present, 61% of patients had hearing preservation, whereas only 27% of patients had hearing preservation with one or more waves absent.[99] Admittedly, papers can be found that dispute any relationship between ABR waveforms and hearing preservation.[120,122,123]

It should be noted that poor ABR waveforms should not be used as a criterion on the basis of which to exclude the possibility of hearing preservation. Stidham and Roberson[124] reported a series of 30 patients undergoing middle fossa craniotomy for hearing preservation. They described 7 patients with hearing improvement, classified as an increase in PTA ≥ 5 dB and/or an improvement in SDS by ≥ 12%. Interestingly, no patient who had normal preoperative ABR experienced a hearing improvement.

Of course, ABR is the most common technique used to monitor hearing intraoperatively (see Chapter 5).

Other Tumors

ABR results for posterior fossa meningiomas have similar rates of sensitivity to those seen for ANs. In the pre-MRI era, House and Brackmann[125] found that only 75% of patients who had non-AN pathology had abnormal ABRs, with 3 out of 10 meningiomas having normal ABR.[125] Laird et al[126] and Granick et al[127] each found that 6 of 6 posterior fossa meningiomas had abnormal ABR. Aiba et al[128] reported abnormal ABR in 8 of 10 cases, and Hart and Lillehie[129] reported abnormal ABR in 5 or 7 cases. Baguley contributed another 25 cases of CPA meningiomas and found abnormal ABR in 100% of tumors.[100] Marangos et al[110] found that 23.5% of meningiomas had normal ABR. Clearly MRI is required to make the diagnosis of this tumor as well.

Epidermoid tumors generally present at an advanced stage with multiple CN deficits and cerebellar signs.[102,103] In the series described by Quaranta,[102] tumors ranged from 3.5 to 7 cm in maximum diameter. The researchers found that ABR was normal in just one case. Absent or delayed waves were present in five cases ipsilateral to the tumor, and four cases had bilateral abnormalities on ABR, so that 90% of their patients had abnormalities on ABR.[102]

Stacked Auditory Brainstem Response

Don et al[130] described a new technique of ABR that they called "stacked ABR." In this test, ABR is obtained using 63 dB nHL clicks in a high-pass noise-making procedure. The wave V amplitude is constructed by temporally aligning wave V of each derived-band ABR and summing the time-shifted responses. Using this technique, the researchers found significantly lower wave V amplitudes in five AN patients who had been missed by conventional ABR technique. These five tumors were all less than 1 cm in their greatest dimension. The researchers proposed this technique as a cost-effective approach to AN screening.

In a further study of stacked ABR, Philibert et al[131] noticed that stacked ABR required a masking technique that might not be readily available. Additionally, they found that the relatively high intensity of the test might be annoying to the patient. Instead, they proposed the use of tone burst to obtain a frequency-specific ABR.

4.3.3 Otoacoustic Emissions

The phenomenon of sound being produced by the ear was first described in 1948,[132] and the definitive paper on otoacoustic emissions (OAEs) was published in 1978.[133] However, it was not until the 1990s that OAE testing became clinically widespread.[134] Otoacoustic emissions testing has enjoyed a significant increase in use as part of a neonatal hearing screening strategy, for monitoring ototoxicity or noise induced hearing loss, and in suspected cases of functional hearing loss.[134]

OAEs are generated by outer hair cells of the cochlea.[135] Although OAEs are not useful as a screening test for ANs or other skull base tumors, they are measures of "cochlear reserve" and have been examined as possible predictors of hearing preservation.[77,99,136]

OAEs are divided into two groups: spontaneous and evoked. Spontaneous emissions are present in roughly 60% of normal ears.[137] Evoked emissions are present in virtually 100% of normal ears.[134] Evoked emissions are divided into distortion product (DPOAE) and transient evoked (TEOAE) otoacoustic emissions (▶ Fig. 4.15).

In a literature review, Robinette et al[99] examined five studies describing 236 AN patients and reported that TEOAEs were present in at least one frequency in 47% of tumor ears.

Brackmann et al[77] described 333 AN patients considered for hearing preservation, 56 of whom patients had DPOAEs measured. Normal DPOAEs were found in 91%.[77]

Ferber-Viart et al[138] examined 168 AN patients who had TEOAEs; 21% had normal preoperative TEOAEs. The researchers did not find an association with tumor size, functional symptoms, PTA, ABR, or ENG response with TEOAEs. Patients who had TEOAEs were an average of 6 years younger than those without. In the subpopulation of 63 patients who underwent hearing conservation surgery, TEOAEs were present in 28% and absent in 72%. Among those who had TEOAEs present, 66% had hearing preserved, compared with only 44% of those who had absent TEOAEs; however, this difference was not statistically significant.[138]

In a more recent study, Kim et al[136] examined 93 patients with AN who were candidates for hearing preservation: 51 had hearing preserved, and 11 (22%) of these had TEOAEs present in all five frequencies tested (1–4 kHz), whereas the remaining 40 (78%) had TEOAE responses in from 0 to 4 of the frequencies

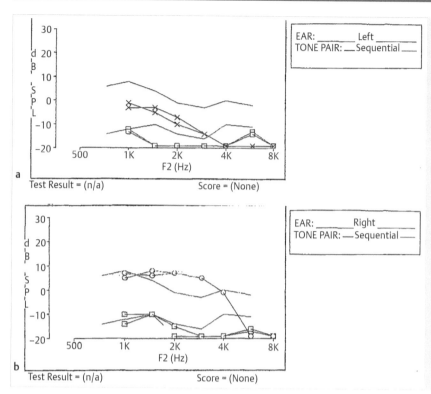

EAR: _____ Left _____
TONE PAIR: __ Sequential __

Fig. 4.15 Distortion product otoacoustic emissions (DPOAE) of intracanalicular acoustic neuroma shown in ▶ Fig. 4.13. **(a)** Left ear (marked with **X**s) emissions are diminished but present from 1 to 3 KHz and are absent for higher frequencies, consistent with the audiometric findings. **(b)** Right ear (marked by circles) DPOAE are normal from 1 to 4 KHz.

Test Result = (n/a)   Score = (None)

EAR: _____ Right _____
TONE PAIR: — Sequential —

Test Result = (n/a)   Score = (None)

tested. In the 42 patients who did not have hearing preserved, only 3 (7%) had positive TEOAE in all five frequency bands, whereas the remaining 39 (93%) had TEOAEs in from 0 to 4 frequency bands ($p < 0.05$). Other positive factors for hearing preservation in their series were small tumor size, tumor within the IAC, better hearing, and shorter latencies on ABR. The researchers concluded that a robust preoperative TEOAE pattern may be used as a favorable indicator for hearing preservation, especially when combined with the other positive factors already listed.[136]

4.3.4 Electronystagmography

Since its introduction in the 1960s, ENG (now often "videonystagmography"), has established itself as the most common test used to evaluate patients who complain of dizziness or vertigo.[139] This test uses a combination of positional testing, optokinetic testing, random saccades and visual pursuit tests, and caloric stimulation to evaluate the VOR and visual tracking centers of the brain. Findings on ENG for peripheral lesions are well described.[140] ENG is an extremely valuable tool for examining the anatomical and functional integrity of the central and peripheral vestibular systems.[141]

The sensitivity of caloric testing for acoustic tumors ranges from 44 to 95%.[83,140,142,143,144] Reduced or absent caloric response is the most frequent finding in AN patients.[140,145,146] The degree of caloric weakness is proportional to the size of the tumor,[140,145,146] although some have disputed this.[92] Different authors use various criteria to describe a significant weakness; these can range from 20%[84] to 25%[77,147] and significantly affect the sensitivity and specificity of a test. The incidence of diminished caloric response by ENG for AN patients is presented in ▶ Table 4.11.

More recently, HSN has been studied as a possible screening test for ANs. Humphriss et al[27] studied 102 AN patients seen preoperatively. They used a passive head-shaking maneuver (1–2 Hz) and recorded eye movements using an ENG system. A significant response was five or more beats of nystagmus with a slow phase of at least 3°/second. In their study, significant caloric paresis was ≥ 25%. All patients had tumors confirmed by MRI and surgery. The researchers found HSN in only 22 patients (i.e., for a sensitivity of 22%). Of these, HSN was contralaterally beating in 19 patients (86%) and ipsilaterally beating in 3 patients (14%) but was absent in the remaining 80 patients. HSN was found more often in patients who had either a greater canal paresis or central vestibular signs than in patients without HSN, but sensitivity still remained low (only 36% sensitivity even with severe [75–100%] canal paresis).[27] A low sensitivity rate (47.6%) for HSN was also reported by Asawavichiangianda et al for ANs.[148]

The range of reported sensitivity and specificity of HSN has been tabulated by Humphriss et al.[27] Sensitivity ranges from 22 to 95%, and specificity for a unilateral vestibular disorder ranges from 53 to 92%. Across the 10 studies reviewed, many different criteria are used for the "gold standard," with ENG canal paresis definitions ranging from greater than 13% to greater than 30% difference. Additionally the methods (active vs. passive) and nature of HSN (e.g., > 3 beats, > 5 beats, > 2.5°/s, > 6°/s) differed across these different studies, underscoring the variable nature of definitions used for HSN.

Optokinetic and smooth pursuit abnormalities, when present, are reliable signs of brainstem compression.[140] Berrettini found a higher frequency of central findings in tumors greater than 3 cm.[83]

Caloric testing has been examined as a predictor of hearing preservation. The horizontal semicircular canal is stimulated

Table 4.11 Incidence of diminished caloric response by electronystagmography

Study	Small		Large	
Linthicum FH, Khalessi MH, Churchill D. Electronystagmographic caloric bithermal vestibular test (ENG): results in acoustic tumor cases. Acoustic tumors 1 1979:237–240	43%		95%	
	Intracanalicular		**Extracanalicular**	
Haapaniemi JJ, Laurikainen ET, Johansson R, Rinne T, Varpula M. Audiovestibular findings and location of an acoustic neuroma. Eur Arch Otorhinolaryngol 2000;257(5):237–241	55%		67%	
	Small tumors (<1 cm)	**Medium (1.1–3 cm)**	**Large tumor (>3 cm)**	
Berrettini S, Ravecca F, Sellari-Franceschini S, Bruschini P, Casani A, Padolecchia R. Acoustic neuroma: correlations between morphology and otoneurological manifestations. J Neurol Sci 1996;144(1–2):24–33	4/5	16/18	16/16	
Naessens B, Gordts F, Clement PA, Buisseret T. Re-evaluation of the ABR in the diagnosis of CPA tumors in the MRI-era. Acta Otorhinolaryngol Belg 1996;50(2):99–102	Overall 62.5%			
Godey B, Morandi X, Beust L, Brassier G, Bourdinière J. Sensitivity of auditory brainstem response in acoustic neuroma screening. Acta Otolaryngol 1998;118(4):501–504	Overall 86%			

through caloric testing, offering insights into the superior vestibular nerve.[144] Small superior vestibular nerve tumors have a more favorable prognosis for hearing preservation.[77,113,149] Accordingly, it is reasoned that patients who have reduced or absent caloric responses have a better chance at hearing preservation, because the superior vestibular nerve is involved.

However, in practice, caloric results are not so clear cut. Linthicum showed that 97.2% of superior nerve tumors had a caloric weakness, whereas only 60% of inferior vestibular nerve tumors had a caloric weakness.[142] Holsinger et al examined 47 AN cases with planned hearing preservation.[150] Their overall rate of measurable hearing postoperatively was 60%. ENG was obtained on 36 patients. Twenty-five patients demonstrated significant unilateral weakness, of whom measurable hearing was preserved in 14 (56%); 11 patients had no caloric weakness, of whom 5 (45%) had hearing preservation.

Brackmann et al published their series of 333 patients with tumors less than 2 cm who were considered candidates for hearing preservation.[77] ENG was performed in 261 patients: 49% had "normal reduced response" (i.e., ≤25% weakness) and 51% had a reduced vestibular response (i.e., >25% weakness). The researchers found similar rates of reduced responses across all hearing categories and found that no significant difference existed between the preserved hearing groups and the no measurable hearing group.[77]

Despite its lack of sensitivity and its inability to discern superior from inferior nerve of origin, ENG might be helpful in identifying patients preoperatively who will have prolonged imbalance postoperatively. Driscoll et al found that central signs seen on ENG in AN patients portended a higher incidence of persistent (>3 months) disequilibrium than those without central signs.[151] Age greater than 55.5 years, female gender, and constant preoperative disequilibrium present for >3.5 months were also associated with prolonged postoperative disequilibrium in their study.

Other Tumors

The literature regarding ENG findings in meningioma is scant compared with that for ANs. Baguley et al compared the results

of 18 of his patients with the tabulated results of caloric testing performed in four previous studies.[100] Overall, abnormal caloric results were found in 55 of 67 (82%) patients, and the incidence of abnormal ABR ranged from 66 to 95% among the five studies.

Marangos et al examined 309 CPA tumors, including 17 meningiomas, found on either CT or MRI.[110] In the four meningiomas with normal ABR, ENG was normal in three; the article does not reveal the ENG results of the other 13 cases.

4.3.5 Rotatory Chair Testing

Rotatory chair testing uses a computer-controlled rotational stimulus of the horizontal VOR (usually from 0.01 to 0.64 Hz). Rotational stimuli produce a reflex slow eye movement in the opposite direction of rotation with a rapid corrective saccade contralaterally.[147] Gain, phase, asymmetry, and failure of visual fixation can be calculated at each test frequency and compared with age-specific normative data. The definition of abnormal findings varies from center to center, but a generally accepted rule is abnormality of gain, phase, or symmetry seen in two frequencies.[147]

As with most balance tests, a "gold standard" is lacking with which to compare sensitivity and specificity. Most reports on dizziness evaluation rely on history and physical findings to indicate "normal" and "abnormal." Because the examining physicians are also the interpreting physicians of the balance test, no blinded comparison reviews are available. Rotary chair has been compared with ENG for its sensitivity and specificity in identifying patients who have vestibulopathy: rotary chair has a higher sensitivity for peripheral vestibular pathology than ENG does, but the specificity of ENG is higher than that of rotary chair.[147]

4.3.6 Computerized Dynamic Posturography

CDP has been clinically available since 1986.[152] This test has two distinct parts: the motor control test (MCT) and the somatosensory organization test (SOT). MCT is a technique used to measure the subject's functional ability to create adequate motor responses to changes in the pitch plane.[58] Three trials are made of small, medium, and large forward and backward movement and the latency, amplitude, and symmetry of neuromuscular response to this movement.[152] Electromyography (EMG) and biomechanical measures can be used to track the patient's responses to each balance perturbation. The commercially available Neurocom MCT uses a strain gauge in the support surface, rather than EMG, to track ankle-torque corrections during balance correction. Normal latencies range from 130 to 160 msec for medium and large perturbations.

The sensory organization test (SOT) measures the relative contributions from the vestibular, proprioceptive, and visual systems to maintenance of balance. This test uses a force platform, which can be stable or referenced to sway (i.e., moved in a horizontal plane or pitched back and forth), and a visual surround, which can be stationary or referenced to sway, to determine the relative importance of visual, somatosensory, and vestibular input.[153,154] Six different testing situations are created by combinations of stationary or moving force plate and stationary or moving visual surrounds (▶ Table 4.12). The computer can change the position of the force plate or visual surround so that it remains in the same position relative to the patient's sway ("sway referenced"). The interested reader is encouraged to consult Allum and Sheperd's excellent review of this topic.[58]

The most commonly recognized pattern in cases of vestibular lesions is abnormalities in situations 5 and 6. Although CDP does not help in localizing a lesion, it does provide a functional measure of a patient's ability to properly use the various input systems to maintain balance.[153,154,155] Sensitivity of CDP to vestibular pathology, in comparison with that of ENG, has been evaluated,[141] but these two modalities provide different types of information. Because not all imbalance results from presence of a vestibular lesion, CDP might certainly be abnormal in a patient who has a normal ENG. Nonetheless, CDP gives information that is helpful in regarding the functional status of the patient and might help in tailoring a rehabilitation program for that patient.[152]

Levine et al used preoperative CDP to determine the nerve of origin for ANs less than 1.5 cm.[156] In a small series, they found that patients who had an inferior vestibular nerve tumor had abnormalities on SOT in conditions 5 and 6, whereas patients whose tumors were from the superior vestibular nerve had normal CDP findings.

Bergson and Sataloff examined 21 patients who had AN using CDP.[157] They found abnormal test results in 81%, usually in conditions 5 and 6. They found no correlation between the presence or severity of preoperative CDP results and postoperative

balance function. Similar findings were reported by El-Kashlan et al.[155]

Collins et al examined changes in balance following AN resection using balance posturography.[158] They found patterns of abnormal sway and prolonged recovery times both pre- and postoperatively, which were most marked 1 month postoperatively.

CDP does have certain limitations: it does not provide lateralizing information, nor indeed any information regarding cause.[153] However, CDP does provide insight into how well patients can use their balance and how imbalance affects their activities of daily living.

4.3.7 Vestibular Evoked Potentials

Vestibular evoked myogenic potentials (VEMPs) are short-latency potentials recorded from surface electrodes over the tonically contracted SCM muscle evoked by high-level acoustic stimuli.[159] The test subject is seated upright and asked to turn the head to the opposite side of the tested muscle. Surface electrodes are placed over the upper half of the SCM, and a ground electrode is placed on the forehead or sternum. Click stimuli sounds are delivered to the ipsilateral ear at intensities of 85 to 100 dB, and EMG is measured. The source of these responses is thought to be saccule.

Matsuzaki et al described two patients with AN who had normal ABR results but abnormal VEMP.[160] The tumors measured 8 and 10 mm. The researchers concluded that VEMP might be useful for early diagnosis of ANs in patients who had normal ABR. In a follow-up study, they reviewed their experience with 87 AN patients, 79% of whom had decreased or absent VEMPs.[161]

Murofishi et al examined 21 patients who had AN and found abnormal or diminished VEMP ipsilateral to the tumor in 80% of patients, whereas all contralateral VEMPs were normal.[162]

Takeichi et al studied 18 patients who had AN and found diminished VEMP on the affected side in 13 patients (72%).[163] They did not find any correlation with disequilibrium, spontaneous nystagmus, canal paresis, or pure-tone hearing.

Tsutsumi et al examined 28 patients who had AN and VEMP.[164] They found no correlation between VEMP and caloric response, nerve of origin, audiometric threshold, or size of tumor.

In a larger study of 170 patients who had AN, Patko et al found abnormally low or absent VEMPs in 78.8% of patients.[165] They did not find any correlation with horizontal canal weakness.

Rauch has shown that VEMP is useful in the diagnosis of superior semicircular canal dehiscence syndrome and Meniere's disease.[166] Additionally, VEMP might provide some insight into brainstem pathology from stroke[167] or multiple sclerosis[168]; however, at the time of this writing, their utility in cases of AN or other skull base tumors is limited.

4.4 Conclusion

The evaluation of patients who have skull base tumors requires a rigorous history and physical examination. Careful evaluation of CN function is demanded. The examining physician should be aware of nontumor conditions that can mimic

Table 4.12 Test conditions in computerized dynamic posturography sensory organization test

Test	Condition
1	Eyes open, fixed support
2	Eyes closed, fixed support
3	Visual surround referenced to sway, fixed support
4	Eyes open, force plate referenced to sway
5	Eyes closed, force plate referenced to sway
6	Force plate and visual surround referenced to sway

the findings of a skull base tumor. Judicious use of ancillary tests of neuro-otologic function helps in determining the extent of disease and plays an important role in deciding treatment methods. Some of these tests can be used to predict postoperative hearing and balance function.

References

[1] Bott L, Thumerelle C, Cuvellier JC, Deschildre A, Vallée L, Sardet A. [Ataxia-telangiectasia: a review]. Arch Pediatr. 2006; 13(3):293–298

[2] Taylor AM, Byrd PJ. Molecular pathology of ataxia telangiectasia. J Clin Pathol. 2005; 58(10):1009–1015

[3] Cross JH. Neurocutaneous syndromes and epilepsy-issues in diagnosis and management. Epilepsia. 2005; 46 Suppl 10:17–23

[4] Kreusel KM. Ophthalmological manifestations in VHL and NF 1: pathological and diagnostic implications. Fam Cancer. 2005; 4(1):43–47

[5] Patel NP, Mhatre AN, Lalwani AK. Molecular pathogenesis of skull base tumors. Otol Neurotol. 2004; 25(4):636–643

[6] Xiao GH, Chernoff J, Testa JR. NF2: the wizardry of merlin. Genes Chromosomes Cancer. 2003; 38(4):389–399

[7] Smith DS, Lee KK, Milczuk HA. Otolaryngologic manifestations of PHACE syndrome. Int J Pediatr Otorhinolaryngol. 2004; 68(11):1445–1450

[8] Comi AM. Pathophysiology of Sturge-Weber syndrome. J Child Neurol. 2003; 18(8):509–516

[9] Freedman SF, Amedee RG, Molony T. Neurotologic manifestations of von Hippel Lindau disease. Ear Nose Throat J. 1992; 71(12):655–658

[10] Brandt T, Strupp M. General vestibular testing. Clin Neurophysiol. 2005; 116 (2):406–426

[11] The control of gaze. In: Kandell E, Schwartz J, Jessell T, eds. Principles of Neural Science. New York: McGraw-Hill; 2000

[12] Mosby's Medical Dictionary. 3rd ed, ed. W. Glanze, St. Louis: C.V. Mosby; 1990

[13] Ross R. How to Examine: The Nervous System. New York: Medical Publishing Co.; 1985

[14] Traccis S, Zoroddu GF, Zecca MT, Cau T, Solinas MA, Masuri R. Evaluating patients with vertigo: bedside examination. Neurol Sci. 2004; 25 Suppl 1: S16–S19

[15] Leigh R, Zee D. The Neurology of Eye Movements. 4th ed. New York: Oxford University Press; 2006

[16] Lee K. The vestibular system and its disorders. In: Lee K, ed. Essential Otolaryngology. New York: Medical Examination Publishing; 1995

[17] Nedzelski JM. Cerebellopontine angle tumors: bilateral flocculus compression as cause of associated oculomotor abnormalities. Laryngoscope. 1983; 93(10):1251–1260

[18] Longridge NS, Mallinson AI. The dynamic illegible E (DIE) test: a simple technique for assessing the ability of the vestibulo-ocular reflex to overcome vestibular pathology. J Otolaryngol. 1987; 16(2):97–103

[19] Herdman SJ, Tusa RJ, Blatt P, Suzuki A, Venuto PJ, Roberts D. Computerized dynamic visual acuity test in the assessment of vestibular deficits. Am J Otol. 1998; 19(6):790–796

[20] Dix MR, Hallpike CS. The pathology symptomatology and diagnosis of certain common disorders of the vestibular system. Proc R Soc Med. 1952; 45 (6):341–354

[21] Halmagyi GM, Curthoys IS. A clinical sign of canal paresis. Arch Neurol. 1988; 45(7):737–739

[22] Schubert MC, Tusa RJ, Grine LE, Herdman SJ. Optimizing the sensitivity of the head thrust test for identifying vestibular hypofunction. Phys Ther. 2004; 84(2):151–158

[23] Foster CA, Foster BD, Spindler J, Harris JP. Functional loss of the horizontal doll's eye reflex following unilateral vestibular lesions. Laryngoscope. 1994; 104(4):473–478

[24] Harvey SA, Wood DJ. The oculocephalic response in the evaluation of the dizzy patient. Laryngoscope. 1996; 106(1 Pt 1):6–9

[25] Harvey SA, Wood DJ, Feroah TR. Relationship of the head impulse test and head-shake nystagmus in reference to caloric testing. Am J Otol. 1997; 18 (2):207–213

[26] Beynon GJ, Jani P, Baguley DM. A clinical evaluation of head impulse testing. Clin Otolaryngol Allied Sci. 1998; 23(2):117–122

[27] Humphriss RL, Baguley DM, Moffat DA. Head-shaking nystagmus in patients with a vestibular schwannoma. Clin Otolaryngol Allied Sci. 2003; 28(6): 514–519

[28] Shockley WW, Stucker FJ, Jr. Squamous cell carcinoma of the external ear: a review of 75 cases. Otolaryngol Head Neck Surg. 1987; 97(3):308–312

[29] Ross DA, Sasaki CT. Cancer of the ear and temporal bone. In: Myers E, Suen J, eds. Cancer of the Head and Neck. Philadelphia, PA: W. B. Saunders; 1996

[30] Clayman GL, Lee JJ, Holsinger FC, et al. Mortality risk from squamous cell skin cancer. J Clin Oncol. 2005; 23(4):759–765

[31] Burkey JM, Lippy WH, Schuring AG, Rizer FM. Clinical utility of the 512-Hz Rinne tuning fork test. Am J Otol. 1998; 19(1):59–62

[32] Vikram KB, Naseeruddin K. Combined tuning fork tests in hearing loss: explorative clinical study of the patterns. J Otolaryngol. 2004; 33(4):227–234

[33] Poe DS, Abou-Halawa A, Abdel-Razek O. Analysis of the dysfunctional Eustachian tube by video endoscopy. Otol Neurotol. 2001; 22(5):590–595

[34] Meyerhoff WL, Anderson RG. Non-auditory presentations of cerebellopontine angle lesions. Laryngoscope. 1984; 94(7):904–906

[35] Nemzek WR. The trigeminal nerve. Top Magn Reson Imaging. 1996; 8(3): 132–154

[36] Saper C. Brain stem, reflexive behavior, and the cranial nerves. In: Kandell E, Schwartz J, Jessell T, eds. Principles of Neural Science. New York: McGraw-Hill; 2000

[37] Carpenter M. Core Text of Neuroanatomy. 3rd ed, Baltimore: Williams and Wilkins; 1985

[38] Doty RL, Mishra A. Olfaction and its alteration by nasal obstruction, rhinitis, and rhinosinusitis. Laryngoscope. 2001; 111(3):409–423

[39] Rombaux P, Collet S, Eloy P, Ledeghen S, Bertrand B. Smell disorders in ENT clinic. B-ENT. 2005 Suppl 1:97–107, quiz 108–109

[40] Hummel T, Welge-Lüessen A. Assessment of olfactory function. Adv Otorhinolaryngol. 2006; 63:84–98

[41] Wrobel BB, Leopold DA. Clinical assessment of patients with smell and taste disorders. Otolaryngol Clin North Am. 2004; 37(6):1127–1142

[42] Schiffman SS. Taste and smell in disease (first of two parts). N Engl J Med. 1983; 308(21):1275–1279

[43] Doty RL, Shaman P, Kimmelman CP, Dann MS. University of Pennsylvania Smell Identification Test: a rapid quantitative olfactory function test for the clinic. Laryngoscope. 1984; 94(2 Pt 1):176–178

[44] Jackson CG, Glasscock ME, III, Hughes G, Sismanis A. Facial paralysis of neoplastic origin: diagnosis and management. Laryngoscope. 1980; 90(10 Pt 1): 1581–1595

[45] House JW, Brackmann DE. Facial nerve grading system. Otolaryngol Head Neck Surg. 1985; 93(2):146–147

[46] Yeh S, Foroozan R. Orbital apex syndrome. Curr Opin Ophthalmol. 2004; 15 (6):490–498

[47] Zaffaroni M, Baldini SM, Ghezzi A. Cranial nerve, brainstem and cerebellar syndromes in the differential diagnosis of multiple sclerosis. Neurol Sci. 2001; 22 Suppl 2:S74–S78

[48] Krasnianski M, Neudecker S, Zierz S. [The Schmidt and Vernet classical syndrome. Alternating brain stem syndromes that do not exist?]. Nervenarzt. 2003; 74(12):1150–1154

[49] Johnston JL. Parasellar syndromes. Curr Neurol Neurosci Rep. 2002; 2(5): 423–431

[50] Schweinfurth JM, Johnson JT, Weissman J. Jugular foramen syndrome as a complication of metastatic melanoma. Am J Otolaryngol. 1993; 14(3):168–174

[51] Paparounas K, Gotsi A, Apostolou F, Akritidis N. Collet-Sicard syndrome disclosing glomus tumor of the skull base. Eur Neurol. 2003; 49(2):103–105

[52] Chacon G, Alexandraki I, Palacio C. Collet-Sicard syndrome: an uncommon manifestation of metastatic prostate cancer. South Med J. 2006; 99(8):898–899

[53] Romberg M. Lehrbuch Der Nervenkrankheiten Des Menschen. Berlin: Duncker; 1846

[54] Weber PC, Cass SP. Clinical assessment of postural stability. Am J Otol. 1993; 14(6):566–569

[55] Fukuda T. Statokinetic Reflexes in Equilibrium and Movement. Tokyo: University of Tokyo Press; 1983

[56] Hickey SA, Ford GR, Buckley JG, Fitzgerald O'Connor AF. Unterberger stepping test: a useful indicator of peripheral vestibular dysfunction? J Laryngol Otol. 1990; 104(8):599–602

[57] Bonanni M, Newton R. Test-retest reliability of the Fukuda Stepping Test. Physiother Res Int. 1998; 3(1):58–68

[58] Allum JH, Shepard NT. An overview of the clinical use of dynamic posturography in the differential diagnosis of balance disorders. J Vestib Res. 1999; 9 (4):223–252

[59] Kuipers-Upmeijer J, Oosterhuis HJ. [Unterberger's test not useful in testing of vestibular function]. Ned Tijdschr Geneeskd. 1994; 138(3):136–139

[60] Horak FB. Clinical measurement of postural control in adults. Phys Ther. 1987; 67(12):1881–1885

[61] El-Kashlan HK, Eisenmann D, Kileny PR. Auditory brain stem response in small acoustic neuromas. Ear Hear. 2000; 21(3):257–262

[62] Gordon ML, Cohen NL. Efficacy of auditory brainstem response as a screening test for small acoustic neuromas. Am J Otol. 1995; 16(2):136–139

[63] Cushing H. Tumors of the Nervus Acusticus and the Syndrome of the Cerebellopontine Angle. Philadelphia: WB Saunders; 1917

[64] Johnson EW. Auditory test results in 110 surgically confirmed retrocochlear lesions. J Speech Hear Disord. 1965; 30(4):307–317

[65] Glasscock ME, III, Levine SC, McKennan KX. The changing characteristics of acoustic neuroma patients over the last 10 years. Laryngoscope. 1987; 97 (10):1164–1167

[66] Jerger J. Clinical experience with impedance audiometry. Arch Otolaryngol. 1970; 92(4):311–324

[67] Jerger J. Impedance terminology. Arch Otolaryngol. 1975; 101(10):589–590

[68] Jerger J, Hayes D. Diagnostic speech audiometry. Arch Otolaryngol. 1977; 103(4):216–222

[69] Hayes D, Jerger J. Impedance audiometry in otologic diagnosis. Otolaryngol Clin North Am. 1978; 11(3):759–767

[70] Clemis JD, Mc Gee T. Brain stem electric response audiometry in the differential diagnosis of acoustic tumors. Laryngoscope. 1979; 89(1):31–42

[71] Dix MR, Hallpike CS. The otoneurological diagnosis of tumours of the VIII nerve. Proc R Soc Med. 1958; 51(11):889–896

[72] Walsh TE, Goodman A. Speech discrimination in central auditory lesions. Laryngoscope. 1955; 65(1):1–8

[73] Hirsch A, Anderson H. Audiologic test results in 96 patients with tumours affecting the eighth nerve. A clinical study with emphasis on the early audiological diagnosis. Acta Otolaryngol Suppl. 1980; 369:1–26

[74] Telischi F. An objective method of analyzing cochlear versus noncochlear patterns of distortion-product otoacoustic emissions in patients with acoustic neuromas. Laryngoscope. 2000; 110(4):553–562

[75] Selesnick SH, Jackler RK. Clinical manifestations and audiologic diagnosis of acoustic neuromas. Otolaryngol Clin North Am. 1992; 25(3):521–551

[76] Committee on Hearing and Equilibrium guidelines for the evaluation of hearing preservation in acoustic neuroma (vestibular schwannoma). American Academy of Otolaryngology–Head and Neck Surgery Foundation, Inc. Otolaryngol Head Neck Surg. 1995; 113(3):179–180

[77] Brackmann DE, Owens RM, Friedman RA, et al. Prognostic factors for hearing preservation in vestibular schwannoma surgery. Am J Otol. 2000; 21(3): 417–424

[78] Anderson H, Barr B, Wedenberg E. The early detection of acoustic tumours by the stapedius reflex test. In: Sensorineural hearing loss. Ciba Found Symp, 1970:275–294

[79] Harner SG, Laws ER, Jr. Clinical findings in patients with acoustic neurinoma. Mayo Clin Proc. 1983; 58(11):721–728

[80] Moffat DA, Hardy DG. Early diagnosis and surgical management of acoustic neuroma: is it cost effective? J R Soc Med. 1989; 82(6):329–332

[81] Thomsen J, Tos M. Acoustic neuroma: clinical aspects, audiovestibular assessment, diagnostic delay, and growth rate. Am J Otol. 1990; 11(1): 12–19

[82] Kanzaki J, Ogawa K, Ogawa S, Yamamoto M, Ikeda S, O-Uchi T. Audiological findings in acoustic neuroma. Acta Otolaryngol Suppl. 1991; 487:125–132

[83] Berrettini S, Ravecca F, Sellari-Franceschini S, Bruschini P, Casani A, Padolecchia R. Acoustic neuroma: correlations between morphology and otoneurological manifestations. J Neurol Sci. 1996; 144(1–2):24–33

[84] Godey B, Morandi X, Beust L, Brassier G, Bourdinière J. Sensitivity of auditory brainstem response in acoustic neuroma screening. Acta Otolaryngol. 1998; 118(4):501–504

[85] Moffat DA, Baguley DM, Hardy DG, Tsui YN. Contralateral auditory brainstem response abnormalities in acoustic neuroma. J Laryngol Otol. 1989; 103(9): 835–838

[86] Beck HJ, Beatty CW, Harner SG, Ilstrup DM. Acoustic neuromas with normal pure tone hearing levels. Otolaryngol Head Neck Surg. 1986; 94(1):96–103

[87] Roland PS, Glasscock ME, III, Bojrab DI, Josey AF. Normal hearing in patients with acoustic neuroma. South Med J. 1987; 80(2):166–169

[88] Selesnick SH, Jackler RK, Pitts LW. The changing clinical presentation of acoustic tumors in the MRI era. Laryngoscope. 1993; 103(4 Pt 1):431–436

[89] Acoustic Neuroma: NIH Consensus Statement, NIH, Editor. 1991:1–24

[90] Morrison A. Acoustic neuroma. In: Management of Sensorineural Hearing Loss. London: Butterworths; 1975:46–79

[91] Telian SA, Kileny PR. Pitfalls in neurotologic diagnosis. Ear Hear. 1988; 9(2): 86–91

[92] Rosenberg SI. Natural history of acoustic neuromas. Laryngoscope. 2000; 110(4):497–508

[93] Schuknecht H. Pathology of the Ear. Cambridge: Harvard University Press; 1974

[94] Graamans K, Van Dijk JE, Janssen LW. Hearing deterioration in patients with a non-growing vestibular schwannoma. Acta Otolaryngol. 2003; 123(1):51–54

[95] Saleh EA, Aristegui M, Naguib MB, Cokesser Y, Landolfi M, Sanna M. Normal hearing in acoustic neuroma patients: a critical evaluation. Am J Otol. 1996; 17(1):127–132

[96] Welling DB, Glasscock ME, III, Woods CI, Jackson CG. Acoustic neuroma: a cost-effective approach. Otolaryngol Head Neck Surg. 1990; 103(3):364–370

[97] Ruckenstein MJ, Cueva RA, Morrison DH, Press G. A prospective study of ABR and MRI in the screening for vestibular schwannomas. Am J Otol. 1996; 17 (2):317–320

[98] Obholzer RJ, Rea PA, Harcourt JP. Magnetic resonance imaging screening for vestibular schwannoma: analysis of published protocols. J Laryngol Otol. 2004; 118(5):329–332

[99] Robinette MS, Bauch CD, Olsen WO, Harner SG, Beatty CW. Nonsurgical factors predictive of postoperative hearing for patients with vestibular schwannoma. Am J Otol. 1997; 18(6):738–745

[100] Baguley DM, Beynon GJ, Grey PL, Hardy DG, Moffat DA. Audio-vestibular findings in meningioma of the cerebello-pontine angle: a retrospective review. J Laryngol Otol. 1997; 111(11):1022–1026

[101] Doyle KJ, De la Cruz A. Cerebellopontine angle epidermoids: results of surgical treatment. Skull Base Surg. 1996; 6(1):27–33

[102] Quaranta N, Chang P, Baguley DM, Moffat DA. Audiologic presentation of cerebellopontine angle cholesteatoma. J Otolaryngol. 2003; 32(4):217–221

[103] Kaylie DM, Warren FM, III, Haynes DS, Jackson CG. Neurotologic management of intracranial epidermoid tumors. Laryngoscope. 2005; 115(6):1082–1086

[104] Jewett DL, Williston JS. Auditory-evoked far fields averaged from the scalp of humans. Brain. 1971; 94(4):681–696

[105] Brackmann DE, Selters WA. Brainstem electric audiometry: acoustic neurinoma detection. Rev Laryngol Otol Rhinol (Bord). 1979; 100(1–2):49–51

[106] Ferguson MA, Smith PA, Lutman ME, Mason SM, Coles RR, Gibbin KP. Efficiency of tests used to screen for cerebello-pontine angle tumours: a prospective study. Br J Audiol. 1996; 30(3):159–176

[107] Bu-Saba NY, Rebeiz EE, Salman SD, Thornton AR, West C. Significance of false-positive auditory brainstem response: a clinical study. Am J Otol. 1994; 15(2):233–236

[108] Hall J. Handbook of Auditory Evoked Responses. Boston: Allyn and Bacon; 1992

[109] Josey AF, Jackson CG, Glasscock ME, III. Brainstem evoked response audiometry in confirmed eighth nerve tumors. Am J Otolaryngol. 1980; 1(4):285–290

[110] Marangos N, Maier W, Merz R, Laszig R. Brainstem response in cerebellopontine angle tumors. Otol Neurotol. 2001; 22(1):95–99

[111] Cueva RA. Auditory brainstem response versus magnetic resonance imaging for the evaluation of asymmetric sensorineural hearing loss. Laryngoscope. 2004; 114(10):1686–1692

[112] Bauch CD, Rose DE, Harner SG. Auditory brain stem response results from 255 patients with suspected retrocochlear involvement. Ear Hear. 1982; 3 (2):83–86

[113] Wilson DF, Hodgson RS, Gustafson MF, Hogue S, Mills L. The sensitivity of auditory brainstem response testing in small acoustic neuromas. Laryngoscope. 1992; 102(9):961–964

[114] Dornhoffer JL, Helms J, Hoehmann DH. Presentation and diagnosis of small acoustic tumors. Otolaryngol Head Neck Surg. 1994; 111(3 Pt 1):232–235

[115] Chandrasekhar SS, Brackmann DE, Devgan KK. Utility of auditory brainstem response audiometry in diagnosis of acoustic neuromas. Am J Otol. 1995; 16 (1):63–67

[116] Zappia JJ, O'Connor CA, Wiet RJ, Dinces EA. Rethinking the use of auditory brainstem response in acoustic neuroma screening. Laryngoscope. 1997; 107(10):1388–1392

[117] Burkey JM, Rizer FM, Schuring AG, Fucci MJ, Lippy WH. Acoustic reflexes, auditory brainstem response, and MRI in the evaluation of acoustic neuromas. Laryngoscope. 1996; 106(7):839–841

[118] Musiek FE, Kibbe K. Auditory brain stem response wave IV-V abnormalities from the ear opposite large cerebellopontine lesions. Am J Otol. 1986; 7(4): 253–257

[119] Rupa V, Job A, George M, Rajshekhar V. Cost-effective initial screening for vestibular schwannoma: auditory brainstem response or magnetic resonance imaging? Otolaryngol Head Neck Surg. 2003; 128(6):823–828

[120] Nadol JB, Jr, Chiong CM, Ojemann RG, et al. Preservation of hearing and facial nerve function in resection of acoustic neuroma. Laryngoscope. 1992; 102 (10):1153–1158

[121] Matthies C, Samii M. Management of vestibular schwannomas (acoustic neuromas): the value of neurophysiology for intraoperative monitoring of auditory function in 200 cases. Neurosurgery. 1997; 40(3):459–466, discussion 466–468

[122] Nadol JB, Jr, Levine R, Ojemann RG, Martuza RL, Montgomery WW, de Sandoval PK. Preservation of hearing in surgical removal of acoustic neuromas of the internal auditory canal and cerebellar pontine angle. Laryngoscope. 1987; 97(11):1287–1294

[123] Kemink JL, LaRouere MJ, Kileny PR, Telian SA, Hoff JT. Hearing preservation following suboccipital removal of acoustic neuromas. Laryngoscope. 1990; 100(6):597–602

[124] Stidham KR, Roberson JB, Jr. Hearing improvement after middle fossa resection of vestibular schwannoma. Otol Neurotol. 2001; 22(6):917–921

[125] House JW, Brackmann DE. Brainstem audiometry in neurotologic diagnosis. Arch Otolaryngol. 1979; 105(6):305–309

[126] Laird FJ, Harner SG, Laws ER, Jr, Reese DF. Meningiomas of the cerebellopontine angle. Otolaryngol Head Neck Surg. 1985; 93(2):163–167

[127] Granick MS, Martuza RL, Parker SW, Ojemann RG, Montgomery WW. Cerebellopontine angle meningiomas: clinical manifestations and diagnosis. Ann Otol Rhinol Laryngol. 1985; 94(1 Pt 1):34–38

[128] Aiba T, et al. Clinical characteristics of rare cerebellopontine angle tumours: comparison with acoustic tumors. in Proceedings of the First International Conference on Acoustic Neuroma. New York: Kugler; 1992

[129] Hart MJ, Lillehei KO. Management of posterior cranial fossa meningiomas. Ann Otol Rhinol Laryngol. 1995; 104(2):105–116

[130] Don M, Masuda A, Nelson R, Brackmann D. Successful detection of small acoustic tumors using the stacked derived-band auditory brain stem response amplitude. Am J Otol. 1997; 18(5):608–621, discussion 682–685

[131] Philibert B, Durrant JD, Ferber-Viart C, Duclaux R, Veuillet E, Collet L. Stacked tone-burst-evoked auditory brainstem response (ABR): preliminary findings. Int J Audiol. 2003; 42(2):71–81

[132] Gold T. Hearing II. The physical basis of the action of the cochlea. Proc Royal Soc Britain. 1948; 135(881):492–498

[133] Kemp DT. Stimulated acoustic emissions from within the human auditory system. J Acoust Soc Am. 1978; 64(5):1386–1391

[134] Hall J. Handbook of Otoacoustic Emissions. San Diego: Singular; 2000

[135] Brownell WE, Bader CR, Bertrand D, de Ribaupierre Y. Evoked mechanical responses of isolated cochlear outer hair cells. Science. 1985; 227(4683):194–196

[136] Kim AH, Edwards BM, Telian SA, Kileny PR, Arts HA. Transient evoked otoacoustic emissions pattern as a prognostic indicator for hearing preservation in acoustic neuroma surgery. Otol Neurotol. 2006; 27(3):372–379

[137] Burns EM, Arehart KH, Campbell SL. Prevalence of spontaneous otoacoustic emissions in neonates. J Acoust Soc Am. 1992; 91(3):1571–1575

[138] Ferber-Viart C, Colleaux B, Laoust L, Dubreuil C, Duclaux R. Is the presence of transient evoked otoacoustic emissions in ears with acoustic neuroma significant? Laryngoscope. 1998; 108(4 Pt 1):605–609

[139] Jongkees LB, Philipszoon AJ. Electronystagmography. Acta Otolaryngol Suppl. 1964; 189: S:uppl: 189:1+

[140] McGee ML. Electronystagmography in peripheral lesions. Ear Hear. 1986; 7 (3):167–175

[141] Amin M, Girardi M, Konrad HR, Hughes L. A comparison of electronystagmography results with posturography findings from the BalanceTrak 500. Otol Neurotol. 2002; 23(4):488–493

[142] Linthicum FH, Khalessi MH, Churchill D. Electronystagmographic caloric bithermal vestibular test (ENG): results in acoustic tumor cases. Acoustic tumors 1 1979:237–240

[143] Naessens B, Gordts F, Clement PA, Buisseret T. Re-evaluation of the ABR in the diagnosis of CPA tumors in the MRI-era. Acta Otorhinolaryngol Belg. 1996; 50(2):99–102

[144] Haapaniemi JJ, Laurikainen ET, Johansson R, Rinne T, Varpula M. Audiovestibular findings and location of an acoustic neuroma. Eur Arch Otorhinolaryngol. 2000; 257(5):237–241

[145] Bergenius J, Magnusson M. The relationship between caloric response, oculomotor dysfunction and size of cerebello-pontine angle tumours. Acta Otolaryngol. 1988; 106(5–6):361–367

[146] Guyot JP, Häusler R, Reverdin A, Berney J, Montandon PB. Diagnosis of cerebellopontine angle tumors. ORL J Otorhinolaryngol Relat Spec. 1992; 54(3): 139–143

[147] Arriaga MA, Chen DA, Cenci KA. Rotational chair (ROTO) instead of electronystagmography (ENG) as the primary vestibular test. Otolaryngol Head Neck Surg. 2005; 133(3):329–333

[148] Asawavichiangianda S, Fujimoto M, Mai M, Desroches H, Rutka J. Significance of head-shaking nystagmus in the evaluation of the dizzy patient. Acta Otolaryngol Suppl. 1999; 540:27–33

[149] Shelton C, Brackmann DE, House WF, Hitselberger WE. Acoustic tumor surgery. Prognostic factors in hearing conversation. Arch Otolaryngol Head Neck Surg. 1989; 115(10):1213–1216

[150] Holsinger FC, Coker NJ, Jenkins HA. Hearing preservation in conservation surgery for vestibular schwannoma. Am J Otol. 2000; 21(5):695–700

[151] Driscoll CL, Lynn SG, Harner SG, Beatty CW, Atkinson EJ. Preoperative identification of patients at risk of developing persistent dysequilibrium after acoustic neuroma removal. Am J Otol. 1998; 19(4):491–495

[152] Voorhees RL. The role of dynamic posturography in neurotologic diagnosis. Laryngoscope. 1989; 99(10 Pt 1):995–1001

[153] Furman JM. Role of posturography in the management of vestibular patients. Otolaryngol Head Neck Surg. 1995; 112(1):8–15

[154] Monsell EM, Furman JM, Herdman SJ, Konrad HR, Shepard NT. Computerized dynamic platform posturography. Otolaryngol Head Neck Surg. 1997; 117 (4):394–398

[155] El-Kashlan HK, Shepard NT, Arts HA, Telian SA. Disability from vestibular symptoms after acoustic neuroma resection. Am J Otol. 1998; 19(1): 104–111

[156] Levine SC, Muckle RP, Anderson JH. Evaluation of patients with acoustic neuroma with dynamic posturography. Otolaryngol Head Neck Surg. 1993; 109 (3 Pt 1):392–398

[157] Bergson E, Sataloff RT. Preoperative computerized dynamic posturography as a prognostic indicator of balance function in patients with acoustic neuroma. Ear Nose Throat J. 2005; 84(3):154–156

[158] Collins MM, Johnson IJ, Clifford E, Birchall JP, O'Donoghue GM. Dynamic assessment of imbalance in acoustic neuroma patients by sway magnetometry. Clin Otolaryngol Allied Sci. 2000; 25(6):570–576

[159] Akin FW, Murnane OD. Vestibular evoked myogenic potentials: preliminary report. J Am Acad Audiol. 2001; 12(9):445–452, quiz 491

[160] Matsuzaki M, Murofushi T, Mizuno M. Vestibular evoked myogenic potentials in acoustic tumor patients with normal auditory brainstem responses. Eur Arch Otorhinolaryngol. 1999; 256(1):1–4

[161] Ushio M, Matsuzaki M, Takegoshi H, Murofushi T. Click- and short tone burst-evoked myogenic potentials in cerebellopontine angle tumors. Acta Otolaryngol Suppl. 2001; 545:133–135

[162] Murofushi T, Matsuzaki M, Mizuno M. Vestibular evoked myogenic potentials in patients with acoustic neuromas. Arch Otolaryngol Head Neck Surg. 1998; 124(5):509–512

[163] Takeichi N, Sakamoto T, Fukuda S, Inuyama Y. Vestibular evoked myogenic potential (VEMP) in patients with acoustic neuromas. Auris Nasus Larynx. 2001; 28 Suppl:S39–S41

[164] Tsutsumi T, Tsunoda A, Noguchi Y, Komatsuzaki A. Prediction of the nerves of origin of vestibular schwannomas with vestibular evoked myogenic potentials. Am J Otol. 2000; 21(5):712–715

[165] Patko T, Vidal PP, Vibert N, Tran Ba Huy P, de Waele C. Vestibular evoked myogenic potentials in patients suffering from an unilateral acoustic neuroma: a study of 170 patients. Clin Neurophysiol. 2003; 114(7): 1344–1350

[166] Rauch SD. Vestibular evoked myogenic potentials. Curr Opin Otolaryngol Head Neck Surg. 2006; 14(5):299–304

[167] Chen CH, Young YH. Vestibular evoked myogenic potentials in brainstem stroke. Laryngoscope. 2003; 113(6):990–993

[168] Alpini D, Pugnetti L, Caputo D, Cornelio F, Capobianco S, Cesarani A. Vestibular evoked myogenic potentials in multiple sclerosis: clinical and imaging correlations. Mult Scler. 2004; 10(3):316–321

[169] Josey AF, Glasscock ME, III, Musiek FE. Correlation of ABR and medical imaging in patients with cerebellopontine angle tumors. Am J Otol. 1988; 9 Suppl:12–16

[170] Weiss MH, Kisiel DL, Bhatia P. Predictive value of brainstem evoked response in the diagnosis of acoustic neuroma. Otolaryngol Head Neck Surg. 1990; 103(4):583–585

[171] Noguchi Y, Komatsuzaki A, Nishida H. Cochlear microphonics for hearing preservation in vestibular schwannoma surgery. Laryngoscope. 1999; 109 (12):1982–1987

5 Anesthesia and Intraoperative Monitoring of Patients with Skull Base Tumors

Walter S. Jellish[†] and Steven B. Edelstein

Summary

Anesthesia support for skull base surgery is complex and is critical for the overall success of the procedure. The anesthesia care team must be aware of the positioning needs of the surgeon and must be able to protect the patient from neurologic injury caused by the abnormal positioning that may be required to access the tumor. In addition, the anesthetic technique must be tailored to ensure a hemodynamically stable patient and a still surgical field without the use of muscle relaxants. Anesthetic technique must also be adjusted to accommodate neurophysiologic monitoring so as to protect patients from neurologic injury during surgical resection. New and modern surgical techniques using minimally invasive technology raise new issues related to hemodynamic stability, fluid status, and overall monitoring of patient homeostasis. These endoscopic procedures offer advantages over open procedures but have their own set of problems that must be addressed by the anesthesiologist. Some of the common problems that anesthesiologists face during skull base surgery, along with methods for preventing and treating these injuries, are presented to help improve outcomes and morbidity after the procedure. Postoperative pain management is also described, including new and novel therapies with which to reduce postcraniotomy pain and headache—all designed to improve recovery and patient well-being after these complex surgeries.

Keywords: anesthesia, skull base surgery, trigeminal cardiac reflex, venous air embolism pneumocephalus, neurophysiologic monitoring

5.1 Introduction

Many issues surround the administration of anesthesia for patients undergoing surgery of the skull base. Not only do difficulties surround exposure of deeply seated anatomic structures, but other issues also involve positioning, prevention of iatrogenic nerve injury, and blood loss. This chapter describes many of the problems encountered with the delivery of anesthesia for skull base surgery and will describe some of the techniques and monitoring used to improve outcomes. The review of this subjective matter is meant to give some insight into the multiple and complex problems faced by the operative team during these procedures.

5.2 Patient Positioning

One of the challenges of skull base surgery concerns patient positioning. The exact approach depends on the patient's anatomy and clinical status as well as on the tumor size. These approaches can be craniofacial, orbitocranial, infratemporal,

suboccipital (transcondylar), and, in some instances, endonasal. Lateral approaches include the retrosigmoid, translabyrinthine, and orbitocranial zygomatic.[1] Each of these approaches is associated with particular positions that have specific challenges and morbidities.

5.2.1 Supine Position

Anterior skull base lesions can be quite difficult to approach surgically, even though the patient is in the supine position. Access to the airway is simple, although the patient may be rotated 180° away from the anesthesia team. There are limited changes in the patient's hemodynamic profile, but there could be significant changes in the pulmonary system, especially related to diaphragmatic elevation. This diaphragmatic position ultimately promotes atelectasis and ventilation-to-perfusion (V/Q) mismatching. The supine position is also used for endonasal endoscopic approaches to the anterior skull base, which includes the sella, cribriform plate, planum sphenoidale, and suprasellar cistern, as well as the clivus, pterygopalatine fossa, and adjacent parasagittal skull base locations.

Lateral approaches such as the retrosigmoid, translabyrinthine, and orbitocranial zygomatic can be accessed via the supine position but require the head to be laterally rotated and fixed. This flexion is sometimes impossible, especially in the elderly, and may be associated with venous obstruction.[2] This positioning reduces the risk of air embolism but can produce brachial plexopathy on the side of the surgery, because the head is turned contralaterally and the ipsilateral shoulder is pushed down to allow access for the surgical approach. Closed claims analysis of brachial injury notes that they usually are associated with general anesthesia, with 10% related to patient positioning (head down, malpositioning of the arms, and sustained neck extension).[3] Retrospective findings from our own surgical database demonstrated a 9% incidence of brachial plexopathy, with 61% ipsilateral to the surgical field. In most cases, these symptoms resolve within two to three days.[1] Care providers should be focused on the initial positioning to protect the patient from overextension and flexion injuries.

5.2.2 Prone Position

The prone position is particularly useful for accessing lesions at or near midline and the fourth ventricle.[4] This positioning is associated with numerous hemodynamic and respiratory changes that must be monitored closely. Significant V/Q mismatching is present in the prone position, and access to the airway is compromised. The anesthesiologist must be vigilant during positioning of the patient, because dislodgement of the endotracheal (ET) tube will require emergency reintubation in suboptimal conditions. Transferring patients from supine to prone positioning produces significant hemodynamic changes secondary to acute changes in preload from either abdominal compression or thoracic impedance. Cardiac dysrhythmias may occasionally

[†] Deceased

occur from changes in preload as a result of this compression, so electrocardiographic (ECG) monitoring is essential.[5] Several types of chest and abdominal rolls composed of fabric or gel, as well as padded square frames that have a large opening for the abdominal contents, have been routinely used to prevent this compression. Other than hemodynamic and respiratory problems, prolonged prone positioning has also been associated with significant facial and tongue edema, orbital/facial swelling, central venous retinal thrombosis, and posterior ischemic optic neuropathy, a disastrous condition that can result in permanent blindness.

5.2.3 Park-Bench Position

The park-bench position (lateral oblique position) is commonly used in skull base procedures involving the posterior fossa (▶ Fig. 5.1). It is a semiprone lateral position with the head flexed and slightly elevated—5 to 10°. It allows both lateral and midline approaches to the posterior fossa.[4] Flexion of the neck may impinge venous circulation, and obstruction might not always be recognized by examination of the external position.[6] This position has less hemodynamic and respiratory effects than the full prone position, but neck flexion may be associated with brachial plexus injuries if care is not taken when assessing

final position. Extreme flexion may compromise spinal cord perfusion and has been associated with quadriplegia.[7] This position offers better surgical exposure and the potential advantages of improved hemostasis. However, the head elevated position brings a higher incidence of venous air embolism (VAE) and pneumocephalus.[8] Open sinuses, noncollapsible bony sinuses, and large veins all heighten risk for VAE.

5.2.4 Lateral Position

The lateral position is frequently used for intracerebellar procedures involving lateral or cerebellar hemispheric lesions, tumors of the clivus, petrous ridge, and anterior and lateral foramen magnum. Typically the retromastoid, transtentorial, and transcondylar surgical approaches require this position (▶ Fig. 5.2).

Again, the position has some significant hemodynamic and pulmonary implications. Significant V/Q mismatching takes place, albeit to far less a degree than for the prone position. Some of the disadvantages of this position include the potential for lateral popliteal nerve palsy in the dependent leg, compression of the dependent shoulder and axillary structures, and presence of the superior shoulder in the surgeon's line of sight.[4] Devices such as axillary rolls (designed to decompress

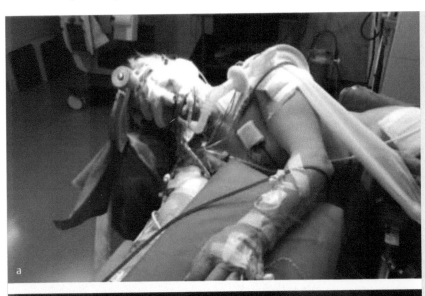

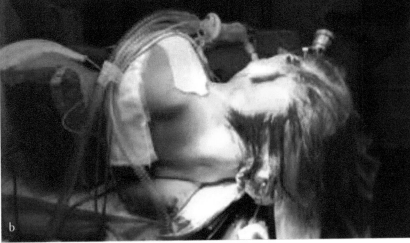

Fig. 5.1 (a, b) Park-bench positioning of patient for lateral and posterior approach to skull base.

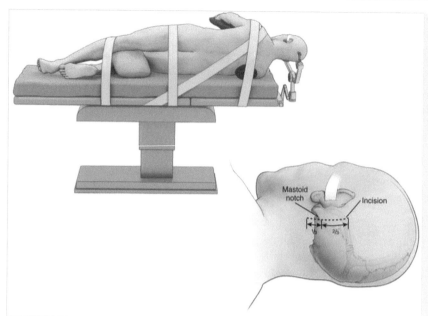

Fig. 5.2 View of patient positioning lateral on the operating table for left-sided tumor resection. Insert demonstrates the incision position for left-sided microvascular decompression for trigeminal neuralgia.

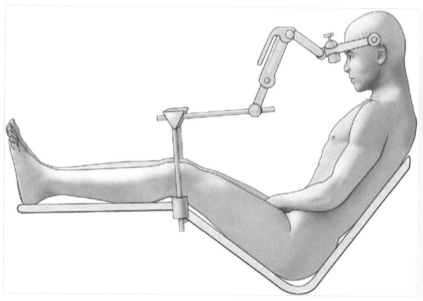

Fig. 5.3 Lateral view of patient placed in sitting position.

dependent axillary neurovascular structures) must be correctly placed, and leg positions and bony protuberances must be padded with foam; in some instances the elbows may be wrapped to avoid ulnar neuropathy from pressure point contact at the ulnar groove. Metal edges should be isolated from the patient, and abnormal flexion or extension of the extremities should be checked for to avoid diminished blood flow and nerve injury. Padding should also be placed under the heels if supine and pillows placed between the knees to avoid peroneal and lateral thigh nerve injury.

5.2.5 Sitting Position

Of all positions used for skull base procedures, the sitting position has undergone the most scrutiny (▶ Fig. 5.3). The theoretical advantage of the sitting position is that it allows for improved cerebral relaxation and promotes gravity drainage of blood and cerebrospinal fluid (CSF).[8] The complications, however, are numerous and include hemodynamic instability, VAE with the possibility of paradoxical air embolism, pneumocephalus, quadriplegia (especially in the presence of extreme neck flexion), and compressive neuropathy.[9,10] Another potential complication includes inadequate cerebral perfusion, but this may be balanced by a reduction in cerebral rate of metabolic oxygen consumption.[11]

Early physiologic studies reveal significant changes when a patient assumes the upright position. Cardiac and systemic vascular resistance are known to increase by 19% and 10%, respectively, and stroke volume and cardiac index may decrease by as much as 21% and 10%, respectively.[12] In the presence of inhalational anesthetic agents, arterial hypotension may be profound, especially because these agents cause vasodilation, with venous pooling in the lower extremities, and cardiovascular depression.[13] It is essential that the anesthesiologist carefully monitor systemic blood pressure as the patient assumes the sitting position. Interventions to maintain blood pressure may include fluid administration, decreasing inhalational agent concentration, compression of distal extremities, and short-term infusions of phenylephrine or other vasoactive drugs.

There is a perceived advantage of the sitting position from the point of view of the respiratory system. Ventilation is unimpeded, because diaphragmatic excursion is greater than in the horizontal position and consequently airway ventilation pressure is lower.[14]

It is important to keep in mind these potential complications when attempting skull base procedures in sitting positions. A vital role for the anesthesiologist who is taking care of the sitting patient is to ensure that the entire care team participates in the careful positioning of the patient. Recent reviews have gone as far as to list contraindications for using this position, including advanced age, hypertonia, chronic obstructive lung disease, and diagnosed patent foramen ovale.[14]

5.3 Complications during Skull Base Procedures

5.3.1 Venous Air Embolism

Venous air embolism (VAE) is one of the complication that concerns physicians most during skull base surgery. Because skull base procedures deal with venous structures that do not collapse and that are typically held open by bone, it is easy to see how venous air can be entrained via one or several of these open venous plexuses. The occurrence of VAE is especially concerning in patients who have a patent foramen ovale (present in 10–30% of the population), in which the potential for paradoxical venous air embolus is high (▶ Fig. 5.4). Matjasko and colleagues have described four grades of VAE seen during sitting craniotomies.[15] These grades (I–IV) relate to changes in precordial Doppler sounds, changes in end-tidal carbon dioxide (ETCO$_2$) levels, ability to aspirate air, and the presence of hemodynamic instability:

- Grade I: characteristic changes in Doppler sounds
- Grade II: changes in the Doppler sound plus fall of end-expiratory CO$_2$ concentration by more than 0.4%
- Grade III: changes in Doppler sounds, fall in end-expiratory CO$_2$ concentration, and aspiration of air through the atrial catheter
- Grade IV: combination of preceding signs with arterial hypotension over 20% and/or arrhythmia or other pathological ECG changes

Factors that play a role in the development of VAE include a pressure gradient between the surgical field and the right atrium, the surgical technique employed, and the amount of air entrained. Moreover, many neurosurgical patients are hypovolemic, which reduces central venous pressure and further increases the risk of a VAE. The bone has been noted to be the source of VAE in 43% of all sitting craniotomies in which an air embolus has occurred. The incidence of neurosurgical skull base VAE has been noted to be 28% for sitting craniotomies, compared with 5% for supine and prone positions.[16] Because many skull base resections could involve the jugular vein and cavernous or sigmoid sinuses, and considering that some positioning requires head elevation, the risk of passive air entrainment is increased. With the translabyrinthine or retrosigmoid approach, the patient is usually supine and no prophylactic measure to monitor or protect for VAE is necessary. Although VAE is frequently detected (a 72% incidence of VAE was detected by transesophageal echocardiography [TEE] in one study[17]), its overall morbidity is currently low, at less than 0.36%.

Monitoring for VAE has been extensively described and usually consists of one or more of the following devices: in descending order of sensitivity, TEE, precordial Doppler (in the right third to sixth intercostal space), pulmonary artery pressure, ETCO$_2$/end-tidal nitrogen, right atrial pressure, ECG, and esophageal stethoscope.[14] Although many clinicians have used a transesophageal echo for detection of VAE, the high sensitivity produces too many false positives, reducing specificity as a monitor for detection of air entrainment.[18] In addition, TEE is expensive and requires that trained personnel be available for

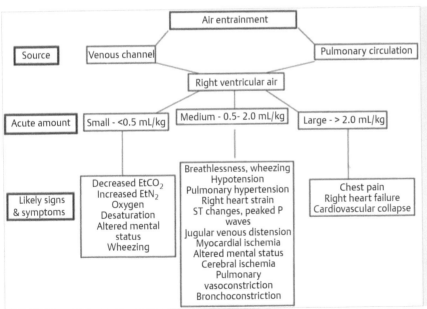

Fig. 5.4 Adverse sequelae from air embolism are dependent on the volume of air as well as the rate of entrainment. Small acute volumes are often well tolerated, whereas larger volumes have substantial effects predominating on cardiovascular, pulmonary and cerebral organ systems. ETCO$_2$ = entitled carbon dioxide; ETNO$_2$ = entitled nitrogen.

Table 5.1 Comparison of methods for detecting vascular air embolism

Method of detection	Sensitivity	Availability	Invasiveness	Limitations
TEE	High (0.02)	Low	High	Expertise required, expensive, invasive
Precordial Doppler	High (0.05)	Moderate	None	Obese patients
PA catheter	High (0.25)	Moderate	High	Fixed distance, small orifice
TCD	High	Moderate	None	Expertise required
ETN$_2$	Moderate (0.5)	Low	None	N$_2$O, hypotension
ETCO$_2$	Moderate (0.5)	Moderate	None	Pulmonary disease
Oxygen saturation	Low	High	None	Late changes
Direct visualization	Low	High	None	No physiologic data
Esophageal stethoscope	Low (1.5)	High	Low	Late changes
ECG	Low (1.25)	High	Low	Late changes

Abbreviations: ECG, electrocardiogram; ETCO$_2$, end-tidal carbon dioxide gas; ETN$_2$, end-tidal nitrogen gas; N$_2$O, nitrous oxide; PA, pulmonary artery; TCD, transcranial Doppler; TEE, transesophageal echocardiography.
Source: Reproduced with permission from Mirski MA, Lele AV, Fitzsimmons L, Toung TJK, Diagnosis and treatment of vascular air embolism, Anesthesiology 2007;106:154–177.

interpretation. TEE has also been associated with vocal cord paralysis from recurrent laryngeal nerve palsy after prolonged use (► Table 5.1).

Recommended therapeutic measures in the event of air entrainment include bilateral compression of the jugular veins, flooding of the wound with saline on the part of the surgeon, discontinuation of nitrous oxide, aspiration of air from a central catheter, and downward tilt of the surgical table. An atrial catheter is usually placed to allow efficient aspiration of trapped air in the heart. Accordingly, it is beneficial for the right atrial catheter to be multiorificed in nature. Bunegin-Albin air aspiration catheters can be difficult to place, for the catheter tip must be in the right atrium, a position that is hard to confirm without use of radiographic imaging or ECG tracing (biphasic P-wave morphology). A trial of placement of right atrial air aspiration catheters noted that the intravenous ECG P-wave morphology that correlated with the right atrial superior vena cava junction, identified by TEE, was the largest monophasic negative P wave without any biphasic component.[19] Another common practice after air entrainment is to attempt to change the patient's position from sitting to left lateral recumbent, but this has been refuted by Geissler and colleagues,[20] who noted that body position had no effect on hemodynamics, nor any on outflow obstruction. Hypotension and a decrease in coronary perfusion pressure appeared to play more of a role in explaining the cardiovascular effects of air emboli.

The role of positive end-expiratory pressure (PEEP) has also come into question. Schmitt and colleagues[17] noted that when PEEP was released, there was a significant occurrence of air emboli as documented by TEE. The group postulates that a sudden decrease of moderate PEEP might decrease right atrial pressure and subsequently increase venous return from cerebral veins. This would result in an increase in air entrainment and possibly an increase in the detectable number of VAE.

5.3.2 Pneumocephalus

Another complication associated with skull base surgery is pneumocephalus, defined as the presence of intraventricular air. In a retrospective review that compared sitting, park-bench, and prone positioning, 100% of the patients in the sitting position, 73% of those in the park-bench position, and 57% of those in the prone position had evidence of intraventricular air.[21] This has been attributed to the large amount of CSF drained as a result of the gravitational effect. A patient in the sitting position is subject to the effects of gravity more than in other positions. As a result, more CSF is ultimately drained, leading to the high incidence of pneumocephalus seen in sitting patients.

Not every case of intraventricular air results in tension pneumocephalus. Historically, approximately 3% of sitting posterior fossa cases were noted to have developed tension pneumocephalus.[9] Postoperative care and length of surgery play a role in the development of tension pneumocephalus, but single contributing factors such as preexisting ventriculoperitoneal shunts, the use of nitrous oxide, and intraoperative diuretics do not appear to play a solitary role.[21]

5.3.3 Macroglossia/Facial Swelling

A rare but potentially catastrophic complication of skull base surgery includes the development of macroglossia. Several case reports describe the occurrence of macroglossia in the immediate postoperative period, but overall incidence is around 1%.[22] Venous drainage of the face, tongue, larynx and orbits enters the internal jugular system, potentially kinking and leading to partial or complete obstruction of the system when the neck is maximally flexed. In the worst case scenario, this may lead to thrombosis of the internal jugular vein.[23]

Other theories regarding the etiology of macroglossia include arterial compression, a neurogenic event, reperfusion injury, and impaired lymphatic drainage.[6,24] Lam and colleagues[6] believe that there is a role for reperfusion injury, for many cases are not associated with cerebral swelling and edema, a condition that might be expected with presence of internal jugular venous obstruction. Obesity, neck flexion, local compression, and long surgical duration have been identified as risk factors and should be kept in mind when patients present for skull base procedures. Regardless of the specific etiology of macroglossia, careful positioning of the head and neck is essential. As a rule, we ensure a space of approximately two fingerbreadths between the mandible and clavicle to prevent venous occlusion. Leaving the patient intubated postoperatively and using steroids will protect the airway and possibly quicken resolution. In cases of severe macroglossia, tracheostomy may be necessary.

5.3.4 Cerebrovascular Complications

Fortunately cerebrovascular accidents and complications are rare during skull base procedures. Injury to the carotid artery is one of the most feared complications and may lead to stroke and other brain injuries. Carotid repair may be required and may include saphenous vein bypass graft from the extracranial carotid artery to the petrous carotid artery and superficial temporal to middle cerebral artery bypass.[25] Usually, when the carotid artery is affected by tumor, a balloon-occlusion test will be performed preoperatively to help identify those patients who would tolerate the sacrifice of the carotid artery if it were to become necessary during the procedure.

"Blowout injury," another carotid vascular complication, is caused when the carotid artery is inadvertently lacerated. Blood loss may be brisk at the time of the injury, and interventions include packing and urgent angiography with balloon occlusion or vascular stenting.[26] Delayed blowout injury can also occur if the carotid artery is exposed in the nasopharynx, but this might be preventable through muscle flap coverage.[25]

Vasospasm has also been reported and may result in stroke. It tends to be seen in younger patients and is thought to be caused by a myogenic reaction in the vessel wall. Vasospasm may result from arterial contact with fresh blood or arterial traction. Treatment usually consists of topical vasodilators such as papaverine, although systemic drugs may also have a role.[27]

5.3.5 Arrhythmias

Because many skull base procedures are in the area of the trigeminal and vagus nerves, as well as the brainstem, arrhythmias during these surgical procedures may be common. Direct stimulation of the vagus may lead to negative chronotropy and inotropy manifested as sinus bradycardia, bradycardia terminating in asystole, asystole with no bradycardia, and arterial hypotension. When the trigeminal nerve is involved, sensory nerve endings send signals to the sensory nuclei of the Gasserian ganglion. These signals ultimately continue along the short internuncial nerve fibers to connect with the motor nuclei efferent pathway of the vagus nerve, producing a cardioinhibitory effect.[28] In this situation, the anesthesiologist should alert the surgeon and may request that the surgeon release traction or choose pharmacologic intervention with a vagolytic substance such as glycopyrrolate or atropine. Atropine, because of its quick onset, may be the drug of choice, but its duration of action is shorter than that of glycopyrrolate. Over time, the reflex tends to decrease in intensity.

This trigeminocardiac reflex (TCR) has garnered much interest in recent years. There seems to be a relationship between light anesthesia (cerebral state index [CSI] > 60) and TCR occurrence.[29] The severity of the response with larger mean arterial pressure (MAP) drops and occurrence of asystole suggests a more severe reflex with a light plane of anesthesia. The best-known anesthetic risk factors for TCR are the fast-acting opioids, such as fentanyl.[30] The effect of propofol, an anesthetic that is currently often used in skull base surgery, has not been fully analyzed. However, studies examining its excitatory postsynaptic potential on cardiovascular neurons in the nucleus ambiguous showed no relative change.[31] At present, a trend toward higher anesthetic doses' having an inhibiting effect on the TCR seems to be real. The prevalence of TCR in a CSI > 60 group was consistently higher than in a CSI 40 to 60 group and a CSI < 40 (deep anesthesia) group. Furthermore, there is a strong trend for light anesthesia to be a risk factor for a more intense asystolic reflex as compared with deeper anesthetic levels. There also seems to be a significant correlation between propofol and the occurrence and intensity of TCR. Evidence suggests that propofol has an inhibitory effect on either the afferent trigeminal neurons or the efferent cardiac vagal neurons.[31] The use of propofol infusions as part of the anesthetic technique will help reduce the incidence and severity of the TCR while producing better anesthetic conditions for other monitoring modalities such as somatosensory evoked potentials (SSEPs) and motor evoked potentials, if they are used.

In most cases, an anticholinergic agent such as glycopyrrate—or, more likely, atropine—will be used to treat the effects of TCR. However, atropine does not totally prevent TCR.[32] In addition, atropine itself can cause severe arrhythmia. Some practitioners now recommend using low-dose epinephrine 10 to 50 μg IV to stabilize cardiovascular function after TCR.

If skull base surgery involves resection of a glomus jugulare or vagale tumor, then one must be aware of the tumor's catecholamine-secreting potential. Glomus jugulare tumors may be considered arteriovenous malformations, may be giant in size, and may be associated with multiple paragangliomas. The incidence of catecholamine secretion is around 4% and can be associated with tachyarrhythmias, hypertension, sweating, myocardial infarction, and cardiovascular collapse, which reflects catecholamine excess. The anesthesiologist should be prepared to treat any hypertensive crisis arising from manipulation of a catecholamine-secreting tumor. Appropriate invasive arterial monitoring is essential, and use of fast- and short-acting vasodilators, such as nitroglycerin, nitroprusside, and, to a lesser extent, phentolamine, is essential. The resection of glomus jugulare tumors may also result in new cranial nerve (CN) injuries, with the highest being of CNs VII and IX.[33]

5.3.6 Blood Loss

Blood loss during resection of skull base tumors may be significant, and the taking of appropriate preoperative measures is essential. Many such tumors are highly vascular, and preoperative assessment is necessary to delineate involvement of the cavernous sinus and jugular bulb. Notably, meningiomas have been shown to produce tissue plasminogen activator, which may lead to increased fibrinolysis during resection.[34]

Preoperative embolization of feeding vessels may lead to decreased blood loss via a decrease in blood flow and pressure within the tumor.[25] Recent studies have evaluated the use of tranexamic acid, a synthetic derivative of the amino acid, lysine, that reversibly blocks lysine-binding sites on plasminogen molecules, preventing conversion to plasmin and inhibiting fibrin clot dissolution.[35] Tranexamic acid may be particularly advantageous in skull base procedures, because even small amounts of bleeding near eloquent cranial base structures could be problematic. The drug has a favorable safety profile but has been noted to increase the risk of cerebral ischemia.[36] It has also been shown to increase the risk of seizures when given in high doses.[37] In several studies, its use with skull base surgery reduced the frequency of transfusion of allogenic blood products, with no apparent increase in seizures or thrombotic complications. The use of this drug may prevent some of the complications of administering large amounts of blood products, including transfusion-associated circulatory overload and transfusion-associated lung injury.

5.3.7 Peripheral Nerve/Cranial Nerve Injuries

Protection from peripheral nerve injuries is of major concern during skull base procedures. All positions, from supine to seated, have at one time or another been associated with nerve injuries. Varying degrees of injury have been noted, with Seddon's classification describing three broad classifications of injury: neurapraxia, axonotmesis, and neurotmesis. Neurapraxia is a mild insult that results in conduction failure across an affected segment; this reversible injury tends to be that most seen during surgical procedures. Axonotmesis occurs when the axon is physically disrupted but the epineurium and perineurium are preserved; recovery depends on the speed of neural regeneration. The worst injuries are those in which neurotmesis has taken place: there is complete disruption of the nerve and support structures, and the prognosis for recovery is exceedingly poor.[38]

Although brachial plexus injuries have been often described due to the contralateral rotation of the head and traction of the ipsilateral shoulder downward,[39] other injuries have been noted, including common peroneal nerve leading to foot drop.[40] Ulnar nerve injuries may also occur, but the complete etiology of their occurrence has yet to be determined. The role of abnormal extension, rotation, obesity, and preexisting disease states, such as diabetes mellitus, have been mentioned as possible contributing factors for ulnar nerve injury. Whatever the etiology, meticulous attention to appropriate intraoperative padding and awareness of the existence of preexisting neurological defects is essential when taking care of these patients.

There has been an increased awareness of neurologic injury to the upper extremities after positioning for these surgical procedures. SSEPs are a proven method of monitoring the spinal cord and brain to prevent neurologic injury and have also been used to monitor the arms and brachial plexus during skull base procedures in which the head is turned contralaterally and the ipsilateral shoulder is pushed down to open the approach for retrosigmoid/translabyrinthine craniotomy. Many studies have found this monitoring modality to be a valid intraoperative tool for monitoring positionally related peripheral nerve injuries in real time.[41,42] It offers 78% sensitivity for detecting upper extremity sensory deficits and 100% sensitivity for detecting combined sensory and motor deficits, with a 98% specificity for predicting normal postoperative function.[43] SSEPs are obtained after the patient is asleep and in a neutral position and are used as a baseline for another set of SSEP waveforms obtained after positioning. If major changes occur, the positioning is readjusted, especially as concerns the affected extremity.

Another set of SSEP values is determined; if improved, the surgery proceeds.

It is plausible that nerve compression and ischemia can be further complicated and more often observed in diabetic patients or those with large body habitus, especially because the most severe injuries are noted in larger individuals. We have extensively studied the technique to monitor for nerve injury during skull base procedures, and based on our results, increased patient body mass index appears to correlate with an increased likelihood of experiencing postoperative peripheral nerve injury due to malpositioning.[44] We believe that this monitoring technique should be used for routine assessment of the brachial plexus during these procedures or at least obtained for high-risk obese patients.

5.4 Monitoring and Anesthesia

Monitoring for skull base procedures depends on the type of procedure to be performed, the vascular and nerve structures involved, and the position in which the patient will be placed for the surgery. In all instances the patient will have standard routine monitoring such as ECG, noninvasive blood pressure, pulse oximetry, capnography, and temperature. Other monitors are added as the complexity, blood loss, surgical trauma, and comorbidities of the patient are factored in. Monitoring for skull base procedures must ensure adequate central nervous system perfusion, maintenance of cardiovascular stability, and the integrity of the neurologic pathways that are being manipulated. Arterial line placement is standard for most intracranial and extracranial procedures of the skull base. Invasive blood pressure monitoring allows closer control of blood pressure and better titration of hyperventilation and blood pH. In addition, hemoglobin levels and electrolyte abnormalities can be easily detected by following serial arterial blood samples obtained from this catheter. Central access with either large-bore single lumen or double lumen catheters is contingent on the length of the surgery, anticipated blood loss, need for estimation of central vascular volume, and position of the patient.

Depending on tumor type and location, neurophysiologic monitoring may also be employed to detect disruption of neural tracts or trauma to CNs that may be near the site of surgery.

Cranial nerve monitoring has markedly decreased postoperative morbidity after skull base surgery. Electromyography (EMG) of the facial, vagus, or trigeminal nerve is used during surgical resection to identify the nerve and preserve neurologic integrity, especially if the nerve is surrounded by a tumor.[45] EMG of CNs provides early recognition of surgical trauma, facilitates tumor excision, identifies nerve dysfunction, and confirms nerve function after the tumor is removed. At any given level of neuromuscular blockade, a facial muscle response is more resistant to neuromuscular blocking agents than a peripheral muscle.[46] This is due to larger motor unit size and the increased number of neuromuscular junctions in the facial muscles. Several studies have demonstrated that neuromuscular blockade, titrated to a T_1 of 25%, still allows adequate response from compound motor action potentials of facial muscles to adequately monitor nerve function.[47] Nerve irritation and tumor infiltration, however, can lead to reduced or blocked conduction. In addition, external or mechanical noise artifacts could mask muscular contraction, and if high-dose inhalational agents are used, muscle activity with nerve stimulation can be further reduced.

If muscle relaxants must be used to facilitate surgical resection, alternative methods for monitoring the facial nerve may be used. The first method stimulates the nerve at the stylomastoid foramen.[48] Antidromic responses are recorded in the operative field. However, this method is awkward to use and does not provide the information obtained by continuous recording. Nerve action potentials can also be recorded at the stylomastoid junction, but this technique is an evoked response. There is no audible feedback compared with EMG and no information concerning this method's sensitivity in detecting injury.

The final method for determining facial nerve integrity in the presence of muscle relaxants is the brainstem facial evoked response[49]; this nerve monitoring method is based on cross-auricular responses to sound that controls ear movement. The facial nerve response is recorded at the mastoid after sound stimulation of the contralateral ear. This technique is technically challenging because of the need for digital computer filtering.

EMG monitoring is important for improved outcomes after skull base surgery. The test relies on measurement of compound muscle action potential (CMAP) generated either by facial muscles or by those of the oropharynx or vocal cords. The motor unit potentials, when summed together, result in the measured CMAP. An adequate assessment of nerve conduction with EMG requires stimulation proximal to the potential site of injury. Nerves suffering from mild to moderate trauma will exhibit reductions in amplitude with increasing amounts of current to elicit a response. After ensuring careful electrode placement for facial nerve electromyographic monitoring (FNEMG) or proper ET tube placement with the nerve integrity monitoring ET tube, both nerves VII and X can be monitored. Prass and Luders described two types of CMAP activity depending on the type of nerve irritation.[50] The first type is the burst potential, which consists of a polyphasic response due to activation of multiple motor units. These are caused by direct contact of the nerve with surgical instruments and are fatigable with repeated nerve contact. The second type of continuous free-running CMAP is a train potential. This could last seconds to minutes and is generated by multiple asynchronous responses from different motor units. Train potentials may be caused by mechanical injury (pressure or stretch) or thermal changes to the nerves. With greater injury to the nerve, a greater intensity and longer duration of nerve potential will be evident. Thermal injury from electrocautery or laser may only become evident on EMG in a delayed manner and may be noted as a gradual increase in baseline but may also be associated with electrical silence. Other causes of nontraumatic train potentials include drill vibration energy transmission to the nerve, temperature irritation from hot or cold irrigants, and hypertonic saline solutions. Even aspiration of CSF from the cerebellopontine angle could produce a drop in temperature, triggering a train response.

Besides assessing for injury, nerve stimulation EMG can be used to identify the nerve within the tumor to help salvage facial function and nerve integrity during the resection. The stimulating probe is touched to or near the nerve, generating a true EMG-stimulated machine gun–sounding response (**Video 5.1**, **Video 5.2**, and **Video 5.3**). Stimulating current levels are normally adjusted from 0.05 to 2 mA. False positives can occur with stimulation-triggered EMG from a phenomenon known as current jump, which happens when volume conduction of current through nearby tissue leads to nerve stimulation. False negative errors can also occur when the presence of CSF or blood in the field produces electrical current shunting away from the nerve of interest. The use of intraoperative EMG has improved outcomes, reducing both facial nerve and vagal injury and reducing morbidity after skull base surgery.

The ability to monitor the adequacy of an anesthetic is important, because it aids in the titration of anesthetic drugs during maintenance periods and, in particular, will prevent movement during stimulation, which can be particularly problematic in unparalyzed patients undergoing skull base procedures. Some have noted bispectral index (BIS) monitoring as an important modality to monitor depth of anesthesia. However, BIS monitors higher-level brain activity and hypnosis and might not be an effective monitor with which to predict post incisional or other movement under anesthesia. FNEMG is usually performed during many skull base procedures, because it helps identify the nerve and reduces iatrogenic injury during tumor resection. We have also noted FNEMG to be an effective monitor of anesthetic depth and a good monitor for predicting and preventing patient movements.[51] FNEMG was highly reliable as a monitor with which to predict movement, having a negative predictive value of 95%. Lack of FNEMG activity is an assurance that the patient will not move. We continuously use FNEMG as a monitor of anesthetic depth during skull base procedures and believe that the use of an opioid infusion as part of the anesthetic technique will prevent movement in nonparalyzed patients undergoing skull base resection.

Brainstem auditory evoked potentials and SSEP monitoring may also be used during resection of skull base tumors, especially if there is possible vascular compromise or ischemia due to temporary occlusion of vascular structures or manipulation of the brainstem. In general, anesthetic effects on Brainstem Auditory Evoked Responses (BAERs) are not dramatic. Slow shifts may be seen as the concentration of inhalational agents increase. Improvement or preservation of hearing may also be accomplished with the use of BAERs. Since these recordings are of small amplitude, thousands of responses must be recorded to acquire an adequate average. Frequently the responses are abnormal and smaller than normal due to the effects of the tumor. Also the time interval required to acquire sufficient responses may reduce the sensitivity of this technique in determining neural injury during tumor removal. Short-latency BAERs are usually resistant to both intravenous and inhalational agents. Increasing blood levels of barbiturates and ketamine will increase interpeak latency. In fact, another hypnotic agent propofol given at 2 mg/kg bolus, followed by an infusion, will increase the latency without changes in amplitude.[52] Inhalational agents such as isoflurane, sevoflurane, and desflurane also increase the latency of the waveform without an appreciable change in amplitude. Conversely, midlatency AEPs are predictably affected in a dose-dependent manner by an increase in latency with a predictable decrease in amplitude.[53,54] Hypercapnia does not change BAERs, but severe hypoxia will depress waveform amplitude.[55] Body temperature will also affect BAERs, with reduced temperature prolonging latency of the observed waveform.[56] In most instances in which changes in waveform resulted from anesthetics, the observations will occur bilaterally. Unilateral decreases in waveform would be indicative of nerve damage secondary to surgical manipulation.

Finally, somatosensory evoked responses may also be used to assess the integrity of the brainstem and other subcortical structures during surgical techniques involving the skull base. SSEP represents reproducible electrical activity of cortical and subcortical structures time-locked to a peripheral nerve stimulus. SSEPs can assess the sensory system from the peripheral nerve through the spinal cord and brainstem to the cerebral cortex. A decrease in amplitude of 50% or greater and an increase in latency of 10% or greater constitutes a significant change that should be investigated.[57] Because SSEPs have a central component to their measurement, they are very sensi-

tive to the effects of anesthetic agents. All volatile anesthetics produce a dose-dependent increase in SSEP latency, an increase in central conduction time, and a decrease in amplitude (▶ Table 5.2).[58] Satisfactory monitoring of early cortical SSEPs is possible with 0.5 to 1.0 minimum alveolar concentration (MAC) isoflurane, desflurane, or sevoflurane, the latter two of which agents permit slightly higher concentrations with satisfactory results.

How volatile anesthetics differ quantitatively is still not entirely known, but sevoflurane and desflurane are associated with less amplitude reduction than isoflurane at a MAC range of 0.7 to 1.3.[59] Intravenous anesthetics generally affect SSEPs less than inhaled anesthetics do. SSEP waveforms are preserved even at high doses of narcotics and barbiturates. Intravenous

Table 5.2 Effects of inhaled anesthetics on somatosensory evoked potentials

Early cortical waveform			
Anesthetic drug/concentration	Latency	Amplitude	Subcortical waveform
Halothane			
• 0.5 MAC + 60% N_2O	<10% ↑	≈ 60% ↓	Negligible
• 1.0 MAC + 60% N_2O	<10% ↑	≈ 70% ↓	Negligible
• 1.5 MAC + 60% N_2O	10–15% ↑	≈ 80% ↓	Negligible
• 1.5 MAC (alone)	10–15% ↑	≈ 70% ↓	Negligible
Isoflurane			
• 0.5 MAC + 60% N_2O	<10% ↑	50–70% ↓	Negligible
• 0.5 MAC (alone)	<15% ↑	<30% ↑	Negligible
• 1.0 MAC + 60% N_2O	10–15% ↑	50–75% ↓	Negligible
• 1.0 MAC (alone)	15% ↑	≈ 50% ↓	Negligible
• 1.5 MAC + 60% N_2O[a]	>15% ↑	>75% ↓	5% ↑ in latency
• 1.6 MAC (alone)[a]	15–20% ↑	60–70% ↓	5% ↑ in latency
			20% ↓ in amplitude
Enflurane			
• 0.5 MAC + 60% N_2O	<10% ↑	≈ 50% ↓	Negligible
• 0.2–0.6 MAC (alone)	<10% ↑	<20% ↓	N/A
• 1.0 MAC + 60% N_2O[a]	20% ↑	≈ 85% ↓	Negligible
• 1.5 MAC + 60% N_2O	Not recordable	Not recordable	Negligible
• 1.5 MAC (alone)[a]	>25% ↑	≈ 85% ↓	Negligible
Sevoflurane			
• 0.5 MAC + 66% N_2O	<5% ↑	38%	Negligible
• 1.0 MAC + 66% N_2O	<10% ↑	≈ 45% ↓	Negligible
• 1.5 MAC + 66% N_2O	<10% ↑	≈ 50% ↓	Negligible
• 1.7–2.5 MAC	10–15% ↑	≈ 100% ↑	N/A
Desflurane			
• 0.5 MAC	<5% ↑	<20% ↓	Negligible
• 1.0 MAC	3–8% ↑	30–40% ↓	Negligible
• 1.5 MAC	≤10% ↑	<50% ↓	Negligible
• Any with 65% N_2O[b]	≥15% ↑	>60% ↓	Negligible
Nitrous oxide			
• 60–65%	No effect	50–55% ↓	Negligible

Abbreviations: ↑, increase; ↓, decrease; MAC, minimum alveolar concentration; N_2O, nitrous oxide; N/A, data not available.

Source: Reproduced from Banoub M, Tetzlaff JE, Schubert A, Pharmacologic and physiologic influences affecting sensory evoked potentials: implications for perioperative monitoring, Anesthesiology 2003;99(3):716–737.

Notes: All data are from humans. A result of "negligible" indicates less than a 5% change in latency.

[a]In a substantial fraction of patients, wave forms were not attainable at this concentration.

[b]Complete loss of wave form observed only with 1.5 MAC desflurane plus 65% N_2O.

agents only modestly affect early and intermediate SSEP components. Most authors report clinically unimportant changes in SSEP latency and amplitude with the administration of opioids given in either anesthetic or analgesic doses. This makes opioids useful as part of the anesthetic when intraoperative physiologic monitoring is used. Propofol affects the SSEP waveform by increasing latency by 8% at a dose of 2.5 mg/kg while having no effect on amplitudes.[60] Total intravenous anesthesia with propofol and sufentanil prolonged cortical latency 10 to 15% and reduced the amplitude by 50%. However, SSEP waveforms stabilized and after 30 minutes were compatible with intraoperative monitoring.[61] Propofol affects synaptic transmission more than axonal conduction. When used as a sedative hypnotic along with opioids, propofol reduces SSEP amplitudes less than N_2O or midazolam. Anesthetics that result in latency prolongation or amplitude depression may confuse the interpretation of SSEP changes and potentially risk either not detecting a critical event or providing excessive false negative interpretations.

In some instances, etomidate or ketamine can be added to the anesthetic regimen to facilitate SSEP waveform measurement. Both can dramatically increase cortical amplitude up to 400% above preinduction baseline in some patients.[62] Subcortical amplitude is reduced by 50%.

The effects of anesthesia on evoked potentials can be greater in neurologically impaired patients than in those without preoperative deficits, so the anesthetic regimen must be adjusted to carefully limit the concentration of volatile anesthetics to less than 1 MAC or to avoid N_2O. If neurophysiologic monitoring will include electrocochleography or SSEP, volatile anesthetics with N_2O should be limited to 0.5 MAC concentrations. Without N_2O, 1-MAC concentrations may be used.

The use of continuous infusions of intravenous anesthetics (propofol) and opioids with low concentrations of background inhalational anesthetics is ideal and recommended for intraoperative neurophysiologic monitoring during skull base procedures. Inhalational agents such as sevoflurane and desflurane have low blood gas partition coefficients and reduced fat solubility. These agents produce rapid induction and emergence with minimal accumulation of anesthetic, even after prolonged anesthesia. In addition, short-acting opioids such as remifentanil are extremely potent and have minimal accumulation when given as an infusion. The half-life is 3 to 8 minutes, and metabolism is produced by nonspecific esterases.

Remifentanil infusions for large skull base procedures may not be an ideal option. The drug produces a rapid emergence from anesthesia with minimal hangover effects and can be easily titrated to reduce acute hemodynamic responses to intense stimulation. It does not accumulate and is ideal for long procedures, especially in patients who have renal compromise. Remifentanil has also been noted to be an ideal agent with which to lessen the risk of movement in the absence of muscle relaxation, a state that occurs in many instances during skull base surgery. Remifentanil, however, also increases the probability of bradycardia, especially at higher doses. This can be problematic during skull base procedures in which the risk of bradycardia or asystole is high from possible TCR. The other significant issue with the use of remifentanil is blood pressure management during the early recovery period. Many patients experience hypertension and tachycardia after discontinuation of remifentanil, most likely due to early analgesic requirements:

the half-life of remifentanil is short, and patients go from a state of intense analgesia to no analgesic effect within 5 minutes. It is likely that the use of remifentanil-based anesthesia will result in lower incidence of emergence hypertension if analgesia for early recovery is provided before emergence.[63]

An advantage to remifentanil is that little or no interaction between residual effects of maintenance opioids and opioid administrated for emergence would be expected. In addition, remifentanil has been associated with hyperalgesia after discontinuation. This may complicate postoperative pain management, though the overall incidence of this complication is unclear. Although we still use remifentanil for some skull base procedures, we do not use the drug when there might be a higher risk of postoperative bleeding due to resections of large tumors that have large vascular beds or feeding vessels. In these situations, longer-acting opioids (fentanyl or sufentanil) are used as background infusions to supplement the inhalational agent. The anesthetic technique that produces the best operating conditions for surgery and CN monitoring uses an anesthetic induction in which propofol and fentanyl are coupled with a short-acting muscle relaxant to facilitate intubation. Maintenance anesthesia is provided with low-dose desflurane or sevoflurane administered in a 50:50 air/O_2 mixture with a background infusion of either fentanyl 2 µg/kg/hour or remifentanil 0.25 to 0.35 µg/kg/minute. No further muscle relaxants are administered.

5.5 Anesthesia Concerns with Vascular Lesions

Skull base surgeries for highly vascular tumors may present many problems related to intraoperative anesthetic management. If the possibility of cerebral hypoperfusion exists, methods of providing cerebral protection must be incorporated into the anesthetic plan. After resection of a tumor involving the carotid, complications are thought to occur by two mechanisms: acute infarction after interruption of blood flow and infarction as a result of clot propagation or embolic phenomenon from static blood. Despite advances in surgical techniques and preoperative assessment, patients are still at risk for transient or permanent stroke, coma, or death from thromboembolic or sustained hypoperfusion. For these reasons, use of perioperative anticoagulation and antiplatelet therapy, plus careful intraoperative blood pressure control with brain protection measures, are important. If the skull base procedure is likely to cause interruption of cerebral blood flow, the intraoperative anesthetic management can be tailored to produce optimal perfusion to the areas affected by the interruption of blood flow. The patient should be hemodiluted prior to interruption of perfusion to reduce blood viscosity and increase blood flow.[64] Hematocrit should be approximately 30% so as to provide the best oxygen transport and cerebral oxygen metabolism. Glucose concentrations are also important if there is a risk of cerebral ischemia. High plasma glucose levels induce anaerobic glycolysis and lactic acidosis, which results in brain edema and microcirculatory dysregulation.[65] In addition, insulin protects against ischemic-initiated excitatory damage, protects mitochondrial oxidation capacity, decreases serum K^+ levels and glucose use, and directly stimulates Na^+/K^+-ATPase.[66]

Tighter control of plasma glucose may be warranted for improving perioperative outcome, but avoidance of hypoglycemia is equally important.

5.6 Anesthesia and Neuroprotection

If temporary vascular occlusion is anticipated, the anesthetic technique should incorporate strategies for augmenting systemic blood pressure. Cerebral ischemia impairs autoregulation of the cerebral vasculature, resulting in resistance blood vessels that are maximally dilated. Blood flow to the ischemic region becomes pressure-passive. Increasing perfusion pressure improves cerebral blood flow and may reduce cell death in the compromised vascular territory by improving collateral circulation.[67] Phenylephrine and norepinephrine are the most commonly used agents. Phenylephrine does not cause direct cerebral vasoconstriction and is often the drug of choice. The ability of phenylephrine to augment cerebral blood flow is probably due to a systemic effect. The tendency for a reflex decrease in heart rate makes the use of phenylephrine particularly useful in patients with coronary artery disease. Another simple but effective measure with which to reduce cerebral ischemia during temporary disruption of blood flow is to elevate the inspired fraction of oxygen. This results in higher tissue levels than expected based on dissolved oxygen in blood. Increasing numbers of studies support the use of normobaric 100% O_2 in the setting of transient focal ischemia.[68]

The neuroprotective effects of hypothermia are not precisely known but probably relate to reduced cerebral oxygen demand (7–8% per 1 °C), decreased release of excitatory neurotransmitters, and increased release of inhibitory neurotransmitters.[69] Evidence indicates that the relationship between brain protection and the degree of hypothermia is not linear and that mild hypothermia (34 °C) may provide protection against cerebral ischemia.[70] Hypothermia to 34 °C is easily achieved intraoperatively by passive cooling and can be reversed after the restoration of blood flow by conventional methods (convection heaters, circulatory water blankets, forced-air warmers, etc.).

In addition to the physiologic manipulations that can be used to preserve the brain during temporary interruption of blood flow, pharmacologic agents may also be used to decrease neuronal activity and metabolic demand. Cerebral protection may be initiated prior to the occurrence of brain ischemia. The sooner the neuroprotective agent is administered, the better. Conventionally, neuroprotection by anesthetics has been considered in terms of their ability to modify cerebral metabolic rate. Anesthetics appear to depress only metabolism associated with neuronal electrical activity. Hypothermia, by depressing the rate of all biochemical reactions, can reduce the energy requirements associated with maintaining cellular integrity and may be neuroprotective, even in the face of an isoelectric electroencephalogram (EEG). The neuroprotective effect of anesthetics may be due to more than just their ability to reduce $CMRO_2$, for anesthetics such as isoflurane produce states of EEG burst suppression similar to that associated with thiopental but do not provide comparable neuroprotection. Many other anesthetic effects may contribute to neuroprotection,[71] including reduction in intracranial pressure (ICP), anticonvulsant action, free radical scavenging, drug-induced inverse steal, antagonism at voltage-sensitive calcium or sodium channel or ligand-gated calcium channels, potentiation of GABAergic transmission, and attenuation of ischemia-induced neurotransmitter release.

The use of thiopental, which is not clinically available in the United States, is known to protect the brain during cardiac bypass.[72] Thiopental, at doses capable of producing EEG burst suppression, should offer protection during short occlusion times, or longer with continuous infusion of the drug. Barbiturates are also thought to enhance gamma-aminobutyric acid activity and antagonize the N-methyl-D-aspartate receptor, which reduces ischemic excitotoxicity.[73] Barbiturate neuroprotection is likely to be most effective in focal ischemia, in which there remains a marginally perfused penumbral zone where O_2 supply is reduced but synaptic activity is still ongoing. Though a good neuroprotectant, its use is hampered by reduced availability of the drug due to reduced production. Propofol, like barbiturates, will induce burst suppression in a dose-dependent fashion. Furthermore, it is metabolized quickly and thus does not accumulate. Although propofol has been shown to be of some benefit, results of animal studies have been inconclusive compared with those for thiopental.[74] Propofol also reduces voltage-activated sodium channel conduction at concentrations within the clinical range. Its antioxidant properties may also be of benefit. Propofol infusions titrated to produce unresponsiveness (8 mg/kg/h) resulted in a 55% depression of cerebral metabolic rate for glucose as measured during positron emission tomography.[70] Etomidate has also been shown to prevent increases in excitatory neurotransmitters during cerebral ischemia, but its protective role compared with other anesthetics is unclear. Studies have demonstrated that etomidate administration, prior to cerebral ischemia, produces a 30% reduction in PaO_2 levels and a 23% increase in $PaCO_2$ concentrations in the cerebral cortex.[75] These changes were thought to be due to etomidate-associated vasoconstriction and a reduction in cerebral blood flow prior to a drop in cerebral metabolic rate. This reduces etomidate's effectiveness as a neuroprotectant even though its short half-life and hemodynamic stability are superior to those of barbiturates. Etomidate has been associated with significant adrenal cortical suppression. Although this could be problematic for most surgeries, its utility is still present for neurosurgical cases in which patients are routinely administered steroids postoperatively.

Volatile anesthetics can also be used to reduce cerebral metabolism, but their ability to dilate arteries and reduce blood pressure makes them a less than optimal choice when attempting to maintain cerebral perfusion to ischemic areas. Other agents, such as calcium channel blockers and local anesthetics, may provide some added benefit through their ability to block ion channels and reduce Na^+/K^+ transmembrane flux, which reduces basal energy expenditures.[76] Other possible mechanisms for cerebral protection by lidocaine include reduction in $CMRO_2$, modulation of leukocyte activity, and reduction of excitotoxin release.[77] Most of the effective neuroprotective techniques used today involve some combination of pharmacologic therapy coupled with some level of hypothermia or other physiologic manipulation.

If neuroprotection is needed or anticipated, EEG monitoring may be helpful for detection of cerebral ischemia or titration of anesthetic agents used to produce burst suppression.

5.7 Anesthesia for Endoscopic Skull Base Surgery

As in most fields of medicine, neurosurgery has seen a movement toward less invasive procedures. As new imaging devices and surgical techniques have been developed, there has been explosive growth in the area of minimally invasive neurosurgical techniques. One area of such development has been endoscopic skull base surgery, especially for acoustic neuromas and pituitary tumors. Other indications include different types of noncommunicating hydrocephalus and intraventricular diseases such as periventricular tumor and colloid and arachnoid cysts. Endoscopic third ventriculostomy is rapidly becoming the treatment of choice for noncommunicating hydrocephalus. It allows the CSF to flow directly from the third ventricle to the basal subarachnoid spaces. The neuroendoscope has also been used to treat infectious hydrocephalus and intraventricular hemorrhage. Endoscopic removal of cysts, biopsies, paraventricular tumors, and hypothalamic hematomas can be removed by this method. The key goal of anesthetic care is to ensure immobility of the patient, who is usually placed in a head fixation device. There should also be a method to detect, prevent, and treat sharp increases in ICP. The anesthetic technique should also allow for rapid emergence and neurologic assessment. Inhalational anesthetics, usually without N_2O, are used. Derbent et al used sevoflurane with an $ETCO_2$ at 30 ± 2 mmHg to reduce the cerebral vasodilatory effect.[78] However, if remifentanil is also administered, care should be taken to avoid hypertension and tachycardia once the drug is stopped. The endoscopic approach requires an image guidance system that may either be CT- or MR-based. The imaging system helps map the area of interest and guide the resection of the tumor. In addition, specific instruments have been created to maximize efficiency in a tight space.[79]

The patient is usually in a semisitting position, rotated away from the anesthesia team, so the airway is removed from the immediate proximity of the anesthesiologist. Endoscopic endonasal approaches to the anterior, clival, and posterior skull base have reduced the need for postoperative analgesic therapy and the surgical trauma that accompanies these procedures. Endoscopic resections of pituitary tumors, craniopharyngiomas, chordoma, and other tumors have been done in recent years through small incisions through the nostril, glabella, and orbital roof by incisions in the eyebrow, superolateral orbit, and subtemporal regions. Because such approaches reduce blood loss and surgical trauma, anesthetic techniques have been modified to adjust to this new emerging surgical technology. The general aims of the anesthesiologist are to provide hemodynamic stability, maintain cerebral oxygenation, provide favorable conditions for surgical exposure, and facilitate rapid emergence.

Every patient should be monitored as if the endoscopic procedure were a major operation rather than a minimally invasive procedure. Beat-to-beat heart rate and MAP monitoring using an indwelling arterial catheter are strongly recommended for all patients. To measure cerebral perfusion pressure, ICP should be measured; one method of doing so is to measure the pressure inside the endoscope. Endoscopic third ventriculotomy is associated with a wide range of hemodynamic effects ranging from minor changes in heart rate and blood pressure to near-fatal cardiac arrest.[80] The possible mechanisms proposed for these changes include hypothalamic stimulation or damage and acute rise in ICP. In some cases this rise in ICP can be due to excess irrigation fluid (either kinking of the irrigation outflow tube or forceful inflows of irrigate fluid).[81]

If the pituitary is involved, hormone replacement therapy should be continued into the postoperative period. In all instances a careful airway evaluation should be performed, especially if the patient has a pituitary tumor and is secreting abnormal amounts of growth hormone. Acromegalics have particularly problematic airways, and depending on the amount of soft tissue overgrowth of the mandible and the amount of tongue enlargement, these patients could be exceedingly problematic to intubate. If awake, fiber-optic intubation cannot be safely performed; a tracheostomy may be done to facilitate control of the airway. With the exception of pituitary tumors, airway control for other endoscopic skull base procedures is routine. For a transnasal endoscopic approach, the surgeon may want to introduce a vasoconstricting agent into each nostril to prevent bleeding. Traditionally a mixture of cocaine and epinephrine has been used. Although the addition of epinephrine limits systemic absorption, the use of cocaine-containing preparations continues to be associated with a risk of arrhythmia and myocardial infarction. Most endoscopic approaches to the skull base are done with the patient in the supine head-up position, with the head tilted or turned to improve access. The choice of anesthetic technique for these procedures is usually determined by personal preference. A total intravenous technique with propofol and remifentanil provides ideal intraoperative conditions with rapid emergence and extubation. Short-acting inhalational agents can also be used in conjunction with remifentanil. Since postoperative pain is minimal, longer–half-life analgesics are not necessary and anesthetic techniques are modified to produce a rapid emergence with minimal hangover effect. With some of the endoscopic approaches there may be periods of intense stimulation. The short-acting opioids should be titrated against blood pressure. At the conclusion of the endoscopic procedure, the patient should be allowed to emerge from anesthesia rapidly and have no evidence of overt bleeding. If the patient remains hemodynamically stable, is breathing spontaneously with adequate respiratory mechanics, and is following commands, then rapid tracheal extubation can occur. Recently, in a study that compared the sublabial transeptal hypophysectomy to the endoscopic approach, significant reduction was seen in the rate of nasal complications and CSF leaks.[82] Others have revealed that purely endoscopic approaches result in less postoperative pain and less blood loss.[83]

Postoperative complications after these procedures are somewhat different from those associated with other skull base approaches and in many instances are related to the irrigation fluids used. Hypothermia can be seen most often in pediatric patients because of the large exchanges of irrigating fluid and ventricular CSF involved.[84] Convulsions have also been reported by several authors, with one case leading to pneumoencephalus.[85] Injury to the hypothalamus may give rise to transient hypothalamic dysfunction with possible syndrome of inappropriate antidiuretic hormone or diabetes insipidus. Postoperative electrolyte changes after intraventricular neuroendoscopy have been reported. Meningeal irritation, headache, and high fever from an inflammatory response to irrigating fluid have been described.[86]

5.8 Postoperative Management

After the completion of the skull base procedure, depending on blood loss and surgical length, the patients who have sufficiently recovered from anesthesia to follow commands and maintain oxygenation while spontaneously breathing are extubated. Recovery from anesthesia is expedited by the use of short-acting low-solubility inhalational agents and infusions of potent opioids. Cranial nerve deficits, including injury to the vagus producing vocal cord paralysis, may occur after skull base surgery. Even though this would produce unilateral vocal cord paralysis, the patient should be awake and able to handle secretions to avoid the risk of aspiration. Pain is an important consideration during the immediate postoperative period. The incidence, magnitude, and duration of acute pain experienced after craniotomy are not well known. Pain after acoustic neuroma surgery, with a posterior fossa approach, has been noted to be severe in 67% of patients and was thought to result from either nuchal dissection or traction on the dura from nuchal musculature.[87] Evidence shows that patients who undergo skull base surgeries experience varying degrees of postoperative pain. Some of this variability may be explained by the different anatomical approaches to the brain and meninges. The proximity of CNs and the chemoreceptor trigger zone to the surgical field may increase the risk of pain and nausea after posterior fossa and skull base surgery. Pain from infratentorial structures is transmitted by efferent fibers in CNs V, IX, and X and the upper three cervical nerves. There is evidence that neurosurgical patients receive inadequate analgesia from currently available regimens.[88] De Beneditis et al demonstrated that patients undergoing surgery by the subtemporal and suboccipital routes have the highest incidence of postoperative pain.[89] Approximately 90% of these patients experienced pain during the first 12 hours after surgery. The pain that occurred was influenced by surgical route and was defined as pulsating or pounding, steady, and sometimes stabbing in nature.

In addition to the acute pain that occurs after the skull base procedure, more and more attention has been focused on the development of postcraniotomy headache that may last for weeks or months after the procedure. Some studies have noted that up to 12% of patients had ongoing headache after 1 year, 25% of which were medically uncontrolled and 33% of which required regular analgesics.[90] Over time, these headaches may take on a daily pattern of occurrence. Increased pericranial muscle tension may contribute to the development of chronic tension headache. Some of these headaches may be produced by scar tissue surrounding the occipital nerves or by fibrous adhesions binding neck muscles directly to the dura.[91] CSF leak or shunt may also cause headache after surgery, even if they sometimes present with normal CSF pressure.[92] Some patients can also present with symptoms of neuropathic pain over the scar, exhibiting allodynia and hyperalgesia.

There are numerous methods of treating postcraniotomy pain, some more successful than others. Scalp blocks have been used for some time to reduce the amount of rescue analgesics needed. The technique described by Pinosky et al[93] involves the injection of local anesthetics through the full thickness of the scalp onto the outer margins of the skull in an area from the postauricular region through the operative preauricular temporal site, then crossing the glabella up to the preauricular postauricular regions of the contralateral sites. Scalp blocks and wound infiltration help by providing transitional anesthesia during the immediate postoperative period. Parenteral opioids, however, are still the cornerstone of therapy after major craniotomy. The mechanism of action is activation of opioid receptors, which leads to inhibition of voltage-gated calcium channels and an increase in potassium influx, reducing neuronal excitability and inhibiting the transmission of painful stimuli.

Nonsteroidal anti-inflammatory drugs (NSAIDs) such as ibuprofen, naproxen, indomethacin, diclofenac, and ketorolac involve the reversible nonselective inhibition of cyclooxygenase Cox-1 and Cox-2 enzymes. Although NSAIDs are effective at providing analgesia, they can also lead to platelet dysfunction and increased bleeding, which could be devastating after skull base surgery. The only injectable option is ketorolac, which has been shown to be an effective analgesic when coupled with fentanyl.[94] Paracetamol's analgesic mechanism of action involves N-acetyl-p-aminophenol central Cox inhibition with weak peripheral effects. It is devoid of the side effects associated with NSAIDs.[95] Intravenous acetaminophen can be used as an adjuvant to other analgesics but may not itself be sufficient to provide adequate analgesia for postcraniotomy pain.[96] Other novel analgesic drugs have been used in an attempt to reduce the incidence of postcraniotomy headache. α2-adrenergic agonists such as dexmedetomidine have been given as an infusion during the surgical procedure and have been associated with an opioid sparing effect by reducing morphine requirements by 60% with a preemptive analgesic effect.[97] NMDA-receptor antagonists have also been noted to reduce analgesic requirements when administered before and during surgery. Low-dose ketamine infusions and dextromethorphan by oral or intramuscular routes have been studied as part of multimodal pain management techniques after craniotomy.[98]

Physiologic evidence suggests that vomiting may be associated more with infratemporal surgery.[88] Because pain is controlled, in most instances, by the judicious use of opioids, postoperative nausea and vomiting (PONV) is addressed with the use of antiemetics. Several methodologies are employed to provide relief from nausea or vomiting, with the antiemetic given as a rescue agent. Anticholinergic medications, such as scopolamine applied as a 1.5 mg scopolamine patch affixed behind the ear on the nonoperative side, may be of value. We have found this method to produce acceptable antiemetic and antinausea function, especially when coupled with ondansetron and dexamethasone. Ondansetron, a serotonin receptor antagonist, has also been used, with limited success, to reduce the incidence and severity of PONV. The addition of dexamethasone (Decadron) to antiemetic regimens seems to reduce the incidence of PONV.[99] Dexamethasone has been demonstrated to be effective for prophylaxis of PONV secondary to prostaglandin metabolism.[100] Others have suggested that dexamethasone's effectiveness may come because a release of endorphins results in mood elevation, a sense of well-being, and appetite stimulation. Corticosteroids may reduce levels of 5-hydroxytryptophan in neural tissue by decreasing tryptophan, its precursor. The anti-inflammatory portion of dexamethasone may prevent release of serotonin in the gut. Finally, dexamethasone may potentiate the main effects of the antiemetics by sensitizing pharmacological receptors. Antiemetics have also been added to patient-controlled analgesia (PCA) solutions to administer these agents simultaneously in conjunction with opioids. Our group demonstrated that patients who undergo craniotomy, especially in the skull base region, have significant postoperative pain.[101] The combination of ondansetron with PCA morphine reduced pain scores in the immediate 24 hours post surgery but had little effect on incidence of PONV and should not be used in combination with PCA morphine. Ondansetron ODT oral treatment given prior to surgery with intraoperative IV dexamethasone, and IV ondansetron was associated with less frequent rescue therapy on the first postoperative day than for patients receiving IV dexamethasone plus placebo.[63] This multimodal treatment may be more effective than single-therapy regimens in reducing nausea and vomiting after skull base procedures in which opioids are administered for analgesia.

5.9 Conclusion

The anesthesia technique used for skull base surgery is instrumental in providing optimum conditions for intraoperative monitoring while enabling the surgeon to accomplish the surgical procedure in a hemodynamically stable patient. The anesthesiologist can also improve postoperative outcomes and reduce morbidity provided that he or she is given information concerning surgical approach, tumor type, and involved vital structures. It is imperative that the neuroanesthesiologist discuss the procedure with the skull base surgical team and be involved in the decisions concerning perioperative management to produce an optimal outcome.

References

[1] Jellish WS, Murdoch J, Leonetti JP. Perioperative management of complex skull base surgery: the anesthesiologist's point of view. Neurosurg Focus. 2002; 12(5):e5

[2] Jung TM, TerKonda RP, Haines SJ, Strome S, Marentette LJ. Outcome analysis of the transglabellar/subcranial approach for lesions of the anterior cranial fossa: a comparison with the classic craniotomy approach. Otolaryngology. 1999; 116(6):642–646

[3] Cheney FW, Domino KB, Caplan RA, Posner KL. Nerve injury associated with anesthesia: a closed claims analysis. Anesthesiology. 1999; 90(4):1062–1069

[4] Smith DS, Osborn I. Posterior fossa: anesthetic consideration. In: Cottrell JE, Smith D, eds. Anesthesia and Neurosurgery. St. Louis: Mosby; 2001:327–331

[5] Faust RJ, Cucchiara RF, Bechtle P. Patient positioning. In: Miller RD, ed. Miller's Anesthesia. Philadelphia: Elsevier;2005:1151–1167

[6] Lam AM, Vavilala MS. Macroglossia: compartment syndrome of the tongue? Anesthesiology. 2000; 92(6):1832–1835

[7] Deem S, Shapiro HM, Marshall LF. Quadriplegia in a patient with cervical spondylosis after thoracolumbar surgery in the prone position. Anesthesiology. 1991; 75(3):527–528

[8] Black S, Ockert DB, Oliver WC. Tumor surgery. In: Cucchiara RF, Michenfelder JD, eds. Clinical Neuroanesthesia. Edinburgh: Churchill Livingstone;1990: 285–308

[9] Standefer M, Bay JW, Trusso R. The sitting position in neurosurgery: a retrospective analysis of 488 cases. Neurosurgery. 1984; 14(6):649–658

[10] Wilder BL. Hypothesis: the etiology of midcervical quadriplegia after operation with the patient in the sitting position. Neurosurgery. 1982; 11(4): 530–531

[11] Hall R, Murdoch J. Brain protection: physiological and pharmacological considerations. Part II: The pharmacology of brain protection. Can J Anaesth. 1990; 37(7):762–777

[12] Ward RJ, Danziger F, Bonica JJ, Allen GD, Tolas AG. Cardiovascular effects of change of posture. Aerosp Med. 1966; 37(3):257–259

[13] Millar RA. Neurosurgical anaesthesia in the sitting position: a report of experience with 110 patients using controlled or spontaneous ventilation. Br J Anaesth. 1972; 44(5):495–505

[14] Porter JM, Pidgeon C, Cunningham AJ. The sitting position in neurosurgery: a critical appraisal. Br J Anaesth. 1999; 82(1):117–128

[15] Matjasko J, Petrozza P, Cohen M, Steinberg P. Anesthesia and surgery in the seated position: analysis of 554 cases. Neurosurgery. 1985; 17(5):695–702

[16] Duke DA, Lynch JJ, Harner SG, Faust RJ, Ebersold MJ. Venous air embolism in sitting and supine patients undergoing vestibular schwannoma resection. Neurosurgery. 1998; 42(6):1282–1286, discussion 1286–1287

[17] Schmitt HJ, Hemmerling TM. Venous air emboli occur during release of positive end-expiratory pressure and repositioning after sitting position surgery. Anesth Analg. 2002; 94(2):400–403

[18] von Gösseln HH, Samii M, Suhr D, Bini W. The lounging position for posterior fossa surgery: anesthesiological considerations regarding air embolism. Childs Nerv Syst. 1991; 7(7):368–374

[19] Kerr RH, Applegate RL, II. Accurate placement of the right atrial air aspiration catheter: a descriptive study and prospective trial of intravascular electrocardiography. Anesth Analg. 2006; 103(2):435–438

[20] Geissler HJ, Allen SJ, Mehlhorn U, Davis KL, Morris WP, Butler BD. Effect of body repositioning after venous air embolism: an echocardiographic study. Anesthesiology. 1997; 86(3):710–717

[21] Toung TJK, McPherson RW, Ahn H, Donham RT, Alano J, Long D. Pneumocephalus: effects of patient position on the incidence and location of aerocele after posterior fossa and upper cervical cord surgery. Anesth Analg. 1986; 65 (1):65–70

[22] Moore JK, Chaudhri S, Moore AP, Easton J. Macroglossia and posterior fossa disease. Anaesthesia. 1988; 43(5):382–385

[23] Tattersall MP. Massive swelling of the face and tongue: a complication of posterior cranial fossa surgery in the sitting position. Anaesthesia. 1984; 39 (10):1015–1017

[24] Kuhnert SM, Faust RJ, Berge KH, Piepgras DG. Postoperative macroglossia: report of a case with rapid resolution after extubation of the trachea. Anesth Analg. 1999; 88(1):220–223

[25] Schwaber MK, Netterville JL, Coniglio JU. Complications of skull base surgery. Ear Nose Throat J. 1991; 70(9):648–654, 659–660

[26] Bogdasarian RS, Kwyer TA, Dauser RC, Chandler WF, Kindt GW. Internal carotid artery blowout as a complication of sphenoid sinus and skull-base surgery. Otolaryngol Head Neck Surg. 1983; 91(3):308–312

[27] Smith PG, Killeen TE. Carotid artery vasospasm complicating extensive skull base surgery: cause, prevention, and management. Otolaryngol Head Neck Surg. 1987; 97(1):1–7

[28] Schaller B. Trigemino-cardiac reflex during microvascular trigeminal decompression in cases of trigeminal neuralgia. J Neurosurg Anesthesiol. 2005; 17 (1):45–48

[29] Meuwly C, Chowdhury T, Sandu N, Reck M, Erne P, Schaller B. Anesthetic influence on occurrence and treatment of the trigemino-cardiac reflex: a systematic literature review. Medicine (Baltimore). 2015; 94(18):e807

[30] Arnold RW, Jensen PA, Kovtoun TA, Maurer SA, Schultz JA. The profound augmentation of the oculocardiac reflex by fast acting opioids. Binocul Vis Strabismus Q. 2004; 19(4):215–222

[31] Wang X, Gorini C, Sharp D, Bateman R, Mendelowitz D. Anaesthetics differentially modulate the trigeminocardiac reflex excitatory synaptic pathway in the brainstem. J Physiol. 2011; 589(Pt 22):5431–5442

[32] Prabhakar H, Ali Z, Rath GP. Trigemino-cardiac reflex may be refractory to conventional management in adults. Acta Neurochir (Wien). 2008; 150(5): 509–510

[33] Al-Mefty O, Teixeira A. Complex tumors of the glomus jugulare: criteria, treatment, and outcome. J Neurosurg. 2002; 97(6):1356–1366

[34] Tsuda H, Oka K, Noutsuka Y, Sueishi K. Tissue-type plasminogen activator in patients with intracranial meningiomas. Thromb Haemost. 1988; 60(3): 508–513

[35] Mebel D, Akagami R, Flexman AM. Use of tranexamic acid is associated with reduced blood product transfusion in complex skull base neurosurgical procedures: a retrospective cohort study. Anesth Analg. 2016; 122(2):503–508

[36] Roos Y, Rinkel G, Vermeulen M, Algra A, van Gijn J. Antifibrinolytic therapy for aneurysmal subarachnoid hemorrhage: a major update of a Cochrane Review. Stroke. 2003; 34(9):2308–2309

[37] Manji RA, Grocott HP, Leake J, et al. Seizures following cardiac surgery: the impact of tranexamic acid and other risk factors. Can J Anaesth. 2012; 59(1): 6–13

[38] Aminoff MJ. Electrophysiologic testing for the diagnosis of peripheral nerve injuries. Anesthesiology. 2004; 100(5):1298–1303

[39] Coppieters MW, Van de Velde M, Stappaerts KH. Positioning in anesthesiology: toward a better understanding of stretch-induced perioperative neuropathies. Anesthesiology. 2002; 97(1):75–81

[40] Sawyer RJ, Richmond MN, Hickey JD, Jarrratt JA. Peripheral nerve injuries associated with anaesthesia. Anaesthesia. 2000; 55(10):980–991

[41] Anastasian ZH, Ramnath B, Komotar RJ, et al. Evoked potential monitoring identifies possible neurological injury during positioning for craniotomy. Anesth Analg. 2009; 109(3):817–821

[42] Uribe JS, Kolla J, Omar H, et al. Brachial plexus injury following spinal surgery. J Neurosurg Spine. 2010; 13(4):552–558

[43] Kamel IR, Drum ET, Koch SA, et al. The use of somatosensory evoked potentials to determine the relationship between patient positioning and impending upper extremity nerve injury during spine surgery: a retrospective analysis. Anesth Analg. 2006; 102(5):1538–1542

[44] Jellish WS, Sherazee G, Patel J, et al. Somatosensory evoked potentials help prevent positioning-related brachial plexus injury during skull base surgery. Otolaryngol Head Neck Surg. 2013; 149(1):168–173

[45] Cheek JC. Posterior fossa intraoperative monitoring. J Clin Neurophysiol. 1993; 10(4):412–424

[46] Lennon RL, Hosking MP, Daube JR, Welna JO. Effect of partial neuromuscular blockade on intraoperative electromyography in patients undergoing resection of acoustic neuromas. Anesth Analg. 1992; 75(5):729–733

[47] Blair EA, Teeple E, Jr, Sutherland RM, Shih T, Chen D. Effect of neuromuscular blockade on facial nerve monitoring. Am J Otol. 1994; 15(2):161–167

[48] Stechison MT. Neurophysiologic monitoring during cranial base surgery. J Neurooncol. 1994; 20(3):313–325

[49] Yingling CD. Intraoperative monitoring of cranial nerves in skull base surgery. In: Jackler RK, Brackmann DE, eds. Neurotology. St. Louis: Mosby; 1994:967–1002

[50] Prass RL, Lüders H. Acoustic (loudspeaker) facial electromyographic monitoring: Part 1. Evoked electromyographic activity during acoustic neuroma resection. Neurosurgery. 1986; 19(3):392–400

[51] Jellish WS, Leonetti JP, Buoy CM, Sincacore JM, Sawicki KJ, Macken MP. Facial nerve electromyographic monitoring to predict movement in patients titrated to a standard anesthetic depth. Anesth Analg. 2009; 109(2):551–558

[52] Chassard D, Joubaud A, Colson A, Guiraud M, Dubreuil C, Banssillon V. Auditory evoked potentials during propofol anaesthesia in man. Br J Anaesth. 1989; 62(5):522–526

[53] Schwender D, Conzen P, Klasing S, Finsterer U, Pöppel E, Peter K. The effects of anesthesia with increasing end-expiratory concentrations of sevoflurane on midlatency auditory evoked potentials. Anesth Analg. 1995; 81(4):817–822

[54] Schwender D, Klasing S, Conzen P, Finsterer U, Pöppel E, Peter K. Midlatency auditory evoked potentials during anaesthesia with increasing endexpiratory concentrations of desflurane. Acta Anaesthesiol Scand. 1996; 40(2):171–176

[55] Sohmer H, Gafni M, Chisin R. Auditory nerve-brain stem potentials in man and cat under hypoxic and hypercapnic conditions. Electroencephalogr Clin Neurophysiol. 1982; 53(5):506–512

[56] Markand ON, Warren CH, Moorthy SS, Stoelting RK, King RD. Monitoring of multimodality evoked potentials during open heart surgery under hypothermia. Electroencephalogr Clin Neurophysiol. 1984; 59(6):432–440

[57] McTaggert-Cowan RA. Somatosensory evoked potentials during spinal surgery. Canadian Journal of Anesthesiology. 1988; 45:387–392

[58] Banoub M, Tetzlaff JE, Schubert A. Pharmacologic and physiologic influences affecting sensory evoked potentials: implications for perioperative monitoring. Anesthesiology. 2003; 99(3):716–737

[59] Rehberg B, Rüschner R, Fischer M, Ebeling BJ, Hoeft A. [Concentration-dependent changes in the latency and amplitude of somatosensory-evoked potentials by desflurane, isoflurane and sevoflurane]. Anasthesiol Intensivmed Notfallmed Schmerzther. 1998; 33(7):425–429

[60] Scheepstra GL, de Lange JJ, Booij LH, Ros HH. Median nerve evoked potentials during propofol anaesthesia. Br J Anaesth. 1989; 62(1):92–94

[61] Borrissov B, Langeron O, Lille F, et al. [Combination of propofol-sufentanil on somatosensory evoked potentials in surgery of the spine]. Ann Fr Anesth Reanim. 1995; 14(4):326–330

[62] Sloan TB, Ronai AK, Toleikis JR, Koht A. Improvement of intraoperative somatosensory evoked potentials by etomidate. Anesth Analg. 1988; 67(6):582–585

[63] Warner DS. Experience with remifentanil in neurosurgical patients. Anesth Analg. 1999; 89(4) Suppl:S33–S39

[64] Wass CT, Lanier WL. Glucose modulation of ischemic brain injury: review and clinical recommendations. Mayo Clin Proc. 1996; 71(8):801–812

[65] Tu YK, Heros RC, Candia G, et al. Isovolemic hemodilution in experimental focal cerebral ischemia. Part 1: Effects on hemodynamics, hemorheology, and intracranial pressure. J Neurosurg. 1988; 69(1):72–81

[66] Voll CL, Auer RN. Insulin attenuates ischemic brain damage independent of its hypoglycemic effect. J Cereb Blood Flow Metab. 1991; 11(6):1006–1014

[67] Wasnick JD, Conlay LA. Induced hypertension for cerebral aneurysm surgery in a patient with carotid occlusive disease. Anesth Analg. 1990; 70(3):331–333

[68] Hoffman WE, Charbel FT, Edelman G. Brain tissue oxygen, carbon dioxide, and pH in neurosurgical patients at risk for ischemia. Anesth Analg. 1996; 82(3):582–586

[69] Minamisawa H, Nordström CH, Smith ML, Siesjö BK. The influence of mild body and brain hypothermia on ischemic brain damage. J Cereb Blood Flow Metab. 1990; 10(3):365–374

[70] Wass CT, Lanier WL. Hypothermia-associated protection from ischemic brain injury: implications for patient management. Int Anesthesiol Clin. 1996; 34(4):95–111

[71] Toner CC, Stamford J. General anesthetics as neuroprotection agents. In: Tidall B, ed. Bailliere's Clinical Anesthesiology International Practice and Research. UK: Sunders; 1996:Vol 10/No 3:515–533

[72] Nussmeier NA, Arlund C, Slogoff S. Neuropsychiatric complications after cardiopulmonary bypass: cerebral protection by a barbiturate. Anesthesiology. 1986; 64(2):165–170

[73] Michenfelder JD, Milde JH, Sundt TM, Jr. Cerebral protection by barbiturate anesthesia: use after middle cerebral artery occlusion in Java monkeys. Arch Neurol. 1976; 33(5):345–350

[74] Zhu H, Cottrell JE, Kass IS. The effect of thiopental and propofol on NMDA- and AMPA-mediated glutamate excitotoxicity. Anesthesiology. 1997; 87(4):944–951

[75] Edelman GJ, Hoffman WE, Charbel FT. Cerebral hypoxia after etomidate administration and temporary cerebral artery occlusion. Anesth Analg. 1997; 85(4):821–825

[76] Lei B, Cottrell JE, Kass IS. Neuroprotective effect of low-dose lidocaine in a rat model of transient focal cerebral ischemia. Anesthesiology. 2001; 95(2):445–451

[77] Mitchell SJ, Pellett O, Gorman DF. Cerebral protection by lidocaine during cardiac operations. Ann Thorac Surg. 1999; 67(4):1117–1124

[78] Lam AM, Manninen PH, Ferguson GG, Nantau W. Monitoring electrophysiologic function during carotid endarterectomy: a comparison of somatosensory evoked potentials and conventional electroencephalogram. Anesthesiology. 1991; 75(1):15–21

[79] Derbent A, Erşahin Y, Yurtseven T, Turhan T. Hemodynamic and electrolyte changes in patients undergoing neuroendoscopic procedures. Childs Nerv Syst. 2006; 22(3):253–257

[80] Manning SC, Bloom DC, Perkins JA, Gruss JS, Inglis A. Diagnostic and surgical challenges in the pediatric skull base. Otolaryngol Clin North Am. 2005; 38 (4):773–794

[81] El-Dawlatly AA, Murshid W, El-Khwsky F. Endoscopic third ventriculostomy: a study of intracranial pressure vs. haemodynamic changes. Minim Invasive Neurosurg. 1999; 42(4):198–200

[82] White DR, Sonnenburg RE, Ewend MG, Senior BA. Safety of minimally invasive pituitary surgery (MIPS) compared with a traditional approach. Laryngoscope. 2004; 114(11):1945–1948

[83] Casler JD, Doolittle AM, Mair EA. Endoscopic surgery of the anterior skull base. Laryngoscope. 2005; 115(1):16–24

[84] Ambesh SP, Kumar R. Neuroendoscopic procedures: anesthetic considerations for a growing trend: a review. J Neurosurg Anesthesiol. 2000; 12(3):262–270

[85] Saxena S, Ambesh SP, Saxena HN, Kumar R. Pneumoencephalus and convulsions after ventriculoscopy: a potentially catastrophic complication. J Neurosurg Anesthesiol. 1999; 11(3):200–202

[86] Oka K, Yamamoto M, Nonaka T, Tomonaga M. The significance of artificial cerebrospinal fluid as perfusate and endoneurosurgery. Neurosurgery. 1996; 38(4):733–736

[87] Schessel DA, Nedzelski JM, Rowed D, Feghali JG. Pain after surgery for acoustic neuroma. Otolaryngol Head Neck Surg. 1992; 107(3):424–429

[88] Irefin SA, Schubert A, Bloomfield EL, DeBoer GE, Mascha EJ, Ebrahim ZY. The effect of craniotomy location on postoperative pain and nausea. J Anesth. 2003; 17(4):227–231

[89] De Benedittis G, Lorenzetti A, Migliore M, Spagnoli D, Tiberio F, Villani RM. Postoperative pain in neurosurgery: a pilot study in brain surgery. Neurosurgery. 1996; 38(3):466–469, discussion 469–470

[90] Kaur A, Selwa L, Fromes G, Ross DA. Persistent headache after supratentorial craniotomy. Neurosurgery. 2000; 47(3):633–636

[91] Hack GD, Hallgren RC. Chronic headache relief after section of suboccipital muscle dural connections: a case report. Headache. 2004; 44(1):84–89

[92] Mokri B, Hunter SF, Atkinson JLD, Piepgras DG. Orthostatic headaches caused by CSF leak but with normal CSF pressures. Neurology. 1998; 51(3):786–790

[93] Rosenberg PH, Veering BT, Urmey WF. Maximum recommended doses of local anesthetics: a multifactorial concept. Reg Anesth Pain Med. 2004; 29(6):564–575, discussion 524

[94] Na HS, An SB, Park HP, et al. Analgesia to manage the postoperative period in patients undergoing craniotomy. Korean J Anesthesiol. 2011; 60(1):30–35

[95] Remy C, Marret E, Bonnet F. State of the art of paracetamol in acute pain therapy. Curr Opin Anaesthesiol. 2006; 19(5):562–565

[96] Verchère E, Grenier B, Mesli A, Siao D, Sesay M, Maurette P. Postoperative pain management after supratentorial craniotomy. J Neurosurg Anesthesiol. 2002; 14(2):96–101

[97] Arain SR, Ruehlow RM, Uhrich TD, Ebert TJ. The efficacy of dexmedetomidine versus morphine for postoperative analgesia after major inpatient surgery. Anesth Analg. 2004; 98(1):153–158

[98] Helmy SA, Bali A. The effect of the preemptive use of the NMDA receptor antagonist dextromethorphan on postoperative analgesic requirements. Anesth Analg. 2001; 92(3):739–744

[99] Hartsell T, Long D, Kirsch JR. The efficacy of postoperative ondansetron (Zofran) orally disintegrating tablets for preventing nausea and vomiting after acoustic neuroma surgery. Anesth Analg. 2005; 101(5):1492–1496

[100] Henzi I, Walder B, Tramèr MR. Dexamethasone for the prevention of postoperative nausea and vomiting: a quantitative systematic review. Anesth Analg. 2000; 90(1):186–194

[101] Jellish WS, Leonetti JP, Sawicki K, Anderson D, Origitano TC. Morphine/ondansetron PCA for postoperative pain, nausea, and vomiting after skull base surgery. Otolaryngol Head Neck Surg. 2006; 135(2):175–181

6 Endoscopic Endonasal Skull Base Surgery

Carl H. Snyderman and Paul A. Gardner

Summary

Endoscopic endonasal surgery (EES) of the skull base has become accepted for the treatment of most ventral skull base lesions. EES is applicable to all patient populations and can be applied to a wide variety of benign and malignant pathologies. Multidisciplinary teamwork is a key feature of EES, and an incremental program for training is proposed. Endonasal approaches can be divided into surgical modules that provide flexibility in tailoring the approach to the patient. They are organized along sagittal and coronal (anterior, middle, and posterior) planes, with the sphenoid sinus at the epicenter. Each module is associated with specific anatomical landmarks. Anatomical limitations of endonasal approaches are established by major neural and vascular structures. The risks of EES are similar to those of transcranial surgery. The most common complication, cerebrospinal fluid leak, has diminished with the use of vascularized flaps (local and regional) for reconstruction.

Keywords: classification, coronal, endonasal, endoscopic, sagittal, skull base, training

6.1 Principles of Endoscopic Endonasal Surgery

The endonasal corridor is just one of multiple corridors that provide access to the skull base. Although the endoscope has enabled surgeons to accomplish more via the endonasal corridor, endoscopic endonasal surgery (EES) of the skull base is predicated on choosing the best approach for the patient, one that accomplishes the goals of surgery with the least chance of morbidity for the patient. Multiple factors are considered in choosing the best approach: tumor size and extent, location, patient comorbidities, risks, morbidity, reconstruction, duration, prior treatment, experience and training of surgical team, and resources.

For many tumors, the endonasal corridor provides the most direct access without displacement of normal neural and vascular tissues. The golden rule of EES is to avoid crossing the plane of nerves and vessels that surround the ventral skull base. If a tumor is on the other side of a major nerve or vessel, an alternative approach should be considered. For some tumors, a multicorridor approach will be necessary to access all parts of the tumor while minimizing manipulation of neurovascular structures.

Unlike other types of collaborative surgery, EES is true team surgery. For much of the operation, surgeons work concurrently rather than sequentially, with one surgeon driving the endoscope and the other surgeon performing bimanual dissection. The benefits of team surgery include superior visualization, increased efficiency, enhanced problem solving, and modulation of enthusiasm. Although the highest-quality endoscopes currently provide a 2D image, 3D visual cues result from the relative movement of instruments. Dynamic endoscopy facilitates the accurate passage of instruments and optimizes the surgical view without hindering bimanual dissection. An experienced cosurgeon is especially critical in a crisis such as a vascular injury for maintenance of a surgical view and active problem solving.

Bimanual access and dissection is key for performing microsurgical resection. The same techniques as would be used with an "open" surgery must be applied to realize the advantages of EES. These include early devascularization, internal debulking, microsurgical blunt and sharp dissection, and early vascular control. In addition, wide exposure allows for freedom of movement and early bony decompression of critical structures. Oncological principles can be preserved with EES for malignant sinonasal tumors.[1] Although en bloc excision is not feasible for many tumors, piecemeal resection does not have an adverse effect on outcomes so long as the final margins are negative. Superior visualization with endoscopy may facilitate complete tumor removal with improved oncological outcomes.

6.2 Indications

EES is indicated for the management of a wide variety of benign and malignant tumors of the nasal cavity, paranasal sinuses, skull base, pituitary, brain and meninges, orbit, and spine in all patient populations, including young pediatric patients.[2] Examples of tumor types are provided in the following descriptions of endonasal approaches.

The limitations of EES are determined by multiple factors, including the experience of the surgical team.[3] Anatomical constraints include major neural and vascular structures: internal carotid artery (ICA), vertebrobasilar arterial system, and cranial nerves (CNs). Further advances in technology and techniques continue to extend the limits of the endoscopic endonasal approach.

6.3 Classification of Endonasal Approaches

Endoscopic endonasal approaches are divided into surgical modules that can be combined like building blocks to create a tailored surgical approach for each tumor (▶ Table 6.1).[4] The classification of endonasal approaches is designed to be intuitive, with orientation in sagittal and coronal anatomical planes. The sphenoid sinus is the starting point for many of these modules, because the sphenoid contains the most critical anatomical structures (carotid arteries and optic nerves), is easily accessible and familiar, and is at the junction of the sagittal and coronal planes.

6.3.1 Sagittal Plane Modules

The sagittal plane is a midline corridor that extends from the frontal sinus to the craniovertebral junction (▶ Fig. 6.1).

Table 6.1 Classification of endonasal approaches to the ventral skull base

- Sagittal plane
  - Transfrontal
  - Transcribriform
  - Transplanum/transtuberculum (suprasellar)
  - Transsellar
  - Transclival
    - Superior: dorsum sellae, posterior clinoid processes
    - Middle: midclivus
    - Inferior: foramen magnum
  - Transodontoid
- Coronal plane
  - Anterior (anterior cranial fossa)
    - Supraorbital
    - Transorbital
  - Middle (middle cranial fossa)
    - Medial transcavernous
    - Medial petrous apex
    - Transpterygoid
    - Contralateral transmaxillary
    - Suprapetrous
    - Meckel's cave
    - Lateral transcavernous
  - Posterior (posterior cranial fossa)
    - Infrapetrous ("far medial")
    - Transjugular tubercle
    - Transcondylar
    - Parapharyngeal space

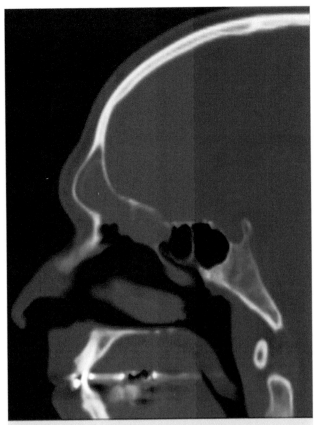

Fig. 6.2 A transfrontal approach was used to remove tumor from the frontal sinus in this patient who had recurrent inverted papilloma. Note remodeling of a septation within the frontal sinus due to upward expansion of the tumor.

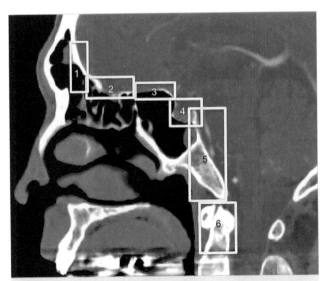

Fig. 6.1 The sagittal plane is a midline corridor divided into modules corresponding to the cranial fossae. Anterior: transfrontal (1), transcribriform (2), and transplanum/transtuberculum (suprasellar) (3). Middle: transsellar (4). Posterior: transclival (5), transodontoid (6).

Transfrontal Approach

The transfrontal approach provides access to the frontal sinus, the posterior table of the frontal sinus, and the crista galli. A Draf 3 frontal sinusotomy is performed to remove the floor of the frontal sinus. The opening is limited posteriorly by the crista galli in the midline, which extends to the anterior cribriform plates. With drilling of the bone anteriorly at the level of the nasion and the use of angled endoscopes and instruments, the posterior table of the frontal sinus is accessible. Lateral access is enhanced by using a binarial approach with creation of a superior septal window.

Common pathologies for this approach include nasal dermoids, fibro-osseous lesions such as osteoma and juvenile ossifying fibroma, and superior extension of sinonasal tumors such as inverted papilloma (▶ Fig. 6.2). Tumor involvement of the anterior table or lateral recesses of the frontal sinus may necessitate an open approach. A transfrontal approach provides the anterior limit of resection for tumors that involve the cribriform plate (esthesioneuroblastoma).

Transcribriform Approach

The transcribriform approach extends from the frontal sinus anteriorly to the planum sphenoidale posteriorly and is accessed through the ethmoid sinuses and bounded by the orbits laterally. The transcribriform approach provides access to the anterior cranial fossa for tumors that arise intracranially (olfactory groove meningioma), tumors that arise from the olfactory sulcus (hamartoma, olfactory schwannoma, and olfactory neuroblastoma), and sinonasal cancers that extend to the anterior cranial base (▶ Fig. 6.3).

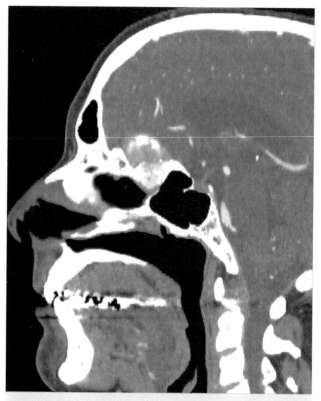

Fig. 6.3 This olfactory grove meningioma is posterior to the crista galli and displays tumor calcification with characteristic hyperostosis of the skull base in the cribriform region.

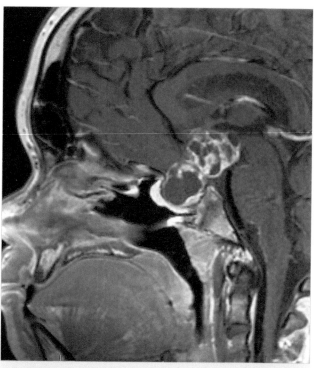

Fig. 6.4 This suprasellar craniopharyngioma with solid and cystic components extends to the third ventricle and requires a combined transplanum and transsellar approach.

The endonasal version of the classic craniofacial resection combines transfrontal, transcribriform, and transplanum approaches and extends from the frontal sinus anteriorly to the planum sphenoidale posteriorly, to the medial walls of the orbit laterally, and to the nasal septum inferiorly.[5] On the lateral aspect of the tumor, the medial wall of the orbit (lamina papyracea) and periorbita may be resected to provide a margin. The cribriform plates are bounded laterally by the anterior and posterior ethmoidal arteries. These may be cauterized and transected on the orbital side of the skull base to devascularize tumors and provide access to the orbital roof.

Transplanum/Transtuberculum (Suprasellar) Approach

The transplanum approach provides access to the suprasellar area through the roof of the sphenoid sinus and is limited by the optic canals posterolaterally and the cribriform plates anteriorly. It is often combined with a transsellar approach for the removal of extrasellar pituitary adenomas, craniopharyngiomas, and tuberculum meningiomas (▶ Fig. 6.4).[6,7] The bone of the sella, tuberculum, and planum is removed as needed by thinning the bone and dissecting it from the underlying dura using dissectors or a Kerrison rongeur. Between the optic canals and parasellar ICAs, access is narrowed but can be improved by removing the bone of the medial opticocarotid recess (mOCR) and even laterally to decompress the medial optic canals. Removal of the tuberculum exposes the superior intercavernous sinus, which

must be cauterized and ligated to provide maximal exposure of the pituitary stalk.

A transplanum approach is also used for decompression of the optic canal. The optic canal is separated from the cavernous ICA and superior orbital fissure by the lateral optic–carotid recess (lOCR). The lOCR represents pneumatization of the optic strut and connects with the anterior clinoid. The optic canal may be decompressed in an anterograde or retrograde direction. With an anterograde approach, a medial orbital decompression is followed posteriorly to the orbital apex and optic canal. With a retrograde approach, the tuberculum is drilled at the sphenoid limbus and removal of bone continues laterally to the optic canal. The ophthalmic artery is inferior to the optic nerve and is at risk for injury intradurally. Drilling of bone superior to the optic canal leads to the anterior clinoid, which cannot be well accessed endonasally. Indications for optic nerve decompression include tuberculum meningiomas that extend laterally to the optic canal, fibrous dysplasia, trauma, and tumors in the orbital apex. Tumors that extend superolateral to the optic nerve or that involve the anterior clinoid may require an alternate or combined approach.

Transsellar Approach

The transsellar approach provides access to tumors of the pituitary gland (pituitary adenomas, Rathke's cleft cysts; ▶ Fig. 6.5).[8] The sella is bounded by the cavernous sinus in all directions and by the cavernous segment of the ICA laterally. Bone overlying the cavernous ICA may be thinned and removed to allow lateral displacement of the ICA and access to the anterior–inferior, superior,

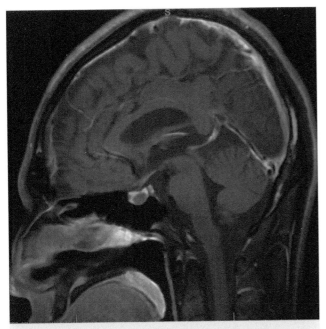

Fig. 6.5 A transsellar approach is used to drain this Rathke's cyst.

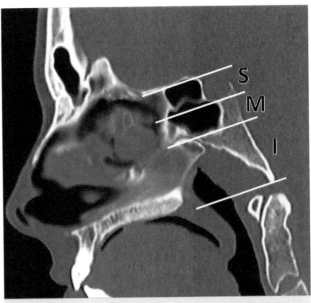

Fig. 6.6 The clivus is divided into three regions (superior [S], middle [M], and inferior [I]) based on the anatomy of the sphenoid sinus. The floor of the sella demarcates the superior and middle clivus, whereas the floor of the sphenoid sinus demarcates the middle and inferior clivus.

and posterior compartments of the cavernous sinus for extrasellar pituitary adenomas.[9]

Transclival Approach

The clivus extends from the posterior clinoids to the foramen magnum. Transclival approaches are divided into three segments (superior, middle, and inferior) (▶ Fig. 6.6).

Superior (Pituitary Transposition)

The superior clivus comprises the dorsum sella and extends from the posterior clinoids to the floor of the sella. Access to the superior clivus requires transposition of the pituitary gland.[10] This is best performed as an interdural dissection through the medial cavernous sinus, leaving the pituitary gland ensheathed in the meningeal layer of dura. The inferior hypophyseal arteries may be sacrificed on one or both sides without loss of pituitary function. Removal of the tuberculum sellae provides additional room for superior displacement of the gland. Care must be taken to avoid damage to the unprotected neurohypophysis, but the gland can be elevated from the fossa with preservation of the superior hypophyseal arterial supply as well as superior and lateral dural venous drainage, thereby preserving function.

The superior clivus is bounded laterally by the parasellar cavernous and clinoidal segments of the ICA. Removal of the dorsum sellae and posterior clinoid processes and subsequent dural opening provides access to the basilar apex. Cranial nerve III (oculomotor) is located between the posterior cerebral artery and the superior cerebellar artery and forms the lateral anatomical boundary.

A pituitary transposition may be necessary for the removal of craniopharyngiomas and meningiomas that arise posterior to the dorsum sellae, infundibulum, or gland. A superior transclival

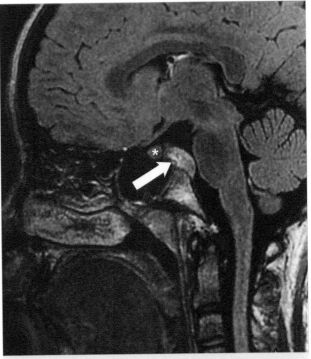

Fig. 6.7 A superior and middle transclival approach with transposition of the pituitary gland (*asterisk*) is necessary to remove this chordoma of the upper clivus (*arrow*).

approach provides access to the posterior clinoids for infiltrative tumors such as chordomas or extrasellar pituitary adenomas and intradural access for tumors such as petroclival meningiomas (▶ Fig. 6.7).

Middle

The middle clivus extends from the floor of the sella to the floor of the sphenoid sinus (clival recess) and is bounded by the pituitary gland superiorly and the paraclival cavernous segments of the ICA laterally. The medial petrous apex is located deep to the paraclival ICA.

Removal of the bone posteriorly and dural opening provides access to the basilar artery. This requires packing of the significant *inter*dural basilar plexus. Cranial nerve VI (abducens) originates from the brainstem at the level of the vertebrobasilar junction inferiorly and courses obliquely deep to the paraclival ICA, where it enters Dorello's canal. It is at risk of injury with drilling of bone deep to the paraclival ICA in the upper third of the midclivus.

The middle transclival approach is most commonly used for chordomas, meningiomas, and extrasellar pituitary adenomas (▶ Fig. 6.7).[11] Chordomas often grow between the periosteal and meningeal layers of the basilar plexus into Dorello's canal. Nasopharyngeal carcinomas can also extend into the midclivus, which can be drilled for a margin.

Inferior

The inferior clivus extends from the floor of the sphenoid sinus to the foramen magnum and is most often combined with a middle transclival approach for infiltrative tumors such as chordomas and chondrosarcomas, as well as for access to meningiomas of the posterior cranial fossa (▶ Fig. 6.8).[12] It can also be combined with a transodontoid approach to access craniocervical junction tumors such as chordomas and foramen magnum meningiomas. Drilling of the inferior clival bone to the underlying dura can provide a margin of resection for nasopharyngeal cancer, for both primary resection and following radiation therapy.

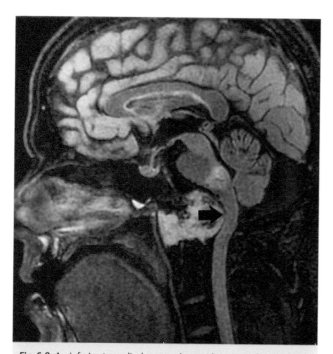

Fig. 6.8 An inferior transclival approach provides access for this large chordoma with brainstem compression (*arrow*).

The inferior clivus is bounded laterally by the lacerum segment of the ICA. The vidian nerve within the pterygoid canal is a landmark for localization of the lacerum and petrous ICA. Removal of the bone posteriorly and dural opening exposes the vertebral and anterior spinal arteries. The hypoglossal nerve courses laterally dorsal to the vertebral arteries.

Transodontoid

The transodontoid approach provides access to the craniovertebral junction from the lower clivus to the body of C2. The nasopalatine line (a line tangential to the inferior edge of the nasal bones and posterior edge of the hard palate) roughly demarcates the inferior limit of access to the spine.[13] Caudal access can be improved by drilling the posterior aspect of the maxillary crest flush with the hard palate. Laterally, ectatic parapharyngeal ICAs may limit dissection of the retropharyngeal soft tissues, especially at the level of C1. Removal of the soft tissues of the nasopharynx between the Eustachian tubes and from the sphenoid rostrum to the plane of the hard palate exposes the anterior arch of C1, which can be drilled to access the odontoid and body of C2. Removal of bone laterally (lateral mass of C1) is limited so as to avoid instability of the spine and avoid injury to the vertebral arteries. Intradurally, access is limited laterally by the vertebral arteries, and care must be taken to protect the caudal continuation of the anterior spinal artery.

A transodontoid approach is most commonly used for the treatment of degenerative or inflammatory bony compression, basilar invagination, or, rarely, significant pannus with brainstem compression but also provides access for tumors at foramen magnum such as meningiomas and chordomas of the craniovertebral junction (▶ Fig. 6.9).[14]

6.3.2 Coronal Plane

The coronal plane is divided into three coronal planes corresponding to the cranial fossae (anterior, middle, and posterior; ▶ Fig. 6.10). The transpterygoid approach is a prerequisite for many of the modules of the middle and posterior coronal planes.

Anterior Fossa

Supraorbital

Removal of the medial wall of the orbit (lamina papyracea) with sacrifice of the ethmoidal arteries and displacement of the orbital contents (subperiosteal plane) reliably provides access to the orbital roof to the midpoint of the orbit. The most common bony tumors in this region are benign fibro-osseous lesions (▶ Fig. 6.11). Removal of the orbital roof allows extended resection of dural margins for tumors such as meningiomas (dural tail or lateral extension) and olfactory neuroblastomas. Access is limited anterior to the anterior ethmoidal artery. Intradurally, there are no critical neurovascular structures in this location, which is lateral to the fronto-orbital branches and olfactory tract.

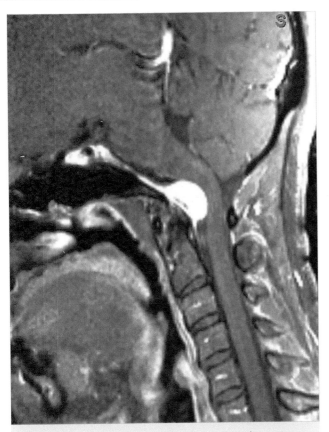

Fig. 6.9 A transodontoid approach provides access to the craniovertebral junction for tumors such as this meningioma of the foramen magnum.

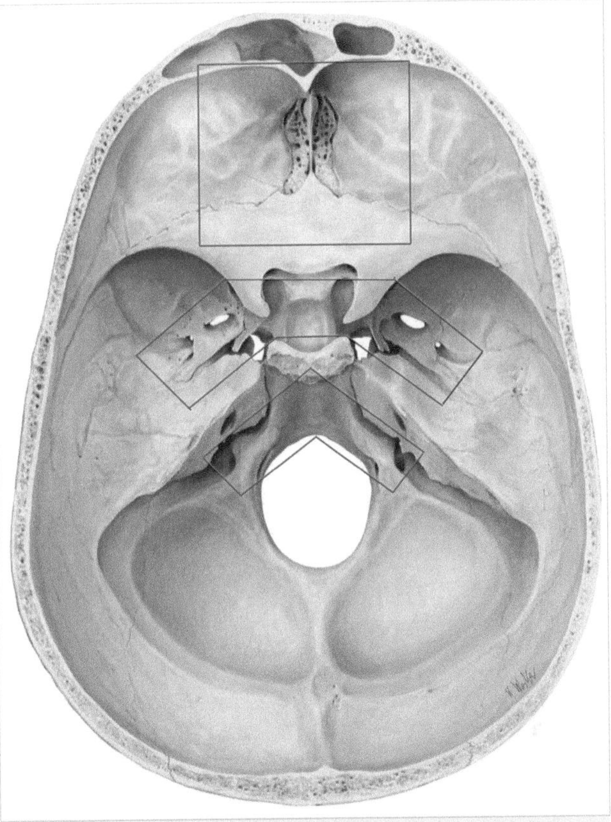

Fig. 6.10 Coronal plane procedures correspond to the respective cranial fossae (anterior, middle, and posterior). (Reproduced with permission from Schuenke M, Schulte E, Schumacher U, Atlas of Anatomy Image Collection: Neck and Internal Organs, New York, NY: Thieme; 2007. Illustration by Karl Wesker/Markus Voll. Illustration by Karl Wesker/Markus Voll.)

Transorbital

Intraconal orbital tumors can be removed using a medial transorbital approach so long as they are inferior and medial to the optic nerve (▶ Fig. 6.12).[15] Following removal of the lamina papyracea, the periorbita is incised and the medial and inferior rectus muscles are identified. Dissection between the muscles provides access to tumors that are medial and inferior to the optic nerve without damaging the nerve supply to the extraocular muscles that lie immediately deep/lateral and deep/superior to the muscles. A smaller dissection window is also available between the medial and superior oblique muscles. A simultaneous transconjunctival approach can facilitate identification of the extraocular muscles, retraction of orbital tissues, and anterior tumor dissection.

The transorbital approach is typically reserved for benign tumors such as vascular tumors (hemangioma, cavernoma) and schwannomas. It also provides an avenue for bony decompression, biopsy, or partial (rarely complete) resection of infiltrative neoplasms (pseudotumor, lymphoma, optic glioma) or optic nerve sheath tumors (meningioma, though only in the presence of an already blind eye). Care is usually taken to preserve the ethmoidal arteries when possible in these cases, for they provide important collateral circulation to the optic nerve. The ophthalmic and central retinal arteries generally run lateral and inferior to the optic nerve, respectively.

Middle Fossa

Medial Transcavernous

A medial approach to the cavernous sinus provides access to the medial (superior and posterior) compartments of the cavernous sinus.[9] Access is enhanced with removal of bone over the cavernous ICA and lateral displacement of the ICA. Depending on tumor extension and patient anatomy, the anterior compartment can sometimes be partially addressed as well. Pituitary adenomas with extension into the cavernous sinus are best followed from the sella, taking the same route as the tumor (▶ Fig. 6.13). The CNs are invested in the dura of the lateral cavernous sinus wall and are generally protected from injury unless this dura is invaded. Recurrent pituitary adenomas may be isolated in a cavernous sinus compartment. Rarely, other tumors (hemangiomas, meningiomas, chordomas) may occur or extend here.[16] Nonadenomas are at much higher risk for resection than softer, less invasive adenomas are.

Medial Petrous Apex

A midclival approach between the floor of the sella and the floor of the sphenoid sinus at the level of the clival recess provides access to the medial petrous apex, which is bounded anteriorly by the petrous and paraclival segments of the ICA and posteriorly by the posterior cranial fossa dura. The medial

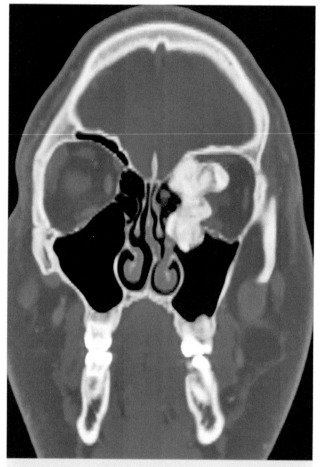

Fig. 6.11 This orbital osteoma is attached to the roof of the ethmoid sinus and orbit. Decompression of the medial orbit and sacrifice of the ethmoidal arteries provides access as far as the midsagittal plane of the orbital roof.

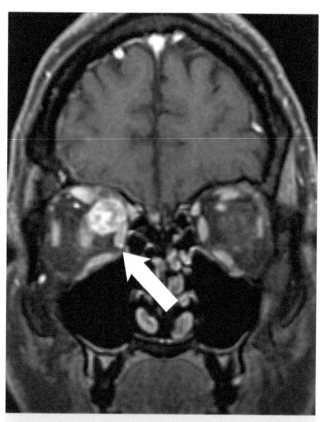

Fig. 6.12 Intraconal orbital lesions that are medial and inferior to the optic nerve can be approached between the medial and inferior rectus muscles (*arrow*) with preservation of function.

triangle (Gardner's triangle) for accessing the petrous apex consists of the window between the paraclival ICA anteriorly, the abducens nerve superiorly, and the petroclival fissure inferiorly. Expansile lesions such as cholesterol granulomas often expand this area, providing easy access, and can even extend into the clival recess (▶ Fig. 6.14).

If additional access is needed, the bone overlying and lateral to the paraclival ICA can be removed to allow lateral displacement of the vessel. Cranial nerve VI (abducens) courses deep to the upper paraclival ICA in Dorello's canal and is susceptible to injury where it runs between the periosteal and meningeal layers of the dura.

In addition to cholesterol granulomas, a medial petrous apex approach can be used for the treatment of petrous apicitis, biopsy of petrous apex tumors (primary and metastatic), and resection of clival tumors that extend laterally (meningioma, chordoma, chondrosarcoma).[17]

Transpterygoid

The transpterygoid approach is a starting point for many of the surgical modules in the middle and posterior coronal planes. It provides access to the lateral recess of the sphenoid

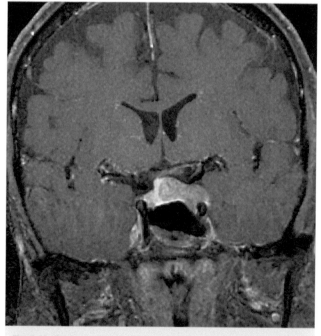

Fig. 6.13 Pituitary adenomas may grow into the compartments of the cavernous sinus. Removal of bone over the parasellar internal carotid artery (ICA) with lateral displacement of the ICA provides direct access with a medial transcavernous approach.

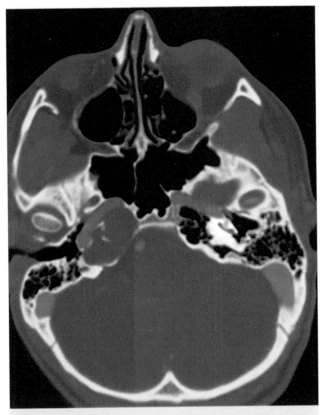

Fig. 6.14 Expansile lesions such as this cholesterol granuloma can be reached with a medial petrous apex approach at the level of the clival recess between the internal carotid artery (petrous and paraclival segments) and brainstem.

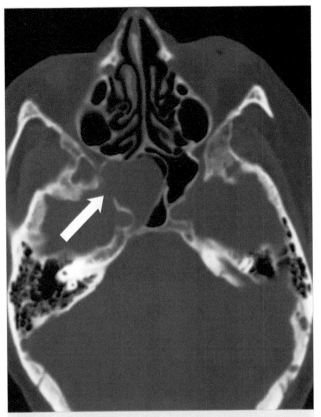

Fig. 6.15 A transpterygoid approach is necessary to reach bone defects (*arrow*) of the lateral recess of the sphenoid sinus as seen with this meningoencephalocele.

sinus, lateral and anterior cavernous sinus compartments, and petrous and lacerum segments of the ICA. A middle meatal antrostomy or medial maxillectomy is followed by sacrifice of the sphenopalatine and palatosphenoidal arteries. The posterior maxillary wall is removed to expose the contents of the pterygopalatine space, which are displaced laterally to expose the base of the pterygoid bone and the pterygoid canal containing the vidian nerve.[18] Foramen rotundum containing the maxillary division (V2) of the trigeminal nerve is located superolaterally. The lateral recess of the sphenoid sinus can now be fully opened between these two foramina with additional removal of bone from the pterygoid base. Further lateral or pterygoid access requires sacrifice of the vidian nerve.

A transpterygoid approach provides access to the lateral recess of the sphenoid sinus for treatment of meningoencephaloceles that typically originate just lateral to the maxillary nerve (▶ Fig. 6.15). Sacrifice of the vidian nerve with drilling of the pterygoid base is essential to fully access these defects or remove all remnants of tumor in patients with angiofibromas.

Contralateral Transmaxillary

Endonasal approaches to the petrous apex are limited anteriorly and laterally by the ICA. Mobilization of the ICA risks injury to the vessel and still does not provide access to the most lateral aspects of the medial petrous apex. A contralateral transmaxillary (CTM) approach improves access to the petrous apex by providing a trajectory that is parallel to the petrous ICA.[19] In comparison with an endonasal approach, the angle is improved by approximately 25° (▶ Fig. 6.16). An anterior maxillotomy (Caldwell-Luc approach) is performed contralateral to the petrous apex of interest and is combined with bilateral sphenoidotomies and removal of sphenoid rostrum. This provides a conduit for suction, dissection, and powered instrumentation, avoiding contact with the ICA and allowing for more lateral access.

The CTM approach greatly enhances the ability to achieve a gross total resection for neoplasms such as chordomas and chondrosarcomas (▶ Fig. 6.17). The approach can be extended superiorly to the cavernous ICA and inferiorly to the parapharyngeal ICA. The deep limits are the cochlea, internal auditory canal, and jugular foramen.

Suprapetrous

Suprapetrous approaches are defined by their relationship above the petrous ICA. They provide access to Meckel's cave, lateral cavernous sinus, and floor of the middle cranial fossa.

Meckel's Cave

Meckel's cave is bounded by the paraclival ICA medially and the petrous ICA inferiorly. Superiorly, CN VI establishes the inferior limit of the lateral cavernous sinus and superior orbital fissure and overlies the ophthalmic branch of the trigeminal nerve. The

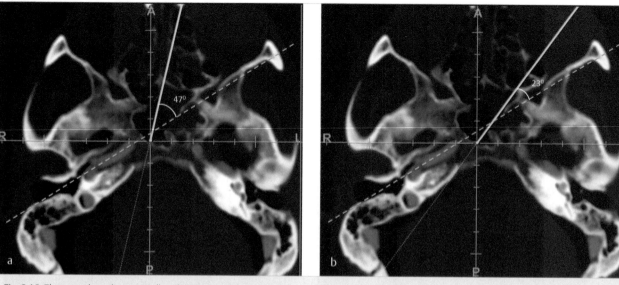

Fig. 6.16 The contralateral transmaxillary (CTM) approach improves the angle of approach to the petrous apex by approximately 25°. **(a)** Contralateral endonasal approach. **(b)** CTM approach.

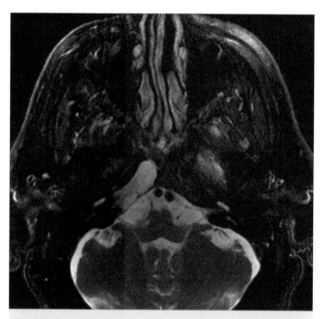

Fig. 6.17 Complete resection of this chondrosarcoma of the right petrous apex is facilitated by a contralateral transmaxillary approach.

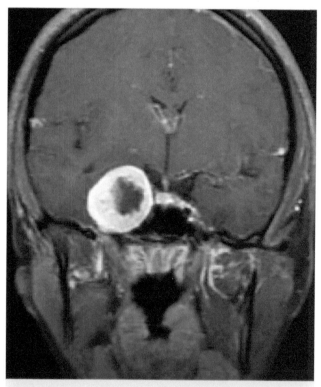

Fig. 6.18 Tumors of Meckel's cave such as this trigeminal schwannoma can be reached using a transpterygoid approach to Meckel's cave, following the course of the vidian nerve and V2, lateral to the paraclival internal carotid artery (ICA) and superior to the petrous ICA.

vidian nerve is an important landmark for localization of the petrous ICA and runs lateral to foramen lacerum to cross the petrous ICA.[18] Sacrifice of the vidian nerve is necessary to gain access to Meckel's cave. The maxillary nerve (second division of the trigeminal nerve) and vidian nerve are separated by the lateral recess of the sphenoid sinus. Increased pneumatization is associated with greater separation of these nerves. These two nerves converge on Meckel's cave. Drilling the pterygoid base inferior and slightly lateral to foramen rotundum will expose the mandibular nerve (third division of the trigeminal nerve) at foramen ovale.

Most tumors involving Meckel's cave are benign: meningiomas and schwannomas (▶ Fig. 6.18). Malignant sinonasal neoplasms (adenoid cystic carcinoma, squamous cell carcinoma) may have perineural extension along the vidian or maxillary nerves to Meckel's cave; resection of the nerve to Meckel's cave can sometimes provide a margin.

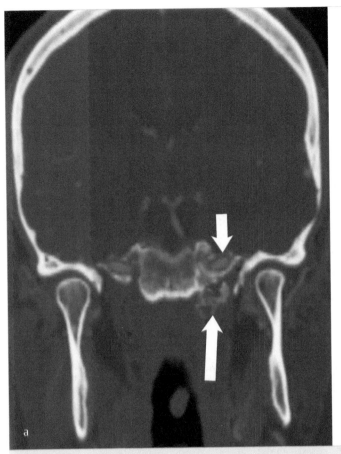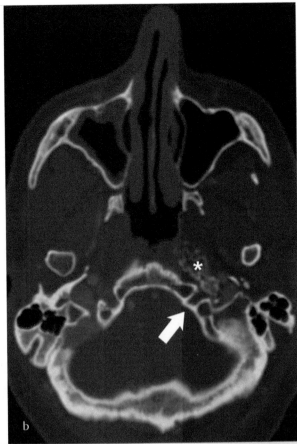

Fig. 6.19 **(a)** Coronal CT demonstrates a chondrosarcoma of the lateral clivus and occipital condyle (*long arrow*). It is inferior to the petrous segment of the internal carotid artery (*short arrow*). **(b)** Tumor (*asterisk*) extends to the hypoglossal canal (*arrow*), which separates the jugular tubercle and occipital condyle.

Lateral Transcavernous

The transpterygoid approach provides lateral access beyond the medial cavernous sinus, allowing resection of tumors in the anterior and lateral compartments.[9] However, indications for operating in the lateral portion of the cavernous sinus are limited.[16] Tumors that invade the lateral cavernous sinus (extrasellar pituitary adenomas, meningiomas) are difficult to dissect without causing loss of CN function, and they have a higher rate of ICA injury. As a result, unless patients are already symptomatic from lateral cavernous sinus invasion or have failed other treatments, residual tumor is often intentionally left in this region.

Posterior Fossa

The posterior coronal plane extends laterally from the lower clivus and craniovertebral junction, below the petrous ICA, and provides access to the skull base above and below the hypoglossal nerve (▶ Fig. 6.10). The lateral limit is the jugular foramen, hypoglossal canal, and parapharyngeal ICA.

Infrapetrous

Infrapetrous approaches to the skull base are inferior to the petrous segment of the ICA. The hypoglossal canal separates the jugular tubercle above (transjugular tubercle approach) from the occipital condyle below (transcondylar approach).[12,20] These approaches are typically associated with clival tumors (chordoma, chondrosarcoma, meningioma) featuring lateral origin or infiltration of the bone (▶ Fig. 6.19). These approaches provide access to the medial portions of the lower cranial base and craniovertebral junction whose lateral portions are accessed from a far lateral approach. Accordingly, they have been analogously called the "far medial" approach.

Transjugular Tubercle

The jugular tubercle is a small triangle of bone situated between the hypoglossal canal and jugular bulb, immediately below foramen lacerum. As its name implies, drilling of the jugular tubercle leads to the jugular bulb/foramen. An endonasal landmark for the level of the hypoglossal canal is a small ridge where the longus capitis muscle attaches to the bone, also known as the supracondylar groove. The jugular tubercle is accessed endonasally by dissecting the upper attachment of the Eustachian tube from foramen lacerum, typically with a tailored mid- or lower clival exposure.[20]

Transcondylar

The occipital condyle articulates with the C1 lateral mass. Clival exposure is extended laterally from the foramen magnum, retracting the torus tubarius of the Eustachian tube and removing or disconnecting the longus capitis muscles.[21] Up to 75% of the occipital condyle on one or both sides can be removed endonasally without loss of cervical stability.[22,23]

Parapharyngeal Space

The parapharyngeal space is one of the most challenging areas in which to operate due to the lack of fixed landmarks and the variable course of the parapharyngeal ICA. In some cases, tortuous parapharyngeal ICAs may approach midline behind the nasopharyngeal mucosa at the level of C1. Preoperative computed tomography angiography is especially useful to identify this ectatic variant, which is most common in elderly patients. Selected tumors at the skull base that are medial to the parapharyngeal ICA may be removed via an endonasal approach. Most commonly, the parapharyngeal ICA is the lateral limit for excision of nasopharyngeal carcinoma and malignant salivary gland tumors (▶ Fig. 6.20). Clival tumors (chordoma, chondrosarcoma) may extend through the petrous bone to the parapharyngeal ICA.

Landmarks for the parapharyngeal ICA include the junction of the cartilaginous and bony Eustachian tube (immediately adjacent), mandibular nerve (V3) at foramen ovale (medial),

and the lateral pterygoid plate (points toward the ICA from an endonasal perspective). The parapharyngeal ICA is behind the stylopharyngeal fascia and immediately lateral to the longus capitis muscle.[24,25]

Proximal control or dissection of the ICA can be achieved by combining an endonasal approach with a transcervical approach.[26] With endoscopic assistance, the parapharyngeal ICA can be dissected to the level of the skull base so as to establish a plane of separation between the ICA and the deep surface of the tumor prior to endonasal resection. A CTM approach can provide improved access for tumors that are infrapetrous and extend to the parapharyngeal ICA where it enters the carotid canal.[19] However, thoughtful case selection should be applied to avoid seeding or tumor contamination of multiple surgical sites.

6.4 Reconstruction

Vascularized reconstructive options for the ventral skull base include local and regional flaps.[27,28] Local flaps include the nasoseptal, middle turbinate, and inferior turbinate (lateral nasal wall) flaps. The nasoseptal flap is the primary choice for most defects, especially sellar, suprasellar, and clival defects. The lateral nasal wall flap is most suitable for small midclival defects because of its limited arc of rotation. Regional flaps include pericranial, temporoparietal, and palatal flaps. Large anterior cranial base defects may be reconstructed with a nasoseptal or extracranial pericranial flap.[29] Larger defects, whether anterior or posterior fossa, are generally best reconstructed with multiple layers, including an inlay graft (collagen or autologous tissue), epidural onlay graft (autologous or allogeneic tissue), and vascularized flap. The addition of intervening fat graft has been shown to lower the risk of pontine encephalocele in the setting of large clival and dural defects.[30]

In addition to the surgical approach, flap selection depends on multiple factors, including patient factors (prior surgery, preoperative embolization, morbidity of reconstruction), tumor factors (location, extent, histology), and surgeon preference. Flap selection based on surgical modules is listed in ▶ Table 6.2.

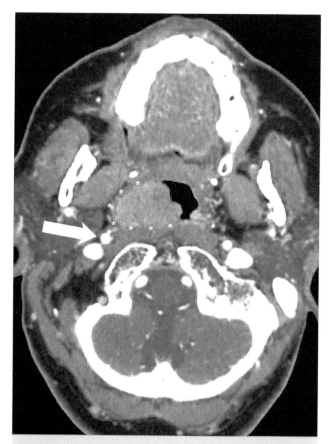

Fig. 6.20 A clear cell carcinoma of the nasopharynx (*outlined with asterisks*) is in close proximity to the parapharyngeal internal carotid artery (ICA) (*arrow*). For this tumor, an endoscopic transcervical approach was used to dissect the ICA from the deep surface of the tumor. Endoscopic resection of the tumor was then performed transnasally.

Table 6.2 Selection of reconstructive flap

Sagittal plane	First choice	Second choice
TF	NSF	PF
TC	NSF	PF
TP	NSF	PF
TF + TC + TP	PF	NSF
Transsellar	NSF	ITF
Transclival	NSF	ITF/TPFF
Transodontoid	NSF	ITF/TPFF
Coronal plane	**First choice**	**Second choice**
Anterior	NSF	PF
Middle	NSF	ITF/TPFF
Posterior	NSF	ITF/TPFF

Abbreviations: ITF, inferior turbinate flap; NSF, nasoseptal flap; PF, pericranial flap; TC, transcribriform; TF, transfrontal; TP, transplanum; TPFF, temporoparietal fascia flap.

It is important to preserve the vascular supply for potential flaps as part of the surgical approach. With a transclival approach, the nasoseptal flap blocks the surgical field and is placed into the maxillary sinus (middle meatal antrostomy) to provide access. With a unilateral transpterygoid approach, a nasoseptal flap is preferentially harvested from the contralateral side. When bilateral transpterygoid approaches are necessary, the flap pedicle can be mobilized by exposing the pterygopalatine fossa. Even if a nasoseptal flap is used, the vascular pedicle for a lateral nasal wall flap is usually preserved on the same side in case the nasoseptal flap fails and a secondary flap is necessary. Other strategies for preserving the blood supply include preserving the vascular pedicle on one side when a reconstructive flap is not anticipated (as a "rescue" flap) or raising a flap and then returning it to the septum if it is not needed.[31] The blood supply to an extracranial pericranial flap is not jeopardized with endonasal approaches and is the preferred reconstructive flap for large anterior cranial base defects when there is neoplastic involvement or other defects of the nasal septum.

6.5 Limitations

Limitations of EES may include patient age (infants), pathology, surgical access, blood loss, reconstruction, duration of surgery, complications, morbidity, training, and resources. Sinus infection

is a contraindication for immediate surgery and should be treated prior to addressing any pathology with potential for dural transgression.

6.5.1 Anatomical

Anatomical limitations to endonasal approaches are primarily the location of major neural and vascular structures (▶ Fig. 6.21). These include the CNs, ICA, and vertebrobasilar arteries. Endoscopic endonasal approaches were developed to provide a ventral/medial corridor for medial tumors that displace these structures laterally or posteriorly. Anatomical limits by surgical module are listed in ▶ Table 6.3.

6.5.2 Training

The learning curve for EES is long, with difficult transitions from extradural to intradural and from sagittal to coronal planes. The learning curve can be approached as five training levels progressing from basic sinus surgery to advanced EES (▶ Table 6.4).[32] The training program is incremental, based on familiarity of anatomy, technical difficulty, risk of neural and vascular injury, intradural and vascular dissection, and type of pathology. Mastery of each level is recommended before advancing to the next. Critical team skills are developed by collaborating on intrasellar pituitary surgeries (hemostasis of cavernous sinus) and repair of cerebrospinal fluid (CSF) leaks (dural reconstruction) with level II procedures. Failure to collaborate on simple procedures misses a key opportunity to gain team proficiency.

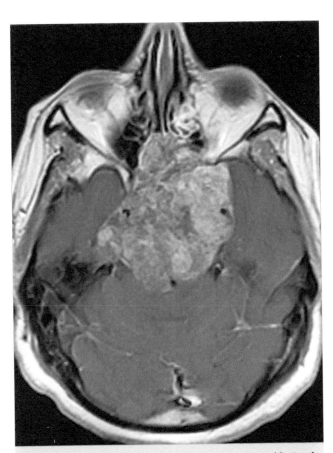

Fig. 6.21 This large chordoma demonstrates the anatomical limits of endoscopic endonasal surgery. It is bounded by the internal carotid arteries and basilar artery as well as the cranial nerves.

Table 6.3 Anatomical limits of surgical modules

Sagittal plane	Cranial nerve	Vessel
Transfrontal (TF)	I	Superior sagittal sinus
Transcribriform (TC)	I	A2/3
Transplanum (TP)	I/II	A1/A2/ACoA
TF + TC + TP	I/II	A1/A2/A3/ACoA
Transsellar	II/VI	ICA
Transclival	VI/XII	ICA/VB/AICA/SCA/PCA
Transodontoid	XII	VA
Coronal plane	**Cranial nerve**	**Vessel**
Anterior	II	N/A
Supraorbital	II	Oph
Transorbital		
Middle	VI	ICA
Medial transcavernous	VI, VII, VIII	ICA
Medial petrous apex	V, VI	ICA (medial/petrous)
Suprapetrous	III, IV, V1	ICA (medial)
Lateral transcavernous		
Posterior	IX, X, XI, XII	ICA
Transjugular tubercle	XII	
Transcondylar		
Parapharyngeal		

Abbreviations: ACoA, anterior communicating artery; AICA, anteroinferior cerebellar artery; ICA, internal carotid artery; Oph, ophthalmic artery; PCA, posterior cerebral artery; SCA, superior cerebellar artery; TC, transcribriform; TF, transfrontal; TP, transplanum; VA, vertebral artery; VB, vertebrobasilar artery junction.

Table 6.4 Training program for endoscopic endonasal surgery

Level I

- Sinus surgery

Level II

- Advanced sinus surgery
- Cerebrospinal fluid leaks
- Sella/pituitary (intrasellar)

Level III

- Sella/pituitary (extrasellar)
- Optic nerve decompression
- Orbital surgery
- Extradural skull base surgery

Level IV

- Intradural skull base surgery

Level V

- Coronal plane (carotid dissection)
- Vascular surgery

6.6 Complications

EES of the skull base is not minimally invasive and has risks similar to those of transcranial surgery.[33,34] The most common complication is a postoperative CSF leak, which occurs in 5 to 10% of patients who have an intraoperative CSF leak. The use of vascularized flaps such as the nasoseptal flap for reconstruction has greatly diminished the risk of a postoperative CSF leak. The risk of postoperative infection (meningitis, brain abscess) is low and is associated with CSF leak. Prompt treatment of postoperative CSF leaks with endoscopic surgical reexploration and repair minimizes the risk of infection. Cranial nerve injury can be avoided with the help of image guidance, neurophysiological monitoring (electromyography),[35] and mastery of surgical anatomy.

Fortunately, the risk of vascular injury is low, with comparable rates noted for endoscopic and microscopic surgery.[36] The ability to repair a vascular injury is limited, however, and endovascular control is often necessary. Treatment algorithms provide a stepwise approach to the management of vascular injuries and help limit morbidity and mortality.[37]

EES is designed to minimize manipulation of brain tissue. Comparisons of endonasal and transcranial approaches for olfactory groove meningiomas demonstrate less radiographic trauma to the frontal lobes with EES.[38] Ongoing studies will address the impact of EES on preservation of neurocognitive function.

6.7 Conclusion

Our classification of endonasal approaches to the ventral skull base provides a logical and systematic method that facilitates preoperative planning and surgery. Organization along sagittal and coronal planes is intuitive and matches radiological imaging. Surgical modules can be combined to create a tailored approach for each patient. Anatomical knowledge provides surgical landmarks that are specific to each module, minimizing surgical morbidity and establishing anatomical constraints for EES. Proper training is necessary to safely perform EES of the skull base.

References

[1] Snyderman CH, Carrau RL, Kassam AB, et al. Endoscopic skull base surgery: principles of endonasal oncological surgery. J Surg Oncol. 2008; 97(8):658–664

[2] Kassam AM, Gardner PA, Prevedello DM, Snyderman CH, Carrau RL. Principles of endoneurosurgery. In: Kassam AB, Gardner PA, eds. Endoscopic Approaches to the Skull Base. Progress in Neurological Surgery. Vol. 26. Basel: Karger; 2012:21–26

[3] Solares CA, Ong YK, Snyderman CH. Transnasal endoscopic skull base surgery: what are the limits? Curr Opin Otolaryngol Head Neck Surg. 2010; 18 (1):1–7

[4] Snyderman CH, Pant H, Carrau RL, Prevedello DM, Gardner PA, Kassam AB. Classification of endonasal approaches to the ventral skull base. In: Stamm AC, ed. Transnasal Endoscopic Skull Base and Brain Surgery. New York: Thieme; 2011:83–91

[5] Pinheiro-Neto CD, Fernandez-Miranda JC, Wang EW, Gardner PA, Snyderman CH. Anatomical correlates of endonasal surgery for sinonasal malignancies. Clin Anat. 2012; 25(1):129–134

[6] Paluzzi A, Fernandez-Miranda JC, Pinheiro-Neto C, et al. Endoscopic endonasal infrasellar approach to the sellar and suprasellar regions: technical note. Skull Base. 2011; 21(5):335–342

[7] Koutourousiou M, Fernandez-Miranda JC, Stefko ST, Wang EW, Snyderman CH, Gardner PA. Endoscopic endonasal surgery for suprasellar meningiomas: experience with 75 patients. J Neurosurg. 2014; 120(6):1326–1339

[8] Paluzzi A, Fernandez-Miranda JC, Tonya Stefko S, Challinor S, Snyderman CH, Gardner PA. Endoscopic endonasal approach for pituitary adenomas: a series of 555 patients. Pituitary. 2014; 17(4):307–319

[9] Fernandez-Miranda JC, Zwagerman NT, Abhinav K, et al. Cavernous sinus compartments from the endonasal endoscopic approach: anatomical considerations and surgical relevance to adenoma surgery. J Neurosurg. 2017; •••:1–12–; [Epub ahead of print]

[10] Fernandez-Miranda JC, Gardner PA, Rastelli MM, Jr, et al. Endoscopic endonasal transcavernous posterior clinoidectomy with interdural pituitary transposition. J Neurosurg. 2014; 121(1):91–99

[11] Koutourousiou M, Gardner PA, Tormenti MJ, et al. Endoscopic endonasal approach for resection of cranial base chordomas: outcomes and learning curve. Neurosurgery. 2012; 71(3):614–624, discussion 624–625

[12] Morera VA, Fernandez-Miranda JC, Prevedello DM, et al. "Far-medial" expanded endonasal approach to the inferior third of the clivus: the transcondylar and transjugular tubercle approaches. Neurosurgery. 2010; 66(6 Suppl Operative):211–19, discussion 219––2–20

[13] de Almeida JR, Zanation AM, Snyderman CH, et al. Defining the nasopalatine line: the limit for endonasal surgery of the spine. Laryngoscope. 2009; 119 (2):239–244

[14] Zwagerman NT, Tormenti MJ, Tempel ZJ, et al. Endoscopic endonasal resection of the odontoid process—clinical outcomes in 34 patients. J Neurosurg. 2017; •••:1–9–; [Epub ahead of print]

[15] Paluzzi A, Gardner PA, Fernandez-Miranda JC, et al. "Round the clock" surgical access to the orbit. J Neurol Surg B Skull Base. 2015; 76(1):12–24

[16] Koutourousiou M, Vaz Guimaraes Filho F, Fernandez-Miranda JC, et al. Endoscopic endonasal surgery for tumors of the cavernous sinus: a series of 234 patients. World Neurosurg. 2017; 103:713–732

[17] Paluzzi A, Gardner P, Fernandez-Miranda JC, et al. Endoscopic endonasal approach to cholesterol granulomas of the petrous apex: a series of 17 patients: clinical article. J Neurosurg. 2012; 116(4):792–798

[18] Pinheiro-Neto CD, Fernandez-Miranda JC, Rivera-Serrano CM, et al. Endoscopic anatomy of the palatovaginal canal (palatosphenoidal canal): a landmark for dissection of the vidian nerve during endonasal transpterygoid approaches. Laryngoscope. 2012; 122(1):6–12

[19] Patel CR, Wang EW, Fernandez-Miranda JC, Gardner PA, Snyderman CH. Contralateral transmaxillary corridor: an augmented endoscopic approach to the petrous apex. J Neurosurg. 2017; •••:1–9–; [Epub ahead of print]

[20] Fernandez-Miranda JC, Morera VA, Snyderman CH, Gardner P. Endoscopic endonasal transclival approach to the jugular tubercle. Neurosurgery. 2012; 71(1 Suppl Operative):ONS146–1–59

[21] Wang WH, Abhinav K, Wang E, Snyderman C, Gardner PA, Fernandez-Miranda JC. Endoscopic endonasal transclival transcondylar approach for foramen magnum meningiomas: surgical anatomy and technical note. Oper Neurosurg (Hagerstown). 2016; 12(2):153–162

[22] Kooshkabadi A, Choi PA, Koutourousiou M, et al. Atlanto-occipital instability following endoscopic endonasal approach for lower clival lesions: experience with 212 cases. Neurosurgery. 2015; 77(6):888–897

[23] Perez-Orribo L, Little AS, Lefevre RD, et al. Biomechanical evaluation of the craniovertebral junction after anterior unilateral condylectomy: implications for endoscopic endonasal approaches to the cranial base. Neurosurgery. 2013; 72(6):1021–1029, discussion 1029–1030

[24] Liu J, Sun X, Liu Q, Wang D, Wang H, Ma N. Eustachian tube as a landmark to the internal carotid artery in endoscopic skull base surgery. Otolaryngol Head Neck Surg. 2016; 154(2):377–382

[25] Simon F, Vacher C, Herman P, Verillaud B. Surgical landmarks of the nasopharyngeal internal carotid using the maxillary swing approach: a cadaveric study. Laryngoscope. 2016; 126(7):1562–1566

[26] Snyderman CH, Gardner PA, Wang EW, Fernandez-Miranda JC. Transcervical endoscopic approach for removal of parapharyngeal space masses. Oper Tech Otolaryngol—Head Neck Surg. 2014; 25:265–273

[27] Bhatki AM, Pant H, Snyderman C, et al. Reconstruction of the cranial base after endonasal skull base surgery: local tissue flaps. Operative Techniques in Otolaryngology. 2010; 21(1):74–82

[28] Bhatki A, Pant H, Snyderman C, et al. Reconstruction of the cranial base following endonasal skull base surgery: regional tissue flaps. Operative Techniques in Otolaryngology. 2010; 21(1):83–90

[29] Zanation AM, Snyderman CH, Carrau RL, Kassam AB, Gardner PA, Prevedello DM. Minimally invasive endoscopic pericranial flap: a new method for endonasal skull base reconstruction. Laryngoscope. 2009; 119(1):13–18

[30] Koutourousiou M, Filho FV, Costacou T, et al. Pontine encephalocele and abnormalities of the posterior fossa following transclival endoscopic endonasal surgery. J Neurosurg. 2014; 121(2):359–366

[31] Rivera-Serrano CM, Snyderman CH, Gardner P, et al. Nasoseptal "rescue" flap: a novel modification of the nasoseptal flap technique for pituitary surgery. Laryngoscope. 2011; 121(5):990–993

[32] Snyderman C, Kassam A, Carrau R, Mintz A, Gardner P, Prevedello DM. Acquisition of surgical skills for endonasal skull base surgery: a training program. Laryngoscope. 2007; 117(4):699–705

[33] Kassam AB, Prevedello DM, Carrau RL, et al. Endoscopic endonasal skull base surgery: analysis of complications in the authors' initial 800 patients. J Neurosurg. 2011; 114(6):1544–1568

[34] Carrau R, Kassam A, Snyderman C, Prevedello D, Mintz A, Massegur YH. Complications of endoscopic skull base surgery. Acta Otorrinolaringol Esp. 2007; 58:106–113

[35] Thirumala PD, Mohanraj SK, Habeych M, et al. Value of free-run electromyographic monitoring of extraocular cranial nerves during expanded endonasal surgery (EES) of the skull base. J Neurol Surg Rep. 2013; 74(1):43–50

[36] Gardner PA, Tormenti MJ, Pant H, Fernandez-Miranda JC, Snyderman CH, Horowitz MB. Carotid artery injury during endoscopic endonasal skull base surgery: incidence and outcomes. Neurosurgery. 2013; 73(2) Suppl Operative:ons261–ons269, discussion ons269–ons270

[37] Gardner PA, Snyderman CH, Fernandez-Miranda JC, Jankowitz BT. Management of major vascular injury during endoscopic endonasal skull base surgery. Otolaryngol Clin North Am. 2016; 49(3):819–828

[38] de Almeida JR, Carvalho F, Vaz Guimaraes Filho F, et al. Comparison of endoscopic endonasal and bifrontal craniotomy approaches for olfactory groove meningiomas: a matched pair analysis of outcomes and frontal lobe changes on MRI. J Clin Neurosci. 2015; 22(11):1733–1741

7 Reconstruction of Skull Base Defects

Parth V. Shah, Gregory Capra, Cristine N. Klatt-Cromwell, Brian D. Thorp, Charles S. Ebert Jr., and Adam M. Zanation

Summary

This chapter describes the multitude of reconstructive options, both endoscopic and open, that have been created in the last twenty years to adapt to the expanding role of endoscopic endonasal surgery for a wide variety of skull base defects and lesions. These reconstructive techniques include grafts, local and regional vascularized flaps, and microvascular free flaps. Indications, advantages, and disadvantages of each reconstructive option are discussed. Details of techniques for harvest and placement of each type of reconstruction are outlined. Patient selection, postoperative care, potential complications, and current data detailing outcomes of these reconstructive options are also described.

Keywords: skull base reconstruction, endoscopic skull base surgery, nasoseptal flap, pericranial flap, temporoparietal flap, free flap, CSF leak

7.1 Introduction

In the past 20 years, endoscopic endonasal surgery has expanded to become an approach for resection of both extradural and intradural skull base lesions. The goals of this approach are to completely resect skull base tumors with negative margins and minimal morbidity, as well as to reconstruct residual skull base defects in a reliable manner. These methods of reconstruction must be watertight if they are to prevent postoperative complications, including cerebrospinal fluid (CSF) leak, meningitis, pneumocephalus, and death.

Reconstruction of the skull base directly correlates with the type and extent of surgical defect that has been created. In the past, these reconstructions were performed primarily using cellular or acellular grafts. However, as endoscopic techniques have expanded and the sizes of these residual defects have increased, such grafts have been unable to provide adequate closure. Accordingly, the harvest of vascularized tissue was explored as an innovative option for reconstruction. Examples of vascularized tissue used in both endoscopic and open techniques include the nasoseptal flap, pericranial flap, and turbinate flaps.

Thus, as the indications for endoscopic skull base resections have expanded, the need for advanced endoscopic reconstructive techniques has increased as well. In this chapter, we discuss various options for endoscopic reconstruction, including cellular and acellular grafts, as well as vascularized regional flaps. In addition, we address open techniques for skull base defects that cannot be repaired endoscopically due to either failure of prior reconstruction or anatomic limitations.

7.2 Goals of Reconstruction

Skull base surgeons must keep in mind several goals of reconstruction when formulating their surgical plan.[1] The primary objective is to separate the cranial cavity and brain from the sinonasal tract while also providing an adequate seal. In addition, the reconstructive choice must protect the brain and intracranial neurovasculature from infection and desiccation. By providing this watertight seal, the reconstructive technique can also help accelerate the healing process. Dead spaces that have been created should be obliterated. Finally, both function and cosmesis should be preserved and/or restored. With these key aspects of reconstruction in mind, the skull base surgeon must choose a proper technique that achieves these goals.

7.3 Types of Defects

The nature of the skull base defect itself is a key factor in the decision of the proper reconstructive technique. First, defects can be categorized by size. Small defects are usually less than 1 cm in size, whereas larger defects are greater than 3 cm in size. For small defects, acellular grafts and nonvascularized tissue grafts are usually adequate for reconstruction. For medium-sized defects, local flaps are a more suitable option. For larger defects, regional or free flaps are generally used.

Next, defects are characterized by their extension.[1,2] Skull base defects can be intradural or extradural. Whereas extradural defects involve resection of skull base with intact dura, and thus without leakage of CSF, intradural defects involve violation of dura and can be divided into two groups: extra-arachnoidal and intra-arachnoidal. By definition, cases of intra-arachnoidal defect involve CSF leak. The distinguishing factor between high- and low-flow CSF leak is whether a cistern was directly opened.

7.4 Patient Selection

The decision to perform endoscopic skull base surgery requires careful patient selection and preoperative planning that includes examination of multiple tumor characteristics, including size, extent, location, and relationship to surrounding structures and neurovasculature. During this planning stage, reconstructive options are addressed. Patient factors that can lead to poor healing outcomes include prior radiation and smoking. Additionally, intracranial hypertension and obesity can increase the difficulty of the reconstruction. Certain defects, depending on their location and size, can be associated with a greater risk of CSF leakage, and the chosen reconstructive option must address this.

7.5 Endoscopic Techniques

After smooth induction of anesthesia and endotracheal intubation, the patient is positioned appropriately for both resection and reconstruction. One of the main concerns to be relayed to the anesthesia team is that of avoiding intraoperative hypertension and hypotension. The patient is kept supine, the head of the bed is slightly elevated, and padding is placed around the heels and elbows to prevent postoperative peripheral neuropathies. All potential reconstructive donor sites are exposed. If a lumbar drain will be used, the neurosurgery team should place it during this preparatory time. Next the image guidance system must be set up and the patient registered into the system. By this point, CT and MRI images should already be loaded. Axial, coronal, and sagittal cuts must be visible and linked. Finally, all surgical sites are sterilely prepped and draped.

7.5.1 Acellular and Cellular Grafts

Acellular and cellular grafts generally have a role in most skull base procedures, but they can be used alone for small defects. Acellular grafting materials can be made from a collagen matrix (Duragen, Integra Life Sciences) or dermal matrix (AlloDerm, LifeCell). Duragen is usually placed in an inlay fashion, either in the epidural or in the subdural plane. To prevent CSF leakage, the graft should be placed 0.5 to 1 cm past the dural margin. If the resection includes areas where there are limited bony edges, or if an inlay graft cannot be placed, AlloDerm can be placed in onlay fashion in the subdural or epidural plane after removal of all underlying mucosa. Multilayer reconstruction and bolstering techniques are described hereafter. The intranasal edges of the AlloDerm are usually bolstered by oxidized cellulose (or absorbable packing), with sequential application of biologic or synthetic glue and absorbable gelatin sponge.

Another graft option is the use of cellular tissue for repair. Examples of cellular grafts include free mucosal grafts, abdominal fat grafts, and dermal fat grafts. Free mucosal grafts are very commonly used and can be taken from the nasal floor, septum, or middle turbinate. The advantage of this graft is that there is no need for a second donor site, so donor site morbidity is rare. The middle turbinate is used quite often for moderate-sized skull base defects. The mucosa of this structure is stripped and then used as a graft. It is placed onto the skull base after the mucosa has been cleared from bony ledges. Although it provides a scaffold for healing, its small size limits its use in larger skull base resections. Another cellular graft that is commonly used is the abdominal free fat graft. Often employed as a bolster of biologic dressing in a multilayered reconstruction technique, it can also be used to obliterate spaces such as the clival recess or a nasopharyngeal defect after tumor resection. Options for donor sites include the periumbilical region, the right or left lower abdominal quadrants, and the lateral hip. Harvest is performed by making a small incision in any one of these regions and circumferentially dissecting an appropriate volume of fat. The specimen is then placed in saline prior to use. Often the dermis is taken along with fat in what is termed a dermal fat graft. To harvest this, an elliptical incision is performed and carried through the dermis without violating the fat. The epidermis is removed, and the specimen is again circumferentially dissected to remove the desired volume of fat while keeping the dermis in continuity. Although these cellular grafts have shown great value in small and sometimes moderate-sized defects, their use in larger resections (i.e., greater than 3 cm in size) has been associated with a higher rate of postoperative CSF leakage, ultimately prompting development of the innovation of vascularized reconstruction.[3]

7.5.2 Nasoseptal Flap

The nasoseptal flap is the primary workhorse for most skull base reconstruction surgery. It was first described by Hadad et al in 2006, in whose retrospective review of 43 patients who underwent endoscopic reconstruction of large anterior dural defects only 5% had postoperative CSF leakage.[3] The vascular supply of this flap is the posterior septal artery, which is a branch of the sphenopalatine artery. The extra length provided by this pedicle allows use of this flap for multiple types of defects. The flap itself is composed of mucoperiosteum and mucoperichondrium.

Harvest of the nasoseptal flap is initiated at the beginning of the case prior to tumor resection because of the location of the pedicle (▶ Fig. 7.1). The flap must be harvested and the vascular supply protected prior to sphenoidotomy and septectomy. First the inferior turbinates are outfractured bilaterally and the ipsilateral middle turbinate is excised. To protect the olfactory epithelium, the superior harvest incision is made 1 to 2 cm from the most superior portion of the septum. The inferior incision is made below the floor of the sphenoid sinus and across the posterior choana. This incision should extend along the nasal floor. Both the superior and inferior incisions are connected with a vertical incision at the level of the head of the inferior turbinate. All incisions should be made prior to elevation of the flap, both to prevent tearing and because orienting the tissue and maintaining tension can be difficult once it has been elevated. Elevation of the flap should begin anteriorly with either a Cottle elevator or suction dissector. The flap is elevated posteriorly to the sphenoid face. After ensuring that the vascular supply is intact following elevation, the nasoseptal flap can be placed in the nasopharynx or ipsilateral maxillary sinus to prevent inadvertent damage during the ablative portion of the procedure.

One of the major advantages of this flap is that there is no need for a second surgical site. However, a significant disadvantage is that it needs to be harvested prior to surgical resection, particularly the sphenoidotomy and septectomy portions of the procedure. To circumvent this problem, the "rescue" technique, or partial harvest, was created.[4] In this technique, the superior incision is made extending from the sphenoid os

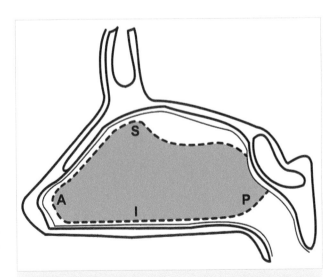

Fig. 7.1 Nasoseptal flap. Sagittal view of the nasal septum with dashed lines indicating incision sites for harvest of the nasoseptal flap. A, anterior; I, inferior; P, posterior; S, superior. (Illustration by Saikat Basu, PhD, University of North Carolina at Chapel Hill.)

to the superior aspect of the septum, about 1 cm below its cranialmost aspect. The incision is then extended 2 cm anteriorly, after which the flap is reflected inferiorly using a Cottle elevator to expose the sphenoid rostrum. The vascular pedicle is protected during this process. Once the partial harvest has been completed, the posterior septectomy and remainder of the resection can be performed without compromising flap viability. Once the flap is placed in proper orientation and position, it is supplemented with a multilayer bolster.

7.5.3 Posterior Pedicled Inferior Turbinate Flap

The nasoseptal flap is not a viable option for skull base reconstruction in certain patients, such as those who have had prior septectomy or wide sphenoidotomies. In these instances, the vascular supply to the nasoseptal flap has been compromised and an alternative solution is required for endoscopic reconstruction. One option is the posterior pedicled inferior turbinate flap (PPITF), which is based on the inferior turbinate artery.[5] This artery arises from a branch of the posterior lateral nasal artery (PLNA), which itself arises from the sphenopalatine artery. The PLNA travels in a descending course over the perpendicular plate of the ascending process of the palatine bone. It gives off a branch that supplies the middle turbinate. The remainder courses inferiorly and enters the inferior turbinate at its superolateral attachment. It then pierces the bone and soft tissue before giving off several branches.

The PPITF should be harvested ipsilateral to the defect. The flap has a much smaller volume than the nasoseptal flap, so the entire inferior turbinate should be harvested to ensure adequate coverage. Harvest begins by identifying the sphenopalatine artery as it exits the sphenopalatine foramen. This is followed distally until the PLNA branches. Two parallel incisions are then made—one just superior to the inferior turbinate and the other following the caudal margin of the turbinate. A vertical incision at the anterior head of the inferior turbinate is made to connect the two parallel incisions. Next the mucoperiosteum of the inferior turbinate is elevated from anterior to posterior. Preserving the vascular pedicle as it enters the superior aspect of the lateral attachment of the inferior turbinate and the PLNA is essential.

When placing the flap, any nonvascularized tissue between the margins of the defect and the flap must be removed. Biologic glue can then be applied, followed by a multilayer bolster. A 16 Fr coudet catheter is placed to provide pressure against the PPITF. A limitation of this flap is its smaller coverage area, which is approximately 60% of the anterior cranial fossa per prior endoscopic analysis.[6] To compensate for this, the flap can be supplemented with free grafts. Bilateral flaps can be used for larger defects. Another disadvantage is the shorter length of the flap and its pedicle, as well as its restricted angle of rotation. Thus this flap is more useful for posterior defects of the sellar, pansellar, and midclival regions.

7.5.4 Posterior Pedicled Middle Turbinate Flap

A third purely endoscopic option for skull base reconstruction is the posterior pedicled middle turbinate flap (PPMTF), which

has been investigated in cadaveric studies.[7] To understand this harvest technique, it is necessary to review the anatomy of the middle turbinate and of the vascular supply to this flap. The middle turbinate inserts into the lateral nasal wall at its anterior and posterior segments. It also attaches to the skull base between these sites at the vertical lamella of the cribriform plate. The vascular supply of the middle turbinate is a branch of the sphenopalatine artery, which traverses its posterior attachment. Harvest begins with a vertical incision at the anterior head of the middle turbinate. Next a horizontal incision is made along the vertical attachment of the middle turbinate just inferior to the skull base, and this is extended from anterior to posterior. The mucoperiosteum of the medial surface of the middle turbinate is then raised from superior to inferior, after which the bone of the middle turbinate is removed. Transection of the vertical attachment of the turbinate to the skull base is then followed by the lateral attachment of the flap to the skull base. The flap is elevated posteriorly and the basal lamella is transected, leaving a posteriorly pedicled flap that originates from the lateral surface of the middle turbinate.

The PPMTF can be used for defects of the planum sphenoidale, sella, and fovea ethmoidalis. It can occasionally be used to cover clival defects. An advantage of this technique is the arc of rotation and greater length of the middle turbinate flap when compared with the inferior turbinate. Its superior position also allows it to provide better coverage of some of the aforementioned defects than the inferior turbinate flap can. One disadvantage is that it becomes increasingly difficult to harvest and use when anatomic sinonasal variations are present.[2] Both turbinate flaps provide options in cases in which the nasoseptal flap cannot be used. In our practice, the PPMTF has become less used because of the difficulty of harvest and the limited surface area for reconstruction.

7.6 Endoscopic-Assisted and Open Techniques

7.6.1 Endoscopic-Assisted Pericranial Flap

Prior to its use in endoscopic skull base surgery, the pericranial flap had been a commonly used reconstructive option employed by neurosurgeons in open anterior cranial base procedures. It was then described by Zanation et al for use in endoscopic skull base reconstruction.[8] This axial flap is based on the supraorbital and supratrochlear arteries and provides a large volume of vascularized tissue that can cover the whole skull base. The first step in harvesting this flap is to create a 2-cm midline incision and a 1-cm lateral port incision along the coronal plane of the scalp (▶ Fig. 7.2).

The two arteries are identified by Doppler ultrasound. The location of these vessels is approximated and a 3-cm-wide flap pedicle is marked at the supraorbital rim. Dissection proceeds in a subgaleal plane through the previously made midline incision and extends to the pedicle. The pericranium is incised to the appropriate width and elevated to the level of the pedicle. A transverse 1-cm incision is made in the glabella and dissection proceeds down through the nasion periosteum into a subperiosteal plane, which is further dissected until it communicates

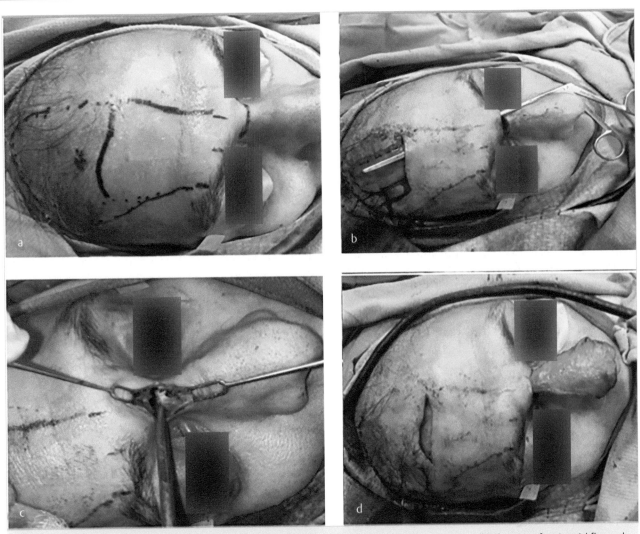

Fig. 7.2 Endoscopic-assisted pericranial flap. **(a)** Outline of pericranial flap geometry and incision over nasion. **(b)** Elevation of pericranial flap and subperiosteal tunnel to site of nasion incision. **(c)** Dissection of nasion down into nasal cavity for transposition of pericranial flap. **(d)** Transposition of pericranial flap through subperiosteal tunnel prior to placement into nasal cavity.

with the subperiosteal plane at the level of the flap pedicle. A drill is used to enter the nasal cavity through the bone of the nasion, and the pericranial flap is transposed via this introduced defect, making sure to keep the flap in proper orientation. The superficial surface of the flap should be placed in contact with the dural defect, and then the flap should be bolstered in place in multilayered fashion, described later. A suction drain may be placed within the scalp to prevent the formation of a hematoma or seroma.

The endoscopic-assisted pericranial flap can be used for reconstruction of cribriform and planar defects, as well as when addressing defects of the sella. The length of the flap is variable and can be extended by placing scalp incisions further posteriorly or by dissecting posterior to the incisions.

7.6.2 Temporoparietal Fascial Flap

The temporoparietal fascial flap is a reconstructive option for defects of the orbit, midface, auricle, and lateral skull base. Its pedicle is composed of the anterior branch of the superficial

temporal artery. This flap is quite pliable and provides a sufficient amount of bulk. Because of its more distant location from the site of tumor, it provides the option of nonradiated tissue for reconstruction after resection of skull base malignancies.[9]

Before its harvest, tumor resection must be completed, after which ipsilateral anterior and posterior ethmoidectomy, as well as maxillary antrostomy, are performed. The sphenopalatine artery and posterior nasal artery are identified and clipped at the level of the sphenopalatine foramen. The pterygopalatine fossa is exposed and the sphenopalatine artery followed proximally. The posterior and lateral walls of the maxillary sinus are resected to enter the infratemporal fossa, with visualization of the internal maxillary artery. The descending palatine artery, which travels inferiorly from the internal maxillary artery, is dissected out from its canal. The contents of the pterygopalatine fossa are retracted inferolaterally to allow visualization of the pterygoid plates. The pterygopalatine ganglion is identified and preserved. Often sacrifice of the vidian nerve is needed to allow displacement of the ganglion. The anterior portion of the pterygoid plates is drilled to enlarge the space for transposition of the flap. Once the preparation for flap transposition has been completed, the external harvest of the flap can begin.

An ipsilateral hemicoronal incision is made to the level of the hair follicles. The superficial temporal artery is at risk of injury due to its position within the subcutaneous tissues, so care must be taken during dissection. The flap is dissected from the subcutaneous tissue, and after adequate exposure, the temporoparietal fascia is incised at its lateral margins. The flap is elevated down to its pedicle from the deep temporal fascia. A vertical incision is made in the superficial layer of the deep temporalis fascia, and a plane is created between fascia and muscle. This plane is followed inferiorly where the periosteum of the zygomatic arch is elevated, thus creating a tunnel beneath the superficial layer of the deep temporalis fascia through which the pedicle will be able to pass. A lateral canthotomy incision is then made to separate the temporalis muscle from lateral orbit and pterygomaxillary fissure. The end result of this dissection is that a continuous tunnel is created that combines the temporal, infratemporal fossa, and transpterygoid approaches. This tunnel is then dilated under endoscopic visualization by threading a guide wire endonasally and passing serial tracheotomy dilators over it. Once dilation is complete, the flap is sutured to the external end of the wire. The wire is then removed via the nostril, pulling the flap through the soft tissue tunnel and into the nasal cavity. It is essential to keep the flap in its proper orientation to prevent twisting and vascular compromise. A collagen matrix graft is placed over the skull base defect in inlay fashion, followed by the temporoparietal fascial flap. A multilayer bolster is then placed, including sealant, absorbable sponges, and sponge packing.

Some risks of using the temporoparietal fascial flap include the potential for injury to the frontal branch of the facial nerve and to the internal maxillary artery during the endoscopic approach. However, the flap does provide a reconstructive option of nonradiated tissue with adequate bulk and pliability for skull base defects.

7.6.3 Palatal Flap

Briefly, a final option for local reconstruction that can be used when other vascularized tissue is not available is the intranasal pedicled palatal mucosal flap.[10] The vascular supply options for this flap are the terminal branches of the sphenopalatine artery or the descending palatine artery. In this technique, mucoperiosteal tissue from the hard palate is tunneled through the greater palatine foramen and transposed into the nasal cavity. Because of the donor site morbidity associated with this flap, it is generally used only when no other options are available.[2]

7.6.4 Microvascular Free Flap

The last vascularized tissue option that will be discussed is the microvascular free flap, which is indicated for use in the reconstruction of large, complex skull base defects.[1] Such flaps can be used in cases of revision surgery and in cases in which the tissue has previously been irradiated. Some commonly used free flaps include the radial forearm, anterolateral thigh, scapular tip, rectus abdominis, and latissimus dorsi. The radial forearm free flap is a fasciocutaneous flap based on the radial artery and vein. It is very pliable and has a long vascular pedicle. The

anterolateral thigh flap is supplied by the lateral femoral circumflex artery and thus provides a long pedicle with a large volume of soft tissue for reconstruction. The scapular tip free flap provides bone for certain skull base defects. Its vascular supply is a branch of the circumflex scapular artery. The rectus abdominis flap is pedicled on the inferior epigastric artery and vein and provides a large skin paddle, whereas the latissimus dorsi flap is a myocutaneous flap supplied by the thoracodorsal artery. Free flaps can provide a large volume of vascularized tissue for complex skull base defects but can also be associated with a number of complications. These include compromise of the vascular anastomosis, leading to flap necrosis, thrombosis of the vascular supply, donor site necrosis, postoperative hematoma/seroma, and poor wound healing.

7.7 Multilayer Bolster and Closure

As alluded to when discussing various vascularized reconstructive options, a multilayer bolster is often necessary to provide support for the repair (▶ Fig. 7.3).[11] Surgicel is usually placed circumferentially around the reconstruction margins, and key regions of the repair can be bolstered with NasoPore. DuraSeal is placed over the entire repair. NasoPore can then be packed in multiple layers to completely cover the region of reconstruction. Finally, nondissolvable packing (e.g., a 16 Fr Coudet catheter) or expandable gelatin sponges can be placed for further bolstering. The expandable sponges are preferred for defects of the planum or ethmoid roof, where pressure against gravity is necessary. The Foley catheter can be used for all types of defects if the optic nerve or chiasm has been exposed. Both types of nondissolvable packing are removed 3 to 5 days after surgery.

7.8 Immediate Postoperative Care

In general, patients who have extensive skull base resections with reconstruction or high-flow intraoperative CSF leaks are admitted to the intensive care unit at least overnight. Because of the increased risk for postoperative leaks in these patients, certain precautions are put into place. They are kept on strict bed rest for 24 to 48 hours from the time of operation. Prophylactic antistaphylococcal antibiotics are administered while packing is in place, and the head of bed is elevated to 30°. In addition, nurses are instructed to prevent nose blowing, sneezing with mouth closed, straining, and the use of straws. Patients are started on a bowel regimen, and a urinary catheter is kept in place to avoid straining during defecation and urination. Once urine output is at an adequate level and there is no concern for diabetes insipidus, the urinary catheter is removed. The remaining precautions are generally maintained throughout the patient's admission and even after discharge until follow-up.

7.9 Lumbar Drains

In the past, lumbar drains were used extensively for most skull base operations, but as techniques for resection and reconstruction have evolved, the use of lumbar drains has become dependent on specific patient factors. Zanation et al described a list of factors that place patients at a higher risk for postoperative CSF

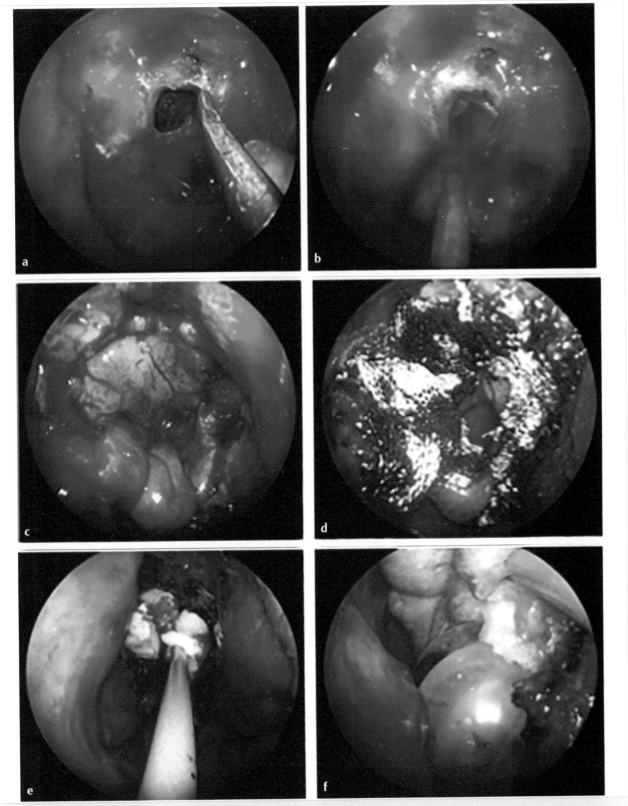

Fig. 7.3 Multilayer reconstruction and bolster. **(a)** Skull base defect. **(b)** Inlay graft using collagen matrix. **(c)** Placement of nasoseptal flap over the entire defect. **(d)** Bolstering of graft with oxidized cellulose absorbable packing. **(e)** Placement of absorbable gelatin sponges. **(f)** Nasal Foley catheter placed for further support.

leak.[2] These include large body habitus; the specific pathology being treated, such as lesions involving the cisterns; entry into the arachnoid cisterns or ventricles; site and size of defects, with those in the anterior cranial base having a greater tendency for postoperative leaks, Cushing's disease, and Adrenocorticotropic hormone-secreting tumors (ACTH)-secreting tumors; and lack of vascularized tissue reconstructive options. Because of the higher risk of CSF leakage in these patients, lumbar drains are placed preoperatively. In cases of high-flow postoperative CSF leak, the patient can be taken back to the operating room for placement of a lumbar drain. Occasionally a ventriculoperitoneal shunt will need to be placed for larger skull base resections or refractory CSF leaks despite lumbar drain placement.[2]

7.10 Outcomes and Postoperative Complications

Regardless of the type of repair, endoscopic and open skull base surgery and reconstruction have multiple risks. Examples include CSF leakage, pneumocephalus, meningitis, infection of reconstructive tissue, and failure of the flap or graft. Pneumocephalus is a postoperative complication that calls for immediate recognition. Symptoms include altered mental status and emesis. Rapid radiologic evaluation can aid in diagnosis, and management may require a return to the operating room for flap/graft inspection and intervention.

Many studies have compared outcomes of endoscopic versus open skull base repairs as well as outcomes of the various endoscopic techniques. In a meta-analysis by Harvey et al, 609 patients who had large dural defects and who had undergone either free graft or vascularized flap reconstructions were included. The CSF leak rate for the free graft group was 15.6% and the leak rate for the vascularized reconstruction group was 6.7%. This difference was found to be statistically significant.[12] Thorp et al performed a retrospective review of 152 vascularized flap skull base reconstructions and found a total of five (3.3%) perioperative CSF leaks.[13] No patients within the cohort experienced flap death or loss. In a different study, Zanation et al assessed 70 skull base reconstructive surgeries for high-flow CSF leakage and obtained a rate of 5.7%.[14] In yet another study, Zanation et al determined that reused nasoseptal flaps were not associated with higher rates of CSF leak or flap death.[15] Finally, Rawal et al investigated outcomes of the nasoseptal rescue flap in seven patients, six of whom had low-flow intraoperative CSF leaks and one of whom had a high-flow CSF leak. Six of the seven patients required use of the rescue flap during the same surgery, and one required its use in a separate procedure about a year later. A 100% success rate was seen in these seven patients, with no recurrent CSF leak or septal perforation.[4]

7.11 Conclusion

The field of skull base surgery has evolved in the last few decades and still continues to advance. To adapt to these changes, techniques for reconstruction have evolved as well. There are now multiple reliable reconstructive options for skull base defects, both endoscopic and open.

References

[1] Hachem RA, Elkhatib A, Beer-Furlan A, Prevedello D, Carrau R. Reconstructive techniques in skull base surgery after resection of malignant lesions: a wide array of choices. Curr Opin Otolaryngol Head Neck Surg. 2016; 24(2): 91–97

[2] Zanation AM, Thorp BD, Parmar P, Harvey RJ. Reconstructive options for endoscopic skull base surgery. Otolaryngol Clin North Am. 2011; 44(5): 1201–1222

[3] Hadad G, Bassagasteguy L, Carrau RL, et al. A novel reconstructive technique after endoscopic expanded endonasal approaches: vascular pedicle nasoseptal flap. Laryngoscope. 2006; 116(10):1882–1886

[4] Rawal RB, Kimple AJ, Dugar DR, et al. Minimizing morbidity in endoscopic pituitary surgery: outcomes of the novel nasoseptal rescue flap technique. Otolaryngology–Head and Neck Surgery. 2012; 147(3):434–437

[5] Fortes FS, Carrau RL, Snyderman CH, et al. The posterior pedicle inferior turbinate flap: a new vascularized flap for skull base reconstruction. Laryngoscope. 2007; 117(8):1329–1332

[6] Harvey RJ, Sheahan PO, Schlosser RJ. Inferior turbinate pedicle flap for endoscopic skull base defect repair. Am J Rhinol Allergy. 2009; 23(5):522–526

[7] Prevedello DM, Barges-Coll J, Fernandez-Miranda JC, et al. Middle turbinate flap for skull base reconstruction: cadaveric feasibility study. Laryngoscope. 2009; 119(11):2094–2098

[8] Zanation AM, Snyderman CH, Carrau RL, Kassam AB, Gardner PA, Prevedello DM. Minimally invasive endoscopic pericranial flap: a new method for endonasal skull base reconstruction. Laryngoscope. 2009; 119(1):13–18

[9] Patel MR, Taylor RJ, Hackman TG, et al. Beyond the nasoseptal flap: outcomes and pearls with secondary flaps in endoscopic endonasal skull base reconstruction. Laryngoscope. 2014; 124(4):846–852

[10] Oliver CL, Hackman TG, Carrau RL, et al. Palatal flap modifications allow pedicled reconstruction of the skull base. Laryngoscope. 2008; 118(12): 2102–2106

[11] Klatt-Cromwell CN, Thorp BD, Del Signore AG, Ebert CS, Ewend MG, Zanation AM. Reconstruction of skull base defects. Otolaryngol Clin North Am. 2016; 49(1):107–117

[12] Harvey RJ, Parmar P, Sacks R, Zanation AM. Endoscopic skull base reconstruction of large dural defects: a systematic review of published evidence. Laryngoscope. 2012; 122(2):452–459

[13] Thorp BD, Sreenath SB, Ebert CS, Zanation AM. Endoscopic skull base reconstruction: a review and clinical case series of 152 vascularized flaps used for surgical skull base defects in the setting of intraoperative cerebrospinal fluid leak. Neurosurg Focus. 2014; 37(4):E4

[14] Zanation AM, Carrau RL, Snyderman CH, et al. Nasoseptal flap reconstruction of high flow intraoperative cerebral spinal fluid leaks during endoscopic skull base surgery. Am J Rhinol Allergy. 2009; 23(5):518–521

[15] Zanation AM, Carrau RL, Snyderman CH, et al. Nasoseptal flap takedown and reuse in revision endoscopic skull base reconstruction. Laryngoscope. 2011; 121(1):42–46

8 Radiotherapy for Skull Base Tumors: Principles and Techniques

Jack Phan, Steven J. Frank, and Paul D. Brown

Summary

This chapter covers radiotherapy principles and modern radiotherapy techniques for skull base tumors. (The clinical applications of radiotherapy in skull base tumors are discussed in Chapter 9.) Radiation physics deals with the properties of photon and particle (e.g., proton) radiation and how they are incorporated into radiation treatment planning, whereas radiobiology covers the basis of dose and fractionation, including hypofractionation and ablative dose delivery, and their effects on tumor and normal tissue biology. Advanced treatment approaches such as intensity-modulated radiation therapy, volumetric arc therapy, carbon ion therapy, intensity-modulated proton therapy, and stereotactic radiosurgery allow highly conformal dose distribution with a steep dose gradient beyond the target volume, thereby reducing the risk of normal tissue damage and widening the therapeutic window. To guide precise and accurate treatment delivery, image-guided radiotherapy incorporating concepts of motion management, target volume delineation, and tracking is discussed.

Keywords: skull base cancer, radiobiology, radiation physics, image-guided radiation therapy, intensity-modulated radiation therapy, volumetric arc therapy, stereotactic radiosurgery, proton therapy

8.1 Introduction

Fractionated radiation therapy and stereotactic radiosurgery (SRS) represent two conceptually different approaches to using ionizing radiation to treat tumors. Fractionated radiation relies on the radiosensitivity difference of the tumor relative to the surrounding normal tissue and is less reliant on precise target localization than radiosurgery is. The concept of fractionation is based on classical radiobiology principles and has been validated clinically in the treatment of head and neck cancers. SRS aims to deliver an ablative dose to the target with a steep dose fall-off outside the target so as to preserve the surrounding normal tissue. SRS was developed by Lars Leksell, a Swedish neurosurgeon, based on the concept of delivering a single high dose of radiation to an intracranial target localized via stereotaxy with high precision and accuracy. Advancements in medical imaging have enabled improved visualization of the tumor and the surrounding anatomy. Corresponding advances in radiation treatment planning and delivery systems have enabled the precise delivery of highly conformal radiation doses to the target so as to minimize collateral damage to adjacent normal organs and preserve normal function.

8.2 History and Principles of Radiation Oncology

The history of radiation therapy began with the discovery of X-rays in 1895 by German physicist Wilhelm Conrad Roentgen.

The first documented therapeutic use of radiation came in 1897, when Professor Leopold Freund demonstrated before the Vienna Medical Society the resolution of a hairy mole after a single exposure to low-dose X-rays. A shift toward fractionated (i.e., involving division of the dose of radiation over a number of treatments) radiotherapy was led by the pioneering work of scientists in Paris, France, who explored the effects of radiation on the testes of rams. They showed that sterilization of the testes in a single dose caused extensive skin sloughing from the scrotum but that when the same dose was fractionated over several weeks, sterilization was achieved with minimal skin damage. This work would eventually establish fractionation as the major form of therapeutic radiation. Other milestone developments in the field included the work of Nobel laureate Hermann Joseph Muller on the genetic effects of radiation, published in 1927, and research performed in the wake of atomic weapons use on Hiroshima and Nagasaki in World War II. Together, these milestones elucidated the biological effects of radiation exposure and radiation-induced carcinogenesis and led to the development of the cell survival curve.

Modern radiation therapy plays a major role in the treatment of skull base neoplasms, both as curative treatment and to palliate tumor-related symptoms. Curative radiotherapy can be delivered as adjuvant therapy, to reduce the risk of tumor recurrence after surgery, and as definitive therapy in which radiation is the primary treatment modality. The ultimate goal of radiotherapy is to achieve 100% tumor control probability (TCP) and thereby prevent local or regional recurrence. Because nearby normal tissues are also exposed to radiation, the normal tissue complication probability (NTCP) increases. The difference between TCP and NTCP is the therapeutic window (▶ Fig. 8.1).

For skull base tumors, this therapeutic window can be narrow, because the tumor is in proximity to critical neural and

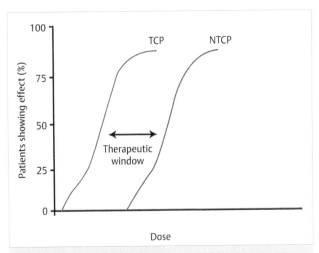

Fig. 8.1 Therapeutic window based on curves for tumor control probability (TCP, *blue line*) and normal tissue complication probability (NTCP, *red line*).

optic structures. Technological advances in radiation therapy, such as conformal radiotherapy, image-guided radiation therapy (IGRT), and SRS, aim to widen this therapeutic window. Radiation physics and radiobiology provide the founding principles of modern radiation delivery methods and understandings of fractionation and of biologic tissues' response to radiation. In addition to discussing the role of radiotherapy in the management of skull base tumors, a goal of this chapter is to provide the reader with an opportunity to become familiar with the

terminology and concepts used in radiation oncology. In the following sections, we briefly introduce several commonly used terms in radiation oncology, with further details provided throughout the chapter.

8.2.1 Target Volumes

There are three main target volumes in radiation treatment planning (▶ Fig. 8.2). The gross tumor volume (GTV) is the visualized gross disease as defined by physical examination and imaging studies. High-quality radiographic imaging is essential for accurate contouring of tumor. The clinical target volume (CTV) is the GTV plus an additional margin to account for microscopic extensions and subclinical disease spread beyond the visualized tumor. For example, pathology studies have shown that in non–small cell lung cancer, a 6-mm CTV margin is required to adequately cover microscopic extension in squamous cell carcinomas, whereas an 8-mm margin is needed for adenocarcinomas.[1] The planning target volume (PTV) is the CTV plus an additional margin to account for uncertainties in treatment planning and delivery, patient setup and positioning, and tumor motion. The PTV, which is largely a geometric expansion based on these uncertainties, is designed to ensure that the intended radiation field covers the entire CTV with each fraction. The organ at risk (OAR) is the volume of a vital organ close to the tumor that should be spared to reduce treatment toxicity.

8.2.2 Alpha/Beta Ratio

The alpha/beta (α/β) ratio is a measure of the radiosensitivity of a tissue type using the ratio of two parameters to describe how a tissue or cell responds to radiation as a function of the dose (▶ Fig. 8.3). The α component is a measure of the intrinsic radiosensitivity of the cell. The β component represents the repairable portion of radiation damage. Tissues that have small α/β ratios are generally less radiosensitive at standard fractionation doses of 2 Gy (i.e., larger β) and imply a large repair

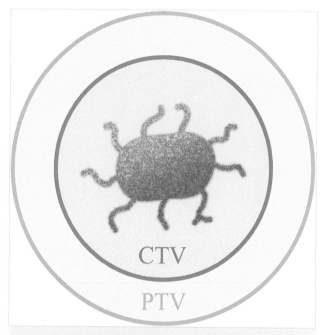

Fig. 8.2 Illustration of visible tumor contoured as gross tumor volume (GTV). Clinical target volume (CTV) encompasses microscopic tumor spread that is subclinical with current imaging scans. Planning target volume (PTV) accounts for uncertainties related to daily patient setup and motion.

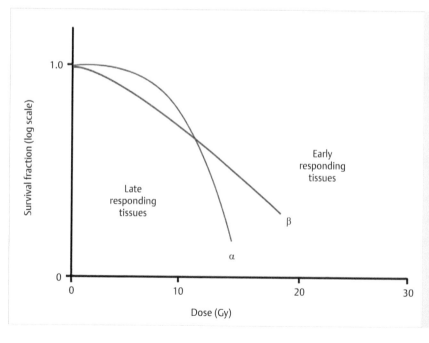

Fig. 8.3 Typical cell survival for early- and late-responding tissues.

capacity (i.e., smaller α). These tissues have a larger sparing effect at standard doses and are typically observed in late-responding tissues, such as nervous tissue. Tissues that have high α/β ratios either imply a poor repair capacity (i.e., smaller β) and/or are more radiosensitive (i.e., larger α). They are typically observed in early-responding tissue, such as skin and mucosal epithelia and most malignant tumors.

8.2.3 Linear Energy Transfer and Relative Biological Effectiveness

Linear energy transfer (LET) is the rate of energy deposited by the charged particles of ionizing radiation. Relative biological effectiveness (RBE) is a term commonly used to compare different types of radiation and their biological effectiveness; it is the RBE of test radiation when compared with a reference radiation that produces the same effect. In most cases, the test radiation refers to protons, neutrons, and carbon ions and the reference radiation is photons or gamma rays. Proton and carbon ion radiation have a higher RBE than photons, because they cause more biological damage at a given dose. As a general rule, radiation having higher LET will also have a higher RBE and thus cause more biological damage.

8.2.4 Fractionation and Sparing Effect

As outlined earlier, fractionation is the concept of breaking up the total dose into smaller daily fractions to give normal tissues time to repair (▶ Fig. 8.4). This approach exploits the radiosensitivity difference between rapidly growing tumor cells and most normal tissues. Thus, when the same radiation dose is given in multiple fractions separated by sufficient time for cell repair (~ 6 h for twice-daily treatments and 24 h for daily treatments), sparing of the tissue (reduction of damage) occurs in a degree depending on the type of radiation used, the dose per fraction given, and the type of tissue irradiated. Standard

(conventional) fractionation doses of 1.8 to 2.0 Gy are typically used to allow for effective sparing of normal tissue.

8.2.5 Altered Fractionation

Altered fractionation refers to various fractionation schemes developed over the past few decades that differ from standard fractionation. *Hyperfractionation* is the breaking up of standard fractionation doses into smaller doses given with higher frequency, with the goal of further exploiting the differences in sensitivity between tumors, which typically have a higher α/β ratio, and normal tissue, which typically has a lower α/β ratio (most parenchymal tissue). The intent of this approach is to lower late toxicity risk in patients who receive conventional radiotherapy. *Accelerated fractionation*, or the shortening of overall treatment time to address the risk of accelerated tumor repopulation that occurs after initiation of oncologic therapy, is often achieved without altering total dose or dose per fraction. A common accelerated fractionation schedule used in head and neck squamous cell carcinoma (HNSCC) is the Danish Head and Neck Cancer Study Group (DAHANCA) regimen of six fractions per week instead of five, which shortens overall treatment time and improves tumor response.[2] Hypofractionation involves increasing the dose per fraction (usually > 3 Gy per day) above the standard fractionation dose. Doing so reduces the number of fractions and shortens the overall course of treatment, results that are logistically and financially favorable. Larger dose per fraction increases the probability of overcoming intrinsic cell resistance and repair capabilities. The increased use of hypofractionation coincides with an increase in stereotactic radiation therapy (SRT) use.

8.2.6 Biologically Effective Dose

The *biologically effective dose (BEDn)* is a summation of the true biological dose delivered as a function of dose per fraction, total dose, and associated α/β ratio (*n*). Often used to determine the

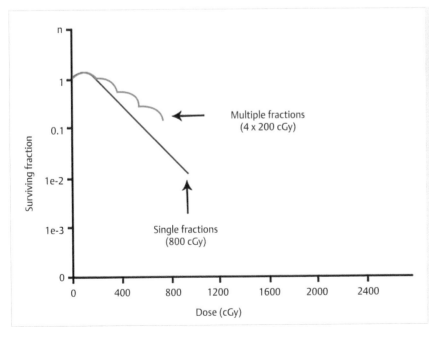

Fig. 8.4 The effect of fractionation on cell survival. Repeated smaller doses of radiation separated by enough time for repair (2 Gy × 4) are less damaging to a sensitive cell than a single fraction (8 Gy × 1) of an equivalent total dose.

optimal dose needed to achieve the same biological effect when deviating from standard fractionation,[3,4] it can be used to increase the TCP, and thus improve tumor control without increasing toxicity, or decrease the NTCP, thereby decreasing treatment complications without compromising tumor control. For example, for HNSCC in which we assume an α/β ratio of 10, the BED_{10} for 70 Gy in 35 fractions is 84 Gy. To achieve a similar BED in 5 fractions, 8.9 Gy per fraction would be required.

8.2.7 Bragg Peak

The *Bragg peak*, a term common in particle therapy, is the depth in tissue at which charged particles release most of their energy to cause a biological effect. The *spread out Bragg peak (SOBP)* is a broader peak, composed of multiple Bragg peaks, that covers the entire tumor. The SOBP is produced using different energies and/or tissue attenuators.

8.2.8 Biologically Equivalent Dose

The *dose equivalent*, which is used to compare charged particles with photons, is the physical dose corrected for biological effectiveness. Different types of particle radiation with differences in LET have different RBE when compared with photons. As a result, the physical dose, in Gray (Gy), of the particle radiation must be multiplied by its RBE and is expressed as Gy (RBE). In many proton studies, the term *cobalt Gray equivalent* is used to refer to a proton RBE of 1.1 with respect to cobalt-60. Note that the biologically equivalent dose is not the same as the BED; biologically equivalent dose is calculated in 2 Gy equivalents and is used to compare the equivalent dose between two different types of radiation, whereas BED is used to compare effective dose between different fractionation schedules of the same radiation type.

8.2.9 Conformal Radiotherapy

The goal of conformal radiotherapy is to best adapt the high-dose field to the shape of the target using advanced computerized radiotherapy planning and delivery systems. Two important benefits emerged from conformal radiotherapy: the ability to reduce dose to normal structures near tumor and the ability to escalate dose to tumor, thus allowing for lower toxicity without compromising dose delivery to the intended target.

8.2.10 Stereotactic Radiation Therapy

SRT is highly conformal radiotherapy that involves the delivery of high doses of radiation in a single session or a few sessions through the use of a special coordinate system for target localization. SRS was originally developed to treat cranial lesions by using a stereotactic head frame to deliver a focal beam of external radiation. Nowadays SRS often refers to the use of SRT in a single session with the goal of delivering a highly focal and ablative dose of radiation with extreme accuracy and precision (typically 0–2-mm PTV margins) and steep dose gradients toward the critical OAR. With the advent of multifraction SRS, the term *fractionated SRT* (FSRT) is sometimes used to distinguish this from single-treatment SRS, although some use the acronym SRS to refer both to single fraction and to a few fractions.

Stereotactic body radiation therapy (SBRT) or stereotactic ablative radiation therapy (SABR) are used when treating extracranial sites with FSRT. SBRT is often delivered in three to six sessions of doses > 6 Gy per session.

8.2.11 Image-Guided Radiation Therapy

IGRT, one of the more significant innovations in radiotherapy, is used together with conformal radiotherapy to reduce the PTV margin by minimizing the positional uncertainty of CTV and OAR targets. IGRT can provide high-resolution 2D, 3D, and 4D images to localize target position and capture motion and volume changes during each treatment, ensuring accurate placement of the radiation field according to the initial radiation treatment plan. IGRT is instrumental for SRT, which involves very small margins.

8.3 Principles of Radiation Physics and Radiobiology

Therapeutic radiation is ionizing radiation (IR), which consists of photons and charged particles. A key characteristic of IR is its capacity for releasing large amounts of local energy to break chemical bonds and produce a biologic effect. Electromagnetic radiation, such as photons, is indirectly ionizing radiation, whereas charged particles such as electrons, protons, and heavily charged ions are directly ionizing radiation.[5]

8.3.1 Electromagnetic Radiation

High-energy X-rays (photons) and gamma rays are the most common type of IR used for radiation therapy. Both photons and gamma rays are indirectly ionizing radiation. As they pass through biologic tissue, they deposit energy that produces electrons that then interact with the target. Photons and gamma rays have similar properties but differ in their origin and their ability to penetrate biologic tissue (▶ Fig. 8.5). Photons are generated by linear accelerators (LINACs) that accelerate electrons at high energy toward a metal target (typically tungsten). The electrons lose kinetic energy when colliding with the metal target, and photons are produced as energy is conserved. Modern LINACs can produce photons that comprise a spectrum of energies expressed in megavolts (MV), where the number (e.g., 6 MV) refers to the maximum energy of the spectrum, which determines the depth of tissue penetration. Photons are the predominant type of radiation used today (e.g., intensity-modulated radiation therapy [IMRT]). Gamma rays are emitted by the nuclear decay of radioactive isotopes and can penetrate biologic tissue to a specific depth. For example, the Gamma Knife (Elekta) system uses cobalt-60 sources to generate gamma rays.

8.3.2 Particle Radiation

Unlike photons, charged particles such as protons, electrons, and other heavy charged ions directly interact with their biologic target. They are clinically useful in the treatment of skull base neoplasms because of their favorable depth-dose distribution characteristics (▶ Fig. 8.6).[6] Protons in particular, because of their relatively large mass, can penetrate tissue with less

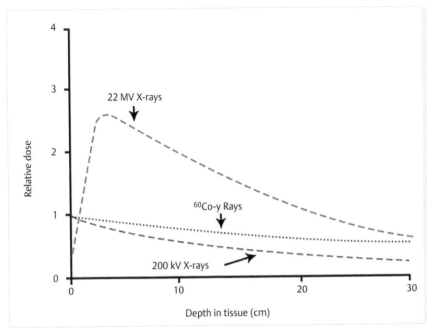

Fig. 8.5 Relative dose as a function of tissue penetration for photons of various energies and gamma ray from cobalt-60 source.

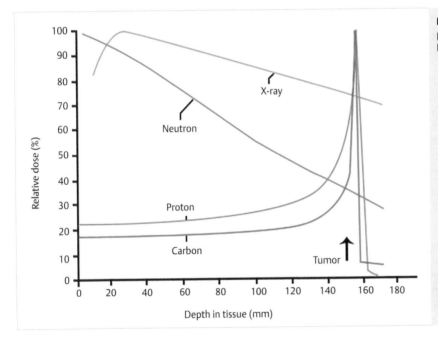

Fig. 8.6 Relative dose as a function of tissue penetration for different particle radiation. Photons (X-rays) are included for comparison.

lateral side scatter than lighter particles such as electrons. This prevents broadening of the proton beam in tissue, so that less unintended dose is delivered to adjacent normal tissue.

Perhaps the most attractive feature of proton therapy is the Bragg peak (▶ Fig. 8.7a), which represents the maximum range of the proton beam, such that few protons penetrate beyond this distance, even by a few millimeters. In clinical use, several energies are used to produce multiple Bragg peaks and thereby create a broader peak called an SOBP, which can be applied to cover the entire tumor (▶ Fig. 8.7b).

Proton beam therapy is useful for skull base tumors such as clival chordomas, as a high dose can be delivered to the tumor, whereas critical structures such as spinal cord or brainstem distal to the proton beam receive minimal to no radiation. Newer

developments include use of a spot scanning technique, which uses a pencil-thin proton beam (typically 5–10 mm wide). Treatment is delivered by scanning and superposition of a pencil-thin proton beam for increased precision and tailoring to the tumor shape. The availability of particle beam therapy is limited to specialized facilities. As of December 2019, 40 medical centers in the United States, and 65 centers in Asia and Europe offer proton beam therapy in accordance with the guidelines of the Particle Therapy Cooperative Group (PTCOG).

Carbon ions are heavier than protons and may bring additional biological advantages while improving dose distribution, owing to their high LET and RBE.[7] Carbon ions are a potential breakthrough in radiotherapy, because their Bragg peak can reach even higher LET values than protons (close to those of

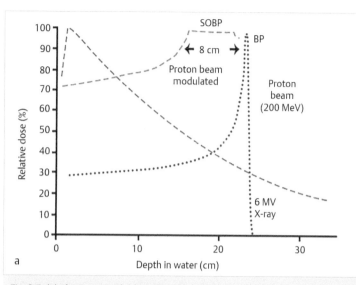
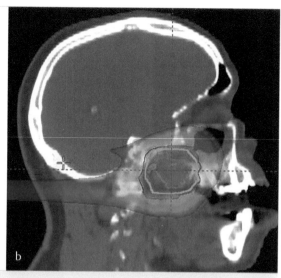

Fig. 8.7 **(a)** The Bragg peak (*dotted purple*) and spread out Bragg peak (SOBP, *dashed green*) of protons. Compared with X-rays (*dashed blue*), the dose for proton builds up slowly in tissue and peaks at the Bragg peak. The SOBP is the aggregate of several individual Bragg peaks produced to cover the entire tumor. **(b)** Proton beam therapy plan for a patient who has a clival chordoma. The entrance dose from the posterior beam is minimal, reducing the radiation dose to brain, brainstem, and spinal cord. The prescribed dose is deposited as an SOBP to cover the tumor.

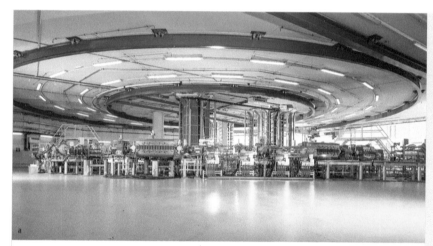
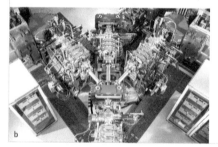
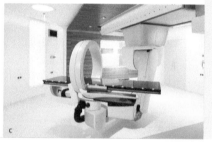

Fig. 8.8 MedAustron Heavy Ion Facility. **(a)** The core of the Synchotron accelerator facility. **(b)** Close-up of heavy ion source of accelerator facility. **(c)** Patient treatment room with robotic couch system and imaging ring for patient. (Courtesy of MedAustron, Wiener Neustadt, Austria.)

alpha particles), producing high levels of irreparable DNA damage independent of free radical production, which is lethal to the cell. In carbon ion therapy, normal tissues are exposed to low-LET radiation similar to that associated with X-rays while the target receives high-LET radiation. As with proton therapy, carbon ion therapy requires expensive particle accelerators (i.e., cyclotrons or synchrotrons) and larger, more complex delivery systems than the more compact and less expensive LINACs (▶ Fig. 8.8). Thus, particle radiation therapy, including IMPT and

heavy ion therapy represent advanced and emerging technologies, albeit are of more limited access compared to photon-based therapies, within the field of radiation oncology aimed to improve cancer treatment.

As of December 2019, there are 13 heavy ion facilities in the world (six in Japan, four in Europe, and three in China). Although heavy ion therapy was developed in Berkeley, California, in the 1960s, the United States currently does not have a heavy ion center. Several multi-ion centers are also in operation, including:

the Heidelberg Ion Therapy center in Germany, the Centro Nazionale di Adroterapia Oncologica in Italy, the Hyogo Ion Beam Medical Center in Japan, the MedAustron Wiener Neustadt in Austria, and the Heavy Ion Center in Shanghai, China. As of 2015, approximately 130,000 patients had been treated using proton therapy and nearly 20,000 with carbon ion therapy, according to the PTCOG website (https://www.ptcog.ch/archive/patient_statistics/Patientstatistics-updateDec2015.pdf).

8.3.3 Interaction with Ionizing Radiation

DNA and phospholipid membranes are widely considered to be the critical targets of ionizing radiation that produces a variety of observed biologic and molecular changes, including cell death, cell division delay, genomic instability, mutation, transformation, bystander effects, and adaptive responses (▶ Fig. 8.9). The clinical manifestation can be tumor cell death or normal tissue toxicity. The type and severity of these effects depend on the energy and type of radiation, the composition of the target tissue, the cellular and molecular response, the duration of exposure, and the cellular microenvironment.

Photons and X-rays are considered *sparsely* ionizing (low-LET) radiation. Their primary mechanism of biological damage occurs indirectly, through production of highly reactive free radicals when the radiation interacts with molecules (mainly water) within the cell (*indirect action*). The most common interaction is with water molecules, producing shorted-lived yet extremely reactive hydroxyl radicals that can damage DNA through cell diffusion. This is the predominant mechanism of cell kill in low-LET radiation such as photons and gamma rays.[5]

Charged particles such as protons are *densely* ionizing (high-LET) radiation and cause cell damage by direct interaction with

DNA and critical targets via the Coulomb force. This leads to ionization or excitation of atoms, causing a chain of physical and chemical effects that eventually produces biologic change that is the main mechanism of cell kill in high-LET radiation such as protons and carbon ions.[5] Thus, for a given tissue type, densely ionizing radiation such as protons and carbon ions will have a higher RBE than sparsely ionizing photons and gamma rays.

8.3.4 Radiation Cell Killing

Cell death, from a radiobiology perspective, is the inability to reproduce indefinitely even if the cell maintains metabolic activity for a period. This phenomenon, which was recognized by radiation biologists for decades as "interphase death," is characterized by an active and orderly process of death. A damaged cell may die at the first cell division after radiation or may undergo a limited number of cell divisions before death. This can be seen histologically when irradiated cells appear morphologically and metabolically intact but then undergo cell death after completing two to three cell divisions.

The mechanism of cell death (i.e., mitotic cell death, apoptosis, necrosis, or autophagy) depends on the radiation dose absorbed and the radiosensitivity of the radiated cell. Mitotic cell death, which occurs when a cell attempts to replicate, is an exponential function of radiation dose; it is considered the dominant mechanism of death, after standard fractionated doses. Radiation-induced apoptosis occurs less frequently and is most evident after lower radiation doses (typically 1.5–5 Gy).

8.3.5 Cell Survival Curve

Cell survival after a single dose of radiation is a probability function of the radiation dose in Gy absorbed. An absorbed dose of 2 Gy is large enough to cause hundreds of lesions in the DNA of an average cell. Most DNA lesions caused by 2 Gy radiation are repairable (*sublethal damage*). Sublethal damage can be repaired, often in hours, and does not lead to cell death. DNA lesions produced by densely ionizing radiation are usually not repairable or reversible (having suffered lethal damage) and eventually lead to cell death.

Cell survival after radiation exposure can be graphically expressed on a logarithmic curve by plotting the portion of surviving cells on the ordinate (*y*-axis) against radiation dose (in Gy) on a linear scale on the abscissa. A typical cell survival curve has a shoulder at the low-dose region followed by a logarithmic decline at the high-dose region (▶ Fig. 8.10). The initial shoulder in the low-dose region is thought to represent sublethal damage (the amount of damage that the tumor cells must overcome with each additional fraction). The steeply sloped portion of the curve represents increased cell death as multiple instances of sublethal damage accumulate.

8.3.6 Linear Quadratic Model

The linear quadratic model is commonly used in radiobiology to explain the cell survival curve (▶ Fig. 8.11). This model assumes that double-helix DNA is the critical target that results in cell kill, with double-strand breaks required for lethal damage. By contrast, a single-strand break in DNA is considered

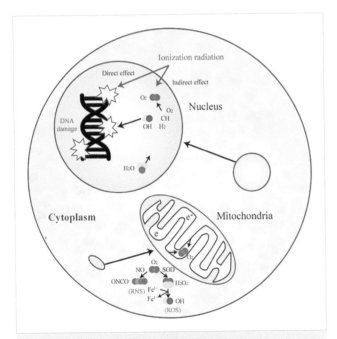

Fig. 8.9 The direct and indirect effects of ionizing radiation, which can cause direct damage to DNA and can also generate reactive oxygen free radicals that can cause DNA and cellular damage.

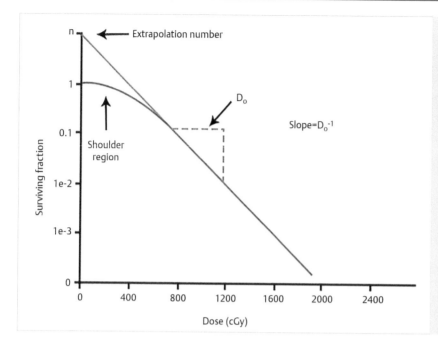

Fig. 8.10 The cell survival curve after radiation exposure. The curve forms an initial shoulder followed by a logarithmic decline. The initial shoulder is caused by sublethal damage.

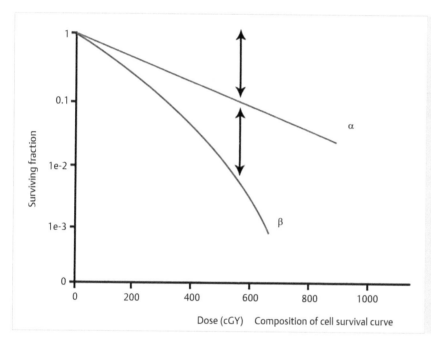

Fig. 8.11 The linear-quadratic model is used to explain the cell survival curve. In this model, a single-strand DNA break is considered repairable, but double strand DNA breaks are not. The alpha–beta ratio is determined from the linear quadratic model.

repairable, sublethal damage. A double-strand break can occur when a single track of radiation breaks both DNA strands or when two individual tracks create two individual single-strand breaks that are close to each other in space and time (▸ Fig. 8.11).

The linear-quadratic model assumes that there are two components to cell killing. The linear (α) component is cell kill from a single event (i.e., one event causing a double strand break) and is a measure of the intrinsic radiosensitivity of the cell. It is proportionate to the dose (αD). The quadratic (β) component is cell kill from the interaction of sublethal events and represents the repairable portion of radiation damage. It is proportionate to the dose squared (βD^2).

The linear-quadratic model is described by the formula

$$\text{Surviving fraction (SF)} = e^{-(\alpha D + \beta D^2)}$$

When radiation is fractionated, the linear-quadratic equation becomes

$$\text{SF} = \text{Number of fractions (n)} \times \left\{ e^{-(\alpha D + \beta D^2)} \right\}$$

8.3.7 α/β Ratio

The linear quadratic model is used to determine the α/β of a given tissue (▸ Fig. 8.12), which represents the relative contribution of α and β components needed to kill a cell using radiation. Each tissue type has its own α/β, so cell survival curves have different shapes for different tissues. It is the difference in

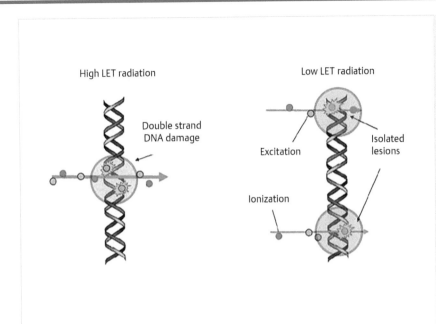

Fig. 8.12 High–linear energy transfer (LET) radiation causes more breaks in DNA per unit track than low-LET radiation does. Double-strand DNA breaks can be caused by a single particle track, as in seen with high-LET radiation (*left*), or by two individual single strand breaks, as seen with low-LET radiation (*right*).

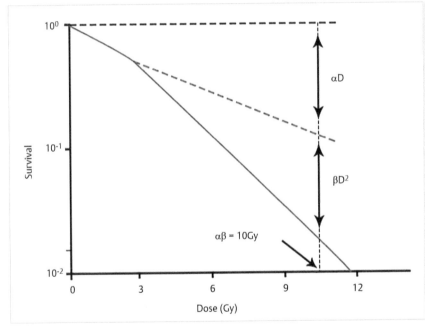

Fig. 8.13 The linear-quadratic model is used to determine the alpha–beta ratio based on the cell survival curve of a cell or tissue type. The ratio is determined by the dose at which the linear and quadratic components of cell killing are equal (10 Gy in the example shown). The linear component is cell kill from a single event, as can occur when a single radiation track damages both DNA strands (*green circle in* ▶ Fig. 8.12) or when two individual radiation tracks damage a single strand of DNA close to each other (*pink circles in* ▶ Fig. 8.12).

α/β between normal tissues and tumor that allows for successful fractionation (▶ Fig. 8.13).

8.3.8 Fractionation and the Four Rs of Radiobiology

In the early 20th century, fractionated radiotherapy replaced single-dose radiation as the major form of therapeutic radiation. The concept of fractionated radiotherapy is based on four well-established radiobiologic principles described by Rod Withers in 1975 as the four Rs of radiobiology: repair of sublethal damage, reassortment, repopulation, and reoxygenation. A fifth R, radiosensitivity, has since been added.[8] The clinical effectiveness of fractionation was demonstrated in head and neck clinical trials developed during the 1970s and 1980s. These trials solidified 2 Gy per fraction per day as the gold standard for fraction size in the majority of malignant skull base tumors.

Fractionation exploits the radiosensitivity difference between rapidly growing tumor cells and most normal tissues (▶ Fig. 8.4). The degree of normal tissue sparing from cancer cells depends on the dose per fraction, the type of tissue irradiated, and the type of radiation used. Hyperfractionation exploits differences in radiation sensitivity between tumor and normal parenchymal tissue to lower late toxicity risk in patients who receive re-irradiation. Accelerated fractionation addresses the risk of accelerated tumor repopulation that occurs after initiation of oncologic therapy. Combination of accelerated fractionation and hyperfractionation, once a common approach, resulted in improved tumor response but also increased acute skin and mucosal toxicity through its effects on the more rapidly proliferating epithelial cells of the skin and mucosa. Consequently, early re-irradiation trials for recurrent HNSCC used four cycles of 1.5 Gy twice daily for 5 days, with a protracted (9-day) treatment break between each cycle to mitigate severe acute toxicity concerns with re-irradiation.[9]

Repair of sublethal damage occurs when there is sufficient time for damage repair between fractions. Each time a radiation dose is fractionated, a shoulder reappears on the cell survival curve. The capacity to repair correlates with the size of the shoulder and is greater in mature, late-responding tissues than in rapidly proliferating tissues. The clinical implication is that decreasing the dose per fraction will increase sparing of late-responding tissues. This principle underlies hyperfractionation theory, which seeks to exploit the difference in repair between early- and late-responding tissues.

Reassortment studies have demonstrated that cells in the G2-M phase of the cell cycle are the most radiosensitive. In reality, cells of any given tissue can be found at various stages of the cell cycle. In an asynchronous population, radiation preferentially kills cells in the most sensitive phase of the cycle. The surviving cells will eventually reach the G2-M phase and consequently become more radiosensitive to the next dose. Reassortment occurs in tissues that have moderate to rapid cell turnover rate and is negligible in late-responding tissues. Fractionation exploits this phenomenon to decrease late-tissue complications and thereby improve the therapeutic ratio.

Repopulation occurs when the tumor cell population is depleted by radiation or cytotoxic treatment and a regenerative response of surviving clonogens (accelerated repopulation) is triggered. The timing and kinetics of regeneration vary by tissue type, with the magnitude depending on the number of remaining cells that retain their proliferative capacity. It is thought that tumor repopulation during radiation treatment breaks, after a subtotal resection surgery, or after chemotherapy accounts for the majority of treatment failures/tumor recurrences. Clinically, Rosenthal et al demonstrated that a total time from surgery to completion of radiotherapy (treatment package time) > 100 days is correlated with decreased local control in patients treated with surgery and adjuvant radiotherapy for head and neck squamous cell carcinoma (SCC).[10] When the regenerative capacity of a tumor exceeds the critical acute-reacting normal tissue tolerance, therapeutic gains can come from shortening the overall course of radiotherapy, in what is called accelerated fractionation (see later this chapter).

Reoxygenation of the tumor microenvironment plays an important role in determining tumor radiosensitivity. In animal models, lack of reoxygenation is a major cause of tumor radiation resistance. Reoxygenation occurs when hypoxic cells closer to the center of the tumor become oxygenated again as a result of tumor shrinkage or reduced oxygen demand. This process is determined by a number of different mechanisms, including changes in interstitial pressure of micro vessels and cell proximity to the blood supply and the presence of certain radiosensitizing systemic agents.

8.4 Radiobiology of Hypofractionation and Skull Base Tumors

According to the classical radiobiologic classification of cranial radiosurgery targets, most skull base tumors are suitable for SRS (▶ Table 8.1). Most malignant skull base tumors (class D) have high α/β.[5] Benign skull base tumors (class B), such as meningiomas, acoustic schwannoma, pituitary adenomas, and craniopharyngiomas, are regarded as late-responding tissues and have lower α/β. When fractionated radiation therapy is used to treat benign tumors, the sparing effects on tumor and normal brain parenchyma and other critical neural structures are similar. In such circumstances, when the radiation dose required to permanently control these tumors exceeds the constraints of normal brain parenchyma and critical structures, the use of a very conformal radiation dose distribution and a very steep dose gradient beyond the tumor volume is critical.

Technological advances in medical imaging and treatment delivery capabilities have enabled precise dose delivery with minimal margins (0–2 mm) and steep dose fall-off outside the target. When a single high dose of radiation such as that used in SRS is used for tumor ablation, the sparing effect of fractionation does not apply. Within the confines of classical radiobiology, the use of a single or extreme hypofractionation regimen of three to five large fractions represents a major paradigm shift. In addition, the clinical success of SBRT or SABR in extracranial sites has challenged the long-standing dogma of fractionation.

In addition to the technological and computer-driven developments, radiobiology developments such as TCP/NTCP modeling and the volume effects for late complications provide

Table 8.1 Classification of skull base radiosurgery targets

Radiosurgical class	Target tissue	Normal tissue	Examples
Class A	*Late-responding tissue*	*Within normal brain/critical neural parenchyma within target*	*Arteriovenous malformation*
Class B (most benign skull base tumors)	Late-responding tissue	Surrounded by normal brain/critical neural parenchyma within target	Paraganglioma, meningioma, acoustic neuroma, pituitary adenoma, and craniopharyngioma
Class C	*Early-responding tissue*	*Within brain/critical neural parenchyma within target*	*Low-grade glioma*
Class D (most malignant skull base tumors)	Early-responding tissue	Surrounded by normal brain/critical neural parenchyma within target	Chordoma, chondrosarcoma, and perineural or direct invasion by squamous cell and nonsquamous carcinomas

theoretical support for larger fraction sizes.[11] Hypofractionation involves increasing the dose per fraction and decreasing the number of fractions, producing a lower total dose and a significantly shorter overall course of treatment. The logistical and financial benefits for the patient are fewer clinic visits and fewer lost work hours. The clinical benefits of hypofractionation have been demonstrated in patients who have breast, prostate, and lung cancer, and this approach has seen increasing use for re-irradiation of head and neck tumors. Compared with standard fractionation, hypofractionated regimens were better tolerated and either clinically equivalent or more effective.[12,13,14,15,16,17] The radiobiological explanation for the increased clinical effectiveness is a widened therapeutic ratio obtained either by increasing TCP (to improve tumor control) without increasing toxicity or by decreasing NTCP (to decrease treatment complications) without compromising tumor control. These calculations are based on α/β estimates with which to determine optimal fraction size and total dose for a given tumor type and their anatomic location. Mechanistically, high fractional doses of radiation (in addition to causing DNA damage) are thought to confer an antiangiogenic effect on the microenvironment vasculature and to elicit an immunogenic response.

8.4.1 Normal Tissue Tolerance of Critical Organs

Many normal tissues can tolerate moderate doses of radiation without losing structural or functional integrity. Distinct radiation-induced tissue injuries occur when a critical number of stem cells is killed, resulting in inadequate replenishment of mature functional cells that are lost through normal physiologic aging. The timing of the damage's manifestation can be acute, subacute, or late and varies by tissue type.

Acute effects can manifest hours to days after radiation injury and are often characterized by inflammation, edema, and denuding of epithelia. Tissues such as skin and mucosa of the head and neck often have a pool of slowly proliferating stem cells and rapidly proliferating progenitor cells. Both pools are depleted in response to radiation, but the mature differentiated cells continue to maintain their function until depleted through normal turnover. As a consequence, acute radiation injury appears at a predictable time point that is determined by the life span of the mature cells. Patchy mucositis and dermatitis typically begin to manifest during the third week of conventionally fractionated radiotherapy, when there are too few progenitor cells to replenish the normal turnover of mature cells.

Subacute (early delayed) effects can manifest several months after radiotherapy. These effects are generally transient and reversible and tend to occur in tissue having longer cell turnover time, such as white matter. Transient diffuse demyelination such as Lhermitte's syndrome or somnolence can occur 3 to 6 months after radiation of the spinal cord and brain tissue, respectively. More severe subacute injuries such as white matter necrosis can resemble tumor progression on contrast-enhanced MRI.[18] This is due to shared characteristics between the tumor and necrosis, such as the presence of contrast enhancement, interval growth, vasogenic edema, and mass effect, as well as proximity to the site of original disease, which is likely to have received the highest radiation dose. Differentiating between radiotherapy-induced toxicity and disease progression is a familiar challenge for neuroradiologists. Care and expertise must be used when evaluating these patients so as to prevent unneeded surgery or discontinuation of otherwise effective systemic therapy when radiation-related MRI changes (pseudoprogression) are mistaken for disease progression. Kumar et al described the differentiating characteristics of radionecrosis after MRI in 150 patients treated for malignant gliomas and coined the terms *soap bubble* and *Swiss cheese* to describe imaging features commonly seen in cases of radionecrosis.[19] Ultimately the gold-standard diagnostic test for radiation necrosis is surgical resection followed by pathologic evaluation.

Chronic effects of radiotherapy can occur months to years after irradiation and can be oncogenic (with radiation-induced soft tissue and bone sarcomas of the skull base known risk factors after radiation exposure).[20] Chronic effects are typically observed in tissues composed of functional parenchymal cells that have very low proliferation rates, such as liver, muscle, and nervous tissue. These tissues contain a population of quiescent stem cells that can rapidly regain proliferative function following tissue loss or damage and thus regenerate the lost tissue. Radiation is thought to produce chronic effects in late tissue types by depleting the population of these stem cells. Time of onset often depends on dose given, and the effects can increase in severity with time as a consequence of an avalanche phenomenon, with the first wave of cell death triggering subsequent proliferation of other injured cells, resulting in progressive and massive cell depletion. Functional tissue/organ failure can occur as a result. Late complications after skull base irradiation include fibrosis, trismus, necrosis of soft tissue and bone, clival necrosis, brain necrosis, hearing impairment, vision loss, and cranial nerve deficit. Temporal lobe necrosis (TLN) is a common late-radiation injury with a radiographic incidence of 10 to 14% after conventional radiation. In patients who receive radiotherapy for nasopharyngeal carcinoma, incidence of TLN can be as high as 35%; the majority are asymptomatic. When the temporal lobes receive less than 60 Gy at 2 Gy per fraction daily, incidence of TLN is < 5%, and indeed it is rarely seen in doses < 50 Gy with standard fractionation.[21] In a published series of T4 nasopharyngeal carcinoma patients treated at MD Anderson Cancer Center, the absolute incidence of radiographic TLN was 14% when median temporal lobe dose exceeded 60 Gy. Approximately 10% of those who had radiographic TLN were symptomatic, exhibiting recurrent headaches, dizziness, short-term memory loss, and cognitive changes.[22]

8.5 Modern Radiation Therapy Techniques for Skull Base Tumors

From a radiotherapy perspective, tumors involving the skull base are among the most difficult to plan and treat. Challenges frequently encountered are submillimeter distance between tumor and a vital OAR structure, the need to simultaneously spare multiple OARs that have varying dose tolerances, and existence of multiple targets requiring differential dose rates. Prior to the advent of highly conformal techniques such as IMRT and IGRT, it was extremely difficult to deliver sufficient tumoricidal doses to many tumor types without exceeding the tolerance of a nearby

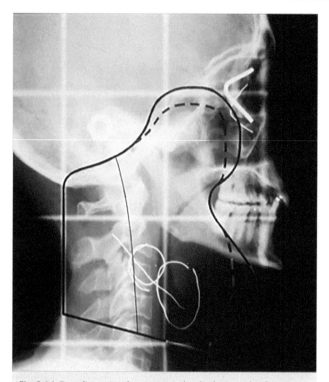

Fig. 8.14 Two-dimensional conventional radiotherapy plan for a patient who has nasopharyngeal carcinoma (NPC), using opposed lateral beams. The initial field was treated to 41.4 Gy, with a superior border at the floor of the pituitary fossa to ensure coverage of sphenoid sinus (*dotted line*). For advanced disease, the superior border included coverage of pituitary fossa, anterior cranial fossa, and sinuses. An off-spinal cord boost field was delivered after 41.4 Gy. The gross disease boosted to 72 Gy, with superior border adjusted to exclude optic apparatus.

critical OAR, such as the optic apparatus, brainstem, or spinal cord.

Significant technological developments in medical imaging, radiation treatment planning, and dose delivery over the past 20 years have made it possible to safely irradiate previously untreatable skull base malignancies. Initial radiotherapy techniques used 2D fluoroscopic imaging (▶ Fig. 8.14). Plans were designed first to ensure generous coverage of target volumes, with sparing of normal tissue a secondary consideration. Because of the simple beam arrangement and emphasis on target coverage over normal tissue protection, a significant amount of brain tissue received the prescribed dose. With the advent of 3D treatment planning that used CT imaging for target delineation, as well as computerized treatment planning and delivery systems (3D-CRT), target volume coverage improved and more normal tissue was spared. Reproducibility of daily treatment setup became more important and consisted of in-room laser alignment to skin marks or tattoos using immobilization devices and periodic setup verification by 2D portal imaging. By today's standards, 2D port imaging quality was poor, but it could identify the location of the isocenter to within 1 to 2 cm using bony landmarks.

8.5.1 Advances in Photon Therapy

More sophisticated conformal techniques such as IMRT using multileaf collimation (MLC) provided greater flexibility and precision in treating irregular tumor volumes with sharper dose gradients and concave dose distributions (▶ Fig. 8.15). In addition, IMRT incorporated inverse planning and allowed for placement of dose constraints on critical structures, improving normal tissue sparing. Studies developed from these data ultimately improved understandings of the dose-volume effects for late complications in critical normal tissues.[23] A newer application of IMRT is volumetric modulated arc therapy (VMAT),

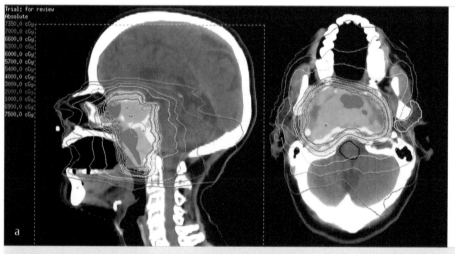
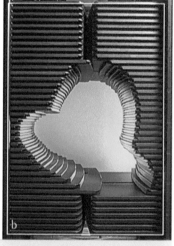

Fig. 8.15 (a) Intensity-modulated radiation therapy plan for a patient who has nasopharyngeal carcinoma (NPC). **(b)** A multileaf collimator (MLC) is a device made of moveable leaflets that can block parts of the radiation beam. The leaflets can move independently in and out of the beam path and conform to the shape of the target. Typical leaves are between 4 and 6 mm in width. Newer high-definition MLCs have leaflets as narrow as 1 to 2.5 mm.

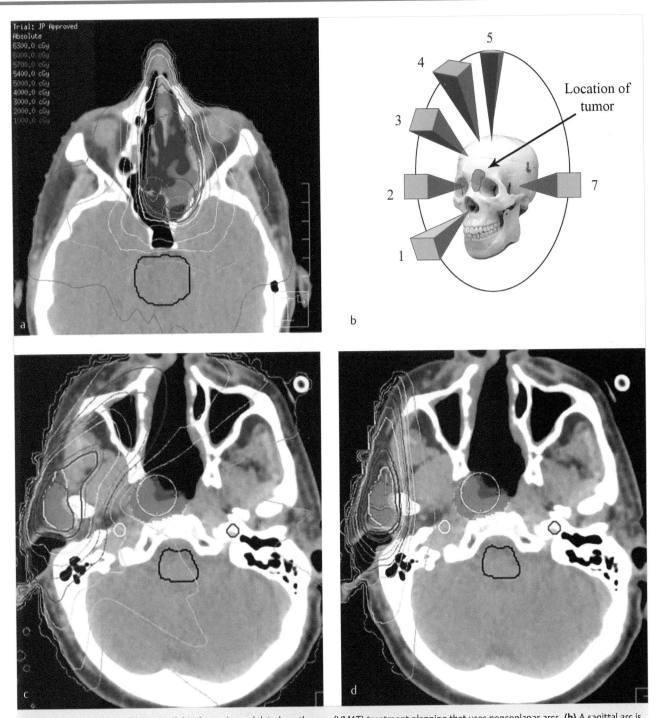

Fig. 8.16 Olfactory neuroblastoma. **(a)** Volumetric modulated arc therapy (VMAT) treatment planning that uses noncoplanar arcs. **(b)** A sagittal arc is used to spare the bilateral orbits, lens, optic nerve, and retina. Comparison of VMAT plan for re-irradiation of a solitary parotid metastasis using **(c)** coplanar and **(d)** noncoplanar approaches.

which delivers radiation in a continuous arc instead of in a static arrangement of a fixed number of beams (typically 6–12 beams) of IMRT. VMAT offers the advantages of shorter treatment delivery time, less radiation exposure, and improved plan quality. The trade-off is potentially increased low-dose exposure to the patient. Novel applications of IMRT and VMAT include use of noncoplanar treatment planning that enables unique dose distributions tailored for skull base tumors (▸ Fig. 8.16).

8.5.2 Advances in Particle Therapy

The Bragg peak is a unique advantage of charged particle therapy in which there is a sharp drop-off in dose beyond the Bragg peak and no exit dose beyond the intended target. Proton beam delivery was initially performed using a passive scatter beam approach, which uses devices such as brass apertures and range compensators to conform and broaden the proton beam so as to create the SOBP. The passive scatter technique

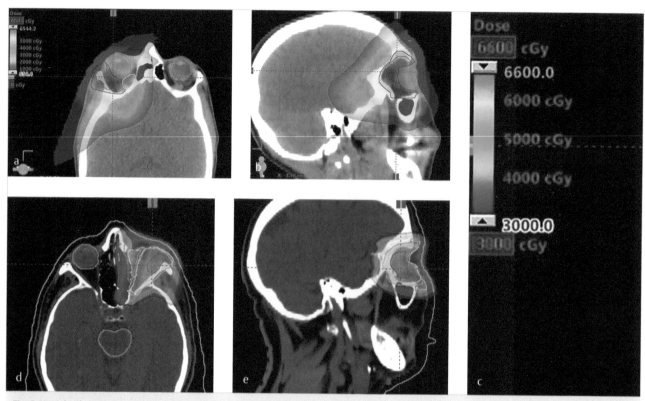

Fig. 8.17 Orbital carcinoma. Comparison of scanning beam proton therapy techniques. Dose distributions are shown for **(a, b)** passive scanning proton therapy and **(c–e)** intensity-modulated proton therapy multifield optimized plans.

(passive scanning proton therapy, or PSPT) is excellent for a well-lateralized target that does not vary significantly in depth. For irregularly shaped tumors, an active scanning beam technique can be used. Together with inverse planning, increased conformality of dose to the target can be achieved. Further optimization of dose distribution can be performed using single-field optimization and multifield optimization approaches. Multifield optimization, also referred to as intensity-modulated proton therapy, is often used for targets that are more complex and that require higher conformality. Example proton plans are illustrated in ▶ Fig. 8.17.

8.5.3 Advances in Radiotherapy Imaging

Radiation oncology is an image-guided intervention, and developments in the field are closely tied to advances in medical imaging. Medical imaging plays two critical roles in modern-day radiotherapy: (1) *image-mediated radiotherapy* and (2) *IGRT*. Image-mediated radiotherapy includes planning images for delineation of target and OAR volumes, evaluation of dose distribution for treatment planning, verification of dose delivery, and evaluation of treatment response. CT planning with IMRT is an example of image-mediated radiotherapy. IGRT, the use of imaging in the treatment room to guide radiation delivery, is a cornerstone of modern radiotherapy.

Like surgery, radiotherapy is local therapy, and it aims to achieve similar goals. Modern surgical skull base procedures enhance direct visualization of targets to eliminate ambiguity in identification, leading to appropriate management. Similarly,

the radiation oncologist seeks to accurately visualize and target tumors while inflicting minimal collateral damage on adjacent normal structures. However, during radiation treatment planning, several assumptions are made that bring inherent disadvantages. The planning CT acquired at simulation is a snapshot, at a single time point, of the tumor and its relation to adjacent normal structures as well as the patient's position. During treatment planning, many suppositions are made regarding the CTV, to estimate the microscopic spread around the tumor, and the PTV, to account for the estimated extent of internal organ motion and setup error. Each treatment is delivered with the assumption that the tumor and patient anatomy, and their positions with respect to the treatment machine, remain unchanged from the time of simulation. IGRT allows the capture of this setup, positioning, and motion information during treatment to ensure that the actual dose delivered matches the prescribed treatment plan. This is done by providing serial snapshots immediately before, and sometimes during, each treatment to verify the accuracy of radiation delivery.

Prior to the introduction of IGRT, PTV margins were the most widely used method of accounting for geometric uncertainties. Typical PTV margins were as large as 1 to 2 cm, which greatly limited the role of radiotherapy for skull base tumors. Modern PTV margins are in the range of 0 to 5 mm, depending on the type of treatment delivery system and IGRT method used. Early IGRT systems consisted of two orthogonal kV-imagers, and setup verification was based on 2D bony anatomy. Volumetric imaging such as cone-beam CT (CBCT) improves on the matching uncertainties when using only 2D planar imaging and provides additional volumetric information based on tumor

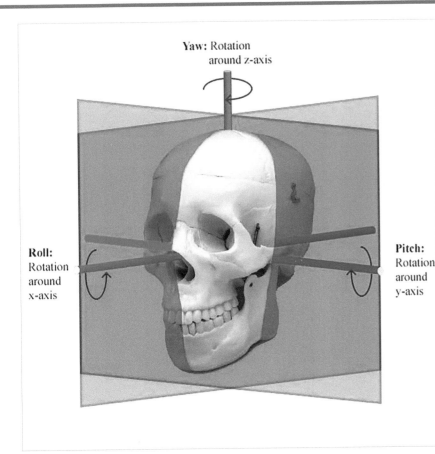

Fig. 8.18 Small rotational displacements in the skull base can result in significant shifts of tumor or critical tissue to or away from the intended dose. Pitch error (chin movement) in particular can exert significant distortion on skull base anatomy.

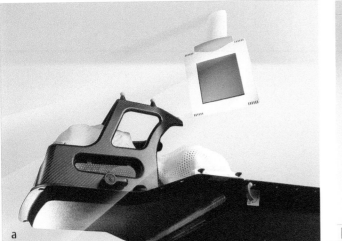
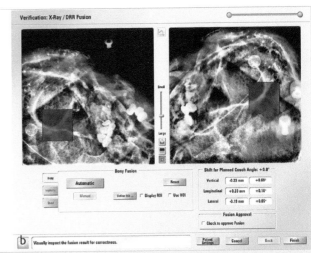

Fig. 8.19 ExacTrac image verification using skull base bony anatomy. **(a)** Illustration of alignment between the immediate pretreatment image and the reference treatment plan image (spyglass) after translational and rotational correction. **(b)** ExacTrac system allows for correction of positional errors with a high degree of precision.

position and the surrounding soft tissue. When organ motion needs to be accounted for, such as for tumors near the lung (respiration) and abdomen/pelvis (bladder filling, bowel effects), gated IGRT systems (4D) that feature real-time tracking can be used. For skull base tumors, correcting for translational (i.e., longitudinal, lateral, and vertical) uncertainties alone is not sufficient when high doses are considered; it is essential to also account for uncertainties in rotational (i.e., pitch, yaw, and roll) motion (▶ Fig. 8.18). Rotational error of as little as 1° can have a significant clinical impact on dose to critical structures in the head and neck and brain (which can result in up to 20% differences in maximum dose to the optic chiasm).[24,25,26,27,28]

For skull base applications, the ability to not only verify but also correct both translation and rotational errors with six degrees of freedom (6D) is critical. In-room IGRT systems such as the Brainlab ExacTrac X-ray 6D system (Brainlab AG) provide high-resolution cranial and spine images for precise 6D fusion based on bony anatomy (▶ Fig. 8.19).

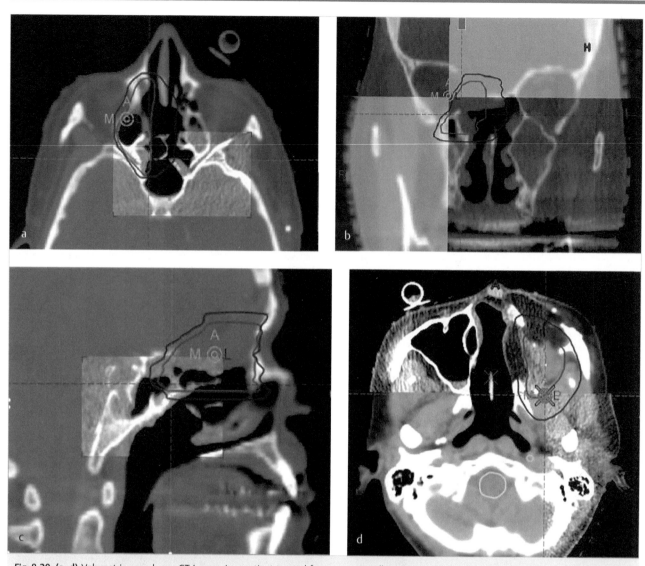

Fig. 8.20 (a–d) Volumetric cone-beam CT images in a patient treated for squamous cell carcinoma (SCC) of the ethmoid sinus with orbital wall involvement. Because of the proximity of high dose to the optic nerve, the need for high-precision image-guided radiation therapy is critical.

Setup verification can be performed before and during each treatment. Together with a 6D robotic couch available on LINAC systems, submillimeter corrections can be made for translational and rotational differences. CBCT is available on many modern LINACs and consists of retractable X-ray detectors mounted either orthogonal to or along the axis of the treatment beam. Whereas the ExacTrac X-ray is useful for targets that are rigidly correlated with bony anatomy, CBCT enables alignment based on both the surrounding soft tissue and bony anatomy (▶ Fig. 8.20). CBCT is especially useful for verifying the position of targets that are nonrigidly correlated with bony structures of the skull base or when alignment to bony structures alone may be suboptimal, such as for tumor or OAR volumes below C1 or near the mandible. CBCT can be used to account for internal organ motion and volume changes during the course of treatment.

8.5.4 Stereotactic Radiation Therapy

Most skull base tumors are extra-axial in location and have a very sharp margin of demarcation with surrounding normal tissue. This makes SRT well suited for the treatment of most skull base tumors. A major goal of the SRT system is to minimize unwanted dose beyond the target volume, which can be achieved through rapid dose fall-off outside the target, accurate localization of the target, and minimization of the uncertainty margins around the target. SRT can be delivered as SRS in which multiple external radiation beams are aimed at an imaging defined target volume to deliver a single high dose of radiation.[29] For tumors that are larger in size and closer to critical structures, FSRT (SBRT or SABR) is often used.[30] Current SRT systems can achieve margins of 0 to 2 mm using a combination of IGRT, head frames or frameless head and neck immobilization devices, and improved treatment planning and delivery software. Several essential considerations determine the quality of SRT: (1) target delineation, (2) setup accuracy and immobilization, (3) image guidance and real-time motion tracking, (4) machine and system capability, (5) evaluation of SRT plan quality, and (6) patient comfort and tolerance.

8.5.5 Target Delineation

It should go without saying that the clinician's expertise in skull base anatomy, interpreting multiple imaging modalities, and understanding tumor behavior and pattern of spread, together with close collaboration with the skull base surgeon or neurosurgeon to identify areas of high risk, is critical for determining accurate target delineation. In the 2D era, knowledge of bony landmarks was sufficient to guide target coverage, but with 3D-CRT, additional anatomic knowledge was required to accurately delineate targets on axial imaging (primarily CT). In the modern era, multiple imaging modalities are available to improve target delineation accuracy. For most applications, CT-based target delineation and treatment planning remains the gold standard. Volumetric MRI sequences, contrast-enhanced dual-energy CT, and PET-CT can provide additional anatomic and biologic information not appreciated on the planning CT (▶ Fig. 8.21).

MRI has the advantage of better discrimination of soft tissue anatomy and is ideal for delineating perineural disease in the skull base. Functional imaging such as PET-CT can help identify tumor activity in regions that may be difficult to assess by

anatomic imaging alone. Planning CT images can be fused with diagnostic images to improve target delineation accuracy. However, co-registration of planning with diagnostic imaging images can be imprecise due to differences in head position and organ displacement. To optimize image fusion quality, MRI or PET-CT images can be obtained with the patient immobilized in the treatment position (▶ Fig. 8.22).

8.5.6 Immobilization, Image Guidance, and Real-Time Motion Tracking

Recent advances in image guidance have allowed delivery of high-dose radiation with increased confidence and safety. Although image guidance is normally used to correct initial setup errors, the robustness of the immobilization device is essential for maintaining the patient's position during actual treatment (intrafractional) so as to maintain the alignment of nonrigid structures such as the cranium, mandible, and cervical spine and to constrain voluntary and involuntary motion.[31,32] A well-developed immobilization system should be highly reproducible during treatment, restrict unwanted motion, be easy to implement, and be comfortable for the patient. Both frame and frameless systems are used in SRT. Stereotactic head frames used in Gamma Knife Stereotactic Radiosurgery (GK-SRS) are fixated to the skull via pins to cranium (▶ Fig. 8.23a). When SRS is fractionated, the use of a head frame is not feasible. Instead, a mouthpiece-assisted frame system can be used to correlate the coordinate frame system to the skull (▶ Fig. 8.23b).

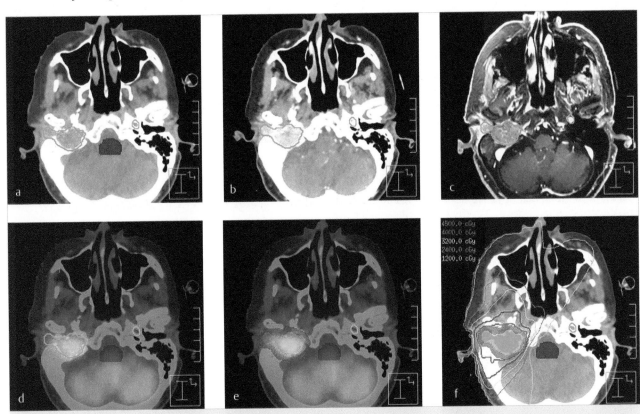

Fig. 8.21 Left skull base metastasis. **(a)** Planning CT co-registered with **(b)** dual-energy CT, **(c)** MRI, and **(d)** PET-CT in treatment planning position creates a composite target volume. **(e)** 2-mm planning target volume expansion and a **(f)** volumetric modulated arc therapy treatment plan showing dose distribution with target in colorwash.

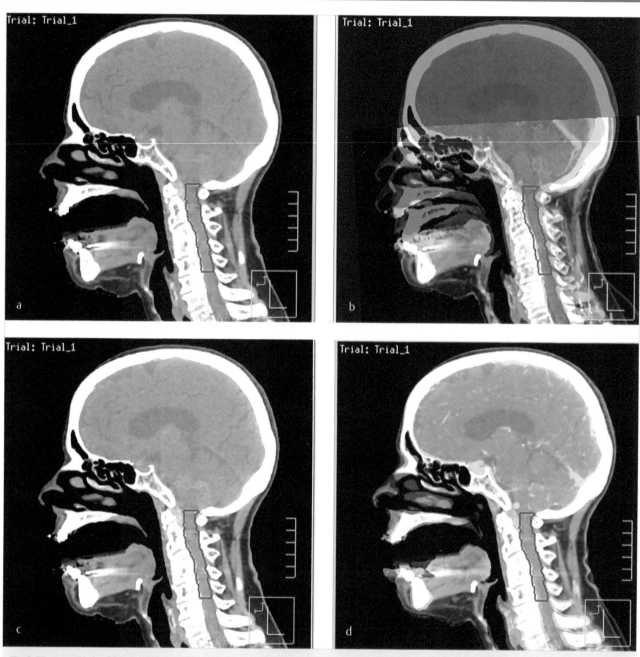

Fig. 8.22 An example of (a) the planning CT (b) fused with a diagnostic CT scan. Notice that differences in head tilt, jaw position, spine curvature, and tongue position limit the usefulness for precise target delineation. (c) Planning CT fused to dual-energy CT with (d) a patient immobilized in the treatment position.

An advantage is the absence of cranium pins and the absence of any need to remove and replace the frame. Disadvantages include the potential difficulty of tolerating this approach as well as its decreased reliability, which requires a larger PTV margin. Frameless systems have the potential advantage of improved patient safety and comfort.

Inter- and intrafractional setup errors for head and neck thermoplastic mask immobilization systems have been extensively investigated. Critical to any immobilization device used for skull base targets is the ability to limit both translational and rotational uncertainties. Published data from Wang et al showed that use of a three-point immobilization system (▶ Fig. 8.23c) together with IGRT can highly restrict patient motion to < 1°

rotational and < 1 mm translational uncertainty, allowing the use of a 2-mm PTV margin with 95% confidence of at least 99% target coverage.[32] For targets below C1 or closer to the mandible, a highly restrictive and robust head and neck immobilization device is necessary to minimize variations in cervical spine curvature and jaw position.

More recently, surface imaging-guided radiosurgery platforms with more comfortable open face masks and optical tracking have been used (▶ Fig. 8.24), with patient positioning monitored in real time through infrared camera tracking of facial topography, providing real-time feedback for necessary corrections. Clinical experience from early adopters demonstrates comparable outcomes to frame-based GK-SRS for treatment of benign

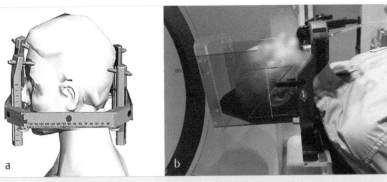
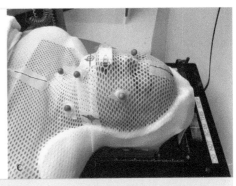

Fig. 8.23 Framed and frameless systems for stereotactic radiotherapy. **(a)** Stereotactic head frames used in Leksell Gamma Knife stereotactic radiosurgery are fixated to the skull via pins to cranium. **(b)** When the use of a head frame is not feasible, a mouthpiece-assisted frame system can be used. The coordinate frame system is correlated to skull position via the hard palate. A special vacuum-assisted bite block with custom prosthesis is used to ensure reliability. **(c)** Frameless three-point immobilization system for linear accelerator (LINAC)-based systems. This consists of a custom posterior cushion, thermoplastic mask, and bite block to fix the hard palate to the mask.

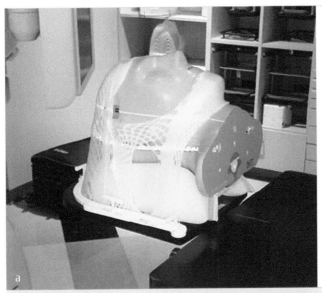
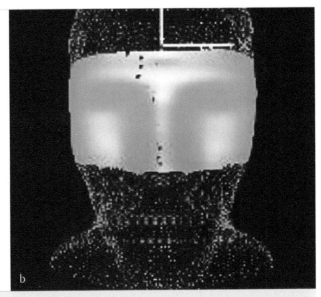

Fig. 8.24 Setup verification using the AlignRT surface guided imaging system. **(a)** Head phantom in an open-face immobilization mask. **(b)** The region of interest defined by skin surface area not obscured by the mask. (Adapted with permission from Paxton AB, Manger RP, Pawlicki T, Kim GY. Evaluation of a surface imaging system's isocenter calibration methods. J Appl Clin Med Phys. 2017 Mar;18(2):85–91.)

skull base tumors.[33] The current geometric accuracy can approach submillimeter precision but is limited to situations in which the external surface is a reliable surrogate for the internal target.

8.5.7 Machine Capability and Stereotactic Radiosurgery Platforms

Technological advances in treatment delivery systems have enabled precise delivery of large doses to the tumor with reduced margins (0–3 mm) and steep dose fall-off outside the tumor. Platforms for delivery of SRS include the Gamma Knife (GK) system, the CyberKnife (CK) system, and LINAC systems such as the Varian TrueBeam STx or Elekta Trilogy. Upgrades and add-ons such as the Varian TrueBeam STx on the Novalis Tx treatment platform are equipped with a 6D couch, integrated third-party in-room IGRT system, and high-definition (2.5 mm or

smaller) MLCs and are well suited for SRS and FSRT applications (▶ Fig. 8.25). The Lekskell GK system consists of ~ 192 noncoplanar collimated beams containing a cobalt-60 source that are arrayed hemispherically to intersect at a single location (isocenter) so as to deliver a highly focal treatment (▶ Fig. 8.26).

In newer systems, each beam has three collimator sizes (4, 8, and 16 mm) providing five sector positions. The target is localized by stereotactic guidance via a temporary stereotactic head frame fixed to the patient's skull. An advantage of the GK system is the shorter distance between the radiation source and target compared with other SRS systems. This can provide more precise treatment featuring smaller beam diameters and less integral dose to normal structures. The Accuray CK robotic radiosurgery system consists of a compact LINAC mounted on an industrial robotic arm that can direct radiation beams to the target from noncoplanar positions based on inputs from two orthogonal stereoscopic X-ray imaging systems (▶ Fig. 8.27).

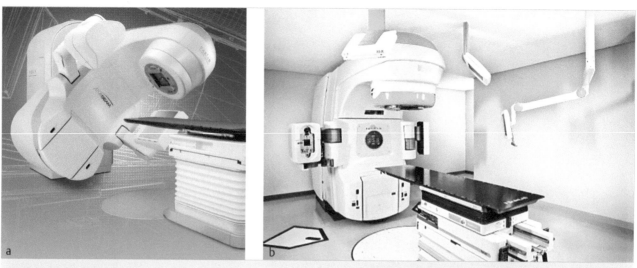

Fig. 8.25 (a) The Varian TrueBeam STx. (b) Linear accelerator outfitted with the Novalis "Brain Lab" frameless stereotactic radiosurgery system.

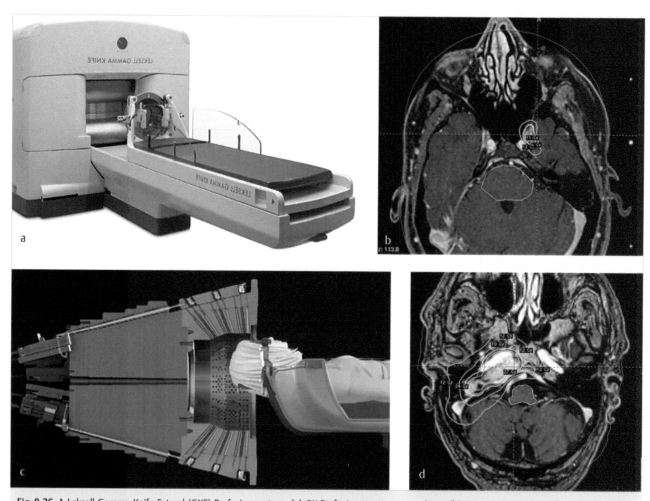

Fig. 8.26 A Leksell Gamma Knife Extend (GKE) Perfexion system. (a) GK Perfexion treatment machine. (b) GK treatment plan delivered in a single session. (c) View of the GK collimator system. (d) GKE treatment plan delivered in three fractions.

Although the robotic arm has nearly 360° freedom of motion, treatment is delivered at discrete sets of positions called nodes. A typical treatment plan may use perhaps 100 to 200 nodes. Images can be acquired at periodic intervals during treatment to guide the robotic treatment head, using 6D tracking of the skull to account for target position and movement. Treatment time can vary based on the number of nodes used and the interval of image acquisition for IGRT during treatment.

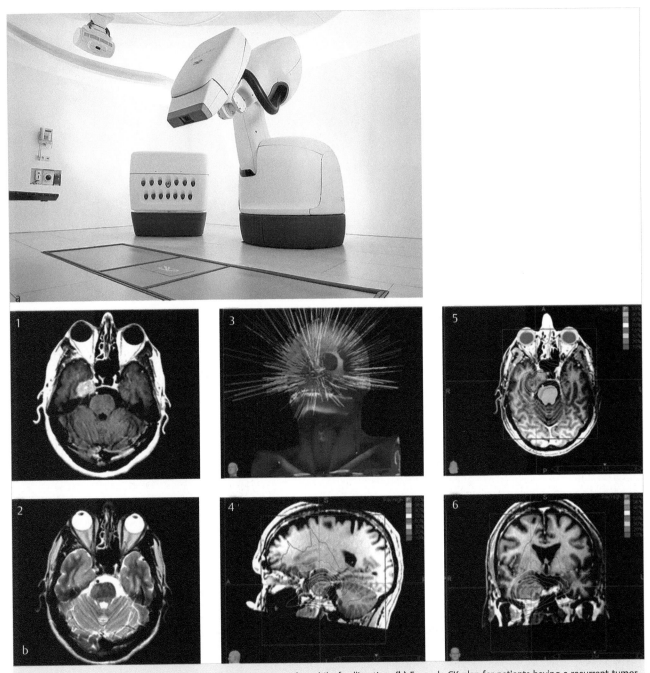

Fig. 8.27 Accuray CyberKnife (CK) system. **(a)** The M6 system with multileaf collimation. **(b)** Example CK plan for patients having a recurrent tumor involving Meckel's cave. (Courtesy of Accuray Incorporated.)

Because of their very favorable physical characteristics and high biological effectiveness, protons can potentially be used for FSRT applications at the skull base.[34] The use of proton SRT can potentially further improve target volume coverage, improve normal tissue sparing, and lower the nontarget integral dose (▶ Fig. 8.28). Proton-based SRT applications are currently being investigated on both the dosimetric and clinical fronts.[35,36]

8.6 Conclusion

Radiotherapy has become an essential tool for the treatment of skull base tumors. Modern-day radiation therapy technologies such as IGRT, VMAT, and SRT have further increased the safety margin around target volumes, allowing for lower normal tissue doses without compromising delivery of tumoricidal doses. Particle therapy such as proton therapy and carbon ion therapy may have added dosimetric and biological advantages. Highly conformal and ablative dose techniques such as SRS and SBRT have challenged the long-standing dogma of fractionation. Furthermore, modern imaging techniques such as MRI can allow for delineation of skull base tumors with submillimeter precision. With the advent of treatment delivery platforms capable of delivering a highly targeted planned dose, it is now possible to achieve a very conformal radiation dose distribution having a

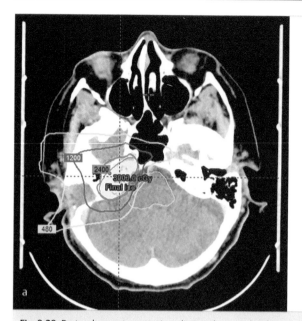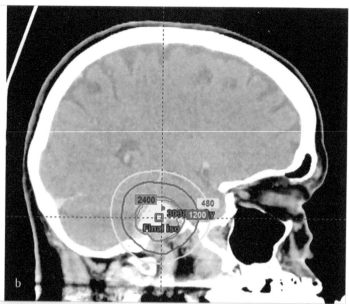

Fig. 8.28 Proton beam stereotactic radiation therapy plan for recurrent carcinoma of the skull base: **(a)** axial and **(b)** sagittal.

steep radiation dose gradient beyond the target volume treated. With these technological advantages, having the clinical expertise with which to accurately identify tumor volume relative to surrounding critical structures is essential to avoid geometric misses or overdose of normal tissue. Proper execution of treatment planning and delivery is necessary to minimize risk of severe complications. Notwithstanding these technological advances, the best management approach for patients who have skull base tumor remains interdisciplinary treatment planning involving the neurosurgeon, head and neck surgeon, radiation oncologist, and other members of the treatment team.

References

[1] Giraud P, Antoine M, Larrouy A, et al. Evaluation of microscopic tumor extension in non-small-cell lung cancer for three-dimensional conformal radiotherapy planning. Int J Radiat Oncol Biol Phys. 2000; 48(4):1015–1024

[2] Overgaard J, Hansen HS, Specht L, et al. Five compared with six fractions per week of conventional radiotherapy of squamous-cell carcinoma of head and neck: DAHANCA 6 and 7 randomised controlled trial. Lancet. 2003; 362 (9388):933–940

[3] Bentzen SM, Dörr W, Gahbauer R, et al. Bioeffect modeling and equieffective dose concepts in radiation oncology–terminology, quantities and units. Radiother Oncol. 2012; 105(2):266–268

[4] Dale RG. The application of the linear-quadratic dose-effect equation to fractionated and protracted radiotherapy. Br J Radiol. 1985; 58(690):515–528

[5] Shrieve DC. Basic principles of radiobiology applied to radiotherapy of benign intracranial tumors. Neurosurg Clin N Am. 2006; 17(2):67–78, v

[6] Loeffler JS, Durante M. Charged particle therapy: optimization, challenges and future directions. Nat Rev Clin Oncol. 2013; 10(7):411–424

[7] Durante M, Loeffler JS. Charged particles in radiation oncology. Nat Rev Clin Oncol. 2010; 7(1):37–43

[8] Steel GG, McMillan TJ, Peacock JH. The 5Rs of radiobiology. Int J Radiat Biol. 1989; 56(6):1045–1048

[9] Spencer SA, Harris J, Wheeler RH, et al. Final report of RTOG 9610, a multi-institutional trial of reirradiation and chemotherapy for unresectable recurrent squamous cell carcinoma of the head and neck. Head Neck. 2008; 30(3): 281–288

[10] Rosenthal DI, Liu L, Lee JH, et al. Importance of the treatment package time in surgery and postoperative radiation therapy for squamous carcinoma of the head and neck. Head Neck. 2002; 24(2):115–126

[11] Nahum AE. The radiobiology of hypofractionation. Clin Oncol (R Coll Radiol). 2015; 27(5):260–269

[12] Whelan TJ, Pignol JP, Levine MN, et al. Long-term results of hypofractionated radiation therapy for breast cancer. N Engl J Med. 2010; 362(6):513–520

[13] Haviland JS, Owen JR, Dewar JA, et al. START Trialists' Group. The UK Standardisation of Breast Radiotherapy (START) trials of radiotherapy hypofractionation for treatment of early breast cancer: 10-year follow-up results of two randomised controlled trials. Lancet Oncol. 2013; 14(11):1086–1094

[14] Dearnaley D, Syndikus I, Sumo G, et al. Conventional versus hypofractionated high-dose intensity-modulated radiotherapy for prostate cancer: preliminary safety results from the CHHiP randomised controlled trial. Lancet Oncol. 2012; 13(1):43–54

[15] Videtic GM, Hu C, Singh AK, et al. A randomized phase 2 study comparing 2 stereotactic body radiation therapy schedules for medically inoperable patients with Stage I peripheral non-small cell lung cancer: NRG oncology RTOG 0915 (NCCTG N0927). Int J Radiat Oncol Biol Phys. 2015; 93(4):757–764

[16] Li Q, Swanick CW, Allen PK, et al. Stereotactic ablative radiotherapy (SABR) using 70 Gy in 10 fractions for non-small cell lung cancer: exploration of clinical indications. Radiother Oncol. 2014; 112(2):256–261

[17] Iyengar P, Kavanagh BD, Wardak Z, et al. Phase II trial of stereotactic body radiation therapy combined with erlotinib for patients with limited but progressive metastatic non-small-cell lung cancer. J Clin Oncol. 2014; 32(34): 3824–3830

[18] Park HH, Hong CK, Jung HH, et al. The role of radiosurgery in the management of benign head and neck tumors. World Neurosurg. 2016; 87: 116–123

[19] Kumar AJ, Leeds NE, Fuller GN, et al. Malignant gliomas: MR imaging spectrum of radiation therapy- and chemotherapy-induced necrosis of the brain after treatment. Radiology. 2000; 217(2):377–384

[20] Milas L, Peters LJ. Conditioning of tissues for metastasis formation by radiation and cytotoxic drugs. Symp Fundam Cancer Res. 1983; 36:321–336

[21] Lawrence YR, Li XA, el Naqa I, et al. Radiation dose-volume effects in the brain. Int J Radiat Oncol Biol Phys. 2010; 76(3) Suppl:S20–S27

[22] Takiar V, Ma D, Garden AS, et al. Disease control and toxicity outcomes for T4 carcinoma of the nasopharynx treated with intensity-modulated radiotherapy. Head Neck. 2016; 38 Suppl 1:E925–E933

[23] Ten Haken RK, Lawrence TS. The clinical application of intensity-modulated radiation therapy. Semin Radiat Oncol. 2006; 16(4):224–231

[24] Lin CC, Lu TW, Wang TM, Hsu CY, Hsu SJ, Shih TF. In vivo three-dimensional intervertebral kinematics of the subaxial cervical spine during seated axial rotation and lateral bending via a fluoroscopy-to-CT registration approach. J Biomech. 2014; 47(13):3310–3317

[25] Takemura A, Togawa K, Yokoi T, et al. Impact of pitch angle setup error and setup error correction on dose distribution in volumetric modulated arc therapy for prostate cancer. Radiological Phys Technol. 2016; 9(2):178–186

[26] Lin MH, Veltchev I, Koren S, Ma C, Li J. Robotic radiosurgery system patient-specific QA for extracranial treatments using the planar ion chamber array and the cylindrical diode array. J Appl Clin Med Phys. 2015; 16(4):290–305

[27] Kim S, Jin H, Yang H, Amdur RJ. A study on target positioning error and its impact on dose variation in image-guided stereotactic body radiotherapy for the spine. Int J Radiat Oncol Biol Phys. 2009; 73(5):1574–1579

[28] Boman E, Kapanen M, Laaksomaa M, Mäenpää H, Hyödynmaa S, Kellokum-pu-Lehtinen PL. Treatment accuracy without rotational setup corrections in intracranial SRT. J Appl Clin Med Phys. 2016; 17(4):86–94

[29] Larson DA, Coffey RJ. Radiosurgery: devices, principles, and rationale. Clin Neurosurg. 1993; 40:429–445

[30] Minniti G, Valeriani M, Clarke E, et al. Fractionated stereotactic radiotherapy for skull base tumors: analysis of treatment accuracy using a stereotactic mask fixation system. Radiat Oncol. 2010; 5:1

[31] Xu F, Wang J, Bai S, Xu QF, Shen YL, Zhong RM. [Interfractional and intrafractional setup errors in radiotherapy for tumors analyzed by cone-beam computed tomography]. Chin J Cancer. 2008; 27(10):1111–1116

[32] Wang H, Wang C, Tung S, et al. Improved setup and positioning accuracy using a three-point customized cushion/mask/bite-block immobilization system for stereotactic reirradiation of head and neck cancer. J Appl Clin Med Phys. 2016; 17(3):180–189

[33] Lau SK, Patel K, Kim T, et al. Clinical efficacy and safety of surface imaging guided radiosurgery (SIG-RS) in the treatment of benign skull base tumors. J Neurooncol. 2017; 132(2):307–312

[34] Hug EB. Review of skull base chordomas: prognostic factors and long-term results of proton-beam radiotherapy. Neurosurg Focus. 2001; 10(3):E11

[35] Amichetti M, Amelio D, Minniti G. Radiosurgery with photons or protons for benign and malignant tumours of the skull base: a review. Radiat Oncol. 2012; 7:210

[36] Register SP, Zhang X, Mohan R, Chang JY. Proton stereotactic body radiation therapy for clinically challenging cases of centrally and superiorly located stage I non-small-cell lung cancer. Int J Radiat Oncol Biol Phys. 2011; 80(4): 1015–1022

9 Clinical Applications of Radiotherapy for Skull Base Tumors

Jack Phan, Steven J. Frank, and Paul D. Brown

Summary

This chapter covers the clinical applications of radiotherapy in skull base tumors. We discuss the role of adjuvant radiotherapy after surgery, definitive radiotherapy when surgery is not recommended, skull base re-irradiation, and palliative radiotherapy. We provide a comprehensive review of clinical outcomes and complications after skull base radiotherapy for benign and malignant tumors. Studies evaluating modern conformal radiotherapy approaches are highlighted. Benign tumors covered in this chapter include pituitary adenoma, acoustic schwannoma, meningioma, craniopharyngioma, and paraganglioma. Malignant tumors covered here include skull base chordoma and chondrosarcoma, nasopharyngeal carcinoma, and sinonasal malignancies. Tables comparing outcomes after conventional fractionation, hypofractionation, and stereotactic radiosurgery are provided. The optimal clinical management and appropriate dose and fractionation for a specific tumor biology and tumor location are discussed.

Keywords: clinical radiotherapy, skull base radiotherapy, normal tissue complications, benign skull base tumors, chordoma, chondrosarcoma, nasopharyngeal carcinoma, paranasal sinus malignancy, re-irradiation

9.1 Introduction

Tumors of the skull base can be categorized by location and/or histologic type. Anatomically, skull base tumors may arise from the following:

- neurovascular structures and meninges of the base of the brain (e.g., schwannoma, meningioma, pituitary adenoma, craniopharyngioma, paraganglioma);
- the base of skull itself (e.g., chordoma, chondrosarcoma, osteosarcoma, plasmacytoma); and
- head and neck structures below the skull base (e.g., nasopharyngeal carcinoma [NPC], paranasal sinus tumor, perineural spread of head and neck tumors).

In addition to a tumor's anatomic location, its subtype often dictates the role and sequence of radiotherapy. Carcinoma arising from the nasopharynx is treated using radiation as the primary modality due to the morbidity associated with resection of tumors arising from this location, whereas carcinoma arising from the paranasal sinus often requires a combination of surgery and radiation therapy to optimize local disease control. Clival chordoma requires very high radiation doses for tumor control and is well suited for proton therapy. High-grade malignant tumors that have a high propensity for nodal recurrence, such as squamous cell carcinomas, have dictated the use of elective nodal irradiation (ENI) fields, whereas benign tumors typically have sharp margins of demarcation from the surrounding normal structures and are amenable to highly conformal local radiation with a steep radiation dose gradient beyond the target.

This chapter covers the clinical radiotherapy applications for skull base tumors. The management of skull base tumors using radiotherapy requires an understanding of both tumor radiobiology and modern treatment planning, delivery, and monitoring techniques; these aspects are discussed in Chapter 8 of this book.

9.2 Normal Tissue Constraints of Critical Organs of the Skull Base

As mentioned in the previous chapter, most skull base tumors are well suited for both fractionated radiotherapy and stereotactic radiosurgery (SRS). Patients who are irradiated for skull base tumors are at risk of developing radiation-induced complications as a result of injury to the normal brain parenchyma and critical structures. ▶ Table 9.1 lists the commonly quoted radiation dose constraints for conventionally fractionated (1.8–2.0 Gy per fraction) radiotherapy (FRT), single fraction SRS, and multisession hypofractionated stereotactic radiotherapy (FSRT). Critical structures at risk include the brain parenchyma, brainstem, spinal cord, optic pathway, and inner ear/cochlea. Significant effort should be made to keep the radiation doses to these critical structures below the constraints during radiation treatment planning so as to minimize the risk of radiation-induced complications.

Table 9.1 Commonly quoted radiation dose constraints for conventionally fractionated and hypofractionated radiation therapy

Critical organ	Conventionally fractionated	Five-fraction fSRS	Three-fraction fSRS	Single-fraction SRS
Brainstem (not medulla)	50–54 Gy	25 Gy Max 23 Gy <0.5 cc	21 Gy Max 18 Gy <0.5 cc	15 Gy Max 10 Gy <0.5 cc
Spinal cord and medulla	45–50 Gy	27 Gy Max 21 Gy <0.35 cc 14.5 Gy <1.2 cc	Under Spinal Cord 3 Fx: 21 Gy Max 18 Gy <0.35 cc 12.3 Gy <1.2 cc	14 Gy Max 10 Gy <0.35 cc 7 Gy <1.2 cc
Optic pathway	50–54 Gy	25 Gy Max 23 Gy <0.2 cc	17.4 Gy Max 15.3 Gy <0.2 cc	8 Gy Max 10 Gy <0.2 cc
Cochlea/inner ear	35–40 Gy	22 Gy Max	17 Gy Max	9 Gy Max

Abbreviations: fSRS, fractionated stereotactic radiosurgery; SRS, stereotactic radiosurgery.

9.3 Pituitary Adenoma

Pituitary adenoma is a broad term for benign primary tumors arising from pituitary glandular tissue. They can be divided into nonsecretory and secretory types. Depending on the type of secretory cells from which they arise, secretory pituitary adenomas can be subdivided into growth hormone (GH)–secreting, prolactin-secreting, adrenocorticotrophic hormone (ACTH)–secreting, gonadotropin-secreting, and thyroid stimulating hormone–secreting tumors. The goals of treatment of pituitary adenomas are tumor control and normalization of the hypersecreted hormone for secretory tumors. Except for prolactinomas, surgical resection is usually recommended because such an approach can decompress the optic apparatus, if it is compressed by the tumor, and can rapidly normalize the hypersecreted hormone in a secretory tumor.[1] When complete surgical resection is not achievable, postoperative radiation therapy is often necessary to stop the growth of the residual tumor and normalize the hypersecreted hormone. Radiation therapy is also indicated for recurrent pituitary adenomas.

9.3.1 Growth Hormone–Secreting Adenoma

There is abundant literature on the use of FRT to treat pituitary adenoma. The typical doses used range from 45 to 54 Gy in conventional fractionation. For nonfunctioning pituitary adenoma, the reported 10-year progression-free survival rate after FRT ranges from 80 to 98%.[2,3,4,5,6,7] For secretory tumors, apart from control of tumor growth, normalization of hypersecreted hormones is one of the main goals of treatment. For GH-secreting tumors, FRT is efficacious in the normalization of GH. However, GH levels tend to fall slowly after treatment and may take years to normalize. Typically, by 10 years, approximately 70 to 90% will have normalized GH levels.[3,4,8]

Multiple studies have evaluated the efficacy of GH normalization rates after SRS and FRT. These studies have yielded no clear significant differences by radiotherapy technique and may be primarily dependent on preradiotherapy GH and insulin-like growth factor (IGF-I) levels.[9] Because of the metabolic effects and cosmetic deformities associated with acromegaly, medical therapy may be given to patients before their GH levels normalize. Colleagues from St. Bartholomew's Hospital reported one of the world's largest series of patients who had acromegaly from pituitary adenoma treated using radiotherapy. GH level decreased to < 2.5 ng/mL in 22%, 60%, and 77% of the 884 patients treated with radiotherapy for acromegaly at 2, 10, and 20 years, respectively.[10] Notably, 63% of patients had a normal IGF-I level by 10 years. Another recent study showed similar findings.[11]

9.3.2 PRL-Secreting Adenoma

When evaluating treatment outcomes, it is important to distinguish between pituitary stalk effect and prolactin hypersecretion. The serum prolactin level is usually lower in the case of stalk effect, which is defined as the loss of hypothalamic inhibition due to compression of the pituitary stalk. Conventional fractionated radiation therapy is usually offered to patients who cannot tolerate bromocriptine or similar medical therapy

or to those who develop disease progression during medical therapy. Normalization of prolactin levels occurs in 50 to 70% of patients after fractionated radiation therapy.[12,13,14,15,16,17,18]

9.3.3 Adrenocorticotrophic Hormone–Secreting Adenoma

Patients who have ACTH-secreting tumors present with Cushing's disease when the tumor is still small and thus usually have microadenomas. Because these tumors are typically very small, they might not be detected on a regular brain MRI. A dynamic MRI or bilateral selective venous sampling of ACTH from the inferior petrosal sinuses can be performed to establish a diagnosis. The metabolic effects of Cushing's disease are very crippling and, if long-standing, can be fatal. Accordingly, the goal of treatment is rapid normalization of the ACTH, and surgical resection is usually the recommended initial treatment. Fractionated radiation therapy is recommended in patients who have residual tumor after surgery and in patients who are medically inoperable. Remission occurs in approximately 50 to 80% of patients after fractionated radiation therapy.[19,20,21]

9.3.4 Stereotactic Radiosurgery for Pituitary Adenoma

SRS has been used in the treatment of pituitary adenomas. Because the optic apparatus is in close to the pituitary gland, a 3- to 5-mm gap between tumor and organ is typically needed to respect the tolerance of the optic chiasm. Abundant data in the literature demonstrate that SRS is a safe and efficacious procedure for the treatment of pituitary adenomas. However, if one anticipates that to deliver an adequate dose to the tumor or target volume, the maximum dose to the optic apparatus cannot be limited to 8 to 10 Gy in a single fraction, then FRT or FSRT in three to five fractions should be recommended instead. SRS is very effective at controlling tumor growth, yielding a tumor control rate of 92 to 100%.[22] The tumor control rate in patients who have endocrine-inactive pituitary tumors treated to lower marginal doses of 14 to 16 Gy is similar to that of patients who have secretory pituitary tumors treated to marginal doses of 14 to 34 Gy. When judging normalization of hormone level, however, inconsistencies in the endpoints used in various studies render interpretation of results difficult. A decrease in hormone hypersecretion can occur within a few months of SRS, but complete normalization can take up to 8 years. Data in the literature suggest that a radiation dose response is involved in normalization of hormone levels. It has also been suggested that the use of antisecretory medications at the time of SRS has a negative impact on the efficacy of the procedure. For endocrine-inactive tumors, a dose of 14 to 16 Gy is usually used; for secretory tumors, a higher dose should be considered.

From the endocrinologist's standpoint, an endocrinological cure of acromegaly is usually defined as a GH level of ≤ 1 ng/mL and a normal IGF-I. A comprehensive review examining the outcomes of SRS for the treatment of acromegaly showed that the rate of endocrine cure ranged from 20 to 82%.[22] This wide variation might be a result of the different percentage of patients receiving antisecretory medications during SRS. For prolactinomas, SRS results in an endocrine cure rate of approximately 30%

and a significant reduction of PRL levels in 29 to 100% of patients.[22] The post-SRS stalk effect may cause PRL to be slightly elevated even when hypersecretion is well controlled.

For ACTH-secreting tumors, reported endocrine cure rates after SRS widely ranged from 10 to 100%.[22,23] However, some of the studies did not specify the criteria for endocrine cure, and other studies used differing criteria. Among the studies having defined criteria of endocrine cure, the rates of endocrine cure ranged from 28 to 100%.[23]

9.3.5 Fractionated Stereotactic Radiotherapy

Recent data on the use of FSRT (typically delivered over three to five fractions) for the treatment of pituitary adenomas is promising. Tumor control rates ranged from 85 to 98%, and reported complication rates were low.[1] Although no direct comparisons of radiotherapy modalities have been performed in a randomized clinical fashion, a recent meta-analysis of eight studies enrolling a total of 634 patients evaluated the efficacy and safety of FSRT ($n = 361$) and SRS ($n = 273$) for treatment of pituitary adenomas.[24] Comparable tumor control rates ranged from 91 to 96%, comparable rates of radiation-induced optic neuropathy ranged from 0 to 2%, and comparable rates of endocrinologic deficits ranged from 1 to 22%. Independent of technique used, whether Gamma Knife (GK)-, CyberKnife (CK)-, or linear accelerator (LINAC)-based, tumors larger than 4 mL were associated with a higher rate of treatment complications (2% vs. 1–2% optic neuropathy; 22% vs. 1–7% pituitary dysfunction) and lower rates of tumor control (91% vs. 96–99%)[24] when compared with those < 4 mL.

9.4 Acoustic Schwannoma

Acoustic schwannomas (vestibular schwannomas) represent the most common cerebellopontine angle tumor (~ 80%). There are four management options for acoustic neuromas: observation, microsurgery, SRS/FSRT, and FRT. Tumor control for all local therapeutic interventions is excellent and focuses on minimizing treatment-related complications, principally hearing preservation and cranial nerve (CN) preservation. In trying to identify the optimal management option, consideration is given to patient age, tumor size, growth rate, symptom burden, and the goals of hearing and CN preservation. Because acoustic schwannomas are slow-growing tumors, some physicians favor close observation for smaller tumors. However, it should be noted that tumor progression can result in permanent loss of hearing function and can increase the risk of complications associated with surgery or radiotherapy. Meta-analyses and prospective data evaluating the natural history of acoustic schwannomas in patients suggest that those having a tumor growth rate > 2.5 mm per year were more likely to lose hearing function.[25,26]

Comparisons have been made between microsurgery and SRS, demonstrating that SRS yields similar tumor control rates but lower incidence of CN deficits. These findings appear to hold as long-term data for SRS emerge.[27,28,29] Acoustic schwannomas are ideal targets for SRS, and the literature contains an abundant clinical data on the use of SRS for acoustic

schwannoma. GK is the SRS modality most commonly used to treat these tumors, but LINAC-based and CK modalities are used as well, with excellent conformality and accuracy. As of 2011, more than 18,000 patients who had acoustic neuroma had been treated using GK.[30] In the past, more rudimentary CT-based planning was used, and plans were typically less conformal, reflecting the state of earlier computer algorithms. Modern treatment planning entails MRI-based planning and the use of a larger number of shots to improve the conformality around the tumor.[31]

9.4.1 Modern Stereotactic Radiosurgery Series for Acoustic Schwannoma

▶ Table 9.2 summarizes the treatment outcomes of selected series for acoustic schwannoma. The prescribed dose for acoustic schwannoma has been lowered since the early 2000s. In earlier studies, marginal doses in the range of 16 to 20 Gy were used.[31,32,33] Reported tumor control rates were excellent, but incidence of radiation-induced hearing loss and CN deficits (mainly trigeminal and facial) was substantial. This prompted investigation of a lower prescribed dose. Modern series using a dose of 12 to 13 Gy did not show inferior tumor control rates,[28,29,31,32,33,34,35,36,37,38,39,40,41,42,43,44,45] and a much higher proportion of patients retained serviceable hearing. There was also lower incidence of trigeminal and facial nerve injury from SRS. One of the largest series of acoustic schwannoma patients treated using GK-SRS ($n = 829$) comes from the University of Pittsburgh. The 10-year tumor control rate was 97%.[33] An update of their 15-year experience showed that facial neuropathy risk was < 1% and that trigeminal symptoms were < 3%, with hearing preservation in up to 77% of patients.[33] A separate report from the same hospital demonstrated that tumor control was not compromised when a reduced dose of 12 to 13 Gy was used.[34] Other series using reduced-dose SRS reported similar high tumor control rates of up to 96%, with up to 88% retention of hearing and little or no facial deficits (0–4%).[37,39,41,42,43] Recently, colleagues at Northwestern reported outcomes for 30 patients treated using GK-SRS to a prescribed dose of 11 Gy. They demonstrated 100% progression-free survival, based on freedom from surgery, and 91% freedom from persistent growth. One patient developed tumor progression requiring resection at 87 months.[44] Similar long-term outcomes using a LINAC-based SRS system was reported by a group from the University of Heidelberg, Germany. Median dose was 13 Gy, prescribed to the 80% isodose line. Median follow-up was 110 months, and 5- and 10-year tumor control rates were 91%.[37] Rates of radiation-induced trigeminal neuralgia and facial weakness were 8 and 5%, respectively, and hearing preservation at 9 years was 55%.

SRS using proton beam has yielded similar excellent results, albeit with a shorter follow-up time. Colleagues from Harvard University reported a 5-year tumor control rate of 95.3%, with a median follow-up of 38.7 months in those receiving proton beam SRS. The prescribed dose was 12 cobalt Gray equivalent (CGE). The trigeminal and facial nerve toxicity rates were 10.6 and 8.9%, respectively. The hearing preservation rate was 33.3%.

Table 9.2 Results of selected modern SRS/FSRT series for acoustic schwannoma

Modality	Patients	Dose	Tumor control (Follow-up)	Hearing preservation	V/VII nerve toxicity
GK-SRS[a,b,c,d,e]	18–313	10–13 Gy	92–98.6% (4–6 y)	52–79%	0–5%/0–4%
Proton SRS[e]	88	12 Gy	93.6% (5 y)	33%	10.6%/8.9%
LINAC SRS[f]	26–49	10–13 Gy	91% - 100% (5–10 y)	55–75%	6–8%/5–7%
LINAC FSRT (Meijer)[f]	80	20–25 Gy 5 Fx	94% (5 y)	2%/3%	0%/0%
LINAC FSRT (Chang)	61	21 Gy 3 Fx	98% (4 y)	98%	0%/0%
LINAC FRT (Chan) (Horan)	42–70	50–54 Gy 30 Fx	97–98% (3–4 y)	73–84%	0–4%/1–3%

Abbreviations: FRT, conventionally fractionated radiotherapy; FSRT, fractionated stereotactic radiotherapy; Fx, fraction; GK-SRS, Gamma Knife–stereotactic radiosurgery; LINAC, linear accelerator; SRS, stereotactic radiosurgery.
[a]Combs SE, Volk S, Schulz-Ertner D, Huber PE, Thilmann C, Debus J. Management of acoustic neuromas with fractionated stereotactic radiotherapy (FSRT): long-term results in 106 patients treated in a single institution. Int J Radiat Oncol Biol Phys 2005;63(1):75–81.
[b]Inoue HK. Low-dose radiosurgery for large vestibular schwannomas: long-term results of functional preservation. J Neurosurg 2005;102(Suppl):111–113.
[c]Iwai Y, Yamanaka K, Shiotani M, Uyama T. Radiosurgery for acoustic neuromas: results of low-dose treatment. Neurosurgery 2003;53(2):282–287, discussion 287–288.
[d]Petit JH, Hudes RS, Chen TT, Eisenberg HM, Simard JM, Chin LS. Reduced-dose radiosurgery for vestibular schwannomas. Neurosurgery 2001;49(6):1299–1306, discussion 1306–1307.
[e]Rowe JG, Radatz MW, Walton L, Hampshire A, Seaman S, Kemeny AA. Gamma knife stereotactic radiosurgery for unilateral acoustic neuromas. J Neurol Neurosurg Psychiatry 2003;74(11):1536–1542.
[f]Meijer OW, Vandertop WP, Baayen JC, Slotman BJ. Single-fraction vs. fractionated LINAC-based stereotactic radiosurgery for vestibular schwannoma: a single-institution study. Int J Radiat Oncol Biol Phys 2003;56(5):1390–1396.

9.4.2 Fractionated Radiotherapy and Fractionated Stereotactic Radiotherapy for Acoustic Schwannoma

Patients who have large acoustic schwannoma not suitable for SRS may be offered FRT; FRT series for acoustic schwannomas have historically consisted of 1.8 to 2.0 Gy daily doses in five fractions per week, for a total dose of 50.4 to 54 Gy. The conventional fractionation schedule was initially developed empirically to provide an optimal "normal tissue sparing effect" between tumor control and treatment toxicity.[47] The largest body of experience with FRT comes from the University of Heidelberg. A total of 106 patients who had acoustic schwannoma were treated to a prescribed dose of 57.5 Gy.[38] The 5-year tumor control rate was 93%, with a median follow-up of 48.5 months. Treatment toxicities were low, with 3.4%, 2.3%, and 6% developing trigeminal nerve, facial nerve, and vestibulocochlear nerve complications, respectively. Investigators from the University of California, Los Angeles and Thomas Jefferson University demonstrated similar results subsequent to FRT. The probability of retaining serviceable hearing in patients who had sporadic tumors was ~ 81%.[45,47] Investigators from Loma Linda University reported proton beam FRT to a prescribed dose of 54 CGE (or 60 CGE for patients who had no serviceable hearing) in 30 fractions.[35] The tumor control rate was 100%, with a median follow-up of 34 months. No trigeminal or facial nerve toxicity was reported. The hearing preservation rate was 31%.

With the advent of intensity modulated radiation therapy (IMRT) and stereotactic localization, FSRT using higher doses per fraction (4–5 Gy in 5 Fx) can be delivered with minimized dose to adjacent critical structures. FSRT fills the gap between SRS and conventional FRT in terms of time commitment and patient selection strategies. FSRT regimens of 3 Gy × 10, 5 Gy × 4, 5 Gy × 5, 4 Gy × 5, 6 Gy × 3, and 7 Gy × 3 have been described for patients who have acoustic schwannoma.[30,46,48,49,50,51] Tumor control rates are comparable, and median follow-up intervals for FSRT studies ranged from 21 to 48.5 months. Investigators from Amsterdam prospectively evaluated 129 patients treated using LINAC-based stereotactic radiotherapy either as a single fraction (10–12.5 Gy prescribed to 80%; n = 49) or FSRT (4–5 Gy × 5 fractions; n = 80). Tumor control (100% SRS vs. 94% FSRT), hearing preservation (75% SRS vs. 61% FSRT), and facial nerve preservation (93% SRS vs. 97% FSRT) were not significantly different between the two groups. There was a slight edge for better trigeminal nerve preservation (92% SRS vs. 98% FSRT; P < 0.05) in the FSRT group.[46] The same group evaluated FSRT for larger acoustic schwannoma. The median tumor size was 9.4 mL (range 8–24). The tumor control rate was 94%, with a median follow-up of 48 months. Hearing was retained in 85% of patients, and 24% experienced a transient enlargement of tumor prior to arrested growth or shrinkage.[52] Overall, outcomes after FSRT demonstrate similar tumor control to FRT, ranging from 94 to 100% with the benefit of lower overall time commitment to patients who had tumors that were not suitable for SRS.

9.4.3 Long-Term Complications after Acoustic Schwannoma Irradiation

The current active area of research is focused on techniques for improving hearing preservation. Unlike hearing preservation, rates of trigeminal and facial nerve toxicity after radiotherapy are low irrespective of the radiation modality used. Hearing preservation after radiotherapy is more varied, with approximately a quarter to a third of patients developing complications related to hearing. The large variation in hearing preservation is partially due to variation in hearing scales and the definition of hearing preservation. In terms of radiotherapy technique, a pooled analysis from three large German centers (Heidelberg, Munich, and Freiburg) evaluated long-term outcomes in 449 patients treated for acoustic schwannomas. Of these, 169 patients received SRS (median dose 13 Gy) and 291 patients received FRT (median dose of 57.6 Gy at 1.8 Gy per fraction). The 10-year local control rate was similar for both groups, at ~ 94%.[36] There was no difference in trigeminal or facial nerve toxicity between FSRT and SRS. Serviceable hearing was preserved in 85% of patients, with loss of useful hearing in 14% of FSRT and 16% of SRS patients. Among those treated using SRS to < 13 Gy, loss of useful hearing was lower, at 13%. Dosimetric studies comparing SRS to FSRT appear to demonstrate an overall advantage to SRS because of the accuracy of a fixed head registration and the steep dose gradient of SRS. However, patients who have preexisting mass effect symptoms are more likely to develop local swelling and worsening of symptoms after SRS. The use of steroids in the immediate post-SRS period can mitigate these potential complications and reduce the need for surgical intervention. Because of its small volume and variable thickness, and the variability of user delineation on imaging, determining the dose-volume limitations for the cochlea is difficult. Several studies have evaluated the association between cochlear dose and persistent hearing loss.[41,53,54]

Pan et al assessed hearing changes in patients after unilateral FRT, using the contralateral ear as standard. A mean cochlear dose of > 44 Gy was associated with > 10 dB increases in bone conduction threshold, whereas the mean dose to the contralateral ear was 4.2 Gy (range 0.4–31.3 Gy).[53] Similarly, other studies found a significant increase in sensorineural hearing loss when the dose received by the cochlea exceeded 45 Gy.[54,55] In a long-term follow-up report, from the Medical University of Vienna, Austria, of 426 patients treated using GK SRS to a median dose of 12 Gy prescribed to 70% isodose line (small intrameatal tumors), 60 to 70% isodose line (Koos grade II) and 50% isodose line (Koos grade III or IV), hearing function prior to treatment and the median dose (> 6 Gy) to the cochlea were independent predictors of serviceable hearing. Studies using MRI-based dose-volume analyses of the cochlea indicate that critical cut-off doses associated with loss of serviceable hearing after SRS were between 3 and 5.3 Gy.[56,57,58] Using bone window CT to delineate the cochlear volume, the median cochlear volume was 80.9 mL (range 51.6–114.2), and hearing preservation was associated with a cochlear dose < 4 Gy in those treated using a fixed-margin dose of 12 Gy.[59] Similarly, in a study evaluating CT-based volumetric cochlear dose and serviceable hearing, 105 patients who had pretreatment serviceable hearing received GK SRS. The authors demonstrated that a mean cochlear dose > 4.9 Gy was associated with time to nonserviceable hearing.[60]

In addition to hearing and CN V and VII function, radiotherapy effects on temporal bone structures are also considered in the radiation treatment plan. Radiation-induced damage to temporal bone structures can manifest as otitis media/externa, mastoiditis, osteoradionecrosis, fibrosis, vertigo, or hearing impairment. It is still too early, owing to SRS dose reduction in the last 10 to 15 years, to draw conclusions about whether FSRT or SRS with lowered prescribed doses has the advantage in terms

of the therapeutic ratio.[30] For tumors up to 3 cm in size, SRS, FSRT, and FRT offer good local control and comparable toxicity. With the advent of IMRT and particle therapy coupled with stereotactic localization, the field of radiotherapy for acoustic schwannoma is rapidly evolving.

9.5 Meningioma

Incidental, asymptomatic, and radiographically stable meningiomas may be observed, with treatment withheld until symptoms and/or growth develops. Skull base meningiomas can be addressed using skull base surgical techniques. Meningiomas tend to infiltrate the critical structures that reside in the region of the skull base and can prevent complete resection from being performed safely, leading to increased risk of tumor progression. To improve tumor control, postoperative radiation therapy is indicated for patients who have subtotally or minimally resected newly diagnosed or recurrent skull base meningiomas.[61] CN complications are in general higher for meningiomas than paragangliomas or schwannomas for a given location of the skull base.

Abundant data in the literature support the use of conventional fractionated 2D and 3D-CRT therapy for management of patients who have subtotally or minimally resected newly diagnosed or recurrent skull base meningiomas.[61] The majority of the series included meningiomas at the skull base as well as in non–skull base locations. In most cases, the typical prescribed dose ranged from 50 to 54 Gy for benign meningiomas. For patients who receive radiation therapy after subtotal resection, it is reasonable to expect a 10-year local control rate of at least 70 to 80% based on the long-term reports in the literature. For patients who have unresectable disease, radiation therapy provides a degree of tumor control and symptomatic relief. In the series from Royal Marsden Hospital, United Kingdom, the reported 5-, 10-, and 15-year disease-free survival rates for patients who had unresectable meningiomas were 53, 47, and 47%, respectively.[62] For patients who had recurrent meningiomas, there was some indication that outcomes were not compromised if radiation therapy was given at the time of recurrence instead of immediately after subtotal tumor resection.[63] However, because of the presence of critical structures such as the optic apparatus, CNs in the cavernous sinus, and brainstem, progression of a skull base meningioma can result in significant neurological morbidity. This question is best answered in a clinical trial setting. The European Organization for Research and Treatment of Cancer is conducting a trial that randomizes patients who have subtotally resected or biopsied World Health Organization grade 1 cerebral meningiomas to observation or postoperative external beam radiation therapy or SRS.

9.5.1 Conformal Radiotherapy for Skull Base Meningioma

Because meningiomas have a sharp margin of demarcation with normal brain parenchyma, they are excellent targets for highly precise radiation techniques such as IMRT, SRS, FSRT, and proton beam therapy (▶ Fig. 9.1). The main advantage of using these techniques is minimizing radiation dose delivery to the areas outside the target volume. IMRT can produce highly conformal

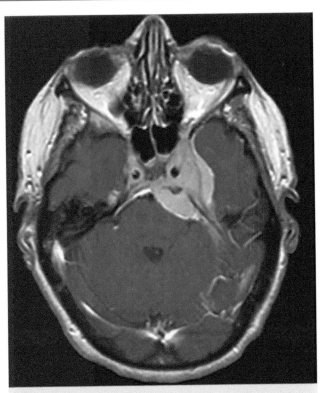

Fig. 9.1 Meningioma involving the cavernous sinus and sphenoid ridge.

isodose distribution around a meningioma target while minimizing dose to surrounding critical structures or organs. It is well suited for targets with complex shapes, such as meningiomas. Colleagues from Baylor College of Medicine treated 40 meningioma patients (32 who had skull base tumors) with IMRT to a dose of 50.4 Gy. For a median follow-up of 30 months, the 5-year tumor control rate was 93%.[64] Acute and late complications were low and occurred in 2.5 and 5% of the patients, respectively. Another study, from the University of Heidelberg, examined the treatment outcomes of 20 patients who had skull base meningiomas treated using IMRT to a prescribed dose of 57.6 Gy. For a median follow-up of 36 months, the tumor control rate was 100%. Approximately 25% of treated tumors showed shrinkage. The incidence of late complications was 10%.[63] A study of 35 patients who had 37 meningiomas treated using IMRT to a prescribed dose of 50.4 Gy at the Cleveland Clinic Foundation showed similar findings. The median follow-up was 19.1 months and the 3-year local control was 97%. No late complications were observed.[65] Although the results are promising, these studies had relatively short follow-up intervals ranging from 19.1 to 36 months. Extended follow-up is required to determine whether IMRT can improve the therapeutic ratio.

9.5.2 Stereotactic Radiosurgery for Meningioma

Data on SRS for the treatment of skull base meningioma have matured in the literature over the past two decades.[61,66,67] The typical prescribed dose was 12 to 18 Gy. Numerous reports demonstrate high efficacy and low toxicity associated with SRS

for treatment of skull base meningioma.[66,68,69,70] Colleagues from Mayo Clinic reported the results of 49 patients who had cavernous sinus meningioma treated using GK-SRS.[70] The mean margin dose was 15.9 Gy. For a median follow-up of 58 months, the tumor control rate was 100%. Symptoms improved for 26% of patients who had preexisting diplopia or facial numbness/weakness. Trigeminal nerve function worsened after treatment in 10% of patients. At the University of Pittsburgh, 129 patients who had cavernous sinus meningioma were treated using GK-SRS. The median margin dose was 13 Gy.[71] Neurologic status remained stable or improved after treatment in 91% of patients. Tumor progression occurred in 6% of patients. Adverse effects occurred in 6.7% of patients. The 5- and 10-year tumor control rates were both 93.1%. At the same institution, 62 patients who had petroclival meningiomas were treated using GK-SRS to a median dose of 11 to 20 Gy.[72] Median follow-up was 37 months, and tumor progression occurred in 8% of the patients. New CN deficits occurred in 8% of patients.

Colleagues from the University of Pittsburg recently published their long-term outcomes in 290 patients treated for meningioma with GK-SRS. The 10- and 20-year freedom from tumor progression rates were 88 and 87%, respectively.[73] Symptoms improved for 20% of patients, and 94% of asymptomatic patients remained asymptomatic. No differences in control rates were found between those who had undergone surgery prior to SRS (89%) versus SRS alone (93%). Treatment toxicity was low, at 3.1%. Other SRS series, either GK- or LINAC-based, showed similar tumor control and toxicity rates for skull base meningioma.[74,75]

FRT can be offered to patients who have skull base meningiomas that are not suitable for treatment using SRS, either due to the size limit or due to their proximity to critical structures such as the optic apparatus. Data on FRT for skull base meningiomas have emerged over the past 10 years. Colleagues from Royal Marsden Hospital, in the United Kingdom, reported their outcomes for patients who had mostly skull base meningiomas treated using FRT.[76] The prescribed dose was 50 to 55 Gy. None of these patients developed any tumor recurrence over the period of follow-up. The group from the University of Heidelberg reported results for one of the largest FRT series for skull base meningiomas. The prescribed dose was 56.8 Gy. The tumor control rate was 98.3% and the complication rate was 1.6%, with a median follow-up of 35 months.[77,78] Other studies using the same approach showed similar tumor control and complication rates.[77,79,80]

9.5.3 Proton Beam Therapy for Skull Base Meningioma

Secondary to the lack of wide availability of proton beam facilities worldwide, protons have not been routinely used in patients who have skull base meningiomas. A few studies have reported on proton beam therapy as the sole modality, or combined with photon beam therapy, for the treatment of skull base meningioma. Investigators from Institut Curie, France, treated 51 skull base meningioma patients with a combination of photon and proton beam therapy.[81] For a median follow-up of 25.4 months, the 4-year local control was 98%. The prescribed dose was 60.6 CGE. Investigators from South Africa treated 23 patients using proton beam radiotherapy, either hypofractionated (31.5 CGE in three fractions) or conventionally fractionated, ranging from 54 CGE in 27 fractions to 61.6 CGE in 16 fractions.[82] For median clinical and imaging follow-ups of 40 and 31 months, respectively, tumor control was achieved in 88% of the patients treated using hypofractionation and in 100% of those treated using conventionally fractionated proton beam therapy. Other proton beam radiotherapy series for meningiomas that included tumors of all locations showed similar outcomes.[83,84] The follow-up times of these studies are relatively short. Considering the indolent nature of benign meningiomas, a prolonged follow-up duration is necessary to determine long-term outcomes with proton beam therapy.

9.6 Craniopharyngioma

Craniopharyngiomas are benign tumors arising from Rathke's pouch. Although they are slow-growing and well circumscribed, their frequent involvement of adjacent structures such as the optic apparatus, pituitary stalk, hypothalamus, and major blood vessels can contribute to significant morbidity and render safe complete surgical resection difficult. Surgical intervention is the standard initial therapy for the purpose of tissue diagnosis and decompression. Attempts at achieving complete surgical resection can be associated with significant morbidity. When complete resection is not possible, limited surgical resection and postoperative radiation therapy can be used to achieve satisfactory rates of tumor control. Conventional fractionated radiation therapy has been shown to be effective in the setting of postoperative treatment as well as for salvage treatment. Because craniopharyngiomas are very well circumscribed tumors, they are very suitable targets for advanced radiation therapy techniques such as IMRT, SRS, FSRT, and proton beam therapy. In patients who have a cystic lesion, intralesional phosphorus-32 (P-32) may be used to treat the tumor.

9.6.1 Fractionated Radiotherapy for Craniopharyngioma

Conventional radiation therapy may be offered in two different settings: for initial treatment of a subtotally resected tumor and for salvage treatment of recurrence after surgical resection. Data in the literature showed that radiation therapy is effective at reducing the risk of recurrence in both settings.[85] The most commonly prescribed dose is 50 to 54 Gy. For patients who received immediate postoperative radiation therapy, 10- and 20-year local control or progression-free survival rates ranged from 57 to 89.1% and from 54 to 79%, respectively.[85] For patients who received postoperative radiation therapy as salvage treatment, similar outcomes were observed. This raises the question of whether delayed instead of immediate radiation therapy should be employed, especially in young children.

Colleagues from Harvard University reported their experience combining photons and protons for treatment of craniopharyngioma.[86] A total of 15 patients, 5 children (median age 15.9 years) and 10 adults (median age 36.2 years), were treated using 160 MeV proton therapy either for the entire course of treatment or in combination with photon beam therapy. The median dose given was 56.9 CGE. For a median follow-up of 11 years, 5- and 10-year local control rates for the 11 surviving

patients were 93 and 85%, respectively. The 10-year overall survival (OS) rate was 72%. None of the 10 adults treated had any change of functional status or working ability. One of the five children had learning difficulties comparable to preradiation therapy level; the remaining children had professional achievements.

9.6.2 SRS for Craniopharyngioma

Both GK- and LINAC-based SRS have been used to treat craniopharyngiomas.[87,88,89,90] Because of the proximity of most craniopharyngiomas to the optic apparatus, there is a risk of radiation-induced visual disturbance if the radiation dose exceeds the tolerance level. Typically, a 3- to 5-mm gap between the tumor and optic apparatus is needed to limit the radiation dose to the structure. Most SRS series showed a local control rate of 86 to 90%.[90,91] In one Swedish series, the rates of tumor progression were 85 and 33% for tumors receiving < 6 Gy and ≥ 6 Gy, respectively.[92] Longer follow-up is needed to determine the efficacy and toxicity of SRS for craniopharyngiomas, because the majority of series had follow-up times of less than 3.5 years. In a few series that had longer-term follow-up, 5-year progression-free survival (PFS) and OS rates were 52 to 68% and 86 to 97%, respectively. Taipei Veterans Hospital recently reported on a 20-year experience treating 137 patients using GK-SRS for craniopharyngiomas.[91] Median follow-up was 45.7 months, and control rates were 73% (solid), 74% (cystic), and 66% (mixed tumors). The 5-year PFS rate was 70%, and 8% had new onset or worsening pituitary deficiency.

9.7 Paraganglioma

A paraganglioma is a tumor that arises from specialized neural crest cells called paraganglia and that can develop from various sites of the body. Clusters of paraganglia are called glomus bodies (or glomus tumors) and are associated with autonomic ganglia. The majority (~ 90%) are benign and sporadic.[93] Approximately 10% of cases are familial and often develop multiple tumors and occur in younger patients.[94] They are associated with mutation of the succinate dehydrogenase gene family, among other genes. Approximately 3% develop within the head and neck, and the main pattern of spread is local. Nodal and distant metastases are rare. Only about 2 to 5% secrete catecholamines. Paragangliomas of the head and neck can originate from four primary sites (▶ Fig. 9.2) and are named by their location:

- Carotid body tumor arises at the bifurcation of the common carotid artery.
- Glomus vagale arises along the extracranial course of the vagus nerve.
- Glomus jugulare arises at the jugular bulb.
- Glomus tympanicum arises in the middle ear from the inferior tympanic branch (Jacobson's nerve) of the glossopharyngeal nerve (CN IX).
- Glomus jugulotympanicum arises from the mastoid branch (Arnold's nerve) of the vagus nerve (CN X) and is found between the middle ear and jugular foramen.

Presentation varies depending on the location of origin and the affected CN. Carotid body tumors are the most common (accounting for 60% of paragangliomas) and often present as a

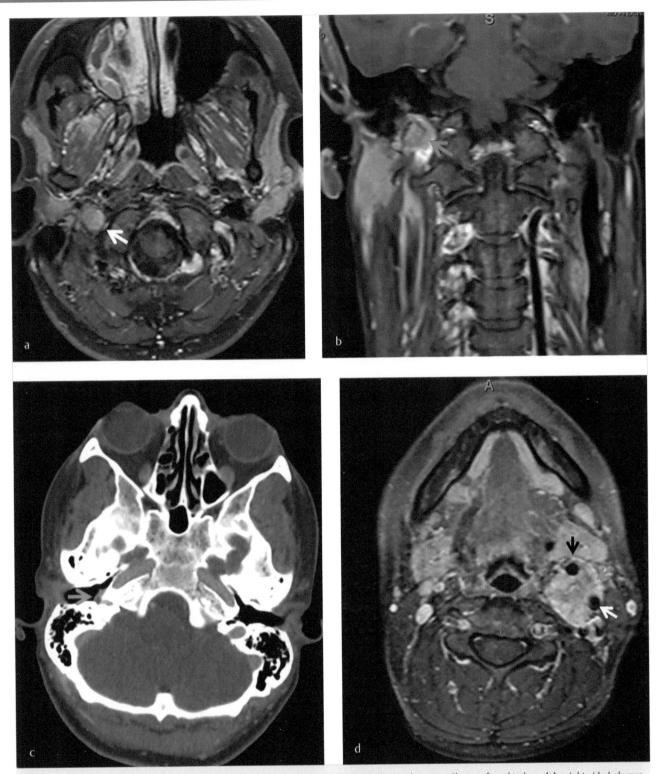

Fig. 9.2 Multiple paraganglioma in a 39-year-old woman who presented with hearing loss and tinnitus. She was found to have **(a)** a right-sided glomus jugulare (*white arrow*) extending to the hypotympanum (**b**; *red arrow*). **(c)** Tumor involving the right hypotympanum (*red arrow*) on CT. **(d)** A third paraganglioma: left-sided carotid body tumor (*red arrow*) showing the splayed internal carotid (*black arrow*) and external carotid (*white arrow*) arteries.

slow-growing, mobile, painless neck mass. Larger tumors can be associated with CN palsies of the vagal (CN X) and hypoglossal (CN XII) nerves and the sympathetic chain. Temporal bone paragangliomas such as glomus jugulare tumors can result in local bone destruction and present with impairment of CNs IX,

X, XI, and XII from mass effect. Glomus tympanicum tumors are associated with hearing loss, pulsatile tinnitus, and disequilibrium and appear as a reddish mass behind the ear drum (known as the "red drum") on physical exam.[95] Glomus vagale tumors are the least common of the head and neck paragangliomas and can present as an intraoral parapharyngeal mass or a painless lateral neck mass behind the angle of mandible; they are associated with dysphagia and hoarseness. Glomus tumors typically grow at a rate of 1 mm per year, with a median doubling time of 4 years.[96] Because these tumors are hypervascular, they are usually demonstrated very well on CT with contrast. CT can be useful to evaluate bone erosion. They also have a characteristic appearance on MRI. Angiography is used to evaluate patients preoperatively.

9.7.1 Radiotherapy for Paraganglioma

The goals of the treatment are tumor and symptomatic control. Treatment options include surgical resection, conventionally fractionated FRT, hypofractionated FSRT, and SRS. Because glomus tumors are rare, even in large medical centers, no consistent treatment algorithm has been developed. The optimal treatment approach depends on tumor location and size as well as on the medical comorbidities of the patient. Surgery is the preferred first-line option, particularly for carotid body tumors, with the goal being a complete resection. However, resection of a skull base paraganglioma such as those of jugulotympanic origin may require sacrifice of one or more CNs, resulting in permanent treatment morbidity. In a study by Fayad et al of 83 patients who had glomus jugulares, a gross total resection was achieved in 81% of cases, but 18.9% of patients developed new CN deficits after surgery. CN injury for larger skull base paragangliomas and vagale tumors can remain high even when using more advanced skull base surgery techniques and preoperative embolization.[97]

In cases in which the risk of surgical resection is too high, or after a subtotal resection, radiation therapy is a safe and effective treatment.[98,99,100,101,102] Historically, radiotherapy was reserved for elderly or debilitated patients who had unresectable or extensive tumors. However, radiotherapy advances and emergence of long-term data have shown that radiotherapy is associated with high rates of tumor control and low rates of long-term complications. Radiotherapy is often considered first-line treatment for paragangliomas located in the skull base or vagale tumors. Unlike the goal of surgery, which is complete tumor removal, the goal of radiotherapy is to stop tumor growth and/or reduce tumor size over time. In terms of target delineation, CT, MRI, and angiography can be used. Because the risk of nodal metastasis is low and tumors are often confined, the clinical target volume typically does not include regional nodes or require extensive subclinical coverage of microscopic infiltration. This makes highly conformal radiotherapy techniques highly attractive for paragangliomas.

9.7.2 Fractionated Radiotherapy for Paraganglioma

FRT delivered to a moderate total dose of 45 to 50 Gy with conventional fractionation (1.8–2.0 Gy per fraction daily) offers excellent tumor control and has the longest and largest experience. In a comprehensive review of all the articles published on radiation therapy for glomus tumors from 1965 to 1988 using a variety of delivery techniques and dosing schedules, the median tumor control was 93%, and the risk of severe complication was 2 to 3%.[103]

▶ Table 9.3 summarizes the treatment outcomes of selected radiation therapy series for glomus tumors. The efficacy and complication rates were not associated with site of origin, whether the carotid body or the vagal ganglia or jugulotympanic in nature. Tumors that recurred typically manifested between 1 and 8 years after treatment. Most of the severe complications were related to use of older 2D and 3D techniques, doses that exceeded current recommendations, and re-irradiation.

Table 9.3 Summary of treatment outcomes for patients treated for glomus tumors using radiotherapy

Series	Patients	Radiotherapy dose	Follow-up	Tumor control
Pemberton[a]	49	37.5–50 Gy in 15–16 days	7.4 y	92%
Krych[b]	23	45 Gy	13.4 y	100%
Wang[c]	15	29–67.5 Gy	5–33 y	80%
Konefal[c]	22	46–55 Gy	10.5 y	91%
Sharma[d]	40	40–50 Gy	13 y	83%
Hinerman[e]	43	37.7–60 Gy	11.1 y	93%
Cummings[f]	45	35 Gy in 3 wk	10 y	93%
Powell[g]	46	35–66 Gy	9 y	85%
Jacob (Mayo)	54	15.3 Gy in 1 Fx	4 y	100%
Scheick (Florida)[h]	11	15 Gy (12.5–15) in 1 Fx	5.3 y	81%
Sheehan[i]	134	Median 15 Gy in 1 Fx	4.2 y	88%

[a]Pemberton LS, Swindell R, Sykes AJ. Radical radiotherapy alone for glomus jugulare and tympanicum tumours. Oncol Rep 2005;14(6):1631–1633.
[b]Krych AJ, Foote RL, Brown PD, Garces YI, Link MJ. Long-term results of irradiation for paraganglioma. Int J Radiat Oncol Biol Phys 2006;65(4):1063–1066.
[c]Wang ML, Hussey DH, Doornbos JF, Vigliotti AP, Wen BC. Chemodectoma of the temporal bone: a comparison of surgical and radiotherapeutic results. Int J Radiat Oncol Biol Phys 1988;14(4):643–648.
[d]Sharma PD, Johnson AP, Whitton AC. Radiotherapy for jugulo-tympanic paragangliomas (glomus jugulare tumours). J Laryngol Otol 1984;98(6):621–629.
[e]Hinerman RW, Mendenhall WM, Amdur RJ, Stringer SP, Antonelli PJ, Cassisi NJ. Definitive radiotherapy in the management of chemodectomas arising in the temporal bone, carotid body, and glomus vagale. Head Neck 2001;23(5):363–371.
[f]Cummings BJ, Beale FA, Garrett PG, et al. The treatment of glomus tumors in the temporal bone by megavoltage radiation. Cancer 1984;53(12):2635–2640.
[g]Powell S, Peters N, Harmer C. Chemodectoma of the head and neck: results of treatment in 84 patients. Int J Radiat Oncol Biol Phys 1992;22(5):919–924.
[h]Scheick SM, Morris CG, Amdur RJ, Bova FJ, Friedman WA, Mendenhall WM. Long-term Outcomes After Radiosurgery for Temporal Bone Paragangliomas. Am J Clin Oncol 2015.
[i]Sheehan JP, Tanaka S, Link MJ, et al. Gamma Knife surgery for the management of glomus tumors: a multicenter study. J Neurosurg 2012;117(2):246–254.

9.7.3 Stereotactic Radiosurgery and Fractionated Stereotactic Radiotherapy for Paraganglioma

Disadvantages of FRT include the longer treatment course (typically 5 weeks), the need for larger planning target volume (PTV) margins to account for daily treatment setup uncertainties, and, in younger patients, the risk of a secondary radiation-induced malignancy. SRS or FSRT offers an attractive alternative, because treatment can be administered in five or fewer fractions with similar local control and complication rates (▶ Fig. 9.3). SRS/FSRT can be used as first-line treatment or as salvage therapy after treatment failure.

Long-term outcomes data after SRS are limited compared with those for surgery and FRT. Follow-up times range from 8 to 12 years for SRS and from 3 to 7 years for FSRT. Across multiple SRS series for glomus jugulare tumors, median tumor control rate was 95% (range 63–100%) and symptomatic improvement rate was

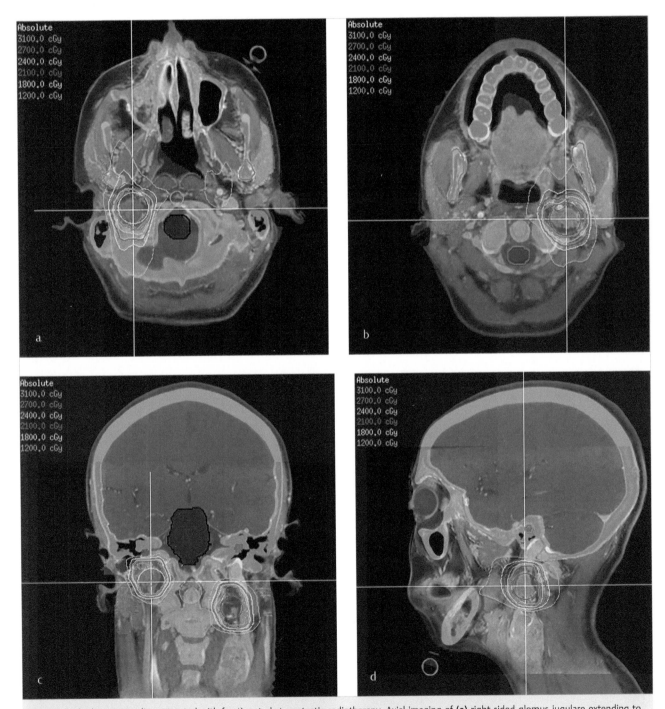

Fig. 9.3 Multiple paraganglioma treated with fractionated stereotactic radiotherapy. Axial imaging of **(a)** right-sided glomus jugulare extending to hypotympanum and **(b)** left-sided glomus vagale. **(c)** Coronal image of treated bilateral tumors. **(d)** Sagittal image. The left carotid body tumor was stable and observed.

40% (range 25–60%).[100,108,109,110,111,112,113,114,115,116,117,118,119,120,121] Complications such as worsening of preexisting CN deficits, tinnitus, and vertigo occurred in 8.5% of patients (range 4–40%), of which 6.5% were transient and 2% permanent. The median dose was ~ 15 Gy (range 12–32 Gy) prescribed to the 50% isodose line in a single session. The use of 13 Gy or less was associated with higher recurrence rates. In a meta-analysis of 19 studies representing 335 patients who had glomus jugulare tumors, performed by Guss et al at John Hopkins, Stanford, and UCSF, the rate of tumor control was 95% among studies with median follow-up of longer than 36 months.[122] There were no differences among SRS systems, with similar high rates of tumor control seen for GK (~ 97%; range 94–99%) and LINAC/CyberKnife (~ 97%; range 92–100%) studies. The authors felt that the clinical outcomes with SRS might be better than reported in the study, because radiosurgery is usually reserved for patients who have contraindications for surgery, residual disease after surgery, or recurrent disease, thus imparting a potential inherent bias whereby tumors that are refractory to surgery may be more aggressive. In a published study by the North American Gamma Knife Consortium (Sheehan et al) on 132 patients from eight GK centers whose paragangliomas were treated to a median dose of 15 Gy, tumor control was 88% at 5 years, with a median follow-up of 50.5 months. Patients demonstrating new or progressive CN deficits were more likely to demonstrate tumor progression ($P = 0.002$). Pulsatile tinnitus improved in 49% of patients, and 11% had improvement in CN deficits. At the Mayo Clinic, 57 patients were treated using SRS between 1990 and 2007 to a mean dose of 15.3 Gy, and local control rates were 100 and 83% at 7 and 10 years, respectively.

Data using FSRT are limited to smaller series with limited follow-up. In general, the tumor volumes treated using FSRT were larger than for single-session SRS series. Several reports used LINAC or CK techniques to doses of 21 to 27 Gy in three fractions or 25 to 30 Gy in five fractions and reported 96 to 100% tumor controls rates with a follow-up duration of ~ 2 years.[123,124,125] Treatment complications rates were minimal, with no new or worsening of preexisting neurologic deficits in all but one study (Wegner and Lieberman), which showed 19% grade 1/2 adverse events (Chun).

Randomized prospective clinical data comparing surgery with FRT or SRS/FSRT are not available. In a systemic literature review by Suarez et al of 2,042 patients who had glomus jugulare and glomus vagale tumors treated using surgery ($n = 1,310$), FRT ($n = 461$), or SRS ($n = 261$), median follow-ups were 66 months, 113 months, and 41 months, respectively. Tumor local control rates were higher with radiotherapy (91.5%) than with surgery (78.1%; $P < 0.05$), and the probability of a major complication was lower with radiotherapy (11%) than with surgery (26%; $P < 0.05$). The authors calculated an iatrogenic cranial neuropathy rate of 1.0 per patient with surgery versus 0.08 per patient with radiotherapy ($P < 0.001$). Local control rates for temporal bone paragangliomas were similar between FRT and newer surgical techniques, but complication rates (CN palsies) were higher with surgery.

An important consideration in the use of radiotherapy for patients who have benign skull base tumors with long-term survivorship is the risk of radiation-induced second malignancies. Although the overall risk is low, development of a radiation-induced sarcoma of the skull base is often fatal. Lalwani et al and Gilbo estimated the rate of radiation-induced sarcoma to be 0.5 to 5% at an average of 8 to 15 years.[126,127] The risk of secondary malignancy with FRT is about 1 in 500, with a latency period of 8 years or longer. The predicted risk of radiation-induced second malignancies with SRS appeared lower. To date, very few cases of radiation-induced malignancy after SRS have been reported, leading some to estimate that the risk of radiation-induced malignancy is negligible with SRS.[108]

Factors that help determine the optimal treatment algorithm for patients who have paraganglioma include tumor location, presenting symptoms, age, comorbidities, tumor volume, imaging characteristics, and rate of growth. Close observation is reasonable for older patients who are asymptomatic and who have comorbidities. Younger patients who have large tumors and significant associated mass effect or high rates of circulating catecholamines may benefit from immediate surgical resection and cytoreduction with consideration of adjuvant radiotherapy based on pathologic risk factors. However, in cases in which CN injury with surgery is likely, radiotherapy can be considered. For paragangliomas of skull base and temporal bone, radiotherapy can be considered as a first-line approach. Good candidates for SRS are those having small- to moderate-volume (< 15 mL) tumors and nonsecreting tumors located above C2. Larger tumors and tumors below the skull base are better suited for FRT. FSRT offers a promising alternative to FRT by combining the advantages of highly precise stereotactic planning and delivery with the convenience of a short-treatment course and the functional sparing advantages of fractionation.

9.8 Chordomas

Chordomas are rare tumors that originate from the remnants of the embryonal notochord. Approximately a third of these tumors occur in the skull base. They are low-grade tumors that grow locally and aggressively, with very high recurrence rates.[128] Local control is the most prognostic factor for survival,[129] and complete surgical resection is the cornerstone to optimal local control, which is the key prognostic factor in survival; however, gross total resection can be challenging due to local infiltration of skull base structures and the proximity of critical neurovasculature. Accordingly, these tumors are most often treated using maximal safe resection and postoperative radiation therapy. Postoperative radiation therapy is employed to reduce the risk of local recurrence. The most common cause of death is uncontrolled local tumor progression, so local tumor control is of utmost importance.[130] Unfortunately, the location of these tumors renders the delivery of a sufficiently high dose of radiation to the area difficult even when using highly conformal techniques that involve photon beam therapy, subsequently resulting in nondurable tumor control. Treatment outcomes achieved with the use of conventional fractionated radiation therapy have been disappointing.

9.8.1 Radiotherapy for Chordoma

The typical prescribed dose for conventional fractionated radiation therapy is 50 to 60 Gy.[131,132,133] Other strategies for intensifying the radiation dose to skull base chordomas, such as SRS and FSRT, have also been used.[133] In the SRS series from Mayo Clinic, for a median follow-up of 4.8 years, 2- and 5-year tumor control rates were 89 and 32%, respectively.[134] The median margin dose was 15 Gy. Patients who had prior fractionated radiotherapy had a higher risk of radiation-induced complications. More recent reports on SRS have suggested that higher biologic radiation doses improve local control. Kano et al from the University of Pittsburgh reported a 5-year control rate of 66%. Other studies also suggested that SRS may be an effective treatment for skull base chordomas.[135,136] FSRT has also been used to treat skull base chordomas. The group from the University of Heidelberg treated patients who had skull base chordomas using FSRT. The prescribed dose was 66.6 Gy. The 2-and 5-year local control rates were 82 and 50%, respectively.[137]

9.8.2 Proton Therapy for Chordoma

Proton radiation therapy is well suited for the treatment of clival chordomas. Because of the absence of an exit dose, a very conformal dose distribution around the target volume can be achieved with proton radiation therapy (PRT). This allows delivery of a higher radiation dose to the tumor so as to improve local control (▶ Fig. 9.4). A large body of experience has been accumulated over the years on the use of PRT for skull base chordoma.[138] In the United States, much of the early clinical experience published on use of PRT for skull base chordomas came from the Lawrence Berkeley National Laboratory, Loma Linda University, and Harvard University. Investigators from Harvard University reported one of the largest experiences (n = 519) using PRT (five fractions per week, four with protons and one with photons) for the treatment of skull base chordoma (n = 290) and low-grade chondrosarcoma (n = 229).[130,139] The prescribed dose was 66 to 83 CGE, conventionally fractionated,

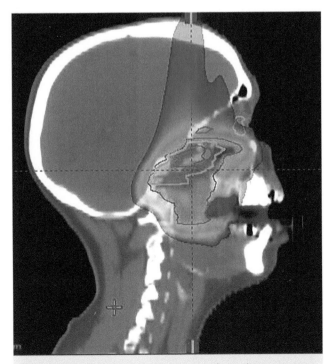

Fig. 9.4 Clival chordoma treated using proton beam therapy. A vertex beam was used in this plan to limit dose to the adjacent brainstem and spinal cord.

and a relative biological effectiveness (RBE) of 1.1 was used. Median follow-up was 41 months, and 5- and 10-year local recurrence-free survival rates were 64 and 42%, respectively. Severe complications occurred in 8% of patients. Hug et al from Loma Linda University treated 58 patients who had skull base chordoma (n = 33) and low-grade chondrosarcoma (n = 25) using proton beam therapy. The median dose was 64.8 to 79.2 CGE.[130] For a mean follow-up period of 33 months, 8 (24%) of 33 patients who had chordomas experienced recurrence. The 3-year local control rate was 67%. The 5-year OS rate was 79%. A group from Institut Curie treated 100 patients who had base of skull or cervical spine chordomas using fractionated radiotherapy that combined photons and protons. A prescribed dose of 67 CGE was given. For a median follow-up of 31 months, a total of 25 patients developed recurrence. The 2- and 4-year tumor control rates were 86.3 and 53.8%, respectively.[140] Colleagues from Boston (Munzenrider et al) published their results from 169 patients treated using combined proton and photon with a median follow-up of 41 months. Their 5- and 10-year local control (LC) rates were 73 and 54%, and corresponding OS rates were 80 and 54% at 10 years after photon–proton combination.[139] The French group (Noel et al) showed 4-year LC and OS rates of 54 and 80% in 100 patients at 31-month follow-up using combined proton and photon (Centre de protonthérapie d'Orsay).[140] Other proton beam radiotherapy series have shown similar results.[141,142,143,144,145]

More recently, spot scanning proton therapy and intensity-modulated proton therapy (IMPT) have been used for treatment of skull base chordomas.[142,143] In contrast to passive scatter, IMPT offers greater control over the proximal aspects of the beam and improved conformality of high-dose regions and allows use of a simultaneous integrated boost technique similar to IMRT for treating multiple target volumes to discrete doses. Investigators from the Paul Scherrer Institute evaluated the use of IMPT for treatment of skull base chordomas and reported a 5-year local control rate of 81% in 64 patients treated to a median dose of 73.5 Gy (RBE), with 94% freedom from grade 3 or 4 toxicity at 5 years.[142] Similarly, at the University of Texas's MD Anderson Cancer Center, IMPT prescribed to a mean dose of 69.8 Gy has been used for treatment of patients who have skull base chordomas, with similar results.[146] Compared with passive scatter plans, IMPT demonstrated improved high-dose conformality and showed better sparing of temporal lobes and brainstem. Given the more favorable outcomes associated with the use of PRT than can be achieved using photon beam irradiation alone, proton beam radiotherapy should be considered in most patients who have skull base chordomas.

9.8.3 Carbon Ion Therapy for Chordoma

Carbon ion therapy combines the physical advantages of protons with the differential increase in relative biologic effectiveness. It is currently not available in the United States and in fact is available only in a few facilities worldwide. Early clinical data from investigators at the University of Heidelberg reported a 3-year tumor control rate of 81% for patients who had chordomas, with no excessive toxicity observed.[147] At the German Ion Research Center (GSI), in a phase I/II trial of carbon ion therapy for the treatment of skull base chordomas and chondrosarcomas, with a median follow-up of 32 months, the 4-year actuarial local control for chordomas was 74%.[148] The prescribed dose was 60 GyE at 3 GyE daily, 7 days a week. These results appeared to be as favorable as those achieved using proton beam therapy. However, longer follow-up is required to determine the long-term efficacy and toxicity associated with the treatment. Uhl et al recently published their long-term data on 155 patients treated with carbon ions using an active raster scanning technique for skull base chordomas.[149,150] The median dose was 60 Gy (RBE 3 Gy), and median follow-up was 72 months. The 5-year LC and OS rates were 72 and 85%, respectively; 10-year rates were 54 and 75%, respectively. Age < 48 and boost volume > 75 mL were associated with improved outcomes. This study represents the largest cohort examined after carbon ion treatment and the second-largest cohort of patients to date with skull base chordoma treated with carbon ion therapy.

Clinical data from other users of particle therapy, including Loma Linda (Hug EB et al),[151] the Paul Scherrer Institut (Ares et al),[143] and the National Institutes of Radiological Science (Mizoe et al),[152] suggest better LC and survival rates than seen with conventional techniques. Currently there are no randomized data comparing use of protons, SRS, and carbon ion therapy.

9.9 Chondrosarcomas

Chondrosarcomas are heterogeneous neoplasms that constitute 10 to 20% of all malignant bone tumors. Those occurring in the head and neck region most commonly arise from the sphenopetrosal and the spheno-occipital synchondroses, the nasal cavity, and the paranasal sinuses. Complete surgical resection is the mainstay of treatment. Postoperative radiation therapy is needed to reduce the risk of recurrence in higher-grade lesions. A high dose of radiation is required to achieve permanent local control. Much like skull base chordomas, skull base chondrosarcomas are subject to the radiation dose constraints of surrounding critical or normal structures, so that the delivery of a high dose of conventional photon beam radiotherapy is often not possible.

9.9.1 Radiotherapy for Chondrosarcoma

Advanced radiation techniques such as conventionally fractionated IMRT, SRS, and FSRT have been used to treat patients who have skull base chondrosarcoma, particularly those who have smaller primary tumor volumes (▶ Table 9.4). At the University of Heidelberg, eight patients were treated for skull base chondrosarcoma using FRT. The prescribed dose was 64.9 Gy. None of the patients developed recurrence after 5 years.[137] In the series from Mayo Clinic, 29 patients who had skull base chordoma (n = 25) and chondrosarcoma (n = 4) were treated using GK-based SRS. All four patients who had skull base chondrosarcoma achieved tumor control with a median follow-up of 4.8 years.[134] Similarly, good results were shown in the study from the University of Pittsburgh.[136] In a study by Hasegawa et al, those who had tumor volumes < 20 mL showed significantly improved tumor control and survival.[153] Iyer et al from Stanford evaluated 22 patients treated with GK-SRS for skull base chondrosarcoma. The 5-year local control and survival rates were 72 and 70%, respectively. Patients who were > 40 years of age and who had no prior radiotherapy showed improved outcomes.[154]

Table 9.4 Summary of results of selected stereotactic radiosurgery series for chondrosarcomas

Series	Patients	Modality/ dose	Tumor volume (mL)	Local control
Krishnan[a]	4	GK/15 Gy × 1	14.4	100% (5 y)
Hasegawa[a]	7	GK/14 Gy × 1	19.7	76% (5 y); 67% (10 y)
Iyer[c]	22	GK/15 Gy × 1	8.0	72% (5 y); 54% (10 y)
Jiang Kondziolka[d] Muthukumar[e] Debus[f]	16	CK/22 Gy × 1, 30 Gy in 5 Fx	35.1	41% (5 y)

Abbreviations: CK, CyberKnife; GK, Gamma Knife.
[a]Krishnan S, Foote RL, Brown PD, Pollock BE, Link MJ, Garces YI. Radiosurgery for cranial base chordomas and chondrosarcomas. Neurosurgery 2005;56(4):777–784.
[b]Hasegawa T, Ishii D, Kida Y, Yoshimoto M, Koike J, Iizuka H. Gamma Knife surgery for skull base chordomas and chondrosarcomas. J Neurosurg 2007;107(4):752–757.
[c]Iyer A, Kano H, Kondziolka D, et al. Stereotactic radiosurgery for intracranial chondrosarcoma. J Neurooncol 2012;108(3):535–542.
[d]Kondziolka D, Lunsford LD, Flickinger JC. The role of radiosurgery in the management of chordoma and chondrosarcoma of the cranial base. Neurosurgery 1991;29(1):38–45, discussion 45–46.
[e]Muthukumar N, Kondziolka D, Lunsford LD, Flickinger JC. Stereotactic radiosurgery for chordoma and chondrosarcoma: further experiences. Int J Radiat Oncol Biol Phys 1998;41(2):387–392.
[f]Debus J, Schulz-Ertner D, Schad L, et al. Stereotactic fractionated radiotherapy for chordomas and chondrosarcomas of the skull base. Int J Radiat Oncol Biol Phys 2000;47(3):591–596.

In a study by Jiang et al, patients were treated using CyberKnife FSRT to a median dose ranging from 22 Gy in a single fraction to 30 Gy in five fractions. FSRT was used for larger tumors. No differences were observed by radiotherapy approach. Tumor control rates in those who had nonrecurrent and recurrent disease were 80 and 50%, respectively. More recently, Kano et al from the University of Pittsburgh published data from the North American Gamma Knife Consortium for skull base chondrosarcomas consisting of seven centers and 46 patients.[155] The median tumor volume was 7.8 mL (range 0.9–41 mL), and median dose was 15 Gy (range 10.5–20 Gy). The 10-year local control and survival rates were 70 and 76%, respectively. Patients who had no prior radiotherapy and smaller tumors were associated with improved outcomes. In fact, those who had no prior radiotherapy and tumor volumes < 5 mL had 100% progression-free survival at 10 years.

9.9.2 Particle Therapy for Chondrosarcoma

High-dose proton beam radiotherapy to treat skull base chondrosarcomas has resulted in excellent local control. Several proton beam radiotherapy studies pertaining to management of skull base chondrosarcoma have been reported. A study from Harvard University of 200 patients treated to a prescribed dose of 72.1 CGE showed a 5-year local control of 99%. Other proton beam studies using similar radiation dose levels showed similar tumor control rates.[139,143]

Carbon ion therapy has been used to treat patients who have skull base chondrosarcomas. Compared with proton beam radiotherapy, carbon ion therapy appears to yield similar tumor control and lower toxicity rate. Fifty-four patients were treated for skull base low- or intermediate-grade chondrosarcoma at GSI in Germany. A dose of 60 CGE (weekly dose 7 × 3 CGE) was prescribed to the tumor volume.[156] For a median follow-up of 33 months, tumor control rates at 3- and 4-years were 96.2 and 89.8%, respectively. The grade 3 late-toxicity rate was 1.9%. In 2010, Uhl et al reported on their carbon ion therapy experience treating 79 patients who had skull base chondrosarcomas to a median dose of 60 CGE at 3 CGE per fraction. Median follow-up was 91 months, the 5- and 1-year local control rates were both 88%, and the 10-year survival rate was 78.9%. Treatment toxicities consisted of vertigo (20%) and hearing deficits (10%). In this study, primary versus recurrent disease did not impact disease control or survival outcomes. Currently, there is an ongoing randomized clinical trial comparing proton to carbon ion radiation therapy in patients who have skull base chordoma, sponsored by Combs et al from Heidelberg University (ClinicalTrials.gov identifier: NCT01182779).[157,158] The estimated enrollment is 319, and the primary outcome is local progression-free survival.

9.10 Nasopharyngeal Carcinoma

NPC is the most common head and neck cancer in Southeast Asia but is relatively rare in the Western Hemisphere. In contrast to the NPC phenotype from Asia, patients who have NPC in the Americas are typically diagnosed at a locally advanced stage, and many tumors are negative for the Epstein-Barr virus phenotype.[159] The nasopharynx is an anatomically complex site in which a surgical resection of tumor in this region can be challenging and can be associated with significant morbidity. Accordingly, NPC is managed primarily using radiation therapy, with or without chemotherapy. The role of surgery is typically limited to neck dissection if there is residual disease after radiation therapy or to salvage therapy for recurrent disease after primary radiotherapy. The typical radiation dose for gross disease is 70 Gy in 33 to 35 fractions. The typical dose for subclinical disease is 59.4 Gy. Because of this cancer's tendency to involve the fissures and the foramina in the skull base, these areas should be included in the radiation field. NPC also carries a high risk of bilateral neck node metastases. Even if there is no clinical evidence of nodal involvement at presentation, elective coverage should include the level II through V and retropharyngeal (RP) nodal basins of the bilateral neck.

Multiple phase III trials have established the role of cisplatin-based concurrent chemoradiation followed by adjuvant cisplatin and 5-fluorouracil therapy in the management of NPC.[160,161,162] Locoregional control (LRC) rates in patients treated with concurrent chemoradiation using IMRT are excellent. The predominant pattern of recurrence is distant metastasis. Several meta-analyses have demonstrated that the addition of adjuvant or neoadjuvant chemotherapy to concurrent chemoradiation in those who have locally advanced NPC provides a small but significant reduction in distant metastasis rate while improving OS.[163]

Nasopharynx cancer treatment has particularly benefited from the rapid evolution of radiotherapy techniques from 2D to 3D-CRT to IMRT and then to proton therapy and MRI-guided radiation therapy. Treatment of NPC initially consisted of conventional 2D radiotherapy (2D-RT) approaches using lateral-opposed fields. This led to satisfactory disease control but high complication rates, particularly for patients who had T3 to T4 disease in which a 72.2 Gy boost to the skull base was used. In the 1990s, 3D-CRT based on CT imaging, which allowed for better target delineation and reduced toxicity to normal tissue, became the standard treatment approach. Because of the complex shape of the target volume and the close proximity of the target volume to various critical structures, IMRT was considered a major advance in the treatment of NPC in terms of improved disease control and reduced toxicity. Randomized clinical studies in NPC treatment have associated IMRT, compared with 3D-CRT, with improved parotid sparing and patient-reported quality of life (QOL) as well as with lower temporal lobe necrosis (TLN) rates.[164] The use of IMRT has also been associated with excellent local control rates of > 85% consistently across multiple studies.[164,165,166,167] In a recent meta-analysis of eight studies comparing patients treated using IMRT ($n = 1,541$) to 2D and 3D conventional techniques ($n = 2,029$), IMRT was associated with better 5-year OS and locoregional control rates as well as lower rates of late xerostomia, trismus, and TLN.[168] In a study from the University of California, San Francisco of NPC patients treated using IMRT, the 4-year local progression-free, local–regional progression-free, and distant metastasis-free rates were 97%, 98%, and 66%, respectively.[169] The 4-year OS was 88%, and toxicity rate was low. Other studies also showed favorable results after IMRT for NPC.[166,170]

9.10.1 Radiotherapy for Stage T3 to T4 Nasopharyngeal Carcinoma

Patients who have stage T3 disease (tumor invasion of the paranasal sinuses, clivus, and other structures of the skull base) or T4 disease (intracranial extension, involvement of CNs, or extension to orbit or infratemporal fossa) present a clinical challenge for the radiation oncologist. The use of IMRT allows the delivery of an adequate tumoricidal dose with an acceptable toxicity risk. ▶ Table 9.5 shows the clinical outcomes of selected series after IMRT for patients who have T4 NPC. Overall, tumor control and survival rates were very good, with acceptable treatment toxicity. Patients from endemic areas represented the majority of studies. The results of non-endemic T4 NPC patients treated using IMRT were reported in a study from the MD Anderson Cancer Center. Takiar et al showed that the results were similar to those for endemic patients.[171] The 5-year locoregional, progression-free survival and OS rates were 80%, 57%, and 69%, respectively. The late grade 3 toxicity rate was 49% at 5 years, with hearing impairment accounting for nearly half (43%) of cases. In this cohort, > 80% of patients received high-dose cisplatin. The incidence of TLN was 14%, of which the majority of cases were subclinical, with 15% of patients with radiographic TLN demonstrating a clinically measurable cognitive impairment.

Table 9.5 Selected IMRT series for T4 nasopharynx carcinoma

Series	Patients	Follow-up (mo)	% T4	Histology	OS	Tumor control	Late toxicity
Lee[a]	67		20%	100% WHO II/III			
Ng[b]	193		19%	100% WHO II/III			
Kwong[c]	50	25	72%	100% WHO II/III	92% (2 y)	93% (2 y LRC)	
Xiao[d]	81	54	40%	100% WHO II/III	75% (5 y)		1 grade 3 fibrosis
Cao[e]	70	27	100%	99% WHO II/III	83% (2 y)	82% (2 y LFFS)	No grade 3/4 xerostomia 50% hearing loss
Huang[f]	30	67	100%	100% WHO II/III	89% (5 y)	75% (5 y LFFS)	
Kong[g]	81	34	100%	100% WHO II/III	90% (3 y)	84% (3 y LFFS)	6 TLN 16 hearing loss 2 CN palsy 4 grade 3 toxicity
Chen[h]	154	53	100%	100% WHO II/III	75% (5 y)	78% (5 y LFFS)	18.5% grade 3 25 hearing loss 8 encephalopathy 3 CN palsy 1 spinal cord injury
Takiar[i]	66	38	100%	80% WHO II/III 20% WHO I	69% (5 y)	80% (5 y LRC)	36% grade 3 (3 y)

Abbreviations: % T4, percent of T4 patients; CN, cranial nerve; IMRT, intensity modulated radiation therapy; LFFS, locoregional failure free survival; LRC, locoregional control; OS, overall survival; TLN, temporal lobe necrosis; WHO, World Health Organization.

[a]Lee N, Xia P, Quivey JM, et al. Intensity-modulated radiotherapy in the treatment of nasopharyngeal carcinoma: an update of the UCSF experience. Int J Radiat Oncol Biol Phys 2002;53(1):12–22.

[b]Ng WT, Lee MC, Hung WM, et al. Clinical outcomes and patterns of failure after intensity-modulated radiotherapy for nasopharyngeal carcinoma. Int J Radiat Oncol Biol Phys 2011;79(2):420–428.

[c]Kwong DL, Pow EH, Sham JS, et al. Intensity-modulated radiotherapy for early-stage nasopharyngeal carcinoma: a prospective study on disease control and preservation of salivary function. Cancer 2004;101(7):1584–1593.

[d]Xiao WW, Huang SM, Han F, et al. Local control, survival, and late toxicities of locally advanced nasopharyngeal carcinoma treated by simultaneous modulated accelerated radiotherapy combined with cisplatin concurrent chemotherapy: long-term results of a phase 2 study. Cancer 2011;117(9):1874–1883.

[e]Cao CN, Luo JW, Gao L, et al. Clinical outcomes and patterns of failure after intensity-modulated radiotherapy for T4 nasopharyngeal carcinoma. Oral Oncol 2013;49(2):175–181.

[f]Huang HI, Chan KT, Shu CH, Ho CY. T4-locally advanced nasopharyngeal carcinoma: prognostic influence of cranial nerve involvement in different radiotherapy techniques. ScientificWorldJournal 2013;2013:439073.

[g]Kong FF, Ying H, Du CR, Huang S, Zhou JJ, Hu CS. Effectiveness and toxicities of intensity-modulated radiation therapy for patients with T4 nasopharyngeal carcinoma. PLoS One 2014;9(3):e91362.

[h]Chen JL, Huang YS, Kuo SH, et al. Intensity-modulated radiation therapy for T4 nasopharyngeal carcinoma. Treatment results and locoregional recurrence. Strahlenther Onkol 2013;189(12):1001–1008.

[i]Takiar V, Ma D, Garden AS, et al. Disease control and toxicity outcomes for T4 carcinoma of the nasopharynx treated with intensity-modulated radiotherapy. Head Neck 2016;38(Suppl 1):E925–E933.

9.10.2 Proton Therapy for Nasopharyngeal Carcinoma

The use of PRT for treatment of NPC is currently under investigation. Dosimetric benefits of PRT over IMRT include decreased beam path toxicity and lower mean doses to the anterior oral cavity, brain, brainstem, and spinal cord without compromise of tumor coverage. PRT can potentially improve radiation-induced nausea and vomiting by delivering lower doses to the area postrema and dorsal vagal complex.[179,180] Clinical data on use of PRT for NPC are emerging. Massachusetts General Hospital (MGH) presented in abstract form early experience with PRT for NPC, demonstrating a 92% local control rate at 3 years for 19 patients who had T4 disease. Preliminary phase II data from MGH evaluating combined photon–proton therapy using a 3D passive scatter PRT technique with concurrent cisplatin and fluorouracil demonstrated > 90% disease control and low toxicity with short follow-up. Similarly, early clinical data from the MD Anderson Cancer Center using IMPT for NPC indicate excellent tumor control and a low treatment toxicity profile and a low treatment toxicity profile. In a 2:1 case-control study of 13 patients treated with IMPT, when compared to IMRT, IMPT was associated with a significantly lower rate of feeding tube dependence (7.7% vs 19.2%), which is likely attributed to lower oral cavity dose.[181,182,183,184]

9.10.3 Proton Therapy for Adenoid Cystic Carcinoma of the Nasopharynx

PRT offers a unique advantage in the treatment of patients who have unresectable adenoid cystic carcinoma (ACC) of the nasopharynx. ACC of the nasopharynx typically presents at a locally advanced stage and is not amenable to surgery. ACC is also an aggressive histology that has a reputation for being somewhat

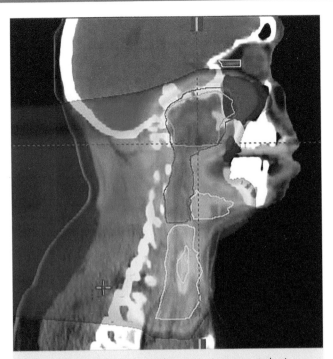

Fig. 9.5 A patient who had nasopharynx carcinoma treated using intensity-modulated proton therapy. Opposed lateral beams allowed complete sparing of the anterior oral cavity while ensuring adequate target coverage and sparing of nearby critical structures such as orbits, brainstem, and spinal cord.

radioresistant. Management strategies that have been used for ACC of the nasopharynx have included high-dose radiotherapy with concurrent chemotherapy (▶ Fig. 9.5). The locoregional control rates in small retrospective studies vary from 9 to 66%. Preliminary clinical data from colleagues at MD Anderson Cancer Center in patients with resectable and unresectable ACC after PRT demonstrate promising local control. In 16 patients with resectable ACC who received adjuvant PRT after surgery, Holliday et al showed local control in 15 (93.7%) patients, with a median follow-up of 24.9 months. Bhattasali et al reported on 8 patients with unresectable ACC of the nasopharynx treated with PRT combined with concurrent cisplatin chemotherapy. Four patients achieved a complete response and 4 patients achieved stabilization of local disease. One patient developed local disease progression. There were 5 acute grade 3 toxicity events and 1 grade 4 optic nerve disorder.[185,186]

9.11 Paranasal Sinus Tumor

Paranasal sinus tumors are rare. Histologic subtypes include epithelial tumors such as squamous cell carcinoma, undifferentiated carcinoma, malignant salivary gland tumors (adenocarcinoma, ACC, and mucoepidermoid carcinoma), and esthesioneuroblastoma, melanoma, rhabdomyosarcoma, plasmacytoma, and lymphoma. For lymphoma and plasmacytoma, low- to moderate-dose (30–50 Gy) radiation therapy, given with or without chemotherapy (depending on histology), is the mainstay of treatment. For other histologies, surgical resection should be considered. The role of radiotherapy in the adjuvant setting is often to enhance tumor control in patients who have high-risk pathology features.

Typically, a high dose of radiation (60 Gy) is required for these tumors. This presents a therapeutic challenge, because the target volume to be treated is often in proximity to critical structures such as the eyes and the optic apparatus, whose maximum tolerated dose is typically below 60 Gy. The staging for paranasal sinus tumor differs according to the histology. Staging for squamous cell carcinoma of the paranasal sinus is based on the site of origin, according to the American Joint Committee on Cancer, for tumors of the maxillary, ethmoid, or nasal cavity. For esthesioneuroblastoma, by contrast, staging is based on anatomic extension as defined by the Kadish system.

Inoperable tumors of the paranasal sinus represent a challenge because of the need to deliver tumorocidal doses in excess of 66 Gy while attempting to spare adjacent critical neurovascular and optic structures. For gross disease, 70 Gy is recommended. A dose of 66 Gy is typically prescribed for gross disease near critical structures when 70 Gy is not achievable (delivered in 2.0 to 2.12 Gy per fraction). For the clinically negative neck, nodal coverage typically includes the level IB (submandibular) and II (subdigastric) and lateral RP regions. For patients who have a lateralized maxillary sinus tumor, coverage includes the ipsilateral IB and II nodes. For those who have nodal metastases at diagnosis, consideration is given to coverage of the entire unilateral neck (levels I–V) or bilateral neck. For tumors crossing midline, the bilateral neck is typically treated. Coverage of facial and buccal nodes should be considered in those who have tumors that involve anterior structures of the nasal cavity and paranasal sinuses, whereas tumors that involve the posterior regions of the nasal cavity and paranasal sinuses often drain to the RP and deep cervical nodes. Nodal metastasis for carcinomas of frontal and sphenoid sinuses is less common. In addition to elective coverage of first- and second-echelon nodes, subclinical dose coverage of perineural pathways, including the skull base, is critical. Common pathways include CNs VII and V1 to V3.

Highly conformal radiotherapy techniques such as IMRT and PRT are the preferred treatment approach for these cases. Troung et al evaluated proton therapy for primary sphenoid sinus cancers and showed an excellent 2-year locoregional control rate of 86%. Oropharyngeal involvement and anterior cranial fossa invasion served as predictors of poor outcome.[187,188]

9.11.1 Squamous Cell Carcinomas

Squamous cell carcinoma of the sinonasal tract is rarer than at other head and neck subsites. For such patients, surgical resection followed by postoperative radiation therapy appears to be the optimal approach.[189,190] However, in cases of very advanced disease that renders surgical resection infeasible, primary radiotherapy can be offered. The prognosis in those who have sinonasal squamous cell carcinoma is poor; carcinomas that arise from Schneiderian papillomas or that are associated with transcriptionally active high-risk human papillomavirus may have a better prognosis.[191] Despite aggressive therapy, clinical outcomes after conventional radiotherapy remain suboptimal, with 5-year tumor control rates below 50% and 5-year survival as low as 27%.[192] The use of highly conformal radiotherapy such as IMRT and GK-SRS can improve local control and reduce treatment morbidity, particularly when the tumor is adjacent to a critical structure. In patients who show no clinical evidence of nodal involvement at diagnosis, high regional nodal failure rates have been reported when elective neck irradiation is not given in those who have squamous cell or high-grade carcinomas.

9.11.2 Sinonasal Mucosal Melanoma

Mucosal melanoma of the paranasal sinus is a rare malignancy that accounts for < 4% of all melanomas.[193] Historically, these tumors are associated with a poor prognosis, both because of their anatomic location and because they are considered radio-resistant to conventional fractionation.[194] Hence the treatment strategy typically involves surgical resection with or without adjuvant radiotherapy. Postoperative radiotherapy is recommended when there is concern about positive surgical margins. However, complications such as dermatitis, mucositis and conjunctivitis, ototoxicity, retinopathy, and osteoradionecrosis are common because of the necessity to deliver a tumorocidal dose. Conformal approaches such as IMRT are preferred over 2D and 3D techniques so as to optimize sparing of adjacent critical structures. Proton therapy can offer additional sparing of critical organs and reduce acute toxicity without compromising local control.[195] Similarly, excellent disease control without unacceptable toxicity has been demonstrated with carbon ion therapy for mucosal melanoma of the paranasal sinus.[196] More recently, fractionated stereotactic radiation therapy (FSRT) delivering a hypofractionated dose of 30 to 35 Gy in three to five fractions has been shown to be an effective salvage strategy for patients previously irradiated to the paranasal sinus.[197,198]

9.11.3 Adenoid Cystic Carcinoma

ACC is a relatively uncommon malignancy, at about 1,200 cases annually in the United States. The majority of cases are locally invasive, but late metastasis can occur years after initial diagnosis and treatment. ACC has an insidious and infiltrative growth pattern, is highly neurotropic, and is known for late hematogenous spreads, particularly to the lung. The main therapeutic approach is surgery. ACC is considered a high-risk histology (NCCN), and postoperative radiation is often recommended to improve locoregional control. The role of chemotherapy and systemic therapy is controversial.

The survival benefit of adjuvant radiotherapy has been inconsistent across multiple studies. According to Schwartz et al, the 5-year absolute survival benefit of adjuvant radiotherapy was 9.5% for those who had pathologic T1 to T2 disease and 11.6% for those who had T3 to T4 disease.[199] Several studies indicate that adjuvant radiotherapy confers a locoregional but not an OS benefit, with 5-year locoregional rates ranging from 77 to 78% after surgery and adjuvant radiotherapy versus 47 to 57% after surgery alone. Those who have a positive margin after surgery benefit the most from adjuvant radiotherapy. However, even with adjuvant radiotherapy, the 10-year recurrence rate is high, prompting reconsideration of the optimal treatment field and dose. In contrast to squamous cell carcinoma, lymphatic spread to the neck is rare among ACC tumors, with a rate of 4% when arising from a major salivary gland.[200] Because of the high propensity for perineural spread, subclinical coverage of CN pathways is imperative.

In unresectable cases, historical local control rates with radiation therapy have been discouraging, ranging from 0 to 44% at 10 years. ACC is often thought of as a chemoresistant and somewhat radioresistant tumor, a view that has prompted investigation of the use of high-LET particle radiation therapy. Results obtained using neutron therapy (a heavy particle similar to carbon ion) showed > 60% local control rates among multiple studies. However, because grade 3 or higher toxicity rates were also high, ranging from 15 to 31%, use of neutrons for ACC involving the skull base has been limited. The results obtained using proton therapy for skull base ACC appear promising, with excellent LRC rates of > 90% and less toxicity than for neutron therapy.[201,202]

SRS is an increasingly used technique for safely providing a boost dose to gross or microscopic disease in the skull base as a component of conventional fractionated approaches. In a study by Douglass et al, an additional dose to perineural disease in the skull base using GK-SRS improved tumor control from 32 to 82% at 40 months compared with absence of GK-SRS boost.[203] Using modern systems, an SRS boost can be integrated as part of the overall radiation treatment plan with reduced uncertainty (▶ Fig. 9.6).

9.11.4 Esthesioneuroblastoma

Esthesioneuroblastoma is a rare neuroectodermal malignancy that arises from the olfactory epithelium lining the roof of the nasal cavity. Standard treatment involves surgical resection followed by postoperative radiation therapy to the tumor bed, which provides very good local disease control. However, the risk of nodal recurrence in the absence of any therapy to the neck can approach 30%.[204,205] Although nodal recurrence risk is high, the role of ENI, particularly among those who have clinically node-negative disease, is more controversial given the long latency period to recurrence and the availability of an effective salvage therapy. A study from the MD Anderson Cancer Center in Texas evaluated 71 clinically node-negative esthesioneuroblastoma patients treated using surgery followed by postoperative radiation, of whom 22 received ENI.[206] For a median follow-up of 82.3 months, the 5-year OS and disease-free survival rates were 87.3 and 68.6%, respectively. The 5-year regional control rate was 100% in patients who received ENI, compared with 82% in those who did not. The observed nodal failure rate in those not receiving ENI was 25%. The majority of nodal recurrences occurred in those who had Kadish C staging and who were of a younger age. For patients who are not candidates for surgery, primary radiation therapy is given. In general, the treatment outcomes associated with primary radiation therapy alone are poor when compared with a complete resection followed by postoperative radiation therapy.[205,207,208] Because late recurrences have been observed in a significant proportion of patients after treatment, the importance of long-term follow-up of these patients cannot be overemphasized.

Because a high dose of radiation (60–70 Gy) is required for the treatment of these tumors, there is a substantial risk of retinopathy and optic neuropathy. To decrease the risk of collateral damage, highly conformal radiotherapy strategies should be used. Multiple studies using IMRT for the treatment of paranasal sinus tumors have been reported in the literature demonstrating reduced toxicity.[209,210]

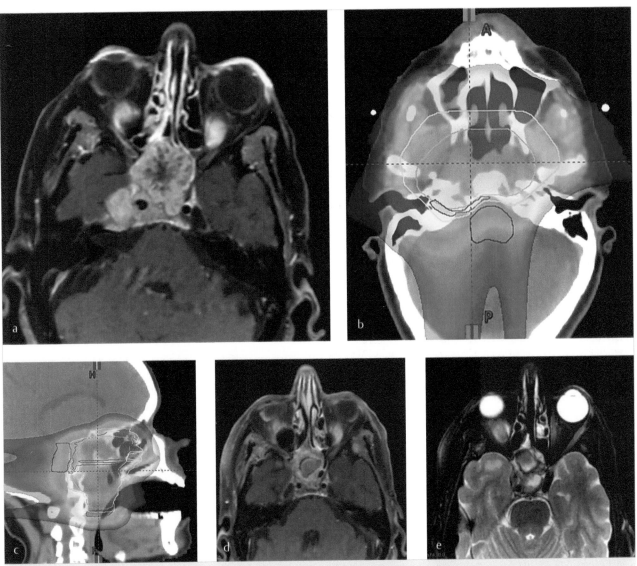

Fig. 9.6 A female who had T4 N0 adenoid cystic carcinoma of the nasopharynx. **(a)** MRI of nasopharyngeal mass extending into the right middle cranial fossa, involving the right cavernous sinus and petrous segments of carotid artery. Posterior tumor extension to clivus. Anterior extension to the planum sphenoidale, superiorly abutting the pituitary gland. **(b,c)** Intensity-modulated proton therapy to 70 cobalt Gray equivalent in 33 fractions with concurrent cisplatin. Maximum surface dose of brainstem was limited to < 60 Gy, and anterior oral cavity was spared. No elective nodal irradiation. **(d)** No evidence of recurrence 2 years post treatment. **(e)** Abnormal T2 signals indicate early signs of right temporal lobe radiation injury.

9.11.5 Sinonasal Undifferentiated Carcinoma

Sinonasal undifferentiated carcinoma (SNUC) is a rare malignancy that runs a very aggressive course. If feasible, patients are frequently managed through surgical resection, with or without adjuvant/neoadjuvant radiation therapy and/or chemotherapy. If the disease is unresectable, definitive radiation therapy with or without chemotherapy can be offered.[211] Reported survival rates after treatment range from 20 to 63%. Given the high risk of cervical nodal metastasis, elective neck irradiation is usually recommended. Definitive radiation therapy for those who have SNUC is extremely challenging. Because of the location, a particular concern is delivery of sufficient dose for tumor control (typically 70 Gy with conventional fractionation) without exceeding the normal tissue tolerance. The use of IMRT or volumetric modulated arc therapy (VMAT) with a robust immobilization system and image guided radiation therapy (IGRT) can reduce the PTV margin. In many cases, this can allow an adequate dose to tumor while respecting the tolerance of the nearby optic apparatus.

▶ Fig. 9.7 illustrates a VMAT plan for a patient who had T4 N0 SNUC with orbital involvement. The patient received two cycles of cisplatin and etoposide with minimal response. This was followed by concurrent chemoradiation to 70 Gy in 33 fractions. The patient was simulated using a three-point custom immobilization system with posterior cushion, bite block, and mask, as described by Wang et al. IGRT consisted of daily ExacTrac and cone-beam CT verification. This allowed use of a reduced PTV margin toward the optic structures. The maximum doses to both the right optic nerve (51.2 Gy) and optic chiasm (50.2 Gy) were below their normal constraints. The left lens could not be

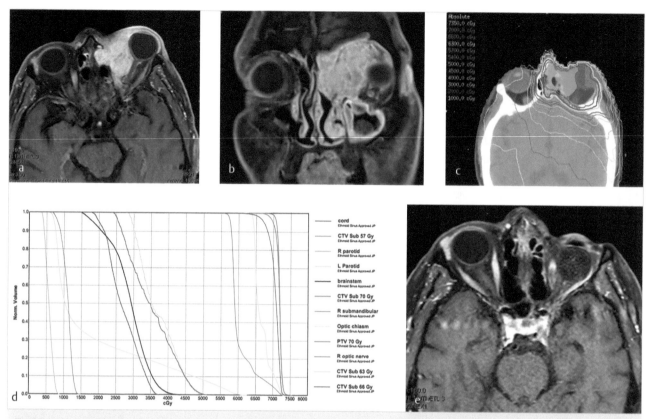

Fig. 9.7 A 63-year-old male who had T4 N0 sinonasal undifferentiated carcinoma. MR showed left orbit invasion on **(a)** axial and **(b)** coronal images. The patient received two cycles of cisplatin and etoposide induction chemotherapy with minimal response followed by concurrent chemoradiation **(c,d)** volumetric modulated arc therapy treatment plan to 70 Gy in 33 fractions using two arcs. Gross disease near brain was treated to 66 Gy with minimal planning target volume expansion toward optic chiasm. The ipsilateral IB and II neck was irradiated electively. This was followed by two additional cycles of chemotherapy. **(e)** MRI 4 years post treatment showed no evidence of disease.

spared, and as expected, the patient required left eye surgery for corneal abrasions 2 years after treatment. Currently, the patient is 4 years posttreatment and shows no evidence of disease. Vision is stable, and performance status is 0; the patient is back to work full-time.

9.12 Skull Base Re-irradiation

Management of recurrent skull base tumors after prior head and neck radiotherapy is a clinical challenge. Historically, surgical resection has been preferred over re-irradiation because of concerns associated with severe toxicity, such as carotid artery rupture (CAR), soft tissue and bone necrosis, TLN, cranial neuropathy, and severe fibrosis. However, a complete surgical resection of a recurrent skull base tumor is often difficult to achieve without incurring significant morbidity. In the past, patients who were not surgical candidates received palliative chemotherapy as the standard of care. Median survival was 6 to 9 months—not much better than for supportive care alone. The advent of highly conformal radiotherapy techniques, however, has reinvigorated interest in curative approach re-irradiation, which may be well suited for the skull base, where surgical options are limited. A potential advantage of skull base re-irradiation is the promise of durable local control in a cohort that has few local therapy options. Furthermore, ablative and

hypofractionated doses can be delivered with "stereotactic precision" to improve local control of tumors refractory to FRT. Treatment using a high dose per fraction was previously not considered an attractive option for re-irradiation of the head and neck because of late complication concerns in a cohort already at high toxicity risk.

The collective experiences from early clinical reports on skull base re-irradiation are promising but consist of small single-institution studies featuring limited long-term follow-up. Cmelak et al. used LINAC-based SRS to re-irradiate 37 patients who had recurrent skull base malignant tumors.[212] The crude local control was 69%, and survival was not reported. Serious treatment complications occurred in five patients. The Mayo Clinic reported experience with GK-SRS in a heterogeneous population of 184 patients, of whom 80% were treated for recurrent disease. SRS was used as a boost to a median dose of 14 Gy in addition to FRT in 49% of patients. In those treated using salvage SRS with curative intent, the 1-year locoregional control rate was 73% and the median OS rate was 15.2 months. Serious late toxicity was low, with 6 and 2% of patients experiencing late grade 3 or 4 toxicity, respectively. Among patients who have recurrent NPC, Chua et al reported on 18 patients who were re-irradiated with SRS to a median dose of 12.5 Gy. The 2-year local control rate was 72%, with one case of TLN. Pollard et al from the MD Anderson Cancer Center evaluated 19 patients re-irradiated for retropharyngeal node recurrence using either conventionally fractionated IMRT or PRT (58%), single fraction SRS, or hypofractionated FSRT (42%; ▸ Fig. 9.8).[213] Median follow-up was 14.7 months. The 1-year local control and survival rates were 100 and 92%, respectively. Three patients experienced acute grade 3 mucositis that required use of narcotics for pain control in the IMRT group. No serious (grade 3 or higher) toxicities were reported.

9.12.1 Stereotactic Radiotherapy for Skull Base Re-irradiation

Recently, FSRT re-irradiation of the skull base has been reported. Coppa et al treated 31 patients who had FSRT to a median dose of 25 Gy in five fractions. The majority of cases were of squamous cell carcinoma (n = 6) and ACC (n = 5) histology. The crude tumor

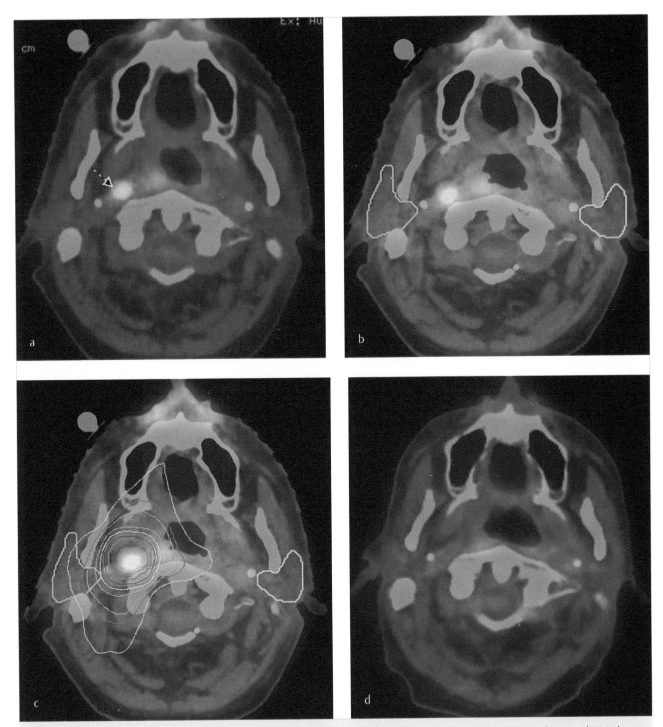

Fig. 9.8 Retropharyngeal (RP) node recurrence in a patient who had esthesioneuroblastoma that had previously been treated using radiation therapy to 60 Gy. **(a)** PET-CT showed a biopsy-proven right RP recurrence. **(b)** Planning CT fused to PET-CT performed in treatment position. **(c)** SBRT treatment plan to a prescribed a dose of 45 Gy in five fractions given on alternating days. Planning considerations included avoiding dose to previously irradiated spinal cord. **(d)** A diagnostic PET-CT 12 months after treatment.

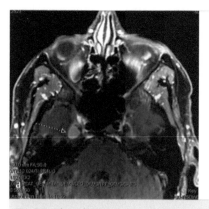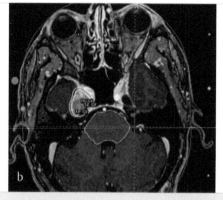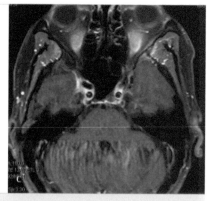

Fig. 9.9 Adenoid cystic carcinoma of floor of mouth previously treated with surgery and chemoradiation. The patient presented with left-sided blurred vision and painful trigeminal neuralgia of cranial nerves V2–V3. **(a)** Pretreatment MRI. **(b)** GK plan consisting of 12 Gy × 1 prescribed to the 50% isodose line. **(c)** MRI 6 months post treatment. Self-reported pain decreased from 7 of 10 to 0 of 10. Baseline Dilaudid requirement decreased from every 2 hours to two to three times per day. Lyrica dose unchanged.

control rate was 74%. In the absence of tumor progression, no complications were related to Stereotactic radiosurgery (SRS). Colleagues from the University of Pittsburgh evaluated 31 patients who had recurrent skull base tumors treated using FSRT to a median dose of 44 Gy in five fractions given on alternating days.[213] The 1-year OS rate was 35%, and crude tumor control was 50%. The median tumor volume was 27 cubic cm, and the predominant histology (55%) was squamous cell carcinoma. Grade 3 toxicity occurred in 15% of patients. There were no grade 4 to 5 toxicities. In all, late toxicity rates from stereotactic body radiation therapy (SBRT) re-irradiation are encouraging, with rates of late grade 3 or high levels of complications ranging from 4 to 22% and rates of late grade 4 ranging from 0 to 9%.[214,215,216,217,218] These appear similar to complication rates in reported IMRT and PRT re-irradiation series, which ranged from 27 to 32% at 2 years in reports featuring actuarial data, with a crude incidence of 15 to 48%. In a 10-year update of institutional experience, the University of Pittsburgh evaluated predictors of toxicity in 291 patients treated using SBRT re-irradiation between 2002 and 2013 for recurrent head and neck cancer (HNC).[219] Incidence of late grade 3 or higher events was 18.9%, whereas incidence of late grade 4 toxicity was 5.1%. On correlative analysis, patients who had larynx or hypopharynx recurrences experienced significantly more late toxicity than those who had recurrences in other sites, including the skull base.

A devastating complication of re-irradiation is CAR. Yamazaki et al reported on 107 patients re-irradiated to a median dose of 30 Gy in five fractions daily. Of the 22 patients (21%) who developed grade 3 or higher toxicities, 11 developed CAR (in 9 of whom it was fatal) at a median time of 5 months. Only patients who had tumor invasion of the carotid > 180° developed CAR, and on multivariate analysis CAR was associated with the presence of ulceration.[220] In two smaller series (*n* = 70 total) using 30 Gy in five fractions daily, incidence of CAR was between 6 and 17%. In one of the studies, CAR occurred in those whose tumor surrounded half or more of the carotid artery wall and when the carotid received 100% of the prescribed dose.[221]

Daily versus alternating-day treatment using SBRT appears to be an important factor in determining toxicity and CAR. The majority of studies reporting higher rates of severe (grade 4 or 5) toxicity used a daily (9.7–17.6%) regimen versus an alternating-day regimen (0–4.5%). From a radiobiology perspective, more than 24 hours are thought to be needed to provide sufficient time for cellular repair when higher fractional doses are given. These results were mirrored in a phase II study by Lartigau et al in which patients were treated to 36 Gy in six fractions, given on alternating days.[222] The reported CAR rate in this study was 2% (1 in 60). More favorable outcomes were reported from the MD Anderson Cancer Center's early SBRT re-irradiation experience by Phan et al.[223] Patients who had a median tumor size of 36.4 mL were treated using SBRT to a median dose of 45 Gy in five fractions, given on alternating days. Most patients (86%) received concurrent cetuximab. The 6-month OS and LRC rates were 79 and 91%, respectively. There were no acute grade 3 or higher toxicities. In a combined analysis, from the same institution, of 63 patients who had smaller skull base tumors (< 60 cm²) re-irradiated with IMRT (30%), PRT (30%), and SBRT (40%), Ng et al (not published) reported 5-year OS and loco-regional failure (LRF) free survival rates of 51 and 67%, respectively. One patient (4%) in the SBRT group and five patients (15%) in the IMRT/PRT group developed grade 3 late toxicity. There were no grade 4 to 5 toxicities.

For symptom palliation, the use of GK-SRS has been shown to reduce trigeminal pain associated with benign and malignant skull base tumors (▶ Fig. 9.9; ▶ Fig. 9.10).[224,225] In a study at the MD Anderson Cancer Center,[226] 27 patients received GK-SRS re-irradiation (median dose 16 Gy) for palliation of trigeminal neuralgia secondary to recurrent malignant skull base tumors. Those without recurrence and with at least a 3-month follow-up (*n* = 19) demonstrated a significant decrease in patient-reported pain and opioid requirement. Of the 13 patients who experienced complete pain relief, 9 were completely off analgesics.

9.13 Conclusion

Skull base tumors present a challenge to neurosurgeons, otolaryngologists, and radiation oncologists. As radiotherapy technology continues to advance, it is important to keep in mind that the best management approach for patients who have a skull

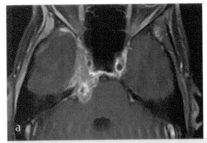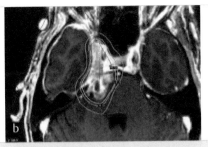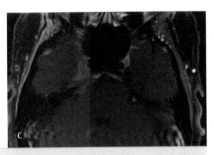

Fig. 9.10 Cutaneous squamous cell carcinoma (SCC) previously treated with surgery and postoperative radiotherapy. Presented with right-sided facial numbness and pain rated at 4 of 10 while taking MS Contin q12 hours, oxycodone q4–6 hours, and gabapentin. Pain was rated at 10 of 10 when off opioids. **(a)** Pretreatment MRI. **(b)** Treatment to 21 Gy in three fractions prescribed to 46% isodose line using Gamma Knife with Extend system. **(c)** MRI 6 months post treatment. Pain was rated at 0 of 10 on gabapentin. Patient is now completely off opioids and is planning to return to work part-time.

base tumor is still interdisciplinary treatment planning. Before initiating any treatment, the treatment team should plan the anticipated extent of surgery and prepare for postoperative radiation therapy as needed. For example, a subtotal skull base tumor resection followed by postoperative radiation therapy can yield outcomes similar to those associated with a complete resection and can lower the risk of operative morbidity and mortality. With modern radiotherapy advances, it is possible to achieve a very conformal radiation dose distribution that exhibits a steep dose gradient beyond the intended target. This can reduce the degree of collateral damage to critical structures and normal brain parenchyma. Furthermore, most skull base tumors have sharp margins of demarcation from the surrounding normal structures, can be localized with high accuracy and precision, and are well suited for conformal radiotherapy techniques. Ideally, increases in the sophistication of surgical and radiation techniques will further improve patient outcomes and help reduce toxicity.

References

[1] Prasad D. Clinical results of conformal radiotherapy and radiosurgery for pituitary adenoma. Neurosurg Clin N Am. 2006; 17(2):129–141, vi

[2] Flickinger JC, Nelson PB, Martinez AJ, Deutsch M, Taylor F. Radiotherapy of nonfunctional adenomas of the pituitary gland: results with long-term follow-up. Cancer. 1989; 63(12):2409–2414

[3] Grigsby PW, Simpson JR, Fineberg B. Late regrowth of pituitary adenomas after irradiation and/or surgery: hazard function analysis. Cancer. 1989; 63(7):1308–1312

[4] Grigsby PW, Simpson JR, Stokes S, Marks JE, Fineberg B. Results of surgery and irradiation or irradiation alone for pituitary adenomas. J Neurooncol. 1988; 6(2):129–134

[5] Tsang RW, Brierley JD, Panzarella T, Gospodarowicz MK, Sutcliffe SB, Simpson WJ. Radiation therapy for pituitary adenoma: treatment outcome and prognostic factors. Int J Radiat Oncol Biol Phys. 1994; 30(3):557–565

[6] McCord MW, Buatti JM, Fennell EM, et al. Radiotherapy for pituitary adenoma: long-term outcome and sequelae. Int J Radiat Oncol Biol Phys. 1997; 39(2):437–444

[7] Brada M, Rajan B, Traish D, et al. The long-term efficacy of conservative surgery and radiotherapy in the control of pituitary adenomas. Clin Endocrinol (Oxf). 1993; 38(6):571–578

[8] Eastman RC, Gorden P, Glatstein E, Roth J. Radiation therapy of acromegaly. Endocrinol Metab Clin North Am. 1992; 21(3):693–712

[9] Minniti G, Scaringi C, Amelio D, Maurizi Enrici R. Stereotactic irradiation of GH-secreting pituitary adenomas. Int J Endocrinol. 2012; 2012:482861

[10] Jenkins PJ, Bates P, Carson MN, Stewart PM, Wass JA. Conventional pituitary irradiation is effective in lowering serum growth hormone and insulin-like growth factor-I in patients with acromegaly. J Clin Endocrinol Metab. 2006; 91(4):1239–1245

[11] Biermasz NR, van Dulken H, Roelfsema F. Long-term follow-up results of postoperative radiotherapy in 36 patients with acromegaly. J Clin Endocrinol Metab. 2000; 85(7):2476–2482

[12] Grigsby PW, Simpson JR, Emami BN, Fineberg BB, Schwartz HG. Prognostic factors and results of surgery and postoperative irradiation in the management of pituitary adenomas. Int J Radiat Oncol Biol Phys. 1989; 16(6):1411–1417

[13] Grigsby PW, Stokes S, Marks JE, Simpson JR. Prognostic factors and results of radiotherapy alone in the management of pituitary adenomas. Int J Radiat Oncol Biol Phys. 1988; 15(5):1103–1110

[14] Littley MD, Shalet SM, Reid H, Beardwell CG, Sutton ML. The effect of external pituitary irradiation on elevated serum prolactin levels in patients with pituitary macroadenomas. Q J Med. 1991; 81(296):985–998

[15] Tsagarakis S, Grossman A, Plowman PN, et al. Megavoltage pituitary irradiation in the management of prolactinomas: long-term follow-up. Clin Endocrinol (Oxf). 1991; 34(5):399–406

[16] Johnston DG, Hall K, Kendall-Taylor P, et al. The long-term effects of megavoltage radiotherapy as sole or combined therapy for large prolactinomas: studies with high definition computerized tomography. Clin Endocrinol (Oxf). 1986; 24(6):675–685

[17] Clarke SD, Woo SY, Butler EB, et al. Treatment of secretory pituitary adenoma with radiation therapy. Radiology. 1993; 188(3):759–763

[18] Hughes MN, Llamas KJ, Yelland ME, Tripcony LB. Pituitary adenomas: long-term results for radiotherapy alone and post-operative radiotherapy. Int J Radiat Oncol Biol Phys. 1993; 27(5):1035–1043

[19] Estrada J, Boronat M, Mielgo M, et al. The long-term outcome of pituitary irradiation after unsuccessful transsphenoidal surgery in Cushing's disease. N Engl J Med. 1997; 336(3):172–177

[20] Howlett TA, Plowman PN, Wass JA, Rees LH, Jones AE, Besser GM. Megavoltage pituitary irradiation in the management of Cushing's disease and Nelson's syndrome: long-term follow-up. Clin Endocrinol (Oxf). 1989; 31(3):309–323

[21] Littley MD, Shalet SM, Beardwell CG, Ahmed SR, Sutton ML. Long-term follow-up of low-dose external pituitary irradiation for Cushing's disease. Clin Endocrinol (Oxf). 1990; 33(4):445–455

[22] Witt TC. Stereotactic radiosurgery for pituitary tumors. Neurosurg Focus. 2003; 14(5):e10

[23] Petrovich Z, Jozsef G, Yu C, Apuzzo ML. Radiotherapy and stereotactic radiosurgery for pituitary tumors. Neurosurg Clin N Am. 2003; 14(1):147–166

[24] Li X, Li Y, Cao Y, et al. Safety and efficacy of fractionated stereotactic radiotherapy and stereotactic radiosurgery for treatment of pituitary adenomas: a systematic review and meta-analysis. J Neurol Sci. 2017; 372:110–116

[25] Stangerup SE, Caye-Thomasen P. Epidemiology and natural history of vestibular schwannomas. Otolaryngol Clin North Am. 2012; 45(2):257–268, vii

[26] Sughrue ME, Yang I, Aranda D, et al. The natural history of untreated sporadic vestibular schwannomas: a comprehensive review of hearing outcomes. J Neurosurg. 2010; 112(1):163–167

[27] Kaylie DM, Horgan MJ, Delashaw JB, McMenomey SO. A meta-analysis comparing outcomes of microsurgery and gamma knife radiosurgery. Laryngoscope. 2000; 110(11):1850–1856

[28] Pollock BE, Driscoll CL, Foote RL, et al. Patient outcomes after vestibular schwannoma management: a prospective comparison of microsurgical resection and stereotactic radiosurgery. Neurosurgery. 2006; 59(1):77–85

[29] Myrseth E, Møller P, Pedersen PH, Vassbotn FS, Wentzel-Larsen T, Lund-Johansen M. Vestibular schwannomas: clinical results and quality of life after microsurgery or gamma knife radiosurgery. Neurosurgery. 2005; 56 (5):927–935

[30] Unger F, Dominikus K, Haselsberger K. [Stereotactic radiosurgery and fractionated stereotactic radiotherapy of acoustic neuromas]. HNO. 2011; 59(1): 31–37

[31] Flickinger JC, Barker FG, II. Clinical results: radiosurgery and radiotherapy of cranial nerve schwannomas. Neurosurg Clin N Am. 2006; 17(2):121–128, vi

[32] Kondziolka D, Lunsford LD, McLaughlin MR, Flickinger JC. Long-term outcomes after radiosurgery for acoustic neuromas. N Engl J Med. 1998; 339 (20):1426–1433

[33] Lunsford LD, Niranjan A, Flickinger JC, Maitz A, Kondziolka D. Radiosurgery of vestibular schwannomas: summary of experience in 829 cases. J Neurosurg. 2005; 102 Suppl:195–199

[34] Flickinger JC, Kondziolka D, Niranjan A, Maitz A, Voynov G, Lunsford LD. Acoustic neuroma radiosurgery with marginal tumor doses of 12 to 13 Gy. Int J Radiat Oncol Biol Phys. 2004; 60(1):225–230

[35] Bush DA, McAllister CJ, Loredo LN, Johnson WD, Slater JM, Slater JD. Fractionated proton beam radiotherapy for acoustic neuroma. Neurosurgery. 2002; 50(2):270–273, discussion 273–275

[36] Combs SE, Engelhard C, Kopp C, et al. Long-term outcome after highly advanced single-dose or fractionated radiotherapy in patients with vestibular schwannomas—pooled results from 3 large German centers. Radiother Oncol. 2015; 114(3):378–383

[37] Combs SE, Thilmann C, Debus J, Schulz-Ertner D. Long-term outcome of stereotactic radiosurgery (SRS) in patients with acoustic neuromas. Int J Radiat Oncol Biol Phys. 2006; 64(5):1341–1347

[38] Combs SE, Volk S, Schulz-Ertner D, Huber PE, Thilmann C, Debus J. Management of acoustic neuromas with fractionated stereotactic radiotherapy (FSRT): long-term results in 106 patients treated in a single institution. Int J Radiat Oncol Biol Phys. 2005; 63(1):75–81

[39] Inoue HK. Low-dose radiosurgery for large vestibular schwannomas: long-term results of functional preservation. J Neurosurg. 2005; 102 Suppl:111–113

[40] Iwai Y, Yamanaka K, Shiotani M, Uyama T. Radiosurgery for acoustic neuromas: results of low-dose treatment. Neurosurgery. 2003; 53(2):282–287, discussion 287–288

[41] Paek SH, Chung HT, Jeong SS, et al. Hearing preservation after gamma knife stereotactic radiosurgery of vestibular schwannoma. Cancer. 2005; 104(3): 580–590

[42] Petit JH, Hudes RS, Chen TT, Eisenberg HM, Simard JM, Chin LS. Reduced-dose radiosurgery for vestibular schwannomas. Neurosurgery. 2001; 49(6): 1299–1306, discussion 1306–1307

[43] Rowe JG, Radatz MW, Walton L, Hampshire A, Seaman S, Kemeny AA. Gamma Knife stereotactic radiosurgery for unilateral acoustic neuromas. J Neurol Neurosurg Psychiatry. 2003; 74(11):1536–1542

[44] Schumacher AJ, Lall RR, Lall RR, et al. Low-dose Gamma Knife radiosurgery for vestibular schwannomas: tumor control and cranial nerve function preservation after 11 Gy. J Neurol Surg B Skull Base. 2017; 78(1):2–10

[45] Selch MT, Pedroso A, Lee SP, et al. Stereotactic radiotherapy for the treatment of acoustic neuromas. J Neurosurg. 2004; 101 Suppl 3:362–372

[46] Meijer OW, Vandertop WP, Baayen JC, Slotman BJ. Single-fraction vs. fractionated LINAC-based stereotactic radiosurgery for vestibular schwannoma: a single-institution study. Int J Radiat Oncol Biol Phys. 2003; 56(5):1390–1396

[47] Andrews DW, Suarez O, Goldman HW, et al. Stereotactic radiosurgery and fractionated stereotactic radiotherapy for the treatment of acoustic schwannomas: comparative observations of 125 patients treated at one institution. Int J Radiat Oncol Biol Phys. 2001; 50(5):1265–1278

[48] Williams JA. Fractionated stereotactic radiotherapy for acoustic neuromas: preservation of function versus size. J Clin Neurosci. 2003; 10(1):48–52

[49] Williams JA. Fractionated stereotactic radiotherapy for acoustic neuromas. Int J Radiat Oncol Biol Phys. 2002; 54(2):500–504

[50] Williams JA. Fractionated stereotactic radiotherapy for acoustic neuromas. Stereotact Funct Neurosurg. 2002; 78(1):17–28

[51] Chang SD, Gibbs IC, Sakamoto GT, Lee E, Oyelese A, Adler JR, Jr. Staged stereotactic irradiation for acoustic neuroma. Neurosurgery. 2005; 56(6):1254–1261, discussion 1261–1263

[52] Casentini L, Fornezza U, Perini Z, Perissinotto E, Colombo F. Multisession stereotactic radiosurgery for large vestibular schwannomas. J Neurosurg. 2015; 122(4):818–824

[53] Pan CC, Eisbruch A, Lee JS, Snorrason RM, Ten Haken RK, Kileny PR. Prospective study of inner ear radiation dose and hearing loss in head-and-neck cancer patients. Int J Radiat Oncol Biol Phys. 2005; 61(5):1393–1402

[54] Chen WC, Jackson A, Budnick AS, et al. Sensorineural hearing loss in combined modality treatment of nasopharyngeal carcinoma. Cancer. 2006; 106 (4):820–829

[55] van der Putten L, de Bree R, Plukker JT, et al. Permanent unilateral hearing loss after radiotherapy for parotid gland tumors. Head Neck. 2006; 28(10): 902–908

[56] Brown M, Ruckenstein M, Bigelow D, et al. Predictors of hearing loss after Gamma Knife radiosurgery for vestibular schwannomas: age, cochlear dose, and tumor coverage. Neurosurgery. 2011; 69(3):605–613, discussion 613–614

[57] Kano H, Kondziolka D, Khan A, Flickinger JC, Lunsford LD. Predictors of hearing preservation after stereotactic radiosurgery for acoustic neuroma: clinical article. J Neurosurg. 2013; 119 Suppl:863–873

[58] Baschnagel AM, Chen PY, Bojrab D, et al. Hearing preservation in patients with vestibular schwannoma treated with Gamma Knife surgery. J Neurosurg. 2013; 118(3):571–578

[59] Massager N, Nissim O, Delbrouck C, et al. Irradiation of cochlear structures during vestibular schwannoma radiosurgery and associated hearing outcome. J Neurosurg. 2007; 107(4) Suppl:733–739

[60] Jacob JT, Carlson ML, Schiefer TK, Pollock BE, Driscoll CL, Link MJ. Significance of cochlear dose in the radiosurgical treatment of vestibular schwannoma: controversies and unanswered questions. Neurosurgery. 2014; 74 (5):466–474

[61] Goldsmith B, McDermott MW. Meningioma. Neurosurg Clin N Am. 2006; 17 (2):111–120, vi

[62] Glaholm J, Bloom HJ, Crow JH. The role of radiotherapy in the management of intracranial meningiomas: the Royal Marsden Hospital experience with 186 patients. Int J Radiat Oncol Biol Phys. 1990; 18(4):755–761

[63] Soyuer S, Chang EL, Selek U, Shi W, Maor MH, DeMonte F. Radiotherapy after surgery for benign cerebral meningioma. Radiother Oncol. 2004; 71 (1):85–90

[64] Uy NW, Woo SY, Teh BS, et al. Intensity-modulated radiation therapy (IMRT) for meningioma. Int J Radiat Oncol Biol Phys. 2002; 53(5):1265–1270

[65] Sajja R, Barnett GH, Lee SY, et al. Intensity-modulated radiation therapy (IMRT) for newly diagnosed and recurrent intracranial meningiomas: preliminary results. Technol Cancer Res Treat. 2005; 4(6):675–682

[66] Kaul D, Budach V, Misch M, Wiener E, Exner S, Badakhshi H. Meningioma of the skull base: long-term outcome after image-guided stereotactic radiotherapy. Cancer Radiother. 2014; 18(8):730–735

[67] Han J, Girvigian MR, Chen JC, et al. A comparative study of stereotactic radiosurgery, hypofractionated, and fractionated stereotactic radiotherapy in the treatment of skull base meningioma. Am J Clin Oncol. 2014; 37(3):255–260

[68] Milker-Zabel S, Zabel-du Bois A, Huber P, Schlegel W, Debus J. Intensity-modulated radiotherapy for complex-shaped meningioma of the skull base: long-term experience of a single institution. Int J Radiat Oncol Biol Phys. 2007; 68(3):858–863

[69] Nutting C, Brada M, Brazil L, et al. Radiotherapy in the treatment of benign meningioma of the skull base. J Neurosurg. 1999; 90(5):823–827

[70] Pollock BE, Stafford SL. Results of stereotactic radiosurgery for patients with imaging defined cavernous sinus meningiomas. Int J Radiat Oncol Biol Phys. 2005; 62(5):1427–1431

[71] Lee JY, Niranjan A, McInerney J, Kondziolka D, Flickinger JC, Lunsford LD. Stereotactic radiosurgery providing long-term tumor control of cavernous sinus meningiomas. J Neurosurg. 2002; 97(1):65–72

[72] Subach BR, Lunsford LD, Kondziolka D, Maitz AH, Flickinger JC. Management of petroclival meningiomas by stereotactic radiosurgery. Neurosurgery. 1998; 42(3):437–443, discussion 443–445

[73] Kondziolka D, Patel AD, Kano H, Flickinger JC, Lunsford LD. Long-term outcomes after Gamma Knife radiosurgery for meningiomas. Am J Clin Oncol. 2016; 39(5):453–457

[74] Spiegelmann R, Nissim O, Menhel J, Alezra D, Pfeffer MR. Linear accelerator radiosurgery for meningiomas in and around the cavernous sinus. Neurosurgery. 2002; 51(6):1373–1379, discussion 1379–1380

[75] Nicolato A, Foroni R, Alessandrini F, Maluta S, Bricolo A, Gerosa M. The role of Gamma Knife radiosurgery in the management of cavernous sinus meningiomas. Int J Radiat Oncol Biol Phys. 2002; 53(4):992–1000

[76] Jalali R, Loughrey C, Baumert B, et al. High precision focused irradiation in the form of fractionated stereotactic conformal radiotherapy (SCRT) for benign meningiomas predominantly in the skull base location. Clin Oncol (R Coll Radiol). 2002; 14(2):103–109

[77] Debus J, Wuendrich M, Pirzkall A, et al. High efficacy of fractionated stereotactic radiotherapy of large base-of-skull meningiomas: long-term results. J Clin Oncol. 2001; 19(15):3547–3553

[78] Milker-Zabel S, Zabel-du Bois A, Huber P, Schlegel W, Debus J. Fractionated stereotactic radiation therapy in the management of benign cavernous sinus meningiomas: long-term experience and review of the literature. Strahlenther Onkol. 2006; 182(11):635–640 [et al]

[79] Litré CF, Colin P, Noudel R, et al. Fractionated stereotactic radiotherapy treatment of cavernous sinus meningiomas: a study of 100 cases. Int J Radiat Oncol Biol Phys. 2009; 74(4):1012–1017

[80] Brell M, Villà S, Teixidor P, et al. Fractionated stereotactic radiotherapy in the treatment of exclusive cavernous sinus meningioma: functional outcome, local control, and tolerance. Surg Neurol. 2006; 65(1):28–33, discussion 33–34

[81] Noël G, Bollet MA, Calugaru V, et al. Functional outcome of patients with benign meningioma treated by 3D conformal irradiation with a combination of photons and protons. Int J Radiat Oncol Biol Phys. 2005; 62(5):1412–1422

[82] Vernimmen FJ, Harris JK, Wilson JA, Melvill R, Smit BJ, Slabbert JP. Stereotactic proton beam therapy of skull base meningiomas. Int J Radiat Oncol Biol Phys. 2001; 49(1):99–105

[83] Weber DC, Lomax AJ, Rutz HP, et al. Swiss Proton Users Group. Spot-scanning proton radiation therapy for recurrent, residual or untreated intracranial meningiomas. Radiother Oncol. 2004; 71(3):251–258

[84] Boskos C, Feuvret L, Noel G, et al. Combined proton and photon conformal radiotherapy for intracranial atypical and malignant meningioma. Int J Radiat Oncol Biol Phys. 2009; 75(2):399–406

[85] Suh JH, Gupta N. Role of radiation therapy and radiosurgery in the management of craniopharyngiomas. Neurosurg Clin N Am. 2006; 17(2):143–148, vi–vii

[86] Luu QT, Loredo LN, Archambeau JO, Yonemoto LT, Slater JM, Slater JD. Fractionated proton radiation treatment for pediatric craniopharyngioma: preliminary report. Cancer J. 2006; 12(2):155–159

[87] Kobayashi T, Tsugawa T, Hatano M, Hashizume C, Mori Y, Shibamoto Y. Gamma Knife radiosurgery of craniopharyngioma: results of 30 cases treated at Nagoya Radiosurgery Center. Nagoya J Med Sci. 2015; 77(3):447–454

[88] Saleem MA, Hashim AS, Rashid A, Ali M. Role of Gamma Knife radiosurgery in multimodality management of craniopharyngioma. Acta Neurochir Suppl (Wien). 2013; 116:55–60

[89] Yomo S, Hayashi M, Chernov M, et al. Stereotactic radiosurgery of residual or recurrent craniopharyngioma: new treatment concept using Leksell Gamma Knife model C with automatic positioning system. Stereotact Funct Neurosurg. 2009; 87(6):360–367

[90] Kobayashi T. Long-term results of Gamma Knife radiosurgery for 100 consecutive cases of craniopharyngioma and a treatment strategy. Prog Neurol Surg. 2009; 22:63–76

[91] Lee CC, Yang HC, Chen CJ, et al. Gamma Knife surgery for craniopharyngioma: report on a 20-year experience. J Neurosurg. 2014; 121 Suppl: 167–178

[92] Ulfarsson E, Lindquist C, Roberts M, et al. Gamma Knife radiosurgery for craniopharyngiomas: long-term results in the first Swedish patients. J Neurosurg. 2002; 97(5) Suppl:613–622

[93] Rinaldo A, Myssiorek D, Devaney KO, Ferlito A. Which paragangliomas of the head and neck have a higher rate of malignancy? Oral Oncol. 2004; 40(5): 458–460

[94] Mendenhall WM, Amdur RJ, Vaysberg M, Mendenhall CM, Werning JW. Head and neck paragangliomas. Head Neck. 2011; 33(10):1530–1534

[95] Phillips GS, LoGerfo SE, Richardson ML, Anzai Y. Interactive Web-based learning module on CT of the temporal bone: anatomy and pathology. Radiographics. 2012; 32(3):E85–E105

[96] Jansen JC, van den Berg R, Kuiper A, van der Mey AG, Zwinderman AH, Cornelisse CJ. Estimation of growth rate in patients with head and neck paragangliomas influences the treatment proposal. Cancer. 2000; 88(12): 2811–2816

[97] Fayad JN, Keles B, Brackmann DE. Jugular foramen tumors: clinical characteristics and treatment outcomes. Otol Neurotol. 2010; 31(2):299–305

[98] Powell S, Peters N, Harmer C. Chemodectoma of the head and neck: results of treatment in 84 patients. Int J Radiat Oncol Biol Phys. 1992; 22 (5):919–924

[99] Wang ML, Hussey DH, Doornbos JF, Vigliotti AP, Wen BC. Chemodectoma of the temporal bone: a comparison of surgical and radiotherapeutic results. Int J Radiat Oncol Biol Phys. 1988; 14(4):643–648

[100] Hinerman RW, Mendenhall WM, Amdur RJ, Stringer SP, Antonelli PJ, Cassisi NJ. Definitive radiotherapy in the management of chemodectomas arising in the temporal bone, carotid body, and glomus vagale. Head Neck. 2001; 23 (5):363–371

[101] Cummings BJ, Beale FA, Garrett PG, et al. The treatment of glomus tumors in the temporal bone by megavoltage radiation. Cancer. 1984; 53(12): 2635–2640

[102] Lightowlers S, Benedict S, Jefferies SJ, et al. Excellent local control of paraganglioma in the head and neck with fractionated radiotherapy. Clin Oncol (R Coll Radiol). 2010; 22(5):382–389

[103] Springate SC, Weichselbaum RR. Radiation or surgery for chemodectoma of the temporal bone: a review of local control and complications. Head Neck. 1990; 12(4):303–307

[104] Pemberton LS, Swindell R, Sykes AJ. Radical radiotherapy alone for glomus jugulare and tympanicum tumours. Oncol Rep. 2005; 14(6):1631–1633

[105] Krych AJ, Foote RL, Brown PD, Garces YI, Link MJ. Long-term results of irradiation for paraganglioma. Int J Radiat Oncol Biol Phys. 2006; 65(4): 1063–1066

[106] Sharma PD, Johnson AP, Whitton AC. Radiotherapy for jugulo-tympanic paragangliomas (glomus jugulare tumours). J Laryngol Otol. 1984; 98(6): 621–629

[107] Scheick SM, Morris CG, Amdur RJ, Bova FJ, Friedman WA, Mendenhall WM. Long-term outcomes after radiosurgery for temporal bone paragangliomas. Am J Clin Oncol. 2015

[108] Sheehan JP, Tanaka S, Link MJ, et al. Gamma Knife surgery for the management of glomus tumors: a multicenter study. J Neurosurg. 2012; 117(2): 246–254

[109] Ibrahim R, Ammori MB, Yianni J, Grainger A, Rowe J, Radatz M. Gamma Knife radiosurgery for glomus jugulare tumors: a single-center series of 75 cases. J Neurosurg. 2016; •••:1–10

[110] Chen PG, Nguyen JH, Payne SC, Sheehan JP, Hashisaki GT. Treatment of glomus jugulare tumors with Gamma Knife radiosurgery. Laryngoscope. 2010; 120(9):1856–1862

[111] Foote RL, Pollock BE, Gorman DA, et al. Glomus jugulare tumor: tumor control and complications after stereotactic radiosurgery. Head Neck. 2002; 24 (4):332–338, discussion 338–339

[112] Ganz JC, Abdelkarim K. Glomus jugulare tumours: certain clinical and radiological aspects observed following Gamma Knife radiosurgery. Acta Neurochir (Wien). 2009; 151(5):423–426

[113] Genç A, Bicer A, Abacioglu U, Peker S, Pamir MN, Kilic T. Gamma Knife radiosurgery for the treatment of glomus jugulare tumors. J Neurooncol. 2010; 97 (1):101–108

[114] Gerosa M, Visca A, Rizzo P, Foroni R, Nicolato A, Bricolo A. Glomus jugulare tumors: the option of Gamma Knife radiosurgery. Neurosurgery. 2006; 59 (3):561–569

[115] Lee CC, Pan DH, Wu JC, et al. Gamma Knife radiosurgery for glomus jugulare and tympanicum. Stereotact Funct Neurosurg. 2011; 89(5):291–298

[116] Liscák R, Vladyka V, Simonová G, Vymazal J, Janousková L. Leksell Gamma Knife radiosurgery of the tumor glomus jugulare and tympanicum. Stereotact Funct Neurosurg. 1998; 70 Suppl 1:152–160

[117] Liscák R, Vladyka V, Wowra B, et al. Gamma Knife radiosurgery of the glomus jugulare tumour—early multicentre experience. Acta Neurochir (Wien). 1999; 141(11):1141–1146

[118] Miller JP, Semaan M, Einstein D, Megerian CA, Maciunas RJ. Staged Gamma Knife radiosurgery after tailored surgical resection: a novel treatment paradigm for glomus jugulare tumors. Stereotact Funct Neurosurg. 2009; 87(1): 31–36

[119] Navarro Martín A, Maitz A, Grills IS, et al. Successful treatment of glomus jugulare tumours with Gamma Knife radiosurgery: clinical and physical aspects of management and review of the literature. Clin Transl Oncol. 2010; 12(1):55–62

[120] Saringer W, Khayal H, Ertl A, Schoeggl A, Kitz K. Efficiency of Gamma Knife radiosurgery in the treatment of glomus jugulare tumors. Minim Invasive Neurosurg. 2001; 44(3):141–146

[121] Sharma MS, Gupta A, Kale SS, Agrawal D, Mahapatra AK, Sharma BS. Gamma Knife radiosurgery for glomus jugulare tumors: therapeutic advantages of minimalism in the skull base. Neurol India. 2008; 56(1):57–61

[122] Guss ZD, Batra S, Limb CJ, et al. Radiosurgery of glomus jugulare tumors: a meta-analysis. Int J Radiat Oncol Biol Phys. 2011; 81(4):e497–e502

[123] Wegner RE, Rodriguez KD, Heron DE, Hirsch BE, Ferris RL, Burton SA. LINAC-based stereotactic body radiation therapy for treatment of glomus jugulare tumors. Radiother Oncol. 2010; 97(3):395–398

[124] Chun SG, Nedzi LA, Choe KS, et al. A retrospective analysis of tumor volumetric responses to five-fraction stereotactic radiotherapy for paragangliomas of the head and neck (glomus tumors). Stereotact Funct Neurosurg. 2014; 92(3):153–159

[125] Schuster D, Sweeney AD, Stavas MJ, et al. Initial radiographic tumor control is similar following single or multi-fractionated stereotactic radiosurgery for jugular paragangliomas. Am J Otolaryngol. 2016; 37(3):255–258

[126] Lalwani AK, Jackler RK, Gutin PH. Lethal fibrosarcoma complicating radiation therapy for benign glomus jugulare tumor. Am J Otol. 1993; 14(4):398–402

[127] Gilbo P, Tariq A, Morris CG, Mendenhall WM. External-beam radiation therapy for malignant paraganglioma of the head and neck. Am J Otolaryngol. 2015; 36(5):692–696

[128] Walcott BP, Nahed BV, Mohyeldin A, Coumans JV, Kahle KT, Ferreira MJ. Chordoma: current concepts, management, and future directions. Lancet Oncol. 2012; 13(2):e69–e76

[129] Noël G, Feuvret L, Ferrand R, Boisserie G, Mazeron JJ, Habrand JL. Radiotherapeutic factors in the management of cervical-basal chordomas and chondrosarcomas. Neurosurgery. 2004; 55(6):1252–1260, discussion 1260–1262

[130] Hug EB. Review of skull base chordomas: prognostic factors and long-term results of proton-beam radiotherapy. Neurosurg Focus. 2001; 10(3):E11

[131] Forsyth PA, Cascino TL, Shaw EG, et al. Intracranial chordomas: a clinicopathological and prognostic study of 51 cases. J Neurosurg. 1993; 78(5):741–747

[132] Catton C, O'Sullivan B, Bell R, et al. Chordoma: long-term follow-up after radical photon irradiation. Radiother Oncol. 1996; 41(1):67–72

[133] Sahgal A, Chan MW, Atenafu EG, et al. Image-guided, intensity-modulated radiation therapy (IG-IMRT) for skull base chordoma and chondrosarcoma: preliminary outcomes. Neuro-oncol. 2015; 17(6):889–894

[134] Krishnan S, Foote RL, Brown PD, Pollock BE, Link MJ, Garces YI. Radiosurgery for cranial base chordomas and chondrosarcomas. Neurosurgery. 2005; 56 (4):777–784

[135] Kondziolka D, Lunsford LD, Flickinger JC. The role of radiosurgery in the management of chordoma and chondrosarcoma of the cranial base. Neurosurgery. 1991; 29(1):38–45, discussion 45–46

[136] Muthukumar N, Kondziolka D, Lunsford LD, Flickinger JC. Stereotactic radiosurgery for chordoma and chondrosarcoma: further experiences. Int J Radiat Oncol Biol Phys. 1998; 41(2):387–392

[137] Debus J, Schulz-Ertner D, Schad L, et al. Stereotactic fractionated radiotherapy for chordomas and chondrosarcomas of the skull base. Int J Radiat Oncol Biol Phys. 2000; 47(3):591–596

[138] Staab A, Rutz HP, Ares C, et al. Spot-scanning-based proton therapy for extracranial chordoma. Int J Radiat Oncol Biol Phys. 2011; 81(4):e489–e496

[139] Munzenrider JE, Liebsch NJ. Proton therapy for tumors of the skull base. Strahlentherapie und Onkologie. Organ der Deutschen Rontgengesellschaft. 1999; 175 Suppl 2:57–63– [et al]

[140] Noël G, Feuvret L, Dhermain F, et al. [Chordomas of the base of the skull and upper cervical spine. 100 patients irradiated by a 3D conformal technique combining photon and proton beams]. Cancer Radiother. 2005; 9 (3):161–174

[141] Noël G, Habrand JL, Mammar H, et al. Combination of photon and proton radiation therapy for chordomas and chondrosarcomas of the skull base: the Centre de Protonthérapie D'Orsay experience. Int J Radiat Oncol Biol Phys. 2001; 51(2):392–398

[142] Weber DC, Rutz HP, Pedroni ES, et al. Results of spot-scanning proton radiation therapy for chordoma and chondrosarcoma of the skull base: the Paul Scherrer Institut experience. Int J Radiat Oncol Biol Phys. 2005; 63(2):401–409

[143] Ares C, Hug EB, Lomax AJ, et al. Effectiveness and safety of spot scanning proton radiation therapy for chordomas and chondrosarcomas of the skull base: first long-term report. Int J Radiat Oncol Biol Phys. 2009; 75 (4):1111–1118

[144] Hug EB, Slater JD. Proton radiation therapy for chordomas and chondrosarcomas of the skull base. Neurosurg Clin N Am. 2000; 11(4):627–638

[145] Hug EB, Loredo LN, Slater JD, et al. Proton radiation therapy for chordomas and chondrosarcomas of the skull base. J Neurosurg. 1999; 91(3):432–439

[146] Grosshans DR, Zhu XR, Melancon A, et al. Spot scanning proton therapy for malignancies of the base of skull: treatment planning, acute toxicities, and preliminary clinical outcomes. Int J Radiat Oncol Biol Phys. 2014; 90 (3):540–546

[147] Schulz-Ertner D, Nikoghosyan A, Thilmann C, et al. Results of carbon ion radiotherapy in 152 patients. Int J Radiat Oncol Biol Phys. 2004; 58(2):631–640

[148] Schulz-Ertner D, Nikoghosyan A, Didinger B, Debus J. Carbon ion radiation therapy for chordomas and low grade chondrosarcomas—current status of the clinical trials at GSI. Radiother Oncol. 2004; 73 Suppl 2:S53–S56

[149] Uhl M, Mattke M, Welzel T, et al. Highly effective treatment of skull base chordoma with carbon ion irradiation using a raster scan technique in 155 patients: first long-term results. Cancer. 2014; 120(21):3410–3417

[150] Durante M, Loeffler JS. Charged particles in radiation oncology. Nat Rev Clin Oncol. 2010; 7(1):37–43

[151] Hug EB, Sweeney RA, Nurre PM, Holloway KC, Slater JD, Munzenrider JE. Proton radiotherapy in management of pediatric base of skull tumors. Int J Radiat Oncol Biol Phys. 2002; 52(4):1017–1024

[152] Mizoe JE, Hasegawa A, Takagi R, Bessho H, Onda T, Tsujii H. Carbon ion radiotherapy for skull base chordoma. Skull Base. 2009; 19(3):219–224

[153] Hasegawa T, Ishii D, Kida Y, Yoshimoto M, Koike J, Iizuka H. Gamma Knife surgery for skull base chordomas and chondrosarcomas. J Neurosurg. 2007; 107(4):752–757

[154] Iyer A, Kano H, Kondziolka D, et al. Stereotactic radiosurgery for intracranial chondrosarcoma. J Neurooncol. 2012; 108(3):535–542

[155] Kano H, Sheehan J, Sneed PK, et al. Skull base chondrosarcoma radiosurgery: report of the North American Gamma Knife Consortium. J Neurosurg. 2015; 123(5):1268–1275

[156] Schulz-Ertner D, Nikoghosyan A, Hof H, et al. Carbon ion radiotherapy of skull base chondrosarcomas. Int J Radiat Oncol Biol Phys. 2007; 67(1):171–177

[157] Nikoghosyan AV, Karapanagiotou-Schenkel I, Münter MW, Jensen AD, Combs SE, Debus J. Randomised trial of proton vs. carbon ion radiation therapy in patients with chordoma of the skull base, clinical phase III study HIT-1-Study. BMC Cancer. 2010; 10:607

[158] Combs SE, Ellerbrock M, Haberer T, et al. Heidelberg Ion Therapy Center (HIT): initial clinical experience in the first 80 patients. Acta Oncol. 2010; 49 (7):1132–1140

[159] Wee J, Nei WL, Yeoh KW, Yeo RM, Loong SL, Qian CN. Why are East Asians more susceptible to several infection-associated cancers (carcinomas of the nasopharynx, stomach, liver, adenocarcinoma of the lung, nasal NK/T-cell lymphomas)? Med Hypotheses. 2012; 79(6):833–842

[160] Al-Sarraf M, LeBlanc M, Giri PG, et al. Chemoradiotherapy versus radiotherapy in patients with advanced nasopharyngeal cancer: phase III randomized Intergroup study 0099. J Clin Oncol. 1998; 16(4):1310–1317

[161] Wei WI, Sham JS. Nasopharyngeal carcinoma. Lancet. 2005; 365(9476):2041–2054

[162] Chen Y, Liu MZ, Liang SB, et al. Preliminary results of a prospective randomized trial comparing concurrent chemoradiotherapy plus adjuvant chemotherapy with radiotherapy alone in patients with locoregionally advanced nasopharyngeal carcinoma in endemic regions of china. Int J Radiat Oncol Biol Phys. 2008; 71(5):1356–1364

[163] OuYang PY, Xie C, Mao YP, et al. Significant efficacies of neoadjuvant and adjuvant chemotherapy for nasopharyngeal carcinoma by meta-analysis of published literature-based randomized, controlled trials. Ann Oncol. 2013; 24(8):2136–2146

[164] Pow EH, Kwong DL, McMillan AS, et al. Xerostomia and quality of life after intensity-modulated radiotherapy vs. conventional radiotherapy for early-stage nasopharyngeal carcinoma: initial report on a randomized controlled clinical trial. Int J Radiat Oncol Biol Phys. 2006; 66(4):981–991

[165] Kam MK, Chau RM, Suen J, Choi PH, Teo PM. Intensity-modulated radiotherapy in nasopharyngeal carcinoma: dosimetric advantage over conventional plans and feasibility of dose escalation. Int J Radiat Oncol Biol Phys. 2003; 56 (1):145–157

[166] Kam MK, Leung SF, Zee B, et al. Prospective randomized study of intensity-modulated radiotherapy on salivary gland function in early-stage nasopharyngeal carcinoma patients. J Clin Oncol. 2007; 25(31):4873–4879

[167] Chen YY, Zhao C, Wang J, et al. Intensity-modulated radiation therapy reduces radiation-induced trismus in patients with nasopharyngeal carcinoma: a prospective study with > 5 years of follow-up. Cancer. 2011; 117(13):2910–2916

[168] Zhang B, Mo Z, Du W, Wang Y, Liu L, Wei Y. Intensity-modulated radiation therapy versus 2D-RT or 3D-CRT for the treatment of nasopharyngeal carcinoma: a systematic review and meta-analysis. Oral Oncol. 2015; 51(11):1041–1046

[169] Lee N, Xia P, Quivey JM, et al. Intensity-modulated radiotherapy in the treatment of nasopharyngeal carcinoma: an update of the UCSF experience. Int J Radiat Oncol Biol Phys. 2002; 53(1):12–22

[170] Wolden SL, Chen WC, Pfister DG, Kraus DH, Berry SL, Zelefsky MJ. Intensity-modulated radiation therapy (IMRT) for nasopharynx cancer: update of the Memorial Sloan-Kettering experience. Int J Radiat Oncol Biol Phys. 2006; 64 (1):57–62

[171] Takiar V, Ma D, Garden AS, et al. Disease control and toxicity outcomes for T4 carcinoma of the nasopharynx treated with intensity-modulated radiotherapy. Head Neck. 2016; 38 Suppl 1:E925–E933

[172] Ng WT, Lee MC, Hung WM, et al. Clinical outcomes and patterns of failure after intensity-modulated radiotherapy for nasopharyngeal carcinoma. Int J Radiat Oncol Biol Phys. 2011; 79(2):420–428

[173] Kwong DL, Pow EH, Sham JS. Intensity-modulated radiotherapy for early-stage nasopharyngeal carcinoma: a prospective study on disease control and preservation of salivary function. Cancer. 2004; 101(7):1584–1593

[174] Xiao WW, Huang SM, Han F, et al. Local control, survival, and late toxicities of locally advanced nasopharyngeal carcinoma treated by simultaneous modulated accelerated radiotherapy combined with cisplatin concurrent chemotherapy: long-term results of a phase 2 study. Cancer. 2011; 117(9): 1874–1883

[175] Cao CN, Luo JW, Gao L, et al. Clinical outcomes and patterns of failure after intensity-modulated radiotherapy for T4 nasopharyngeal carcinoma. Oral Oncol. 2013; 49(2):175–181

[176] Huang HI, Chan KT, Shu CH, Ho CY. T4-locally advanced nasopharyngeal carcinoma: prognostic influence of cranial nerve involvement in different radiotherapy techniques. ScientificWorldJournal. 2013; 2013:439073

[177] Kong FF, Ying H, Du CR, Huang S, Zhou JJ, Hu CS. Effectiveness and toxicities of intensity-modulated radiation therapy for patients with T4 nasopharyngeal carcinoma. PLoS One. 2014; 9(3):e91362

[178] Chen JL, Huang YS, Kuo SH, et al. Intensity-modulated radiation therapy for T4 nasopharyngeal carcinoma. Treatment results and locoregional recurrence. Strahlenther Onkol. 2013; 189(12):1001–1008

[179] Ciura K, McBurney M, Nguyen B, et al. Effect of brain stem and dorsal vagus complex dosimetry on nausea and vomiting in head and neck intensity-modulated radiation therapy. Med Dosim. 2011; 36(1):41–45

[180] Kocak-Uzel E, Gunn GB, Colen RR, et al. Beam path toxicity in candidate organs-at-risk: assessment of radiation emetogenesis for patients receiving head and neck intensity modulated radiotherapy. Radiother Oncol. 2014; 111(2):281–288

[181] Lewis GD, Holliday EB, Kocak-Uzel E, et al. Intensity-modulated proton therapy for nasopharyngeal carcinoma: decreased radiation dose to normal structures and encouraging clinical outcomes. Head Neck. 2016; 38 Suppl 1: E1886–E1895

[182] Holliday EB et al. Proton therapy reduces treatment-related toxicities for patients with nasopharyngeal cancer: a case-match control study of intensity-modulated proton therapy and intensity-modulated photon therapy. Int J Part Ther 2015;2(1):19–28

[183] Holliday E, Frank S. Proton therapy for nasopharyngeal carcinoma. Chinese Clinical Oncology 2016;5(2):13

[184] Holliday E et al. Gastrostomy tube rates decrease by over 50% in patients with nasopharyngeal cancer treated with intensity modulated proton therapy (IMPT): a case–control study. Int J Rad Oncol 2014;90(1):S528

[185] Bhattasali O et al. Definitive proton radiation therapy and concurrent cisplatin for unresectable head and neck adenoid cystic carcinoma: A series of 9 cases and a critical review of the literature. Head Neck 2016;38:E1472–E1480

[186] Holliday E et al. Postoperative intensity-modulated proton therapy for head and neck adenoid cystic carcinoma. Int J Part Ther 2016;2(4):533–543

[187] Patel SH et al. Charged particle therapy versus photon therapy for paranasal sinus and nasal cavity malignant diseases: a systematic review and meta-analysis. The Lancet Oncology 2014; 15(9):P1027–1038

[188] Truong MT, Kamat UR, Liebsch NJ, et al. Proton radiation therapy for primary sphenoid sinus malignancies: treatment outcome and prognostic factors. Head Neck. 2009; 31(10):1297–1304

[189] Parsons JT, Kimsey FC, Mendenhall WM, Million RR, Cassisi NJ, Stringer SP. Radiation therapy for sinus malignancies. Otolaryngol Clin North Am. 1995; 28(6):1259–1268

[190] Llorente JL, López F, Suárez C, Hermsen MA. Sinonasal carcinoma: clinical, pathological, genetic and therapeutic advances. Nat Rev Clin Oncol. 2014; 11 (8):460–472

[191] Lewis JS, Jr. Sinonasal squamous cell carcinoma: a review with emphasis on emerging histologic subtypes and the role of human papillomavirus. Head Neck Pathol. 2016; 10(1):60–67

[192] Blanco AI, Chao KS, Ozyigit G, et al. Carcinoma of paranasal sinuses: long-term outcomes with radiotherapy. Int J Radiat Oncol Biol Phys. 2004; 59(1): 51–58

[193] Roth TN, Gengler C, Huber GF, Holzmann D. Outcome of sinonasal melanoma: clinical experience and review of the literature. Head Neck. 2010; 32 (10):1385–1392

[194] Khan N, Khan MK, Almasan A, Singh AD, Macklis R. The evolving role of radiation therapy in the management of malignant melanoma. Int J Radiat Oncol Biol Phys. 2011; 80(3):645–654

[195] Zenda S, Kawashima M, Nishio T, et al. Proton beam therapy as a nonsurgical approach to mucosal melanoma of the head and neck: a pilot study. Int J Radiat Oncol Biol Phys. 2011; 81(1):135–139

[196] Mizoe JE, Tsujii H, Kamada T, et al. Organizing Committee for the Working Group for Head-And-Neck Cancer. Dose escalation study of carbon ion radiotherapy for locally advanced head-and-neck cancer. Int J Radiat Oncol Biol Phys. 2004; 60(2):358–364

[197] Iwata H, Tatewaki K, Inoue M, Yokota N, Sato K, Shibamoto Y. Salvage stereotactic reirradiation using the CyberKnife for the local recurrence of nasal or paranasal carcinoma. Radiother Oncol. 2012; 104(3):355–360

[198] Ozyigit G, Cengiz M, Yazici G, et al. Robotic stereotactic body radiotherapy in the treatment of sinonasal mucosal melanoma: report of four cases. Head Neck. 2013; 35(3):E69–E73

[199] Lee A, Givi B, Osborn VW, Schwartz D, Schreiber D. Patterns of care and survival of adjuvant radiation for major salivary adenoid cystic carcinoma. Laryngoscope. 2017; 127(9):2057–2062

[200] International H, International Head and Neck Scientific Group. Cervical lymph node metastasis in adenoid cystic carcinoma of the sinonasal tract, nasopharynx, lacrimal glands and external auditory canal: a collective international review. J Laryngol Otol. 2016; 130(12):1093–1097

[201] Dagan R, Bryant C, Li Z, et al. Outcomes of sinonasal cancer treated with proton therapy. Int J Radiat Oncol Biol Phys. 2016; 95(1):377–385

[202] Frank SJ, Cox JD, Gillin M, et al. Multifield optimization intensity modulated proton therapy for head and neck tumors: a translation to practice. Int J Radiat Oncol Biol Phys. 2014; 89(4):846–853

[203] Douglas JG, Goodkin R, Laramore GE. Gamma Knife stereotactic radiosurgery for salivary gland neoplasms with base of skull invasion following neutron radiotherapy. Head Neck. 2008; 30(4):492–496

[204] Demiroz C, Gutfeld O, Aboziada M, Brown D, Marentette LJ, Eisbruch A. Esthesioneuroblastoma: is there a need for elective neck treatment? Int J Radiat Oncol Biol Phys. 2011; 81(4):e255–e261

[205] Monroe AT, Hinerman RW, Amdur RJ, Morris CG, Mendenhall WM. Radiation therapy for esthesioneuroblastoma: rationale for elective neck irradiation. Head Neck. 2003; 25(7):529–534

[206] Jiang W, Mohamed AS, Fuller CD, et al. The role of elective nodal irradiation for esthesioneuroblastoma patients with clinically negative neck. Pract Radiat Oncol. 2016; 6(4):241–247

[207] Chao KS, Kaplan C, Simpson JR, et al. Esthesioneuroblastoma: the impact of treatment modality. Head Neck. 2001; 23(9):749–757

[208] Gruber G, Laedrach K, Baumert B, Caversaccio M, Raveh J, Greiner R. Esthesioneuroblastoma: irradiation alone and surgery alone are not enough. Int J Radiat Oncol Biol Phys. 2002; 54(2):486–491

[209] Diaz EM, Jr, Johnigan RH, III, Pero C, et al. Olfactory neuroblastoma: the 22-year experience at one comprehensive cancer center. Head Neck. 2005; 27 (2):138–149

[210] Duprez F, Madani I, Morbée L, et al. IMRT for sinonasal tumors minimizes severe late ocular toxicity and preserves disease control and survival. Int J Radiat Oncol Biol Phys. 2012; 83(1):252–259

[211] Mendenhall WM, Mendenhall CM, Riggs CE, Jr, Villaret DB, Mendenhall NP. Sinonasal undifferentiated carcinoma. Am J Clin Oncol. 2006; 29(1):27–31

[212] Cmelak AJ, Cox RS, Adler JR, Fee WE, Jr, Goffinet DR. Radiosurgery for skull base malignancies and nasopharyngeal carcinoma. Int J Radiat Oncol Biol Phys. 1997; 37(5):997–1003

[213] Pollard C, III, Nguyen TP, Ng SP, et al. Clinical outcomes after local field conformal reirradiation of patients with retropharyngeal nodal metastasis. Head Neck. 2017; 39(10):2079–2087

[214] Xu KM, Quan K, Clump DA, Ferris RL, Heron DE. Stereotactic ablative radiosurgery for locally advanced or recurrent skull base malignancies with prior external beam radiation therapy. Front Oncol. 2015; 5:65

[215] Roh KW, Jang JS, Kim MS, et al. Fractionated stereotactic radiotherapy as reirradiation for locally recurrent head and neck cancer. Int J Radiat Oncol Biol Phys. 2009; 74(5):1348–1355

[216] Siddiqui F, Patel M, Khan M, et al. Stereotactic body radiation therapy for primary, recurrent, and metastatic tumors in the head-and-neck region. Int J Radiat Oncol Biol Phys. 2009; 74(4):1047–1053

[217] Rwigema JC, Heron DE, Ferris RL, et al. The impact of tumor volume and radiotherapy dose on outcome in previously irradiated recurrent squamous cell carcinoma of the head and neck treated with stereotactic body radiation therapy. Am J Clin Oncol. 2011; 34(4):372–379

[218] Cengiz M, Özyiğit G, Yazici G, et al. Salvage reirradiaton with stereotactic body radiotherapy for locally recurrent head-and-neck tumors. Int J Radiat Oncol Biol Phys. 2011; 81(1):104–109

[219] Unger KR, Lominska CE, Deeken JF, et al. Fractionated stereotactic radiosurgery for reirradiation of head-and-neck cancer. Int J Radiat Oncol Biol Phys. 2010; 77(5):1411–1419

[220] Ling DC, Vargo JA, Ferris RL, et al. Risk of severe toxicity according to site of recurrence in patients treated with stereotactic body radiation therapy for recurrent head and neck cancer. Int J Radiat Oncol Biol Phys. 2016; 95(3): 973–980

[221] Yamazaki H, Ogita M, Himei K, et al. Reirradiation using robotic image-guided stereotactic radiotherapy of recurrent head and neck cancer. J Radiat Res (Tokyo). 2016; 57(3):288–293

[222] Lartigau EF, Tresch E, Thariat J, et al. Multi institutional phase II study of concomitant stereotactic reirradiation and cetuximab for recurrent head and neck cancer. Radiother Oncol. 2013; 109(2):281–285

[223] Phan J, Garden AS, Gunn GB, et al. Linear accelerator-based stereotactic ablative radiation therapy reirradiation for unresectable recurrent head and neck cancer. Int J. Radiat Oncol Biol Phys; 94:932–933

[224] Reddy GD, Wagner K, Phan J, DeMonte F, Raza SM. Management of skull base tumor-associated facial pain. Neurosurg Clin N Am. 2016; 27(3):337–344

[225] Squire SE, Chan MD, Furr RM, et al. Gamma Knife radiosurgery in the treatment of tumor-related facial pain. Stereotact Funct Neurosurg. 2012; 90(3):145–150

[226] Phan J, Pollard C, Brown PD, et al. Stereotactic radiosurgery for trigeminal pain secondary to recurrent malignant skull base tumors. J Neurosurg. 2018; 130(3):812–821

10 Management of Benign Skull Base Tumors in Neuro-oncology: Systemic Cytotoxic and Targeted Therapies

Sophie Tailibert and Marc C. Chamberlain

Summary

The treatment of benign tumors of the skull base relies mainly on a surgical approach whose purpose is to obtain a maximal safe resection as well as, if possible, a complete resection. However, the proximity of functional neurovascular structures such as cranial nerves and the brainstem to skull-based tumors results in frequent inability to obtain a complete resection, leading to frequent local recurrences, significant neurologic disabilities, and decreased survival. Most benign skull-based tumors display a slow growth rate, which often results in intrinsic radioresistance and chemoresistance. Though biologically defined as "benign," these tumors are ultimately complicated by clinical evolution that is far from "benign," being mainly caused by the therapeutic limitations and high risk of recurrence already noted. Nevertheless, considerable progress has been achieved recently in understanding the underlying genetic, epigenetic, molecular, and cellular signaling mechanisms of these tumors, opening a pathway to potentially new therapeutic strategies. Nonetheless, the clinical development of targeted drugs for the different types of benign tumors of the skull base is at an early stage. Limitations such as the rarity of several of these tumors, the lack of preclinical animal model, and the lack of understanding of their clinical relevant biology remain to be addressed. The current review focuses on those benign skull-based tumors that exhibit the genetic and molecular understandings most promising for targeted therapies. The review provides an update on the current management, pathogenesis, and recent therapeutic advances of these tumors.

Keywords: skull base, benign tumors, WHO grade I meningioma, chordoma, craniopharyngioma, giant cell tumor of the bone, chemotherapy, targeted therapy, molecular pathway

10.1 Introduction

Tumors of the skull base are categorized and defined as "benign" according to their pathologic and biologic behavior. Nevertheless, their anatomical location in proximity to critical neurovascular structures such as the cerebral vasculature, cranial nerves, and brainstem generally does not safely permit optimal surgical treatment. The absence of complete resection leads to high local recurrence rates, significant neurologic disabilities, compromised quality of life, and decreased overall survival. A comprehensive approach is thus necessary for management of benign skull base tumors, which often involves multiple therapeutic modalities. The slow growth rate that characterizes "benign tumors" is in large part responsible for their commonly seen intrinsic radioresistance and chemoresistance. This chapter provides an update on the pathogenesis and current neuro-oncology management of these tumors, including the related therapeutic advances from 2018 and earlier. Some benign tumors of the skull base, such as

chondroma, paraganglioma, and pituitary adenoma, are not discussed, whether because they are discussed elsewhere or because there are insufficient data regarding active systemic cytotoxic or targeted treatment. The current review focuses on the benign skull-based tumors that are candidates for new systemic therapeutic approaches based on recently identified genetic and molecular targets. These tumors mainly comprise World Health Organization (WHO) grade I meningioma, chordoma, craniopharyngioma, and giant cell tumor of the bone.

10.2 WHO Grade I Meningioma

10.2.1 Introduction and Treatment

Benign or WHO grade I meningioma, when located in the skull base area, remains a challenge for complete and safe surgical resection; consequently, residual tumor remains postoperatively and there is often a significant risk of neurologic morbidity due to proximity to adjacent eloquent brain. The 2007 WHO classification, updated in 2016, did not change the grading of meningioma except to include existence of brain invasion with a mitotic count ≥ 4 that now categorizes WHO grade II or atypical meningioma.[1] It was previously established that the prognosis and clinical evolution of grade I meningioma with brain invasion was like those characterized as grade II lesions.[2]

Skull base WHO grade I meningioma has a typically indolent onset, with minimal symptoms until tumors become large enough to compromise adjacent functional neurovascular structures. The slow onset results in a delay in diagnosis and presentation, often at an advanced stage.[3] Depending on the location of the WHO grade I meningioma in the skull base, presenting deficits are usually referable to proximate cranial nerves.

Meningiomas of the skull base originate from the olfactory groove, sphenoid wing, suprasellar and parasellar regions, petroclival, cerebellopontine angle, and foramen magnum.[4] Imaging is often characteristic, although radiographic findings may vary among patients. On CT, meningiomas are hyperdense and sometimes calcified. On MRI, meningiomas often are isointense with gray matter on all sequences, and contrast enhancement is intense and homogenous, although necrotic areas may be observed in large lesions.[4]

Meningiomas are highly vascularized tumors that have high relative cerebral blood volume (rCBV) values on MR perfusion. MR perfusion may assist in the differential diagnosis of skull-based lesions.[5,6,7] Diffusion tensor imaging provides additional information about the tumor's cellular content and may help differentiate among atypical, fibroblastic, and benign meningiomas.[4,8,9] High alanine and low N-acetylaspartate peaks are observed on MR spectroscopy (MRS), but bone artifacts in the skull base often limit the use of MRS except for large lesions.[10]

The initial management of patients who have WHO grade I meningioma of the skull base usually consists of surgery, surgery plus radiation therapy (RT), RT alone, or observation.[3,11,12]

Observation is an option in asymptomatic and small lesions, those defined by National Comprehensive Cancer Network (NCCN) guidelines as having a diameter of less than 3 cm, but an observation-only approach is predicated in part on the tumor's anatomical proximity to neurovascular structures. Surgery is recommended for symptomatic lesions whenever possible if it can be performed without sustaining functional morbidity. In instances of incomplete resection, postsurgical RT is often administered.[3,11,12] Differing methods of RT may be used, including conformal external fractionated RT, stereotactic radiosurgery (SRS), stereotactic radiotherapy, intensity-modulated RT (IMRT), and volumetric-modulated arc RT.[13,14,15,16,17] As of 2019, systemic treatment does not have an indication in the frontline treatment of meningioma. Particularly with skull-based WHO grade I meningioma, recurrence is frequent, and surgery or RT are most often deployed again as first salvage therapy. A variety of systemic therapies have been evaluated in surgical and RT refractory meningiomas, including chemotherapy, hormonal therapy, immunotherapy, and targeted therapies. These therapies are discussed hereafter. Regardless, most systemic treatments show modest activity. Recent identification of several molecular and druggable targets may allow development of more active systemic therapies in the future.

In all grades of meningioma, the prognosis is related to extent of resection (Simpson grade), patient characteristics such as gender (unfavorable for male), and tumor pathologic profile, such as WHO grade, Ki67/MIB-1 index, percentage of tumor cells in the S phase, p53 overexpression, telomerase activity, and telomerase reverse transcriptase (TERT) promoter mutation status (unfavorable when mutated).[18,19,20]

10.2.2 Pathogenesis, Genetics, Molecular, and Cellular Biology

Nearly 60% of WHO grade I meningiomas exhibit mutations of the NF2 gene on chromosome 22 (location: q12.2).[21,22,23,24] The NF2 gene codes for the protein merlin, which belongs to the 4.1 family of structural proteins, and behaves as a tumor suppressor. Merlin is named for its similarity to moesin, ezrin and radixin-like protein. Variable levels of merlin loss are observed in different subtypes of grade I meningiomas (lower loss in the meningothelial type than in fibrous and other).[25] Merlin localizes to the cell membrane and is involved in controlling cell–cell contact and cell motility.

The following proteins show some degree of interaction with merlin: CD44 and β1-integrin, βII-spectrin, paxillin, actin, and syntenin. These proteins are involved in cytoskeleton dynamics, sodium–hydrogen exchange regulatory factor, hepatocyte growth factor–receptor regulation, and endocytosis.[26] Merlin downregulates the Yes-associated protein (YAP), a protein that controls cellular proliferation. NF2 mutations result in increased proliferation of arachnoid cap cells and meningioma development.[27]

Besides merlin loss, other protein 4.1 family members are also downregulated in grade I meningiomas. Up to 50% of WHO grade I meningiomas display a dual loss of protein 4.1B (DAL-1) and merlin expression.[28] In up to 85% of sporadic meningioma, loss of TSLC-1 gene (tumor suppressor gene for lung cancer-1) is observed, triggering dysfunctional interactions between its protein and DAL-1.[29] In normal conditions, the protein of the TSLC-1 gene (tumor suppressor gene for lung cancer-1) interacts with DAL-1, which is present in the plasma membrane, close to cell–cell contact points. Both proteins are spectrin–actin-binding proteins, and when they interact by direct binding, they influence cell motility through actin reorganization.[30]

The therapeutic targeting of TSLC-1 and DAL-1 might be part of a future strategy of anti-invasion and antimigration in meningiomas that exhibit intact expression of these two proteins.[26,31] AKT1 mutation is found almost exclusively in skull-based grade I meningiomas and has become another potential therapeutic target since the development of AKT inhibitors.[32,33]

Multiple growth factors and their cognate receptors are observed in meningiomas and likely determine, at least in part, progression through overexpression and dysregulation. These include platelet-derived growth factor BB (PDGF-BB), epidermal growth factor receptor (EGFR), vascular endothelial growth factor (VEGF), transforming growth factor alpha and beta (TGF-alpha and -beta), SDF1 and receptor CXCR, bone morphogenic protein, insulin growth factor I and II (IGF), HER2, somatostatin, fibroblast growth factor, placental growth factor, and cyclo-oxygenase-2 Cox-2 (34–36). EGFR and platelet-derived growth factor receptor beta are both overexpressed in WHO grade I meningiomas.[34]

Meningiomas show alterations of chromosomes 1, 9, 10, 14, and 22, and their proliferation has been associated with mutations of genes in chromosomes 2, 4, 7, 8, 11, 12, and 16, leading to the activation of multiple signaling pathways. The most prominent ones are summarized hereafter.[26,35] The Wnt/β catenin pathway is involved in grade I meningiomas, in which deletions of the tumor suppressor APC gene are observed.[36,37] A third meningiomas of all grades display losses of E-cadherin function, leading to increased invasiveness and higher recurrence rates.[37] The Notch pathway is an intracellular signaling pathway mediated by the transmembrane proteins Notch 1–4.[38,39] Hes-1 is a protein that is a target of the Notch signaling pathway, and its expression is found in all grades of meningioma and related to an overexpression of the Jagged ligand, Notch 1, and Notch 2. TLE2/TLE3 are enhancers that increase the activity of the Split family (co-repressors) and that modulate Hes-1, a NOTCH signaling protein but appear to be upregulated in high-grade meningiomas only.[39]

The hedgehog (Hh)/patch (PTCH) pathway is involved in cell growth and is regulated by the (Smoothened) SMO gene. When Hh binds to PTCH, it activates SMO, leading to the activation of GLI transcription factors such as GLI1 (growth activator), GLI2 (growth activator), and GLI3 (growth repressor). The Hh pathway is also involved in angiogenesis, matrix remodeling, and stem cell homeostasis.[26] A recent large series demonstrated that 28% of SMO mutations (L412F or W535L) and 15% of AKT1E17K mutations are seen in meningiomas of the olfactory groove.[40] Among WHO grade I meningiomas, the group having SMO mutations had a significantly poorer prognosis. Meningiomas in the SMO-mutant group had an overall 36% recurrence rate, significantly higher than in the AKT1-mutant group (16%) and the "SMO and AKT1 wildtype" group (11%). All late recurrences, defined as 5 years after diagnosis, occurred in the SMO-mutant group. The authors suggest that the high frequency of SMO mutations in meningiomas arising from the anterior and medial skull base might be explained by the central role of the sonic hedgehog pathway in craniofacial development during embryogenesis. These results support the systematic determination of SMO mutations, both for prognosis and for potential inclusion of patients in future trials targeting this pathway using Hh inhibitors. The p53/pRB pathway controls the G1 to S phase cell cycle transition through the tumor suppressor gene pRB and is involved in meningioma progression and development of the anaplastic grade.[26]

The PI3K/AKT and mitogen-activated protein kinase (MAPK) are two pathways involved in grade II/III meningiomas only, in which high levels of phosphorylated Akt (PI3K/Akt) are found.[21,41,42,43,44] Decreased levels of MAPK lead to higher recurrence rate. Other pathways, such as the phospholipase A2-arachadonic acid cyclo-oxygenase pathway, the PLC-gamma1-PKC pathway, and the transforming growth factor-beta (TGF-b)-SMAD signaling pathway, have all been related to meningioma pathogenesis.[45,46,47] The levels of expression of cox-2 and of tumor necrosis factor–related apoptosis-inducing ligand receptor 4 (TRAIL-R4) seem correlated to the grade of meningioma.[48] KIT expression is upregulated in 20.6% of meningiomas and is another potential druggable target.[18] TERT promoter mutations, which are correlated to a decreased time to progression and a higher risk of recurrence, are present in only 1.7% of WHO grade I meningiomas.[47]

10.2.3 Systemic Therapies

An accurate assessment of the therapeutic efficacy in meningiomas has not been possible until recently, mainly because of the heterogeneity of response criteria used in different series. The Response Assessment in Neuro-Oncology (RANO) working group recently proposed use of the 6-month progression-free survival (PFS-6) as the standard in clinical trials in recurrent meningiomas.[49] The weighted PFS-6 of WHO grade I meningioma determined by the RANO authors was 29% (95% confidence interval: 20.3–37.7%). The authors concluded that a new therapeutic compound should demonstrate a PFS-6 > 50% in WHO grade I meningioma if it is to be considered a therapy of interest.[49] Nevertheless, there is still a lack of standardization regarding the optimal response criteria. Due to the complex shape of meningioma, the potential superiority of volumetric measures as compared with 2D McDonald criteria has been highlighted.[50]

Chemotherapy

Hydroxyurea (HU), temozolomide, and irinotecan have been evaluated in phase II trials, retrospective cohorts, and case studies in patients having recurrent WHO grade I meningiomas.[20,51,52,53,54,55,56,57,58,59,60,61,62] The reported median PFS ranged from 4 to 90 months.[54,55,58,59] PFS-6 was retrospectively assessed in one series of 60 patients and was only 10%.[59] Using a combination of HU and fractionated conformal RT in 13 patients who had recurrent or progressive lesions, median PFS-12 was 84%, but the specific contribution of HU cannot be disentangled from the effects of radiotherapy.[56] A phase II trial did not show any efficacy of temozolomide in 16 patients with a PFS-6 of 0%.[60] Similarly, irinotecan did not display activity in a series of 16 patients with a reported PFS-6 of 6%.[61] Trabectidin, a novel marine-derived antineoplastic agent, has shown a significant cytotoxic activity in grade II/III meningioma in preclinical studies.[63] Synergy with HU, cisplatin, and doxorubicin was

observed as well. These results led to the development of a phase II clinical trial in recurrent high-grade meningioma, but WHO grade I meningioma are currently excluded.

Hormonal Therapy

Thirty percent and 70% of meningiomas express receptors to estrogen and progesterone, respectively.[45,64,65,66,67] Although PFS-6 is lacking in most published studies, the reported data fail to show any compelling efficacy of any antiestrogen or progesterone agents in recurrent and surgery-naive meningioma WHO grade I. Tamoxifen has been assessed in recurrent meningioma, including a single phase II trial, without significant effect.[45,64,65,66,67,68] No radiographic responses were observed, although prolonged stabilization was seen in some studies.[69,70] The progesterone-targeting agents megestrol acetate, medroxyprogesterone acetate, and mifepristone (RU-486) have been evaluated in grade I meningioma at recurrence or in meningiomas for which there was no prior surgery.[71,72,73,74,75] Like antiestrogen-targeting agents, these agents achieved, at best, long-lasting disease stabilizations.[71,74] Mifepristone was reported to have resulted in limited prolonged volumetric reductions in a few cases but had no significant impact when assessed in a randomized double-blind phase III study in grade I nonsurgical meningioma.[75]

Somatostatin Analogs

Ninety percent of meningiomas express somatostatin receptors, mostly of the sst2A subtype[76] Several retrospective cohorts and phase II studies have assessed the effect of somatostatin analogs such as somatostatin, pasireotide, octreotide (Novartis), Sandostatin LAR (Novartis), pasireotide (Novartis), 90Y-DOTATOC (Abbott), 177Lu-DOTATOC (Novartis) on progressive or recurrent meningiomas of all grades.[50,76,77,78,79,80] Some studies report global PFS-6 rates for tumors of all grades between 32 and 44%.[50,76] A PFS-6 of 50% was observed in recurrent or progressive grade I meningiomas with pasireotide LAR, albeit without any objective radiographic response.[50] The activity of these agents seems limited, notwithstanding a subpopulation of responders' appearing to benefit from somatostatin-based therapy. Factors such as differing expression of somatostatin receptors (sst2 and 3) and level of octreotide uptake might be predictors of response and longer PFS and survival.[50,76,77,78,80]

Interferon Alpha

An encouraging PFS-6 rate of 54% was obtained in a phase II trial of patients who had refractory WHO grade I meningioma treated using interferon-alpha, an active agent in vitro.[45,67,81,82,83] Although no objective radiological response was reported, 74% of patients were stabilized with a median PFS of 7 months and a median overall survival of 8 months (range 3–28 mo).[81]

Molecular Targeted Therapies

The lack of current effective treatment in recurrent or progressive WHO grade I meningioma is related in part to an insufficient understanding of the molecular pathogenesis of these tumors.[26] Despite the identified overexpression of multiple growth factors, including platelet-derived growth factor (PDGF),

Epidermal growth factor (EGF), vascular endothelial growth factor (VEGF), insulin-like growth factor (IGF), transforming growth factor-beta (TGF-β), and their receptor tyrosine kinases, and the dysregulation of their downstream signaling pathways, including the RAS/MAPK, PI3K/Akt, PLC-γ1-PKC, and TGF-β-SMAD pathways, their respective importance is poorly understood, and druggable targets need to be identified.[26] Moreover, other approaches involving insulin-like growth factor receptor 2 (IGFR-2), histone deacetylase, NFκB, HSP90, JAK/STAT, immune checkpoint inhibitor, telomerase inhibitors, BRAF inhibitors, Src kinase, focal adhesion kinase (FAK), and hypoxia-inducible factor 1α might lead to potential new treatments.[26,84,85]

Sixty percent of meningiomas express EGFR.[86,87] A phase II trial evaluating either gefitinib or erlotinib showed poor efficacy in recurrent meningioma WHO grade I patients who had a PFS-6 rate of 25%, 13 months of median overall survival, and 9 weeks median PFS.[88] Most meningiomas of all grades express platelet-derived growth factor (PDGF)-b receptor and manifest an increased level of PDGF.[89,90] In vitro, meningioma cell proliferation is inhibited by anti-PDGF antibodies.[91,92] Imatinib, an inhibitor of PDGF receptor (PDGFR), was given as a single agent in a phase II trial.[93] It showed limited efficacy, with a PFS-6 of 45% in recurrent and progressive WHO grade I meningioma. When combined with HU in the same setting, PFS-6 reached 87.5%.[94] In a small randomized study of recurrent meningioma (all grades) that compared HU with HU + imatinib, PFS-9 (9-month PFS) was 0% and 75%, respectively.[95]

Meningiomas of all grades are highly vascularized and express VEGF and VEGF-R at variable levels related to grade (increased levels with higher grade).[46,96,97,98,99,100] This pathway is involved in tumor growth vis-à-vis angiogenesis as well as in induction of peritumoral edema.[45,66,83,101] Sunitinib (SU011248), a small molecule inhibitor that targets VEGF, PDGF, c-KIT, FLT, RET, macrophage colony–stimulating factor (CSF-1R), and valatinib (PTK787/ZK22584), a VEGFR 1–3 inhibitor, was ineffective in recurrent grade I meningiomas.[102] Bevacizumab, a monoclonal antibody targeting VEGF, has been evaluated mostly in the retrospective setting and is often coadministered with either temozolomide or etoposide.[99,100,103,104] In a phase II trial, bevacizumab was given to patients who had recurrent meningioma who were not otherwise considered candidates for local treatment. Results were encouraging in meningioma WHO grade I: PFS-6 of 87%, median PFS of 22.5 months, median overall survival of 35.6 months, and 100% tumor stabilization.[105] Additionally, bevacizumab appears to have a mitigating effect on peritumoral edema and meningioma growth rate.[106]

Preclinical data show inhibiting activity of temsirolimus, an mTOR inhibitor, in meningioma in which the pathway is activated. Furthermore, a synergistic effect was seen when octreotide was added to everolimus.[107,108] Consequently, this combination is being pursued in all grades of recurrent meningioma patients in a clinical trial with PFS-6 as the primary objective (CEVOREM/NCT02333565).

The therapeutic potential of TRAIL agonists has been evaluated in meningioma cell lines.[108] TRAIL-induced apoptosis was seen in 29.7% of cell lines, but native TRAIL receptor expression was not predictive of TRAIL agonist sensitivity. The coadministration of bortezomib, which induces NOXA expression and downregulation of c-FLIP, may increase sensitivity to TRAIL-induced apoptosis.[109] FAK inhibitors that target NF2 and merlin loss seen in up to 60% of sporadic meningiomas represent another trial in progress in patients who have recurrent meningiomas.[110,111]

The FAK inhibitor GSK2256098 and vismodegib, a hedgehog pathway inhibitor, are being studied in progressive meningiomas with SMO/AKT/NF2 mutations. A histone deacetylase inhibitor and its impact on suppression of p-AKT are also being explored.[18,112]

Some of the numerous potential targets may preferentially be expressed in high-grade rather than low-grade meningiomas. For example, programmed death-1 ligand (PD-L1) is frequently expressed in higher-grade tumors, indicating that it may play a biological role in the aggressive phenotype of meningiomas and may be targetable by PD-1 and PDL-1.[113]

Other approaches, such as gene silencing, supplementation of lost genetic factors, regulation of YAP levels in NF2 mutated tumors, and addressing of deficient intrinsic and extrinsic pathways, may improve management of recurrent and progressive meningiomas.[26]

Insufficient understandings of the evolution of grade I meningiomas and the lack of a preclinical reliable animal model are significant barriers to the development of novel active therapies. The RANO criteria will help standardize results of future trials in recurrent meningioma.

10.3 Chordomas

10.3.1 Introduction to Chordomas and Treatment Overview

Chordomas of the skull base are rare, slow-growing, locally aggressive, and destructive bony tumors derived from embryonic remnants of the notochord. Chordomas located in the skull base represent a third of all chordomas and are most frequently located in the spheno-occipital region.[114] Headaches and intermittent diplopia are the predominant clinical features at onset, followed by additional cranial nerves palsies that differ according to the topography of the chordoma (e.g., supra- or infraclival). Delays in diagnosis are frequently caused by nonspecific symptoms such as nasal congestion or dysphagia that are related to cranial nerve involvement but not always initially identified as being so.

CT imaging is the best technique for assessing bone destruction; it may show characteristic ring-forming calcifications.[115] MRI better shows the extent of tumor, including soft tissue components and dural extension.[116] Chordomas on MRI are hypo- or isointense on T1-weighted and hyperintense on T2-weighted MRI sequences. Contrast enhancement is heterogeneous, with a lobulated "honeycomb" appearance, reflecting the liquid and gelatinous mucoid components and necrotic-hemorrhagic areas.[117] A fusion of CT and MRI ideally provides the most accurate assessment of the anatomical relation between soft tissue tumor components surrounding normal soft tissue and bone.

Though chordomas are classified as benign tumors, their prognosis is more akin to that of a malignant lesion, with high local recurrence rates, including systemic metastases (40% incidence overall, 12.5% from skull base chordoma), largely responsible for tumor-related lethality.[118,119,120,121,122] The median survival rate is approximately 6.29 years with 5-year OS and PFS rates of 78.4 and 50.8%, respectively.[114,121,123]

Histologically, chordomas, like the notochord, are composed of large vacuolated physaliphorous cells surrounded by an extracellular myxoid matrix.[118,124] Chordomas comprise three subgroups: conventional chordomas, chondroid chordomas, and dedifferentiated chordomas (i.e., those with sarcomatous transformation). Conventional chordomas, which comprise chordomatous features only, are most frequent, followed by chondroid chordomas, which comprise additional chondromatous features. Both entities share the same prognosis, unlike dedifferentiated or sarcomatous chordomas, which behave in a more malignant manner.[114,125] Most chordomas stain positive for cytokeratin, and 80% are epithelial membrane antigen–positive. A limited number in addition are S100 protein–positive.[126,127,128] Routine immunohistochemical staining for brachyury, a key transcription factor in notochord development that is overexpressed by chordomas, is a sensitive and specific diagnostic tool that also rules out cartilaginous tumors.[129,130,131,132,133]

The treatment of chordoma is continually evolving owing to continued progress in understanding underlying biology. Chordomas are radioresistant to standard radiation protocols and chemoresistant to classic cytotoxic therapies, in part as a result of their slow-growing kinetics. Standard radiation to the skull base is also limited by the radiosensitivity of the brainstem and other proximate intracranial neurovascular structures that increase the risk of radiation-related injury.[134,135]

For localized disease, consensus guidelines published in 2015 recommend a complete surgical resection with tumor-free margins.[136] Classic open skull base approaches and less invasive endoscopic approaches are used to maximize the resection.[121,122,137,138,139,140,141,142] When residual disease is remaining, often having a relationship to adjacent neurovascular structures, radiotherapy is recommended.[143,144,145,146] Definitive (proton beam) RT is the preferred alternative in instances in which resection is not feasible. Recent advances in heavy particle RT, such as proton and carbon ion beam, are promising in the adjuvant setting of skull base chordomas.[147,148,149] Adjuvant proton therapy, when added to maximal safe resection in skull base chordomas, led to 5-year local control rates of 75.8% and improved survival.[147,148] Adjuvant carbon ion radiation provided similar local 5-year control rates of 70.0%.[149] Image-guided IMRT (IG-IMRT) is also under evaluation for skull base chordoma.[150] Cytotoxic chemotherapy or other systemic therapies have no proven efficacy and are thus not recommended in any line of treatment according to current guidelines.[136,151] Nevertheless, several molecular therapies targeting essential pathways in chordomas are currently under evaluation and are discussed hereafter.

10.3.2 Pathogenesis, Genetics, and Molecular and Cellular Pathways

Advances in the molecular understanding of chordomas have led to the identification of promising prognostic markers and targetable pathways. These include genetic and epigenetic alterations that involve brachyury, downstream pathways, and receptor tyrosine kinases (RTKs). The brachyury or T gene located on chromosome 6q27 encodes a transcription factor essential for the development of the notochord.[152] Normally silenced, brachyury is reexpressed at high levels in chordoma cells. Several lines of evidence also suggest a causative role of brachyury overexpression in chordoma formation. Further brachyury might be involved in the metastatic process by facilitating the epithelial–mesenchymal transition.[153,154,155,156] As already mentioned, the expression of brachyury is very helpful for pathologic diagnosis, but its level does not seem correlated with prognosis.[157]

Other genetic alterations in chordomas include loss of p16, *PTEN*, *CDKN2a/CDKN2b*, and *PDCD4*.[158,159,160,161,162,163,164,165,166,167,168] Losses on chromosome 1p and the *FHIT* gene and gains on 1q and 2p have been detected in skull base chordomas.[152,160] Loss of chromosome 1p36, 9p loss of heterozygosity, and an elevated Ki67 proliferative index are associated with shorter OS in skull base chordomas.[152,161] Additionally, loss of chromosome 1q, gain of 2p, and aberrant brachyury copy number are associated with recurrence.

Many alterations in the signaling pathways and growth factors are involved in chordoma biology as well. Both the *PI3K/AKT/TSC1/TSC2/mTOR* and STAT3 pathways are activated.[162] STAT3 level of expression has reported prognostic value. Changes in *EGFR* signaling, activation of *IGF1R*, and loss of *MTAP* have also been identified.[118,163,164]

Protein tyrosine kinases (PTKs) mediate phosphorylation of selected tyrosine residues, resulting in functional activation of many proteins and thus playing a crucial role in cancer development. RTKs are specialized transmembrane PTKs that mediate signaling via sampling of the external environment. RTKs are composed of extracellular domains that bind cognate environmental ligands and of an intracellular domain that mediates the signaling event via dimerization and binding to other signaling molecules. EGFR overexpression is observed in 69 to 79.6% of chordomas and is related to tumor aggressiveness.[144,163,165,166,167] PDGFR expression is also observed in chordoma. Although PDGFR promotes chordoma cell proliferation through activation of the PI3K/AKT, RAS/ERK, and STAT pathways, PDGFRβ is observed in the stromal component of the tumor and is likely involved in microenvironmental regulation.[144,165,168,169,170,171]

Increased expression of angiogenesis-related factors such as VEGF, hypoxia-inducible factor-1α (HIF-1α) and matrix metalloproteinase (MMP)-2 and -9 has been identified in chordoma tissue and cell lines.[172,173] MMP-9 expression is correlated with higher rates of local recurrence and poor prognosis.[173]

Epigenetic alterations, especially modifications of the expression of microRNA (miRNA) have been identified in chordomas, and may be therapeutically targetable as illustrated in vitro.[174,175,176,177,178,179] For example, the administration of nonselective histone deacetylase inhibitors significantly triggers apoptosis in chordomas cells.[174] Similarly, the blockade of the constitutive downregulation of microRNA-1 in chordomas inhibits cellular proliferation, migratory and invasive properties, and the expression of the oncoprotein SLUG as well.[176,177] The restoration of two constitutively downregulated miRNAs targeting *EGFR*, *MET*, and *Bcl-xL* block cell proliferation.[175]

10.3.3 Systemic Therapies

As already mentioned, cytotoxic chemotherapy has not proven efficacious and thus is not recommended in any line of treatment of chordomas. Brachyury based on its determinant role in notochord development and selective reexpression in chordoma makes this an attractive and potential target.[145] This is illustrated in vitro by the differentiation and senescence of chordoma cells, triggered by silencing the brachyury gene.[180] Currently no treatment directly targets brachyury. An alternative approach would be instead to target downstream or interacting signaling pathways such as FGFR/MEK/ERK signal-transduction and EGFR signaling pathways.[181,182] Immunotherapy may be promising, as illustrated by the partial responses observed in advanced chordoma patients treated with an immune-stimulating therapeutic cancer vaccine designed to elicit brachyury-specific T-cell responses.[183]

Multiple PTKs are posited to be involved in chordoma development and progression, some of which are functionally redundant. Therapeutic strategies comprise simultaneous inhibition of different PTKs or blocking of downstream signaling pathways. In chordomas, the PI3K/AKT/mTOR pathway is activated and PTEN is inhibited.[162,168,169,184] It was hypothesized that therapeutic activity might be seen with inhibition of signaling mediated by EGFR and PDGFR, both of which converge on the PI3K/AKT/mTOR pathway. Some data suggest a potential therapeutic role for combined *AKT* and *mTOR* inhibitors, such as rapamycin.[162]

Preclinical use of the combination of a mTORC1 (rapamycin), mTOR (MLN0128), and PI3K/AKT/mTOR (PI-103) inhibitors presaged clinical activity seen with both mTOR and PDGFR as single agents in recurrent chordoma. The combined clinical efficacy of the combination of an mTOR inhibitor and imatinib in imatinib-resistant patients who had chordomas illustrates another possible strategy.[184,185,186,187] Improved activity-based molecular profiling of a patient's tumor and identification of specific aberrant signaling pathways is likely the most effective approach, as illustrated by the spectacular efficacy of rapamycin on tumors having aberrant mTOR-pathway signaling.[188,189]

PDGFR inhibition with imatinib mesylate (alone or combined with sirolimus) has shown some antitumoral activity in case series and one phase II trial in chordoma patients, including several who had skull base chordomas.[170,185,190,191] An overall clinical benefit of 64% and stabilization rate of 70% were observed in advanced chordoma patients during the phase II trial.[190] Sorafenib, a dual inhibitor targeting PDGF and VEGF pathways, has also been prospectively assessed in a phase II trial of patients who had advanced and metastatic chordomas.[192] The response rate was low (3.7%), although the 9-month PFS was 73% and the 12-month OS 86.5%. The modest efficacy of PDGFR inhibition probably reflects the limitation of drug delivery into the chordoma and thus drug exposure.[144,145,169,192] EGFR inhibition has also shown responses and clinical improvement in a few case series and in a single phase II trial in patients who had recurrent chordoma, including skull base tumors.[145,193,194,195,196,197] Anti-EGFR monoclonal antibodies such as cetuximab, and EGFR tyrosine kinase inhibitors such as gefitinib, erlotinib, and lapatinib, have been studied.[145,193,194,195,196,197] Median PFS was 8 months in a phase II trial of lapatinib,

suggesting the need for a larger trial to establish the role of this strategy.[193]

Inhibition of proangiogenic growth factors such as VEGF is another option for recurrent chordomas. In a small clinical series including patients who had skull base tumors, the combined use of erlotinib and bevacizumab, a humanized anti-VEGF antibody, led to disease stabilization.[198] Small numbers of patients have been treated with the VEGF inhibitors pazopanib or sunitinib.[120] One partial response was achieved with sunitinib, and 50% of patients benefited clinically from pazopanib, exhibiting 14- to 15-month disease stabilization. These data need further confirmation to confirm the place of anti-VEGF therapy in chordomas. Other potential therapeutic targets in chordomas, such as the inhibition of STAT3 with SD-1029, or the selective de novo purine synthesis inhibitor in *MTAP*-deficient chordomas, have shown promise in preclinical studies.[164,199,200]

Although epidemiologic data show an improvement over time in the management of chordomas, with improved survival and local control, this effect is related mostly to earlier diagnosis made possible by improved imaging techniques, to improved surgical resection using endoscopic endonasal approaches, and to recent developments in radiation techniques.[118,121,136,138,139] The place of systemic therapies remains suboptimal and is confined to the recurrent setting when no other options are available. Multiple targeted therapies have been tried with modest results. These approaches need further development based on an improved understanding of the underlying molecular pathways relevant to chordoma and on the increasing use of molecular characterization of chordomas that match the molecular target with a targeted therapy.

10.4 Craniopharyngioma

10.4.1 Introduction to Craniopharyngiomas and Treatment Overview

Craniopharyngiomas (CPs) are rare slow-growing solid or mixed solid–cystic tumors that arise from remnants of Rathke's pouch found along the midline from the nasopharynx to the diencephalon. These epithelial tumors commonly occur close to the optic chiasm in the suprasellar area but may also be observed within the sella, the third ventricle, and the optic system.[201,202,203,204,205] CP often decrease life span and can consequently be considered low-grade malignancies. These tumors show no gender predilection and have a bimodal occurrence between 5 and 14 years in children and 50 and 75 years in adults.[206]

Clinical presentation is variable, depending on the tumor location, and may consist of visual acuity and field disturbances, a wide range of endocrinopathies, headaches caused by compression or hydrocephalus or meningeal spread, and depression. Growth retardation in children and sexual dysfunction in adults are the most frequent endocrine manifestations. Diabetes insipidus is also frequent. Endocrine and visual assessments, including visual field testing, are part of the systematic presurgical and postsurgical usual and customary evaluations. Neuroimaging most often shows a calcified cystic mass in the parasellar region, but both characteristics may be lacking in up to 25% of cases. Based on histological patterns, adamantinomatous and papillary CP are separate entities in the WHO classification.[207] Both subtypes seem to share the same evolution in terms of treatment efficacy and survival.[208,209]

Surgery is the primary and major component of initial treatment. Surgery provides a diagnosis as well as relief of symptoms. Maximal safe resection is advocated, but cyst aspiration followed by partial resection is an alternative in some cases considering that the expected benefits of surgery should be balanced with potential surgical morbidities.

RT is indicated after partial resections and at recurrence.[210] Stereotactic RT and RSR, IMRT, and proton beam RT are most often employed.[210,211,212,213,214,215,216]

Compressive cysts need to be addressed when causing hydrocephalus or visual or hypothalamic disturbances. Percutaneous aspiration or aspiration via an Ommaya reservoir, intracavitary irradiation with stereotactic administered radioisotopes, and intracavitary chemotherapy may be used for this purpose.[217,218,219,220,221,222,223,224,225,226,227,228,229] Surgery and RT may result in a wide range of endocrine, visual, neurological, and cerebrovascular side effects that may appear early or late, depending on clinical context. These treatment-related deficits include panhypopituitarism and related complications such as obesity, diabetes insipidus, sleep and temperature regulation disorders, visual field impairment, cognitive and behavioral disorders, arterial stenosis and ischemic strokes, cerebral cavernomas and aneurysm, moyamoya syndrome, meningioma, and high-grade glioma.[230,231,232,233]

10.4.2 Pathogenesis, Genetics, Molecular and Cellular Overview

The two histologic subtypes of CP show distinct molecular genetics. Activation of the Wnt signaling pathway via activation of mutations in the gene encoding β-catenin (CTNNB1) are reported in 96% of adamantinomatous CP (ACP), a subtype of CP seen mostly in the pediatric population.[234,235,236,237,238,239] This driver mutation leads to accumulation of the protein β-catenin, which plays a role in cell signaling and cell adhesion. The Wnt signaling pathway promotes cell proliferation and differentiation. When the Wnt pathway is activated, β-catenin localizes to the cytoplasm and nucleus and can be detected through standard immunochemistry and used as a marker of CTNNB1 mutation status.[235,236,239,240]

In one study using whole-exome sequencing, mutations of BRAF V600E oncogene were reported in 95% of papillary CP (PCP), which are commonly observed in the adult population and are not found in ACP.[239] In another study using targeted Sanger sequencing, the BRAF V600E mutation was shown in 81% of PCP and in 12.5% of ACP displaying the CTNNB1 mutation as well. These data suggest that these mutations are not mutually exclusive but rather tend to be predominant in one specific subtype of CP.[240] Immunohistochemistry provides the same sensitivity for detection of the BRAF V600E mutation as sequencing and is much more widely available.[235,236,239,240] Circulating BRAF V600E DNA has been detected in blood during treatment with a BRAF inhibitor, indicating that "liquid biopsy" may become a tool in the diagnosis and response to treatment of BRAF V600E mutated CP.[235] The

activating mutation BRAF may serve as a potential therapeutic target.

10.4.3 Systemic Therapies

Intracavitary Chemotherapy

An alternative approach to managing cystic CP is administration of intracystic bleomycin by way of an implanted catheter and reservoir such as an Ommaya device.[228] Experience is more limited than with intracavitary irradiation, but in one series of 17 children, intracystic bleomycin was well tolerated, with five complete remissions and a median progression-free interval of 1.8 years.[229] This approach may have a role in delaying RT or aggressive surgery.

Biological Therapy

The intracystic administration of IFN-α via an intracystic catheter connected to an Ommaya reservoir was assessed in more than 75 patients.[241,242,243] Three million units of IFN-α were administered three times per week. One cycle was defined as 4 weeks of therapy and a total of 36 million units. Patients received from one to nine cycles. In all studies, tolerance to therapy was good, no drug interruption occurred, and significant clinical and radiologic responses were observed in the majority of patients.

Targeted Therapies

The use of BRAF inhibitors in BRAF-mutated PCP may become a new therapeutic option, as suggested by dramatic isolated responses.[244,245,246] Nevertheless, when vemurafenib was used, regrowth was observed as soon as the targeted therapy was interrupted.[244] Combination of a BRAF inhibitor (dabrafenib) and a MEK inhibitor (trametinib) is the new standard treatment in BRAF-mutated melanoma, providing optimal inhibition of the MAPK kinase (MEK) and RAS pathways with a significantly reduced risk of death compared with that seen for use of vemurafenib alone.[247] This approach combining dabrafenib and trametinib has recently been tried successfully in patients who have BRAF-mutated CP and will be further studied in a National Cancer Institute–sponsored multicenter clinical trial.[235,245,246,248]

Future trials are needed to confirm the value of targeted therapies in CPs with respect both to time of implementation (neoadjuvant to facilitate resection, adjuvant after incomplete resection or at relapse) and to overall activity in the multidisciplinary approach of these tumors.[249]

10.5 Giant Cell Tumor of the Bone

10.5.1 Introduction to Giant Cell Tumor of the Bone and Treatment Overview

Giant cell tumor of the bone (GCTB) is a rare, benign, slow-growing but locally destructive intraosseous and osteolytic tumor of skeletally mature young adults in their second to fourth decade, predominant in females and Asians. There is an increased incidence of GCTB of the skull in Paget's disease.

Although GCTB is considered a benign lesion, its evolution is unpredictable. Neurologic deficits often result from local invasive and compressive effects of the tumor. Prognosis is impacted by recurrence, malignant transformation, and the rare (< 5%) occurrence of metastases, predominantly to lungs. The local recurrence rate is high in cases of incomplete surgery, mostly within 2 years of surgery. The recommended follow-up period is 5 years only, because recurrences after that period are quite rare. Clinically, patients present with multiple cranial nerves palsies and headaches. Minimal work-up should include serum calcium and phosphorous, serum parathyroid hormone, bone scan, chest X-ray, contrast brain CT, and MRI. Additionally, some investigators advise performance of a chest CT, at least at time of recurrence, because lung metastases are most common at recurrence but on occasion may be inaugural.

A lytic lesion resulting from an intratumoral hemorrhage is evocative but not pathognomonic of the diagnosis by either skull film or CT scan.[250,251] CT imaging is more accurate for assessment of bone architecture and MRI for the surrounding neurovascular structures. Either may show a hypervascularized and cystic lesion.[252,253] The Campanacci classification categorizes GCTB into three grades (I, II, III), based on clinical and radiological features, but does not correlate with pathology, nor is it prognostic.[254]

GCTB consist of three cell-types: neoplastic giant cell tumor stromal cells, which have high proliferative activity; recruited mononuclear histiocytic cells; and multinuclear giant cells. The histologic heterogeneity of GCTB increases the difficulty of diagnosis, which is compounded by the limited sampling associated with core or fine-needle biopsies. It can be challenging to identify the atypical neoplastic stromal cells among the reactive giant cells and thus to distinguish between benign and malignant GCTB.[255,256]

Until now, surgery has been the mainstay of local treatment, achieving generally good local control rates when resection is complete. Recent advances in the understanding of the molecular pathogenesis of GCTB, and improvements in RT, have led to new and better-tolerated therapeutic options. Nevertheless, to preserve the adjacent neurovascular structures and minimize surgery-related injury, resection is often incomplete and adjuvant therapy thus required. To decrease the risk of post-RT malignant transformation, the NCCN has recommended RT as the last adjuvant option notwithstanding the established radiosensitivity of GCTB and its excellent local control rate. Stereotactic radiosurgery and IMRT have been recently used as adjuvant therapies but require further validation.[251,257,258] Denosumab, a monoclonal antibody targeting the receptor activator of nuclear factor-κB ligand (RANKL), was approved by the FDA in 2013 for the treatment of GCTB.[255,256] Other systemic therapies are discussed hereafter.[259,260]

10.5.2 Pathogenesis, Genetics, and Molecular and Cellular Pathways

The proliferative fraction of GCTB is thought to be derived from the stromal compartment, but the absence of cytologic aspects of malignancy in stromal cells, combined with the lack of clonal cytogenetic structural aberrations in GCTB in most studies, suggests that these cells may be reactive and not neoplastic.[261,262,263,264] However, neoplastic stromal cells

and mesenchymal stem cells share similar differentiation characteristics. When present, the overexpression of p53 and centrosome amplification are correlated with a high risk of recurrence, and the overexpression of p53 is also associated with an increased risk of metastases. Centrosome amplification is more frequent in recurrent and malignant GCTB.[265,266] Fifty-four percent of GCTBs have 20q11 amplifications.[267] Genetic instability is also suggested by the presence of a driver mutation in H3F3A, exclusively in the stromal cells in > 90% of GCTB.[268] Furthermore, telomere dysregulation is present in up to 70% of GCTB, with a telomere protective-capping mechanism permitting telomere length maintenance.[269,270,271] Telomere maintenance markers such as human telomerase reverse transcriptase and promyelocytic leukemia body-related antigens are expressed by GCTB.[271,272,273] A telomeric fusion in chromosomes 11p, 13p, 15p, 18p, 19p, and 21p is present in more than 80% of GCTB, predominantly in grade III tumors.[274]

The multinucleated giant cells in GCTB result from the recruitment of CD68-positive monocytes attracted by SDF-1 and MCP-1, which are produced by stromal cells, and by the VEGF present in the stromal environment, because these monocytes express VEGFR1 (Flt1) among other macrophage markers.[250] At a molecular level, RANKL (receptor activator of nuclear factor kappa B [NF-kB] ligand) plays a major functional role in the molecular pathogenesis of GCTB. The osteoblast-like mononuclear stromal cells display a high rate of expression of RANKL.[255,262,275,276,277,278]

Receptor activator of nuclear factor-kappa beta (RANK) ligand (RANKL) interactions and macrophage colony–stimulating factor (M-CSF) stimulate recruitment of osteoclastic cells from normal mononuclear preosteoclast cells that become multinucleated osteoclast-like giant cells.[279,280,281,282,283] Through a cathepsin K- and MMP-13–mediated process, these giant cells cause the characteristic bone destruction observed in these lesions.[284,285,286] Runx2 may be a driver in cytokine-mediated MMP-13 expression in GCTB stromal cells.[287] CCAAT/enhancer binding protein beta(C/EBPbeta), by activating RANKL promoter, seems to be a significant factor in GCTB pathophysiology.[288] Given the predominant role of RANKL in the genesis of these multinucleated giant cells, the inhibition of RANKL signaling by the use of the targeted antibody denosumab has proven highly effective.

The CD33 + phenotype of the giant cells in GCTB may also in the future be targetable using an anti-CD33 antibody such as gemtuzumab.[282,283] Some cells also are positive for PDGFA, C-kit, and EGFR, all of which can be therapeutically targeted using commercial drugs.[289,290] The EGFR is expressed by neoplastic stromal cells and plays a role in their proliferation, in osteoclastogenesis, and likely in the progression of the disease.[289]

Less prominent RANKL-independent pathways are involved in GCTB osteoclastogenesis and may represent another druggable target.[279] These RANKL-independent pathways include tumor necrosis factor-α, interleukin-6, tumor growth factor-β, a proliferation-inducing ligand, B-cell activating factor, nerve growth factor, insulin-like growth factor I (IGF-I), and IGF-II. Further understanding of GCTB molecular pathogenesis will further inform the development of novel molecular-based therapies.

10.5.3 Systemic Therapies

Chemotherapy

There is limited evidence regarding the benefit of chemotherapy in benign GCTB, and because more efficient and better-tolerated systemic alternatives exist, it is usually not prescribed in these tumors except in cases of malignant GCTB. Doxorubicin, cisplatin, methotrexate, ifosfamide, and cyclophosphamide have been used in advanced aggressive, unresectable tumors, although in non-randomized studies only.[261,291,292,293,294,295,296,297]

Interferon Alpha

Limited retrospective data suggest activity of IFNα in the treatment of aggressive GCTB but at the cost of poor patient tolerance—a common side effect of systemic interferon-based therapy.[296,297,298,299] Consequently, the benefits and risks of IFNα should be balanced in clinical situations in which there are no alternatives.

Biphosphonates

Biphosphonates, with their antiosteoclastic properties, have shown activity in vitro in GCTB.[300,301] However, clinical data are scarce, with limited case reports, retrospective series, and one phase II trial having assessed zoledronic acid.[302,303,304,305] Modest clinical benefit and long-term local disease control have been reported in the adjuvant setting but without any significant preventive effect on local recurrence.[250,300,302,303,304,305,306]

Little information regarding the utility of calcitonin and sunitinib has been reported, but they represent other potential treatment options for recurrent GCTB.[250,307,308] Local control is occasionally seen with oral steroids in patients who have Paget's disease and GCTB.[309,310]

Denosumab

Denosumab is a fully human monoclonal antibody against RANKL. Its clinical benefit has been shown in phase II trials involving recurrent or unresectable GCTB.[260,311,312] Reported objective response rates of 86% are seen along with a reduced need for resective surgery. Long-lasting responses are seen in most patients (96% PFS at a median follow-up of 15 months), which combined with a favorable toxicity profile (1% incidence of osteonecrosis) make denosumab the therapy of first choice in patients who have GCTB (▶ Fig. 10.1).[251,312]

Based on results in 305 patients from two phase II trials, denosumab has been approved for patients who have unresectable

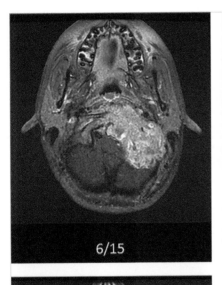
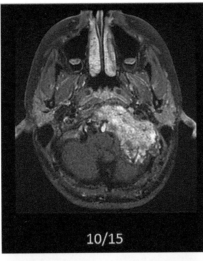
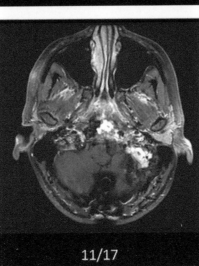

Fig. 10.1 Axial postcontrast T1-weighted MRIs of a 13-year-old girl who had a large skull base giant cell tumor. After the 6/15 scan, she was started on denosumab at 120 mg subcutaneous injection on days 1, 8, and 15 and then every 4 weeks. Scans show continuing response to therapy.

GCTB or in whom a surgery would result in significant functional morbidity. NCCN guidelines emphasize indication for use of denosumab in instances of unresectable tumor. However, there are no data regarding the optimal duration or dose schedule of denosumab. Additionally, the optimal timing for the use of denosumab is also not well defined. Denosumab use has been proposed in the neoadjuvant setting, when surgery is expected to be incomplete, and when disease is clinically aggressive or is associated with a low performance status (PS) and impaired quality of life.[273] The goals are to improve the resectability of the tumor by reducing its size (i.e., downstage) and to further achieve improvement in performance status (PS) and quality of life (QoL). Potential benefits in the adjuvant setting after surgery, to reduce local recurrence, is also under evaluation.[312]

There are limited data on the long-term safety of denosumab, especially relating to the most serious treatment-related adverse event, mandibular osteonecrosis. New challenges come with new therapies, and response assessment in GCTB is no exception. Postdenosumab treatment pathology can be challenging to interpret in some cases.[313] Most often seen is a significant reduction of giant cells and neoplastic stromal cells, with some degree of bone reformation. However, cellular atypia and some patterns of ossification may suggest osteosarcoma or an undifferentiated pleomorphic sarcoma.[255,260,313] Correlation of posttreatment pathology with clinical and imaging data is often necessary to achieve a correct diagnosis.

Although the role of (18F-FDG) PET scanning is not clear at time of diagnosis in GCTB, FDG-PET does appear to be a sensitive marker of early response to denosumab, as changes in standardized uptake values reflect tumor metabolism and angiogenesis.[314,315,316,317] Nevertheless, MRI should not be replaced by FDG-PET; rather, the latter provides correlative information that may augment MRI findings.

The introduction of denosumab has profoundly altered the management of GCTB of the skull base, providing a new treatment option that augments surgery. However, because many questions remain unanswered regarding the practical aspects and timing of denosumab treatment, further prospective randomized trials are needed.

10.6 Conclusion

"Benign" tumors of the skull base are characterized by a high local recurrence rate and attendant consequences, including diminished QOL and decreased survival. In some of these tumors, such as chordomas, improvements in global management have been observed over time with earlier diagnosis and better local control as a result of improved imaging and surgical techniques. Nevertheless, management of these tumors remains challenging, and despite the recent making of considerable progress in understandings of their genetics and molecular pathogenesis, many limitations remain with respect to current systemic therapies.

Because these tumors are rare, treatment of numbers of patients large enough to allow determination of the benefits of novel targeted therapies can be difficult. As a result, most studies of targeted agents have involved a single institution and comprised small numbers of patients. Furthermore, and as has become increasingly apparent in other tumor types, molecular

characterization and matching of actionable targets with targeted therapies are essential to best determining the role of these new therapies. Studies such as these will require multi-institutional efforts and likely also industry sponsors to provide access to novel targeted therapies. The application of precision or personalized oncology based on the molecular profiling of aberrant pathways in individual patients holds great promise for advancing the treatment of patients who have skull-based benign tumors.

References

[1] Louis DN, Perry A, Reifenberger G, et al. The 2016 World Health Organization Classification of Tumors of the Central Nervous System: a summary. Acta Neuropathol. 2016; 131(6):803–820

[2] Perry A, Stafford SL, Scheithauer BW, Suman VJ, Lohse CM. Meningioma grading: an analysis of histologic parameters. Am J Surg Pathol. 1997; 21(12):1455–1465

[3] Black PM, Villavicencio AT, Rhouddou C, Loeffler JS. Aggressive surgery and focal radiation in the management of meningiomas of the skull base: preservation of function with maintenance of local control. Acta Neurochir (Wien). 2001; 143(6):555–562

[4] Mathur A, Jain N, Kesavadas C, Thomas B, Kapilamoorthy TR. Imaging of skull base pathologies: role of advanced magnetic resonance imaging techniques. Neuroradiol J. 2015; 28(4):426–437

[5] Hakyemez B, Erdogan C, Bolca N, Yildirim N, Gokalp G, Parlak M. Evaluation of different cerebral mass lesions by perfusion-weighted MR imaging. J Magn Reson Imaging. 2006; 24(4):817–824

[6] Zimny A, Sasiadek M. Contribution of perfusion-weighted magnetic resonance imaging in the differentiation of meningiomas and other extra-axial tumors: case reports and literature review. J Neurooncol. 2011; 103(3):777–783

[7] Kremer S, Grand S, Rémy C, et al. Contribution of dynamic contrast MR imaging to the differentiation between dural metastasis and meningioma. Neuroradiology. 2004; 46(8):642–648

[8] Zhang H, Rödiger LA, Shen T, Miao J, Oudkerk M. Preoperative subtyping of meningiomas by perfusion MR imaging. Neuroradiology. 2008; 50(10):835–840

[9] Jolapara M, Kesavadas C, Radhakrishnan VV, et al. Role of diffusion tensor imaging in differentiating subtypes of meningiomas. J Neuroradiol. 2010; 37(5):277–283

[10] Cho YD, Choi GH, Lee SP, Kim JK. (1)H-MRS metabolic patterns for distinguishing between meningiomas and other brain tumors. Magn Reson Imaging. 2003; 21(6):663–672

[11] Mendenhall WM, Morris CG, Amdur RJ, Foote KD, Friedman WA. Radiotherapy alone or after subtotal resection for benign skull base meningiomas. Cancer. 2003; 98(7):1473–1482

[12] NCCN Clinical Practice Guidelines in Oncology [Internet]. Available from: http://www.nccn.org/professionals/physician_gls/f_guidelines.asp#cns

[13] Milker-Zabel S, Zabel-du Bois A, Huber P, Schlegel W, Debus J. Intensity-modulated radiotherapy for complex-shaped meningioma of the skull base: long-term experience of a single institution. Int J Radiat Oncol Biol Phys. 2007; 68(3):858–863

[14] Minniti G, Amichetti M, Enrici RM. Radiotherapy and radiosurgery for benign skull base meningiomas. Radiat Oncol. 2009; 4:42

[15] Lee JY, Niranjan A, McInerney J, Kondziolka D, Flickinger JC, Lunsford LD. Stereotactic radiosurgery providing long-term tumor control of cavernous sinus meningiomas. J Neurosurg. 2002; 97(1):65–72

[16] Spiegelmann R, Cohen ZR, Nissim O, Alezra D, Pfeffer R. Cavernous sinus meningiomas: a large LINAC radiosurgery series. J Neurooncol. 2010; 98(2):195–202

[17] Skeie BS, Enger PO, Skeie GO, Thorsen F, Pedersen PH. Gamma Knife surgery of meningiomas involving the cavernous sinus: long-term follow-up of 100 patients. Neurosurgery. 2010; 66(4):661–668, discussion 668–669

[18] Sahm F, Schrimpf D, Olar A, et al. TERT promoter mutations and risk of recurrence in meningioma. J Natl Cancer Inst. 2015; 108(5):djv377

[19] Yew A, Trang A, Nagasawa DT, et al. Chromosomal alterations, prognostic factors, and targeted molecular therapies for malignant meningiomas. J Clin Neurosci. 2013; 20(1):17–22

[20] Le Rhun E, Taillibert S, Chamberlain MC. Systemic therapy for recurrent meningioma. Expert Rev Neurother. 2016; 16(8):889–901

[21] Newton HB. Molecular neuro-oncology and development of targeted therapeutic strategies for brain tumors. Part 2: PI3K/Akt/PTEN, mTOR, SHH/PTCH and angiogenesis. Expert Rev Anticancer Ther. 2004; 4(1):105–128

[22] Kim WY, Lee HY. Brain angiogenesis in developmental and pathological processes: mechanism and therapeutic intervention in brain tumors. FEBS J. 2009; 276(17):4653–4664

[23] Wellenreuther R, Kraus JA, Lenartz D, et al. Analysis of the neurofibromatosis 2 gene reveals molecular variants of meningioma. Am J Pathol. 1995; 146 (4):827–832

[24] Mawrin C, Perry A. Pathological classification and molecular genetics of meningiomas. J Neurooncol. 2010; 99(3):379–391

[25] Pavelin S, Bečić K, Forempoher G, et al. The significance of immunohistochemical expression of merlin, Ki-67, and p53 in meningiomas. Appl Immunohistochem Mol Morphol. 2014; 22(1):46–49

[26] Miller R, Jr, DeCandio ML, Dixon-Mah Y, et al. Molecular targets and treatment of meningioma. J Neurol Neurosurg. 2014; 1(1):1000101

[27] Perry A, Gutmann DH, Reifenberger G. Molecular pathogenesis of meningiomas. J Neurooncol. 2004; 70(2):183–202

[28] Saraf S, McCarthy BJ, Villano JL. Update on meningiomas. Oncologist. 2011; 16(11):1604–1613

[29] Striedinger K, VandenBerg SR, Baia GS, McDermott MW, Gutmann DH, Lal A. The neurofibromatosis 2 tumor suppressor gene product, merlin, regulates human meningioma cell growth by signaling through YAP. Neoplasia. 2008; 10(11):1204–1212

[30] Wang H, Xu M, Cui X, et al. Aberrant expression of the candidate tumor suppressor gene DAL-1 due to hypermethylation in gastric cancer. Sci Rep. 2016; 6:21755

[31] Pervaiz S. Anti-cancer drugs of today and tomorrow: are we close to making the turn from treating to curing cancer? Curr Pharm Des. 2002; 8(19): 1723–1734

[32] Clark VE, Erson-Omay EZ, Serin A, et al. Genomic analysis of non-NF2 meningiomas reveals mutations in TRAF7, KLF4, AKT1, and SMO. Science. 2013; 339(6123):1077–1080

[33] Sahm F, Bissel J, Koelsche C, et al. AKT1E17K mutations cluster with meningothelial and transitional meningiomas and can be detected by SFRP1 immunohistochemistry. Acta Neuropathol. 2013; 126(5):757–762

[34] Dickinson PJ, Surace EI, Cambell M, et al. Expression of the tumor suppressor genes NF2, 4.1B, and TSLC1 in canine meningiomas. Vet Pathol. 2009; 46(5): 884–892

[35] Ragel BT, Jensen RL. Aberrant signaling pathways in meningiomas. J Neurooncol. 2010; 99(3):315–324

[36] Saydam O, Shen Y, Würdinger T, et al. Downregulated microRNA-200a in meningiomas promotes tumor growth by reducing E-cadherin and activating the Wnt/beta-catenin signaling pathway. Mol Cell Biol. 2009; 29(21): 5923–5940

[37] Zhou L, Ercolano E, Ammoun S, Schmid MC, Barczyk MA, Hanemann CO. Merlin-deficient human tumors show loss of contact inhibition and activation of Wnt/β-catenin signaling linked to the PDGFR/Src and Rac/PAK pathways. Neoplasia. 2011; 13(12):1101–1112

[38] Fernandez-Valle C, Tang Y, Ricard J, et al. Paxillin binds schwannomin and regulates its density-dependent localization and effect on cell morphology. Nat Genet. 2002; 31(3):354–362

[39] Cuevas IC, Slocum AL, Jun P, et al. Meningioma transcript profiles reveal deregulated Notch signaling pathway. Cancer Res. 2005; 65(12):5070–5075

[40] Boetto J, Bielle F, Sanson M, Peyre M, Kalamarides M. SMO mutation status defines a distinct and frequent molecular subgroup in olfactory groove meningiomas. Neuro-oncol. 2017; 19(3):345–351

[41] Santarius T, Kirsch M, Nikas DC, Imitola J, Black PM. Molecular analysis of alterations of the p18INK4c gene in human meningiomas. Neuropathol Appl Neurobiol. 2000; 26(1):67–75

[42] Cai SL, Tee AR, Short JD, et al. Activity of TSC2 is inhibited by AKT-mediated phosphorylation and membrane partitioning. J Cell Biol. 2006; 173(2):279–289

[43] Vander Haar E, Lee SI, Bandhakavi S, Griffin TJ, Kim DH. Insulin signalling to mTOR mediated by the Akt/PKB substrate PRAS40. Nat Cell Biol. 2007; 9(3): 316–323

[44] Xie J, Johnson RL, Zhang X, et al. Mutations of the PATCHED gene in several types of sporadic extracutaneous tumors. Cancer Res. 1997; 57(12): 2369–2372

[45] Chamberlain MC. The role of chemotherapy and targeted therapy in the treatment of intracranial meningioma. Curr Opin Oncol. 2012; 24(6): 666–671

[46] Mawrin C, Chung C, Preusser M. Biology and clinical management challenges in meningioma. Am Soc Clin Oncol Educ Book ASCO Am Soc Clin Oncol Meet. 2015; 35:e106–e115

[47] Preusser M, Berghoff AS, Hottinger AF. High-grade meningiomas: new avenues for drug treatment? Curr Opin Neurol. 2013; 26(6):708–715

[48] Kato Y, Nishihara H, Mohri H, et al. Clinicopathological evaluation of cyclooxygenase-2 expression in meningioma: immunohistochemical analysis of 76 cases of low and high-grade meningioma. Brain Tumor Pathol. 2014; 31 (1):23–30

[49] Kaley T, Barani I, Chamberlain M, et al. Historical benchmarks for medical therapy trials in surgery- and radiation-refractory meningioma: a RANO review. Neuro-oncol. 2014; 16(6):829–840

[50] Norden AD, Ligon KL, Hammond SN, et al. Phase II study of monthly pasireotide LAR (SOM230C) for recurrent or progressive meningioma. Neurology. 2015; 84(3):280–286

[51] Schrell UM, Rittig MG, Anders M, et al. Hydroxyurea for treatment of unresectable and recurrent meningiomas. II. Decrease in the size of meningiomas in patients treated with hydroxyurea. J Neurosurg. 1997; 86(5):840–844

[52] Mason WP, Gentili F, Macdonald DR, Hariharan S, Cruz CR, Abrey LE. Stabilization of disease progression by hydroxyurea in patients with recurrent or unresectable meningioma. J Neurosurg. 2002; 97(2):341–346

[53] Rosenthal MA, Ashley DL, Cher L. Treatment of high risk or recurrent meningiomas with hydroxyurea. J Clin Neurosci. 2002; 9(2):156–158

[54] Newton HB, Scott SR, Volpi C. Hydroxyurea chemotherapy for meningiomas: enlarged cohort with extended follow-up. Br J Neurosurg. 2004; 18 (5):495–499

[55] Loven D, Hardoff R, Sever ZB, et al. Non-resectable slow-growing meningiomas treated by hydroxyurea. J Neurooncol. 2004; 67(1–2):221–226

[56] Hahn BM, Schrell UMH, Sauer R, Fahlbusch R, Ganslandt O, Grabenbauer GG. Prolonged oral hydroxyurea and concurrent 3D-conformal radiation in patients with progressive or recurrent meningioma: results of a pilot study. J Neurooncol. 2005; 74(2):157–165

[57] Weston GJ, Martin AJ, Mufti GJ, Strong AJ, Gleeson MJ. Hydroxyurea treatment of meningiomas: a pilot study. Skull Base. 2006; 16(3):157–160. 820

[58] Kim M-S, Yu D-W, Jung Y-J, Kim SW, Chang CH, Kim OL. Long-term follow-up result of hydroxyurea chemotherapy for recurrent meningiomas. J Korean Neurosurg Soc. 2012; 52(6):517–522

[59] Chamberlain MC, Johnston SK. Hydroxyurea for recurrent surgery and radiation refractory meningioma: a retrospective case series. J Neurooncol. 2011; 104(3):765–771

[60] Chamberlain MC, Tsao-Wei DD, Groshen S. Temozolomide for treatment-resistant recurrent meningioma. Neurology. 2004; 62(7):1210–1212. 835

[61] Chamberlain MC, Tsao-Wei DD, Groshen S. Salvage chemotherapy with CPT-11 for recurrent meningioma. J Neurooncol. 2006; 78(3):271–276

[62] Swinnen LJ, Renkin C, Rushing EJ, et al. Proceedings SNO, annual meeting of the Society of Neuro-oncology, 18–21 Nov 2010, 830 Montreal, QC. Ongoing clinical trials. Abstract OT-08: iv70. Neuro-oncol. 2010; 12 suppl4:iv69–iv78

[63] Preusser M, Spiegl-Kreinecker S, Lötsch D, et al. Trabectedin has promising antineoplastic activity in high-grade meningioma. Cancer. 2012; 118(20): 5038–5049

[64] Chamberlain M. What constitutes activity of systemic therapy in recurrent meningioma? Neurology. 2015; 85:1090

[65] Rockhill J, Mrugala M, Chamberlain MC. Intracranial meningiomas: an overview of diagnosis and treatment. Neurosurg Focus. 2007; 23(4):E1

[66] Norden AD, Drappatz J, Wen PY. Advances in meningioma therapy. Curr Neurol Neurosci Rep. 2009; 9(3):231–240

[67] Sioka C, Kyritsis AP. Chemotherapy, hormonal therapy, and immunotherapy for recurrent meningiomas. J Neurooncol. 2009; 92(1):1–6

[68] Goldsmith B, McDermott MW. Meningioma. Neurosurg Clin N Am. 2006; 17 (2):111–120, vi

[69] Markwalder T-M, Seiler RW, Zava DT. Antiestrogenic therapy of meningiomas—a pilot study. Surg Neurol. 1985; 24(3):245–249

[70] Goodwin JW, Crowley J, Eyre HJ, Stafford B, Jaeckle KA, Townsend JJ. A phase II evaluation of tamoxifen in unresectable or refractory meningiomas: a Southwest Oncology Group study. J Neurooncol. 1993; 15(1):75–77

[71] Grunberg SM, Weiss MH. Lack of efficacy of megestrol acetate in the treatment of unresectable meningioma. J Neurooncol. 1990; 8(1):61–65

[72] Grunberg SM, Weiss MH, Spitz IM, et al. Treatment of unresectable meningiomas with the antiprogesterone agent mifepristone. J Neurosurg. 1991; 74 (6):861–866

[73] Grunberg SM, Weiss MH, Russell CA, et al. Long-term administration of mifepristone (RU486): clinical tolerance during extended treatment of meningioma. Cancer Invest. 2006; 24(8):727–733

[74] Jääskeläinen J, Laasonen E, Kärkkäinen J, Haltia M, Troupp H. Hormone treatment of meningiomas: lack of response to medroxyprogesterone acetate (MPA). A pilot study of five cases. Acta Neurochir (Wien). 1986; 80 (1–2):35–41

[75] Touat M, Lombardi G, Farina P, Kalamarides M, Sanson M. Successful treatment of multiple intracranial meningiomas with the antiprogesterone receptor agent mifepristone (RU486). Acta Neurochir (Wien). 2014; 156(10):1831–1835

[76] Chamberlain MC, Glantz MJ, Fadul CE. Recurrent meningioma: salvage therapy with long-acting somatostatin analogue. Neurology. 2007; 69 (10):969–973

[77] Johnson DR, Kimmel DW, Burch PA, et al. Phase II study of subcutaneous octreotide in adults with recurrent or progressive meningioma and meningeal hemangiopericytoma. Neuro-oncol. 2011; 13(5):530–535

[78] Simó M, Argyriou AA, Macià M, et al. Recurrent high-grade meningioma: a phase II trial with somatostatin analogue therapy. Cancer Chemother Pharmacol. 2014; 73(5):919–923

[79] Gerster-Gilliéron K, Forrer F, Maecke H, Mueller-Brand J, Merlo A, Cordier D. 90Y-DOTATOC as therapeutic option for complex recurrent or progressive meningiomas. J Nucl Med. 2015; 56(11):1748–1751

[80] Marincek N, Radojewski P, Dumont RA, et al. Somatostatin receptor-targeted radiopeptide therapy with 90Y-DOTATOC and 177Lu-DOTATOC in progressive meningioma: long-term results of a phase II clinical trial. J Nucl Med. 2015; 56(2):171–176

[81] Chamberlain MC, Glantz MJ. Interferon-alpha for recurrent World Health Organization grade 1 intracranial meningiomas. Cancer. 2008; 113(8): 2146–2151

[82] Chamberlain MC. IFN-α for recurrent surgery- and radiation-refractory high-grade meningioma: a retrospective case series. CNS Oncol. 2013; 2(3): 227–235

[83] Wen PY, Quant E, Drappatz J, Beroukhim R, Norden AD. Medical therapies for meningiomas. J Neurooncol. 2010; 99(3):365–378

[84] Mordechai O, Postovsky S, Vlodavsky E, et al. Metastatic rhabdoid meningioma with BRAF V600E mutation and good response to personalized therapy: case report and review of the literature. Pediatr Hematol Oncol. 2015; 32(3): 207–211

[85] Gelerstein E, Berger A, Jonas-Kimchi T, et al. Regression of intracranial meningioma following treatment with nivolumab: case report and review of the literature. J Clin Neurosci. 2017; 37:51–53

[86] Johnson M, Toms S. Mitogenic signal transduction pathways in meningiomas: novel targets for meningioma chemotherapy? J Neuropathol Exp Neurol. 2005; 64(12):1029–1036

[87] Simon M, Boström JP, Hartmann C. Molecular genetics of meningiomas: from basic research to potential clinical applications. Neurosurgery. 2007; 60(5):787–798

[88] Norden AD, Raizer JJ, Abrey LE, et al. Phase II trials of erlotinib or gefitinib in patients with recurrent meningioma. J Neurooncol. 2010; 96(2):211–217

[89] Chamberlain MC. Is there effective systemic therapy for recurrent surgery- and radiation-refractory meningioma? CNS Oncol. 2013; 2(1):1–5

[90] Pietras K, Sjöblom T, Rubin K, Heldin CH, Ostman A. PDGF receptors as cancer drug targets. Cancer Cell. 2003; 3(5):439–443

[91] Johnson MD, Woodard A, Kim P, Frexes-Steed M. Evidence for mitogen-associated protein kinase activation and transduction of mitogenic signals by platelet-derived growth factor in human meningioma cells. J Neurosurg. 2001; 94(2):293–300

[92] Todo T, Adams EF, Fahlbusch R, Dingermann T, Werner H. Autocrine growth stimulation of human meningioma cells by platelet-derived growth factor. J Neurosurg. 1996; 84(5):852–858, discussion 858–859

[93] Wen PY, Yung WKA, Lamborn KR, et al. Phase II study of imatinib mesylate for recurrent meningiomas (North American Brain Tumor Consortium study 01–08). Neuro-oncol. 2009; 11(6):853–860

[94] Reardon DA, Norden AD, Desjardins A, et al. Phase II study of Gleevec® plus hydroxyurea (HU) in adults with progressive or recurrent meningioma. J Neurooncol. 2012; 106(2):409–415

[95] Mazza E, Brandes A, Zanon S, et al. Hydroxyurea with or without imatinib in the treatment of recurrent or progressive meningiomas: a randomized phase II trial by Gruppo Italiano Cooperativo di Neuro-Oncologia (GICNO). Cancer Chemother Pharmacol. 2016; 77(1):115–120

[96] Nassehi D, Dyrbye H, Andresen M, et al. Vascular endothelial growth factor A protein level and gene expression in intracranial meningiomas with brain edema. APMIS. 2011; 119(12):831–843

[97] Preusser M, Hassler M, Birner P, et al. Microvascularization and expression of VEGF and its receptors in recurring meningiomas: pathobiological data in favor of anti-angiogenic therapy approaches. Clin Neuropathol. 2012; 31(5): 352–360

[98] Baumgarten P, Brokinkel B, Zinke J, et al. Expression of vascular endothelial growth factor (VEGF) and its receptors VEGFR1 and VEGFR2 in primary and recurrent WHO grade III meningiomas. Histol Histopathol. 2013; 28(9): 1157–1166

[99] Lou E, Sumrall AL, Turner S, et al. Bevacizumab therapy for adults with recurrent/progressive meningioma: a retrospective series. J Neurooncol. 2012; 109(1):63–70

[100] Nayak L, Iwamoto FM, Rudnick JD, et al. Atypical and anaplastic meningiomas treated with bevacizumab. J Neurooncol. 2012; 109(1):187–193

[101] Kaley TJ, Wen P, Schiff D, et al. Phase II trial of sunitinib for recurrent and progressive atypical and anaplastic meningioma. Neuro-oncol. 2015; 17(1): 116–121

[102] Raizer JJ, Grimm SA, Rademaker A, et al. A phase II trial of PTK787/ZK 222584 in recurrent or progressive radiation and surgery refractory meningiomas. J Neurooncol. 2014; 117(1):93–101

[103] Nunes FP, Merker VL, Jennings D, et al. Bevacizumab treatment for meningiomas in NF2: a retrospective analysis of 15 patients. PLoS One. 2013; 8(3): e59941

[104] Alanin MC, Klausen C, Caye-Thomasen P, et al. Effect of bevacizumab on intracranial meningiomas in patients with neurofibromatosis type 2—a retrospective case series. Int J Neurosci. 2016; 126(11):1002–1006

[105] Grimm S, Kumthekar P, Chamberlain M, et al. Phase II trial of bevacizumab in patients with surgery and radiation refractory progressive meningioma. Neuro-Oncol. 2015; 17(Suppl 5):v130. (abstract MNGO-04)

[106] Furtner J, Schöpf V, Seystahl K, et al. Kinetics of tumor size and peritumoral brain edema before, during, and after systemic therapy in recurrent WHO grade II or III meningioma. Neuro-oncol. 2016; 18(3):401–407

[107] Pachow D, Andrae N, Kliese N, et al. mTORC1 inhibitors suppress meningioma growth in mouse models. Clin Cancer Res. 2013; 19(5):1180–1189

[108] Graillon T, Defilles C, Mohamed A, et al. Combined treatment by octreotide and everolimus: octreotide enhances inhibitory effect of everolimus in aggressive meningiomas. J Neurooncol. 2015; 124(1):33–43

[109] Koschny R, Boehm C, Sprick MR, et al. Bortezomib sensitizes primary meningioma cells to TRAIL-induced apoptosis by enhancing formation of the death-inducing signaling complex. J Neuropathol Exp Neurol. 2014; 73(11): 1034–1046

[110] Domingues P, González-Tablas M, Otero Á, et al. Genetic/molecular alterations of meningiomas and the signaling pathways targeted. Oncotarget. 2015; 6(13):10671–10688

[111] Shah NR, Tancioni I, Ward KK, et al. Analyses of merlin/NF2 connection to FAK inhibitor responsiveness in serous ovarian cancer. Gynecol Oncol. 2014; 134(1):104–111

[112] Du Z, Abedalthagafi M, Aizer AA, et al. Increased expression of the immune modulatory molecule PD-L1 (CD274) in anaplastic meningioma. Oncotarget. 2015; 6(7):4704–4716

[113] Han SJ, Reis G, Kohanbash G, et al. Expression and prognostic impact of immune modulatory molecule PD-L1 in meningioma. J Neurooncol. 2016; 130 (3):543–552

[114] McMaster ML, Goldstein AM, Bromley CM, Ishibe N, Parry DM. Chordoma: incidence and survival patterns in the United States, 1973–1995. Cancer Causes Control. 2001; 12(1):1–11

[115] Rassekh CH, Nuss DW, Kapadia SB, Curtin HD, Weissman JL, Janecka IP. Chondrosarcoma of the nasal septum: skull base imaging and clinicopathologic correlation. Otolaryngol Head Neck Surg. 1996; 115(1):29–37

[116] Meyers SP, Hirsch WL, Jr, Curtin HD, Barnes L, Sekhar LN, Sen C. Chondrosarcomas of the skull base: MR imaging features. Radiology. 1992; 184 (1):103–108

[117] Doucet V, Peretti-Viton P, Figarella-Branger D, Manera L, Salamon G. MRI of intracranial chordomas. Extent of tumour and contrast enhancement: criteria for differential diagnosis. Neuroradiology. 1997; 39(8):571–576

[118] Youssef C, Aoun SG, Moreno JR, Bagley CA. Recent advances in understanding and managing chordomas. F1000 Res. 2016; 5:2902

[119] Gulluoglu S, Turksoy O, Kuskucu A, Ture U, Bayrak ÖF. The molecular aspects of chordoma. Neurosurg Rev. 2016; 39(2):185–196

[120] Lipplaa A, Dijkstra S, Gelderblom H. Efficacy of pazopanib and sunitinib in advanced axial chordoma: a single reference centre case series. Clin Sarcoma Res. 2016; 6:19

[121] Di Maio S, Temkin N, Ramanathan D, Sekhar LN. Current comprehensive management of cranial base chordomas: 10-year meta-analysis of observational studies. J Neurosurg. 2011; 115(6):1094–1105

[122] Yasuda M, Bresson D, Chibbaro S, et al. Chordomas of the skull base and cervical spine: clinical outcomes associated with a multimodal surgical resection combined with proton-beam radiation in 40 patients. Neurosurg Rev. 2012; 35(2):171–182, discussion 182–183

[123] McMaster M. Update on the epidemiology of chordoma: SEER registry data 1973–2007. Poster presented at: Third International Chordoma Research Workshop, March 17–19, 2011; Bethesda, MD

[124] Adson AW, Kernohan JW, Woltman HW. Cranial and cervical chordomas—a clinical and histologic study. Arch Neurol Psychiatry. 1935; 33(2):247–261

[125] Hruban RH, Traganos F, Reuter VE, Huvos AG. Chordomas with malignant spindle cell components: a DNA flow cytometric and immunohistochemical study with histogenetic implications. Am J Pathol. 1990; 137(2):435–447

[126] Mitchell A, Scheithauer BW, Unni KK, Forsyth PJ, Wold LE, McGivney DJ. Chordoma and chondroid neoplasms of the spheno-occiput: an immunohistochemical study of 41 cases with prognostic and nosologic implications. Cancer. 1993; 72(10):2943–2949

[127] Abenoza P, Sibley RK. Chordoma: an immunohistologic study. Hum Pathol. 1986; 17(7):744–747

[128] Meis JM, Giraldo AA. Chordoma: an immunohistochemical study of 20 cases. Arch Pathol Lab Med. 1988; 112(5):553–556

[129] Vujovic S, Henderson S, Presneau N, et al. Brachyury, a crucial regulator of notochordal development, is a novel biomarker for chordomas. J Pathol. 2006; 209(2):157–165

[130] Song W, Gobe GC. Understanding molecular pathways and targets of brachyury in epithelial-mesenchymal transition (EMT) in human cancers. Curr Cancer Drug Targets. 2016; 16(7):586–593

[131] Tirabosco R, Mangham DC, Rosenberg AE, et al. Brachyury expression in extra-axial skeletal and soft tissue chordomas: a marker that distinguishes chordoma from mixed tumor/myoepithelioma/parachordoma in soft tissue. Am J Surg Pathol. 2008; 32(4):572–580

[132] Oakley GJ, Fuhrer K, Seethala RR. Brachyury, SOX-9, and podoplanin, new markers in the skull base chordoma vs chondrosarcoma differential: a tissue microarray-based comparative analysis. Mod Pathol. 2008; 21(12):1461–1469

[133] Schwab JH, Boland PJ, Agaram NP, et al. Chordoma and chondrosarcoma gene profile: implications for immunotherapy. Cancer Immunol Immunother. 2009; 58(3):339–349

[134] Terahara A, Niemierko A, Goitein M, et al. Analysis of the relationship between tumor dose inhomogeneity and local control in patients with skull base chordoma. Int J Radiat Oncol Biol Phys. 1999; 45(2):351–358

[135] Catton C, O'Sullivan B, Bell R, et al. Chordoma: long-term follow-up after radical photon irradiation. Radiother Oncol. 1996; 41(1):67–72

[136] Stacchiotti S, Sommer J, Chordoma Global Consensus Group. Building a global consensus approach to chordoma: a position paper from the medical and patient community. Lancet Oncol. 2015; 16(2):e71–e83

[137] Di Maio S, Rostomily R, Sekhar LN. Current surgical outcomes for cranial base chordomas: cohort study of 95 patients. Neurosurgery. 2012; 70(6):1355–1360, discussion 1360

[138] Chibbaro S, Cornelius JF, Froelich S, et al. Endoscopic endonasal approach in the management of skull base chordomas—clinical experience on a large series, technique, outcome, and pitfalls. Neurosurg Rev. 2014; 37(2):217–224, discussion 224–225

[139] Fernandez-Miranda JC, Gardner PA, Snyderman CH, et al. Clival chordomas: a pathological, surgical, and radiotherapeutic review. Head Neck. 2014; 36(6):892–906

[140] Zhang Q, Kong F, Yan B, Ni Z, Liu H. Endoscopic endonasal surgery for clival chordoma and chondrosarcoma. ORL J Otorhinolaryngol Relat Spec. 2008; 70(2):124–129

[141] Fatemi N, Dusick JR, Gorgulho AA, et al. Endonasal microscopic removal of clival chordomas. Surg Neurol. 2008; 69(4):331–338

[142] Saito K, Toda M, Tomita T, Ogawa K, Yoshida K. Surgical results of an endoscopic endonasal approach for clival chordomas. Acta Neurochir (Wien). 2012; 154(5):879–886

[143] Stacchiotti S, Gronchi A, Fossati P, et al. Best practices for the management of local-regional recurrent chordoma: a position paper by the Chordoma Global Consensus Group. Ann Oncol. 2017; 28(6):1230–1242

[144] Di Maio S, Yip S, Al Zhrani GA, et al. Novel targeted therapies in chordoma: an update. Ther Clin Risk Manag. 2015; 11:873–883

[145] Di Maio S, Kong E, Yip S, Rostomily R. Converging paths to progress for skull base chordoma: review of current therapy and future molecular targets. Surg Neurol Int. 2013; 4:72

[146] Tzortzidis F, Elahi F, Wright D, Natarajan SK, Sekhar LN. Patient outcome at long-term follow-up after aggressive microsurgical resection of cranial base chordomas. Neurosurgery. 2006; 59(2):230–237

[147] Weber DC, Malyapa R, Albertini F, et al. Long term outcomes of patients with skull-base low-grade chondrosarcoma and chordoma patients treated with pencil beam scanning proton therapy. Radiother Oncol. 2016; 120(1):169–174

[148] Matloob SA, Nasir HA, Choi D. Proton beam therapy in the management of skull base chordomas: systematic review of indications, outcomes, and implications for neurosurgeons. Br J Neurosurg. 2016; 30(4):382–387

[149] Schulz-Ertner D, Karger CP, Feuerhake A, et al. Effectiveness of carbon ion radiotherapy in the treatment of skull-base chordomas. Int J Radiat Oncol Biol Phys. 2007; 68(2):449–457

[150] Sahgal A, Chan MW, Atenafu EG, et al. Image-guided, intensity-modulated radiation therapy (IG-IMRT) for skull base chordoma and chondrosarcoma: preliminary outcomes. Neuro-oncol. 2015; 17(6):889–894

[151] Colia V, Stacchiotti S. Medical treatment of advanced chordomas. Eur J Cancer. 2017; 83:220–228

[152] Kitamura Y, Sasaki H, Kimura T, et al. Molecular and clinical risk factors for recurrence of skull base chordomas: gain on chromosome 2p, expression of brachyury, and lack of irradiation negatively correlate with patient prognosis. J Neuropathol Exp Neurol. 2013; 72(9):816–823

[153] Miettinen M, Wang Z, Lasota J, Heery C, Schlom J, Palena C. Nuclear brachyury expression is consistent in chordoma, common in germ cell tumors and small cell carcinomas, and rare in other carcinomas and sarcomas: an immunohistochemical study of 5229 cases. Am J Surg Pathol. 2015; 39(10):1305–1312

[154] Palena C, Roselli M, Litzinger MT, et al. Overexpression of the EMT driver brachyury in breast carcinomas: association with poor prognosis. J Natl Cancer Inst. 2014; 106(5):106 pii

[155] Du R, Wu S, Lv X, Fang H, Wu S, Kang J. Overexpression of brachyury contributes to tumor metastasis by inducing epithelial-mesenchymal transition in hepatocellular carcinoma. J Exp Clin Cancer Res. 2014; 33:105

[156] Yoshihama R, Yamaguchi K, Imajyo I, et al. Expression levels of SOX2, KLF4 and brachyury transcription factors are associated with metastasis and poor prognosis in oral squamous cell carcinoma. Oncol Lett. 2016; 11(2):1435–1446

[157] Zhang L, Guo S, Schwab JH, et al. Tissue microarray immunohistochemical detection of brachyury is not a prognostic indicator in chordoma. PLoS One. 2013; 8(9):e75851

[158] Yang C, Hornicek FJ, Wood KB, et al. Characterization and analysis of human chordoma cell lines. Spine. 2010; 35(13):1257–1264

[159] Rinner B, Froehlich EV, Buerger K, et al. Establishment and detailed functional and molecular genetic characterisation of a novel sacral chordoma cell line, MUG-Chor1. Int J Oncol. 2012; 40(2):443–451

[160] Diaz RJ, Guduk M, Romagnuolo R, et al. High-resolution whole-genome analysis of skull base chordomas implicates FHIT loss in chordoma pathogenesis. Neoplasia. 2012; 14(9):788–798

[161] Horbinski C, Oakley GJ, Cieply K, et al. The prognostic value of Ki-67, p53, epidermal growth factor receptor, 1p36, 9p21, 10q23, and 17p13 in skull base chordomas. Arch Pathol Lab Med. 2010; 134(8):1170–1176

[162] Presneau N, Shalaby A, Idowu B, et al. Potential therapeutic targets for chordoma: PI3K/AKT/TSC1/TSC2/mTOR pathway. Br J Cancer. 2009; 100(9):1406–1414

[163] Shalaby A, Presneau N, Ye H, et al. The role of epidermal growth factor receptor in chordoma pathogenesis: a potential therapeutic target. J Pathol. 2011; 223(3):336–346

[164] Sommer J, Itani DM, Homlar KC, et al. Methylthioadenosine phosphorylase and activated insulin-like growth factor-1 receptor/insulin receptor: potential therapeutic targets in chordoma. J Pathol. 2010; 220(5):608–617

[165] Fasig JH, Dupont WD, LaFleur BJ, Olson SJ, Cates JM. Immunohistochemical analysis of receptor tyrosine kinase signal transduction activity in chordoma. Neuropathol Appl Neurobiol. 2008; 34(1):95–104

[166] Weinberger PM, Yu Z, Kowalski D, et al. Differential expression of epidermal growth factor receptor, c-Met, and HER2/neu in chordoma compared with 17 other malignancies. Arch Otolaryngol Head Neck Surg. 2005; 131(8):707–711

[167] Ptaszyński K, Szumera-Ciećkiewicz A, Owczarek J, et al. Epidermal growth factor receptor (EGFR) status in chordoma. Pol J Pathol. 2009; 60(2):81–87

[168] Tamborini E, Virdis E, Negri T, et al. Analysis of receptor tyrosine kinases (RTKs) and downstream pathways in chordomas. Neuro-oncol. 2010; 12(8):776–789

[169] Tamborini E, Miselli F, Negri T, et al. Molecular and biochemical analyses of platelet-derived growth factor receptor (PDGFR) B, PDGFRA, and KIT receptors in chordomas. Clin Cancer Res. 2006; 12(23):6920–6928

[170] Casali PG, Messina A, Stacchiotti S, et al. Imatinib mesylate in chordoma. Cancer. 2004; 101(9):2086–2097

[171] Orzan F, Terreni MR, Longoni M, et al. Expression study of the target receptor tyrosine kinase of Imatinib mesylate in skull base chordomas. Oncol Rep. 2007; 18(1):249–252

[172] Li X, Ji Z, Ma Y, Qiu X, Fan Q, Ma B. Expression of hypoxia-inducible factor-1α, vascular endothelial growth factor and matrix metalloproteinase-2 in sacral chordomas. Oncol Lett. 2012; 3(6):1268–1274

[173] Chen KW, Yang HL, Lu J, et al. Expression of vascular endothelial growth factor and matrix metalloproteinase-9 in sacral chordoma. J Neurooncol. 2011; 101(3):357–363

[174] Scheipl S, Lohberger B, Rinner B, et al. Histone deacetylase inhibitors as potential therapeutic approaches for chordoma: an immunohistochemical and functional analysis. J Orthop Res. 2013; 31(12):1999–2005

[175] Zhang Y, Schiff D, Park D, Abounader R. MicroRNA-608 and microRNA-34a regulate chordoma malignancy by targeting EGFR, Bcl-xL and MET. PLoS One. 2014; 9(3):e91546

[176] Osaka E, Kelly AD, Spentzos D, et al. MicroRNA-155 expression is independently predictive of outcome in chordoma. Oncotarget. 2015; 6(11):9125–9139

[177] Osaka E, Yang X, Shen JK, et al. MicroRNA-1 (miR-1) inhibits chordoma cell migration and invasion by targeting slug. J Orthop Res. 2014; 32(8):1075–1082

[178] Duan Z, Shen J, Yang X, et al. Prognostic significance of miRNA-1 (miR-1) expression in patients with chordoma. J Orthop Res. 2014; 32(5):695–701

[179] Duan Z, Choy E, Nielsen GP, et al. Differential expression of microRNA (miRNA) in chordoma reveals a role for miRNA-1 in Met expression. J Orthop Res. 2010; 28(6):746–752

[180] Hsu W, Mohyeldin A, Shah SR, et al. Generation of chordoma cell line JHC7 and the identification of brachyury as a novel molecular target. J Neurosurg. 2011; 115:760–769

[181] Hu Y, Mintz A, Shah SR, Quinones-Hinojosa A, Hsu W. The FGFR/MEK/ERK/brachyury pathway is critical for chordoma cell growth and survival. Carcinogenesis. 2014; 35(7):1491–1499

[182] Nelson AC, Pillay N, Henderson S, et al. An integrated functional genomics approach identifies the regulatory network directed by brachyury (T) in chordoma. J Pathol. 2012; 228(3):274–285

[183] Heery CS, Marte H, Madan J, et al. NCI experience using yeast-brachyury vaccine (GI-6301) in patients (pts) with advanced chordoma. J Clin Oncol. 2014; 32:3081–3081

[184] Schwab J, Antonescu C, Boland P, et al. Combination of PI3K/mTOR inhibition demonstrates efficacy in human chordoma. Anticancer Res. 2009; 29(6):1867–1871

[185] Stacchiotti S, Marrari A, Tamborini E, et al. Response to imatinib plus sirolimus in advanced chordoma. Ann Oncol. 2009; 20(11):1886–1894

[186] Han S, Polizzano C, Nielsen GP, Hornicek FJ, Rosenberg AE, Ramesh V. Aberrant hyperactivation of akt and mammalian target of rapamycin complex 1 signaling in sporadic chordomas. Clin Cancer Res. 2009; 15(6):1940–1946

[187] Davies JM, Robinson AE, Cowdrey C, et al. Generation of a patient-derived chordoma xenograft and characterization of the phosphoproteome in a recurrent chordoma. J Neurosurg. 2014; 120(2):331–336

[188] Ricci-Vitiani L, Runci D, D'Alessandris QG, et al. Chemotherapy of skull base chordoma tailored on responsiveness of patient-derived tumor cells to rapamycin. Neoplasia. 2013; 15(7):773–782

[189] Shrager J, Tenenbaum JM. Rapid learning for precision oncology. Nat Rev Clin Oncol. 2014; 11(2):109–118

[190] Stacchiotti S, Longhi A, Ferraresi V, et al. Phase II study of imatinib in advanced chordoma. J Clin Oncol. 2012; 30(9):914–920

[191] Hindi N, Casali PG, Morosi C, et al. Imatinib in advanced chordoma: a retrospective case series analysis. Eur J Cancer. 2015; 51(17):2609–2614

[192] Bompas E, Le Cesne A, Tresch-Bruneel E, et al. Sorafenib in patients with locally advanced and metastatic chordomas: a phase II trial of the French Sarcoma Group (GSF/GETO). Ann Oncol. 2015; 26(10):2168–2173

[193] Stacchiotti S, Tamborini E, Lo Vullo S, et al. Phase II study on lapatinib in advanced EGFR-positive chordoma. Ann Oncol. 2013; 24(7):1931–1936

[194] Hof H, Welzel T, Debus J. Effectiveness of cetuximab/gefitinib in the therapy of a sacral chordoma. Onkologie. 2006; 29(12):572–574

[195] Lindén O, Stenberg L, Kjellén E. Regression of cervical spinal cord compression in a patient with chordoma following treatment with cetuximab and gefitinib. Acta Oncol. 2009; 48(1):158–159

[196] Launay SG, Chetaille B, Medina F, et al. Efficacy of epidermal growth factor receptor targeting in advanced chordoma: case report and literature review. BMC Cancer. 2011; 11:423

[197] Singhal N, Kotasek D, Parnis FX. Response to erlotinib in a patient with treatment refractory chordoma. Anticancer Drugs. 2009; 20(10):953–955

[198] Asklund T, Danfors T, Henriksson R. PET response and tumor stabilization under erlotinib and bevacizumab treatment of an intracranial lesion noninvasively diagnosed as likely chordoma. Clin Neuropathol. 2011; 30(5):242–246

[199] Yang C, Schwab JH, Schoenfeld AJ, et al. A novel target for treatment of chordoma: signal transducers and activators of transcription 3. Mol Cancer Ther. 2009; 8(9):2597–2605

[200] Lubin M, Lubin A. Selective killing of tumors deficient in methylthioadenosine phosphorylase: a novel strategy. PLoS One. 2009; 4(5):e5735

[201] Laws ER, Jr. Transsphenoidal microsurgery in the management of craniopharyngioma. J Neurosurg. 1980; 52(5):661–666

[202] Northfield DW. Rathke-pouch tumours. Brain. 1957; 80(3):293–312

[203] Rush JA, Younge BR, Campbell RJ, MacCarty CS. Optic glioma: long-term follow-up of 85 histopathologically verified cases. Ophthalmology. 1982; 89(11):1213–1219

[204] Bollati A, Giunta F, Lenzi A, Marini G. Third ventricle intrinsic craniopharingioma: case report. J Neurosurg Sci. 1974; 18(3):216–219

[205] Cashion EL, Young JM. Intraventricular craniopharyngioma: report of two cases. J Neurosurg. 1971; 34(1):84–87

[206] Bunin GR, Surawicz TS, Witman PA, Preston-Martin S, Davis F, Bruner JM. The descriptive epidemiology of craniopharyngioma. J Neurosurg. 1998; 89(4):547–551

[207] Louis DN, Ohgaki H, Wiestler OD, Cavenee WK, eds. Craniopharyngioma. In: World Health Organization Classification of Tumours of the Nervous System, Editorial and Consensus Conference Working Group, Lyon, France: IARC Press; 2007

[208] Weiner HL, Wisoff JH, Rosenberg ME, et al. Craniopharyngiomas: a clinico-pathological analysis of factors predictive of recurrence and functional outcome. Neurosurgery. 1994; 35(6):1001–1010, discussion 1010–1011

[209] Crotty TB, Scheithauer BW, Young WF, Jr, et al. Papillary craniopharyngioma: a clinicopathological study of 48 cases. J Neurosurg. 1995; 83(2):206–214

[210] Minniti G, Esposito V, Amichetti M, Enrici RM. The role of fractionated radiotherapy and radiosurgery in the management of patients with craniopharyngioma. Neurosurg Rev. 2009; 32(2):125–132

[211] Combs SE, Thilmann C, Huber PE, Hoess A, Debus J, Schulz-Ertner D. Achievement of long-term local control in patients with craniopharyngiomas using high precision stereotactic radiotherapy. Cancer. 2007; 109(11):2308–2314

[212] Kobayashi T. Long-term results of Gamma Knife radiosurgery for 100 consecutive cases of craniopharyngioma and a treatment strategy. Prog Neurol Surg. 2009; 22:63–76

[213] Niranjan A, Kano H, Mathieu D, Kondziolka D, Flickinger JC, Lunsford LD. Radiosurgery for craniopharyngioma. Int J Radiat Oncol Biol Phys. 2010; 78(1):64–71

[214] Fitzek MM, Linggood RM, Adams J, Munzenrider JE. Combined proton and photon irradiation for craniopharyngioma: long-term results of the early cohort of patients treated at Harvard Cyclotron Laboratory and Massachusetts General Hospital. Int J Radiat Oncol Biol Phys. 2006; 64(5):1348–1354

[215] Luu QT, Loredo LN, Archambeau JO, Yonemoto LT, Slater JM, Slater JD. Fractionated proton radiation treatment for pediatric craniopharyngioma: preliminary report. Cancer J. 2006; 12(2):155–159

[216] Bishop AJ, Greenfield B, Mahajan A, et al. Proton beam therapy versus conformal photon radiation therapy for childhood craniopharyngioma: multi-institutional analysis of outcomes, cyst dynamics, and toxicity. Int J Radiat Oncol Biol Phys. 2014; 90(2):354–361

[217] McMurry FG, Hardy RW, Jr, Dohn DF, Sadar E, Gardner WJ. Long term results in the management of craniopharyngiomas. Neurosurgery. 1977; 1(3):238–241

[218] Ignelzi RJ, Squire LR. Recovery from anterograde and retrograde amnesia after percutaneous drainage of a cystic craniopharyngioma. J Neurol Neurosurg Psychiatry. 1976; 39(12):1231–1235

[219] Gutin PH, Klemme WM, Lagger RL, MacKay AR, Pitts LH, Hosobuchi Y. Management of the unresectable cystic craniopharyngioma by aspiration through an Ommaya reservoir drainage system. J Neurosurg. 1980; 52(1):36–40

[220] Manaka S, Teramoto A, Takakura K. The efficacy of radiotherapy for craniopharyngioma. J Neurosurg. 1985; 62(5):648–656

[221] Huk WJ, Mahlstedt J. Intracystic radiotherapy (90Y) of craniopharyngiomas: CT-guided stereotaxic implantation of indwelling drainage system. AJNR Am J Neuroradiol. 1983; 4(3):803–806

[222] Julow J, Lányi F, Hajda M, et al. The radiotherapy of cystic craniopharyngioma with intracystic installation of 90Y silicate colloid. Acta Neurochir (Wien). 1985; 74(3–4):94–99

[223] Voges J, Sturm V, Lehrke R, Treuer H, Gauss C, Berthold F. Cystic craniopharyngioma: long-term results after intracavitary irradiation with stereotactically applied colloidal beta-emitting radioactive sources. Neurosurgery. 1997; 40(2):263–269, discussion 269–270

[224] Pollock BE, Lunsford LD, Kondziolka D, Levine G, Flickinger JC. Phosphorus-32 intracavitary irradiation of cystic craniopharyngiomas: current technique and long-term results. Int J Radiat Oncol Biol Phys. 1995; 33(2):437–446

[225] Backlund EO, Johansson L, Sarby B. Studies on craniopharyngiomas. II. Treatment by stereotaxis and radiosurgery. Acta Chir Scand. 1972; 138(8):749–759

[226] Van den Berge JH, Blaauw G, Breeman WA, Rahmy A, Wijngaarde R. Intracavitary brachytherapy of cystic craniopharyngiomas. J Neurosurg. 1992; 77(4):545–550

[227] Barriger RB, Chang A, Lo SS, et al. Phosphorus-32 therapy for cystic craniopharyngiomas. Radiother Oncol. 2011; 98(2):207–212

[228] Zhang S, Fang Y, Cai BW, Xu JG, You C. Intracystic bleomycin for cystic craniopharyngiomas in children. Cochrane Database Syst Rev. 2016; 7: CD008890

[229] Hukin J, Steinbok P, Lafay-Cousin L, et al. Intracystic bleomycin therapy for craniopharyngioma in children: the Canadian experience. Cancer. 2007; 109(10):2124–2131

[230] Olsson DS, Andersson E, Bryngelsson IL, Nilsson AG, Johannsson G. Excess mortality and morbidity in patients with craniopharyngioma, especially in patients with childhood onset: a population-based study in Sweden. J Clin Endocrinol Metab. 2015; 100(2):467–474

[231] Lo AC, Howard AF, Nichol A, et al. Long-term outcomes and complications in patients with craniopharyngioma: the British Columbia Cancer Agency experience. Int J Radiat Oncol Biol Phys. 2014; 88(5):1011–1018

[232] Liu AK, Bagrosky B, Fenton LZ, et al. Vascular abnormalities in pediatric craniopharyngioma patients treated with radiation therapy. Pediatr Blood Cancer. 2009; 52(2):227–230

[233] Enchev Y, Ferdinandov D, Kounin G, Encheva E, Bussarsky V. Radiation-induced gliomas following radiotherapy for craniopharyngiomas: a case report and review of the literature. Clin Neurol Neurosurg. 2009; 111(7):591–596

[234] Oikonomou E, Barreto DC, Soares B, De Marco L, Buchfelder M, Adams EF. Beta-catenin mutations in craniopharyngiomas and pituitary adenomas. J Neurooncol. 2005; 73(3):205–209

[235] Martinez-Gutierrez JC, D'Andrea MR, Cahill DP, Santagata S, Barker FG, II, Brastianos PK. Diagnosis and management of craniopharyngiomas in the era of genomics and targeted therapy. Neurosurg Focus. 2016; 41(6):E2

[236] Kato K, Nakatani Y, Kanno H, et al. Possible linkage between specific histological structures and aberrant reactivation of the Wnt pathway in adamantinomatous craniopharyngioma. J Pathol. 2004; 203(3):814–821

[237] Sekine S, Shibata T, Kokubu A, et al. Craniopharyngiomas of adamantinomatous type harbor beta-catenin gene mutations. Am J Pathol. 2002; 161(6):1997–2001

[238] Buslei R, Nolde M, Hofmann B, et al. Common mutations of beta-catenin in adamantinomatous craniopharyngiomas but not in other tumours originating from the sellar region. Acta Neuropathol. 2005; 109(6):589–597

[239] Brastianos PK, Taylor-Weiner A, Manley PE, et al. Exome sequencing identifies BRAF mutations in papillary craniopharyngiomas. Nat Genet. 2014; 46(2):161–165

[240] Larkin SJ, Preda V, Karavitaki N, Grossman A, Ansorge O. BRAF V600E mutations are characteristic for papillary craniopharyngioma and may coexist with CTNNB1-mutated adamantinomatous craniopharyngioma. Acta Neuropathol. 2014; 127(6):927–929

[241] Cavalheiro S, Di Rocco C, Valenzuela S, et al. Craniopharyngiomas: intratumoral chemotherapy with interferon-alpha: a multicenter preliminary study with 60 cases. Neurosurg Focus. 2010; 28(4):E12

[242] Cavalheiro S, Dastoli PA, Silva NS, Toledo S, Lederman H, da Silva MC. Use of interferon alpha in intratumoral chemotherapy for cystic craniopharyngioma. Childs Nerv Syst. 2005; 21(8–9):719–724

[243] Dastoli PA, Nicácio JM, Silva NS, et al. Cystic craniopharyngioma: intratumoral chemotherapy with alpha interferon. Arq Neuropsiquiatr. 2011; 69(1):50–55

[244] Aylwin SJ, Bodi I, Beaney R. Pronounced response of papillary craniopharyngioma to treatment with vemurafenib, a BRAF inhibitor. Pituitary. 2016; 19(5):544–546

[245] Brastianos PK, Shankar GM, Gill CM, et al. Dramatic response of BRAF V600E mutant papillary craniopharyngioma to targeted therapy. J Natl Cancer Inst. 2015; 108(2):djv310

[246] Roque A, Odia Y. BRAF-V600E mutant papillary craniopharyngioma dramatically responds to combination BRAF and MEK inhibitors. CNS Oncol. 2017; 6(2):95–99

[247] Robert C, Karaszewska B, Schachter J, et al. Improved overall survival in melanoma with combined dabrafenib and trametinib. N Engl J Med. 2015; 372(1):30–39

[248] Brastianos PK, Santagata S. Endocrine tumors: BRAF V600E mutations in papillary craniopharyngioma. Eur J Endocrinol. 2016; 174(4):R139–R144

[249] Tritos NA. Is there a role for targeted medical therapies in patients with craniopharyngiomas? Future Oncol. 2015; 11(24):3221–3223

[250] Singh AS, Chawla NS, Chawla SP. Giant-cell tumor of bone: treatment options and role of denosumab. Biologics. 2015; 9:69–74

[251] Guajardo JH, de la Peña C, Gonzalez MF, et al. Giant cell tumour of the skull base treated with surgery, stereotactic radiosurgery and denosumab: case report and review of literature. Open Access Library Journal.. 2017; 4:e3571

[252] Murphey MD, Nomikos GC, Flemming DJ, Gannon FH, Temple HT, Kransdorf MJ. From the archives of AFIP. Imaging of giant cell tumor and giant cell reparative granuloma of bone: radiologic-pathologic correlation. Radiographics. 2001; 21(5):1283–1309

[253] Kwon JW, Chung HW, Cho EY, et al. MRI findings of giant cell tumors of the spine. AJR Am J Roentgenol. 2007; 189(1):246–250

[254] Campanacci M, Baldini N, Boriani S, Sudanese A. Giant-cell tumor of bone. J Bone Joint Surg Am. 1987; 69(1):106–114

[255] Thomas DM. RANKL, denosumab, and giant cell tumor of bone. Curr Opin Oncol. 2012; 24(4):397–403

[256] Lacey DL, Boyle WJ, Simonet WS, et al. Bench to bedside: elucidation of the OPG-RANK-RANKL pathway and the development of denosumab. Nat Rev Drug Discov. 2012; 11(5):401–419

[257] Roeder F, Timke C, Zwicker F, et al. Intensity modulated radiotherapy (IMRT) in benign giant cell tumors—a single institution case series and a short review of the literature. Thieke C, Bischof M, Debus J, Huber PE

[258] Kim IY, Jung S, Jung TY, et al. Gamma Knife radiosurgery for giant cell tumor of the petrous bone. Clin Neurol Neurosurg. 2012; 114(2):185–189

[259] Colia V, Provenzano S, Hindi N, Casali PG, Stacchiotti S. Systemic therapy for selected skull base sarcomas: chondrosarcoma, chordoma, giant cell tumour and solitary fibrous tumour/hemangiopericytoma. Rep Pract Oncol Radiother. 2016; 21(4):361–369

[260] Thomas D, Henshaw R, Skubitz K, et al. Denosumab in patients with giant-cell tumour of bone: an open-label, phase 2 study. Lancet Oncol. 2010; 11(3):275–280

[261] Osaka S, Toriyama M, Taira K, Sano S, Saotome K. Analysis of giant cell tumor of bone with pulmonary metastases. Clin Orthop Relat Res. 1997 (335):253–261

[262] Morgan T, Atkins GJ, Trivett MK, et al. Molecular profiling of giant cell tumor of bone and the osteoclastic localization of ligand for receptor activator of nuclear factor kappaB. Am J Pathol. 2005; 167(1):117–128

[263] Schwartz HS, Jenkins RB, Dahl RJ, Dewald GW. Cytogenetic analyses on giant-cell tumors of bone. Clin Orthop Relat Res. 1989(240):250–260

[264] Haque AU, Moatasim A. Giant cell tumor of bone: a neoplasm or a reactive condition? Int J Clin Exp Pathol. 2008; 1(6):489–501

[265] Papanastassiou I, Ioannou M, Papagelopoulos PJ, et al. P53 expression as a prognostic marker in giant cell tumor of bone: a pilot study. Orthopedics. 2010; 33(5):33

[266] Moskovszky L, Dezsö K, Athanasou N, et al. Centrosome abnormalities in giant cell tumour of bone: possible association with chromosomal instability. Mod Pathol. 2010; 23(3):359–366

[267] Smith LT, Mayerson J, Nowak NJ, et al. 20q11.1 amplification in giant-cell tumor of bone: array CGH, FISH, and association with outcome. Genes Chromosomes Cancer. 2006; 45(10):957–966

[268] Behjati S, Tarpey PS, Presneau N, et al. Distinct H3F3A and H3F3B driver mutations define chondroblastoma and giant cell tumor of bone. Nat Genet. 2013; 45(12):1479–1482

[269] Rao UN, Goodman M, Chung WW, Swalski P, Pal R, Finkelstein S. Molecular analysis of primary and recurrent giant cell tumors of bone. Cancer Genet Cytogenet. 2005; 158(2):126–136

[270] Gorunova L, Vult von Steyern F, Storlazzi CT, et al. Cytogenetic analysis of 101 giant cell tumors of bone: nonrandom patterns of telomeric associations and other structural aberrations. Genes Chromosomes Cancer. 2009; 48(7): 583–602

[271] Forsyth RG, De Boeck G, Bekaert S, et al. Telomere biology in giant cell tumour of bone. J Pathol. 2008; 214(5):555–563

[272] Schwartz HS, Dahir GA, Butler MG. Telomere reduction in giant cell tumor of bone and with aging. Cancer Genet Cytogenet. 1993; 71(2):132–138

[273] van der Heijden L, Dijkstra PDS, van de Sande MAJ, et al. The clinical approach toward giant cell tumor of bone. Oncologist. 2014; 19(5):550–561

[274] Matsuo T, Hiyama E, Sugita T, et al. Telomerase activity in giant cell tumors of bone. Ann Surg Oncol. 2007; 14(10):2896–2902

[275] Atkins GJ, Haynes DR, Graves SE, et al. Expression of osteoclast differentiation signals by stromal elements of giant cell tumors. J Bone Miner Res. 2000; 15(4):640–649

[276] Skubitz KM, Cheng EY, Clohisy DR, Thompson RC, Skubitz AP. Gene expression in giant-cell tumors. J Lab Clin Med. 2004; 144(4):193–200

[277] Huang L, Xu J, Wood DJ, Zheng MH. Gene expression of osteoprotegerin ligand, osteoprotegerin, and receptor activator of NF-kappaB in giant cell tumor of bone: possible involvement in tumor cell-induced osteoclast-like cell formation. Am J Pathol. 2000; 156(3):761–767

[278] Roux S, Amazit L, Meduri G, Guiochon-Mantel A, Milgrom E, Mariette X. RANK (receptor activator of nuclear factor kappa B) and RANK ligand are expressed in giant cell tumors of bone. Am J Clin Pathol. 2002; 117(2): 210–216

[279] Hemingway F, Taylor R, Knowles HJ, Athanasou NA. RANKL-independent human osteoclast formation with APRIL, BAFF, NGF, IGF I and IGF II. Bone. 2011; 48(4):938–944

[280] Liao TS, Yurgelun MB, Chang SS, et al. Recruitment of osteoclast precursors by stromal cell derived factor-1 (SDF-1) in giant cell tumor of bone. J Orthop Res. 2005; 23(1):203–209

[281] Clézardin P. [The role of RANK/RANKL/osteoprotegerin (OPG) triad in cancer-induced bone diseases: physiopathology and clinical implications]. Bull Cancer. 2011; 98(7):837–846

[282] Forsyth RG, De Boeck G, Baelde JJ, et al. CD33 + CD14- phenotype is characteristic of multinuclear osteoclast-like cells in giant cell tumor of bone. J Bone Miner Res. 2009; 24(1):70–77

[283] Maggiani F, Forsyth R, Hogendoorn PC, Krenacs T, Athanasou NA. The immunophenotype of osteoclasts and macrophage polykaryons. J Clin Pathol. 2011; 64(8):701–705

[284] Lau YS, Sabokbar A, Gibbons CL, Giele H, Athanasou N. Phenotypic and molecular studies of giant-cell tumors of bone and soft tissue. Hum Pathol. 2005; 36(9):945–954

[285] Lindeman JH, Hanemaaijer R, Mulder A, et al. Cathepsin K is the principal protease in giant cell tumor of bone. Am J Pathol. 2004; 165(2):593–600

[286] Mak IW, Seidlitz EP, Cowan RW, et al. Evidence for the role of matrix metalloproteinase-13 in bone resorption by giant cell tumor of bone. Hum Pathol. 2010; 41(9):1320–1329

[287] Mak IW, Cowan RW, Popovic S, Colterjohn N, Singh G, Ghert M. Upregulation of MMP-13 via Runx2 in the stromal cell of giant cell tumor of bone. Bone. 2009; 45(2):377–386

[288] Ng PK, Tsui SK, Lau CP, et al. CCAAT/enhancer binding protein beta is upregulated in giant cell tumor of bone and regulates RANKL expression. J Cell Biochem. 2010; 110(2):438–446

[289] Balla P, Moskovszky L, Sapi Z, et al. Epidermal growth factor receptor signalling contributes to osteoblastic stromal cell proliferation, osteoclastogenesis and disease progression in giant cell tumour of bone. Histopathology. 2011; 59(3):376–389

[290] Patibandla MR, Thotakura AK, Rao MN, et al. Clival giant cell tumor—a rare case report and review of literature with respect to current line of management. Asian J Neurosurg. 2017; 12(1):78–81

[291] Dominkus M, Ruggieri P, Bertoni F, et al. Histologically verified lung metastases in benign giant cell tumours—14 cases from a single institution. Int Orthop. 2006; 30(6):499–504

[292] Anract P, De Pinieux G, Cottias P, Pouillart P, Forest M, Tomeno B. Malignant giant-cell tumours of bone. Clinico-pathological types and prognosis: a review of 29 cases. Int Orthop. 1998; 22(1):19–26

[293] Bertoni F, Present D, Enneking WF. Giant-cell tumor of bone with pulmonary metastases. J Bone Joint Surg Am. 1985; 67(6):890–900

[294] Faisham WI, Zulmi W, Halim AS, Biswal BM, Mutum SS, Ezane AM. Aggressive giant cell tumour of bone. Singapore Med J. 2006; 47(8):679–683

[295] Maloney WJ, Vaughan LM, Jones HH, Ross J, Nagel DA. Benign metastasizing giant-cell tumor of bone: report of three cases and review of the literature. Clin Orthop Relat Res. 1989(243):208–215

[296] Stewart DJ, Belanger R, Benjamin RS. Prolonged disease-free survival following surgical debulking and high-dose cisplatin/doxorubicin in a patient with bulky metastases from giant cell tumor of bone refractory to "standard" chemotherapy. Am J Clin Oncol. 1995; 18(2):144–148

[297] Zorlu F, Selek U, Soylemezoglu F, Oge K. Malignant giant cell tumor of the skull base originating from clivus and sphenoid bone. J Neurooncol. 2006; 76(2):149–152

[298] Kaiser U, Neumann K, Havemann K. Generalised giant-cell tumour of bone: successful treatment of pulmonary metastases with interferon alpha, a case report. J Cancer Res Clin Oncol. 1993; 119(5):301–303

[299] Kaban LB, Troulis MJ, Wilkinson MS, Ebb D, Dodson TB. Adjuvant antiangiogenic therapy for giant cell tumors of the jaws. J Oral Maxillofac Surg. 2007; 65(10):2018–2024

[300] Chang SS, Suratwala SJ, Jung KM, et al. Bisphosphonates may reduce recurrence in giant cell tumor by inducing apoptosis. Clin Orthop Relat Res. 2004 (426):103–109

[301] Cheng YY, Huang L, Lee KM, Xu JK, Zheng MH, Kumta SM. Bisphosphonates induce apoptosis of stromal tumor cells in giant cell tumor of bone. Calcif Tissue Int. 2004; 75(1):71–77

[302] Martin-Broto J, Cleeland CS, Glare PA, et al. Effects of denosumab on pain and analgesic use in giant cell tumor of bone: interim results from a phase II study. Acta Oncol. 2014; 53(9):1173–1179

[303] Tse LF, Wong KC, Kumta SM, Huang L, Chow TC, Griffith JF. Bisphosphonates reduce local recurrence in extremity giant cell tumor of bone: a case-control study. Bone. 2008; 42(1):68–73

[304] Balke M, Campanacci L, Gebert C, et al. Bisphosphonate treatment of aggressive primary, recurrent and metastatic giant cell tumour of bone. BMC Cancer. 2010; 10:462

[305] Yu X, Xu M, Xu S, Su Q. Clinical outcomes of giant cell tumor of bone treated with bone cement filling and internal fixation, and oral bisphosphonates. Oncol Lett. 2013; 5(2):447–451

[306] Arpornchayanon O, Leerapun T. Effectiveness of intravenous bisphosphonate in treatment of giant cell tumor: a case report and review of the literature. J Med Assoc Thai. 2008; 91(10):1609–1612

[307] George S, Merriam P, Maki RG, et al. Multicenter phase II trial of sunitinib in the treatment of nongastrointestinal stromal tumor sarcomas. J Clin Oncol. 2009; 27(19):3154–3160

[308] Nouri H, Hedi Meherzi M, Ouertatani M, et al. Calcitonin use in giant cell bone tumors. Orthop Traumatol Surg Res. 2011; 97(5):520–526

[309] De Chiara A, Apice G, Fazioli F, Silvestro P, Carone G, Manco A. Multicentric giant cell tumor with viral-like inclusions associated with Paget's disease of bone: a case treated by steroid therapy. Oncol Rep. 1998; 5(2): 317–320

[310] Ziambaras K, Totty WA, Teitelbaum SL, Dierkes M, Whyte MP. Extraskeletal osteoclastomas responsive to dexamethasone treatment in Paget bone disease. J Clin Endocrinol Metab. 1997; 82(11):3826–3834

[311] Chawla S, Henshaw R, Seeger L, et al. Safety and efficacy of denosumab for adults and skeletally mature adolescents with giant cell tumour of bone: interim analysis of an open-label, parallel-group, phase 2 study. Lancet Oncol. 2013; 14(9):901–908

[312] Rutkowski P, Ferrari S, Grimer RJ, et al. Surgical downstaging in an open-label phase II trial of denosumab in patients with giant cell tumor of bone. Ann Surg Oncol. 2015; 22(9):2860–2868

[313] Roitman PD, Jauk F, Farfalli GL, Albergo JI, Aponte-Tinao LA. Denosumab-treated giant cell tumor of bone: its histologic spectrum and potential diagnostic pitfalls. Hum Pathol. 2017; 63:89–97

[314] Skubitz K, Thomas D, Chawla S, Staddon A. Response to treatment with denosumab in patients with giant cell tumor of bone (GCTB): FDG PET results from two phase 2 trials. J Clin Oncol. 2014; 32(5) Suppl:10505

[315] McKinney AM, Reichert P, Short J, et al. Metachronous, multicentric giant cell tumor of the sphenoid bone with histologic, CT, MR imaging, and positron-emission tomography/CT correlation. AJNR Am J Neuroradiol. 2006; 27(10): 2199–2201

[316] Aoki J, Watanabe H, Shinozaki T, et al. FDG PET of primary benign and malignant bone tumors: standardized uptake value in 52 lesions. Radiology. 2001; 219(3):774–777

[317] Strauss LG, Dimitrakopoulou-Strauss A, Koczan D, et al. 18F-FDG kinetics and gene expression in giant cell tumors. J Nucl Med. 2004; 45(9):1528–1535

11 Rehabilitation of Speech and Swallowing of Patients with Tumors of the Skull Base

Jaimie Payne, Denise A. Barringer, and Jan S. Lewin

Summary

Skull base tumors place patients at risk for the development of communication and swallowing deficits because of their proximity to cranial nerves, regardless of the site of the lesion or pathology. Over the past decade, the focus of treatment has shifted from surgical ablation despite functional impact to more thoughtful consideration of treatments that minimize cranial nerve injury and associated communication and swallowing impairments. Accordingly, thorough evaluation by expert multidisciplinary teams that include a speech-language pathologist knowledgeable in the evaluation and management of patients with skull base tumors is essential. This chapter highlights critical components in the evaluation and rehabilitation of patients who have dysphagia, dysarthria, and dysphonia, the differential diagnoses of which remain the cornerstone of successful recovery of patients who have skull base tumors. A discussion of normal speech and swallowing function provides the reader with a foundation for comparison, after which disorders are identified by site of lesion (anterior, middle, and posterior fossa). Important diagnostic tools used by speech-language pathologists to assess speech, swallowing, and vocal function are reviewed. Finally, a brief synopsis of rehabilitative techniques completes the chapter.

Keywords: dysphagia, dysarthria, cranial nerves, speech-language pathology, swallowing, speech, voice, aspiration, dysphonia, function

11.1 Introduction

The inabilities to communicate and to eat normally are two of the most disturbing outcomes of brain tumors that are often not appreciated until they are lost.[1] Both communication and swallowing are complex processes that require a highly specific interplay between the efferent signals from the cortex, subcortex, and brainstem and the afferent signals from the structures of the aerodigestive tract, including the pharynx, larynx, and oral cavity. Skull base tumors, regardless of the site or pathology of the lesion, put patients at risk for the development of a variety of communication and/or swallowing deficits.[2] Over the past decade, the focus of treatment has shifted from surgical resection despite the functional impact to ensuring that the selected treatment minimizes cranial nerve injury and the subsequent impairments.[3] However, any treatment that affects structures within the skull base, whether directly or, because of collateral insult, indirectly, increases the risk for lower cranial nerve injury and thus disorders of speech, swallowing, and voice production.

Recent data suggest that 9.8% of patients who undergo surgical resection of a skull base tumor will have cranial nerve injury,[4] of whom 29 to 31% will experience postoperative swallowing impairments, or dysphagia[5,6]; up to 30% will experience deficits that affect speech production, or dysarthria[7]; and 10% will experience problems that affect the quality of the voice, or dysphonia.[8] It is important to remember that, although less prevalent, some patients may also present with worsened neurocognitive function after surgery.[9] Thus early preoperative consultation by speech-language pathologists who are expert in the management of patients with skull base tumors is critical. Data show that optimal recovery is facilitated when the patient and family receive important information regarding the disease and its effect on survival and posttreatment quality of life.[10] Furthermore, critical information provided by an experienced speech-language pathologist has been shown to help the medical team prepare patient and family for the potential delayed effects of treatment on speech and swallowing function.[11] Anecdotal experience demonstrates that patients who are knowledgeable are often better able to accept their treatment and the potential for functional consequences. Accordingly, patients who have skull base tumors, and their families as well, should thoroughly understand both the impact on function and the crucial need for posttreatment rehabilitation.

This chapter highlights critical components in the evaluation and rehabilitation of patients who have communication and swallowing disorders associated with tumors of the skull base. Accordingly, we have divided the chapter into three areas of focus: (1) normal neurophysiology of swallowing and communication, (2) common swallowing and communication disorders associated with tumors of the base of skull and their treatment, and (3) assessment and treatment of communication and swallowing disorders in patients who have tumors of the base of skull.

11.2 Normal Neurophysiology of Swallowing and Communication

11.2.1 Swallowing Neurophysiology

Swallowing is a complex interaction of biomechanical, neurophysiological, and behavioral events that occur in strict hierarchical sequence and that depend on intact sensory awareness and basic recognition of the act of eating. Historically, swallowing was considered solely a brainstem function of sensory and motor integration coordinated by the reticular nuclei within the pons and medulla.[12,13] However, ongoing research using functional magnetic resonance imaging (fMRI) has shown broad cortical involvement during swallowing, with the most prominent centers of activity located within the lateral precentral and postcentral gyri and the right insula.

Sensory innervation to the mouth, pharynx, and larynx is generally provided by the trigeminal (cranial nerve V), glossopharyngeal (cranial nerve IX), and vagus (cranial nerve X) nerves. Each of these nerves provides important sensory information that helps initiate and control the act of swallowing.

Table 11.1 Speech and swallowing impairments associated with each cranial nerve

Nerve	Disordered physiology	Swallowing symptoms	Speech symptoms
V	↓ Jaw movement ↓ Face, mouth, and jaw sensation	↓ Mastication ↓ Oral containment	Unilateral: insignificant Bilateral: severely ↓ articulatory precision
VII	↓ Facial movement and sensation ↑ Salivation	Residue in the lateral sulci Drooling	Mild distortion of b, p, f, v
VIII	↓ Hearing ↓ Balance	Not applicable	Distortion of resonance ↓ Articulatory precision of all sounds over time
IX	Delayed pharyngeal trigger ↓ Velopharyngeal closure ↓ Laryngeal elevation	Aspiration before and during swallow	Hypernasality
X	↓ Palatal, pharyngeal, laryngeal excursion ↓ True vocal cord abduction and/or adduction ↓ Pharyngeal sensation	Stasis/residue in the valleculae, posterior pharyngeal wall, and pyriform sinuses Aspiration during or after swallow Inability to cough	Hypernasality Breathiness and hoarseness ↓ Pitch range ↓ Vocal loudness
XII	↓ Lingual range of motion and strength	↓ Bolus consolidation ↓ Anterior to posterior movement of the bolus Oral residue	Imprecise articulation of l, t, d, s, z, sh, ch, k, g

Although the sequence of muscle activity in swallowing generally occurs once the pharyngeal swallow has been triggered, sensory feedback may alter the precise occurrences of muscle contractions. Motor innervation in swallowing is mediated primarily via cranial nerves V, IX, X, and XII.[14]

▶ Table 11.1 summarizes the impact to physiology and speech and swallowing symptoms associated with cranial nerve injury. Many of the techniques used for swallowing rehabilitation rely on this sensorimotor interrelationship, using sensory pathways to stimulate motor function.[15]

Swallowing generally occurs in four phases or stages: oral preparatory, oral, pharyngeal, and esophageal. The sequence of these stages is generally predictable, although the relative timing varies depending on the size and texture of the food being swallowed. Swallowing has been recognized as largely reflexive, because only the oral preparatory and oral phases are purely voluntary. The oral preparatory phase initiates the process of swallowing. During this phase, smooth coordination and transition between mastication and manipulation prepares and forms the food into a cohesive, manageable bolus that is ultimately propelled posteriorly to the oropharynx.

The next phase of swallowing, the pharyngeal phase, combines both voluntary and involuntary control and occurs with the initiation or "trigger" of the swallowing reflex. Generally, the area between the anterior faucial arches and the point at which the tongue base crosses the rim of the mandible is considered to be the key location for initiation of the pharyngeal swallow. The swallow trigger primarily depends on cranial nerve IX. In synchrony with the onset of the swallow reflex, the soft palate elevates and retracts to close the velopharyngeal port, thereby preventing nasal regurgitation of swallowed material. The base of tongue makes contact with the bulging posterior pharyngeal wall to help propel the food through the pharynx, while the hyoid and larynx bone move superiorly and anteriorly to prevent food from entering the airway, thereby directing the bolus posteriorly into the cervical esophagus. The elevation and anterior movements of the hyolaryngeal complex are essential to the opening of the upper esophageal sphincter, or cricopharyngeus muscle, which allows the bolus to enter the cervical esophagus without aspiration.

11.2.2 Communication Neurophysiology

It is important to remember that communication is more than simply the articulation of sounds and syllables into meaningful utterances, or speech. Communication begins within the cerebral cortex and subcortex as a thought that is then organized and converted into language within the perisylvian region of the dominant hemisphere, specifically Broca's area and the insula. The motor program or plan is transferred from the premotor cortex to the lower portion of the motor cortex through tracts to the cranial nerves that activate the muscles of the respiratory tract, larynx, and oral cavity for speech production.[16] As a result, any disruption or injury to these regions or tracts will result in communication problems.

11.3 Common Disorders of Swallowing

Swallowing disorders associated with tumors of the skull base are not generally the result of a single cause; rather, they are the culmination of multiple insults resulting from the tumor itself, the surgical resection, the surgical approach, and/or the adjuvant treatments used to treat the disease. In general, tumors that affect the posterior skull base will result in more profound swallowing dysfunction, because the cranial nerves that are critical to swallowing originate in this region. The consequences of damage to these nerves are often devastating, and many patients require the long-term use of a gastrostomy tube for nutrition and a permanent tracheotomy tube because of chronic aspiration that can eventually lead to aspiration pneumonia, a frequent and serious problem in patients who have base of skull tumors.[5,8,17] In addition to the functional insult caused by tumors of the skull base, the anterior and middle regions of the skull base also have specific tumor- and treatment-associated swallowing disorders.

11.3.1 Anterior Skull Base

Swallowing disorders associated with anterior skull base tumors occur as a result of anatomical alterations rather than cranial nerve dysfunction. The surgical exposure of anterior skull base tumors may require resection of structures such as the maxilla or mandible that provide important structural support during swallowing. As a result, functional deficits most commonly occur in the oral preparatory and/or oral phases of swallowing. In general, anterior skull base tumors do not affect the pharyngeal stage of swallowing.

Labial sensory and motor loss resulting from splitting of the maxilla often renders patients unable to maintain a labial seal, leading to drooling and food loss from the mouth. More extensive surgical approaches such as total maxillectomy cause palatal defects that hinder oral transit, lingual movements and contacts, often resulting in velopharyngeal incompetency and nasal regurgitation. Current advances in endoscopic surgical approaches to anterior skull base tumors have shown improved speech and swallowing outcomes, because they are less invasive and thus result in fewer injuries to the structures critical for swallowing. Fewer lower cranial nerve injuries are thus associated with this approach than are associated with open anterior craniotomy (0% vs. 23.5%, $p = 0.04$, respectively).[18]

11.3.2 Middle Skull Base

Like tumors of the anterior skull base, tumors of the middle base of skull are more apt to affect the oral preparatory and oral phases of swallowing than they are the pharyngeal phase. Damage to the middle skull base can result in unilateral or bilateral impairment of cranial nerves V and/or VII, which control the ability to open the mouth and masticate as well as the ability to maintain facial tone and symmetry. Data have shown a 41% incidence of facial nerve palsy in patients after cerebellopontine angle (CPA) surgery.[19] Generally patients are able to compensate for unilateral damage, but when the patient experiences facial nerve involvement, patient surveys report lower quality of life measures, including by describing eating as challenging, especially in social settings.[19]

11.3.3 Posterior Skull Base

Although anterior and middle skull base tumors can cause significant swallowing difficulties and impede the speed, adequacy, and efficiency of oral intake, patients can usually compensate for these deficits. However, tumors that affect the posterior skull base generally result in far more severe deficits and present greater challenges for rehabilitation of swallowing function because of the effect on the involuntary pharyngeal phase of swallowing. Dysphagia has been reported in 29% of patients after posterior fossa surgery, 41.1% of whom aspirate.[6]

In most cases, injuries to cranial nerves IX and X occur together, because both nerves exit the base of skull through the jugular foramen. Researchers found that nearly half of a population of 181 patients who experienced unilateral vagal palsy after CPA surgery also experienced pharyngeal palsy.[8] When injury occurs to cranial nerve IX, the pharyngeal swallowing reflex, pharyngeal contraction, and velopharyngeal competency are generally affected. Subsequently, patients may present with delayed or even absent swallow reflex, resulting in aspiration, pharyngeal stasis of food, and nasal regurgitation.[5] Injury to the vagus nerve often results in more severe swallowing impairment, as this nerve is responsible for several physiologic activities that work in concert with the pharyngeal trigger of swallowing. High vagal injuries, especially those associated with skull base surgeries, result in the most serious problems, because they affect all three branches of the nerve—the pharyngeal, superior laryngeal, and recurrent laryngeal nerves[20]—and can thus significantly affect both voice and swallowing. Patients may require a tracheostomy tube[8,17] because of airway compromise, and vocal fold medialization in cases of vocal fold paralysis (10–29%),[8,19] to restore phonation and an efficient cough. In the most severe cases, placement of an enteral feeding tube has been reported in 5 to 66% of patients.[5,8,17] In addition, because of the significant morbidity associated with skull base surgeries, patients often require longer hospital stays, which reduce emotional well-being and quality of life.[5,8,21]

Insult at any level of the vagus nerve may result in aspiration because of decreased laryngeal sensation, impaired pharyngeal contraction, or reduced airway closure.[22] Clinically, the superior and recurrent laryngeal branches of the vagus nerve are most important for glottic airway protection, whereas the pharyngeal branch ensures adequate pharyngeal contraction via innervation to the pharyngeal constrictor musculature. Injury to the superior laryngeal nerve can leave patients insensate to aspirate, causing them to silently, without coughing or any indication of awareness, aspirate food or liquid into the trachea. Damage to the recurrent laryngeal nerve usually results in paresis or paralysis of one or both of the true vocal cords, depending on the level of injury, impairing glottic valving in response to the aspirate. Clinicians should be advised that patients who have vagal injuries are at high risk for aspiration, with up to a 67% incidence rate reported.[5,8] It is important to remember that a lack of patient reaction should not be equated with safe swallowing in this population, whose members are at high risk for silent aspiration.

One of the most important cranial nerves involved in the oropharyngeal swallow is cranial nerve XII, the hypoglossal nerve, which innervates the tongue muscles. Any damage to the hypoglossal nerve, whether unilateral or bilateral, affects the lingual movements critical to the manipulation and transport of food from the anterior portion of the oral cavity to the pharynx. Patients who have hypoglossal nerve injuries will have difficulty maintaining a cohesive food bolus during the oral stage of swallowing, resulting in oral residue after the swallow.[22] More important, base of tongue retraction to the posterior pharyngeal wall helps propel the food through the pharynx. If this movement is impaired, then a significant amount of food collects within the valleculae, making swallowing laborious and inefficient, so that patients may expend inordinate effort for little nutritional gain. In addition, these patients remain at risk for aspiration, because food left in the pharynx after the swallow may easily fall into an airway at test.

Aspiration and dysphagia resulting from surgical damage to lower cranial nerves has been found to be the most dangerous complication related to resection of skull base tumors.[4] Alternatively, patients who have gradual tumor progression generally demonstrate the best potential for compensation of swallowing deficits, whereas patients who experience acute insults often have more severe problems, because they have not had the benefit of time to adjust to their swallowing problems.[2,21] It is critical that patients who have cranial nerve dysfunction be referred to a speech-language pathologist for baseline evaluation of dysphagia to maintain oral nutrition and reduce complications.

11.4 Common Disorders of Communication

The most common disorders of communication associated with base of skull lesions and their treatment are those that affect the motor aspects of speech production rather than semantics or language. Dysarthria remains the primary communication impairment in this patient population: a group of neurological motor speech disorders characterized by weakness, paralysis, incoordination, sensory deprivation, and alterations in muscle tone.[23] Dysarthric speech is often described as slurred and imprecise. The type of dysarthria is distinguished on the basis of its auditory perceptual characteristics, which in turn have diagnostic implications for lesion localization.[24]

11.4.1 Anterior Skull Base

Similar to swallowing, communication impairments associated with the anterior skull base are generally a function of damage to the anatomical structures. For example, maxillectomy results in a palatal defect that mostly impairs vocal resonance, or the quality of speech, but that can also affect speech intelligibility because of the loss of articulatory contact. Palatal prostheses or obturators that fill the defect and reestablish anatomical continuity are generally the best way to manage these types of problems.

Although less common, larger lesions of the anterior skull base that require retraction of the frontal lobes may also result in cognitive–linguistic disorders. The most common of these are aphasia and right hemisphere disorder (RHD). Aphasia is a language disorder that affects verbal expression, writing, auditory comprehension, and reading. In a majority of patients, it is an outcome of insult to the perisylvian cortex of the dominant left hemisphere.[25] In contrast, RHD is a cognitive disorder that affects memory, problem solving, attention, and social use of language, among other things. Unlike patients who have aphasia or dysarthria, patients who have RHD articulate well and use appropriate grammar and words. However, they present with impaired social pragmatics, resulting in communication that is often irrelevant and disconnected, and they lack appropriate affect.[26] The impact of such deficits may appear subtle but can be devastating to interpersonal relationships.

11.4.2 Middle and Posterior Skull Base

Flaccid Dysarthria

The most common communication disorder associated with middle or posterior skull base tumors is flaccid dysarthria secondary to cranial nerve dysfunction. Patients who have flaccid dysarthria demonstrate imprecise articulation with reduced speech intelligibility because of weakness of important speech muscles.[24] Much as for swallow, the critical nerves for articulation and speech production are cranial nerves V, VII, IX, X, and XII. Hypernasality and audible nasal emission are consequences

of velopharyngeal incompetency when the pharyngeal branch of the vagus nerve is damaged.

Unilateral lesions that include the superior and recurrent laryngeal branches often result in breathiness or aphonia, reduced vocal intensity, and limited pitch range because of impairment to vocal fold function. Lesions of the superior laryngeal nerve that spare the pharyngeal and recurrent branches are most often associated with an inability to change the pitch of the voice. Unilateral recurrent laryngeal nerve lesions resulting in impaired true vocal fold motion most often cause a weak, breathy, and hoarse voice because of impaired vocal fold approximation during phonation. Vocal fold augmentation is often performed using temporary injection procedures or permanent medialization thyroplasty to restore vocal fold approximation. These procedures have been shown to benefit patients who have temporary or permanent voice and swallowing impairments by restoring the glottic valving mechanism.[17,19] Bilateral vocal fold damage is likely the most severe consequence of vagal nerve injury, which may cause inhalatory stridor or total airway obstruction. These problems are much harder to correct, and in many cases patients require a tracheostomy tube to breathe.

Damage to cranial nerve XII results in lingual weakness that can significantly affect speech production. The overriding speech characteristic of cranial nerve XII lesions is imprecise articulation, specifically of sounds involving the tongue.

Ataxic Dysarthria

Direct or indirect damage to the cerebellum or surrounding regions, including the cerebellar pontine angle and the dentate nucleus, frequently result in ataxic dysarthria. Patients who have ataxic dysarthria demonstrate irregular speech movements that include altered speech prosody, prolongation of sounds, and prominent fluctuations in pitch and loudness, commonly described as "drunken" speech.[24]

Cerebellar Mutism Syndrome

One of the more unusual communication disorders that occurs as a result of posterior skull base tumors is cerebellar mutism syndrome (CMS). This disorder mainly affects children, without associated cranial nerve damage or long tract signs. CMS is characterized by a transient mutism that occurs 12 to 96 hours after surgery and typically resolves after a few weeks or months.[27] Unfortunately, CMS is a surprisingly common complication in children who have posterior fossa tumor resection. Investigators reported mutism in 33% (9 of 27) of cases after posterior fossa tumor removal, 67% of whom presented with dysarthria once speech was regained.[27]

11.5 Assessment and Intervention in Swallowing and Communication Disorders

Evaluation of swallowing and communication should be performed as early as possible in patients who have pretreatment tumor-related deficits and, preferably, before treatment begins in patients who are at high risk for treatment-related dysfunction or who already demonstrate baseline deficits. A comprehensive evaluation should include a thorough review of the patient's history, a patient/family interview, a neurological screening that includes an examination of the oral mechanism, and a motor speech examination. Formal measures provide additional information for differential diagnosis and lesion localization. Additionally, patient-reported outcome measures are a critical component that provide the patient's own perception of his or her speech and swallowing deficits and should be included in any formal test battery of speech and swallowing function.[3,19,22] The results from these examinations are carefully analyzed, and an individually tailored treatment plan specific to the presenting communication and swallowing symptoms is designed.

11.5.1 Clinical Assessment

The clinical or bedside swallowing examination allows observation of important events in the oropharyngeal stages of swallowing. It affords an opportunity to observe the patient's reactions to swallowing and to assess the parameters that are visible, such as labial closure, coughing, and laryngeal elevation, that are key indicators of swallowing safety. The impact of behaviors such as attention, impulsivity, and judgment must be taken into consideration when making recommendations regarding the patient's safety for eating and drinking. Clinical assessments of swallowing are not reliable indicators of pharyngeal physiology or aspiration and thus should not be used as a replacement for objective swallowing measures. Clinical swallowing examinations are good indicators of the need for objective swallowing assessments, such as the modified barium swallow study or the fiberoptic endoscopic evaluation of swallowing.

Phonatory function is also an important consideration that should be evaluated, for it is often associated with specific communication and swallowing problems, particularly those caused by vocal fold paralysis. Maximum phonation time is a simple tool that provides indirect information regarding the efficiency of glottic closure, as shorter phonatory durations may be suggestive of vocal fold dysfunction.

11.5.2 Instrumental Assessments

There are two main instrumental studies of swallowing: MBS and FEES. The indications for use of each test depends on the presenting swallowing problem and the patient's ability to undergo a radiographic examination.

Modified Barium Swallow Study

Perhaps the most widely used tool for evaluating oropharyngeal swallowing is the videofluoroscopic examination, or MBS study.[28] The MBS study is different from the standard barium swallow in that it shows the entire oropharyngeal swallow, including all four stages of swallowing. It provides information regarding all events, allowing diagnosis of specific swallowing disorders and causes of aspiration. A further benefit is that it gives the clinician the opportunity to attempt specific therapeutic techniques during the study with a view to determining his or her ability to alleviate the swallowing deficit. Refer to **Video 11.1**, which shows normal swallowing function as assessed via MBS.

Fiberoptic Endoscopic Evaluation of Swallowing

FEES is a videoendoscopic tool that can be used at the bedside or in the clinic by a single clinician.[29] It is the key assessment tool for visualization of aspiration, airway protection, and laryngeal sensation. However, two distinct disadvantages are associated with FEES. First, inability to visualize the oral stage of swallowing prevents evaluation of oral phase events during FEES. Second, much of the oropharyngeal physiology of swallowing must be inferred because of the limitations of endoscopy. Refer to **Video 11.2**, which shows normal swallowing function as assessed via MBS. ▶ Fig. 11.1 compares aspiration as evaluated via MBS and FEES.

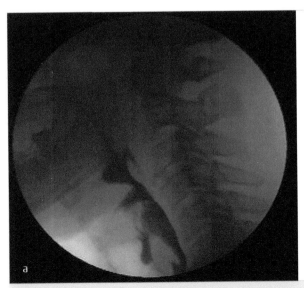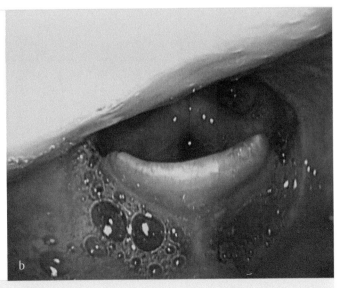

Fig. 11.1 (a) Aspiration on an MBS study. **(b)** Aspiration on a FEES examination.

Laryngeal Videostroboscopy

Laryngeal videostroboscopy is a clinical evaluation tool that allows the examiner to directly observe vocal fold mobility and vibration. Videostroboscopy is easily performed in a clinic setting using either a rigid or flexible fiberoptic endoscope. Although indirect laryngoscopy provides a clear image of laryngeal anatomy, pathology, and true vocal fold mobility, only laryngeal videostroboscopy can show the patterns of movement, closure, and mucosal vibration that are critical determinants of vocal function. It thus is a very useful examination with which to detect early recovery of vocal fold motion in patients who have vocal fold paralysis.

11.5.3 Communication Examination

The examination of communication includes a combination of formal standardized test batteries and informal perceptual measures that are selected on the basis of the patient's presenting problems. Informal test measures that evaluate the rate, rhythm, and precision of speech production may include the repetition of sounds in isolation and the production of rapidly sequenced syllables. These measures, along with examination of the oral mechanism, are the most useful tools for differentially diagnosing speech disorders and flaccid versus ataxic dysarthria, and they often help identify associated neurological disease processes.[24]

Disorders of cognition and language such as aphasia and RHD are best evaluated using standardized tests that rely less on perceptual, subjective judgments and more on the objective analysis and documentation of semantic and syntactic errors that commonly occur in patients who have language disorders.

11.5.4 Treatment

In general, treatment for speech and swallowing disorders either restores function or compensates for dysfunction. Therapeutic exercises that improve the strength and coordination of the oropharyngeal musculature are important restorative techniques for both speech and swallowing disorders. Exercises should be tailored to the patient's deficits so as to maximize functional recovery.[22] Recent advances in swallowing rehabilitation have incorporated mass practice in a hierarchical arrangement of increasingly difficult to swallow foods so as to improve swallowing efficiency.[30] Additionally, device-driven therapy programs that use biofeedback to strengthen critical swallowing and respiratory musculature have shown promising outcomes for patients who have impaired swallowing and vocal function.[31] Finally, vocal fold augmentation with injection or surgical medialization thyroplasty may be indicated in cases of unilateral vocal fold paralysis to improve phonation and coughing by restoring glottic closure that indirectly provides swallowing benefit.[32]

Alternatively, compensatory strategies give patients the ability to maintain function in the short term while working on long-term functional improvement.[22] Compensatory strategies become the focus of treatment when full restoration of normal function is not a realistic goal. In cases of swallowing impairment, compensatory approaches control the flow of food and eliminate the patients' symptoms, such as aspiration, but do not

necessarily change the physiology of the patient's swallow.[15] Examples of such approaches include postural changes, diet modifications, feeding techniques, and the use of intraoral prosthetic devices. Patients with communication impairments, such as dysarthria, benefit from compensatory strategies such as a slow rate of speech or the use of an alternative communication device, a picture board, or a voice-generated system to improve listener understanding and reduce frustration.

11.6 Conclusion

Patients who have base of skull tumors present significant diagnostic, treatment, and rehabilitative challenges that require the unique expertise of a strong multidisciplinary team of specialists.[19] The acute effects of a skull base tumor often prevent normal communication, impede the ability to eat by mouth, and severely disrupt normal patient and family interactions, to frequently overwhelming effect. Whether the deficits are acute or long-term, the speech pathologist plays a critical role in educating, rehabilitating, and preserving as close to normal function as possible. Speech pathologists who are expert in the management of patients who have skull base tumors provide appropriate intervention that may allow oral nutrition while avoiding medical complications such as aspiration. It is thus important that a speech pathologist be consulted early in the patient's course of evaluation and treatment, at the time of diagnosis, to reduce fears and misconceptions, maintain realistic expectations about functional recovery, and optimize communication and swallowing outcomes in patients who have skull base tumors.[5]

11.7 Case Report 1

The patient is a 55-year-old right-handed female who was diagnosed (1972) with anaplastic ependymoma of the fourth ventricle. She is status post three subtotal resections as well as radiation treatment to the posterior fossa, for a total of 54 Gy (1991). The patient was eating a regular diet, including both solids and liquids. She subsequently underwent percutaneous fluoroscopic gastrostomy in November 1995 due to persistent dysphagia and recurrent episodes of pneumonia. She presented to the speech pathology service a year later (1996), complaining of a progressive decline in speech and swallowing. An MBS study and speech assessment were performed.

Clinical assessment revealed multiple cranial nerve palsies (III, V, VII, IX, X, and XII) characterized by articulatory imprecision due to lingual weakness, hypernasality, irregular prosody, and dysphonia. Conversational speech was approximately 50% intelligible. Results revealed a moderate to severe mixed flaccid–ataxic dysarthria. Refer to **Video 11.3**. The patient was taught to use compensatory speech strategies to improve her intelligibility so that she could communicate her needs to family members.

The MBS study showed impaired lingual strength and coordination, decreased bolus formation, delayed initiation of the swallow reflex, reduced base of tongue retraction, and reduced hyolaryngeal excursion. Silent aspiration occurred before, during, and after swallows of thin liquids. Refer to **Video 11.4**. Compensatory strategies and diet modifications were unsuccessful in alleviating aspiration. Objective swallowing examination resulted in a diagnosis of a moderately severe oropharyngeal dysphagia. Recommendations included omission of oral intake of liquids. Swallowing was judged adequate for other food consistencies. No further episodes of aspiration pneumonia were documented.

11.8 Case Report 2

The patient, a 56-year-old right-handed female diagnosed with a right jugular foramen tumor, presented with an 8-month history of tinnitus and progressive swallowing difficulties. Cranial nerve examination revealed atrophy of the right side of her tongue, with deviation to the right upon protrusion (XII), and uvular elevation toward the left, with absent gag on the right (IX and X). Baseline videostroboscopic examination of vocal function and an MBS study showed adequate function despite a mild paresis of the right true vocal fold (X).

The patient underwent a transtemporal approach for resection of a vagal schwannoma of the right CPA. Postoperative indirect endoscopy demonstrated a right vocal fold paralysis in a lateralized position with glottic incompetency for voice production. Refer to **Video 11.5**. Note the salivary residue within the right pyriform sinus and the bowing of the right vocal fold. Videostroboscopy demonstrated bilateral vibration with good evidence of preserved mucosal wave. Postoperative MBS revealed a moderate oropharyngeal dysphagia characterized by significant pharyngeal residue resulting from unilateral pharyngeal and lingual weakness. No evidence of aspiration was visualized. The patient demonstrated poor pharyngeal contraction on the right, with significant postswallowing residue that was reduced using a right head turn, chin tuck, and thin liquid swallow to facilitate swallowing through the unimpaired side. Refer to **Video 11.6**. The patient underwent an injection laryngoplasty, then a medialization thyroplasty. Videostroboscopic imaging shows a well-medialized right vocal fold 3 years after surgical augmentation, with excellent glottic closure for voice and airway protection. Refer to **Video 11.7**. MBS revealed a safe swallow without aspiration and mild pharyngeal residue that was well compensated.

References

[1] Yorkston KM, Miler RM, Stand EA. Management of Speech and Swallowing in Degenerative Diseases. Austin, TX: Pro-Ed, Inc.; 1995

[2] Levine TM. Swallowing disorders following skull base surgery. Otolaryngol Clin North Am. 1988; 21(4):751–759

[3] Rivas A, Boahene KD, Bravo HC, Tan M, Tamargo RJ, Francis HW. A model for early prediction of facial nerve recovery after vestibular schwannoma surgery. Otol Neurotol. 2011; 32(5):826–833

[4] Ramina R, Maniglia JJ, Fernandes YB, et al. Jugular foramen tumors: diagnosis and treatment. Neurosurg Focus. 2004; 17(2):E5

[5] Starmer HM, Best SR, Agrawal Y, et al. Prevalence, characteristics, and management of swallowing disorders following cerebellopontine angle surgery. Otolaryngol Head Neck Surg. 2012; 146(3):419–425

[6] Wadhwa R, Toms J, Chittiboina P, et al. Dysphagia following posterior fossa surgery in adults. World Neurosurg. 2014; 82(5):822–827

[7] Cho YS, So YK, Park K, et al. Surgical outcomes of lateral approach for jugular foramen schwannoma: postoperative facial nerve and lower cranial nerve functions. Neurosurg Rev. 2009; 32(1):61–66

[8] Best SR, Starmer HM, Agrawal Y, et al. Risk factors for vagal palsy following cerebellopontine angle surgery. Otolaryngol Head Neck Surg. 2012; 147(2):364–368

[9] Dijkstra M, van Nieuwenhuizen D, Stalpers LJ, et al. Late neurocognitive sequelae in patients with WHO grade I meningioma. J Neurol Neurosurg Psychiatry. 2009; 80(8):910–915

[10] Portnoy RK. Head and Neck Cancer. New York, NY: Plenum Press; 1995

[11] Peterson KL, Fenn J. Treatment of dysphagia and dysphonia following skull base surgery. Otolaryngol Clin North Am. 2005; 38(4):809–817, xi

[12] Carptenter DO. Central nervous system mechanisms in deglutition and emesis. In: Wood JD, ed. Handbook of Physiology. Gastrointestinal System Control of Food and Water Intake. Vol. 1. Bethesda, MD: American Physiological Society; 1989:685–714

[13] Jean A. Brainstem control of swallowing: localization and organization of the central pattern generator for swallowing. In: Taylor A, ed. Neurophysiology of the Jaws and Teeth. London: MacMillan; 1990:294–321

[14] Bhatnagar SC. Neuroscience for the Study of Communicative Disorders. 2nd ed. Baltimore, MD: Lippincott Williams & Wilkins; 2002

[15] Logemann J. Evaluation and Treatment of Swallowing Disorders. 2nd ed. Austin, TX: Pro-Ed; 1998

[16] Love RJ, Webb WG. Neurology for the Speech-Language Pathologist. 3rd ed. Boston, MA: Butterworth-Heinemann; 1996

[17] Bielamowicz S, Gupta A, Sekhar LN. Early arytenoid adduction for vagal paralysis after skull base surgery. Laryngoscope. 2000; 110(3 Pt 1):346–351

[18] Jeswani S, Nuño M, Wu A, et al. Comparative analysis of outcomes following craniotomy and expanded endoscopic endonasal transsphenoidal resection of craniopharyngioma and related tumors: a single-institution study. J Neurosurg. 2016; 124(3):627–638

[19] Starmer HM, Ward BK, Best SR, et al. Patient-perceived long-term communication and swallow function following cerebellopontine angle surgery. Laryngoscope. 2014; 124(2):476–480

[20] Eibling DE, Boyd EM. Rehabilitation of lower cranial nerve deficits. Otolaryngol Clin North Am. 1997; 30(5):865–875

[21] Fang TJ, Tam YY, Courey MS, Li HY, Chiang HC. Unilateral high vagal paralysis: relationship of the severity of swallowing disturbance and types of injuries. Laryngoscope. 2011; 121(2):245–249

[22] Cheesman AD, Kelly AM. Rehabilitation after treatment for jugular foramen lesions. Skull Base. 2009; 19(1):99–108

[23] Dworkin JP. Motor Speech Disorders: A Treatment Guide. St. Louis, MO: Mosby; 1991

[24] Duffy JR. Motor Speech Disorders: Substrates, Differential Diagnosis, and Management. St. Louis, MO: Mosby-Year Book, Inc; 1995

[25] Rosenbek JC, LaPointe LL, Wertz RT. Aphasia: A Clinical Approach. Boston, MA: College-Hill Press; 1989

[26] Myers PS. Right Hemisphere Damage: Disorders of Communication and Cognition. San Diego, CA: Singular Publishing Group, Inc; 1999

[27] Mei C, Morgan AT. Incidence of mutism, dysarthria and dysphagia associated with childhood posterior fossa tumour. Childs Nerv Syst. 2011; 27(7):1129–1136

[28] Logemann J. Manual for the Videofluorographic Study of Swallowing. 2nd ed. Austin, TX: Pro-Ed; 1993

[29] Langmore SE, Schatz K, Olson N. Endoscopic and videofluoroscopic evaluations of swallowing and aspiration. Ann Otol Rhinol Laryngol. 1991; 100(8):678–681

[30] Crary MA, Carnaby GD, LaGorio LA, Carvajal PJ. Functional and physiological outcomes from an exercise-based dysphagia therapy: a pilot investigation of the McNeill Dysphagia Therapy Program. Arch Phys Med Rehabil. 2012; 93(7):1173–1178

[31] Sapienza CM. Respiratory muscle strength training applications. Curr Opin Otolaryngol Head Neck Surg. 2008; 16(3):216–220

[32] Kupferman ME, Acevedo J, Hutcheson KA, Lewin JS. Addressing an unmet need in oncology patients: rehabilitation of upper aerodigestive tract function. Ann Oncol. 2011; 22(10):2299–2303

12 Neuropsychological Assessment of Patients with Skull Base Tumors

Mariana E. Bradshaw

Summary

This chapter provides readers with information regarding the nature of neurocognitive impairment in adult patients who have skull base tumors and underscores the importance of neuropsychological evaluation in the multidisciplinary care of patients who have skull base tumors. While the current literature is limited, it suggests that the proximity of skull base tumors to critical brain structures leaves some patients vulnerable to neurocognitive impairment. Necessary treatments, including surgery and radiation, can also give rise to neurocognitive dysfunction. Patients may also exhibit symptoms of affective distress. Ideally, assessment of neurocognitive function should begin prior to intervention and extend well beyond treatment and should use reliable and repeatable measures that are sensitive to even subtle changes, with particular attention to the domains of memory, attention, processing speed, and executive functioning, as well as changes in a patient's overall mood state. Such an approach helps capture both tumor- and treatment-related neurocognitive sequelae that can impact patients' independent functioning and successful management of life roles. It also allows for early implementation of interventions, if necessary, that can be personalized to reduce the impact of neurocognitive impairment and improve patients' quality of life.

Keywords: cognition, neuropsychological assessment, skull base tumors

12.1 Introduction

Although neurocognitive compromise has historically been overlooked, a growing body of literature suggests that it is not uncommon in patients who have skull base tumors and that it can arise either secondary to the tumor itself or as a result of subsequent interventions. Neuropsychological evaluation is increasingly being recognized as an important component of the multidisciplinary care required for patients who have tumors of the skull base.[1,2] Advances in treatment have resulted in longer survival times and lower rates of recurrence, but these successes are not always achieved without some risk of damage to critical proximal neuroanatomical structures, including the frontal and temporal cortices, frontal–subcortical circuits, hypothalamus, and mammillary bodies. There is relatively limited literature regarding the neurocognitive and neurobehavioral sequelae associated with tumors of the skull base, and the majority of data reviewed in this chapter are gleaned from studies that had small sample sizes. However, available data do suggest that patients who have tumors of the skull base are vulnerable to development of a variety of neurocognitive deficits, particularly in the domains of memory and executive functioning. Even when neurocognitive impairment is relatively subtle, impacts on functional well-being can be significant. A mean loss of health-related work productivity of 6.15%, as assessed by the Work Limitations Questionnaire, was reported in one study of patients who had skull base tumors.[3] Although overall mean neurocognitive performance was within one standard deviation of normative expectation, there was a significant association between lower learning/memory and greater work productivity loss. In addition, although very few participants reported symptoms that met the criteria for clinical depression, there was also an association between higher levels of reported depressive symptoms and greater work productivity loss. These findings highlight the need for identification of and interventions for the neurocognitive sequelae of skull base tumors.

12.2 Neurocognitive Impairment Associated with Skull Base Tumors

12.2.1 Tumor-Related Neurocognitive Impairment

It is well established that patients who have primary supratentorial brain tumors are very likely to exhibit neurocognitive impairment, even prior to treatment with surgery, chemotherapy, or radiation; in fact, neurocognitive complaints are secondary only to headache as a presenting symptom.[4] Indeed, 60 to 100% of patients who have supratentorial brain tumors exhibit at least some degree of neurocognitive impairment prior to intervention, with variability in the nature and severity of this impairment depending on lesion location and lesion momentum, or tumor growth rate. In patients who have brain metastases, pretreatment neurocognitive impairment has been observed in up to 90% of patients, with volume (rather than number) of metastases being an important factor in the severity of impairment.[5] The location of many skull base tumors also leaves patients at inherent risk for the development of neurocognitive impairment secondary to the compression or impingement of critical proximal brain structures as tumors in and around the cranial vault grow and crowd healthy brain tissue.

Evidence of pretreatment neurocognitive impairment has been documented in multiple small studies of patients who had tumors in the anterior and middle cranial fossae. In a group of nine patients who had nasopharyngeal carcinoma and who underwent neuropsychological evaluation before receiving paranasal sinus radiation, several patients exhibited abnormal performance even prior to treatment.[6] Another study of patients who had craniopharyngioma revealed that half ($n = 6$ of 12) exhibited significant impairments in memory and executive functioning prior to surgical resection, hypothesized to be related to interruption of frontal–hypothalamic connections.[7] In a 2016 study, patients with meningiomas in the skull base (anterior and middle fossa, $n = 26$) were compared with patients who had meningiomas in the convexity ($n = 28$), as well as to a control group of matched healthy volunteers ($n = 52$). At preoperative baseline, overall patient performance was significantly lower than for the control group across measures assessing delayed recall, verbal fluency, and executive functioning. Patients who had skull base meningioma exhibited greater difficulty with memory than those who had convexity tumors, and those who had tumors in the middle cranial fossa exhibited even greater memory impairment than those who had tumors in the anterior cranial fossa, likely reflecting the proximity of the middle cranial fossa to the temporal lobes, which are known to be critical for memory function.[8]

A case study provided evidence of the untoward effects of damage due to compression by a skull base tumor: a 57-year-old man was found to have a cystic lesion above the suprasellar region (later identified as a craniopharyngioma) that compressed the base of the hypothalamus and damaged the mammillary bodies. Formal neuropsychological evaluation conducted prior to any intervention revealed an isolated but dense anterograde amnesia.[9] These reports suggest that even without invasion of brain tissue, skull base tumors result in neurocognitive dysfunction secondary to compression of critical brain structures, including the temporal lobes, hypothalamus, and mammillary bodies, or to disruption of subcortical networks.

12.2.2 Treatment-Related Neurocognitive Impairment

Surgical Morbidity

Detecting and understanding the neurocognitive impact of surgical resection requires an understanding of the potential transient hazards associated with these procedures as well as of the potentially chronic effects secondary to either focal damage of nearby structures or more diffuse dysfunction related to disruption of larger distributed networks. Fortunately, acute postoperative declines are often due primarily to reactive edema and therefore are transient in nature. This appeared to be the case in results reported by Ichimura et al in 2010; they described transient decline on both traditional paper-and-pencil neuropsychological measures of learning/memory and on computerized tests of reaction time 1 month after resection of posterior cranial fossa tumors via the middle fossa. These changes had recovered by 3-month follow-up.[10]

If healthy tissue is damaged during the surgical procedure, however, some long-term neurocognitive impairment is possible, and at least some studies have raised concerns about neurocognitive impairment after surgery for resection of skull base tumors. Steinvorth et al observed abnormally slowed speed of processing in a study of 40 patients who had base of skull meningiomas assessed after surgery but prior to initiation of radiation therapy. They also reported that patients who had undergone three or more surgical resections exhibited greater difficulty on tests that assessed attention than did the group as a whole.[11] Schick et al reported that 1 to 6 years after middle fossa vestibular schwannoma surgery, approximately 35% of patients exhibited evidence of memory impairment, with particularly poor performance noted for a patient who had evidence of temporal lobe gliosis.[12] Dijkstra et al reported that an average of 3.4 years after treatment, patients who had surgically treated skull base meningiomas performed significantly worse on tests assessing verbal memory, information

processing, and psychomotor speed than did patients who had convexity meningiomas.[13] Not only neurocognitive functioning but also behavioral functioning may be affected after surgical resection. Evaluation of patients who had anterior skull base meningiomas after resection found that those patients who had lesions involving the ventromedial prefrontal cortex were rated as having a greater decline in adaptive functioning (i.e., employment, independence, and self-care).[14] In patients who had craniopharyngioma, it appears that hypothalamic involvement leaves patients at greater risk for cognitive impairment, including memory loss, attentional deficits, and reduced information processing speed.[15]

It has been argued that patients who have tumors in the skull base may be more vulnerable to neurocognitive change than those who have meningiomas in the convexity secondary to the inherently difficult nature of the surgery.[13] It must be noted, however, that the aforementioned studies did not include preoperative baseline evaluations; thus it cannot be determined with certainty whether the neurocognitive impairment noted postoperatively truly resulted from the surgical resection or rather had been present preoperatively, secondary to the effect of the tumor on surrounding brain tissue. Prospective studies that include preoperative baseline evaluations have provided needed insight into the nature of postoperative impairment. One such study evaluated 58 patients who had skull base meningioma evaluated prior to and at intervals after resection. Results revealed that compared with preoperative baseline performance, patients exhibited acute declines in verbal memory, working memory, and executive functioning that were noted at the follow-up evaluation 3 to 5 months postoperatively. These declines were generally transient, with the majority of patients' performance being stable to improved relative to baseline 1 year after surgery; only a small minority exhibited persistent deficits.[16]

Another prospective study of skull base meningioma patients found no neurocognitive decline relative to preoperative baseline 1 year after resection and in fact found improvement on tasks assessing verbal fluency, processing speed, and fine motor dexterity. However, impairments in memory that were present preoperatively persisted.[8] This suggests that much of the neurocognitive impairment observed postoperatively is likely secondary to the impact of the tumor itself rather than an untoward effect of surgical resection, and it stresses the importance of baseline neuropsychological evaluation to appropriately interpret the presence and nature of neurocognitive impairment for skull base tumor patients.

Taken together, these studies provide evidence that although patients can recover from the acute effects of surgical resection, neurocognitive deficits may persist if damage to healthy brain occurred preoperatively secondary to the tumor itself or if the required surgical approach injures surrounding tissue.

Radiation-Induced Morbidity

Radiation therapy for skull base tumors may also pose a risk to neurocognitive function, as some treatment plans necessarily include exposure to structures critical for neurocognitive functioning. Of particular concern is late-delayed toxicity, which can develop months to years after completion of radiation therapy. Several factors have been identified as being associated with greater risk for the development of radiation-induced neurocognitive impairment, including age (younger than 5 or older than 60), dose per fraction (greater than 2 Gy), higher total dose, hyperfractionated schedules, shorter overall treatment time, comorbid vascular risk factors, concurrent or subsequent chemotherapy, and greater total volume of brain exposed to radiation.[17] With regard to memory specifically, an association has been reported between greater exposure to the bilateral hippocampi and greater impairment in long-term memory.[18] Studies investigating the neurocognitive impact of radiation therapy for skull base tumors have yielded mixed findings, perhaps in part due to the heterogeneity of skull base tumors and associated treatment plans, with different tumor types involving different risk to critical brain structures. In 1997 Glosser et al found only a mild decline in motor speed in the chronic and delayed periods after irradiation for chondrosarcoma (mean 25.4 and 47.4 months, respectively). They otherwise reported no evidence of adverse neurocognitive effects despite radiation dose of 50 to 60 CGE involving midline and temporal lobe structures.[19] A prospective 1-year follow-up study of 40 patients who had skull base meningiomas also suggested the relative safety of radiation therapy. This study showed a significant but transient decline in memory after the first radiation fraction. No further declines were noted thereafter; rather, improvements were noted in attention after the first radiation fraction, with further significant improvements in attention and memory after 6 months and still further improvements at 1 year.[11]

In contrast to the preceding findings, in 2000 Meyers et al reported that patients who completed radiation for tumors of the paranasal sinus exhibited impairment in memory, executive functioning, and motor functioning in a pattern suggestive of frontal–subcortical dysfunction. Degree of impairment was associated with total dose of radiation therapy and time since treatment; average time since radiation to testing was 6 years.[6] Notably, Steinvorth et al[11] followed patients for only up to 1 year, so late delayed effects might not yet have developed. Although Glosser et al[19] had a longer follow-up time, that study also eliminated patients who had radiation necrosis and thus failed to account for those patients who might have experienced the most toxic effects of their radiation therapy.

Much of the available literature regarding neurocognitive functioning after radiation therapy for skull base tumors involves patients who have nasopharyngeal carcinoma, as these patients are particularly vulnerable to the development of temporal lobe necrosis after treatment due to exposure of the temporal lobe(s) to radiation.[20] In a study of 30 patients treated using intensity-modulated radiation therapy, 76.7% exhibited significant declines in neurocognitive functioning compared with pretreatment performance on tests assessing memory, language, and verbal fluency. Higher dose generally, and to the temporal lobes specifically, was associated with worse neurocognitive outcome.[21] In 2000 Cheung et al compared patients who had nasopharyngeal carcinoma who developed radiation-induced temporal lobe necrosis with those who did not as well as with healthy controls, finding that although patients who did not have necrosis tended to perform worse than controls did, there was not a statistically significant difference. Patients who had necrosis performed significantly worse than both

controls and patients who did not have necrosis on tests of memory as well as across measures assessing language, motor functioning, and executive functioning.[20]

In summary, patients who undergo radiation therapy may be at risk for development of neurocognitive dysfunction if the dose distribution includes critical brain structures; particular concern is raised for late delayed effects, which might not develop until months to years after therapy. In addition to clearly identified radiation necrosis, other imaging biomarkers may be associated with these neurocognitive changes. Alterations in functional network connectivity were identified in patients who had nasopharyngeal carcinoma after radiation therapy using fMRI and were associated with degree of neurocognitive impairment.[22] In patients who developed radiation necrosis, a higher number of temporal cerebral microbleeds was also identified as being associated with greater neurocognitive impairment.[23]

12.3 Affective Distress in Patients Who Have Skull Base Tumors

In addition to neurocognitive changes, patients who have skull base tumors may experience mood disturbance. There is a dearth of strong literature regarding the prevalence of depression and anxiety in cases of skull base tumor. A report on 18 patients who had malignant tumors of the skull base found that post treatment a third reported possible or probable anxiety or depression, as measured by the Hospital Anxiety and Depression Scale (HADS).[24] Similarly, 29% of patients who had skull base chordoma and who had undergone surgery and/or radiation were found to have moderate or severe depression, as measured by the Patient Health Questionnaire (PHQ-9).[25] Slightly higher estimates were reported in 2008 by Lue et al, who found that of 43 patients posttreatment for nasopharyngeal carcinoma, 51.2% reported significant symptoms of anxiety (as measured by the Beck Anxiety Inventory) and 44.2% reported significant symptoms of depression (as measured by the Beck Depression Inventory–II).[26]

There is some evidence to suggest that affective distress in patients who have tumors of the skull base may stabilize and/or decline through the disease course. A prospective study investigating neuropsychological functioning in patients who had chordomas and low-grade chondrosarcomas of the skull base found improvements in self-reported symptoms of depression and anxiety over time, with a tendency for mood to stabilize approximately 1 year after radiation therapy.[19] Similarly, a study assessing neuropsychological outcomes in patients who had skull base meningiomas after fractionated stereotactic radiotherapy found improvements in overall mood states 6 weeks after completion of treatment, with stabilization thereafter.[11] In 2017 Zweckberger et al also reported that in patients who had skull base meningiomas, self-reported symptoms of depression and anxiety remained stable after resection in more than 90% of cases.[16] As neurocognitive impairment persisted even in the context of improved mood, these findings suggest that affective distress does not explain the observed neurocognitive impairments in this patient population.

12.4 Neuropsychological Assessment of Patients Who Have Skull Base Tumors

Neuropsychological evaluation is beneficial in determining the impact of the tumor on neurocognitive functioning, as well as to monitor for possible treatment-related changes. Assessment is also helpful in determining the presence and/or impact of neuromedical or psychological/psychiatric comorbidities. Unfortunately, the diagnosis of a skull base tumor does not preclude additional diagnosis of, for example, a comorbid neurodegenerative condition. Neuropsychological assessment may be diagnostically relevant in determining whether observed neurocognitive changes reflect tumor/treatment effects or are secondary to another process.

12.4.1 Clinical Interview

As with any neuropsychological evaluation, the assessment of cognition is incomplete without a thorough clinical interview that can provide context for the acquired neurocognitive test results. Although pretreatment baseline evaluations are ideal, it is not uncommon for patients to present for their first evaluation after the initiation or completion of some treatment. Thus the clinical interview should address factors relevant to a patient's level of premorbid functioning; this will include information regarding educational and occupational attainment, any developmental delays, and relevant medical comorbidities. In addition to obtaining this background information, the clinician should acquire information from the patient and a collateral informant, if available, regarding the patient's subjective baseline level of functioning and the chronology of any perceived changes, including the perceived impact on the patient of the tumor and its treatment. The interview is also used to garner information regarding current relative need for supervision and assistance, as well as any functional difficulties in personal and/or occupational responsibilities. This is also a time for identification of any mood or personality changes, as well as discussion of changes to family or occupational roles that might cause distress.

12.4.2 Neurocognitive Test Selection

Screening measures, such as the Mini Mental State Examination (MMSE), generally fail to provide the breadth and sensitivity needed to capture the neurocognitive sequelae of tumors and associated treatment.[27] An appropriate neuropsychological assessment is often broad in scope but has a particular focus on those cognitive skills that may be particularly vulnerable to tumor and treatment effects. There is no one "correct" assessment battery that must be used to properly evaluate these abilities, but certain standards of practice should be followed. An objective test robust to brain insult is typically included in the first evaluation to further inform estimates of premorbid functioning. As already noted, patients who have tumors of the skull base may be particularly vulnerable to changes in the domains of memory and executive functioning. Further test selection may thus weigh more heavily in these domains. Accordingly, tests of memory should include both verbal and visual information and should assess multiple aspects of memory, including learning, retrieval, and consolidation. Tests assessing executive functioning often include those tapping working memory, cognitive flexibility, and reasoning. Additional measures may assess basic naming abilities, verbal fluency, visuospatial skills (from simple to complex), processing speed, and fine motor dexterity. The choice of how many tests to administer must take into account the patient's physical well-being. Fatigue is perhaps the most commonly reported cancer-related symptom, and it is also a common complaint among patients who have skull base tumors.[28,29] Test batteries must therefore be selected with the patient's stamina in mind, and/or assessment may need to be distributed across multiple testing sessions.

With these considerations taken into account, neurocognitive assessment is generally well tolerated by patients, as has been demonstrated in clinical trials.[30] The possibility of sensory change secondary to tumor effects must also be considered. For example, some skull base tumors may result in visual field deficits or diplopia, whereas others may lead to significant tinnitus and/or hearing loss. If these deficits are severe enough to interfere with a patient's ability to perform tasks involving visual or auditory stimuli, this will necessarily change the clinician's test selection to those that can be adequately presented. Clinical experience suggests that skull base tumor–related sensory deficits are rarely so severe as to entirely preclude assessment through one modality or another; however, the clinician should use information regarding any such limitations to guide test selection and interpretation. For example, a visual field deficit is unlikely to prevent administration of all visually mediated measures. However, this may slow performance on speed of processing tasks requiring visual scanning and/or may have an untoward impact on reading abilities. Interpretation in such a case would need to be made accordingly to ensure that potentially weak performance in these other domains is not overinterpreted, with test data perhaps needing to be supplemented by additional information from the clinical interview, behavioral observations, and complementary measures to ensure appropriate clinical analysis. As when evaluating other brain tumor patients, chosen measures should have well-established reliability and validity. Tests that have alternate forms are preferred when available so as to allow for more frequent evaluation with a reduced risk of practice effects.

12.4.3 Mood and Quality of Life Assessment

Examination of affective distress is typically also included in a thorough neuropsychological evaluation. Affective distress has the potential to impact neurocognitive performance but, of equal importance, requires assessment and management to optimize patient care, well-being, and functioning. Aspects of attention and memory are particularly vulnerable to symptoms of depression and anxiety.[31,32] Information regarding a patient's affective state is gathered during the clinical interview. In addition, patient-reported outcome measures are commonly used to determine the severity of mood disturbance. As when selecting a neurocognitive test, the clinician may choose from a variety of measures relying on the particular question of interest, psychometric properties, and normative data to inform interpretation.

Cognitive, affective, and physical symptoms may all have an untoward impact on overall patient quality of life. There is no one correct tool for measuring these factors, but several measures have been developed specifically to assess quality of life in patients who have cancer generally and skull base tumors specifically. Interested readers are referred to Chapter 14 for further information regarding quality of life and outcome measures in this patient population.

12.4.4 Care Path

The clinical care path for patients who have skull base tumors may vary depending on the referral question. As already noted, ideally a preoperative baseline evaluation should be made. In addition to accurately establishing whether any observed impairment is secondary to the tumor itself or is treatment-related, early (pretreatment) evaluations prevent misclassification errors in which patients are erroneously labeled as cognitively intact compared with normative standards even when comparison with their own personal baseline would in fact reveal significant changes from premorbid levels of functioning.[33] Establishing these baselines is certainly critical for research design, but even in clinical work it is ideal to comprehend the level of a patient's neurocognitive functioning prior to intervention. In cases of severe neurocognitive disorders (e.g., anterograde amnesia), it is also critical to identify potential capacity for medical decision-making issues and acute patient care/safety issues.

Postoperative follow-up is ideally scheduled after the patient has been discharged from inpatient care but prior to initiation of any adjuvant therapy this offers an opportunity to identify neurocognitive changes associated with surgery that may benefit from interventions, as well as to establish a new "baseline" prior to receipt of adjuvant therapies such as radiation. Recommendations regarding neuropsychological surveillance after radiation therapy may vary depending on the aggressiveness of the tumor, need for further treatment, stability of neurocognitive functioning, and relevant clinical questions (such as return to work or school). Given that delayed effects of radiation may not occur for years after completion of treatment, continued monitoring is recommended; if both the tumor and neurocognitive functioning remain stable, follow-up intervals may be extended over time.

12.5 Management of Neurocognitive and Affective Symptoms in Skull Base Tumors

When neurocognitive impairments emerge and or persist after treatment for skull base tumors, information gleaned from neuropsychological evaluation can yield recommendations regarding personalized intervention strategies with which to reduce the untoward impact of neurocognitive dysfunction and improve patient quality of life. There is limited evidence to support techniques aimed at restoration of neurocognitive function in brain tumor patients. One randomized, controlled trial in 140 glioma patients found that patients who participated in a program incorporating both computer-based attention retraining

and compensatory skills training performed significantly better on tests of attention and verbal memory at 6-month follow-up compared with waitlist controls. They also reported subjective improvements in mental fatigue.[34] It remains to be seen whether these findings can be generalized to patients who have skull base tumors. The majority of neuropsychological interventions have focused largely on compensatory strategy training, which might include use of specific external cues, including organized written reminders, as well as on metacognitive strategies for increasing self-awareness and self-correcting as needed. Such an approach is described in a case report of a woman who had been treated with surgery and radiation for a craniopharyngioma as an adult and who described cognitive difficulties predating these interventions. Neuropsychological assessment revealed impairments in attention, executive functioning, and memory. Intervention used goal management training in which she was taught to interrupt non–goal-related behavior and refocus attention. Following intervention, she was observed to improve on objective tests requiring attention and organization, and she reported subjective improvements in her functional well-being at work as well.[35]

Pharmacologic interventions have also been developed with which to address neurocognitive symptoms. There is modest evidence of benefit from stimulant agents for improving neurocognitive functioning and symptoms of fatigue in patients who have brain tumors, including medulloblastoma[36,37]; however, further research is needed to determine the efficacy of these treatments in patients who have skull base tumors specifically. In the event of severe radiation-induced toxicity (e.g., temporal lobe radionecrosis), preliminary evidence indicates that high-dose alpha-tocopheral (vitamin E) may be beneficial in ameliorating associated impairments in memory and executive functioning.[38]

In addition to use of pharmacologic treatments and personalized compensatory strategy training to address cognitive dysfunction, referrals may be recommended to address factors that could be relevant to both neurocognitive functioning and overall patient well-being, including affective distress, pain, and fatigue. Ultimately, a multidisciplinary team approach using both pharmacologic and nonpharmacologic interventions to address the neurocognitive, affective, and somatic symptoms resulting from skull base tumors and their treatment is often necessary. Although not all patients might return to their premorbid level of functioning, goals should be centered on minimizing the impact of both tumor and treatment on patient well-being and optimizing daily functioning.

12.6 Conclusion

Patients who have tumors of the skull base may be vulnerable to neurocognitive impairment secondary to untoward effects of the tumor itself or as an unfortunate result of necessary treatments. Advances in treatment approaches may lessen treatment toxicity; minimally invasive surgeries may reduce the likelihood of complications secondary to damage to healthy tissue,[39] and advances in both radiation techniques, including use of proton therapy, may limit exposure of normal brain structures to unnecessary radiation.[40] More work is needed to determine which treatment approaches provide the greatest tumor control while posing the least possible risk to neurocognition. Patients may nevertheless be left with neurocognitive impairment that reduces functional well-being and overall quality of life. Thorough neuropsychological evaluation may be used to establish the nature and severity of any such neurocognitive deficits, to monitor change over time, and to facilitate the development and implementation of multidisciplinary interventions that minimize the impact of neurocognitive changes, with the ultimate goal of improving patient quality of life and functional well-being.

Acknowledgment

The author gratefully acknowledges Dr. Jeffrey S. Wefel for his editorial contributions to this chapter.

References

[1] Komotar RJ, Roguski M, Bruce JN. Surgical management of craniopharyngiomas. J Neurooncol. 2009; 92(3):283–296

[2] Zoicas F, Schöfl C. Craniopharyngioma in adults. Front Endocrinol (Lausanne). 2012; 3:46

[3] Nugent BD, Weimer J, Choi CJ, et al. Work productivity and neuropsychological function in persons with skull base tumors. Neurooncol Pract. 2014; 1(3): 106–113

[4] Tucha O, Smely C, Preier M, Lange KW. Cognitive deficits before treatment among patients with brain tumors. Neurosurgery. 2000; 47(2):324–333, discussion 333–334

[5] Meyers CA, Smith JA, Bezjak A, et al. Neurocognitive function and progression in patients with brain metastases treated with whole-brain radiation and motexafin gadolinium: results of a randomized phase III trial. J Clin Oncol. 2004; 22(1):157–165

[6] Meyers CA, Geara F, Wong PF, Morrison WH. Neurocognitive effects of therapeutic irradiation for base of skull tumors. Int J Radiat Oncol Biol Phys. 2000; 46(1):51–55

[7] Donnet A, Schmitt A, Dufour H, Grisoli F. Neuropsychological follow-up of twenty two adult patients after surgery for craniopharyngioma. Acta Neurochir (Wien). 1999; 141(10):1049–1054

[8] Liouta E, Koutsarnakis C, Liakos F, Stranjalis G. Effects of intracranial meningioma location, size, and surgery on neurocognitive functions: a 3-year prospective study. J Neurosurg. 2016; 124(6):1578–1584

[9] Tanaka Y, Miyazawa Y, Akaoka F, Yamada T. Amnesia following damage to the mammillary bodies. Neurology. 1997; 48(1):160–165

[10] Ichimura S, Ohira T, Kobayashi M, et al. Assessment of cognitive function before and after surgery for posterior cranial fossa lesions using computerized and conventional tests. Neurol Med Chir (Tokyo). 2010; 50(6):441–448 (Tokyo)

[11] Steinvorth S, Welzel G, Fuss M, et al. Neuropsychological outcome after fractionated stereotactic radiotherapy (FSRT) for base of skull meningiomas: a prospective 1-year follow-up. Radiother Oncol. 2003; 69(2):177–182

[12] Schick B, Greess H, Gill S, Pauli E, Iro H. Magnetic resonance imaging and neuropsychological testing after middle fossa vestibular schwannoma surgery. Otol Neurotol. 2008; 29(1):39–45

[13] Dijkstra M, van Nieuwenhuizen D, Stalpers LJ, et al. Late neurocognitive sequelae in patients with WHO grade I meningioma. J Neurol Neurosurg Psychiatry. 2009; 80(8):910–915

[14] Abel TJ, Manzel K, Bruss J, Belfi AM, Howard MA, III, Tranel D. The cognitive and behavioral effects of meningioma lesions involving the ventromedial prefrontal cortex. J Neurosurg. 2016; 124(6):1568–1577

[15] Fjalldal S, Holmer H, Rylander L, et al. Hypothalamic involvement predicts cognitive performance and psychosocial health in long-term survivors of childhood craniopharyngioma. J Clin Endocrinol Metab. 2013; 98(8):3253–3262

[16] Zweckberger K, Hallek E, Vogt L, Giese H, Schick U, Unterberg AW. Prospective analysis of neuropsychological deficits following resection of benign skull base meningiomas. J Neurosurg. 2017; 127(6):1242–1248

[17] Crossen JR, Garwood D, Glatstein E, Neuwelt EA. Neurobehavioral sequelae of cranial irradiation in adults: a review of radiation-induced encephalopathy. J Clin Oncol. 1994; 12(3):627–642

[18] Gondi V, Hermann BP, Mehta MP, Tomé WA. Hippocampal dosimetry predicts neurocognitive function impairment after fractionated stereotactic radiotherapy for benign or low-grade adult brain tumors. Int J Radiat Oncol Biol Phys. 2012; 83(4):e487–e493

[19] Glosser G, McManus P, Munzenrider J, et al. Neuropsychological function in adults after high dose fractionated radiation therapy of skull base tumors. Int J Radiat Oncol Biol Phys. 1997; 38(2):231–239

[20] Cheung M, Chan AS, Law SC, Chan JH, Tse VK. Cognitive function of patients with nasopharyngeal carcinoma with and without temporal lobe radionecrosis. Arch Neurol. 2000; 57(9):1347–1352

[21] Hsiao KY, Yeh SA, Chang CC, Tsai PC, Wu JM, Gau JS. Cognitive function before and after intensity-modulated radiation therapy in patients with nasopharyngeal carcinoma: a prospective study. Int J Radiat Oncol Biol Phys. 2010; 77 (3):722–726

[22] Ma Q, Wu D, Zeng LL, Shen H, Hu D, Qiu S. Radiation-induced functional connectivity alterations in nasopharyngeal carcinoma patients with radiotherapy. Medicine (Baltimore). 2016; 95(29):e4275

[23] Shen Q, Lin F, Rong X, et al. Temporal cerebral microbleeds are associated with radiation necrosis and cognitive dysfunction in patients treated for nasopharyngeal carcinoma. Int J Radiat Oncol Biol Phys. 2016; 94(5): 1113–1120

[24] Martinez-Devesa P, Barnes ML, Alcock CJ, Kerr RS, Milford CA. Evaluation of quality of life and psychiatric morbidity in patients with malignant tumours of the skull base. J Laryngol Otol. 2006; 120(12):1049–1054

[25] Diaz RJ, Maggacis N, Zhang S, Cusimano MD. Determinants of quality of life in patients with skull base chordoma. J Neurosurg. 2014; 120(2):528–537

[26] Lue BH, Huang TS, Chen HJ. Physical distress, emotional status, and quality of life in patients with nasopharyngeal cancer complicated by post-radiotherapy endocrinopathy. Int J Radiat Oncol Biol Phys. 2008; 70(1):28–34

[27] Meyers CA, Wefel JS. The use of the mini-mental state examination to assess cognitive functioning in cancer trials: no ifs, ands, buts, or sensitivity. J Clin Oncol. 2003; 21(19):3557–3558

[28] Hanna EY, Mendoza TR, Rosenthal DI, et al. The symptom burden of treatment-naive patients with head and neck cancer. Cancer. 2015; 121(5): 766–773

[29] Kaul D, Budach V, Misch M, Wiener E, Exner S, Badakhshi H. Meningioma of the skull base: long-term outcome after image-guided stereotactic radiotherapy. Cancer Radiother. 2014; 18(8):730–735

[30] Meyers CA, Hess KR. Multifaceted end points in brain tumor clinical trials: cognitive deterioration precedes MRI progression. Neuro-oncol. 2003; 5(2): 89–95

[31] Eysenck MW, Derakshan N, Santos R, Calvo MG. Anxiety and cognitive performance: attentional control theory. Emotion. 2007; 7(2):336–353

[32] Kizilbash AH, Vanderploeg RD, Curtiss G. The effects of depression and anxiety on memory performance. Arch Clin Neuropsychol. 2002; 17(1):57–67

[33] Wefel JS, Lenzi R, Theriault RL, Davis RN, Meyers CA. The cognitive sequelae of standard-dose adjuvant chemotherapy in women with breast carcinoma: results of a prospective, randomized, longitudinal trial. Cancer. 2004; 100 (11):2292–2299

[34] Gehring K, Sitskoorn MM, Gundy CM, et al. Cognitive rehabilitation in patients with gliomas: a randomized, controlled trial. J Clin Oncol. 2009; 27 (22):3712–3722

[35] Metzler-Baddeley C, Jones RW. Brief communication: cognitive rehabilitation of executive functioning in a case of craniopharyngioma. Appl Neuropsychol. 2010; 17(4):299–304

[36] Meyers CA, Weitzner MA, Valentine AD, Levin VA. Methylphenidate therapy improves cognition, mood, and function of brain tumor patients. J Clin Oncol. 1998; 16(7):2522–2527

[37] Gehring K, Patwardhan SY, Collins R, et al. A randomized trial on the efficacy of methylphenidate and modafinil for improving cognitive functioning and symptoms in patients with a primary brain tumor. J Neurooncol. 2012; 107 (1):165–174

[38] Chan AS, Cheung MC, Law SC, Chan JH. Phase II study of alpha-tocopherol in improving the cognitive function of patients with temporal lobe radionecrosis. Cancer. 2004; 100(2):398–404

[39] Barzaghi LR, Spina A, Gagliardi F, Boari N, Mortini P. Trans-frontal-sinus-subcranial approach to olfactory groove meningiomas: surgical results, clinical and functional outcome in a consecutive series of 21 patients. World Neurosurg. 2017:pii: S1878-8750(17)30201-30202. [Epub ahead of print]

[40] Noel G, Gondi V. Proton therapy for tumors of the base of the skull. Chin Clin Oncol. 2016; 5(4):51

13 Cerebrovascular Management in Skull Base Tumors

Anoop P. Patel, Sabareesh K. Natarajan, Basavaraj Ghodke, and Laligam N. Sekhar

Summary

Skull base tumors represent a particular challenge with regard to management of cerebrovascular structures, as they often displace, encase, or invade vital blood vessels during their growth. Surgical management of these tumors requires intimate knowledge of their association with blood vessels as well as of appropriate management strategies. The goal of this chapter is to discuss cerebrovascular management during surgery for skull base tumors with emphasis on understanding patterns of vascular involvement and how such considerations are important for preoperative planning. We also address revascularization for challenging cases, including indications, techniques, and outcomes.

Keywords: subarachnoid encasement, bypass, revascularization, vessel injury, venous reconstruction, radial artery graft, saphenous vein graft, vasospasm

13.1 Introduction

Skull base tumors are some of the most challenging lesions for surgeons to deal with. Involvement of critical vascular structures is one of the reasons surgery for these tumors is particularly difficult. Knowledge of vascular management during these operations is important for ensuring optimal patient outcomes while maximizing surgical resection. This chapter focuses on various aspects of vascular management during skull base surgery, including preoperative evaluation and embolization, arterial and venous preservation and reconstruction, management of intraoperative vascular injury, and postoperative management of vasospasm.

13.2 Preoperative Imaging

Typical imaging for skull base tumors includes an MRI, in which T2-weighted sequences are often most useful for delineating the relationship of the tumor to the vasculature. Important things to note on preoperative MRI include degree of encasement or involvement of a vessel (partial vs. circumferential), presence of a cerebrospinal fluid (CSF) or arachnoid plane on T2-weighted imaging, and any evidence of arterial or venous narrowing related to the mass. Postcontrasted images can be useful for looking at the extent of the tumor but in many cases do not allow for distinction between vascular structures and enhancing tumor.

Cerebral angiography is the gold standard for evaluating vascular involvement of skull base tumors. Angiography allows simultaneous visualization of degree of stenosis of arterial or venous structures, collateralization, and evaluation of compensatory flow via balloon test occlusion and compression studies. The relative sizes and contributions of the internal carotid arteries, completeness of the circle of Willis, and comparative size of the vertebral arteries (VA) should all be noted. Variant anatomy (such as atretic segments, fetal configurations, and duplicated arteries) should

be clearly visualized and integrated into the surgeon's vascular management plan.

In cases of internal carotid artery (ICA) encasement, we perform angiography with ipsilateral common carotid artery compression. In a patient in whom surgical occlusion is planned, a carotid compression arteriogram with contralateral carotid and vertebral injection is performed to evaluate collateral flow through the anterior communicating artery (Acom) or the posterior communicating artery (Pcom). This information is used to decide whether the external carotid artery (ECA; no cross flow) or ICA (cross flow present) should be used as the donor artery for bypass, and it gives the surgeon vital information about collateral sources and tolerance for temporary occlusion during bypass or reconstruction.

Venous phase angiography is a must for any tumors that involve or are adjacent to the large venous outflow structures, such as the torcula, transverse and sigmoid sinuses, vein of Labbé, and straight sinus. The size and dominance of the transverse or sigmoid sinus and collateralization through the torcula can alter the surgical approach by revealing a very large sigmoid sinus or high-riding jugular bulb, either of which can significantly affect the amount of exposure. If there is complete occlusion and collateralization of venous drainage, this typically means that the venous structure can be sacrificed in the region adjacent to the tumor. If there is flow through a major venous channel with little evidence of collateralization, effort should be made to preserve this so as to prevent venous hypertension and infarct postoperatively. This can be accomplished either by leaving tumor behind or by aggressive resection and venous reconstruction.

Configuration, relative sizes, and anastomotic relationships of the veins draining the temporal lobe are particularly important. In most patients, the veins of Labbé and the superficial middle cerebral veins have an inverse relationship. The most common configuration is one in which they are relatively equal in size, but in some cases a particularly large vein of Labbé is accompanied by small middle cerebral veins, or vice versa. The consequences of occluding a large or dominant vein must be factored into surgical planning to avoid venous infarction. Knowledge of Labbé drainage is particularly important for subtemporal and presigmoid approaches, for opening the dura along the floor of the temporal fossa can compromise the vein of Labbé if its location is not known preoperatively.[1,2,3,4]

As a result, preoperative angiography is critically important for understanding both arterial and venous relationships during skull base surgery. In situations in which angiography is not available or is contraindicated, CT or MRI angiography and/or venography can provide useful adjunctive information but rarely replaces the value of a complete cerebral angiogram.

13.3 Preoperative Embolization

Preoperative angiography also provides an opportunity for embolization. It is our practice to attempt embolization for all cranial base meningiomas so as to reduce blood loss and operative time, as has been reported in prior studies.[5,6,7] Decreasing vascularity to the tumor has the dual advantage of improving visualization during resection and, in some cases, causing the tumor to necrose and soften, allowing for easier removal and decreasing the forces transmitted to adjacent neural structures.

The arteries commonly embolized include the meningohypophyseal branch of the ICA; the branches of the ECA—the sphenopalatine artery, middle meningeal artery, accessory meningeal artery, internal maxillary artery, ascending pharyngeal artery, and others; and, rarely, the meningeal branches of the VA.

Tumor embolization is performed under local (ECA branches) or general (ICA branches) anesthesia. To facilitate the selective catheterization of the small branches, a Renegade (Boston Scientific; for larger pedicles, such as ascending pharyngeal artery) or Marathon (ev3; for smaller pedicles, such as meningohypophyseal trunk) microcatheter is used. A manual injection of undiluted, nonionic contrast agent is performed with a 1.0 mL syringe, very slowly until the contrast agent becomes visible, after which the rate of injection is increased slowly. If tumor vascularity is apparent, the injection is repeated, with the rate of injection increased to possibly identify reflux into the carotid siphon. Filming is biplane so as to evaluate potential cross-filling of contralateral branches. An idea of the force required to cause reflux into cerebral arteries is thus obtained prior to the embolization procedure.

Embolization is ideally performed 3 to 7 days before the planned procedure. The goal of embolization is to permeate the interstices of the tumor with particles, occluding the feeding arteries at the very end if they are large. Embolization material consists of particles of polyvinyl acetyl foam (PVA) suspended in undiluted, nonionic contrast agent, injected slowly. The size of the particle used depends on the potential for reflux and supply to cranial nerves (CNs) from the pedicle being embolized. The average size of the particles used for embolization is 150 to 250 μm, with larger particles 250 to 400 μm being used for the embolization of the ascending pharyngeal artery to avoid occlusion of branches feeding CNs X and XI. Additionally, small Gelfoam pledgets are used to block arteries at the end of the procedure. In hypervascular tumors, liquid embolic agents such as Onyx, n-BCA, or coils are used for flow reduction.

The risks of embolization, including skin necrosis, CN dysfunction, stroke, and blindness, should be weighed against the perioperative and postoperative advantages. Embolization of some large or giant tumors may result in tumor swelling, which may precipitate emergent surgery.

13.4 Management of Arterial Encasement

Intracranial skull base tumors frequently encase the basal arteries, ICA, VA, basilar artery (BA), and their branches. Most tumors that encase vessels in the subarachnoid segment of the artery respect the arachnoid planes around the tumor and vessel. As a result, they can often be dissected away safely after adequate debulking. The most important factors that determine whether a tumor will be resectable from around a vessel are presence of perforators, evidence of vessel narrowing (indicating vessel invasion), and

overall consistency of the tumor.[8] The arachnoid planes are typically absent in cases of prior surgery or radiotherapy, rendering this dissection less feasible; arterial or venous injury is much more common in such cases. Extradural involvement of an artery can also be managed by microdissection of the tumor from the artery or vein if the pathology involved is benign. For example, schwannomas, cavernous hemangiomas, and benign meningiomas are almost always amenable to dissection. Instances of recurrent or higher-grade meningiomas or more malignant pathology (head and neck malignancy, sarcomas, adenoid cystic carcinoma) in which the arterial wall is invaded and the artery is narrowed represent situations in which intraoperative injury would be likely if dissection were attempted.

Management of these situations should be taken on a case-by-case basis. If the pathology in question can be treated using adjuvant chemotherapy or radiation, the management strategy will typically involve leaving tumor behind on the vessel and treatment with adjuvant techniques. However, when alternative therapies have been exhausted (recurrences) or the pathology is by nature highly malignant (e.g., adenoid cystic carcinoma), vascular sacrifice and aggressive resection should be considered with or without reconstruction or bypass, depending on the situation. Although the use of bypasses for skull base tumors has declined in frequency owing to advances in adjuvant treatment techniques, bypass and primary reconstruction techniques remain valuable tools in the management of skull base tumors such as recurrent meningiomas, recurrent chordomas, chondrosarcomas, and other malignant tumors.[9,10,11,12,13]

13.4.1 Operative Technique in a Tumor with Subarachnoid Encasement

Proximal control of the exposed artery is obtained, followed by exposure of the tumor while minimizing brain retraction and then distal exposure of the artery beyond the encasement. The artery is then traced through the tumor from both sides, with frequent debulking. Suction, bipolar cautery, fine dissectors, and microscissors are used for dissection of the artery. In case of an artery that has multiple perforators, the surface without perforators is dissected first, followed by the portion containing perforating branches.

13.4.2 Decision to Bypass in Cases of Vascular Occlusion or Sacrifice

The need for bypass in cases in which sacrifice of the ICA or VA is planned is somewhat controversial and depends on many patient-specific factors. Information obtained from preoperative balloon occlusion tests, coupled with monitoring of cerebral blood flow by single photon emission computed tomography (SPECT), transcranial dopplers (TCD), or angiography, can provide insights into whether a vessel can be sacrificed without the need for bypass. The success of this selective bypass approach depends on the accuracy of preoperative testing.

Based on a review of a series of patients operated on by the senior author (LNS) who were not revascularized and who suffered strokes, as well as the reports of other surgeons who had similar experiences,[14,15,16,17] we currently practice a universal bypass approach if the ICA must be occluded for tumor cases. For posterior circulation, bypass is not necessary for a markedly nondominant VA. However, if the VA is equal or dominant, we do perform a reconstruction or bypass. The BA should always be reconstructed if injured, although patients can tolerate distal basilar occlusion if there is significant PCom flow. In the event of unexpected intraoperative injury to major arteries, it is best to reconstruct the vessel using either a local, regional, or extraintracranial bypass technique, because the adequacy of collateral circulation cannot be determined.

Indications for bypass in the modern era of skull base surgery can be summarized as follows[18]:

- Benign tumor encasing a major artery and the tumor cannot be dissected free for complete resection without damaging the artery. Bypass is typically pursued with recurrent and previously radiated benign tumors. As an alternative, a small amount of tumor can be left behind and re-irradiated if allowable.
- Malignant tumor involving a major artery: complete resection is the goal set preoperatively based on the principles of oncologic treatment, whereby negative margins are imperative for optimal tumor control.
- A major artery already occluded by the tumor and the patient is having ischemic symptoms, or there is preoperative evidence of significantly reduced cerebrovascular reserve.
- Unplanned intraoperative injury to a major artery that cannot be directly repaired or sutured.

13.4.3 Choice of Bypass Grafts

Bypasses may be divided into two groups: replacement bypasses (e.g., radial artery graft [RAG]/saphenous vein graft [SVG] to replace the ICA/VA) and augmentation bypasses (e.g., STA–MCA bypass performed in a patient who has brain ischemia secondary to ICA occlusion, or occipital artery [OA] to posteroinferior cerebellar artery [PICA] for a patient who has VA occlusion). Most of the bypasses performed for skull base tumors are replacement bypasses using RAG, SVG, or rarely,

the superficial temporal artery (STA). Local repair of an injured artery may also be performed in some cases.

The radial artery provides flow rates between 50 and 150 mL/minute acutely, and flow can increase significantly over the ensuing days, as measured by duplex ultrasound.[19] We perform preoperative mapping of the arterial tree of the arm as well as an Allen's test to ensure adequate collateral perfusion. Although the radial artery is easier to harvest than the saphenous vein is, postoperative vasospasm in RAG is an important concern but has been largely alleviated by use of the pressure distention technique, which significantly lowers rates of postoperative vasospasm in arterial grafts.[9,20,21]

SVGs are an alternative to RAG for high-flow replacement bypasses. We use the saphenous vein when the radial artery is smaller than 1.5 mm or is unavailable for any reason (e.g., prior harvest, insufficiency of palmar arch). In children younger than 12, the radial artery is typically too small, mandating the use of SVG if needed. Flow rates in SVGs are typically higher than in RAGs, in the range of 100 to 250 mL/minute.[19] These high flow rates can cause flow mismatches and/or hyperperfusion syndromes when anastomosed to the middle cerebral artery (MCA) or posterior cerebral artery (PCA). Moreover, vein grafts are more technically challenging to anastomose and can be prone to kinking. Accordingly, a RAG that has been pressure-distended to decrease postoperative vasospasm is our graft conduit of choice.

13.4.4 Anesthesia, Monitoring, and Preparation

When a bypass may be needed, preoperative duplex imaging of the radial arteries and saphenous veins and an Allen's test are performed to facilitate graft selection based on the parameters already outlined (▶ Fig. 13.1). We also monitor pulse oximetry intraoperatively to ensure adequate perfusion of the hand after temporary occlusion of the radial artery prior to harvest. The patient is given 325 mg of aspirin preoperatively. Intraoperative

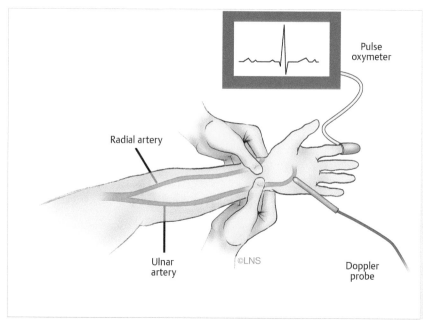

Pulse oxymeter

Radial artery

Ulnar artery

©LNS

Doppler probe

Fig. 13.1 The Allen's test for evaluating patency of the palmar arch prior to harvesting radial artery.

monitoring of electroencephalogram, somatosensory evoked potentials, and motor evoked potentials is employed. Total intravenous anesthesia is used to allow monitoring of motor evoked potentials. If a bypass is performed, the anesthesiologist is asked to raise the patient's mean arterial pressure by about 20% during temporary occlusion to facilitate collateral perfusion and then places the patient in burst suppression with propofol for brain protection. Approximately 3,000 to 5,000 units of heparin are also administered just prior to vascular occlusion. We do not reverse heparinization at the end of the procedure. Meticulous hemostasis is required prior to heparin dosing to prevent bleeding that can obscure the operative field.

13.4.5 High-Flow (Replacement) Bypass Technique

High-flow bypass techniques are important when major arteries (ICA, dominant VA) must be sacrificed during tumor resection. Replacement of 100 to 250 mL/minute of blood flow can be accomplished using this technique. For a tumor involving the ICA, an ECA or cervical ICA to MCA–M2 segment bypass is preferred (▶ Fig. 13.2). If the MCA vessels are particularly small, the supraclinoid ICA may be used as a recipient vessel. If the proximal ECA or ICA is unavailable for bypass because of tumor involvement, then the V2–V3 segment of the VA can be used as a proximal anastomosis site (▶ Fig. 13.3).

The cervical ICA is exposed in the neck. The tumor is exposed after a craniotomy and an orbital or orbitozygomatic osteotomy. Our practice is to inspect the tumor and determine whether bypass will be needed—a judgment that sometimes requires removal of some of the tumor along the vessel to determine whether the plane is favorable. When there is no clear plane or when vascular invasion is evident, we proceed with bypass prior to aggressive resection of the tumor.

Accordingly, the radial artery (the entire artery from the brachial artery bifurcation to the anterior wrist) or the saphenous vein (in the upper leg and lower thigh) is removed, flushed with heparinized saline, and distended under pressure to relieve vasospasm. The distal anastomosis is performed first, to the MCA (M1 bifurcation or M2 segment) or to the supraclinoid ICA. This is followed by the proximal anastomosis to the ECA (if collateral circulation is poor) or to the ICA (if some collaterals are present). If flow through the grafts is satisfactory as assessed by Doppler/intraoperative angiography, then the ICA is trapped between the cervical and supraclinoid segment, proximal to the bypass. The operation is stopped at this stage and a postoperative angiogram obtained to ensure patency of the bypass.

For VA replacement, an extreme lateral retrocondylar or partial transcondylar approach is used. Proximal anastomosis to the VA is done in the V3 segment extradurally, most commonly as the VA traverses the sulcus arteriosus of C1 and prior to the dural entry point. If the distal anastomosis is distal to the PICA, then the PICA may be reimplanted or a PICA-to-PICA anastomosis performed. Alternatively, the PICA may be occluded if there is good collateral flow from the distal vessel. For BA injury, VA or ECA to PCA–P2 segment bypass is performed using RAG or SVG. A temporal craniotomy with a zygomatic osteotomy or a petrosal approach is used to expose the PCA.

13.4.6 Low-/Moderate-Flow (Augmentation) Bypass Techniques

When the patient has some compensatory flow from collateral circulation, a flow-augmenting bypass such as an STA–MCA may be used to add 25 to 100 mL/minute of perfusion. In the posterior circulation, this can be accomplished using an OA–PICA bypass. The more common technique of STA–MCA bypass is discussed here.

The STA is exposed by a direct cut-down technique. The course of the vessel is traced by Doppler ultrasound or frameless neuronavigation and marked on the scalp. Working under the operating microscope, dissection is started distally and the vessel traced proximally. A small cuff of connective tissue is left around the artery. The vessel is left in situ until the bypass procedure. A T-incision is created from the skin incision made to expose the artery so as to facilitate muscle dissection and a small pterional craniotomy. A middle cerebral branch in the distal sylvian fissure (M3 branch), the largest temporal or parietal cortical branch relatively free of perforators, is used for anastomosis. Ideally the recipient vessel should be at least 1.5 mm in diameter, but it can be as narrow as 1.0 mm. The recipient vessel is dissected free of its arachnoidal covering,

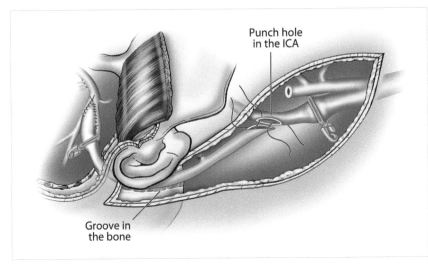

Punch hole
in the ICA

Groove in
the bone

Fig. 13.2 Cervical internal carotid artery (ICA) to supraclinoid ICA bypass.

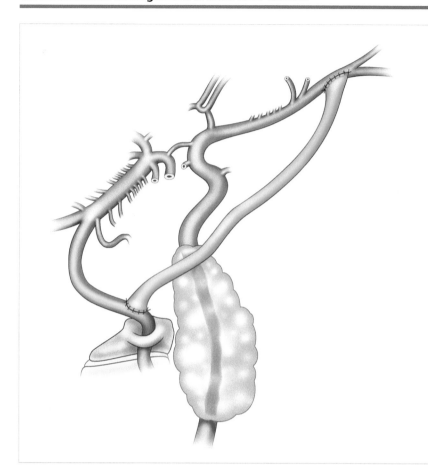

Fig. 13.3 V3 segment vertebral artery to supra-clinoid internal carotid artery bypass.

and a small rubber dam is placed under the artery. The STA is divided, and an oblique arteriotomy and slight fish-mouthing of the STA is done (▶ Fig. 13.4a). Anastomosis to the MCA is done using diametrically opposing sutures at the ends and either running or interrupted 9-0 or 10-0 nylon sutures (▶ Fig. 13.4b,c,d,e). Prior to the tying of the last suture, the lumen is flushed with heparinized saline and the suture tightened. Flow through the STA is checked using a Doppler probe.

13.4.7 Staged Operations

Our typical practice is to stage operations in which a bypass is needed. Craniotomy, exposure osteotomies, and bypass are done during the first surgery, followed by tumor resection 3 to 7 days later. This delay allows some degree of hemodynamic equilibrium and graft maturity after bypass is performed and allows the tumor resection to be done after heparinization has worn off. In addition, tumor resection and skull base repair can be lengthy. The tumor resection and the skull base repair are lengthy and to couple them after the exposure, osteotomy and bypass would make a longer procedure.

13.4.8 Postoperative Management

Postoperative monitoring of graft patency is usually done by Doppler evaluation. An angiogram is performed in the immediate postoperative period or within 24 hours of surgery. If this is not possible, a CT angiogram is obtained to ensure graft patency.

Patients are maintained on 325 mg of aspirin. Patients who have SVG are maintained on subcutaneous heparin, 5,000 U every 8 hours for 3 days, in addition to aspirin. Duplex ultrasound studies are performed to follow the volume flow through the graft. The systolic blood pressure should be maintained below 140 mm Hg for 2 to 3 days.

Graft occlusion is most common at the time of surgery or within 24 hours of surgery. If occlusion is noted intraoperatively, it is corrected as needed. Typically the anastomotic sites at the proximal and distal end are examined for thrombus and are reexplored to resolve any kinking or flow-related stasis in the vessel. Further heparinization can be employed if clot continues to form despite good flow. If the graft occludes in the postoperative period, the patient is typically taken back to the operating room for reexploration. Our general practice is not to employ endovascular thrombolysis in these cases, because some mechanical reason for thrombus formation typically needs to be dealt with to ensure long-term patency. Vasospasm occurs occasionally with RAG (despite use of the intraoperative pressure distention technique) and can be successfully treated by endovascular angioplasty or administration of intra-arterial vasodilators such as nicardipine. Following discharge (7–10 days), patients are kept on aspirin for life in case of vein graft and for at least 1 year in cases of RAG. We typically obtain duplex flow measurements and CT angiogram or MR angiogram at 3 months, 1 year, and then subsequently every 1 to 2 years, depending on the situation.

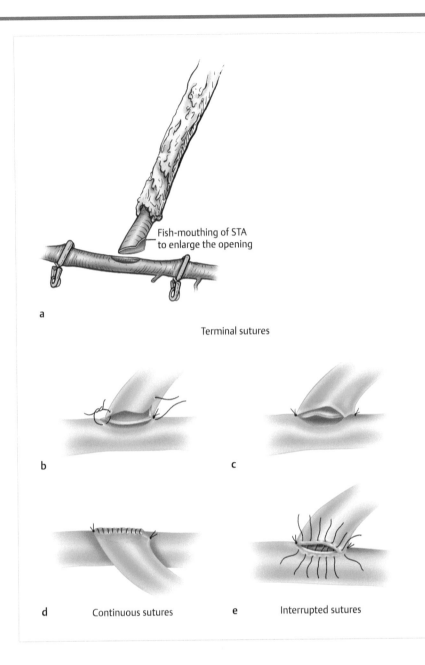

Fish-mouthing of STA to enlarge the opening

a

Terminal sutures

b   c

d   Continuous sutures   e   Interrupted sutures

Fig. 13.4 **(a)** The superficial temporal artery is fish-mouthed to enlarge the opening and compensate for size mismatch prior to end-to-side anastomosis. **(b,c)** Terminal stitches are placed at the heel and the diametrically opposite end of the anastomosis. **(d)** One side is anastomosed with continuous sutures and **(e)** the opposite side with interrupted sutures.

13.4.9 Results

From 1988 to 2006, 130 patients underwent bypasses for tumors (79 for skull base meningiomas, 7 for chondrosarcomas, 7 for chordomas, and 5 for adenoid cystic carcinomas, in addition to other tumors such osteogenic sarcoma, schwannoma, hemangiomas, and hemangiopericytomas; ▶ Table 13.1). The immediate patency rate for bypasses was 95.4%, and gross total resection was achieved in 82 (63%) patients, with 29 RAGs and 101 SVGs used. Two patients had delayed graft occlusions (after 2 years), which were revised. Sixteen patients had disease progression or recurrence and died. One patient, who was wheelchair-bound and had multiple lower CN palsies, died 8 months after surgery. One patient had a major stroke despite functioning of the graft and died after 7 days.

As already noted, modern practice patterns have led to a decrease in the number of tumors treated using aggressive resection

and bypass. The senior author examined his modern series of 20 bypasses in 18 patients operated on for skull base tumors between 2003 and 2012.[18] Mean age was 41 years, with 14 anterior circulation bypasses and 4 posterior circulation bypasses. Long-term patency was 100%, although one patient did require a revision of the graft after stenosis was found on surveillance imaging. Seventy-seven percent of patients had had prior treatment, whether surgery or radiation therapy. In this series of largely recurrent or radiated tumors, gross total resection (GTR) was possible in 72% of patients. Long-term outcomes were good for 14 of the patients (mRS < 2), with a mean follow-up of 47 months. One patient died during the perioperative period from complications related to aspiration pneumonia. Of the five patients operated on for malignant disease involving a major artery, three died from progression of their disease (osteosarcoma, synovial sarcoma, chordoma). Similarly poor long-term survival results with highly malignant head and neck disease have been reported by other

Table 13.1 Revascularization for tumors 1988–2006

Number of patients	130
• Meningiomas	79
• Chondrosarcoma	7
• Chordoma	7
• Adenoid cystic carcinoma	5
• Miscellaneous	32
Type of graft	
• Radial artery graft	29
• Saphenous vein graft	101
Extent of resection	
• Gross total resection	82 (63%)
• Incomplete resection	48 (37%)
Graft patency	
• Immediate patency rate	124/130 (95.4%)
• Delayed graft occlusion	2 (managed by revision, patent at follow-up)
Mortality	
• Due to surgery	2/130 (1.5%)
• Major stroke despite patent graft	1
• Preoperative deficits and morbidity after surgery	1
• Due to disease progression/recurrence	17/130 (13.1%)

authors.[22] Accordingly, bypass and aggressive resection in cases of highly malignant disease should be considered on a case-by-case basis.

Treatment of the majority of benign lesions or recurrent/higher-grade meningiomas resulted in excellent long-term outcomes. These results have been borne out in several smaller case series of skull base lesions from other institutions.[23,24,25] Accordingly, bypass for the management of complex skull base tumors involving major vessels can be beneficial with good patient selection and surgical technique that minimizes morbidity.

13.5 Preservation and Reconstruction of Veins and Sinuses

Major cerebral veins are usually at risk during surgery for skull base tumors owing to displacement of veins from fixed drainage sites in the brain and/or their division to approach a lesion. Veins have thinner walls, and skull base operations frequently involve putting bridging veins on stretch, making them prone to rupture. This can be avoided by minimizing extent of brain retraction or by mobilizing veins from arachnoid or adhesions to the skull base.

When venous outflow is compromised by a lack of adequate collateral circulation, venous infarction follows, bringing swelling, hemorrhage, and neuronal death. The clinical consequences, which can often be disastrous, will depend on the region of brain involved and the size of the venous structure occluded. The consequences of cerebral venous sinus occlusion also depend on the availability of collateral circulation. When such collaterals are not available, papilledema, visual loss, and pseudotumor cerebri syndrome are observed in milder cases, whereas severe diffuse brain swelling, coma, and death may be observed in severe cases. Acute venous or venous sinus occlusion is potentially very dangerous, whereas slow and chronic venous or venous sinus occlusion is far better tolerated. Even in such patients, some neurologic manifestations may follow when the collaterals are poor. As such, detailed preoperative study of the venous phase cerebral angiogram is very helpful in determining the extent of venous collateralization and the anatomy of venous drainage patterns. This can often provide insight into whether major venous sinus occlusion has already occurred and which veins can be sacrificed.

In the majority of patients, the temporal tip draining veins can be divided without adverse consequences. However, if the superficial middle cerebral (sylvian) vein is large and the vein of Labbé is either absent due to prior surgery or atretic because of an anatomic variation, the superficial middle cerebral vein should be preserved. The vein(s) of Labbé can vary in the location of their drainage and are at risk for injury during subtemporal and transpetrosal approaches. Presigmoid approaches such as the retrolabyrinthine (with or without petrous apicectomy) and translabyrinthine and total petrosectomy all move the surgeon anteriorly from the drainage point of the vein of Labbé. However, in some patients, these strategies might not prevent excessive stretching of the vein, in which case the surgeon can consider dividing the tentorium and placing the retractor on the mobilized free edge rather than the temporal lobe itself to minimize venous stretching. When the vein is very large and dominant, having an anterior drainage site, the surgical approach may have to be modified accordingly, to a retrosigmoid (or retrosigmoid + orbitozygomatic with frontotemporal craniotomy) approach, so as to prevent venous injury and postoperative infarction, particularly on the dominant side.

13.5.1 Venous Reconstruction

Indications for venous reconstruction include accidental injury to a large vein or venous sinus, brain swelling noted after occlusion of a venous structure, or injury to any deep vein. The simplest reconstruction method is typically direct repair using 8–0 nylon sutures. Dural mobilization can be used to release tension on the anastomosis if necessary. Direct repair is usually successful even if the repaired vein is slightly stenotic. When a segment of the vein is missing and direct repair is difficult, a segment of saphenous vein, a vein from the forearm or neck, or the radial artery may be used as an interposition graft.[26] Postoperative thrombosis is the main problem with venous reconstruction and may occur because of injury to the endothelium of the transplanted vein and the slow blood flow through the vein in general. To prevent this, we give patients 4,000 U of intravenous heparin during the reconstruction procedure, subcutaneous heparin during the first 7 postoperative days (5,000 U q8h), and aspirin 325 mg daily thereafter for 2 to 3 months.

13.5.2 Cerebral Venous Sinuses

Cerebral venous sinuses transmit a large volume of venous blood from the brain. The patency of the venous sinuses is very important to preserve the functional integrity of the brain.

The only venous sinuses that may safely be occluded in most patients are the cavernous sinuses, the superior petrosal sinuses, and the nondominant, well-collateralized transverse and sigmoid sinuses. Occlusion of the cavernous sinus can usually be performed without adverse effects on vision and the orbit due to the presence of many collateral drainage channels from the orbit.

13.5.3 Intraoperative Sinus Occlusion Test

To determine whether a venous structure can be occluded at the time of surgery, we perform an intraoperative sinus occlusion test with venous pressure monitoring (▶ Fig. 13.5). Venous pressure is measured by inserting a 20-gauge butterfly needle connected to a standard pressure transducer. Normal venous sinus pressure should be less than 15 mm Hg, depending on the position of the head. After a stable reading is obtained, a temporary clip is applied on the venous sinus at the appropriate point of expected occlusion. We closely monitor the brain and/or cerebellum for swelling and evoked potentials and intrasinus pressure for at least 5 minutes. Although venous pressure is the most sensitive indicator of venous hypertension, cerebellar swelling can also occur very rapidly. If brain swelling

occurs, evoked potentials change, or intrasinus pressure increases by more than 5 mm Hg, then the temporary clip is removed and the decision is made not to sacrifice the sinus. If the initial intrasinus pressure is above 15 mm Hg but there is no significant increase in the pressure on occlusion, then sacrifice may be considered, but pressure must be continuous monitored during the rest of the operation, because a delayed increase in intrasinus pressure may occur and necessitate reconstruction. Preoperative occlusion tests of the venous sinuses are not safe, because the clinical response is delayed and the effects are not fully reversible.

13.5.4 Reconstruction of Venous Sinuses

Direct Repair

If a small portion of the circumference of a venous sinus is involved by a tumor, direct repair is recommended. In such patients, the tumor is excised and the sinus is repaired using 5–0 or 6–0 Prolene sutures, by direct suturing if possible. If the defect is too large or if direct suturing will cause significant stenosis, then the venous sinus can be reconstructed using either a dural flap from adjacent dura (▶ Fig. 13.6) or a free dural patch

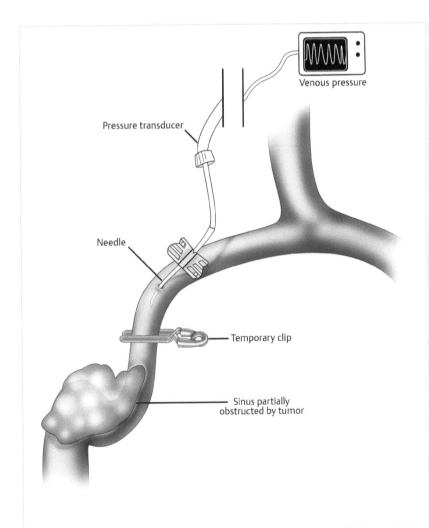

Venous pressure

Pressure transducer

Needle

Temporary clip

Sinus partially obstructed by tumor

Fig. 13.5 Technique of the intraoperative sinus occlusion test. A butterfly needle is inserted into the sinus following placement of temporary clip to occlude the sinus and the pressure is monitored. An increase of greater than 5 mm Hg at any time is considered a failed test.

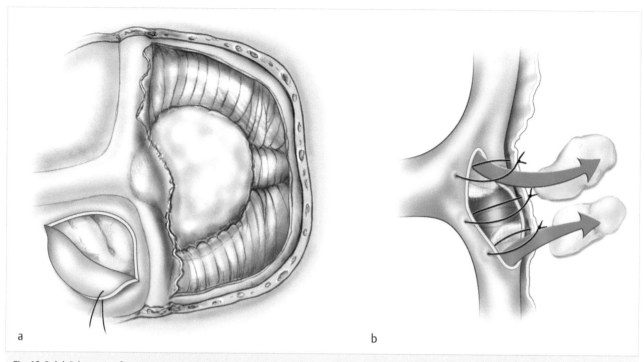

Fig. 13.6 (a) Schematic of a meningioma invading the torcula. **(b)** Removal of the tumor and reconstruction with a dural flap from adjacent dura.

(▶ Fig. 13.7). Typically, the graft is anchored to the sinus wall on one side before removal of the tumor, facilitating easier closure after the resection has been completed.

Once the tumor has been removed, management of venous bleeding during repair depends on the situation. The sinus can be allowed to bleed if it is a small rent, occluded with finger pressure or temporary clips if some collaterals exist, or occluded with a balloon shunt if high flow exists through the sinus (▶ Fig. 13.8). If the repair is likely to take more than 10 minutes, the patient needs to be heparinized. In retrosigmoid/presigmoid approaches, it is sometimes advantageous to ligate the sigmoid sinus for better exposure of the tumor. In these cases, we perform a direct repair of the sinus using 6–0 Prolene sutures at the end of the operation.

Graft Reconstruction

Graft reconstruction of the sinus is performed in cases of total segmental defect,[26] which cannot be repaired directly. The indications for such sinus repair are shown in ▶ Table 13.2. When the sinus to be repaired is large (≥ 1 cm diameter), the saphenous vein extracted from the thigh is used (▶ Fig. 13.9). If the sinus has been previously partially occluded by the tumor, the radial artery is used, because it tends to stay open even while the flow rate is low. Because of the discrepancy in size, an end-to-side technique is used for RAG (▶ Fig. 13.10), whereas an end-to-end technique is used for SVG.

13.5.5 Results for Tumors Involving Cerebral Veins and Venous Sinuses

The decision to aggressively manage tumors that invade the major venous sinuses is a controversial one. Most would agree that aggressive resection with en bloc removal of the sinus can be done safely when there is complete occlusion preoperatively and the collateralized veins are preserved. Controversy arises in cases of partial occlusion, in which the risk of recurrence from leaving residual is balanced against the possibility of intraoperative or postoperative complications from aggressive removal of tumor and sinus reconstruction. Although some advocate GTR only in cases of complete occlusion preoperatively,[27] others have suggested that reconstruction can be performed with good outcome. Sindou and Alvernia presented a series of 100 patients who had meningiomas involving the major sinuses and reported a mortality rate of 3% and venous-related morbidity of 8%.[28] Their recurrence rate was 4%, and there was a statistically significant decrease in venous morbidity in favor of those who had undergone venous reconstruction. They concluded that in their series, aggressive resection coupled with venous reconstruction resulted in a lower recurrence rate and better outcomes overall. Similarly, DiMeco et al reported a series of 108 patients in whom they aggressively resected tumor from the superior sagittal sinus.[29] Although their overall recurrence rate was higher, they confirmed Simpson grading as an independent predictor of recurrence, advocating for an aggressive resection approach.

The principles that we follow in managing patients with tumors involving the cerebral veins and venous sinuses are as follows:

- Meningiomas involving the venous sinuses are treated when symptomatic or demonstrate interval growth. They are otherwise observed or considered for radiation.
- Two options are considered and presented to the patient: radical resection along with the involved sinus or conservative resection and radiosurgery. The decision to go ahead with radical resection involves the basic principles of any tumor

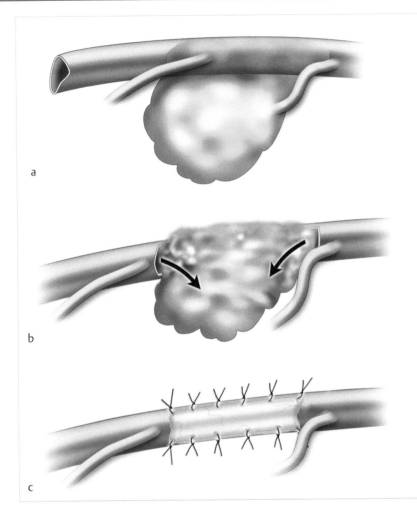

a

b

c

Fig. 13.7 Repair of a superior sagittal sinus using a free dural patch. **(a)** Tumor invading the sinus. **(b)** Removal of tumor creating a defect in the lateral wall of the sinus. **(c)** Reconstruction using a free dural patch sutured in place with interrupted sutures. Typically one limb of the patch is sutured in place prior to tumor removal so that the patch can be more easily and quickly secured after the tumor is removed.

resection, such as age, comorbidities, and regions involved; major cranial vascular; and CN involvement. Once the decision is made to do a radical resection with the sinus, the principles of whether reconstruction is required are followed as already described.

- Peeling of the tumor from the sinus can be done if only one of the walls is involved and the wall is reconstructed as previously described.
- If two walls are involved, the tumor may be still removed and repaired using a dural or venous patch.
- If three walls or more than 50% of the sinus is involved, sinus reconstruction with graft may be required.
- If the sinus is completely occluded preoperatively, no repair is needed. However, when flow is present intraoperatively, the surgeon must be prepared for reconstruction, because occlusion in cases of partial flow often results in venous hypertension.
- Radiosurgery may cause delayed sinus thrombosis with brain edema and seizures. Accordingly, all veins should be preserved intraoperatively to maximize venous collateral drainage.

The senior author has published his series of outcomes on patients with meningiomas that invaded the major venous sinuses.[30] Between 2003 and 2013, a total of 38 patients were treated with tumors involving the sagittal sinus (26 patients), torcula (5 patients), transverse (5 patients) and sigmoid sinus

(2 patients). Tumors were World Health Organization (WHO) grade I in 71% of patients and WHO grade II in 29% of patients, and GTR was achieved in 86.9%. Tumors involving the sinuses were divided into four groups: (I) complete occlusion ($n = 13$), (II) subtotal occlusion, 50 to 95% ($n = 9$), (III) partial occlusion, < 50% ($n = 14$), and (IV) lesion attached to outer wall ($n = 2$). Of the 38 patients, 21 underwent attempted sinus reconstruction (13 primarily, 8 with a patch of either dura or Gore-Tex). Of the 21 attempted reconstructions, 18 remained patent, with 3 occlusions. Two of these patients had no related complications, and one developed focal right-hand seizures in the postoperative period, which resolved with antiepileptics. There were no deaths, and two patients had recurrent disease in the follow-up period of 26 months.

13.5.6 Vasospasm after Cranial Base Tumor Resection

Cerebral vasospasm is well known to occur after various cerebral neurosurgical events that cause subarachnoid hemorrhage. Cerebral vasospasm can also occur after cranial base tumor resection.[31] Vasospasm manifests clinically 7 to 30 days postoperatively. For unclear reasons, pituitary tumors and craniopharyngiomas have a higher incidence of vasospasm. Delayed neurologic deterioration in a patient who has undergone cranial base tumor surgery not explained by an intracranial mass

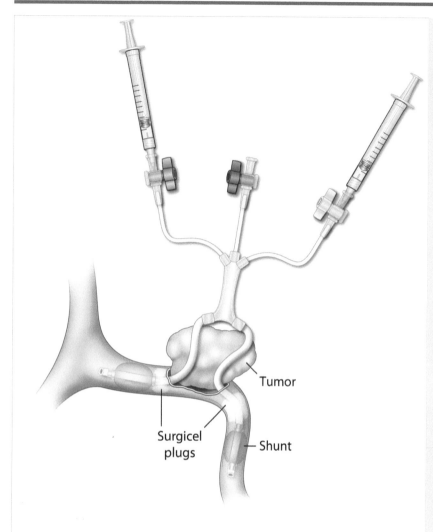

Tumor

Surgicel plugs

Shunt

Table 13.2 Indications for reconstruction of cerebral venous sinuses

Status	Decision
Collaterals	
• Excellent collaterals	Reconstruction unnecessary; provides practice for surgeons
• Marginal collaterals	Reconstruction recommended
• Poor or no collaterals	Occlusion dangerous; reconstruction if there is accidental injury
Sinus occlusion	
• One wall involved, sinus occlusion < 50%	Resection, resuture or a small patch
• Two walls involved, sinus occlusion > 50%	Resection possible, vein patch for repair, preserve collaterals
• Three walls involved, sinus occlusion > 90%	Test occlusion with pressure monitoring, sinus repair if pressure increases > 5 mm Hg

lesion should be promptly investigated using angiography. If vasospasm is diagnosed, it should be treated aggressively with hypertensive, hypervolemic therapy and, if necessary, endovascular angioplasty.

13.6 Case Study 1

Meningioma with subarachnoid vascular encasement: A 43-year old woman presented with headaches and diplopia and was discovered to have a very large clival meningioma with severe brainstem compression (▶ Fig. 13.11). She underwent preoperative embolization successfully through the meningohypophyseal artery as well as the ascending pharyngeal artery (▶ Fig. 13.12). She then underwent gross total resection of the tumor through a retrolabyrinthine, transpetrosal approach (▶ Fig. 13.13). The BA and the anterior inferior cerebellar artery were encased by the tumor, but the plane was favorable and the tumor was dissected free safely. Postoperatively, the patient had a partial CN VI palsy but was otherwise intact. Pathology was consistent with WHO grade I meningioma. She had recovered completely at follow-up 6 months after surgery, and her MRI showed no tumor recurrence (▶ Fig. 13.14).

13.7 Case Study 2

Recurrent giant cell tumor treated with SVG interposition graft for the VA: A 16-year-old boy presented with a recurrent giant

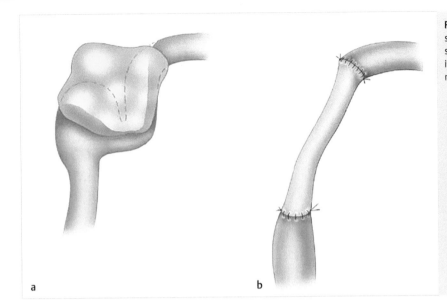

Fig. 13.9 **(a)** Tumor encased and invaded the sigmoid sinus to narrow the sinus. **(b)** Part of the sinus was resected along with the tumor, and an interposition graft (saphenous vein) was used for reconstruction (end-to-end anastomosis).

a

b

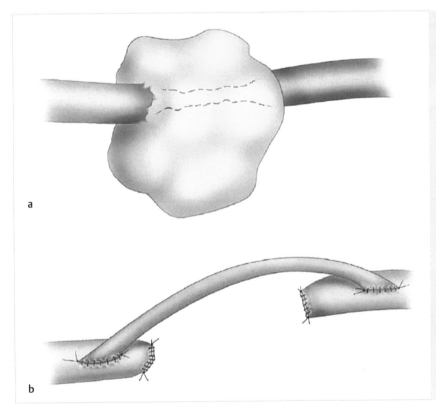

Fig. 13.10 **(a)** Tumor invading sinus. **(b)** Tumor resected with sinus and interposition graft (radial artery) placed (end-to-side anastomoses).

a

b

cell tumor of the lower clivus, C1, occipital condyle, and foramen magnum area on the left side 4 years after initial resection (▶ Fig. 13.15). An extreme lateral, complete transcondylar approach was performed and the tumor gross totally resected. Tumor was filling the jugular bulb, occluding the sigmoid sinus, and encasing the hypoglossal nerve (▶ Fig. 13.16). Dissection was tedious, and the extracranial left VA was encased by tumor. In addition, the tumor had parasitized several branches of the artery itself. During attempted dissection of the encased portion of the artery, the VA was damaged irreparably. A saphenous vein interposition graft was used to replace the damaged portion of the artery, which was excised along with the specimen (▶ Fig. 13.17). An additional area of tumor involvement was found at the dural penetration point of the VA (V3–V4 junction). This segment was excised and a primary end-to-end reanastomosis was performed. The patient recovered well after the operation but had persistent voice hoarseness that ultimately required vocal cord medial-

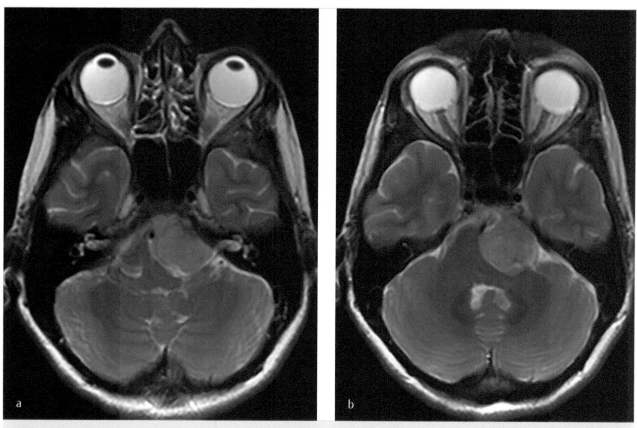

Fig. 13.11 (a, b) Preoperative MRI images showing a large petroclival meningioma, with severe brainstem compression displacing and encasing the basilar artery and several of its branches.

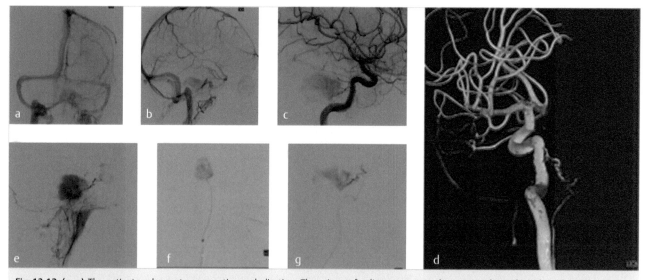

Fig. 13.12 (a–g) The patient underwent preoperative embolization. The primary feeding artery was the meningohypophyseal trunk, with some additional contribution from the ascending pharyngeal artery. Both arteries were embolized.

ization to improve voice quality. Postoperative angiogram demonstrated patency of the VA reconstruction (▶ Fig. 13.18). Because of the unilateral condylar resection, occiput–C3 fusion and fixation in halo traction was performed until the patient was adequately fused. The patient remains free of tumor 10 years after surgery.

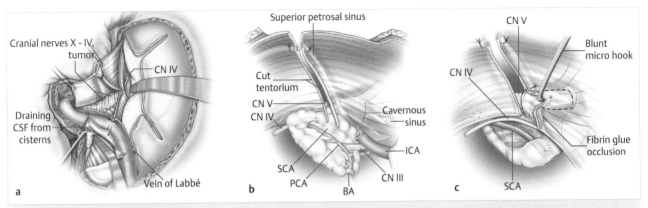

Fig. 13.13 **(a)** A retrolabyrinthine transpetrosal approach was used to expose the tumor. The tumor clearly encased the anteroinferior cerebellar artery as well as several cranial nerves (CNs). **(b)** The arachnoid planes around the CNs and the encased arteries were preserved, and the tumor consistency was soft, allowing for safe removal of the tumor from around critical structures. The basilar artery was adjacent to the posterior aspect of the tumor but was able to be dissected free. **(c)** The proximal portion of Meckel's cave was opened to remove the tumor extending into that area.

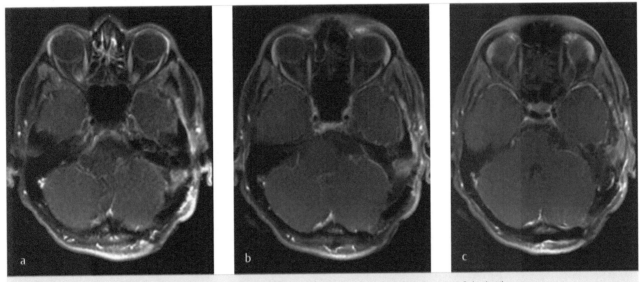

Fig. 13.14 **(a–c)** Postoperative MRI images showing gross total resection of the tumor with preservation of the basilar artery.

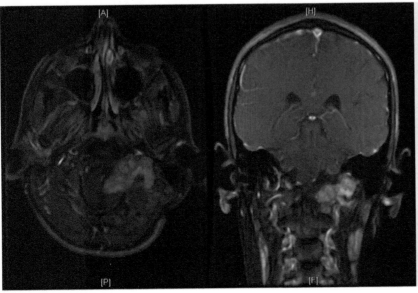

Fig. 13.15 Preoperative MRI showing recurrent giant cell tumor involving the lower clivus, occipital condyle, and foramen magnum.

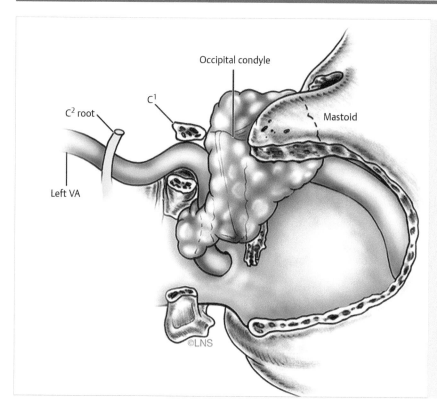

Fig. 13.16 The tumor had occluded the sigmoid sinus and was encasing the extracranial vertebral artery as well as the hypoglossal nerve. The occipital condyle has been largely destroyed by tumor infiltration as well.

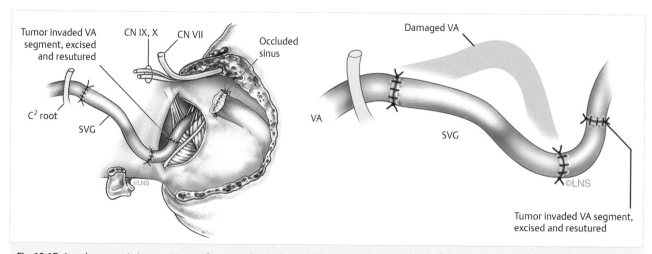

Fig. 13.17 A saphenous vein interposition graft was used to replace the damaged segment of the vertebral artery (VA). In addition, there was an area of VA involvement more distally at the point of dural penetration which was excised. The artery was then reanastomosed primarily at that site.

13.8 Case Study 3

Recurrent chordoma with emergent ECA–M2 bypass with radial artery interposition: A 45-year-old woman presented with a recurrent chordoma (▶ Fig. 13.19) involving the cavernous sinus and brainstem. Her primary symptom was declining vision in her left eye. She was unwilling to accept blood transfusions. She underwent a frontotemporal craniotomy with orbitozygomatic osteotomy and transcavernous approach to the tumor. The cavernous segment of the ICA was invaded with tumor and irreparably damaged during resection (▶ Fig. 13.20a). A RAG was placed from the ECA to the M2 MCA, and the operation was stopped (▶ Fig. 13.20b).

The patient recovered without any deficits or imaging evidence of stroke. Postoperative angiogram showed a patent bypass and good filling of the intracranial circulation (▶ Fig. 13.21). A week later, she underwent a second-stage operation to remove tumor from the cavernous sinus, petrous apex, and brainstem. She did completely lose vision in her left eye but was otherwise neurologically intact postoperatively. She had a near total resection with a small amount of residual in the area of Meckel's cave (▶ Fig. 13.22). The patient had radiosurgery for the remaining tumor and remains progression-free after 13 years.

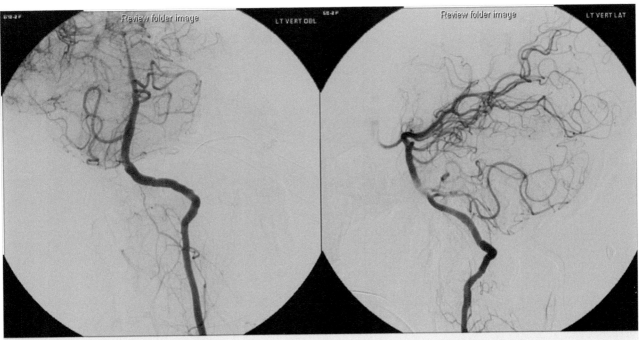

Fig. 13.18 Postoperative angiogram demonstrating patency of the saphenous vein graft and good flow through the posterior circulation.

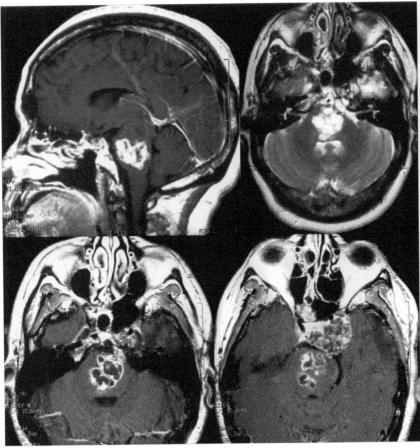

Fig. 13.19 Preoperative MRIs showing chordoma involving the cavernous sinus and infiltrating the brainstem.

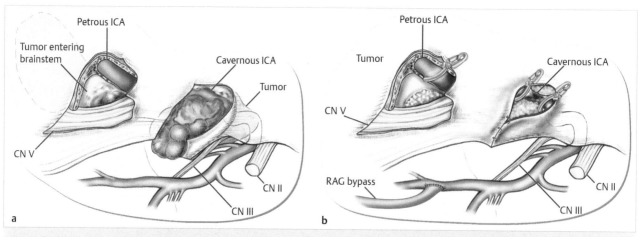

Fig. 13.20 **(a)** The cavernous portion of the internal carotid artery (ICA) was invaded by tumor, which extended through Meckel's cave and into the posterior fossa and brainstem. **(b)** A radial artery bypass to the middle cerebral artery was performed, and the involved portion of the ICA was trapped prior to tumor removal in a second stage.

13.9 Case Study 4

Parasagittal meningioma with direct repair of superior sagittal sinus: A 41-year-old woman had undergone a craniotomy and subtotal resection of a WHO grade II left parasagittal meningioma invading the superior sagittal sinus and adjacent to the motor cortex (▶ Fig. 13.23) 3 years earlier by another neurosurgeon. Postoperatively she had Cyber Knife (Accuray) radiation for the residual tumor. She presented to us 3 years later with recurrence of seizures. Her MRI revealed recurrence of the tumor adjacent to the motor cortex, with peritumoral edema and narrowing of the superior sagittal sinus (▶ Fig. 13.23b). Preoperative angiogram showed that the sinus was patent at the junction of the posterior and middle third, with prominent cortical veins draining on either side (▶ Fig. 13.24). She underwent bilateral frontoparietal craniotomy, gross total microsurgical resection of the tumor, and partial direct reconstruction of the superior sagittal sinus (▶ Fig. 13.25). Postoperative computerized tomographic venogram (CTV) showed patency of the superior sagittal sinus (SSS) (▶ Fig. 13.26). MRI at 6-week follow-up showed GTR with a patent SSS (▶ Fig. 13.27). Pathology was consistent with WHO grade II meningioma, but considering the presence of GTR and her prior radiation therapy, additional radiation was deferred at that time. She continues to be tumor-free 2 years after surgery.

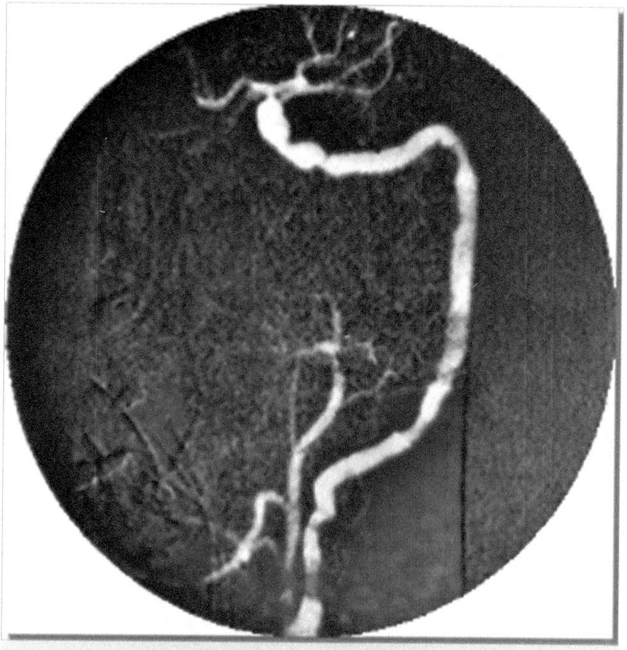

13.10 Case Study 5

Glomus tumor with sigmoid sinus reconstruction using SVG. A 62-year-old man presented with worsening seizure, right-sided tinnitus, and swallowing disturbances. On examination, he had 20% hearing loss in his right ear, was unable to perform tandem walk, and had nystagmus. MRI scan showed a highly vascular glomus jugulare tumor in the right jugular foramen, filling the region of right jugular bulb (▶ Fig. 13.28). The tumor encased the petrosal segment of the ICA, bowing it forward. The sigmoid and transverse sinuses were larger on the right side but were subtotally occluded by the tumor. There was a good communication between the two sinuses at the torcular Herophili (▶ Fig. 13.29), suggesting that occlusion during surgery should

Fig. 13.21 Postoperative angiogram demonstrating flow through the bypass and opacification of the middle cerebral artery through an external carotid artery injection.

be safe. During the operation, intrasinus pressure was measured prior to sinus occlusion and excision of the tumor. Although the intrasinus pressure was initially unchanged after occlusion, the pressure increased steadily during the operation to > 35 torr, mandating sinus reconstruction using a saphenous vein interposition graft (▶ Fig. 13.30). A 5-cm-long vein graft was sutured from the sigmoid sinus to the internal jugular vein. Patency of the graft was verified by postoperative angiography (▶ Fig. 13.31). The patient subsequently developed communicating hydrocephalus that required shunt placement. He also had a transient postoperative facial nerve palsy, which recovered completely. The patient is 6 years postsurgery and is doing well, with no neurologic deficits and no evidence of recurrent tumor.

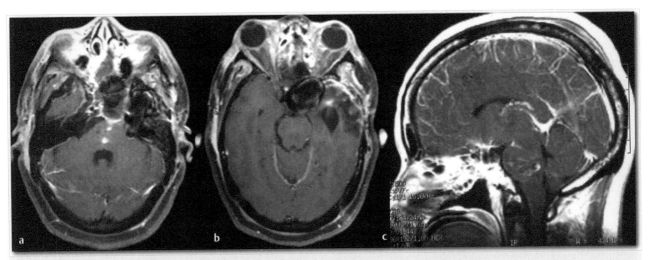

Fig. 13.22 (a, b) Axial and (c) sagittal contrast-enhanced T1 images of an MRI scan showing near total resection of the tumor with some residual in Meckel's cave.

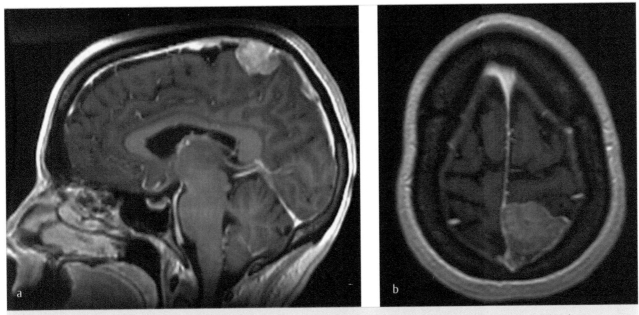

Fig. 13.23 (a, b) Preoperative imaging demonstrating a recurrent parasagittal meningioma with involvement of the superior sagittal sinus.

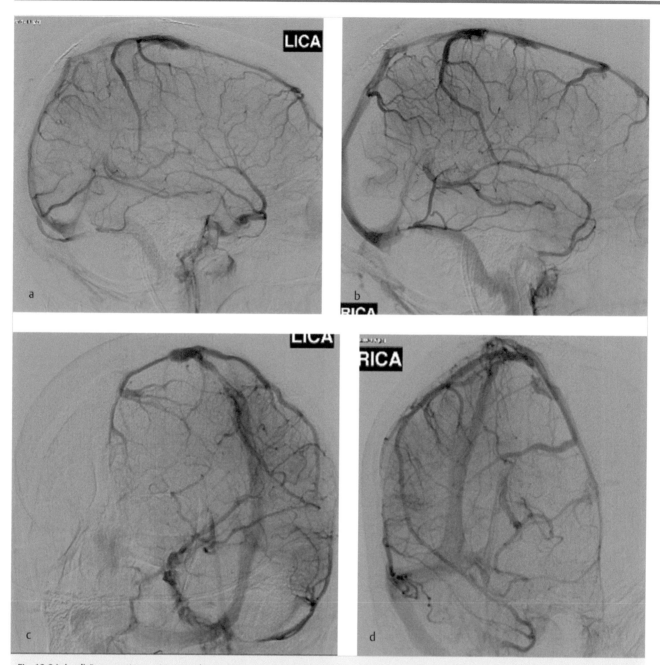

Fig. 13.24 (a–d) Preoperative angiograms demonstrating a narrowed but patent superior sagittal sinus. Several large draining veins were present in the region adjacent to the narrowing, suggesting some collateralization of the venous drainage.

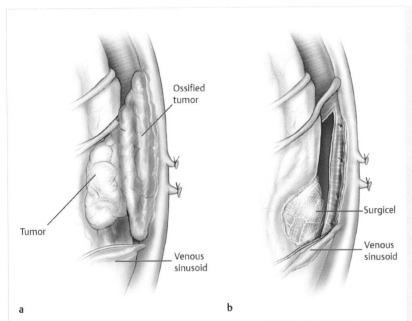

Fig. 13.25 (a) The tumor had invaded both the sinus and the surrounding brain. **(b)** It was removed completely and the sinus repaired directly. Flow was confirmed using Doppler insonation at the time of surgery.

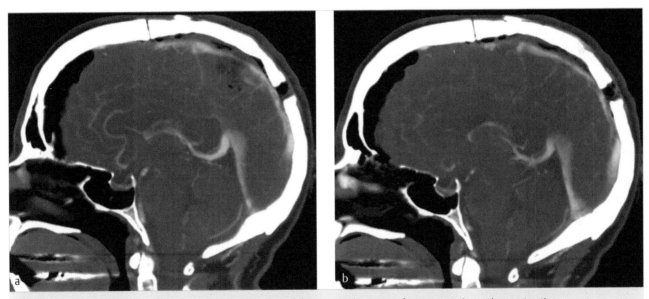

Fig. 13.26 (a, b) Postoperative MR venogram showing patency of the sinus in the region of tumor resection and reconstruction.

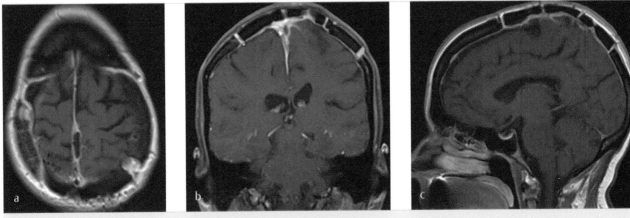

Fig. 13.27 (a–c) Six-week follow-up MRI showing continued patency of the sinus.

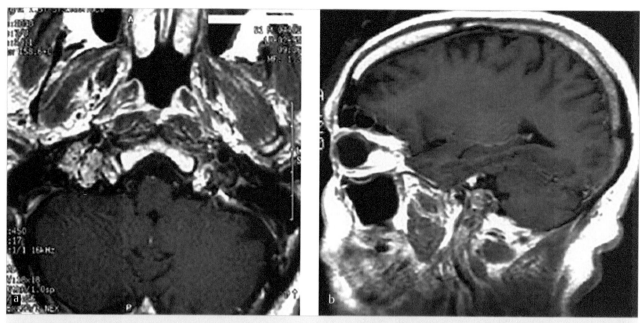

Fig. 13.28 (a, b) Preoperative MRIs showing a right-sided glomus tumor involving the jugular foramen.

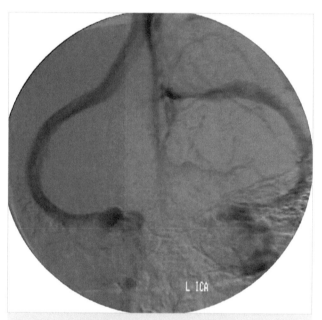

Fig. 13.29 Preoperative angiography showing a patent venous system with bilateral drainage from the superior sagittal sinus. Mild narrowing of the right sigmoid and transverse sinuses was present, but there was still significant drainage through the right side.

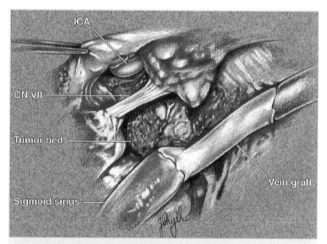

Fig. 13.30 The saphenous vein graft, cranial nerve VII, the tumor bed, and the petrous internal carotid artery.

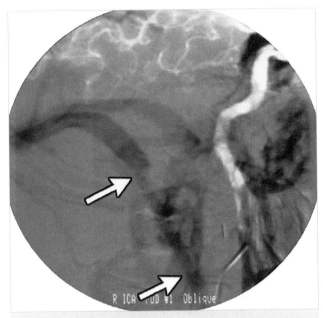

Fig. 13.31 Postoperative angiography demonstrating patency of the vein graft (*arrows*).

References

[1] Guppy KH, Origitano TC, Reichman OH, Segal S. Venous drainage of the inferolateral temporal lobe in relationship to transtemporal/transtentorial approaches to the cranial base. Neurosurgery. 1997; 41(3):615–619, discussion 619–620

[2] Koperna T, Tschabitscher M, Knosp E. The termination of the vein of "Labbé" and its microsurgical significance. Acta Neurochir (Wien). 1992; 118(3–4):172–175

[3] Kyoshima K, Oikawa S, Kobayashi S. Preservation of large bridging veins of the cranial base: technical note. Neurosurgery. 2001; 48(2):447–449

[4] Lustig LR, Jackler RK. The vulnerability of the vein of Labbé during combined craniotomies of the middle and posterior fossae. Skull Base Surg. 1998; 8(1):1–9

[5] Borg A, Ekanayake J, Mair R, et al. Preoperative particle and glue embolization of meningiomas: indications, results, and lessons learned from 117 consecutive patients. Neurosurgery. 2013; 73(2) Suppl Operative:ons244–ons251, discussion ons252

[6] Raper DM, Starke RM, Henderson F, Jr, et al. Preoperative embolization of intracranial meningiomas: efficacy, technical considerations, and complications. AJNR Am J Neuroradiol. 2014; 35(9):1798–1804

[7] Shah AH, Patel N, Raper DM, et al. The role of preoperative embolization for intracranial meningiomas. J Neurosurg. 2013; 119(2):364–372

[8] Ishikawa M, Nishi S, Aoki T, et al. Predictability of internal carotid artery (ICA) dissectability in cases showing ICA involvement in parasellar meningioma. J Clin Neurosci. 2001; 8(4) Suppl 1:22–25

[9] Mohit AA, Sekhar LN, Natarajan SK, Britz GW, Ghodke B. High-flow bypass grafts in the management of complex intracranial aneurysms. Neurosurgery. 2007; 60(2) Suppl 1:ONS105–ONS122, discussion ONS122–ONS123

[10] Natarajan SK, Sekhar LN, Schessel D, Morita A. Petroclival meningiomas: multimodality treatment and outcomes at long-term follow-up. Neurosurgery. 2007; 60(6):965–979, discussion 979–981

[11] Sekhar LN, Kalavakonda C. Cerebral revascularization for aneurysms and tumors. Neurosurgery. 2002; 50(2):321–331

[12] Sekhar LN, Tzortzidis FN, Bejjani GK, Schessel DA. Saphenous vein graft bypass of the sigmoid sinus and jugular bulb during the removal of glomus jugulare tumors: report of two cases. J Neurosurg. 1997; 86(6):1036–1041

[13] Tzortzidis F, Elahi F, Wright D, Natarajan SK, Sekhar LN. Patient outcome at long-term follow-up after aggressive microsurgical resection of cranial base chordomas. Neurosurgery. 2006; 59(2):230–237

[14] Larson JJ, Tew JM, Jr, Tomsick TA, van Loveren HR. Treatment of aneurysms of the internal carotid artery by intravascular balloon occlusion: long-term follow-up of 58 patients. Neurosurgery. 1995; 36(1):26–30

[15] McIvor NP, Willinsky RA, TerBrugge KG, Rutka JA, Freeman JL. Validity of test occlusion studies prior to internal carotid artery sacrifice. Head Neck. 1994; 16(1):11–16

[16] Origitano TC, al-Mefty O, Leonetti JP, DeMonte F, Reichman OH. Vascular considerations and complications in cranial base surgery. Neurosurgery. 1994; 35(3):351–362, discussion 362–363

[17] Sekhar LN, Patel SJ. Permanent occlusion of the internal carotid artery during skull-base and vascular surgery: is it really safe? Am J Otol. 1993; 14(5):421–422

[18] Yang T, Tariq F, Chabot J, Madhok R, Sekhar LN. Cerebral revascularization for difficult skull base tumors: a contemporary series of 18 patients. World Neurosurg. 2014; 82(5):660–671

[19] Morton RP, Moore AE, Barber J, et al. Monitoring flow in extracranial-intracranial bypass grafts using duplex ultrasonography: a single-center experience in 80 grafts over 8 years. Neurosurgery. 2014; 74(1):62–70

[20] Evans JJ, Sekhar LN, Rak R, Stimac D. Bypass grafting and revascularization in the management of posterior circulation aneurysms. Neurosurgery. 2004; 55(5):1036–1049

[21] Sekhar LN, Bucur SD, Bank WO, Wright DC. Venous and arterial bypass grafts for difficult tumors, aneurysms, and occlusive vascular lesions: evolution of surgical treatment and improved graft results. Neurosurgery. 1999; 44(6):1207–1223, discussion 1223–1224

[22] Kalani MY, Kalb S, Martirosyan NL, et al. Cerebral revascularization and carotid artery resection at the skull base for treatment of advanced head and neck malignancies. J Neurosurg. 2013; 118(3):637–642

[23] Couldwell WT, Taussky P, Sivakumar W. Submandibular high-flow bypass in the treatment of skull base lesions: an analysis of long-term outcome. Neurosurgery. 2012; 71(3):645–650, discussion 650–651

[24] Rangel-Castilla L, McDougall CG, Spetzler RF, Nakaji P. Urgent cerebral revascularization bypass surgery for iatrogenic skull base internal carotid artery injury. Neurosurgery. 2014; 10(4) Suppl 4:640–647, discussion 647–648

[25] Wanibuchi M, Akiyama Y, Mikami T, et al. Radical removal of recurrent malignant meningeal tumors of the cavernous sinus in combination with high-flow bypass. World Neurosurg. 2015; 83(4):424–430

[26] Morita A, Sekhar LN. Reconstruction of the vein of Labbé by using a short saphenous vein bypass graft: technical note. J Neurosurg. 1998; 89(4):671–675

[27] Caroli E, Orlando ER, Mastronardi L, Ferrante L. Meningiomas infiltrating the superior sagittal sinus: surgical considerations of 328 cases. Neurosurg Rev. 2006; 29(3):236–241

[28] Sindou MP, Alvernia JE. Results of attempted radical tumor removal and venous repair in 100 consecutive meningiomas involving the major dural sinuses. J Neurosurg. 2006; 105(4):514–525

[29] DiMeco F, Li KW, Casali C, et al. Meningiomas invading the superior sagittal sinus: surgical experience in 108 cases. Neurosurgery. 2004; 55(6):1263–1272, discussion 1272–1274

[30] Mantovani A, Di Maio S, Ferreira MJ, Sekhar LN. Management of meningiomas invading the major dural venous sinuses: operative technique, results, and potential benefit for higher grade tumors. World Neurosurg. 2014; 82(3–4):455–467

[31] Bejjani GK, Sekhar LN, Yost A-M, Bank WO, Wright DC. Vasospasm after cranial base tumor resection: pathogenesis, diagnosis, and therapy. Surg Neurol. 1999; 52(6):577–583, discussion 583–584

14 Quality of Life and Measures of Outcome for Patients with Skull Base Tumors

John R. De Almeida and Dan M. Fliss

Summary

Skull base tumors are a heterogeneous group of tumors with variable anatomic extension, histopathology, and treatment approaches. Because of these tumors' proximity to critical neurovascular structures, both disease and treatment factors may have a significant impact on health-related quality of life. Although generic quality of life instruments may be used to assess quality of life for patients who have skull base tumors, disease-specific quality of life instruments may help better compare patients' quality of life. Several physical and nonphysical domains of quality of life may be affected by these tumors. Specific measurement of nasal, visual, endocrine, and neurologic physical domains is important in assessing the full impact on the disease and treatment on physical function. With the emergence of endoscopic cranial base surgery and new radiotherapy techniques such as proton beam therapy, patients may experience greater improvements in their quality of life after treatment than with more traditional techniques, although large prospective studies are still needed.

Keywords: quality of life, endoscopic skull base surgery, open skull base surgery, radiotherapy, functional outcomes

14.1 Introduction

Skull base tumors and their treatment may have a significant impact on health-related quality of life. The skull base is an anatomically complex partition that structurally separates the cranial cavity from the remainder of the head and neck. Critical neurovascular structures such as cranial nerves, the spinal cord, carotid and vertebral arteries, and jugular veins traverse the skull base. It is intimate with sensory organs, such as the eye and the olfactory and auditory apparatuses, as well as with neuroendocrine structures, such as the pituitary gland. Tumors of the skull base and their treatment may result in injury to any of these structures. Moreover, the skull base and craniofacial skeleton are intimately linked to facial appearances, and treatment of tumors in this location may be associated with disfigurement and an alteration of one's identity. All these consequences may affect patients' physical functioning and have a far-reaching impact on their position in life.

Over the past several decades, a better understanding of treatment-related impact on quality of life and functional outcomes has been born from the development of validated measurement instruments as well as from research aimed at better quantifying treatment morbidity. The improved understanding of the impact of treatment on quality of life and functional outcomes has spawned newer surgical and nonsurgical techniques that purport to ameliorate treatment morbidity. The development of endoscopic endonasal approaches to selected anterior skull base tumors and newer radiotherapy modalities such as proton beam and intensity modulated radiotherapy are some examples of techniques that may improve quality of life. Despite many advances, however, patients still suffer from their disease and treatment. Measuring quality of life and functional outcomes in patients who have skull base tumors may aid treating clinicians as they counsel patients on the impact of treatment, assess and compare the effectiveness of different treatment modalities, and identify patients who are at risk for a loss of quality of life while serving as important outcomes in clinical trials. This chapter focuses on the impact that treatment of skull base tumors has on quality of life, as well as on the measurement tools used to quantify that impact.

14.2 Challenges in Assessing Quality of Life in Patients Who Have Skull Base Tumors

The very nature of the construct of quality of life is one that is inherently difficult to measure. This multidimensional construct is defined by the World Health Organization as individuals' perception of their position in life in the context of the culture and value systems in which they live and in relation to their goals, expectations, standards, and concerns. It is a broad ranging concept affected in a complex way by the person's physical health, psychological state, level of independence, social relationships, personal beliefs and their relationship to salient features of their environment.[1]

Experts have suggested that a quality of life instrument should include among its dimensions physical function, emotional function, social function, role performance, pain, and other disease-specific symptoms.[2] Any instrument used to measure quality of life must assess these various dimensions of quality of life.

The complexities of the definition of quality of life pose several challenges when measuring this concept. To better illustrate this point, consider two hypothetical patients who have similar skull base tumors treated in the same fashion. The first has chronic nasal crusting after surgery but adapts to this limitation and remains socially active and emotionally well-adjusted. The second patient suffers a cranial nerve VI palsy after surgery and avoids driving and social interaction as a result. A single summary score of the various dimensions of quality of life would be helpful for comparing the quality of life of these individuals. However, a summary score would require a weighting of the relative importance of these very disparate problems. Unfortunately, weighting separate dimensions is not a simple task and may be fraught with problems. The relative importance of one issue to one individual may not be the same as for another individual. For these reasons, experts recommend avoiding complex weighting schemes when measuring quality of life.[3,4] Realistically, however, no two issues are of equal importance, particularly with skull base tumors. Simple scoring schemes that equally weight items may be preferable

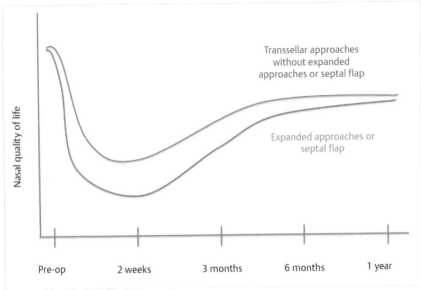

Fig. 14.1 Nasal quality of life after skull base surgery.

to more complex schemes that do not capture the full depth of individual patient problems.[4]

Perhaps the biggest challenge in measuring quality of life for skull base tumors is the enormous variability of histopathologies, treatments, and dimensions of life that are affected by treatment. This variability makes comparing quality of life between populations very difficult. For these reasons, instruments used to measure quality of life must have good measurement properties (reliability and validity), and disease-specific instruments may be preferable. In comparison with generic quality of life instruments, disease-specific instruments may be more sensitive to change, better tolerated by patients because the dimensions are more relevant, and more responsive to detecting subtle treatment effects.[4]

14.3 Symptom-Specific Quality of Life and Functional Outcomes Following Skull Base Surgery

14.3.1 Nasal Outcomes

Nasal outcomes have been studied extensively in patients who have skull base tumors, particularly in patients who have undergone endoscopic endonasal surgery for pituitary and sellar pathology (▶ Fig. 14.1). Several studies have highlighted the acute nasal morbidity after surgery, followed by a gradual recovery of function.[5,6,7,8] This temporary nasal morbidity includes an acute subjective loss of smell, nasal crusting/discharge, and postnasal drip that in most cases resolves by 6 months.[5] Many of the nasal complaints following endoscopic endonasal approaches, particularly nasal crusting, are more pronounced with the use of the nasoseptal flap in reconstruction.[7]

The impact of surgical approach on nasal morbidity has also been studied. One systematic review compared the endoscopic and microscopic (sublabial or transseptal) approaches for sellar tumors.[9] The authors noted that there were insufficient data in published series to conclusively identify any differences in olfactory disturbances or nasal crusting between approaches.

Table 14.1 Nasal-specific quality of life instruments for skull base tumors

	Items	Validated for skull base tumors?	Reliability	Validity
SNOT-22	22	No	Internal consistency, test–retest	Known group differences; responsiveness
ASK Nasal–12	12	Yes	Internal consistency, test–retest	Concurrent validity, discriminant validity
SBI Nasal Domain	4	Yes	Internal consistency, test–retest	Construct validity (known group differences)

The review also noted indications of increased rate of rhinologic complications, such as septal perforations, synechiae, epistaxis, and postoperative deviated septums, in patients undergoing a microscopic approach.

Nasal symptom specific quality of life in skull base surgery has been evaluated using a number of validated instruments (▶ Table 14.1). Many of these instruments are relevant to patients who have inflammatory sinus disease. Although not validated specifically for patients who have skull base tumors, the Sinonasal Outcomes Test–22 questionnaire (SNOT-22) has been used to evaluate nasal morbidity after endoscopic endonasal approaches for skull base tumors.[10] This instrument comprises 22 items and has been extensively validated and cross-validated in many languages. Internal consistency, test–retest reliability, responsiveness, and construct validity (i.e., known group differences), and minimally important clinical differences have been demonstrated.[10] Other instruments have also been used to evaluate nasal dysfunction after skull base surgery. The Anterior Skull Base Nasal Inventory (ASK-Nasal 12) has been developed to quantify nasal-related quality of life changes in patients undergoing skull base surgery.[11] This 12-item instrument has demonstrated internal consistency, test–retest reliability, concurrent validity, and discriminant validity. Finally, the Skull Base Inventory (SBI) nasal domain is a four-item domain in a larger disease-specific instrument that has been shown to be reliable, with good internal consistency and test–retest reliability, and valid, with good construct validity.[12]

These instruments have been used to demonstrate the immediate decrease, followed by gradual improvement, in nasal quality of life for patients who have skull base tumors. The SNOT-22 was used to demonstrate that patients who had endoscopic skull base surgery experienced loss of smell and taste, nasal obstruction, postnasal discharge, and nighttime wakefulness.[13] The authors demonstrated a poorer nasal-related quality of life in patients who had nasoseptal flaps than in those who did not. The temporal trend demonstrates gradual improvement over time after surgery, reaching a plateau roughly 6 months after surgery. Using the ASK-Nasal 12 in a large multi-institutional prospective study, another group demonstrated that nasal quality of life reaches a nadir at 2 weeks, followed by recovery at roughly 3 months after surgery.[14] In this study, the use of nasal splints predicted poor quality of life at 2 weeks after surgery, with the presence of ongoing symptoms of sinusitis predicting poor nasal quality of life at 3 months after surgery. This general trend in nasal dysfunction and gradual recovery is corroborated in many studies (▶ Fig. 14.2).[5,13,14]

The use of the nasoseptal flap adversely affects nasal quality of life following endoscopic endonasal skull base surgery. Following surgery, patients who undergo a nasoseptal flap for reconstruction experience clinical deterioration, as evidenced by endoscopic examination.[15,16] The septal flap is associated with complications such as cartilage necrosis, prolonged crusting, and septal perforation.[17] The use of a nasoseptal flap may further contribute to nasal morbidity by the loss of olfaction, even if only transient.[18] Using a historical cohort as a comparison and the SNOT-22 instrument as a measurement tool, one group demonstrated improved nasal quality of life scores after discontinuing use of the nasoseptal flap and limiting unnecessary sinus mucosal manipulation by reducing antrostomies

and turbinate resections.[19] Some authors have suggested techniques for reducing the morbidity of the septal flap by applying a free mucosal graft to the denuded septum.[20] Although this technique has been shown to reduce postoperative crusting, whether it may reduce olfactory deficits related to the nasoseptal flap has not yet been determined. Furthermore, it is often difficult to predict whether a septal flap is indeed required. For example, if a cerebrospinal fluid (CSF) leak is encountered, a septal flap maybe necessary to reduce the risk of a postoperative leak but might not be needed if no leak is encountered. One potential way of avoiding the morbidity of the flap for pituitary surgery is to use the "rescue" nasoseptal flap. This technique preserves the vascular pedicle of the flap over the face of the sphenoid without harvesting the flap from the septum. Thus the morbidity of the flap harvest may be avoided.[21]

14.3.2 Visual Outcomes

Not all skull base tumors necessarily affect visual outcomes. Visual outcomes are most relevant to sellar and parasellar skull base tumors proximate to the optic nerves or malignancies featuring direct involvement of orbital contents. Pituitary adenomas, meningiomas of the tuberculum sella, planum sphenoidale, and olfactory groove, as well as sinonasal malignancies, can all affect visual outcomes. Large single-institution studies demonstrated excellent visual acuity and visual field outcomes for endoscopic transsphenoidal pituitary surgery.[23,24,25,26] As many as 73 to 80% of patients experienced an improvement in their preoperative visual acuity, and only 2 to 5% experienced a decline in vision, mainly as a result of postoperative hemorrhage.[23,24,25,26] Young age, preoperative visual function, and craniocaudal dimension of tumors have been shown to be predictive factors for visual recovery.[23] Visual fields are similarly favorable. Roughly 62 to 95% of patients experienced an improvement in their visual field defect, and no patients experienced a decline in visual field after surgery.[23,24,25,26]

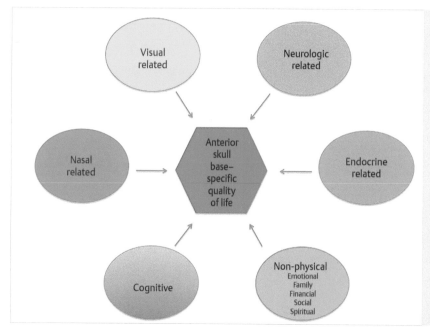

Fig. 14.2 Anterior skull base–specific quality of life.

Visual outcomes are an important metric when comparing effectiveness of the endoscopic endonasal approach and traditional transcranial approaches for skull base meningiomas. A recent systematic review of traditional transcranial approaches for tuberculum sella meningiomas demonstrated that vision improved, worsened, or remained unchanged in 65.5%, 10.4%, or 24.7%, respectively.[27] In comparison, a large single-institution study evaluating the endoscopic endonasal approach for tuberculum meningiomas demonstrated that 85.7% of patients who had preoperative visual acuity deficits improved.[28] Similar outcomes have been demonstrated in patients who had olfactory groove meningiomas. Over 86% of patients had improvement in their visual symptoms.[29] The authors suggest that in comparison with open approaches, the endoscopic approach offers superior visualization of the vascular supply to the optic apparatus, the ability to decompress both optic canals, and avoidance of brain and optic nerve retraction. One study directly compared visual outcomes using the endoscopic ($n = 17$) and transcranial approaches ($n = 15$) for tuberculum sellae and planum sphenoidale meningiomas amenable to either approach, demonstrating a superior rate of visual improvement in the endoscopic group (93% vs. 56%, $p = 0.049$).[30] The improved visual outcomes seen when using the endoscopic approach compared with traditional transcranial approaches has been corroborated in a systematic review that showed an increased postoperative visual improvement with the endoscopic endonasal approach (OR 1.5, $p = 0.05$).[31] These findings still remain controversial, however,[32] and must be weighed against the likely increased risk of CSF leak, the surgical expertise available, and the ability to fully access the tumor.

In patients who have sinonasal malignancies of the skull base, vision is affected by direct orbital extension more commonly than by optic nerve compression. Involvement of the orbit by tumor extension may necessitate orbital exenteration for complete tumor resection. Loss of an eye may have a significant impact on quality of life by limiting binocular vision, removing the ability to drive in many patients, as well as by impacting cosmetic appearance. The oncologic adequacy of orbital preservation has been investigated by many groups, some of which have advocated for orbital preservation with involvement of lamina papyracea or periorbita and, in some instances, limited involvement of orbital fat without ocular globe or extraocular muscle involvement.[33,34,35,36] The effects on visual outcomes attributable to surgery include diplopia, globe malposition, and enophthalmos, whereas the effects on visual outcome attributable to radiation include impaired visual acuity, dry eye, keratopathy, and visual field defect.[36] The advent of intensity modulated radiotherapy may improve visual outcomes by sparing the optic nerves.[37,38]

14.3.3 Endocrine Outcomes

Endocrine outcomes are important to health-related quality of life and are particularly relevant to many skull base tumors that involve the hypothalamic–pituitary axis, such as pituitary adenomas and craniopharyngiomas. Emerging evidence also suggests that patients receiving radiotherapy for malignancies of the skull base are at increased risk for endocrinologic abnormalities. Pituitary insufficiency following surgery for sellar tumors or endocrinopathies associated with functioning

adenomas may affect physical function and quality of life in a number of ways, ranging from the need to supplement hormone levels with medication to the need to manage symptoms related to endocrinopathies.

Several systematic reviews have reported endocrine outcomes for patients undergoing either endoscopic endonasal or microscopic approaches to pituitary adenomas.[9,39,40,41,42] In one review, remission rates of hypersecreting functioning adenomas after surgery were comparable to those seen for the endoscopic and microscopic approaches (66% vs. 60%, $p = 0.35$).[40] A subgroup analysis demonstrated that surgical approach did not affect outcomes for various functioning adenomas, including patients who had acromegaly, prolactinomas, and Cushing's disease. However, postoperative diabetes insipidus was less common in patients undergoing the endoscopic approach (15 vs. 28%, $p = 0.003$).[40] The increased likelihood of diabetes insipidus with transcranial and microscopic approaches in comparison with endoscopic endonasal approaches was also demonstrated in another systematic review (9.1% and 8.7% vs. 4.7%).[41] Hypopituitarism after an open transcranial approach or transsphenoidal microscopic approach was also shown to be greater than with the endoscopic endonasal approach (9.1% and 9.9% vs. 1.1%, $p < 0.05$ for both comparisons).[41] Li et al corroborated these findings in their systematic review, reporting a 22% risk reduction in diabetes insipidus after surgical intervention in patients undergoing endoscopic endonasal approaches compared with transsphenoidal microscopic approaches in 1,350 patients across 17 studies.[42]

In cases of craniopharyngioma, endocrine dysfunction after surgery is directly related to the extent of resection. In a systematic review, patients undergoing a gross total resection or subtotal resection had significantly more anterior pituitary lobe dysfunction than those undergoing biopsy (59% and 55% vs. 21%, $p < 0.001$).[43] The same study showed a similar increase in the risk of diabetes insipidus (25% and 10% vs. 6%, $p < 0.001$) and panhypopituitarism (16% and 14% vs. 2%, $p < 0.006$). Overall the authors noted fewer long-term complications with subtotal removal and adjuvant therapy than with gross total removal and thus advocate consideration of subtotal removal to minimize long-term sequelae and impact on quality of life. Surgical approach was also a predictor of poor endocrine function in one study that showed higher rates of panhypopituitarism in patients undergoing pterional craniotomy to access craniopharyngiomas, compared with the transsphenoidal approach.[44] Preservation of the pituitary stalk is necessary to minimize endocrine dysfunction.[45]

Patients who have sinonasal malignancies affecting the skull base may also be at risk for endocrine abnormalities. Although direct surgical resection of the hypothalamic pituitary axis for sinonasal malignancy would be unlikely, the effects of adjuvant or definitive radiotherapy may be underrecognized.[46,47] In one study, 62% of patients who had sinonasal malignancies treated using radiotherapy had hormonal disturbances, with 24% having multiple hormonal deficiencies.[47]

14.3.4 Neurologic Outcomes

Neurological, neuropsychiatric, and cognitive outcomes are of particular concern for patients who have skull base tumors. Although in many instances these symptoms can be subtle and difficult to measure, the impact on health-related quality of life can be significant and may indeed impact the ability to carry out day-to-day functions.[48] The impact of skull base tumors and their treatment on neurological and neuropsychiatric symptoms depends on tumor location, with anterior skull base lesions impacting cognitive function, executive functions, and memory but tumors of the clivus, sella, and parasellar region primarily affecting cranial nerves.

Anterior skull base meningiomas have been studied extensively with regard to neurological outcomes. Zweckberger et al showed that 23% of all patients who have meningiomas and who undergo surgery have temporary—and 12% have permanent—neurological deficits.[49] In this study the authors recorded cranial nerve deficits, gait disturbances, vision impairment, speech impairment, depression, anxiety, verbal learning, memory, cognition, visuomotor processing, and working memory. Interestingly, short-term memory was not affected by surgery, but significant impairment in verbal learning capacity was noted in 9% of patients in the short term.[49] Similarly, visual memory significantly deteriorated in 6%. Further tests were used to measure cognitive speed and concentration, and 6% significantly deteriorated. Nonsurgical approaches such as Gamma Knife radiosurgery may be associated with similar outcomes.[50]

Endoscopic endonasal approaches for meningiomas offer a theoretical benefit of reducing brain retraction while potentially reducing the risk of frontal lobe injury. Although there are no current studies comparing objective outcomes or patient-reported neurocognitive outcomes, one study showed reduced radiographic evidence of frontal lobe changes on MRI in patients undergoing an endoscopic endonasal approach compared with bifrontal craniotomy, in a matched paired analysis.[51]

Lesions of the central skull base are typically associated with a different morbidity profile than anterior skull base lesions are. With advances in endoscopic cranial base surgery, most tumors in the central skull base are accessible endoscopically. One large series of chordomas managed through an endoscopic endonasal approach demonstrated new cranial neuropathies in 6.7% patients and new long tract symptoms, such as quadriparesis in one (1.7%) patient secondary to pontine hemorrhage.[52] A recent meta-analysis compared outcomes achieved through anterior midline approaches, such as the endoscopic endonasal approach, with those achieved through transcranial approaches, showing that incidence of new cranial nerve deficits was lower with the former (7.7% vs. 16.1%), although no statistical analyses were performed.[53]

14.4 Disease-Specific Quality of Life Instruments for Skull Base Pathology

The impact of skull base tumors on patients' health-related quality of life is unique to these diseases. Because of their potential impact on sensory organs, neurological structures, and cosmesis, tumors in this location carry a unique morbidity profile. Hence disease-specific instruments are needed to capture the impact of these tumors on quality of life. To capture the breadth of these illnesses, disease-specific instruments must possess a wide variety of domains to comprehensively measure the patient experience. Although generic quality of life instruments are useful in comparing a broad range of diseases, they might not be as useful for measuring the unique quality of life impact of skull base tumors. Disease-specific instruments, by contrast, comprehensively cover various domains associated with quality of life for skull base tumors. They may be used to compare different modalities of treatment or different surgical approaches. They may also be used to assess changes over time after treatment and to assess responses to treatment or other interventions.

We recently reviewed all disease-specific quality of life instruments for anterior skull base tumors[54,55] and identified nine disease-specific instruments, of which seven were designed to measure quality of life changes associated with specific types of functioning pituitary adenoma. Only two disease-specific instruments, the SBI[56] and the Anterior Skull Base Questionnaire,[57] were designed to measure quality of life for general anterior skull base pathology (▶ Table 14.2).

The SBI is a 41-item disease-specific instrument covering five physical (endocrine, nasal, neurologic, visual, other) and six nonphysical (cognitive, emotional, family, financial, social, spiritual) domains, of which 22 items are disease-specific. Preliminary reliability (internal consistency 0.7–0.95; test–retest reliability [> 0.70]), content validity, and construct validity have been demonstrated.[12,56] The instrument has been validated in patients who have undergone both open and endoscopic approaches.

The Anterior Skull Base Questionnaire is a 35-item disease-specific instrument that includes 7 disease-specific items. It was originally validated in patients undergoing open skull base surgical approaches[57] but has since undergone preliminary field

Table 14.2 Disease-specific quality of life instruments for anterior skull base pathology

	Items	Domains	Applicability	Reliability	Validity
Anterior Skull Base Quality of Life Questionnaire	35	6: Performance Physical function Vitality Pain Influence on Emotions Specific symptoms	Open and endoscopic skull base surgery Anterior and central skull base tumors	Internal consistency, test–retest reliability	Construct validity
Skull Base Inventory	41	11: (5 Physical) Endocrine Nasal Neurologic Visual Other (6 Nonphysical) Cognitive Emotional Family Financial Social Spiritual	Open and endoscopic skull base surgery Anterior and central skull base tumors	Internal consistency, test–retest reliability	Content validity, construct validity

testing in patients undergoing endoscopic approaches.[58] The authors demonstrated good internal consistency (0.8), test–retest reliability (0.9), and construct validity.

Both disease-specific instruments have notable strengths and broad applications for patients who have skull base tumors. The SBI was designed with input from patient focus groups consisting of patients who had undergone open and endoscopic approaches. Covering a significant breadth of disease-specific items and physical and nonphysical domains, this instrument is designed to measure QOL in all skull base tumors. Because it captures content related to visual, nasal, neurologic, endocrine, and cognitive change, it is ideal for assessing quality of life changes for anterior skull base tumors. Its limitations include a limited focus on endocrine disturbances and limited field testing to date. The Anterior Skull Base Questionnaire has undergone significant validation and has been broadly used since its original description. Its original intent was to capture quality of life in patients undergoing open approaches, so its ability to measure QOL in patients undergoing endoscopic approaches might be limited. Furthermore, because it contains seven disease-specific items, it might lack some discriminative ability in patients who have skull base tumors. However, both instruments have demonstrated utility in measuring quality of life in patients who have skull base tumors.

14.5 Quality of Life Following Treatment of Skull Base Tumors

14.5.1 Open Surgical Approaches

Because of the dramatic impact that treating skull base tumors can have on quality of life, there has been considerable interest in research in skull base quality of life over the past couple decades. New instruments have enabled clinicians to better evaluate quality of life outcomes while comparing surgical techniques and other treatment modalities. In the era of primarily open skull base surgical approaches, early quality of life research reported some humbling results. Fukuda et al studied 13 patients who underwent open skull base approaches, of whom 89% had long-term complaints and 63% were dissatisfied with their condition after surgery.[59] These findings of poor quality of life after use of open skull base surgical approaches were corroborated by Woertgen et al, who noted that overall quality of life scores were poor (mean score 42 out of 100) among survivors who had anterior skull base malignancies.[60] The authors noted that only 45% of survivors had returned to work and observed that concerns about employment played a significant role in the overall low scores. In a study of 27 patients who had anterior skull base tumors, nearly half (48%) experienced depression related to their treatment, and 7% had suicidal ideation following surgery.[62]

By contrast, Gil et al demonstrated that 74% of patients had stable quality of life whereas 26% worsened after surgery.[61] These findings helped elucidate the quality of life challenges experienced by patients whose skull base tumors have been managed using open surgical approaches. The full scope of the quality of life impact might not always be fully recognized by treating clinicians. In one study, although patient- and caregiver-reported quality of life scores seemed to correlate reasonably well, surgeon- and patient-reported quality of life scores did not, with surgeons tending to overestimate the quality of life experienced by their patients.[63] Despite these demonstrated challenges with open surgical approaches, such approaches are often still indicated and indeed required, particularly in patients who have extensive tumor involvement.

14.5.2 Endoscopic Endonasal Surgical Approaches

The purported improvement in health-related quality of life was a large impetus for the development and adoption of endoscopic endonasal approaches to the skull base. Although this has not been fully borne out in large-scale comparative studies, the immediate differences are often readily apparent. The early quality of life studies examining endoscopic endonasal approaches demonstrated very good postoperative scores after endoscopic endonasal approaches.[64] Pant et al demonstrated improvement in quality of life scores by 3 months after surgery. Patients who underwent secondary surgeries and those who had nasoseptal flaps seemed to do worse than patients who underwent primary surgeries and those who did not have flaps, respectively. This early work also demonstrated that nasal dysfunction was a large contributor to disease-related quality of life impairment and might persist up to 6 to 12 months after surgery. McCoul et al used the Anterior Skull Base Questionnaire and the SNOT-22 to measure quality of life in patients undergoing endoscopic endonasal approaches for pituitary and nonpituitary pathology and noted that sinonasal morbidity and impaired sinonasal quality of life were self-limited.[65,66] These subjective differences in nasal function using patient-reported instruments have been further substantiated using objective measures. One study demonstrated no significant loss of objective smell using the University of Pennsylvania Smell Identification Test after endoscopic skull base surgery.[67] Although nasal-related quality of life often deteriorates after endoscopic surgery, visual-related quality of life tends to improve—not surprisingly, this often being the goal of these operations.[5]

Studies have shown that each histopathology can uniquely affect quality of life. Patients who have functioning pituitary adenomas may suffer impairment of their quality of life related to their endocrine disturbances.[68] For these patients, it seems that subtotal resection of their disease may adversely affect their quality of life.[69] Similarly, patients who have craniopharyngiomas may experience a decline in their quality of life related to hypopituitarism and endocrinopathies in addition to visual disturbances.[70] Patients who have meningioma of the anterior skull base, particularly older patients (> 55), may have a decline in their quality of life.[71] Surprisingly, not all malignant tumors have a lasting impact on quality of life. Castelnuovo et al demonstrated that patients can recover their overall quality of life up to a year after surgery despite having malignant tumors of the anterior skull base.[72]

14.5.3 Endoscopic versus Open Surgical Approaches

The evolution of endoscopic techniques for cranial base surgery has generally been associated with comparable survival,[73,74,75]

247

fewer complications,[76,77,78] shorter hospital stay,[79] and a perception among treating clinicians that these techniques are associated with improved quality of life. However, large cohort studies comparing quality of life outcomes are still needed.

Abergel et al compared quality of life in patients who underwent endoscopic endonasal approaches ($n=41$) with that of those who underwent open subcranial approaches ($n=37$). Using the Anterior Skull Base Questionnaire, the authors demonstrated significantly higher scores in physical function as well as impact on emotions in the endoscopic endonasal group.[80] Interestingly, no significant differences were shown between approaches in disease-specific symptoms such as impairment in smell, nasal secretions, cosmesis, appetite, epiphora, or visual disturbances. However, the study measured quality of life scores in both populations in a cross-sectional study with a general bias in timing since surgery: more time had elapsed from surgery to completion of questionnaire for patients who had undergone open approaches.

A recent systematic review looking at quality of life outcomes following skull base surgery concluded that patients undergoing endoscopic approaches tend to have earlier recovery of quality of life than those undergoing open approaches and recover to a greater extent, with no long-term deleterious effects in sinonasal outcomes, than seen with open approaches.[81]

Little et al compared quality of life in patients undergoing microscopic and endoscopic transsphenoidal approaches for pituitary lesions in a prospective cohort study.[82] The authors found that with regard to sinonasal specific quality of life, there were no significant differences in outcomes, although patients undergoing an endoscopic approach had more frequent nasal debridement postoperatively. Both groups experienced a transient decline at 2 weeks, with eventual return to normal at 3 months.

14.5.4 Radiotherapy

Several studies have shown that radiotherapy is an adverse predictor of quality of life. Palme et al noted poorer quality of life scores in patients who had anterior skull base tumors undergoing radiotherapy using the FACT-HN instrument.[62] In patients undergoing endoscopic endonasal approaches, the addition of radiotherapy tends to adversely affect overall quality of life outcomes and the return to normal sinonasal health.[12,69,83,84] Newer techniques such as proton beam therapy are purported to improve health-related quality of life by minimizing radiation dose to critical structures taking advantage of a energy fall-off known as the Bragg peak. Although no comparative studies exist to substantiate a correlation with improved quality of life compared with that seen using preexisting techniques such as intensity-modulated radiotherapy, one study indicates good quality of life outcomes in patients treated with proton beam therapy as adjuvant therapy for chordomas or chondrosarcomas.[85] In this study patients did not experience a significant decline in quality of life during treatment, as measured by the EORTC QLQ-C30 questionnaire. However, further studies comparing quality of life of patients undergoing different modalities of radiotherapy are needed.

14.6 Conclusion

Over the past few decades, quality of life research has helped improve understandings of the experience of patients who have skull base tumors. These patients experience a significant impact in their physical well-being and impairment in their physical function. Impairment in nasal, visual, endocrine, and neurologic function is not uncommon in patients who have skull base tumors. Disease-specific quality of life instruments may be useful in measuring skull base tumors' effect on quality of life. Although patients who have skull base tumors may experience a decline in their quality of life as a result of their treatment, newer surgical and nonsurgical approaches might help ameliorate the negative impact on quality of life.

References

[1] World Health Organization (WHO). Rehabilitation after cardiovascular diseases, with special emphasis on developing countries: report of a WHO expert committee. WHO Technical Report Series 831. Geneva: WHO;1993

[2] Fitzpatrick R, Fletcher A, Gore S, Jones D, Spiegelhalter D, Cox D. Quality of life measures in health care. I: Applications and issues in assessment. BMJ. 1992; 305(6861):1074–1077

[3] Jenkinson C, Ziebland S, Fitzpatrick R, Mowat A. Sensitivity to change of weighted and unweighted versions of two health status measures. Int J Health Sci. 1991; 2:189–194

[4] Fletcher A, Gore S, Jones D, Fitzpatrick R, Spiegelhalter D, Cox D. Quality of life measures in health care. II: Design, analysis, and interpretation. BMJ. 1992; 305(6862):1145–1148

[5] Bedrosian JC, McCoul ED, Raithatha R, Akselrod OA, Anand VK, Schwartz TH. A prospective study of postoperative symptoms in sinonasal quality-of-life following endoscopic skull-base surgery: dissociations based on specific symptoms. Int Forum Allergy Rhinol. 2013; 3(8):664–669

[6] Balaker AE, Bergsneider M, Martin NA, Wang MB. Evolution of sinonasal symptoms following endoscopic anterior skull base surgery. Skull Base. 2010; 20(4):245–251

[7] de Almeida JR, Snyderman CH, Gardner PA, Carrau RL, Vescan AD. Nasal morbidity following endoscopic skull base surgery: a prospective cohort study. Head Neck. 2011; 33(4):547–551

[8] Sowerby LJ, Gross M, Broad R, Wright ED. Olfactory and sinonasal outcomes in endoscopic transsphenoidal skull-base surgery. 2013; 3(3):217–220

[9] Rotenberg B, Tam S, Ryu WHA, Duggal N. Microscopic versus endoscopic pituitary surgery: a systematic review. Laryngoscope. 2010; 120(7):1292–1297

[10] Hopkins C, Gillett S, Slack R, Lund VJ, Browne JP. Psychometric validity of the 22-item Sinonasal Outcome Test. Clin Otolaryngol. 2009; 34(5):447–454

[11] Little AS, Kelly D, Milligan J, et al. Prospective validation of a patient-reported nasal quality-of-life tool for endonasal skull base surgery: the Anterior Skull Base Nasal Inventory-12. J Neurosurg. 2013; 119(4):1068–1074

[12] Larjani S, Monteiro E, Witterick I, et al. Preliminary cross-sectional reliability and validity of the Skull Base Inventory (SBI) quality of life questionnaire. J Otolaryngol Head Neck Surg. 2016; 45(1):45

[13] Pant H, Bhatki AM, Snyderman CH, et al. Quality of life following endonasal skull base surgery. Skull Base. 2010; 20(1):35–40

[14] Little AS, Kelly D, Milligan J, et al. Predictors of sinonasal quality of life and nasal morbidity after fully endoscopic transsphenoidal surgery. J Neurosurg. 2015; 122(6):1458–1465

[15] Harvey RJ, Malek J, Winder M, et al. Sinonasal morbidity following tumour resection with and without nasoseptal flap reconstruction. Rhinology. 2015; 53(2):122–128

[16] Hanson M, Patel PM, Betz C, Olson S, Panizza B, Wallwork B. Sinonasal outcomes following endoscopic anterior skull base surgery with nasoseptal flap reconstruction: a prospective study. J Laryngol Otol. 2015; 129 Suppl 3:S41–S46

[17] Soudry E, Psaltis AJ, Lee KH, Vaezafshar R, Nayak JV, Hwang PH. Complications associated with the pedicled nasoseptal flap for skull base reconstruction. Laryngoscope. 2015; 125(1):80–85

[18] Kim BY, Kang SG, Kim SW, et al. Olfactory changes after endoscopic endonasal transsphenoidal approach for skull base tumors. Laryngoscope. 2014; 124(11):2470–2475

[19] Thompson CF, Suh JD, Liu Y, Bergsneider M, Wang MB. Modifications to the endoscopic approach for anterior skull base lesions improve postoperative sinonasal symptoms. J Neurol Surg B Skull Base. 2014; 75(1):65–72

[20] Kimple AJ, Leight WD, Wheless SA, Zanation AM. Reducing nasal morbidity after skull base reconstruction with the nasoseptal flap: free middle turbinate mucosal grafts. Laryngoscope. 2012; 122(9):1920–1924

[21] Rawal RB, Kimple AJ, Dugar DR, Zanation AM. Minimizing morbidity in endoscopic pituitary surgery: outcomes of the novel nasoseptal rescue flap technique. Otolaryngol Head Neck Surg. 2012; 147(3):434–437

[22] de Almeida JR, Witterick IJ, Gullane PJ, et al. Physical morbidity by surgical approach and tumor location in skull base surgery. Head Neck. 2013; 35(4):493–499

[23] Barzaghi LR, Medone M, Losa M, Bianchi S, Giovanelli M, Mortini P. Prognostic factors of visual field improvement after trans-sphenoidal approach for pituitary macroadenomas: review of the literature and analysis by quantitative method. Neurosurg Rev. 2012; 35(3):369–378, discussion 378–379

[24] Gnanalingham KK, Bhattacharjee S, Pennington R, Ng J, Mendoza N. The time course of visual field recovery following transphenoidal surgery for pituitary adenomas: predictive factors for a good outcome. J Neurol Neurosurg Psychiatry. 2005; 76(3):415–419

[25] Juraschka K, Khan OH, Godoy BL, et al. Endoscopic endonasal transsphenoidal approach to large and giant pituitary adenomas: institutional experience and predictors of extent of resection. J Neurosurg. 2014; 121(1):75–83

[26] Paluzzi A, Fernandez-Miranda JC, Tonya Stefko S, Challinor S, Snyderman CH, Gardner PA. Endoscopic endonasal approach for pituitary adenomas: a series of 555 patients. Pituitary. 2014; 17(4):307–319

[27] Turel MK,. sermoulas G, Yassin-Kassab A, et al. Tuberculum sellae meningiomas: a systematic review of transcranial approaches in the endoscopic era. J Neurosurg Sci. 2016:[epub ahead of print]

[28] Koutourousiou M, Fernandez-Miranda JC, Stefko ST, Wang EW, Snyderman CH, Gardner PA. Endoscopic endonasal surgery for suprasellar meningiomas: experience with 75 patients. J Neurosurg. 2014; 120(6):1326–1339

[29] Koutourousiou M, Fernandez-Miranda JC, Wang EW, Snyderman CH, Gardner PA. Endoscopic endonasal surgery for olfactory groove meningiomas: outcomes and limitations in 50 patients. Neurosurg Focus. 2014; 37(4):E8

[30] Bander ED, Singh H, Ogilvie CB, et al. Endoscopic endonasal versus transcranial approach to tuberculum sellae and planum sphenoidale meningiomas in similar cohort of patients. J Neurosurg. 2017:[epub ahead of print]

[31] Clark AJ, Jahangiri A, Garcia RM, et al. Endoscopic surgery for tuberculum sellae meningiomas: a systematic review and meta-analysis. Neurosurg Rev. 2013; 36(3):349–359

[32] Komotar RJ, Starke RM, Raper DM, Anand VK, Schwartz TH. Endoscopic endonasal versus open transcranial resection of anterior midline skull base meningiomas. World Neurosurg. 2012; 77(5–6):713–724

[33] Neel GS, Nagel TH, Hoxworth JM, Lal D. Management of orbital involvement in sinonasal and ventral skull base malignancies. Otolaryngol Clin North Am. 2017; 50(2):347–364

[34] Lisan Q, Kolb F, Temam S, Tao Y, Janot F, Moya-Plana A. Management of orbital invasion in sinonasal malignancies. Head Neck. 2016; 38(11):1650–1656

[35] Muscatello L, Fortunato S, Seccia V, Marchetti M, Lenzi R. The implications of orbital invasion in sinonasal tract malignancies. Orbit. 2016; 35(5):278–284

[36] Rajapurkar M, Thankappan K, Sampathirao LM, Kuriakose MA, Iyer S. Oncologic and functional outcome of the preserved eye in malignant sinonasal tumors. Head Neck. 2013; 35(10):1379–1384

[37] Chi A, Nguyen NP, Tse W, Sobremonte G, Concannon P, Zhu A. Intensity modulated radiotherapy for sinonasal malignancies with a focus on optic pathway preservation. J Hematol Oncol. 2013; 6:4

[38] Duprez F, Madani I, Morbée L, et al. IMRT for sinonasal tumors minimizes severe late ocular toxicity and preserves disease control and survival. Int J Radiat Oncol Biol Phys. 2012; 83(1):252–259

[39] Strychowsky J, Nayan S, Reddy K, Farrokhyar F, Sommer D. Purely endoscopic transsphenoidal surgery versus traditional microsurgery for resection of pituitary adenomas: systematic review. J Otolaryngol Head Neck Surg. 2011; 40(2):175–185

[40] Goudakos JK, Markou KD, Georgalas C. Endoscopic versus microscopic transsphenoidal pituitary surgery: a systematic review and meta-analysis. Clin Otolaryngol. 2011; 36(3):212–220

[41] Komotar RJ, Starke RM, Raper DM, Anand VK, Schwartz TH. Endoscopic endonasal compared with microscopic transsphenoidal and open transcranial resection of giant pituitary adenomas. Pituitary. 2012; 15(2):150–159

[42] Li A, Liu W, Cao P, Zheng Y, Bu Z, Zhou T. Endoscopic versus microscopic transsphenoidal surgery in the treatment of pituitary adenoma: a systematic review and meta-analysis. World Neurosurg. 2017; 101:236–246–; [epub ahead of print]

[43] Clark AJ, Cage TA, Aranda D, et al. Treatment related morbidity and the management of pediatric craniopharyngioma. J Neurosurg Pediatrics. 2012; 10:293–301

[44] Gautier A, Godbout A, Grosheny C, et al. Craniopharyngioma Study Group. Markers of recurrence and long-term morbidity in craniopharyngioma: a systematic analysis of 171 patients. J Clin Endocrinol Metab. 2012; 97(4):1258–1267

[45] Li K, Lu X, Yang N, Zheng J, Huang B, Li L. Association of pituitary stalk management with endocrine outcomes and recurrence in microsurgery of craniopharyngiomas: a meta-analysis. Clin Neurol Neurosurg. 2015; 136:20–24

[46] Sathyapalan T, Dixit S. Radiotherapy-induced hypopituitarism: a review. Expert Rev Anticancer Ther. 2012; 12(5):669–683

[47] Snyers A, Janssens GO, Twickler MB, et al. Malignant tumors of the nasal cavity and paranasal sinuses: long-term outcome and morbidity with emphasis on hypothalamic-pituitary deficiency. Int J Radiat Oncol Biol Phys. 2009; 73(5):1343–1351

[48] Ausman JI. A revolution in skull base surgery: the quality of life matters! Surg Neurol. 2006; 65(6):635–636

[49] Zweckberger K, Hallek E, Vogt L, Giese H, Schick U, Unterberg AW. Prospective analysis of neuropsychological deficits following resection of benign skull base meningiomas. J Neurosurg. 2017; 127(6):1242–1248

[50] Starke R, Kano H, Ding D, et al. Stereotactic radiosurgery of petroclival meningiomas: a multicenter study. J Neurooncol. 2014; 119(1):169–176

[51] de Almeida JR, Carvalho F, Vaz Guimaraes Filho F, et al. Comparison of endoscopic endonasal and bifrontal craniotomy approaches for olfactory groove meningiomas: a matched pair analysis of outcomes and frontal lobe changes on MRI. J Clin Neurosci. 2015; 22(11):1733–1741

[52] Koutourousiou M, Gardner PA, Tormenti MJ, et al. Endoscopic endonasal approach for resection of cranial base chordomas: outcomes and learning curve. Neurosurgery. 2012; 71(3):614–624, discussion 624–625

[53] Labidi M, Watanabe K, Bouazza S, et al. Clivus chordomas: a systematic review and meta-analysis of contemporary surgical management. J Neurosurg Sci. 2016; 60(4):476–484

[54] de Almeida JR, Vescan AD. Outcomes and quality of life following skull base surgery. Curr Otorhinolaryngol Rep. 2013; 1(4):214–220

[55] de Almeida JR, Witterick IJ, Gullane PJ, et al. Quality of life instruments for skull base pathology: systematic review and methodologic appraisal. Head Neck. 2013; 35(9):1221–1231

[56] de Almeida JR, Vescan AD, Gullane PJ, et al. Development of a disease-specific quality-of-life questionnaire for anterior and central skull base pathology—the Skull Base Inventory. Laryngoscope. 2012; 122(9):1933–1942

[57] Gil Z, Abergel A, Spektor S, Shabtai E, Khafif A, Fliss DM. Development of a cancer-specific anterior skull base quality-of-life questionnaire. J Neurosurg. 2004; 100(5):813–819

[58] Cavel O, Abergel A, Margalit N, Fliss DM, Gil Z. Quality of life following endoscopic resection of skull base tumors. J Neurol Surg B Skull Base. 2012; 73(2):112–116

[59] Fukuda K, Saeki N, Mine S, et al. Evaluation of outcome and QOL in patients with craniofacial resection for malignant tumors involving the anterior skull base. Neurol Res. 2000; 22(6):545–550

[60] Woertgen C, Rothoerl RD, Hosemann W, Strutz J. Quality of life following surgery for malignancies of the anterior skull base. Skull Base. 2007; 17(2):119–123

[61] Gil Z, Abergel A, Spektor S, et al. Quality of life following surgery for anterior skull base tumors. Arch Otolaryngol Head Neck Surg. 2003; 129(12):1303–1309

[62] Palme CE, Irish JC, Gullane PJ, Katz MR, Devins GM, Bachar G. Quality of life analysis in patients with anterior skull base neoplasms. Head Neck. 2009; 31(10):1326–1334

[63] Gil Z, Abergel A, Spektor S, Khafif A, Fliss DM. Patient, caregiver, and surgeon perceptions of quality of life following anterior skull base surgery. Arch Otolaryngol Head Neck Surg. 2004; 130(11):1276–1281

[64] Pant H, Bhatki AM, Snyderman CH, et al. Quality of life following endonasal skull base surgery. Skull Base. 2010; 20(10):35–40

[65] McCoul ED, Anand VK, Bedrosian JC, Schwartz TH. Endoscopic skull base surgery and its impact on sinonasal-related quality of life. Int Forum Allergy Rhinol. 2012; 2(2):174–181

[66] McCoul ED, Anand VK, Schwartz TH. Improvements in site-specific quality of life 6 months after endoscopic anterior skull base surgery: a prospective study. J Neurosurg. 2012; 117(3):498–506

[67] Sowerby LJ, Gross M, Broad R, Wright ED. Olfactory and sinonasal outcomes in endoscopic transsphenoidal skull-base surgery. Int Forum Allergy Rhinol. 2013; 3(3):217–220

[68] Georgalas C, Badloe R, van Furth W, Reinartz S, Fokkens WJ. Quality of life in extended endonasal approaches for skull base tumours. Rhinology. 2012; 50 (3):255–261

[69] McCoul ED, Bedrosian JC, Akselrod O, Anand VK, Schwartz TH. Preservation of multidimensional quality of life after endoscopic pituitary adenoma resection. J Neurosurg. 2015; 123(3):813–820

[70] Patel KS, Raza SM, McCoul ED, et al. Long-term quality of life after endonasal endoscopic resection of adult craniopharyngiomas. J Neurosurg. 2015; 123 (3):571–580

[71] Jones SH, Iannone AF, Patel KS, et al. The impact of age on long-term quality of life after endonasal endoscopic resection of skull base meningiomas. Neurosurgery. 2016; 79(5):736–745

[72] Castelnuovo P, Lepera D, Turri-Zanoni M, et al. Quality of life following endoscopic endonasal resection of anterior skull base cancers. J Neurosurg. 2013; 119(6):1401–1409

[73] Meccariello G, Deganello A, Choussy O, et al. Endoscopic nasal versus open approach for the management of sinonasal adenocarcinoma: a pooled-analysis of 1826 patients. Head Neck. 2016; 38 Suppl 1:E2267–E2274

[74] Farquhar D, Kim L, Worrall D, et al. Propensity score analysis of endoscopic and open approaches to malignant paranasal and anterior skull base tumor outcomes. Laryngoscope. 2016; 126(8):1724–1729

[75] Fu TS, Monteiro E, Muhanna N, Goldstein DP, de Almeida JR. Comparison of outcomes for open versus endoscopic approaches for olfactory neuroblastoma: a systematic review and individual participant data meta-analysis. Head Neck. 2016; 38 Suppl 1:E2306–E2316

[76] Ganly I, Patel SG, Singh B, et al. Complications of craniofacial resection for malignant tumors of the skull base: report of an international collaborative study. Head Neck. 2005; 27(6):445–451

[77] Nicolai P, Battaglia P, Bignami M, et al. Endoscopic surgery for malignant tumors of the sinonasal tract and adjacent skull base: a 10-year experience. Am J Rhinol. 2008; 22(3):308–316

[78] Hanna E, DeMonte F, Ibrahim S, Roberts D, Levine N, Kupferman M. Endoscopic resection of sinonasal cancers with and without craniotomy: oncologic results. Arch Otolaryngol Head Neck Surg. 2009; 135(12):1219–1224

[79] Wood JW, Eloy JA, Vivero RJ, et al. Efficacy of transnasal endoscopic resection for malignant anterior skull-base tumors. Int Forum Allergy Rhinol. 2012; 2 (6):487–495

[80] Abergel A, Cavel O, Margalit N, Fliss DM, Gil Z. Comparison of quality of life after transnasal endoscopic vs open skull base tumor resection. Arch Otolaryngol Head Neck Surg. 2012; 138(2):142–147

[81] Kirkman MA, Borg A, Al-Mousa A, Haliasos N, Choi D. Quality-of-life after anterior skull base surgery: a systematic review. J Neurol Surg B Skull Base. 2014; 75(2):73–89

[82] Little AS, Kelly DF, Milligan J, et al. Comparison of sinonasal quality of life and health status in patients undergoing microscopic and endoscopic transsphenoidal surgery for pituitary lesions: a prospective cohort study. J Neurosurg. 2015; 123(3):799–807

[83] Harrow BR, Batra PS. Sinonasal quality of life outcomes after minimally invasive resection of sinonasal and skull-base tumors. Int Forum Allergy Rhinol. 2013; 3(12):1013–1020

[84] Deckard NA, Harrow BR, Barnett SL, Batra PS. Comparative analysis of quality-of-life metrics after endoscopic surgery for sinonasal neoplasms. Am J Rhinol Allergy. 2015; 29(2):151–155

[85] Srivastava A, Vischioni B, Fiore MR, et al. Quality of life in patients with chordomas/chondrosarcomas during treatment with proton beam therapy. J Radiat Res (Tokyo). 2013; 54 Suppl 1:i43–i48

15 Pediatric Skull Base Surgery

Nidal Muhanna, Alon Pener Tesler, and Dan M. Fliss

Summary

The pediatric population presents with a variety of different skull base pathologies than are seen in adults. The treatment of such pathologies is also different owing to this population's different anatomy and to concerns over long-term outcomes. Because sarcomas and middle cranial fossa tumors are more common in the pediatric population, surgery can cause significant functional and aesthetic issues, impacting the psychological development of the child. These surgeries typically require the use of a multidisciplinary team, including specialists in neurosurgery, otorhinolaryngology, plastic and reconstructive surgery, maxillofacial surgery and prosthodontics, pediatric critical care, radiology, and pediatric oncology, as well as social workers or other child life specialists. Fortunately, thanks to technological advances made in the surgical field, more radical tumor extirpations can be performed that have a greater impact on long-term survival and reduced morbidity in pediatric patients. This chapter provides a brief introduction to the types of skull base tumors commonly found in the pediatric population. We describe several approaches for the surgical treatment of such tumors, as well as the principles of skull base reconstruction.

Keywords: pediatric surgery, skull base tumor, pediatric tumor, neurosurgery, otorhinolaryngology

15.1 Pathology

One of the key differences between pediatric skull base surgery and adult skull base surgery is the type of pathology being addressed. Overall, skull base tumors are less common in the pediatric population than in the adult, with benign tumors being significantly more common.[1] Children are also more likely to be affected by congenital abnormalities and tumors associated with genetic conditions, which surgeons should keep in mind, for such patients are likely to have more than one system affected. In ▶ Table 15.1 we present some of the more common lesions found in the pediatric population.

15.1.1 Benign Lesions

Although benign lesions generally have a better prognosis than malignant lesions, many of these lesions can compress important neuronal structures, requiring surgery to relieve the pressure. In the pediatric population, however, the age of the patient can affect the decision of whether to perform surgery. The risks of surgery and anesthesia on the developing brain must be considered, along with the benefits of performing surgery while the skull is still developing.

The most common benign tumors are craniopharyngiomas, which originate in Rathke's pouch and can lead to increased intracranial pressure, bitemporal hemianopsia, and hypothalamic disturbances.[2] Juvenile nasal angiofibromas (JNAs) are benign vascular tumors caused by an incomplete regression of the first branchial arch artery, affecting only males.[3] Fibro-osseous lesions are a group of tumors in which normal bone is replaced by connective tissue composed of fibroblasts excreting matrix and cementlike elements. Conditions for development of these lesions include fibrous dysplasia, aneurysmal bone cysts, giant granulomas, ossifying fibromas, giant cell tumors, osteoma, osteoblastoma, osteosarcoma, and the like.[4,5,6] Langerhans cell histiocytosis (LCH), a clonal proliferation of dendritic cells, is the most common type of histiocytosis.[7]

Some of these tumors are related to genetic conditions, such as neurofibromatosis types 1 and 2 (NF1 and NF2, respectively). NF1 may present with optic gliomas or neurofibromas. Optic gliomas are low-grade pilocytic or pilomyxoid astrocytomas, with rare instances of more advanced neoplasms in young adults.[8] Neurofibromas arise from nonmyelinating Schwann cells. The majority of NF1 patients will develop neurofibromas, which can be either cutaneous or plexiform with various morphological types.[9] NF2 may present with schwannomas—slow-growing tumors originating from the nerve sheath of peripheral nerves. Schwannomas of the vestibular nerve are the most common type, almost all of which are related to neurofibromatosis type 2 (NF2).[10]

Not all the lesions seen in the pediatric population result from neoplasms, however; many are congenital abnormalities. These include encephaloceles—neural tube defects in which cranial vault content protrudes through gaps in the cranium. The content of the sac may include the meninges (meningocele), brain matter (meningoencephalocele), and parts of the ventricles (hydroencephalocele). Dermoid and epidermoid cysts are benign, low-grade lesions originating in remnants of ectodermal tissue and infiltrating the neural tube or pharyngeal arches during the third to fifth weeks of development.[11] Finally, mucoceles—cystic lesions of the paranasal sinuses that form due to blockage or stricture of the ostia, causing an accumulation of secretions in a cyst lined by upper respiratory epithelium—are rare in children and are usually associated with cystic fibrosis, nasal polyposis, trauma, or surgery.[12]

Table 15.1 Classification of pediatric skull base lesions

Lesion	Classification
Craniopharyngiomas	Benign neoplasm
Juvenile nasal angiofibromas	Benign neoplasm
Fibro-osseous lesions	Benign neoplasm
Langerhans cell histiocytosis	Benign neoplasm
Optic gliomas	Benign neoplasm
Neurofibromas	Benign neoplasm
Schwannomas[a]	Benign neoplasm
Encephaloceles	Congenital abnormality
Dermoid and epidermoid cysts	Congenital abnormality
Mucoceles	Congenital abnormality
Sarcomas	Malignant neoplasm
Esthesioneuroblastoma	Malignant neoplasm

[a]Note that schwannomas may, rarely, become malignant neoplasms.

15.1.2 Malignant Lesions

The most common of the malignant lesions in children are sarcomas. These include the following subtypes: rhabdomyosarcoma (RMS; 48%), malignant fibrous histiocytoma (11%), osteosarcoma (8%), Ewing's sarcoma (6%), chordoma (4%), malignant nerve sheath tumor (4%), chondrosarcoma (3%), and synovial sarcoma (2%).[13]

RMS, a sarcoma derived from striated muscle, is the most common soft tissue sarcoma of childhood. Fifty percent of patients are diagnosed in the first decade of life, and they often present with advanced disease.[14,15] RMS can be classified histologically as either embryonal or alveolar. Embryonal RMS typically occurs in children under age 10, often in the head and neck. Alveolar RMS occurs more commonly in adolescents and young adults, affecting the trunk and extremities. Embryonal RMS has a more favorable prognosis than alveolar RMS.[16] Chordomas are slow-growing, locally aggressive, malignant bone tumors arising from notochord remnants along the spinal cord. Clival chordomas are locally aggressive and commonly involve adjacent structure such as the suprasellar area, cavernous sinus, parapharyngeal space, temporal bone, and fossa.[17]

Neuroectodermal tumors include esthesioneuroblastoma, Ewing's sarcoma, and malignant nerve sheath tumor (a.k.a. malignant schwannoma). Esthesioneuroblastoma (or olfactory neuroblastoma) is a rare malignant tumor of the olfactory nerve found in the nasal cavity. Eight percent of cases occur before the age of 25, but very rarely (< 1%) before the age of 10.[18] Ewing's sarcoma, a highly malignant neoplasm of the bone, includes classic Ewing's sarcoma, Askin's tumor, and peripheral primitive neuroectodermal tumor.[19] Although they accounts for 10% of all primary bone malignancies, only 1 to 6% of Ewing's sarcomas occur in the skull.[20] Schwannomas have already been described, as they are usually benign. In rare instances, however, they may become malignant, in which case they have a poor prognosis and a high rate of recurrence (40–50%).[21]

15.1.3 Cytogenetic Variations

Malignant pathologies can arise from genetic aberrations in the cell's DNA, which can be tumor-specific or nonspecific, resulting in deletions and gains. In stepwise genetic transformations, one genetic alteration may increase a cell's growth and replication abilities, encouraging more genetic changes that can increase tumor invasion and metastases.[22] These cytogenetic variations can be diagnostic and can help determine the prognosis for some tumors.

Some tumors that show complex karyotype changes include squamous cell carcinoma, chordomas, and RMS.[22] It has been shown that half of nonkeratinizing squamous cell carcinomas have an abnormal karyotype.[23] In chordomas, frequent chromosomal aberrations have been discovered, often involving losses in chromosomes 3, 4, 10, and 13.[24] Approximately 75% of RMS tumors are estimated to involve complex karyotypes. These frequently involve translocation breakpoints in the 1p11–q11 region, translocations of 13q14, gains of chromosomes 2, 7, 8, 12, and 13, and losses at chromosome 11p15.5.[23,25,26]

Additionally, some tumors are associated with specific chromosomal changes. Approximately 78% of patients who have Ewing's sarcoma have a translocation of t(11;22)(q24;q12).[22] Synovial sarcoma has a translocation of t(X;18) in more than 90% of cases, with a third of cases having this as the sole chromosomal abnormality.[27] With such specific tumor markers, a simple biopsy of a suspicious mass can make the diagnosis and treatment plan easy to determine.

15.2 Principles of Pediatric Skull Base Surgery

15.2.1 Surgical Techniques

Although numerous surgical techniques are available to treat skull base tumors, most such techniques have been developed for use in adults, most likely due to the paucity of tumors in the pediatric population. Nonetheless, various approaches have been successfully performed in children and are described here.

Anterior Skull Base Open Approaches

Several open approaches are tried and true methods for anterior skull base tumor extirpation, including the following: subcranial, subfrontal, transfacial/transmaxillary, midface degloving, orbitozygomatic, and fronto-orbital. The subcranial approach is often combined with other approaches if a large tumor invades adjacent structures such as the orbit, pterygomaxillary fossa, or maxilla.

Subcranial

The goal of this approach is to gain access to the anterior skull base from the medial orbital rims along the ethmoid roof to the planum sphenoidale and superior clivus.[28,29] The subcranial approach is applied when lesions involve the central anterior skull base, such as in the cribriform plate and the frontal sinus, and for lesions extending far into the paranasal sinus, nasal cavity, or orbits, including esthesioneuroblastomas, meningoencephaloceles, gliomas, and nasal dermoid cysts. This technique can only be performed if the lesion does not have extensions to adjacent bony structures or fossae. If such extensions are found, additional approaches are combined, such as transfacial, midface degloving, orbitozygomatic, transorbital, Le Fort I, pterional, and the like.

A bicoronal incision is made from one supra-auricular area to the other on the contralateral side 2 cm behind the hairline (▶ Fig. 15.1; ▶ Fig. 15.2). A subperiosteal pericranial flap is raised anteriorly, exposing the periorbita down to the nasal bone and laterally to the temporalis fascia. Then the flap is reflected anteriorly to expose the area to be resected. An osteotomy may be performed either by type A osteotomy, which includes the anterior wall of the frontal sinus, or by type B osteotomy, which includes the posterior wall of the frontal sinus. In both types the segment is extracted en bloc, with the nasal bone and superior medial walls of the orbits as a single segment that is stored in saline for reinsertion after tumor extirpation. Bilateral ethmoidectomy and sphenoidotomy are performed to complete the exposure with possible unilateral preservation of the cribriform plate so as to preserve olfaction.

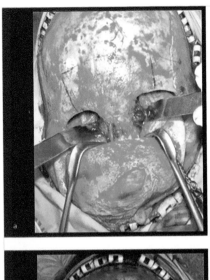
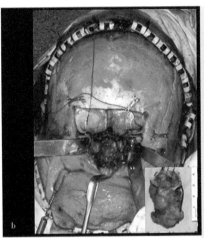
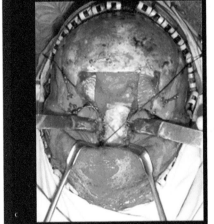
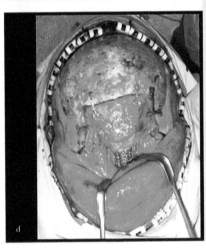

Fig. 15.1 A 14-year-old boy suffering from esthesioneuroblastoma with intracranial involvement. The subcranial approach was performed via a bicoronal incision, with the raising of a subperiosteal pericranial flap deflected anteriorly. **(a)** A type B osteotomy was performed that included the posterior wall of the frontal sinus. **(b)** The naso-fronto-orbital segment is extracted en bloc, followed by an ethmoidectomy, sphenoidectomy, and extirpation of the tumor (seen at the inferior right edge). **(c)** Reconstruction of the orbits with titanium mesh, centripetal tension sutures of the medial canthi, and packing of the nasal cavity with a Vaseline gauze. **(d)** Inset of the naso-fronto-orbital segment wrapped in anterior lateral thigh free flap and titanium mesh reconstruction of the nasal bone.

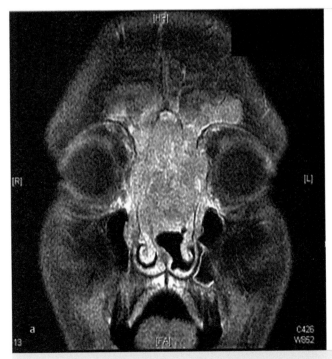
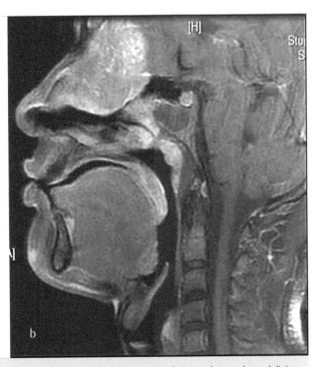

Fig. 15.2 Preoperative **(a)** coronal and **(b)** sagittal T2-weighted, gadolinium-enhanced MRI scans show a hyperintense lesion with irregular gadolinium uptake invading the nasal cavity, lamina papyracea bilaterally, and anterior skull base.

Subfrontal

The subfrontal approach gains access to anterior skull base tumors with intracranial extension while providing wide exposure, enabling minimal brain manipulation.[30,31] This can be useful for large tumors, such as craniopharyngiomas and JNAs. A bicoronal incision is made from the zygoma along the hairline to the contralateral zygoma. A subperiosteal pericranial flap is raised and reflected anteriorly, followed by a craniotomy involving both anterior and posterior walls of the frontal sinus, osteotomy of the nasolacrimal suture, and the roof of the orbits in one or two segments.

Transfacial

The transfacial approach is typically used to provide adequate access to the skull base, giving a wide operative view of deep lesions. The benefits include minimizing intraoperative brain traction, avoiding piecemeal resection, and reducing damage to neural and vascular structures.[32,33] The transfacial approach includes transfacial swing osteotomy, transnasomaxillary, and transpalatal, as well as a few others. Transfacial swing osteotomy and frontopterional approach can be used to access the clivus, requiring a Weber-Ferguson incision, which can result in a large scar.[32] The transnasomaxillary approach allows for exposure of the entire midline skull base region for large nasopharyngeal and clival lesions, such as chondrosarcomas, meningoencephaloceles, and gliomas. It is performed through a modified Weber-Ferguson incision, directing the incision across the radix and along the opposite subciliary margin of the lower lid.[34] The transpalatal approach is often used for skull base herniations, including meningoceles and encephaloceles, particularly in neonates who are unable to undergo transnasal endoscopic approaches. The transpalatal approach can provide better visualization in neonates than the transnasal endoscopic approach can and is associated with less morbidity than open craniotomy is.[35] The procedure begins with a U-shaped incision in the hard palate, 5 mm from the dental arch. The subperiosteal flap is raised to gain access to the nasopharynx, allowing visualization of the vomer for its removal. The lateral atretic plates are removed, and the flap is closed using a two-layered closure.[36]

Midfacial Degloving

Midfacial degloving offers access to nasal cavity and paranasal sinus lesions without leaving an external scar on the face.[37] In this procedure, a transfixion incision and a bilateral intercartilaginous incision are performed, through which nasal dorsum tissues, anterior wall of the maxillary sinus, glabella, and frontal bone are lifted. The surgeon then extends them laterally toward the nasal cavity floor to touch the caudal portion of the transfixion incision. A sublabial incision is made from the first molar to the contralateral tooth, incising the mucoperiosteum. The tissues are raised bilaterally to the inferior orbital rim using a periosteum elevator. The flap is then raised to the glabella, medial cantus region, and forehead so as to expose the midfacial skeleton, allowing for removal of the tumor, which can include inverted papillomas and nasopharyngeal angiofibromas.[38]

Maxillectomy

A maxillectomy, which may be partial or total, involves removal of the maxilla to access tumors in the hard palate. Suprastructure maxillectomy involves an osteotomy above the malar eminence and through the inferior–lateral wall of the orbit. If combined with the subcranial approach, reconstruction of the orbit is warranted either by titanium mesh or split calvarial bone graft and a vascularized flap. In cases involving extensive loss of volume, a large complex defect, total maxillectomy with orbital exenteration, or radiation therapy (adjuvant or neoadjuvant), a vascularized free flap is preferred, usually from the anterolateral thigh or rectus abdominis.

Transorbital

Tumors invading the content of the anterior orbit or the orbital apex necessitate orbital exenteration.[39] If the tumor does not involve the maxilla, a transorbital approach may suffice with or without sparing of the eyelid, oncological margins permitting. If a tumor involves the skull base, orbital content, and walls of the maxilla, a combined subcranial–total maxillectomy is indicated, which includes orbital exenteration.[40]

Le Fort I

The combined subcranial–Le Fort I osteotomy entails freeing of the alveolus ridge so as to gain access to the lower clivus when it is not attainable by other open approaches or endoscopically.[41] A gingivobuccal incision is performed and a facial flap raised to the level of the infraorbital nerves and laterally to the pterygomaxillary junction. Then a Le Fort I osteotomy is performed, followed by a partial maxillectomy.[40] This approach may harm the buds of the permanent denture in children younger than 10 years old and thus should be avoided in such patients if possible. Some tumors that can be removed through this technique include angiofibromas, hemangiomas, giant cell tumors, and malignant fibrous histiocytoma.[42]

Lateral Approaches

Lateral approaches are used when lesions, often chordomas, invade the temporal bone, middle cranial fossa, or cavernous sinus and are subdivided into anterolateral (subtemporal), lateral (transpetrous), and posterolateral.[43] The anterolateral approach entails a question mark incision following the hairline (▶ Fig. 15.3; ▶ Fig. 15.4), removal of the zygomatic process, and raising of a temporalis muscle flap, thus exposing the infratemporal fossa and pterionic area, followed by a craniotomy with anterior (pterygoid) or posterior (petrous) extension as needed.[30] The lateral (transpetrous) approaches are commonly used for tumors of the petrous bone and include presigmoid, retrolabyrinthine, translabyrinthine, transcochlear, and total or radical temporal bone resection (petrosectomy), depending on the area of the temporal bone involved.

Preoperative hearing and facial nerve function are crucial considerations when assessing the appropriate lateral approach, as these may need to be sacrificed. Benign lesions usually do not necessitate such measures.[44] The skin incision is a C-shaped retroauricular incision with possible extension and obliteration of the external auditory canal. The posterior–lateral

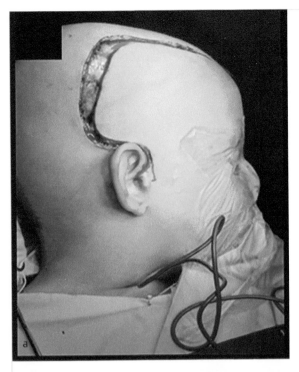
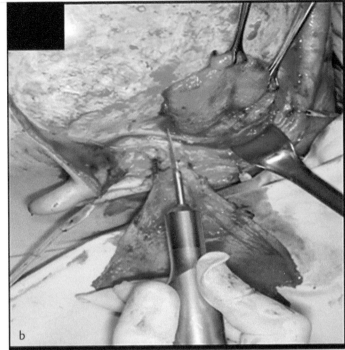
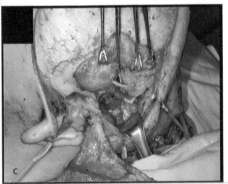
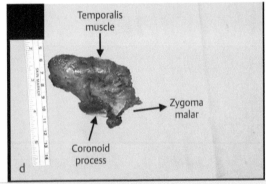
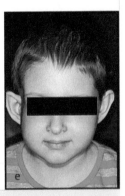

Fig. 15.3 A 10-year-old girl suffering from spindle cell sarcoma (nonrhabdoid) of the right infratemporal fossa space involving the mandible, masseter muscle, and pterygoid muscles. The surgery was followed by systemic chemotherapy with ifosfamide and Adriamycin. **(a)** Surgical extirpation of the tumor was performed via question mark incision. **(b)** The resection included the raising of a pericranial flap and detachment and deflection of the temporal muscle, gaining superior access to the infratemporal fossa. The tumor is seen held by Babcock forceps. **(c)** The zygomatic arch is freed en bloc with the tumor, which is held by Babcock forceps. Reconstruction was performed using a pericranial local flap. **(d)** The tumor ex vivo, including part of the temporalis muscle, the zygomatic arch, and the coronoid process. **(e)** Anterior view of the patient 347 days post, with reasonable cosmetic and functional results.

or retrosigmoid approach gains access to cerebellopontine angle tumors by exposing the lateral aspect of the posterior fossa at the junction of the sigmoid and transverse sinuses. Exposure is gained superiorly to the level of the tentorium and inferiorly to the jugular foramen, with possible extension by drilling of the petrous bone into the internal acoustic meatus, Meckel's cave, and cavernous sinus.

Subcranial–Pterional Approach

This combined approach was been first detailed at our institute by Zucker, Fliss, et al[45] and is a combination of two well-described approaches: the subcranial approach developed by

Raveh et al[28] and the pterional approach described by Yasargil et al.[46] Lesions that suit this approach are tumors of the anterolateral fossa (zone II), tumors involving the posterior or lateral aspect of the orbit, parasellar tumors extending to the cavernous sinus, and meningiomas having orbital or nasal extensions. The incision and bicoronal flap are performed in the same fashion as the subcranial approach, which may be extended to include a "hockey stick" incision if concomitant neck metastases are found. The flap is extended unilaterally to the level of the zygomatic arch while preserving the frontal branch of the facial nerve. The type B subcranial osteotomy is extended laterally with added bur holes at the temporal squama and an osteotomy made lateral to the orbital rim.

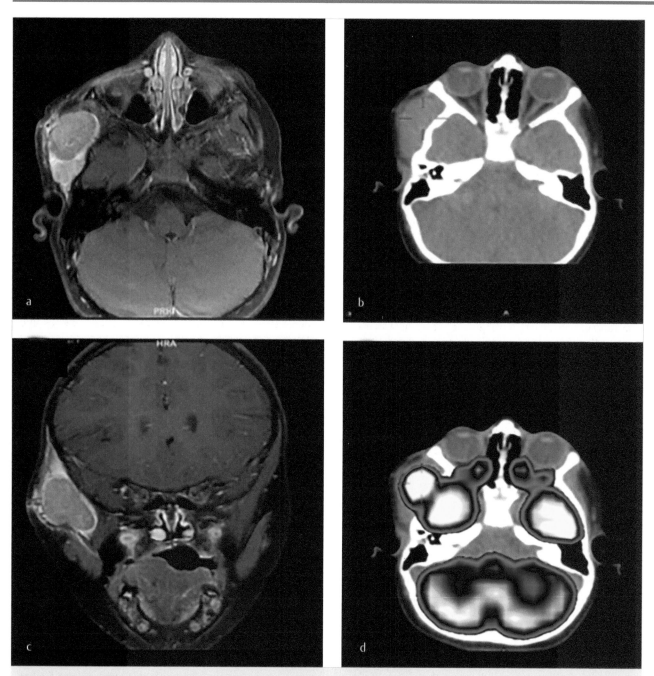

Fig. 15.4 (a) Axial and (b) coronal T1-weighted, gadolinium-enhanced MRI scans showing a lesion measuring 58 mm vertically and 19.5 mm wide with irregular contrast uptake involving the temporal muscle, extending to the external auditory canal, and involving the zygoma and ramus of the mandible. (c) Axial view of CT scan showing an isointense soft tissue lesion of the right temporal fossa measuring 37 × 39 mm. (d) CT/PET exhibiting marked pathological FDG uptake of the lesion. No distant or regional metastases were identified.

The Endoscopic Endonasal Approach

The endoscopic endonasal approach has proved to be highly effective for the treatment of lesions of the nasal cavity, para-nasal sinuses, ventral skull base, and clivus, including cranio-pharyngiomas, angiofibromas, chordomas, and dermoid and epidermoid cysts. Among its many advantages are its minimally invasive nature and midline corridor, which enables minimiza-tion of the manipulation of neurovasculature structures and brain tissue.[47] Nevertheless, larger lesions that infiltrate the anterior or lateral fossae, lateral frontal sinus, anterior maxilla, orbit, or lower clivus are not amenable for a purely endoscopic approach. Furthermore, children younger than 7 years, and especially toddlers younger than 2 years, pose a significant technical challenge, as their nasal aperture is significantly narrower.[48]

The endonasal approaches are divided into sagittal and coronal.[49] Sagittal approaches include the transfrontal, tran-scribriform, transplanum, transsphenoidal, transclival, and transodontoid. Coronal approaches include the transorbital, petrous apex, lateral transcavernous, transpetrous, and trans-condylar–parapharyngeal. Combination of an endoscopic approach with a subcranial or subfrontal approach (termed the cranioendoscopic approach) is usually indicated in extensive disease (T3–T4) exhibiting intracranial origin or skull base involvement, with acceptable results.[50] Knowledge of the development of the skull base and its relevant implications on endoscopic surgical anatomy is imperative, for pneumatization patterns of the paranasal sinuses vary wildly with age.

15.2.2 Pediatric Skull Base Reconstruction

Complete cerebrospinal fluid (CSF) leak prevention is a major part of surgical success in skull base reconstruction, as the risk of meningitis is substantial (approximately 10%/y) irrespective of size or location.[51] Defects that involve the arachnoid matter above cisterns or ventricles result in "high-flow" leaks, whereas other locations usually result in "low-flow" leaks. High-flow leaks call for reconstruction with pedicled flaps, whereas low-flow leaks may be managed using multilayered, nonvascularized flaps, with comparable results.[52] Whenever possible—usually when the defect is small (less than 1.0–1.5 cm)—primary closure should be attempted or a nonvascularized flap used to cover. Medium-sized low-flow defects can be managed using an underlay of temporalis fascia, and bigger defects are repaired using fascia lata grafts. In cases of larger complex defects, local pedicled flaps or vascularized free flaps should be applied in a multilayered fashion. Multilayered reconstruction is preferred to single-layered repairs,[52,53,54] although there have been recent reports of single-layered repairs even in cases of large anterior defects.[55] The "underlay" part is inset in one or two parts: first, collagen matrix may be inserted to the intradural space to provide volume support; second, a cover of fascia or acellular dermis graft is inset between the arachnoid or dura matter and the bony defect, or over the bone if the shape of the defect is not amenable to complete underlying. Accordingly, the harvested graft should be radially larger than the bony defect by 5 to 10 mm.[53] Afterward, an "overlay" of fascia lata, pedicled flap, or another free flap is sutured over the defect, taking care to ensure sufficient size and the facing of the mucosal side outward for optimal adhesion and prevention of accumulation of secretions in the potential space between the layers.[54] CSF leaks can be managed successfully endoscopically using a nasoseptal flap or inferior or middle turbinate flaps.

15.2.3 Potential Complications

As with any surgical procedure, complications are a potential outcome that bears consideration. Vascular injury can occur to the cavernous sinus, the carotid artery, or intracranial vessels, leading to intracranial hemorrhaging. Cerebral vascular accidents and strokes also pose risks. If the dura is involved in the surgery, CSF leak can occur, increasing the risk of meningitis and hydrocephalus.[56] Sinusitis is also a potential complication and may be more likely to occur in the pediatric population than the adult owing to incomplete sinus pneumatization or anatomical variations.[57]

Damage to the pituitary gland can result in complications ranging from diabetes insipidus to panhypopituitarism, a life-threatening syndrome without proper treatment.[30,56,57] Cranial nerve injuries can result in vision loss, diplopia, facial numbness, facial nerve palsy, dysphagia, dysphonia, and the like.[56,57,58] Although these complications may also occur in adults, children are sometimes more likely to suffer from them. For example, children under age 3 might not have a fully developed mastoid tip, so that the facial nerve is more superficial than in adults.[30] Skull base procedures do not, however, appear to have any effect on facial growth in children.[58] Finally, the possible effects of anesthesia and the risk of aspiration pneumonia should be considered for a child undergoing any surgical procedure.

15.3 Conclusion

Tumors of the skull base in pediatric patients present a unique surgical challenge. The pathology and anatomy found in these patients is markedly different from those of the adult, thus affecting the treatment approach. Furthermore, treatment should take into account not only the location of the lesion but also the cytogenetics and the long-term outcome for the patient, including aesthetic and psychological factors as well as mortality and morbidity. Although the potential complications of the surgical procedures discussed herein should be considered with an experienced, multidisciplinary surgical team, skull base lesions in children can be successfully and safely treated.

References

[1] Teo C, Dornhoffer J, Hanna E, Bower C. Application of skull base techniques to pediatric neurosurgery. Childs Nerv Syst. 1999; 15(2–3):103–109

[2] Müller HL. Craniopharyngioma. Endocr Rev. 2014; 35(3):513–543

[3] López F, Triantafyllou A, Snyderman CH, et al. Nasal juvenile angiofibroma: current perspectives with emphasis on management. Head Neck. 2017; 39 (5):1033–1045

[4] Mehta D, Clifton N, McClelland L, Jones NS. Paediatric fibro-osseous lesions of the nose and paranasal sinuses. Int J Pediatr Otorhinolaryngol. 2006; 70(2): 193–199

[5] Ciniglio Appiani M, Verillaud B, Bresson D, et al. Ossifying fibromas of the paranasal sinuses: diagnosis and management. Acta Otorhinolaryngol Ital. 2015; 35(5):355–361

[6] Stapleton AL, Tyler-Kabara EC, Gardner PA, Snyderman CH. Endoscopic endonasal surgery for benign fibro-osseous lesions of the pediatric skull base. Laryngoscope. 2015; 125(9):2199–2203

[7] Gadner H, Minkov M, Grois N, et al. Histiocyte Society. Therapy prolongation improves outcome in multisystem Langerhans cell histiocytosis. Blood. 2013; 121(25):5006–5014

[8] Komotar RJ, Burger PC, Carson BS, et al. Pilocytic and pilomyxoid hypothalamic/chiasmatic astrocytomas. Neurosurgery. 2004; 54(1):72–79, discussion 79–80

[9] Wise JB, Cryer JE, Belasco JB, Jacobs I, Elden L. Management of head and neck plexiform neurofibromas in pediatric patients with neurofibromatosis type 1. Arch Otolaryngol Head Neck Surg. 2005; 131(8):712–718

[10] Ruggieri M, Praticò AD, Serra A, et al. Childhood neurofibromatosis type 2 (NF2) and related disorders: from bench to bedside and biologically targeted therapies. Acta Otorhinolaryngol Ital. 2016; 36(5):345–367

[11] Caldarelli M, Colosimo C, Di Rocco C. Intra-axial dermoid/epidermoid tumors of the brainstem in children. Surg Neurol. 2001; 56(2):97–105

[12] Nicollas R, Facon F, Sudre-Levillain I, Forman C, Roman S, Triglia JM. Pediatric paranasal sinus mucoceles: etiologic factors, management and outcome. Int J Pediatr Otorhinolaryngol. 2006; 70(5):905–908

[13] Peng KA, Grogan T, Wang MB. Head and neck sarcomas: analysis of the SEER database. Otolaryngology–Head and Neck Surgery. 2014; 151(4):627–633

[14] Shern JF, Yohe ME, Khan J. Pediatric rhabdomyosarcoma. Crit Rev Oncog. 2015; 20(3–4):227–243

[15] Reilly BK, Kim A, Peña MT, et al. Rhabdomyosarcoma of the head and neck in children: review and update. Int J Pediatr Otorhinolaryngol. 2015; 79(9):1477–1483

[16] Gil Z, Fliss DM. Skull-base surgery in children and adolescents. In: Stucker FJ, de Souza C, Kenyon GS, Lian TS, Draf W, Schick B, eds. Rhinology and Facial Plastic Surgery. Berlin, Heidelberg: Springer Berlin Heidelberg; 2009:469–476

[17] Guinto G, Guinto-Nishimura Y. Clivus chordomas: role of surgery. World Neurosurg. 2014; 81(5–6):688–689

[18] Jethanamest D, Morris LG, Sikora AG, Kutler DI. Esthesioneuroblastoma: a population-based analysis of survival and prognostic factors. Arch Otolaryngol Head Neck Surg. 2007; 133(3):276–280

[19] Balamuth NJ, Womer RB. Ewing's sarcoma. Lancet Oncol. 2010; 11(2):184–192

[20] Moschovi M, Alexiou GA, Tourkantoni N, et al. Cranial Ewing's sarcoma in children. Neurol Sci. 2011; 32(4):691–694

[21] Amirian ES, Goodman JC, New P, Scheurer ME. Pediatric and adult malignant peripheral nerve sheath tumors: an analysis of data from the surveillance, epidemiology, and end results program. J Neurooncol. 2014; 116(3):609–616

[22] Gil Z, Fliss DM. Cytogenetic analysis of skull base tumors: where do we stand? Curr Opin Otolaryngol Head Neck Surg. 2012; 20(2):130–136

[23] Gil Z, Orr-Urtreger A, Voskoboinik N, Trejo-Leider L, Shomrat R, Fliss DM. Cytogenetic analysis of 101 skull base tumors. Head Neck. 2008; 30(5):567–581

[24] Sandberg AA, Bridge JA. Updates on the cytogenetics and molecular genetics of bone and soft tissue tumors: chondrosarcoma and other cartilaginous neoplasms. Cancer Genet Cytogenet. 2003; 143(1):1–31

[25] Gordon T, McManus A, Anderson J, et al. United Kingdom Children's Cancer Study Group, United Kingdom Cancer Cytogenetics Group. Cytogenetic abnormalities in 42 rhabdomyosarcoma: a United Kingdom Cancer Cytogenetics Group study. Med Pediatr Oncol. 2001; 36(2):259–267

[26] Kullendorff CM, Donner M, Mertens F, Mandahl N. Chromosomal aberrations in a consecutive series of childhood rhabdomyosarcoma. Med Pediatr Oncol. 1998; 30(3):156–159

[27] Sandberg AA, Bridge JA. Updates on the cytogenetics and molecular genetics of bone and soft tissue tumors: synovial sarcoma. Cancer Genet Cytogenet. 2002; 133(1):1–23

[28] Raveh J, Laedrach K, Speiser M, et al. The subcranial approach for fronto-orbital and anteroposterior skull-base tumors. Arch Otolaryngol Head Neck Surg. 1993; 119(4):385–393

[29] Raveh J, Turk JB, Lädrach K, et al. Extended anterior subcranial approach for skull base tumors: long-term results. J Neurosurg. 1995; 82(6):1002–1010

[30] Gil Z, Constantini S, Spektor S, et al. Skull base approaches in the pediatric population. Head Neck. 2005; 27(8):682–689

[31] Ducic Y, Coimbra C. The subfrontal approach to the anterior skull base. Oper Tech Otolaryngol–Head Neck Surg. 2010; 21(1):9–18

[32] Kim SR, Lee JW, Han YS, Kim HK. Transfacial surgical approaches to secure wide exposure of the skull base. Arch Craniofac Surg. 2015; 16(1):17–23

[33] Nabili V, Kelly DF, Fatemi N, St John M, Calcaterra TC, Abemayor E. Transnasal, transfacial, anterior skull base resection of olfactory neuroblastoma. Am J Otolaryngol. 2011; 32(4):279–285

[34] Weinzweig J. Plastic Surgery Secrets. 2nd ed. Philadelphia, PA: Mosby/Elsevier; 2010

[35] Hoff SR, Edwards MS, Bailey CM, Koltai PJ. The transpalatal approach to repair of congenital basal skull base cephaloceles. J Neurol Surg B Skull Base. 2014; 75(2):96–103

[36] Puri P, Höllwarth ME. Pediatric Surgery: Diagnosis and Management. Springer Berlin Heidelberg; 2009

[37] Jeon SY, Jeong JH, Kim HS, Ahn SK, Kim JP. Hemifacial degloving approach for medial maxillectomy: a modification of midfacial degloving approach. Laryngoscope. 2003; 113(4):754–756

[38] Ferreira LM, Rios AS, Gomes EF, Azevedo JF, Araújo RdeP, Moraes RB. Midfacial degloving—access to nasal cavity and paranasal sinuses lesions. Rev Bras Otorrinolaringol (Engl Ed). 2006; 72(2):158–162

[39] Jurdy L, Merks JH, Pieters BR, et al. Orbital rhabdomyosarcomas: a review. Saudi J Ophthalmol. 2013; 27(3):167–175

[40] Fliss DM, Abergel A, Cavel O, Margalit N, Gil Z. Combined subcranial approaches for excision of complex anterior skull base tumors. Arch Otolaryngol Head Neck Surg. 2007; 133(9):888–896

[41] Sasaki CT, Lowlicht RA, Astrachan DI, Friedman CD, Goodwin WJ, Morales M. Le Fort I osteotomy approach to the skull base. Laryngoscope. 1990; 100(10 Pt 1):1073–1076

[42] Lewark TM, Allen GC, Chowdhury K, Chan KH. Le Fort I osteotomy and skull base tumors: a pediatric experience. Arch Otolaryngol Head Neck Surg. 2000; 126(8):1004–1008

[43] George B, Bresson D. Skull base approaches in children. In: Özek MM, Cinalli G, Maixner W, Sainte-Rose C, eds. Posterior Fossa Tumors in Children. Cham: Springer International Publishing; 2015:209–218

[44] Grinblat G, Prasad SC, Fulcheri A, Laus M, Russo A, Sanna M. Lateral skull base surgery in a pediatric population: a 25-year experience in a referral skull base center. Int J Pediatr Otorhinolaryngol. 2017; 94:70–75

[45] Zucker G, Nash M, Gatot A, Amir A, Fliss DM. The combined subcranial-pterional approach to the anterolateral skull base. Oper Tech Otolaryngol–Head Neck Surg. 2000; 11(4):286–293

[46] Yasargil MG, Antic J, Laciga R, Jain KK, Hodosh RM, Smith RD. Microsurgical pterional approach to aneurysms of the basilar bifurcation. Surg Neurol. 1976; 6(2):83–91

[47] Zwagerman NT, Zenonos G, Lieber S, et al. Endoscopic transnasal skull base surgery: pushing the boundaries. J Neurooncol. 2016; 130(2):319–330

[48] Tatreau JR, Patel MR, Shah RN, et al. Anatomical considerations for endoscopic endonasal skull base surgery in pediatric patients. Laryngoscope. 2010; 120 (9):1730–1737

[49] Snyderman C, Kassam A, Carrau R, Mintz A, Gardner P, Prevedello DM. Acquisition of surgical skills for endonasal skull base surgery: a training program. Laryngoscope. 2007; 117(4):699–705

[50] Hanna E, DeMonte F, Ibrahim S, Roberts D, Levine N, Kupferman M. Endoscopic resection of sinonasal cancers with and without craniotomy: oncologic results. Arch Otolaryngol Head Neck Surg. 2009; 135(12):1219–1224

[51] Bernal-Sprekelsen M, Rioja E, Enseñat J, et al. Management of anterior skull base defect depending on its size and location. BioMed Res Int. 2014(4): 346873

[52] Soudry E, Turner JH, Nayak JV, Hwang PH. Endoscopic reconstruction of surgically created skull base defects: a systematic review. Otolaryngology–Head and Neck Surgery. 2014; 150(5):730–738

[53] Zanation A, Carrau R, Snyderman C, et al. Endoscopic reconstruction of anterior skull base defects. In: Kassam AB, Gardner PA, eds. Endoscopic Approaches to the Skull Base. 2012;26:168–181

[54] Zuniga MG, Turner JH, Chandra RK. Updates in anterior skull base reconstruction. Curr Opin Otolaryngol Head Neck Surg. 2016; 24(1):75–82

[55] Yoo F, Wang MB, Bergsneider M, Suh JD. Single layer repair of large anterior skull base defects without vascularized mucosal flap. J Neurol Surg B Skull Base. 2017; 78(2):139–144

[56] Walz PC, Elmaraghy CA, Jatana KRY. Endoscopic skull base surgery in the pediatric patient. In: Amornyotin S, ed. Endoscopy—Innovative Uses and Emerging Technologies. 2015:ch. 13

[57] Chivukula S, Koutourousiou M, Snyderman CH, Fernandez-Miranda JC, Gardner PA, Tyler-Kabara EC. Endoscopic endonasal skull base surgery in the pediatric population. J Neurosurg Pediatr. 2013; 11(3):227–241

[58] Tsai EC, Santoreneos S, Rutka JT. Tumors of the skull base in children: review of tumor types and management strategies. Neurosurg Focus. 2002; 12(5):e1

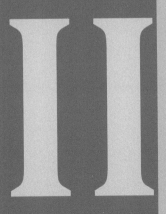

16 Surgical Management of Tumors of the Nasal Cavity, Paranasal Sinuses, Orbit, and Anterior Skull Base

Ehab Y. Hanna, Shaan M. Raza, Shirley Su, Michael E. Kupferman, and Franco DeMonte

Summary

This chapter discusses surgical anatomy, regional pathology, and clinical assessment, including imaging and biopsy of tumors of the nasal cavity, paranasal sinuses, orbit, and anterior skull base. The chapter describes in great detail the surgical management of these tumors, including preoperative assessment, indications, contraindications, surgical approaches (open and endoscopic), extent of resection, management of the orbit, and reconstructive strategies. Finally, the chapter discusses the outcomes and prognosis of patients who have sinonasal cancers.

Keywords: sinus cancers, skull base cancers, endoscopic resection, maxillectomy, ethmoidectomy, craniofacial resection, orbit, paranasal sinuses, nasal cavity, anterior skull base

16.1 Introduction

During the past two decades, significant advances have been made in both the diagnosis and the management of cancer of the nasal cavity and paranasal sinuses. The most significant advances in diagnosis are office endoscopy and high-resolution imaging. These diagnostic tools have allowed more accurate delineation of the extent of sinonasal tumors and thus improved treatment planning. Significant advances in treatment include progress made in cranial base surgery allowing for safe excision of tumors involving the cranial base. In addition, the development of microvascular free tissue transfer has made possible effective reconstruction of more extensive surgical defects. Advances have also been made in both planning and delivery of radiotherapy, such as intensity-modulated radiation therapy (IMRT) and proton therapy. Both modalities allow optimal radiation dosimetry to the tumor while sparing normal surrounding tissue. Various new combinations of effective cytotoxic chemotherapeutic and targeted biologic agents are also being increasingly incorporated in the overall management of patients who have sinonasal cancer.

Recent advances made in diagnosis and treatment of patients who have sinonasal cancer have clearly impacted our ability to control the disease and improve survival. Over the past 50 years, survival rates have improved, from 25 to 40% in the 1960s to 65 to 75% in the past decade. Despite this improvement, a significant number of patients die of their disease. The rarity of these tumors, and their presenting symptoms' similarity to those of more common benign conditions, coupled with the propensity for early spread and involvement of surrounding critical structures, are reflected in the fact that most patients still present with advanced-stage disease. This has clearly hampered attempts to further improve prognosis. In this chapter, we present current trends in diagnosis, classification, staging, and surgical treatment of patients who have cancers of the nasal cavity and paranasal sinuses.

16.2 Surgical Anatomy

16.2.1 Nasal Cavity

The nasal cavity is bounded by the bony pyriform aperture and the external framework of the nose (▶ Fig. 16.1). The nasal cavity opens anteriorly through the skin-lined nasal vestibule into the nares and communicates posteriorly through the choanae with the nasopharynx (▶ Fig. 16.2a). The nasal cavity is divided in the midline by the *nasal septum*, which includes both cartilaginous and bony components (▶ Fig. 16.2b). The cartilage of the septum is quadrilateral in shape and is thicker at its margins than at its center. Its anterior margin is connected with the nasal bones and

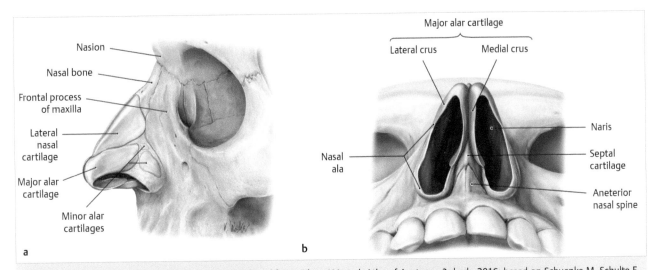

Fig. 16.1 (a, b) Anatomy of the external nose. (Reproduced from Gilroy AM et al, Atlas of Anatomy, 3rd ed., 2016; based on Schuenke M, Schulte E, Schumacher U, Thieme Atlas of Anatomy: Head, Neck, and Neuroanatomy, illustrations by Voll M and Wesker K, 2nd ed., New York: Thieme Medical Publishers; 2016.)

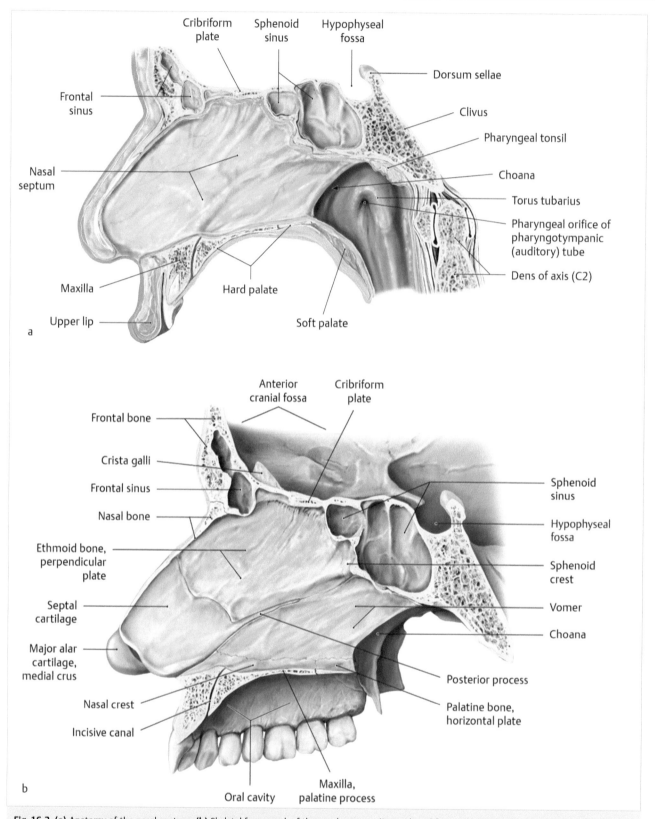

Fig. 16.2 **(a)** Anatomy of the nasal septum. **(b)** Skeletal framework of the nasal septum. (Reproduced from Gilroy AM et al, Atlas of Anatomy, 3rd ed., 2016; based on Schuenke M, Schulte E, Schumacher U, Thieme Atlas of Anatomy: Head, Neck, and Neuroanatomy, illustrations by Voll M and Wesker K, 2nd ed., New York: Thieme Medical Publishers; 2016.)

is continuous with the anterior margins of the lateral cartilages; below, it is connected to the medial crura of the greater alar cartilages by fibrous tissue (▶ Fig. 16.1). Its posterior margin is connected with the perpendicular plate of the ethmoid; its inferior margin is connected with the vomer and the palatine process of the maxilla.

On the *lateral nasal wall* are the superior, middle, and inferior nasal turbinates, and below and lateral to each turbinate (concha) is the corresponding nasal passage or meatus (▶ Fig. 16.3). Above the superior turbinate is a narrow recess, the sphenoethmoidal recess, into which the sphenoid sinus opens. The superior meatus is a short oblique passage extending about halfway along the upper

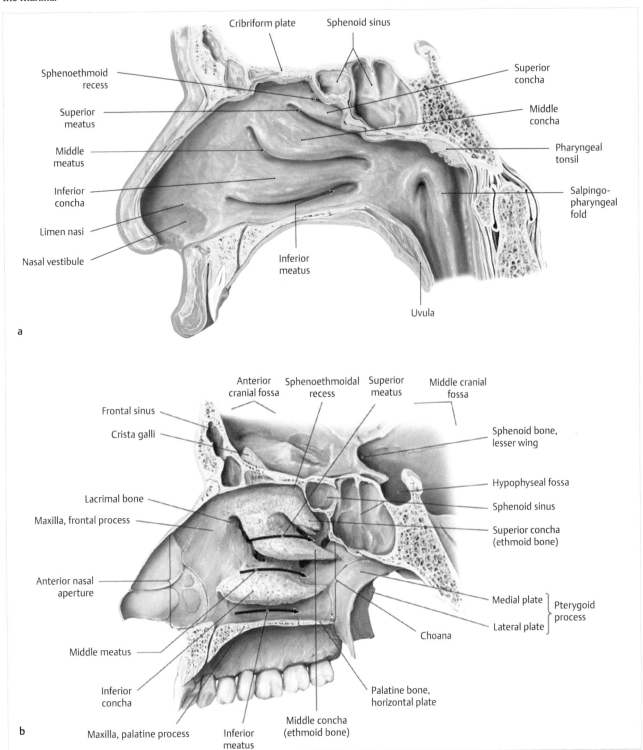

Fig. 16.3 (a) Anatomy of the lateral nasal wall. (b) Skeletal framework the lateral nasal wall. (Reproduced from Gilroy AM et al, Atlas of Anatomy, 3rd ed., 2016; based on Schuenke M, Schulte E, Schumacher U, Thieme Atlas of Anatomy: Head, Neck, and Neuroanatomy, illustrations by Voll M and Wesker K, 2nd ed., New York: Thieme Medical Publishers; 2016.) *(Continued)*

(Continued)

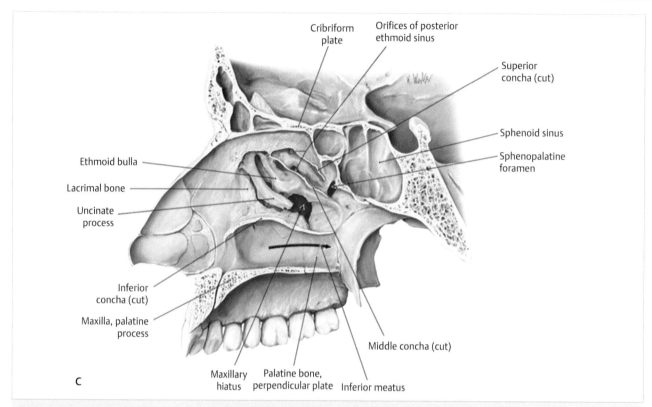

Cribriform plate

Orifices of posterior ethmoid sinus

Superior concha (cut)

Sphenoid sinus

Sphenopalatine foramen

Ethmoid bulla

Lacrimal bone

Uncinate process

Inferior concha (cut)

Maxilla, palatine process

Middle concha (cut)

Maxillary hiatus

Palatine bone, perpendicular plate

Inferior meatus

C

Fig. 16.3 *(Continued)* **(c)** Removal of the middle turbinate demonstrates the anatomy of the middle meatus. (Reproduced from Gilroy AM et al, Atlas of Anatomy, 3rd ed., 2016; based on Schuenke M, Schulte E, Schumacher U, Thieme Atlas of Anatomy: Head, Neck, and Neuroanatomy, illustrations by Voll M and Wesker K, 2nd ed., New York: Thieme Medical Publishers; 2016.)

border of the middle turbinate; the posterior ethmoid cells open into the front part of this meatus. The middle meatus is below and lateral to the middle turbinate. The anatomy of the middle meatus is fully displayed by removing the middle turbinate.

The bulla ethmoidalis is the most prominent anterior ethmoid air cell. The hiatus semilunaris is a curved cleft lying below and in front of the bulla ethmoidalis. It is bounded inferiorly by the sharp concave margin of the uncinate process of the ethmoid bone and leads into a curved channel, the infundibulum, bounded above by the bulla ethmoidalis and below by the lateral surface of the uncinate process of the ethmoid. The anterior ethmoid air cells open into the front part of the infundibulum. The frontal sinus drains through the nasofrontal duct, which in approximately 50% of subjects will also drain into the infundibulum. However, when the anterior end of the uncinate process fuses with the front part of the bulla, this continuity is interrupted and the nasofrontal duct then opens directly into the anterior end of the middle meatus. Below the bulla ethmoidalis, partly hidden by the inferior end of the uncinate process, is the ostium of the maxillary sinus. An accessory ostium from the maxillary sinus is frequently present below the posterior end of the middle nasal concha. The inferior meatus is below and lateral to the inferior nasal turbinate. The nasolacrimal duct opens into the inferior meatus under cover of the anterior part of the inferior turbinate.

The *roof of the nasal cavity* is narrow from side to side and slopes downward (at about a 30° angle) from front to back. The cribriform plate, which transmits the filaments of the olfactory nerve, forms the roof of the nasal cavity medial to the superior attachment of the middle turbinate. Lateral to the middle turbinate,

the fovea ethmoidalis forms the roof of the ethmoid sinuses. Careful assessment of the anatomy of the nasal roof, especially the relationship of the cribriform plate to the fovea ethmoidalis, is critical in avoiding a cerebrospinal fluid (CSF) leak during transnasal surgery in this region. The cribriform plate is usually at a slightly lower horizontal plane than the fovea ethmoidalis, forming a shallow olfactory groove. This configuration is described as Keros type I (▶ Fig. 16.4). However, the cribriform plate may be moderately or significantly lower than the fovea ethmoidalis, resulting in a medium (Keros type II) or deep (Keros type III) olfactory groove. The topography of the roof may also be asymmetrical.[1]

The *floor of the nasal cavity* is concave from side to side and almost horizontal anteroposteriorly. The palatine process of the maxilla forms the anterior three-fourths, and the horizontal process of the palatine bone the posterior fourth, of the nasal floor (▶ Fig. 16.2b).

The majority of the nasal cavity is lined by pseudostratified ciliated columnar epithelium, which contains mucous and serous glands (respiratory epithelium). Specialized olfactory epithelium lines the most superior portion of the nasal cavity and has direct connections with the olfactory tracts through openings in the cribriform plate.

The *arteries of the nasal cavities* are the anterior and posterior ethmoidal branches of the ophthalmic artery, which supply the ethmoid and frontal sinuses and the roof of the nose. The sphenopalatine artery supplies the mucous membrane covering the lateral nasal wall. The septal branch of the superior labial artery supplies the anteroinferior septum. The veins form a close cavernous plexus beneath the mucous membrane. This plexus is

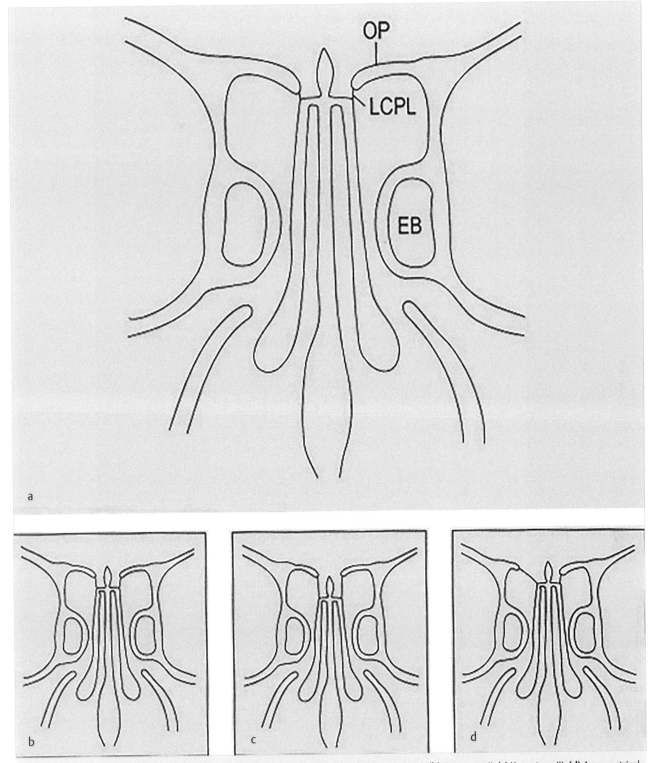

Fig. 16.4 Anatomy of the ethmoid roof and lateral lamella of the cribriform plate. **(a)** Keros type I. **(b)** Keros type II. **(c)** Keros type III. **(d)** Asymmetrical ethmoid roof. Note that the right lateral lamella of the cribriform plate is very thin and long and is obliquely oriented, including much of the right ethmoid roof. OP, orbital plate of frontal bone; LCPL, lateral cribriform plate lamella; EB, ethmoid bulla.

especially well marked over the lower part of the septum and over the middle and inferior turbinates. *Venous drainage* follows a pattern similar to arterial supply. The lymphatic drainage from the anterior part of the nasal cavity, similar to that of the external nose, is to the submandibular group of lymph nodes (Level I). *Lymphatics* from the posterior two-thirds of the nasal cavities and from the paranasal sinuses drain to the upper jugular (Level II) and retropharyngeal lymph nodes.

The *sensory nerves of the nasal cavity* transmit either somatoautonomic or olfactory sensation. *Somatoautonomic nerves* include

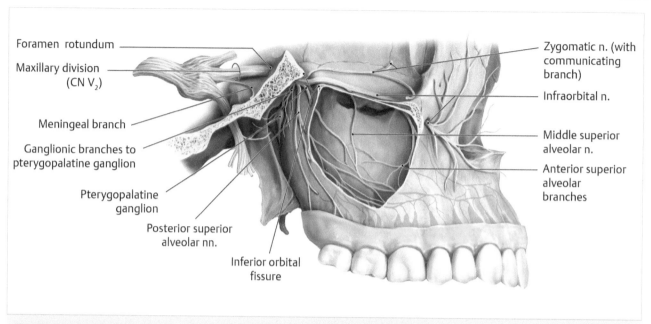

Fig. 16.5 Anatomy of the maxillary sinus (lateral wall removed). (Reproduced from Gilroy AM et al, Atlas of Anatomy, 3rd ed., 2016; based on Schuenke M, Schulte E, Schumacher U, Thieme Atlas of Anatomy: Head, Neck, and Neuroanatomy, illustrations by Voll M and Wesker K, 2nd ed., New York: Thieme Medical Publishers; 2016.)

the nasociliary branch of the ophthalmic, which supplies the anterior septum and lateral wall. The anterior alveolar nerve, a branch of the maxillary (V2), provides sensory innervation to the inferior meatus and inferior turbinate. The nasopalatine nerve supplies the middle of the septum. The anterior palatine nerve supplies the lower nasal branches to the middle and inferior turbinates. The nerve of the pterygoid canal (vidian) and the nasal branches from the sphenopalatine ganglion supply the upper and posterior septum and the superior turbinate. The *olfactory nerve* fibers arise from the bipolar olfactory cells and unite in fasciculi, which form a plexus beneath the mucous membrane and then ascend, passing into the skull through the foramina in the cribriform plate. Intracranially, olfactory nerve fibers enter the under surface of the olfactory bulb, in which they ramify and form synapses with the dendrites of the mitral cells of the olfactory tract.

16.2.2 Maxillary Sinus

The maxillary sinus (*antrum of Highmore*), the largest of the accessory sinuses of the nose, is a pyramidal cavity in the body of the maxilla (▶ Fig. 16.5; ▶ Fig. 16.6). Its base is formed by the lateral wall of the nasal cavity, and its apex extends into the zygomatic process. Its roof or orbital wall is frequently ridged by the infraorbital canal, whereas its floor is formed by the alveolar process of the maxilla and is usually 1 to 10 mm below the level of the floor of the nose (▶ Fig. 16.6). Projecting into the floor are several conical elevations corresponding with the roots of the first and second molar teeth; in some cases the floor is perforated by one or more of these roots. The natural ostium of the maxillary sinus is partially covered by the uncinate process and communicates with the lower part of the hiatus semilunaris of the lateral nasal wall (▶ Fig. 16.3; ▶ Fig. 16.5). An accessory ostium is frequently seen in, or immediately behind, the hiatus. The maxillary sinus appears as a shallow groove on the medial surface of the bone about the

fourth month of fetal life but does not reach its full size until after the second dentition.

16.2.3 Ethmoid Sinus

The ethmoidal air cells consist of numerous thin-walled cavities situated in the ethmoidal labyrinth and bounded by the frontal, maxillary, lacrimal, sphenoid, and palatine bones. They lie in the upper part of the nasal cavity, between the orbits (▶ Fig. 16.6). The ethmoid sinuses are separated from the orbital cavity by a thin bony plate, the lamina papyracea. On either side they are arranged in three groups: anterior, middle, and posterior. The anterior and middle groups open into the middle meatus of the nose—the former by way of the infundibulum, the latter on or above the bulla ethmoidalis (▶ Fig. 16.3). The posterior cells open into the superior meatus under cover of the superior nasal concha. Sometimes one or more ethmoid air cells extends over the orbital cavity (supraorbital ethmoid cells) or the optic nerve (Onodi cell). The ethmoidal cells begin to develop during fetal life.

16.2.4 Frontal Sinus

The paired frontal sinuses appear to be outgrowths from the most anterior ethmoidal air cells. They are situated behind the superciliary arches and are rarely symmetrical, and the septum between them frequently deviates to one or the other side of the midline. Absent at birth, the frontal sinuses are generally fairly well developed between the seventh and eighth years but reach their full size only after puberty. The frontal sinus is lined with respiratory epithelium and drains into the anterior part of the corresponding middle meatus of the nose through the nasofrontal duct, which traverses the anterior part of the labyrinth of the ethmoid. The soft tissues of the forehead are located anteriorly, the orbits are located inferiorly, and the anterior cranial fossa is located posteriorly

(▶ Fig. 16.3). Blood and neural supply is from the supraorbital and supratrochlear neurovascular bundles.

16.2.5 Sphenoid Sinus

The sphenoid sinus begins at the most posterior and superior portion of the nasal cavity (▶ Fig. 16.3). This midline structure, which is contained within the body of the sphenoid bone, is irregular and often has an eccentrically located intersinus septum. When exceptionally large, the sphenoid sinus may extend into the roots of the pterygoid processes or great wings and may pneumatize the basilar part of the occipital bone. The sphenoid sinus ostium is located on the anterior wall of the sinus and communicates directly with the sphenoethmoidal recess above and medial to the superior turbinate. The sphenoid sinuses are present as minute cavities at birth, but their main development takes place after puberty. The posterosuperior wall of the sphenoid sinus displays the forward convexity caused by the floor of the sella turcica, which contains the pituitary gland.

The optic nerve and the internal carotid artery are closely related to the superior lateral wall of the sphenoid sinus, and their bony canals may be dehiscent within the sinus cavity (▶ Fig. 16.7). Vascular and neural supplies come from the sphenopalatine and posterior ethmoidal arteries and the branches of the sphenopalatine ganglion, respectively.

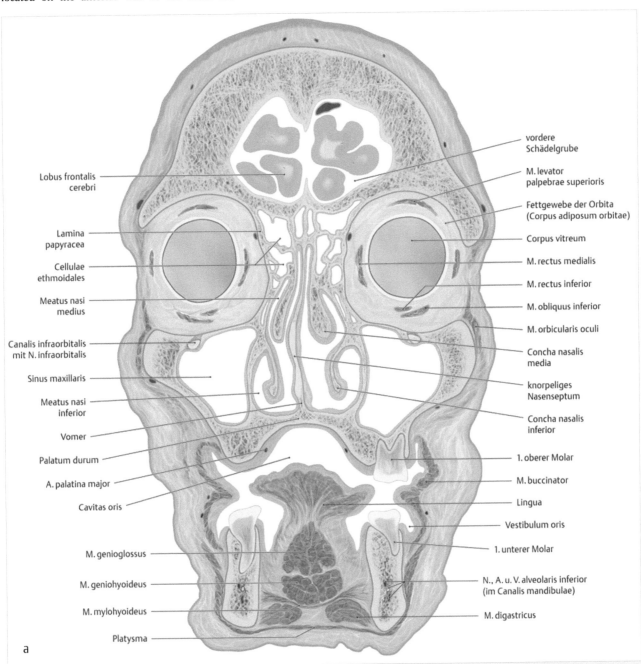

Fig. 16.6 (a, b) Anatomy of the ethmoid and maxillary sinuses (coronal sections). (Reproduced from Schuenke M, Schulte E, Schumacher U, Thieme Atlas of Anatomy: Head, Neck, and Neuroanatomy, illustrations by Voll M and Wesker K, 2nd ed., New York: Thieme Medical Publishers; 2016.) *(Continued)*

(Continued)

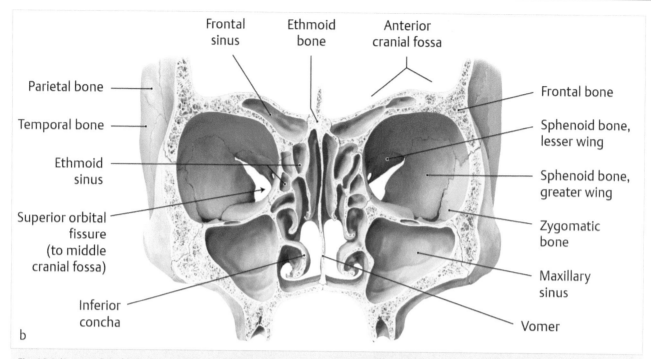

Fig. 16.6 (Continued) (a, b) Anatomy of the ethmoid and maxillary sinuses (coronal sections). (Reproduced from Schuenke M, Schulte E, Schumacher U, Thieme Atlas of Anatomy: Head, Neck, and Neuroanatomy, illustrations by Voll M and Wesker K, 2nd ed., New York: Thieme Medical Publishers; 2016.)

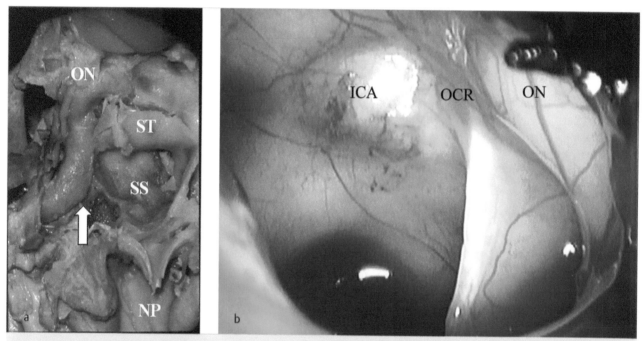

Fig. 16.7 (a) Cadaver dissection of the sphenoid sinus (SS). The sinus is located in the midline superior to the nasopharynx (NP). The sella turcica (ST) forms a convexity in the posterosuperior wall. The internal carotid artery (arrow) courses through the lateral wall of the sinus and is related superiorly to the optic nerve (ON). (b) Endoscopic view of the left sphenoid sinus. Note the internal carotid artery (ICA) and ON impressions on the lateral and superior walls. A bony septum within the sinus inserts into the opticocarotid recess (OCR).

16.2.6 Infratemporal Fossa

The infratemporal fossa is an irregularly shaped space situated below and medial to the zygomatic arch. It is bounded anteriorly by the posterior surface of the maxilla, superiorly by the greater wing of the sphenoid and the undersurface of the squamous portion of the temporal bone, medially by the lateral pterygoid plate, and laterally by the ramus of the mandible. It contains the inferior aspect of the temporalis muscle as well as the medial and lateral pterygoid muscles (▶ Fig. 16.8). It also contains branches of the internal maxillary vessels, including the middle meningeal artery, and the mandibular (V3) nerves, including the lingual, inferior alveolar,

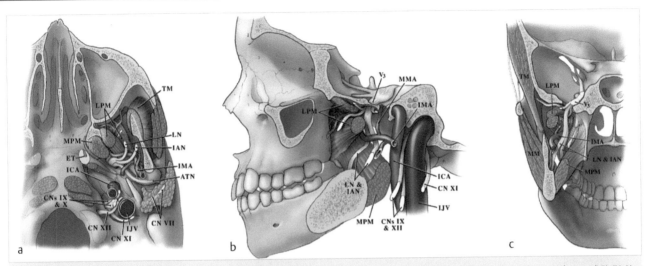

Fig. 16.8 Anatomy of the infratemporal fossa: **(a)** inferior, **(b)** lateral, and **(c)** anterior views. ATN, auriculotemporal nerve; CN, cranial nerve (VII, IX, X, XI, and XII); ET, Eustachian tube; IAN, inferior alveolar nerve; ICA, internal carotid artery; IJV, internal jugular vein; IMA, internal maxillary artery; LN, lingual nerve; LPM, lateral pterygoid muscle; MM, masseter muscle; MMA, middle meningeal artery; MPM, medial pterygoid muscle; TM, temporalis muscle; V3, third division of the trigeminal nerve.

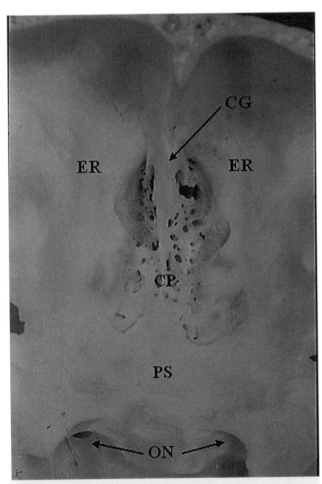

Fig. 16.9 The floor of the anterior cranial fossa. The cribriform plate (CP) is characterized by the presence of foramina for the olfactory nerves on each side of the crista galli (CG), which is seen in the midline. Lateral to the CP are the ethmoidal roof and, even more lateral, the roof of the orbit. Posterior to the cribriform plate is the planum sphenoidale (PS). The optic nerves (ON) form the optic chiasm behind the planum sphenoidale.

and auriculotemporal nerves. The foramen ovale and foramen spinosum open on its roof and the alveolar canals on its anterior wall. The inferior orbital and pterygomaxillary fissures communicate with and may act as routes of spread of cancer to the infratemporal fossa. The infratemporal fossa also contains the upper carotid sheath, including the internal carotid artery, the internal jugular vein, and the last four cranial nerves.

16.2.7 Pterygopalatine Fossa

The pterygopalatine fossa is a small triangular space situated behind the maxillary sinus, in front of the pterygoid plates, and beneath the apex of the orbit. This fossa communicates with the orbit by the inferior orbital fissure, with the nasal cavity by the sphenopalatine foramen, and with the infratemporal fossa by the pterygomaxillary fissure (▶ Fig. 16.5). Five foramina open into it, of which three are on the posterior walls: the foramen rotundum, the pterygoid canal, and the pharyngeal canal, in this order downward and medial. On the medial wall is the sphenopalatine foramen, and below is the superior orifice of the pterygopalatine canal. The fossa contains the maxillary nerve, the sphenopalatine ganglion, and the terminal part of the internal maxillary artery. The fissures and foramina of the pterygopalatine fossa serve as "highways" for spread of cancer from the sinonasal region to the orbit, infratemporal fossa, and cranial base.

16.2.8 Anterior Cranial Fossa

The floor of the anterior fossa is formed by the orbital plates of the frontal bone, the cribriform plate of the ethmoid, and the lesser wings and front part of the body of the sphenoid. In the midline it presents, from anterior to posterior, the frontal crest for the attachment of the falx cerebri; the foramen cecum, which usually transmits a small vein from the nasal cavity to the superior sagittal sinus (SSS); and the crista galli, the free margin of which affords attachment to the falx cerebri (▶ Fig. 16.9).

On either side of the crista galli is the olfactory groove formed by the cribriform plate, which supports the olfactory

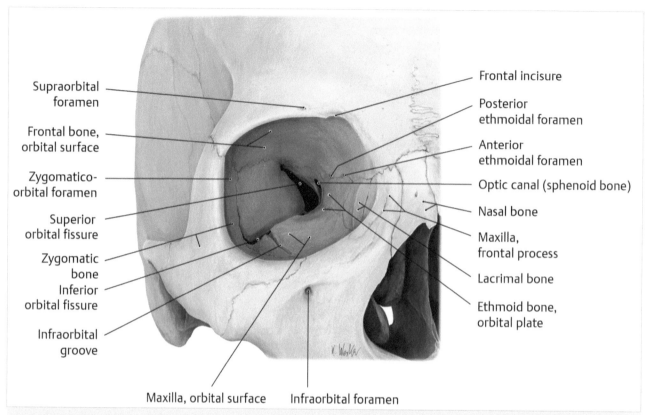

Fig. 16.10 Anatomy of the right orbit. (Reproduced from Gilroy AM et al, Atlas of Anatomy, 3rd ed., 2016; based on Schuenke M, Schulte E, Schumacher U, Thieme Atlas of Anatomy: Head, Neck, and Neuroanatomy, illustrations by Voll M and Wesker K, 2nd ed., New York: Thieme Medical Publishers; 2016.)

bulb and presents foramina for the transmission of the olfactory nerves. Lateral to either olfactory groove are the internal openings of the anterior and posterior ethmoidal foramina. The anterior, situated about the middle of the lateral margin of the olfactory groove, transmits the anterior ethmoidal vessels and the nasociliary nerve. The nerve runs in a groove along the lateral edge of the cribriform plate. The posterior ethmoidal foramen opens at the back part of this margin under cover of the projecting lamina of the sphenoid and transmits the posterior ethmoidal vessels and nerve. More laterally, the cranial floor forms the orbital roof and supports the frontal lobes of the cerebrum. Further back, in the middle, are the planum sphenoidale, forming the roof of the sphenoid sinus, and the anterior margin of the chiasmatic groove, running laterally on either side to the upper margin of the optic foramen (▶ Fig. 16.9).

16.2.9 Orbit

The orbits are two quadrilateral pyramidal cavities, their bases directed forward and lateral and their apices backward and medial so that their long axes diverge at a 45° angle and would meet over the body of the sphenoid if continued backward. The orbit is anatomically defined by seven bones (▶ Fig. 16.10)—frontal, zygomatic, maxillary, lacrimal, ethmoid, sphenoid, and palatine—and by the orbital septum, which originates at the arcus marginalis, fusing with the levator aponeurosis above and the capsulopalpebral fascia below. It is bounded by the ethmoid and sphenoid sinuses at its medial aspect, the frontal sinus superomedially, the cranial vault superiorly and posteriorly, the temporal fossa

laterally, and the maxillary sinus inferiorly. Each orbital cavity has a roof, a floor, a medial and a lateral wall, a base, and an apex.

The roof is formed anteriorly by the orbital plate of the frontal bone and posteriorly by the lesser wing of the sphenoid. It presents *medially* the trochlear fovea for the attachment of the cartilaginous pulley of the superior oblique muscle and *laterally* the lacrimal fossa for the lacrimal gland.

The floor is formed mainly by the orbital surface of the maxilla: anteriorly and *laterally* by the orbital process of the zygomatic bone and posterior and *medially*, to a small extent, by the orbital process of the palatine bone. At its medial angle is the superior opening of the nasolacrimal canal, immediately to the lateral side of which is a depression for the origin of the inferior oblique muscle. Running anteriorly near the middle of the floor is the infraorbital canal, ending anterior to the maxilla in the infraorbital foramen and transmitting the infraorbital nerve and vessels.

The medial wall is formed from anterior to posterior by the frontal process of the maxilla, the lacrimal bone, the lamina papyracea of the ethmoid, and a small part of the body of the sphenoid anterior to the optic foramen. Anteroinferiorly, the lacrimal sac is situated between the anterior and posterior lacrimal crests at the junction between the medial wall and the floor. The lacrimal part of the orbicularis oculi arises from the posterior lacrimal crest. At the junction of the medial wall and the roof, the frontoethmoidal suture presents the anterior and posterior ethmoidal foramina, the former transmitting the nasociliary nerve and anterior ethmoidal vessels and the latter the posterior ethmoidal nerve and vessels. These foramina indicate the level of the cranial base within the orbit.

The lateral wall is formed by the orbital process of the zygomatic and the orbital surface of the greater wing of the sphenoid. On the orbital process of the zygomatic bone are the orbital tubercle (Whitnall's) and the orifices of one or two canals, which transmit the branches of the zygomatic nerve. Between the roof and the lateral wall, near the apex of the orbit, is the superior orbital fissure (SOF). Through this fissure the oculomotor, the trochlear, the ophthalmic division of the trigeminal (V1), and the abducent nerves enter the orbital cavity, as do also some filaments from the cavernous plexus of the sympathetic and the orbital branches of the middle meningeal artery. Passing posteriorly through the fissure are the ophthalmic vein and the recurrent branch from the lacrimal artery to the dura mater. The lateral wall and the floor are separated posteriorly by the inferior orbital fissure, which transmits the maxillary nerve (V2) and its zygomatic branch, the infraorbital vessels, and the ascending branches from the sphenopalatine ganglion.

The base of the orbit (orbital rim), quadrilateral in shape, is formed superiorly by the supraorbital arch of the frontal bone, in which is the supraorbital notch or foramen for the passage of the supraorbital vessels and nerve; inferiorly by the zygomatic bone and maxilla, united by the zygomaticomaxillary suture; *laterally* by the zygomatic bone and the zygomatic process of the frontal joined by the zygomaticofrontal suture; and *medially* by the frontal bone and the frontal process of the maxilla, united by the frontomaxillary suture.

The apex is situated in the posterior aspect of the orbit. The optic foramen is a short, cylindrical canal through which passes the optic nerve and ophthalmic artery.

The extraocular muscles—four rectus muscles and two obliques—control movement of the eye. Cranial nerve III innervates all but the lateral rectus and the superior oblique muscles, which are innervated by cranial nerves VI and IV, respectively. The rectus muscles originate at the annulus of Zinn and insert on the globe, forming a muscle cone, which is the central anatomic space in the orbit.

The lacrimal system comprises secretory and drainage systems. Secretory glands (the glands of Moll, Kraus, and Wolfring) may be found along the margin of the eyelid. The lacrimal gland, with its palpebral and orbital lobes, is located in the superotemporal orbit (▶ Fig. 16.11). The lacrimal drainage system, located in the inferonasal orbit, is represented by the puncta, canaliculi, lacrimal sac,

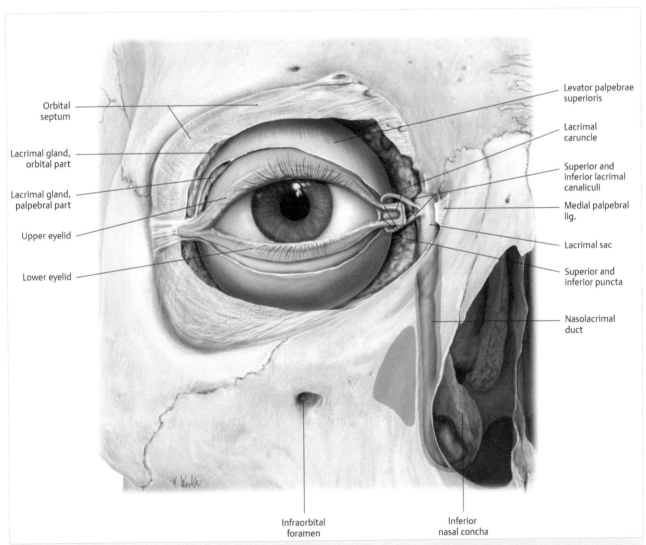

Fig. 16.11 Anatomy of the lacrimal system. (Reproduced from Gilroy AM et al, Atlas of Anatomy, 3rd ed., 2016; based on Schuenke M, Schulte E, Schumacher U, Thieme Atlas of Anatomy: Head, Neck, and Neuroanatomy, illustrations by Voll M and Wesker K, 2nd ed., New York: Thieme Medical Publishers; 2016.)

and nasolacrimal duct. Tumor involvement of the lacrimal system may present with epiphora.

The skin of the eyelid is continuous with the palpebral and bulbar conjunctivae, which are, in turn, contiguous with the globe. Each of these epithelial surfaces represents a potential site of origin for cancer.

16.3 Regional Pathology and Differential Diagnosis

16.3.1 Tumors of the Nasal Cavity and Paranasal Sinuses

The mucosal lining of the nose—*the Schneiderian membrane*—is derived from ectoderm. This is uniquely different from the mucosa of the rest of the upper respiratory tract, which is derived from endoderm. Olfactory neuroepithelium lines the superior portion of the nasal cavity and the roof of the nose and gives rise to neuroectodermal tumors, such as olfactory neuroblastoma and neuroendocrine carcinoma.[2,3,4] The sinonasal epithelium also has minor salivary glands and gives rise to salivary gland tumors, such as adenoid cystic carcinoma and mucoepidermoid carcinoma.[5,6,7,8] However, the most common epithelial neoplasms of the sinonasal tract are those arising from "metaplastic" squamous epithelium, namely squamous cell carcinoma, and those originating from the seromucinous glands of the mucosal lining, collectively known as adenocarcinomas.[9] The unique histology of this region is reflected in the histogenesis of a complex variety of epithelial and non-epithelial tumors (▶ Table 16.1). These tumors have a wide range of biologic behavior, and a few arise only in the sinonasal tract (e.g., inverted papilloma, olfactory neuroblastoma). Non-epithelial tumors are similar to those in other regions in the head and neck. The details of some of these tumors, such as squamous and non-squamous carcinoma, melanoma, esthesioneuroblastoma, sarcomas, and angiofibromas and fibro-osseous lesion, are discussed in more detail in other chapters in Section III of the book.

Overall, sinonasal cancer accounts for about 1% of all malignancies and approximately 3% of cancers of the head and neck. It shows a male predominance (▶ Fig. 16.12a) and a strong predilection for Caucasians (▶ Fig. 16.12b). The majority of patients are older than 50 years at the time of diagnosis (▶ Fig. 16.12c). The most common malignant tumor of the nasal cavity and paranasal sinuses is squamous cell carcinoma (▶ Fig. 16.12d). Although the maxillary antrum is the most commonly involved sinus (▶ Fig. 16.12e), anterior skull base invasion is most frequently encountered with malignant neoplasms of the nasal cavity and ethmoid sinus. Upward extension of these neoplasms toward the cribriform plate or fovea ethmoidalis is not uncommon, and it heralds intracranial extension.[10] Primary carcinoma of the frontal sinus is uncommon, and those arising in the sphenoid sinus are rare.[11] Unfortunately, despite significant improvement in diagnostic techniques such as nasal endoscopy and high-resolution imaging, most patients present with advanced-stage disease (▶ Fig. 16.12f).

16.3.2 Tumors of the Orbit

The majority of malignant tumors involving the orbit represent direct extension of tumors of the sinonasal tract. Cancers arising

Table 16.1 Tumors of the sinonasal tract

Benign
- Epithelial
  - Papilloma
  - Adenoma
  - Dermoid
- Non-epithelial
  - Fibroma
  - Chondroma
  - Osteoma
  - Neurofibroma
  - Hemangioma
  - Lymphangioma
  - Nasal glioma

Intermediate
- Schneiderian papilloma
  - Inverted
  - Papillary
  - Cylindrical
- Angiofibroma
- Ameloblastoma
- Fibrous dysplasia
- Ossifying fibroma
- Giant cell tumor

Malignant
- Epithelial
  - Squamous cell carcinoma
    - Differentiated (well, moderately, poorly)
    - Basaloid squamous
    - Adenosquamous
  - Nonsquamous cell carcinoma
    - Adenoid cystic carcinoma
    - Mucoepidermoid carcinoma
    - Adenocarcinoma
    - Neuroendocrine carcinoma
    - Hyalinizing clear cell carcinoma
  - Melanoma
  - Olfactory neuroblastoma
  - Sinonasal undifferentiated carcinoma (SNUC)
- Non-epithelial
  - Chordoma
  - Chondrosarcoma
  - Osteogenic sarcoma
  - Soft tissue sarcoma
    - Fibrosarcoma
    - Malignant fibrous histiocytoma
    - Hemangiopericytoma
    - Angiosarcoma
    - Kaposi's sarcoma
    - Rhabdomyosarcoma
  - Lymphoproliferative
    - Lymphoma
    - Polymorphic reticulosis
    - Plasmacytoma
- Metastatic

Source: Data from Hanna EY, et al, Cancer of the nasal cavity, paranasal sinuses, and orbit, in: Myers EN, ed., Cancer of the Head and Neck, 4th ed., Philadelphia: Saunders; 2003:155–206.

primarily within the orbit are less common and may be classified broadly into pediatric and adult groups. Further subclassification may be according to site of origin or histologic type or both.

The most common intraocular tumor seen in children is *retinoblastoma*, which usually presents by age 3. Other common tumors in the orbit in children include rhabdomyosarcoma, neuroblastoma, lymphoma, and leukemia. *Rhabdomyosarcoma*

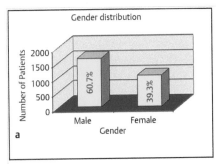
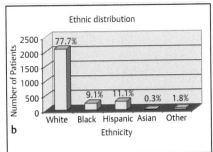
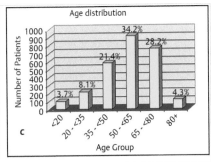
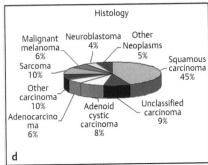
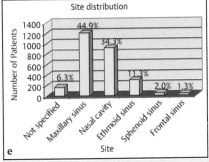
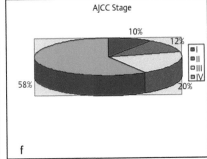

Fig. 16.12 **(a–f)** Patients who have sinonasal cancer, seen at the Department of Head and Neck Surgery of MD Anderson Cancer Center between 1944 and April 2007 (N = 2,698 patients).

is the most common primary and *neuroblastoma* the most common metastatic cancer to the orbit in children. *Granulocytic sarcoma* as a primary orbital neoplasm may precede or follow systemic leukemia. Primarily found in children with myelogenous leukemia, this tumor rarely occurs in adults.[12]

In adults, approximately 65% of orbital tumors are malignant. The most common benign tumors are vascular malformations and pleomorphic adenoma of the lacrimal gland. Malignant tumors of the *lacrimal gland* are most commonly lymphomas or tumors of salivary gland origin. Overall, lymphoma is the most common tumor of the orbit in adults. The main differential diagnoses are lymphoid hyperplasia and orbital pseudotumor. Malignant salivary gland tumors of the lacrimal gland include adenoid cystic carcinoma, malignant mixed cell tumor, and mucoepidermoid carcinoma. Neoplasms of the *lacrimal sac* include squamous cell carcinoma, adenocarcinoma, transitional cell carcinoma, salivary gland carcinoma, and poorly differentiated carcinoma. Cancer of the skin of the *lid* includes basal cell carcinoma, squamous cell carcinoma, sebaceous cell carcinoma, and malignant melanoma, any of which may invade the orbit. Tumors arising from the *conjunctiva* may also invade the orbit, including malignant melanoma, squamous carcinoma, and lymphoma. Choroidal melanoma is the most common *intraocular* malignancy and is biologically distinct from conjunctival or cutaneous melanoma.[12]

Primary *intraorbital* malignancies in adults are rare. Malignant neurogenic tumors of the orbit are uncommon, but those of peripheral nerve sheath origin predominate. They most commonly represent malignant degeneration in patients who have multiple benign neurofibromatosis. Other sarcomas that infrequently arise within the orbit include osteosarcoma, chondrosarcoma, malignant fibrous histiocytoma, hemangiopericytoma, and liposarcoma. Multiple myeloma may present in the orbit as a solitary plasmacytoma, or the orbit may be involved as part of

disseminated disease. Hematogenous *metastasis* to the orbit most commonly originates from a primary in the lung or prostate in males. In females, carcinoma of the breast is the most common source of metastasis to the orbit.[12]

16.4 Clinical Assessment

Clinical evaluation of patients who have cancer of the nasal cavity, paranasal sinuses, and orbit should help achieve three objectives: (1) establishment of the diagnosis, (2) determination of the extent and stage of disease, and (3) development of a plan for treatment. These objectives are usually achieved through a detailed history, comprehensive clinical examination of the head and neck, imaging, and biopsy.

16.4.1 History and Clinical Examination

The signs and symptoms of *early* sinonasal tumors are very subtle and nonspecific. Early lesions are often completely asymptomatic or mimic more common benign conditions, such as chronic sinusitis, allergy, or nasal polyposis. Because early detection of sinonasal tumors is probably the most important factor in improving prognosis, a high degree of suspicion is necessary to diagnose smaller lesions. Common symptoms include nasal obstruction, "sinus pressure" or pain, nasal discharge that may be bloody, anosmia, or epistaxis. Failure of these symptoms to respond to adequate medical therapy or the presence of unilateral signs and symptoms should alert the physician to the possibility of malignancy and warrants further investigation using high-resolution imaging. Comprehensive examination of the nasal cavity should be done after topical decongestion and anesthesia using rigid or flexible endoscopy (▶ Fig. 16.13; **Video 16.1** and **Video 16.2**).

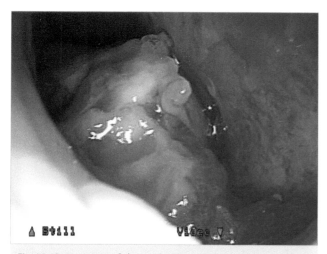

Fig. 16.13 Carcinoma of the nasal cavity: endoscopic view showing a tumor arising from the floor of the right nasal cavity. Biopsy revealed squamous cell carcinoma.

The presence of intranasal masses, ulcers, or areas of contact bleeding may indicate a malignant tumor. Although unilateral "polyps" may be inflammatory, they are more commonly neoplastic. Tumors may also present as submucosal masses without changes in the mucosa other than displacement. Any suspicious lesions should be biopsied, preferably after high-resolution imaging has been obtained to avoid severe bleeding and/or CSF leak, as discussed hereafter.

Extension of sinonasal tumors to adjacent structures renders the diagnosis obvious but is a late manifestation of the disease. Soft tissue swelling of the face may indicate tumor extension through the anterior bony confines of the nose and sinuses (▶ Fig. 16.14).

Inferior extension toward the oral cavity may present with an ulcer or a submucosal mass in the palate or the alveolar ridge (▶ Fig. 16.15). Middle ear effusion may indicate tumor involvement of the nasopharynx, Eustachian tube, pterygoid plates, or tensor veli palatini muscle. Extension to the skull base may lead to involvement of the cranial nerves, causing anosmia, blurred vision, diplopia, or hypoesthesia along the

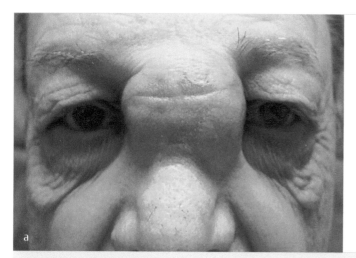
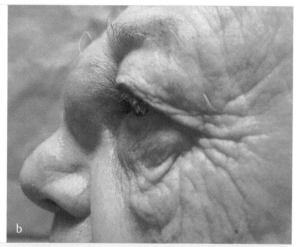

Fig. 16.14 (a, b) Advanced ethmoid carcinoma, with clinical photographs showing the mass centered on the nasion and causing widening of the interpalpebral distance (telecanthus). The mass shows involvement of the overlying skin and destruction of the underlying nasal bone.

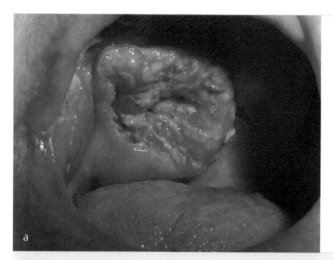
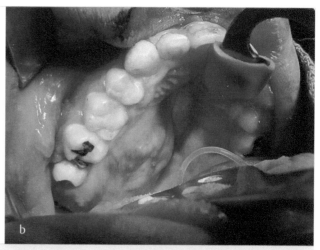

Fig. 16.15 (a, b) Carcinoma of the maxillary sinus may extend inferiorly and destroy the palate, presenting as **(a)** an ulcer or **(b)** a submucosal mass.

branches of the trigeminal nerves. The presence of associated neck masses usually represents metastatic disease in the cervical lymph nodes.

Orbital involvement is common in patients who have cancer arising from the ethmoid, maxillary sinuses, frontal, or sphenoid sinuses, in descending order of frequency. Less commonly, the orbit is involved with a primary tumor of the eye or its adnexa. Signs and symptoms of tumors in the orbit are usually due to mass effect or neuromuscular dysfunction. The patient may complain of proptosis, irregular shape of the eyelid, or blepharoptosis. Epiphora usually indicates involvement of the nasolacrimal duct (▶ Fig. 16.11). Double vision may result from compression or infiltration of ocular nerves or muscles. Visual loss secondary to optic nerve involvement is usually a late sign, although more subtle signs of optic nerve dysfunction are more frequently encountered, among them afferent pupillary defect, loss of color vision, and visual field defect. Finally, orbital involvement may be asymptomatic and is discovered only on CT or MRI evaluation of patients who have sinonasal complaints.

Evaluation of patients who have suspected primary or secondary malignancy in the orbit should include a *detailed neuro-ophthalmologic examination*. This usually includes detailed assessment of visual acuity, visual fields, and ocular motility. Other ophthalmologic evaluation includes careful pupillary examination for afferent pupillary defect or anisocoria as well as external examination, including Hertel's exophthalmometry and marginal reflex distance as an indicator of eyelid position. Slit lamp examination of the conjunctivae, cornea, anterior chamber, and lens is appropriate. Finally, detailed examination of the fundus may reveal compressive effect, intraocular malignancy, or an unrelated reason for visual loss. Formal testing of color vision and automated visual fields are commonly appropriate.

16.5 Imaging

16.5.1 Indications

Imaging of the nasal cavity, paranasal sinuses, and orbit is indicated whenever there is clinical suspicion of a neoplastic process. Imaging is also indicated for obtaining pretreatment information regarding the location, size, extent, and invasiveness of the primary tumor, as well as the presence of regional and distant metastasis. Such information is crucial in deciding on therapeutic options and for proper preoperative planning of the optimal surgical approach. Imaging also plays an important role in posttreatment follow-up, indicating areas of residual or recurrent disease and defining suspicious areas for biopsy.

16.5.2 Imaging Modalities

Both CT and MRI may be needed for optimal radiologic assessment of sinonasal malignancy, particularly in assessing the cranial base, orbit, and pterygopalatine and infratemporal fossae. Coronal images best delineate involvement of the orbital walls and invasion of the skull base, particularly the cribriform plate. Axial images are particularly helpful in demonstrating tumor extension through the posterior wall of the maxillary sinus into the pterygopalatine fossa and infratemporal fossae. Sagittal images are particularly helpful in evaluating extension along the cribriform plate, planum sphenoidale, and clivus (▶ Fig. 16.16). The main advantage of *CT scans* is in delineating the architecture of the bones, especially in "bone windows."

The addition of contrast enhancement increases tumor definition from adjacent soft tissue, especially intracranially. Bone destruction and soft tissue invasion suggest an aggressive lesion, usually a malignant neoplasm. Widening or sclerosis of the foramina of the infraorbital, vidian, mandibular, or maxillary nerves may indicate perineural spread (▶ Fig. 16.17).

MRI is unsurpassed in delineating soft tissue detail, both intra- and extracranially (▶ Fig. 16.16). Obliteration of fat planes in the pterygopalatine fossa, infratemporal fossa, and nasopharynx usually indicates tumor transgression along these boundaries. Dural thickening or enhancement is usually an indication of tumor involvement, and evaluation of critical structures such as the brain and carotid artery is best delineated by MRI. Similarly, enhancement or thickening of cranial nerves indicates perineural spread, which is better detected on MRI than on CT (▶ Fig. 16.17).[13] Perhaps one of the most significant advantages of MRI is the ability to distinguish tumor from retained secretions secondary to obstruction of sinus drainage (▶ Fig. 16.18).

MRI is also particularly helpful in monitoring patients during the postoperative follow-up period, although this role may be supplanted in the near future by PET scans because of their ability to distinguish between tumor recurrence and posttreatment fibrosis. *PET-CT* is also helpful in delineating regional and distant metastasis (▶ Fig. 16.19).

Angiography is not indicated in the routine assessment of patients who have neoplasms of the nose, paranasal sinuses, and orbit. In certain selected cases, however, angiography may be necessary. These cases include vascular neoplasms of the sinonasal region, in which angiography not only delineates tumor's extent and blood supply but also permit the use of selective embolization of the vascular supply to the tumor (▶ Fig. 16.20). This reduces intraoperative blood loss, facilitating surgical resection.

16.6 Biopsy

16.6.1 Nasal Cavity and Paranasal Sinuses

The definitive diagnosis of a neoplasm of the nasal cavity and paranasal sinuses relies on expert histopathologic review of any biopsy specimens by a head and neck pathologist to confirm the exact diagnosis prior to treatment. This is critical, for the treatment and prognosis of sinonasal cancer is greatly influenced by histology.[14]

The vast majority of sinonasal neoplasms are accessible for biopsy through a strictly endonasal approach. A wide variety of rigid nasal endoscopes offer superb visualization of intranasal lesions with a high degree of optical resolution and bright illumination (▶ Fig. 16.13). The application of topical anesthetics and decongestants improves visualization and allows thorough examination of the nasal cavity. The site of origin of the lesion and its relation to the nasal walls (septum, floor, roof, and lateral nasal wall) should be noted. An adequate specimen should be

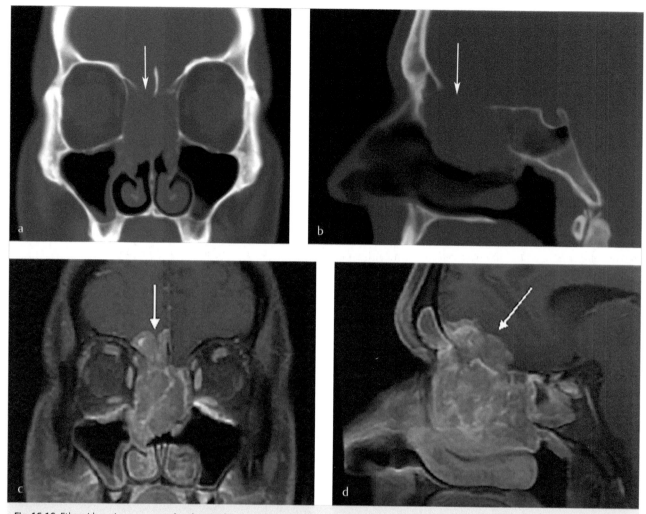

Fig. 16.16 Ethmoid carcinoma: coronal and sagittal images showing **(a, b)** bony destruction on CT scan and **(c, d)** intracranial invasion on T1-MRI with contrast.

obtained, avoiding crushing of tissue, and should be submitted for histopathologic examination. If a diagnosis of lymphoma is suspected, fresh tissue should be sent in saline rather than fixed in formalin. Most endonasal biopsies can be performed in the outpatient setting with minimal discomfort to the patient. In certain cases, the diagnosis of a highly vascular neoplasm, such as angiofibroma, may be suspected on clinical grounds. Under these circumstances, it is prudent not to perform the biopsy until imaging and angiography (possibly with embolization) are performed (▶ Fig. 16.20). Preoperative biopsy can then be performed in the operating room under controlled conditions to confirm the diagnosis before surgical resection. If a nasal mass is suspected to have an intracranial communication such as an encephalocele, meningocele, or nasal glioma, this should be confirmed with imaging so as to avoid inadvertent CSF leak and subsequent meningitis (▶ Fig. 16.21).

16.6.2 Orbit

In most cases of primary intraorbital tumors, the approach used to obtain a biopsy is dictated by the location of the tumor. Lesions in the superior orbit may be addressed by a coronal flap or through a brow incision (modified Kronlein or Stallard-Wright incision). Lateral orbital lesions may require removal of the orbital rim. The transconjunctival approach, with detachment of the lateral canthal tendon, provides access to the orbital floor. The medial orbit may be entered through a modified Lynch-type or transcaruncular incision. Lesions within the muscle cone may be addressed by elevating conjunctiva and Tenon's capsule from the globe and detaching the necessary rectus muscle. Lacrimal gland lesions are best approached through the upper lid crease.[1]

16.7 Preoperative Preparation

A thorough preoperative assessment should determine the candidacy of a patient for surgical management of his or her neoplasm. This involves a careful "mapping" of the tumor's extent as well as of the patient's general medical condition and functional status, usually accomplished by a detailed history and physical examination and a comprehensive examination of the head and neck region, including through endoscopy of the sinonasal region. Cranial nerve examination and ophthalmologic evaluation should be done to evaluate cranial base and orbital

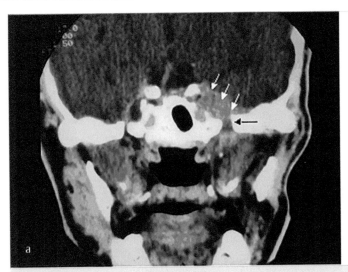
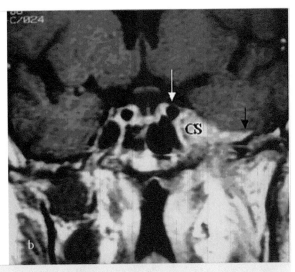

Fig. 16.17 Perineural spread of adenoid cystic carcinoma along the third division of the trigeminal nerve (V3). **(a)** A coronal CT with IV contrast showing widening of the left foramen ovale (*black arrow*) compared with the right. There is also enhancement and thickening along the left Meckel's cave (*white arrows*). **(b)** A coronal T1-weighted MRI with gadolinium showing marked thickening and enhancement of V3, trigeminal ganglion, and lateral cavernous sinus (CS). The tumor abuts the cavernous carotid artery (*white arrow*). There is enhancement of the dura along the floor of the middle cranial fossa (*black arrow*). This "dural tail" is usually a sign of dural involvement with tumor.

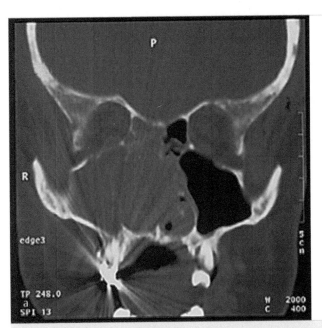
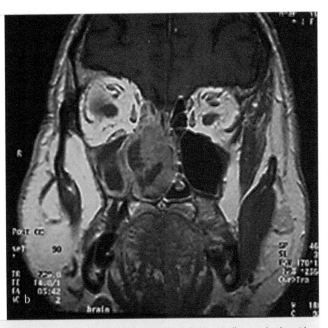

Fig. 16.18 Sinonasal melanoma. **(a)** Coronal CT scan demonstrating opacification of the right nasal cavity as well as of the maxillary and ethmoid sinuses. There appears to be destruction of the lateral nasal wall and the nasal septum. The lesion abuts the orbital floor and the cribriform plate, but whether these structures are involved is unclear. **(b)** Coronal T1-weighted MRI with gadolinium of the same patient, revealing that the lesion is limited to the nasal cavity and ethmoid sinuses and that the changes in the maxillary sinuses are due to retained secretions secondary to obstruction of the ostium rather than soft tissue involvement. It also demonstrates that the lesion does not invade the orbit or the cranial base. The presence of low-signal areas within the lesion gives it a heterogeneous appearance characteristic of sinonasal melanoma.

extension, respectively. High-resolution imaging should be obtained using CT or MRI, or both, to accurately assess the tumor extent. In certain cases, angiography will be needed to determine the extent of carotid arterial involvement. The balloon occlusion test should be performed if carotid artery resection or reconstruction is contemplated. Preoperative embolization may be indicated in certain vascular tumors.

Neurosurgical consultation is needed if a combined craniofacial approach is anticipated. If free vascularized flaps will be used for reconstruction, expertise with microvascular surgery is needed, and appropriate consultation should be obtained. Evaluation by a maxillofacial prosthodontist is required in most patients to obtain preoperative dental impressions and design surgical obturators or splints for maintenance of proper dental

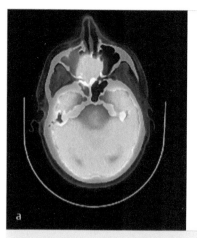
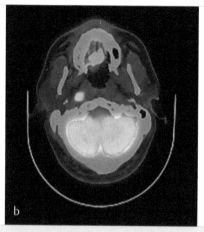
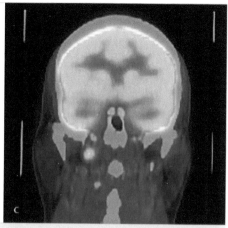

Fig. 16.19 PET-CT of head and neck: images from the same patient whose CT and MRI are depicted in Fig. 16.16. The fused PET-CT images show ethmoid carcinoma (a) with metastasis to the retropharyngeal lymph nodes, (b, c) not detected on CT or MRI.

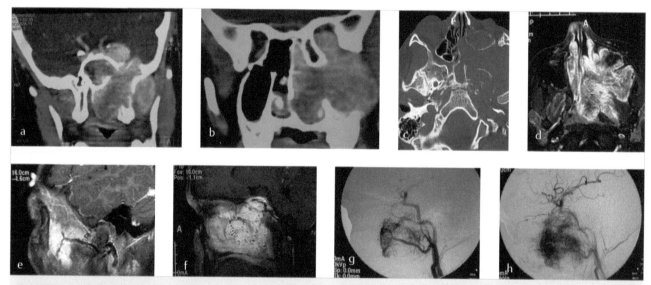

Fig. 16.20 Juvenile nasopharyngeal angiofibroma. (a, b) Coronal and (c) axial CT with contrast and (d) axial T1–axial MRI with contrast showing the mass in the nasal cavity, maxillary sinus, nasopharynx, sphenoid sinus, pterygoid plates, and pterygopalatine and infratemporal fossa. The mass involves the floor of the middle cranial fossa and extends intracranially to the cavernous sinus. T1–sagittal MRI shows flow voids of increased extensive vascular supply coming from the (e) internal maxillary artery and (f) internal carotid artery. (g) Early-phase angiogram showing the blood supply and contribution from the internal maxillary artery and (h) late-phase angiogram showing significant tumor vascular blush and contribution from the internal carotid artery.

occlusion and oral rehabilitation. Similar expertise is essential in cases requiring prosthetic orbital, nasal, or facial rehabilitation. Consultations with ophthalmology should be considered for detailed neuro-ophthalmologic examination of all patients who are known or suspected to have orbital involvement. If orbital exenteration is contemplated, visual function of the contralateral eye should be carefully assessed.

Medical and radiation oncology colleagues should be consulted with a view to considering incorporation of chemotherapy or radiation in the treatment plan. Radiation and/or chemotherapy may be used preoperatively as induction (neoadjuvant) therapy or postoperatively as adjuvant therapy. This is particularly important in patients who have advanced-stage disease (e.g., dural or orbital involvement) or high-grade lesions (e.g., sinonasal undifferentiated carcinoma [SNUC]). In certain cases, chemotherapy or radiation may be a reasonable alternative to surgery, but such decisions are best discussed in the format of a multidisciplinary tumor board. If surgery is chosen as a treatment modality, the plan for the surgical approach, the extent of resection, and reconstructive options should then be formulated, with the resulting plan communicated clearly among the various members of the surgical team, particularly the otolaryngologists–head and neck surgeons, neurosurgeons, and plastic and reconstructive surgeons.

Careful assessment of the patient's general medical condition should be carried out prior to surgery. Preoperative chest radiograph, blood counts, liver and renal function tests, blood sugar and electrolyte levels, coagulation studies, and electrocardiogram (ECG) should be performed routinely. Appropriate consultations from medical colleagues should be obtained to optimize

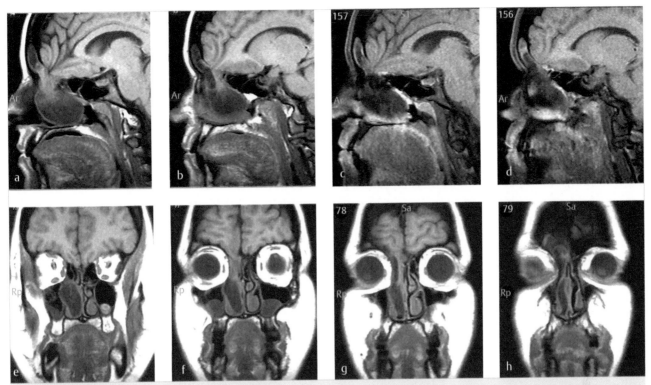

Fig. 16.21 Meningoencephalocele. **(a–d)** Sagittal and **(e–g)** coronal T1-MRI with gadolinium showing a defect in the anterior cranial base at the right fovea ethmoidalis and cribriform plate. There is herniation of a meningoencephalocele, which presented as a nasal mass. Inadvertent biopsy of such lesions may lead to cerebrospinal fluid leaks and should be avoided.

the patient's medical status before surgery and help with management postoperatively. The patient's nutritional status should be evaluated, and enteral or parenteral feeding may be considered if indicated. High-resolution imaging for metastatic work-up is not routinely performed unless indicated by history, clinical examination, chest radiograph results, or blood test abnormalities.

Finally, the surgical team should discuss with the patient and family the nature of the disease, the evaluation, and the indications, risks, possible complications, sequelae, and alternatives for therapy. The expected postoperative course should be described, including length of stay in the hospital, feeding, rehabilitation, and need for adjunctive therapy. This ongoing communication should be maintained in a clear, honest, and sympathetic fashion throughout the course of patient care.

16.8 Surgery

16.8.1 Indications and Contraindications

Surgery is indicated when there is adequate evidence that the tumor can be completely resected with acceptable morbidity. For early-stage disease (T1–T2), surgery alone may be adequate treatment, but for more advanced-stage resectable disease, postoperative adjuvant radiation or chemoradiation is commonly used to improve tumor control.[15] The development of new combined craniofacial approaches has extended the indications of surgery to include some patients who have skull base and even intracranial extension.[16,17] The advent of new reconstructive techniques, including microvascular free flaps, pericranial flaps, and prosthetic rehabilitation, has reduced morbidity and improved rehabilitation after extensive resection of advanced sinonasal cancer.[18,19,20] In the presence of tumor extension to the cavernous sinus, internal carotid artery, or optic chiasm; extensive brain parenchymal involvement; or distant metastasis, surgery is usually contraindicated. However, in selected cases, surgery with proper adjuvant therapy may still offer the most effective local disease palliation even in the presence of extensive disease.

16.8.2 Surgical Principles

When dealing with the subject of surgical treatment of sinonasal cancer, a distinction must be made between the terminology used to describe the surgical approach and the extent of resection. A surgical approach describes the various incisions, soft tissue dissection, and skeletal osteotomies required to expose the tumor and adjacent structures so as to perform a complete and safe resection. By contrast, the extent of tumor resection describes the various structures that must be surgically extirpated to achieve total tumor removal with tumor-free margins. Obviously, both the surgical approach and the extent of resection are closely related and depend on the extent of tumor as well as its aggressiveness and related critical structures. The various surgical approaches and extent of resection are listed in ▶ Table 16.2.[12]

The choice of surgical approach and extent of resection generally depends on the location and extent of the tumor. In some cases, different approaches may be equally effective for resection of a particular tumor. For example, a tumor of the nasal cavity, lateral nasal wall, ethmoid, sphenoid, and medial maxillary sinus that requires a medial maxillectomy and a total sphenoethmoidectomy may be adequately resected using a transfacial, endoscopic, or sublabial approach (▶ Fig. 16.18;

▶ Fig. 16.22). However, the following principles should always guide the surgeon in choosing the optimal approach and extent of resection for all patients undergoing surgical treatment of sinonasal cancer:
- Adequate oncologic resection
- Minimal brain retraction
- Protection of critical neurovascular structures
- Meticulous reconstruction of the skull base
- Optimal esthetic outcome

Table 16.2 Surgical treatment of sinonasal cancers

Surgical approach

Endoscopic

Lateral rhinotomy and Weber-Furgesson

Transoral–transpalatal

Facial "degloving"

Craniofacial

Extent of resection

Ethmoidectomy

Inferior maxillectomy

Medial maxillectomy

Total maxillectomy

Anterior cranial base resection

Infratemporal fossa dissection

Orbital exenteration

16.8.3 Surgical Approach

Endonasal Approaches

Endoscopic endonasal approaches (EEA) are increasingly being used for surgical excision of selected tumors of the sinonasal tract, either alone or in combination with open approaches. Endoscopic surgery avoids craniofacial soft tissue dissection, skeletal disassembly and brain retraction. Other advantages of EEA include direct bilateral access to the tumor; superior illumination, magnification, and visualization of the surgical field (▶ Fig. 16.7); wider angles of vision using angled endoscopes; and relatively less morbidity than with open surgical approaches.

When endoscopic endonasal surgery was first advocated for the treatment of sinonasal malignancies, concerns were raised regarding the oncological soundness of the procedure.[21]

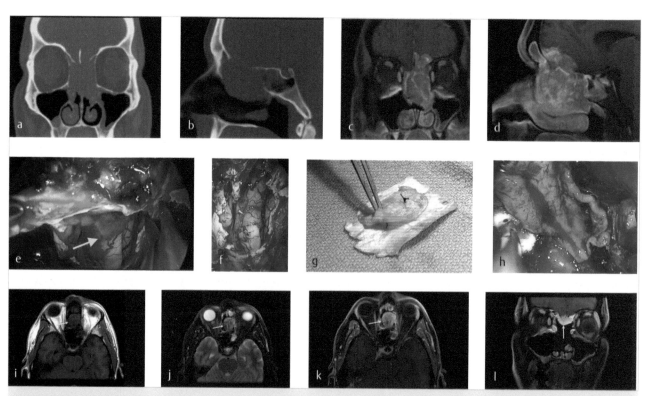

Fig. 16.22 Endoscopic resection of sinonasal tumor. **(a,b)** Preoperative CT and **(c,d)** MRI of a patient who has olfactory neuroblastoma. **(e)** Intraoperative endoscopic view. The dura is opened and the tumor is seen to arise from the olfactory bulb (*arrow*). **(f)** Tumor resection is complete, and the dural defect is shown. **(g)** Multilayer graft reconstruction. Fascia lata graft is harvested. A double layer is created, with the smaller one to be placed intradurally and the larger to be placed extradurally but underneath the bony defect of the skull base (intracranially). Both layers are sutured together to stabilize them during placement and obliterate any dead space between them. **(h)** A contralateral vascularized nasoseptal flap based on the posterior septal branch of the sphenopalatine artery is rotated to cover the double layer graft. **(i–l)** Postoperative MRI showing the enhancing nasoseptal flap in place (*arrows*).

Criticisms have centered on the inability of the endoscopic approach to perform an en bloc resection. Proponents of the endoscopic technique argue that unless the tumor is small, en bloc resection is rarely achievable using open surgery.[22,23] Several studies have shown that the method of resection (en bloc vs. piecemeal) does not significantly impact oncological outcomes, as well as that achieving negative resection margins is paramount regardless of the surgical approach.[24,25]

Over the past decade, increasing evidence has come to light regarding the safety and oncological effectiveness of these techniques. Several institutions have reported their experience with endoscopic surgery and have shown reduced morbidity, shorter hospital stay, better quality of life, and equivalent survival outcomes to those of open surgery in carefully selected patients.[26]

The keys to achieving adequate oncologic results using EEA are good selection of patients and the surgeon's experience using this approach. EEA are most suited for central tumors involving the nasal septum, nasal cavity and lateral nasal wall, ethmoid and sphenoid sinuses, and clivus (▶ Fig. 16.22a,b). Tumors with extension into the facial soft tissue, involvement of the anterior wall of the frontal sinus, deep orbital invasion, lateral supraorbital extension, or significant brain parenchymal invasion are not readily accessible using EEA and require the addition of an open approach.

The surgical technique of EEA to the sinonasal region and the anterior skull base has been described in detail.[23] The standard endoscopic endonasal "craniofacial" resection starts with debulking of the intranasal tumor, identifying the attachment of tumor origin and resection of the sinonasal component. A posterior septectomy provides a binasal approach for the surgeon and the assistant, allowing a four-hand technique for dissection. If not involved with tumor, a vascularized nasal septal flap is developed contralaterally based on the posterior septal branch of the sphenopalatine artery. In some cases when the tumor does not involve the septum, this flap can be developed ipsilaterally or bilaterally. A complete anterior and posterior ethmoidectomy are then performed, and the sphenoid sinuses are opened bilaterally. The bony skull base is skeletonized bilaterally from the frontal sinus anteriorly to the planum sphenoidale posteriorly. The medial orbital walls are also skeletonized bilaterally, delineating the lateral extent of the surgical corridor. After control of vascular supply from the anterior and posterior ethmoid arteries, the lamina papyracea, fovea ethmoidalis, cribriform plate, crista galli, and planum sphenoidale can be removed using a high-speed diamond drill, using copious irrigation to avoid heat injury to critical neural structures. After removal of the bone of the anterior central skull base, the dura, olfactory bulbs and tracts, and periorbita can be resected depending on the extent of tumor involvement (▶ Fig. 16.22c,d).

Reconstruction of the skull base in the early stages of EEA's development was a major challenge but has significantly evolved over the past decade. Early reconstructive experience was associated with CSF leak rates of 20 to 30% for EEA of the anterior skull base.[27,28] Multilayer reconstruction of the dural defect using fascia lata is performed with one layer intradurally and a second layer extradurally (▶ Fig. 16.22e). The application of a nasoseptal flap placed extradurally has lowered leak rates to 5% (▶ Fig. 16.22f,g).[29] When there is tumor involvement of the superior nasal septum, the "extended nasoseptal flap" can be harvested from the lower septum and extended onto the floor and lateral wall of the nasal cavity.[30] Other vascularized reconstructive alternatives for the anterior skull base include minimally invasive pericranial flap,[31] the middle turbinate flap for small defects, and the transpterygoid temporoparietal fascia flap.[32,33] The inferior turbinate flap, though robust, has limited reach and is best suited to clival defects.[34] Other flaps described in the literature, such as the palatal flap,[35] the buccinator myomucosal flap,[36] and the occipital galeopericranial flap,[37] may be considered.

Some investigators have achieved favorable results using non-vascularized reconstructive options. Gil et al described a double-layered tensor fascia lata repair that had a CSF leak rate of 0.8%.[38] Histological examination of resected fascia lata in patients who received a second operation shows evidence of neovascularization of the fibrous tissue, even without the presence of a vascularized flap. Villaret et al proposed a three-layer reconstruction using the iliotibial tract[39] and reported postoperative CSF leak rates of around 4%. When the skull base and dural defect are too large for purely endoscopic reconstruction, an open approach may provide the safest way to achieve reliable cranionasal separation and avoid CSF leak and the risk of meningitis.[40,41]

The limitations of EEA include lack of binocular vision and depth perception, which is important when dealing with critical neurovascular structures. Ergonomic limitations include the inability of the primary surgeon to control the endoscope and two instruments simultaneously, hence the reliance on a surgical assistant for camera control during two-handed surgery. The major limitation of EEA is the inability to repair or patch dural defects using suture techniques, which limits reconstructive options after endoscopic resection of intradural tumors. We continue to explore novel applications in robotic endoscopic skull base surgery with a view to overcoming some of these limitations (▶ Fig. 16.23; Video 16.3).[42,43,44,45] The oncologic outcomes of EEA in the treatment of sinonasal cancers are discussed at the end of this chapter, in the section on outcomes and prognosis.

Transfacial Approaches: Lateral Rhinotomy and Weber-Fergusson

Transfacial approaches are the most commonly used surgical approaches for resection of locally advanced sinonasal tumors. They allow adequate exposure of the nasal cavity, maxillary sinus, pterygopalatine fossa, pterygoid plates, ethmoid sinuses, medial and inferior orbital walls, sphenoid sinus, nasopharynx, clivus, and medial aspect of the infratemporal fossa.

The *lateral rhinotomy* is the standard incision for exposure of sinonasal tumors through a transfacial approach (▶ Fig. 16.24). It can be used alone, or various extensions of the basic incision may be added for further exposure depending on the extent of tumor.[12] The *Weber-Fergusson* incision adds a lip-splitting and subciliary incision for added exposure of the maxillary bone. We prefer to extend the lateral rhinotomy toward the medial brow, using a Lynch-type extension, and avoid the subciliary incision of the classic Weber-Fergusson so as to minimize eye lid complications, as discussed further under the section on total maxillectomy.

The basic lateral rhinotomy incision provides adequate exposure when performing a medial maxillectomy. Elevation of the soft tissues of the cheek is done in a subperiosteal plane over the

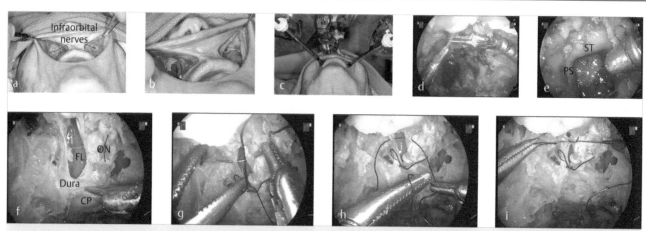

Fig. 16.23 Robotic-assisted endoscopic surgery of the anterior skull base (cadaveric dissection). **(a)** Soft tissue approach: bilateral sublabial incisions and soft tissue flap elevation. **(b)** Bilateral anterior maxillary antrostomies. **(c)** Robotic ports placement. The camera port is placed into the right nostril and the right and left surgical arm ports through the respective anterior, then middle antrostomies. **(d)** Bimanual sharp dissection of the mucosa covering the fovea ethmoidalis and cribriform plate. **(e)** Wide sphenoidotomy with excellent access to the sella turcica (ST) and parasellar region (PS). **(f)** The cribriform plate (CP) is removed bilaterally, and the cut edges of the olfactory nerves (ON) are shown. The dura is incised or resected to expose the inferior surface of the frontal lobes (FL) intracranially. **(g–i)** Dural repair: suturing the dural edges, making a loop, and tightening the knot. (Reproduced with permission from Hanna EY, Holsinger C, DeMonte F, Kupferman M, Robotic endoscopic surgery of the skull base: a novel surgical approach, *Arch Otolaryngol Head Neck Surg*, 2007;133(12):1209–1214.)

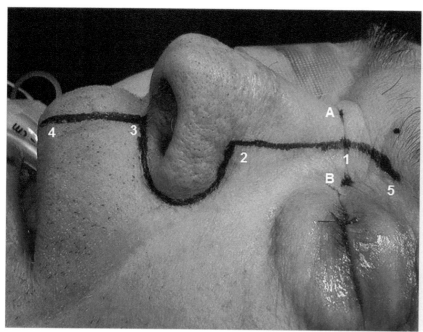

Fig. 16.24 (1,2,3) Lateral rhinotomy incision and **(4,5)** its extensions. A temporary tarsorrhaphy protects the ipsilateral globe. The basic lateral rhinotomy incision is outlined by connecting three surface points. **(1)** The first point is marked halfway between **(A)** the nasion and **(B)** the medial canthus. **(2)** The second point is where the alar crease begins, and **(3)** the third point is at the base of the columella. The basic incision provides adequate exposure for a medial maxillectomy. The basic incision may be extended to include **(4)** a lip-splitting extension or **(5)** a Lynch-type extension if further exposure is necessary. The extended incision provides adequate exposure for a total maxillectomy.

maxilla and around the inferior orbital nerve (▶ Fig. 16.25a). The attachment of the medial canthal tendon to the nasal bone is released. The periorbita is elevated over the medial orbital wall, exposing the lacrimal crest, the lamina papyracea, and the frontoethmoidal suture. This suture serves as a landmark for the position of the floor of the anterior cranial fossa and when followed posteriorly leads to the anterior and posterior ethmoidal foramina.

The anterior and posterior ethmoidal arteries are cauterized with bipolar electrocautery, clipped or ligated, and transected (▶ Fig. 16.25b). The optic nerve is located 4 to 5 mm posterior to the posterior ethmoidal artery. The orbital floor should be dissected as far lateral as the inferior orbital fissure. The lacrimal sac

is identified in its fossa between the anterior and posterior lacrimal crests. If a medial maxillectomy is performed, the lacrimal sac is elevated from the fossa, the lacrimal duct transected, and the sac marsupialized into the nasal cavity to provide adequate drainage of the lacrimal system and to prevent stenosis (▶ Fig. 16.25c).

Midfacial Degloving and Sublabial Approaches

The midfacial degloving approach is most commonly used in the management of large benign lesions of the sinonasal region and skull base, such as juvenile nasopharyngeal angiofibroma;

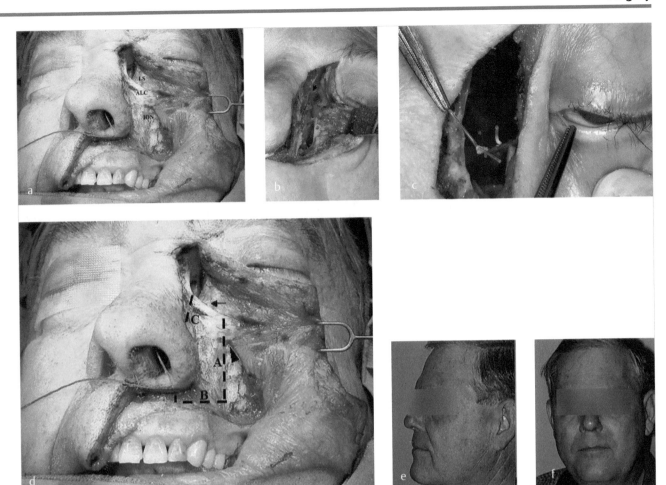

Fig. 16.25 Lateral rhinotomy and medial maxillectomy. **(a)** Elevation of the soft tissues of the cheek is done in a subperiosteal plane over the maxilla, as well as around the inferior orbital nerve (ION). The periorbita is elevated over the anterior lacrimal crest (ACL) to expose the lacrimal sac (LS). **(b)** Dissection of the medial periorbita over the lamina papyracea reveals the anterior ethmoid artery (*arrow*) at the level of the frontoethmoid suture line, which marks the level of the anterior cranial floor. The artery is coagulated by bipolar electrocautery, clipped or ligated, then transected. **(c)** After the lacrimal sac is transected, it is marsupialized into the surgical cavity as a dacryocystorhinostomy. Silicone stents are placed through the upper and lower canaliculi and brought into the nasal cavity to prevent postoperative epiphora. These stents are removed in about 3 to 6 months. **(d)** Medial maxillectomy. Osteotomies: **(A)** vertically medial to the infraorbital foramen (*arrowhead*), **(B)** horizontally above the level of dental roots and into the pyriform aperture, and **(C)** obliquely along the nasomaxillary suture line. If the lateral nasal wall is to be resected, then the lacrimal sac (*arrow*) is transected and marsupialized into the nasal cavity. **(e, f)** Postoperative appearance of a lateral rhinotomy incision.

for selected malignancies in the same area; and to afford access to the nasopharynx and infratemporal fossa. The main advantage of the "degloving" approach is that an external facial incision is avoided. Another advantage is providing simultaneous exposure bilaterally to the inferior and medial maxilla (▶ Fig. 16.26)—particularly helpful when approaching tumors with bilateral involvement of the nasal cavity and maxillary sinus. A major disadvantage, however, is the limited superior and posterior exposure, as well as the need for constant retraction of the soft tissue envelope to ensure continued adequate exposure.

The midfacial degloving approach requires a basic level of proficiency and understanding of closed rhinoplasty incisions. It involves a complete transfixion incision of the membranous septum. This is joined endonasally with a bilateral intercartilaginous incision, with soft tissue elevation over the nasal dorsum as far superior as the nasal root. The nasal skeleton is thus "degloved" from overlying soft tissues as far lateral as the pyriform aperture. A gingivobuccal incision extends bilaterally across the midline to both

maxillary tuberosities laterally. Subperiosteal dissection is continued cephalad over the face of both maxillae. The dissection joins the nasal degloving using sharp dissection over the pyriform aperture attachments (▶ Fig. 16.26).

The sublabial approach may also be used to access tumors of the sphenoclival region such as chordoma, particularly if the lesion extends lower than the horizontal plane of the palate, such as to the lower third of the clivus and craniovertebral junction (▶ Fig. 16.27). A Le Fort I osteotomy is done, and the maxilla is displaced inferiorly after posterior osteotomies separate the maxilla from the pterygoid plates. We prefer a combination of unilateral or half a Le Fort I osteotomy with a median or paramedian palatal osteotomy for better displacement of the maxilla inferiorly and laterally. This offers wider exposure, because it avoids the cantilever effect of the posterior maxilla upward, restricting exposure with inferior displacement of the anterior maxillary segment when the bilateral (complete) Le Fort osteotomy is used.

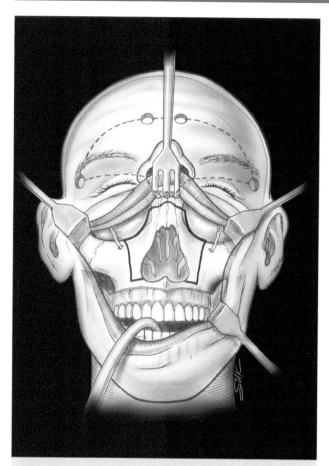

Fig. 16.26 Sublabial "facial degloving" approach. In addition to avoiding facial incisions, the sublabial approach has the advantage of providing bilateral access the medial and inferior maxillary segments.

16.8.4 Extent of Resection

Medial Maxillectomy

The most common indication for medial maxillectomy is in treatment of tumors of the nasal cavity, lateral nasal wall, and medial maxillary sinus (▶ Fig. 16.18). Medial maxillectomy includes removal of the lateral nasal wall as well as of the medial maxillary segment bounded laterally by the infraorbital nerve. In addition, a complete sphenoethmoidectomy is usually performed.

The incision most commonly used for exposure is the lateral rhinotomy (▶ Fig. 16.24). Alternatively, a midfacial degloving, as described later, may be used—and indeed is preferable if bilateral medial maxillectomy is needed (▶ Fig. 16.26). Endonasal endoscopic medial maxillectomy and sphenoethmoidectomy may be also performed for appropriately selected tumors (▶ Fig. 16.22).

If the lateral rhinotomy is performed and soft tissue exposure is completed as discussed in the previous section, *osteotomies* are done as shown in ▶ Fig. 16.25d and the anterior wall of the maxillary sinus above the level of dental roots and medial to the infraorbital nerve is removed. Lateral to the infraorbital foramen, the anterior wall antrostomy may be enlarged to expose the zygomatic recess of the antrum.

Resection of the lateral nasal wall begins with an inferior osteotomy along the nasal floor below the attachment of the inferior turbinate, starting at the pyriform aperture, and carried posteriorly to the posterior maxillary wall. With the orbit retracted laterally and protected by a malleable brain retractor, the lamina papyracea is identified and, if necessary, resected. A complete sphenoethmoidectomy is done, staying below the level of the frontoethmoidal suture to avoid injury to the floor of the anterior cranial fossa. The superior attachment of the middle turbinate is then transected along the roof of the nose. Posteriorly, the lateral nasal wall cuts are connected with right-angled scissors behind the turbinates. The specimen is thus delivered and examined for margins using frozen section control. If the tumor involves the nasal septum, it should be included in the resection specimen by adding appropriate septal cuts to allow for tumor-free margins.

Closure begins by reattachment of the medial canthal tendon to the nasal bone in its anatomic position. Meticulous multilayered closure of the lateral rhinotomy is performed and usually results in excellent healing and acceptable postoperative appearance (▶ Fig. 16.25e). If a sublabial approach is done, the mucosal incisions are closed with absorbable suture. Nonadherent nasal packing may be left for 1 to 2 days.

Inferior Maxillectomy

This procedure involves resection of the inferior maxillary sinus below the plane of the infraorbital nerve. It is most commonly used for neoplasms of the alveolar process of the maxilla having minimal extension to the maxillary antrum. Similarly, lesions of the hard palate sparing the antrum can be treated by an inferior maxillectomy. A combination of sublabial and palatal incisions is usually used for exposure, with osteotomies done around the lesion, ensuring an adequate margin of resection (▶ Fig. 16.28). Alternatively, a midfacial degloving can be used for lesions crossing the midline and involving the inferior maxilla bilaterally.

Total Maxillectomy

If the extent of resection requires a total maxillectomy, then the lateral rhinotomy incision may be extended by adding lip-splitting, gingivobuccal, and palatal incisions inferiorly. The lip-splitting incision, which may be done along the philtrum or in the midline, connects the lateral rhinotomy with the sublabial incision, allowing more lateral elevation of the facial flap. The gingivobuccal incision starts from the lip-splitting incision and extends as far laterally as the region of the first molar and over the lateral surface of the maxillary tuberosity. In patients undergoing total maxillectomy, a median or paramedian palatal incision is performed over the hard palate, extending from an interincisor space anteriorly to the junction of the soft and hard palate posteriorly. The incision then continues laterally between the hard and the soft palate to curve posterolaterally around the maxillary tuberosity, meeting the gingivobuccal incision (▶ Fig. 16.29).

In patients undergoing total maxillectomy with orbital preservation, we prefer to extend the lateral rhinotomy superiorly beneath the medial brow rather than laterally through a subciliary incision used in the classic Weber-Fergusson approach (▶ Fig. 16.29b). We described several advantages to

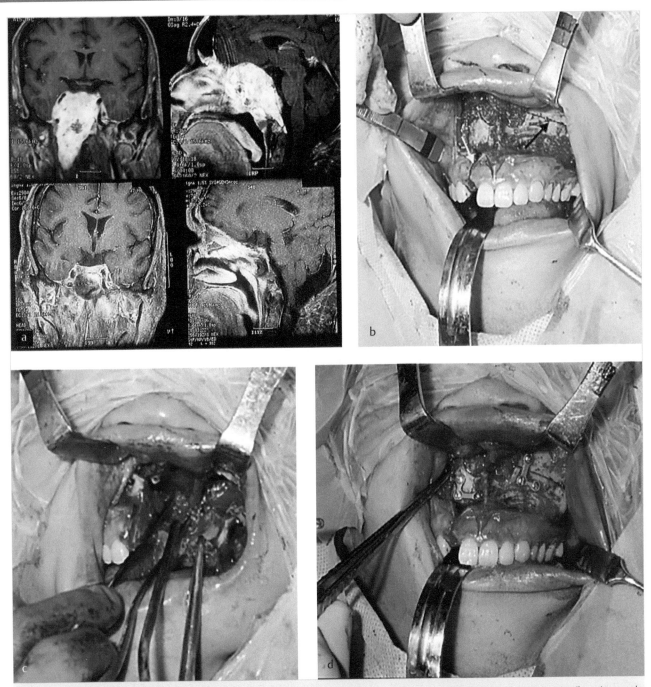

Fig. 16.27 Sublabial approach and inferior maxillotomy for access to sphenoclival region. **(a)** Preoperative (upper) and postoperative (lower) coronal and sagittal MRI of a patient with clival chordoma. **(b)** Le Forte I osteotomy (*black arrow*) is done on one side only and connects the pyriform aperture. A second paramedian palatal osteotomy is performed (*white arrow*). **(c)** Inferior displacement of the maxilla (maxillotomy) to expose the sphenoid sinus, nasopharynx, and clivus. **(d)** Rigid fixation of the maxillary segments using "preregistered" titanium microplates to avoid any malocclusion.

this modification.[46] First, avoiding a subciliary incision eliminates any disruption to the lower lid skin–muscle–tarsus complex, minimizing lower eyelid complications, particularly ectropion and prolonged eyelid edema. Another advantage is avoiding trifurcation of the incision, reducing the risk of skin breakdown at the medial canthal area. This is especially important for previously irradiated patients, who are more prone to develop medial canthal skin dehiscence. Similarly, because the vascularity of the thin lower eyelid skin is not

affected with the extended lateral rhinotomy incision, patients who undergo orbital floor reconstruction with implants such as titanium mesh have less chance to develop wound breakdown and implant exposure. Although the extended lateral rhinotomy incision has several functional and cosmetic advantages, it does not compromise exposure and provides an adequate approach for a safe oncologic resection. The extension of the lateral rhinotomy incision beneath the medial eyebrow shifts the fulcrum of rotation of the soft tissue flap

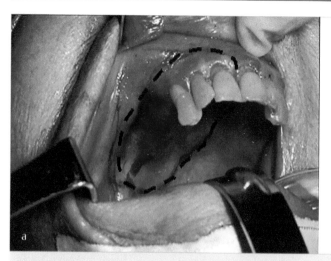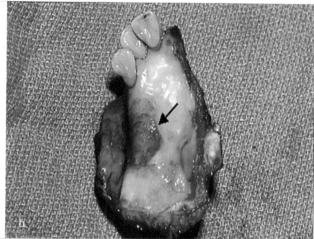

Fig. 16.28 Inferior maxillectomy. (a) Gingivobuccal and palatal incisions and osteotomies are done around the lesion. If there is adequate space between the central incisors, then the osteotomy may be performed using a microreciprocating saw in the interincisor space. Otherwise, the ipsilateral central incisor should be extracted and the osteotomy placed in the tooth socket in order to avoid loss of bony support to the remaining contralateral incisor. (b) Inferior maxillectomy specimen showing adequate surgical margins around an upper alveolar ridge carcinoma (*arrow*).

superiorly and laterally, enhancing lateral exposure, which is not less than that obtained with a classic Weber-Fergusson incision (▶ Fig. 16.29b). Transection of the infraorbital nerve allows even more lateral and posterior elevation of the soft tissues, exposing the entire maxillary bone as far lateral as its zygomatic extension and posteriorly to the pterygomaxillary fissure and over the pterygoid plates. Additionally, its postoperative cosmetic appearance is superior to that achieved using the Weber-Fergusson incision (▶ Fig. 16.25e).

Regardless of the incision used, elevation of the facial flap is usually done in the subperiosteal plane. However, if the tumor has invaded the anterior wall of the maxillary antrum, a supraperiosteal plane is used. Occasionally, the cheek skin overlying the maxilla is included with the specimen if it is involved with tumor. With the globe protected by a temporary tarsorrhaphy stitch, the periorbita is dissected along the medial, inferior, and lateral orbital walls.

Lateral osteotomies are performed along the frontal and temporal processes of the zygoma (▶ Fig. 16.29b). Medial osteotomies are done along the frontal process of the maxilla and along the medial orbital wall just below the frontoethmoidal suture, extending posteriorly to the level of the posterior ethmoidal foramen. The medial and lateral osteotomies are then connected superiorly across the orbital floor along the inferior orbital fissure. Inferiorly, a midline sagittal osteotomy is made across the hard palate. The ipsilateral central incisor should be preserved, if possible, to enhance prosthesis retention. Finally, after the internal maxillary artery is identified at its entrance through the pterygomaxillary fissure, ligated, and transected, a posterior osteotomy is done to disarticulate the maxilla from the pterygoid plates. The maxilla is delivered by anteroinferior traction, and remaining soft tissue attachments are cut using curved heavy scissors. Bleeding, which is usually encountered at this point, is controlled by temporary packing of the cavity, followed by electrocoagulation of bleeding mucosal surfaces or ligature of bleeding points. The pterygoid plexus of veins may be a source of persistent bleeding but can be managed by hemostatic figure-of-eight sutures and Surgicel packing. Bleeding is usually minimized if the internal maxillary artery

is ligated before the posterior osteotomy is done along the pterygomaxillary fissure.

Total maxillectomy usually involves removal of the entire maxillary bone, including the palate and the orbital floor (▶ Fig. 16.29c). Preservation of the orbital floor (subtotal maxillectomy) or the palate (suprastructure maxillectomy) may be possible if these structures are not involved with tumor. Depending on the extent of the lesion, resection may extend beyond the posterior wall to the pterygopalatine fossa and pterygoid plates. Perineural spread of tumor along V2 may be resected by following the nerve through foramen rotundum and into Meckel's cave (▶ Fig. 16.30).[47]

Craniofacial Resection

Surgical resection of the *anterior* cranial base is commonly indicated for patients who have sinonasal tumors involving the cribriform plate or fovea ethmoidalis. This is done, by definition, for most cases of esthesioneuroblastoma as well as for carcinoma of the ethmoid or maxillary sinuses approaching or involving the anterior cranial base (▶ Fig. 16.16). Tumors transgress the cribriform plate either by direct bony invasion or by perineural spread along the filaments of the olfactory nerves. The dura of the anterior cranial fossa forms a barrier that delays, to a certain extent, brain invasion. Dural resection in patients who have intracranial but extradural disease or patients who have limited dural involvement often provides an adequate oncologic margin. However, malignant tumors that transgress the dural barrier and involve the underlying brain parenchyma are usually associated with poor prognosis.[25] However, even in some cases featuring limited frontal lobe involvement, anterior craniofacial resection may still be indicated for local control of the disease.

Resection of the floor of the *middle* cranial fossa is sometimes performed in patients who have sinonasal tumors so as to achieve tumor-free surgical margins for lesions extending to the roof of the infratemporal fossa or for those tumors that exhibit perineural spread along the branches of the trigeminal nerve to the Gasserian ganglion, most commonly adenoid cystic carcinoma.

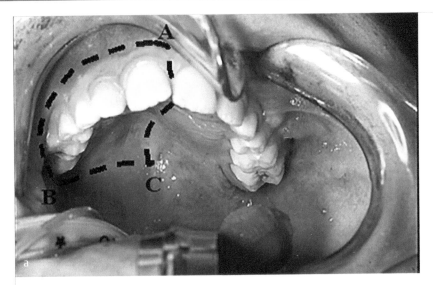
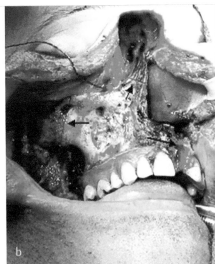
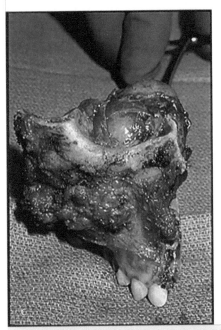
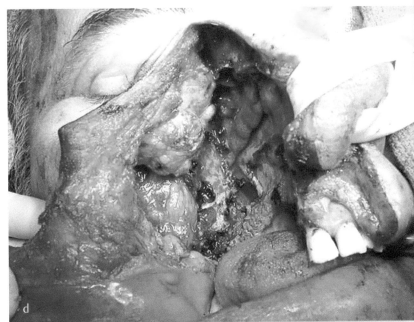

Fig. 16.29 Total maxillectomy. **(a)** Intraoral incisions. **(b)** The exposure offered through an extended lateral rhinotomy shown in this figure is not less than that offered by the Weber-Fergusson incision. The advantage of the former is its ability to avoid subciliary incision and its potential for lower eyelid ectropion and edema. Osteotomies have been performed as indicated by the arrows. **(c)** En bloc resection specimen. Note tumor involvement of the orbital floor, which required resection. Because the tumor did not transgress the periorbita, the eye was preserved. **(d)** Total maxillectomy defect with removal of the orbital floor and periorbita.

Craniofacial approaches combine extra- and intracranial access to the anterior and lateral skull base. Extracranial approaches may include transfacial, sublabial, and endonasal approaches, as previously described (▶ Fig. 16.31).

The *bicoronal incision* starts in a preauricular crease anterior to the tragus. The superficial temporal artery should be dissected and preserved. The scalp incision is extended in the coronal plane, staying behind the hairline along its entire course, to the contralateral preauricular region. We prefer to gently curve the incision anteriorly at the midline (▶ Fig. 16.32a,b). The scalp flap is elevated in a subgaleal plane superficial to the pericranium between the superior temporal lines bilaterally. Lateral and inferior to the superior temporal lines, an incision is made

through both the superficial and deep layers of the temporalis fascia 1.0 to 1.5 cm posterior to the superior orbital rim and extends posteriorly parallel to the course of the zygomatic arch (▶ Fig. 16.32c). Dissection proceeds below the plane of the deep layer of the temporalis fascia to preserve the frontal branch of the facial nerve, which is superficial to the fascia. The scalp flap is elevated anteriorly toward the superior orbital rims and posteriorly toward the vertex.

Pericranial incisions are made as far posteriorly as necessary to provide adequate length for the pericranial flap and along the superior temporal lines bilaterally. The pericranial flap is dissected free from the underlying bone and reflected anteriorly (▶ Fig. 16.32d). Careful dissection and preservation of the

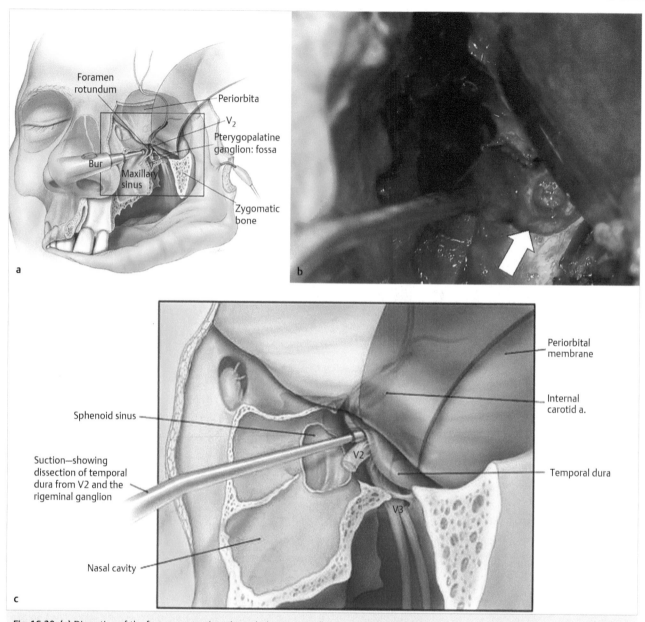

Fig. 16.30 **(a)** Dissection of the foramen rotundum through the transmaxillary route and **(b)** close-up schematic. **(c)** Intraoperative view of thickened V2 within the foramen rotundum (*arrow*).

supraorbital neurovascular pedicles is necessary to provide a well-vascularized pericranial flap for reconstruction of the cranial base defect. The supraorbital nerves and vessels are located along the medial third of the superior orbital rim. Elevation of the supraorbital rim periosteum begins laterally and proceeds medially until the margin of the supraorbital groove is carefully exposed with a fine elevator. The nerve and vessels may exit the skull either through a notch or a true foramen. If a notch is present, then the nerve can be dissected free without difficulty. If a foramen rather than a notch is found, the floor of the foramen is removed with a fine osteotome. This liberates the pedicle and further elevation of the superior periorbita is then achieved.

Frontal, temporal, or frontotemporal craniotomy is then performed to allow access to the floor of the anterior or middle

cranial fossa or both, respectively. For a *frontal craniotomy*, bilateral bur holes are then placed in the depression posterior to the frontal–zygomatic sutures (MacCarty's keyhole) after reflection of the temporalis muscle, leaving a cuff of fascia at the superior temporal line for reattaching the muscle during closure (▶ Fig. 16.32e). These anatomic keyholes provide access to the anterior fossa dura and by inferior enlargement of the periorbita if needed. A bur hole is then placed on the SSS, well anterior to the coronal suture, exposing the dura on both sides of the sinus. The bifrontal craniotomy is performed between the bur holes. The craniotomy may be extended inferiorly to the level of the frontonasal suture.

Compared with frontal craniotomy, *subfrontal approaches* have the advantage of minimizing brain retraction by providing wider and more direct exposure of the floor of the anterior

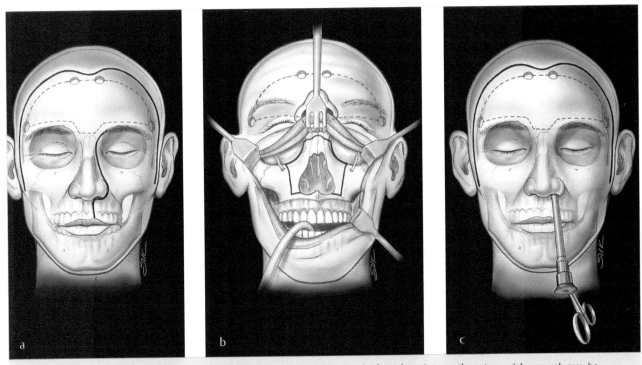

Fig. 16.31 Anterior craniofacial resection: extracranial approaches. In addition to the frontal craniotomy, the extracranial approach may be **(a)** transfacial, **(b)** sublabial, or **(c)** endonasal.

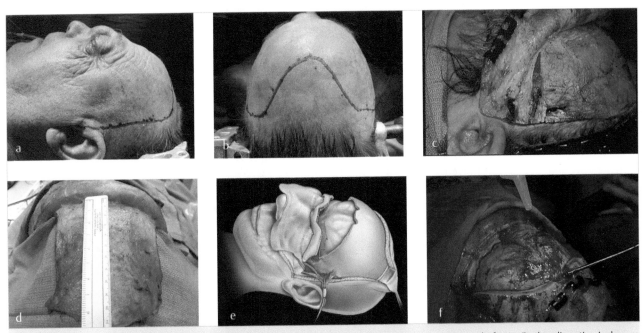

Fig. 16.32 Frontal craniotomy. **(a,b)** Bicoronal incision. **(c)** Incision of the superficial layer of the deep temporalis fascia. Further dissection is done deep to this plane to preserve the frontal branch of the facial nerve. **(d)** The pericranial flap. Adequate length and good vascular supply of the flap are prerequisites for effective reconstruction of the skull base defect. **(e)** Schematic of frontal craniotomy. **(f)** Intraoperative photograph of frontal craniotomy.

cranial fossa (▶ Fig. 16.33). This is especially helpful in more posteriorly located lesions such as those involving the planum sphenoidale, clivus, orbital apex, and optic chiasm (▶ Fig. 16.34).

The subfrontal approach is done by adding osteotomies that allow incorporation of the superior orbit and/or nasal bone to the craniotomy. These skeletal elements may be removed in several subunits or as a single bone flap (▶ Fig. 16.35).[10] Bilateral *nasal*

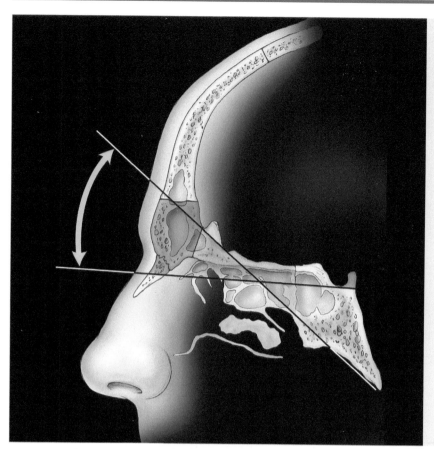

Fig. 16.33 Subfrontal approach. Note the increased basal exposure provided by the subfrontal approach by incorporating the supraorbital rim, glabella, and nasal bone with the frontal craniotomy.

osteotomies are done along the lower border of the nasal bones and then along the suture line between the nasal and lacrimal bones (▶ Fig. 16.35c). The osteotomies are connected across the midline below the frontoethmoid suture line and in front of the anterior ethmoidal vessels. This avoids injury to the cribriform plate and olfactory nerves. After the dura and periorbita have been carefully dissected from the bone, the lateral wall and roof of each orbit are removed in separate *orbital osteotomies* (▶ Fig. 16.35c). Under direct visualization, taking care to protect the periorbita and dura, an anteroposterior cut is made at the medial aspect of the orbital roof, staying lateral to the ethmoid sinus. A second anteroposterior cut is made at the inferior aspect of the lateral orbital wall. These cuts are connected posteriorly, with protection of the tissues of the SOF. The bone flap consisting of the frontal bone, orbital roof, superior–lateral orbital rims, and nasal bones can be removed for wide exposure (▶ Fig. 16.35d,e).

After completing the craniotomy, brain "relaxation" is achieved by opening the dura and allowing release of CSF or by withdrawing CSF from a lumbar subarachnoid drain, hypocapnia through controlled hyperventilation, mannitol diuresis, or steroids. This also lessens the need for brain retraction, which minimizes postoperative brain edema. Next, the *dura* is carefully dissected along the floor of the anterior cranial fossa to expose the crista galli and olfactory grooves. The *olfactory nerves* are transected to expose the cribriform plate. Dural elevation is continued to expose the fovea ethmoidalis and orbital roofs. Posteriorly, the planum sphenoidale and the base of the anterior clinoid process may be exposed as dictated by the extent of the tumor. If the dura is involved with the tumor, intradural exposure is

achieved and dura incisions are made around the tumor, and the dissection proceeds in a subdural plane and the dura, and even brain tissue if involved, is resected along with the tumor.

With simultaneous exposure provided superiorly through the intracranial approach and inferiorly through the extracranial approach, osteotomies of the cranial floor around the tumor can be safely completed. Malleable retractors are used to protect the brain and the orbit as osteotomies are made. The placement of osteotomies and the extent of resection are dictated by the extent of tumor involvement and are tailored in each case. Typically, however, osteotomies are made from the planum sphenoidale, along the roof of the ethmoid, and forward to the front of the cribriform plate (▶ Fig. 16.36). Frozen section control of the margins should be done to ensure the adequacy of resection.

Management of the Orbit

Sinonasal Tumors

Every effort should be made to preserve the eye as long as preservation does not compromise the adequacy of oncologic resection. However, attempts at orbital preservation in the face of gross residual disease usually result in poor disease control and ultimate loss of orbital function. Most studies have shown that if orbital invasion is limited to the bony orbit or the periorbita, orbital preservation is possible without compromising oncologic outcome.[12] Orbital exenteration is usually indicated when there is gross invasion of the periorbital fat, extraocular muscles, or optic nerve. The presence of proptosis or diplopia may be due to displacement

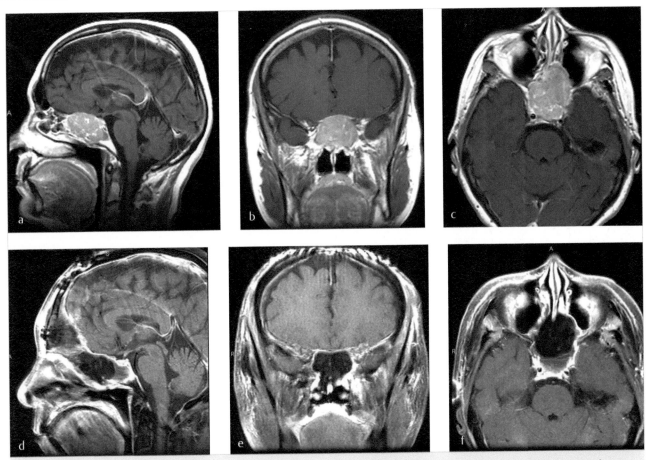

Fig. 16.34 Pre- **(a–c)** and postoperative **(d–f)** MRI of tumor involving the planum sphenoidale and upper two-thirds of the clivus removed via a subfrontal approach.

rather than invasion of the intraorbital contents. Decreased visual acuity or visual fields or the presence of an afferent pupillary defect usually indicate gross invasion of the orbit. Orbital invasion by perineural spread rather than direct extension may be missed unless careful examination of the cranial nerves, especially V1 and V2, is done. Detailed neuro-ophthalmologic examination should be conducted on all patients who have suspected or confirmed orbital involvement by sinonasal or other skull base tumors. If orbital exenteration is contemplated, always ensure that the patient has useful vision in the contralateral eye.

In the absence of any ocular signs or symptoms, however, evaluation of the extent of orbital involvement relies mainly on imaging. High-resolution CT and MRI are complementary and provide critical information regarding the extent of orbital bony and soft tissue involvement, respectively. CT scans obtained at 1- to 3-mm slices with detailed bone windows are best for evaluating bony involvement of the orbital walls. MRI is best used to evaluate the extent of soft tissue invasion beyond the periorbita (▶ Fig. 16.37). MRI is also useful in detecting perineural spread proximally beyond the orbital apex and into the cavernous sinus or optic chiasm, which compromises surgical margins, local disease control, and survival, and thus is a contraindication for surgical resection.[13] Even using the best imaging techniques, the definitive and most accurate assessment of the extent of orbital invasion and whether the eye can be preserved has to be made intraoperatively. This needs to be clearly

discussed with the patient and family, and informed consent for possible exenteration needs to be obtained in high-risk cases.

There is an evolving role for induction chemotherapy and concurrent chemoradiation in the management of patients who have orbital invasion by advanced sinonasal cancers (▶ Fig. 16.37). The role of such neoadjuvant treatment in enhancing the chances of orbital preservation continues to be investigated.[48]

If a decision is made to exenterate the orbit, then supra- and subciliary incisions are made around the upper and lower eyelids, respectively. This allows for preservation of the eyelids, which can be used to line the orbit. If the eyelids are involved with cancer, they must be included in the resection (▶ Fig. 16.38). The periorbita is incised over the superior and lateral orbital rims. Dissection continues along the roof of the orbit and lateral walls until the SOF and the optic foramen are exposed. Lidocaine is injected around these structures to block any autonomic-induced cardiac arrhythmias. To prevent troublesome bleeding, the neurovascular structures in the SOF are slowly and carefully isolated, ligated or clipped, and transected. The optic nerve and the ophthalmic artery are then managed in similar fashion. The extraocular muscles are transected at their origin in the orbital apex. The medial and inferior orbit may be left attached to the specimen if en bloc resection of the eye in patients who have sinonasal cancer is indicated. Osteotomies are done as previously described for total maxillectomy, except that the orbital bony cuts are connected at the orbital apex rather than at the inferior orbital fissure.

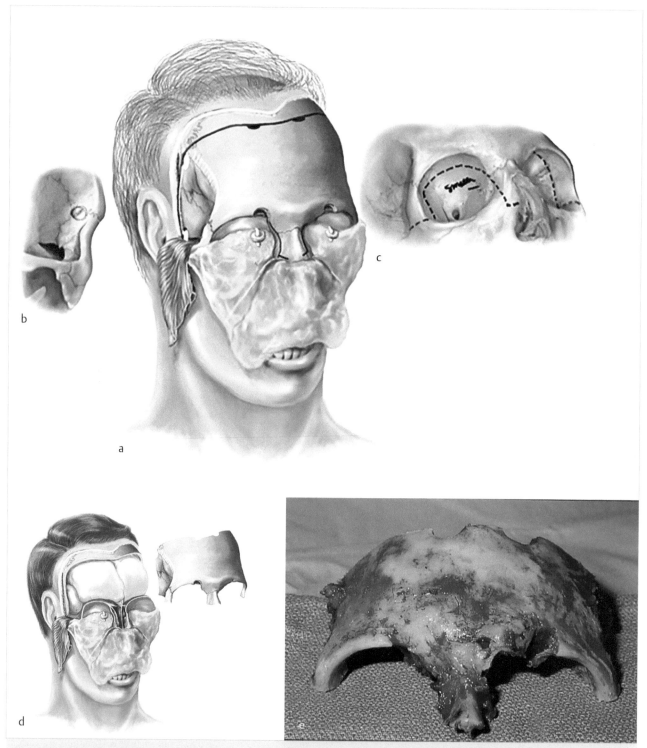

Fig. 16.35 Subfrontal approach. **(a)** Bicoronal incision and soft tissue dissection. The scalp flap is reflected anteriorly down to the level of the nasal bones. The supraorbital nerves were surrounded by complete foramina rather than a notch. Osteotomies around the foramina allow downward reflection of the nerves with the soft tissue flap. Bur holes are placed on either side of the superior sagittal sinus, anterior to the coronal suture. **(b)** Bilateral bur holes are placed posterior to the frontal–zygomatic sutures. These anatomic keyholes provide access to the anterior fossa dura and periorbita, separated by the bony orbital roof. **(c)** Orbital and nasal osteotomies. The cranio-orbital-nasal bone flap is removed as a single unit as illustrated by **(d)** the drawing and **(e)** intraoperative photograph.

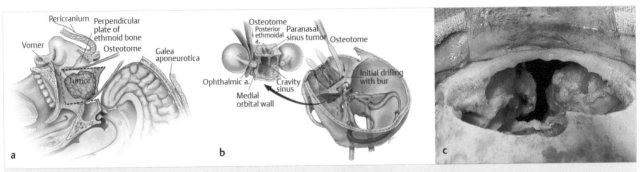

Fig. 16.36 Resection of the floor of the anterior cranial fossa. **(a, b)** Osteotomies along the floor of the anterior cranial fossa. **(c)** Intraoperative photograph showing resection of the floor of the anterior cranial fossa and the medial orbital walls.

Table 16.3 Reconstruction of surgical defects

Defect	Goals of reconstruction
Palate	Oronasal separation
Cranial base	Cranionasal separation
Orbital–maxillary	Eye and cheek support
Dental	Restoration of dentition and occlusion
Facial	Restoration of facial defects and cosmesis

Primary Orbital Tumors

Surgery for primary orbital tumors will depend on whether the tumor is benign or malignant. Examples of benign tumors include vascular malformation, neurofibroma, osteoma, and pleomorphic adenoma of the lacrimal gland (▶ Fig. 16.39; ▶ Fig. 16.40; ▶ Fig. 16.41; ▶ Fig. 16.42).

Examples of malignant tumors include lymphoma, which is the most common, and salivary gland tumors of the lacrimal gland, such as adenoid cystic carcinoma (▶ Fig. 16.43).

In most cases of primary intraorbital tumors, the surgical approach is largely dictated by the location of the tumor. Tumors of the medial orbit may be removed through a transethmoid modified Lynch approach (▶ Fig. 16.41). The transconjunctival approach, with detachment of the lateral canthal tendon, provides access to the orbital floor. Tumors of the lateral orbit are best approached through a lateral orbitotomy, using either a brow incision (modified Kronlein or Stallard-Wright incision) or a hemi- or bicoronal approach. The advantages of the hemi- or bicoronal approaches include wider exposure for tumor resection, avoidance of periocular incisions, and excellent cosmetic results (▶ Fig. 16.42). Tumors of the superior orbit or tumors invading intracranially are best resected through a cranio-orbito-zygomatic approach (▶ Fig. 16.43).

Reconstruction, Complication Avoidance, and Rehabilitation

Meticulous reconstruction of surgical defects resulting from resection of sinonasal and orbital tumors is essential to preventing complications and to optimizing surgical and functional outcome. The goals and strategies of reconstruction will depend on the extent and location of the surgical defect. ▶ Table 16.3 summarizes the major areas of reconstruction and their respective goals.

Palatal Reconstruction: Oronasal Separation

Effective separation between the oral and nasal cavities is essential for effective speech and deglutition. Palatal defects resulting from a maxillectomy are simply and effectively sealed using a prosthetic obturator. Preoperatively, the oromaxillofacial prosthodontist takes dental impressions and designs a *surgical* obturator, which is used at the end of surgery to seal the palatal defect (▶ Fig. 16.44).[49] The surgical obturator can be slightly modified intraoperatively to custom-fit the defect. The advantages of this immediate reconstruction are early postoperative restoration of normal speech and oral feeding, minimizing the early postoperative morbidity of surgery and obviating the need for enteral feeding. Preoperatively, clear communication between the head and neck surgeon and the maxillofacial prosthodontist about the anticipated maxillary defect is required for optimal results. An additional advantage of the surgical obturator is its ability to support the surgical packing used to immobilize the skin graft lining the cheek flap. This epithelial lining, when completely healed, minimizes granulation tissue formation, provides a smooth mucosal lining, reduces scar contracture of the cheek, provides a scar band to support the obturator, and facilitates cavity hygiene (▶ Fig. 16.44a).

At the end of the first postoperative week, and after removal of the surgical packing, the surgical obturator is replaced with an *interim* obturator (▶ Fig. 16.44b). This is used for several weeks after discharging the patient from the hospital and after completion of adjuvant therapy, allowing the surgical cavity to heal completely. Patients are instructed to remove the obturator periodically and clean the cavity with saline irrigation. During follow-up visits, the obturator is removed and cleaned of any crusts or debris. Finally, a *permanent* obturator is designed to custom-fit the cavity after it matures to its final shape and dimensions. The acrylic dome incorporated into its design provides some cheek support (▶ Fig. 16.44c,d). In addition to being a simple and effective method of reconstructing palatal defects, use of permanent obturators can also provide full dental restoration. At follow-up visits, removal of the obturator allows easy inspection of the cavity for any evidence of recurrent disease.

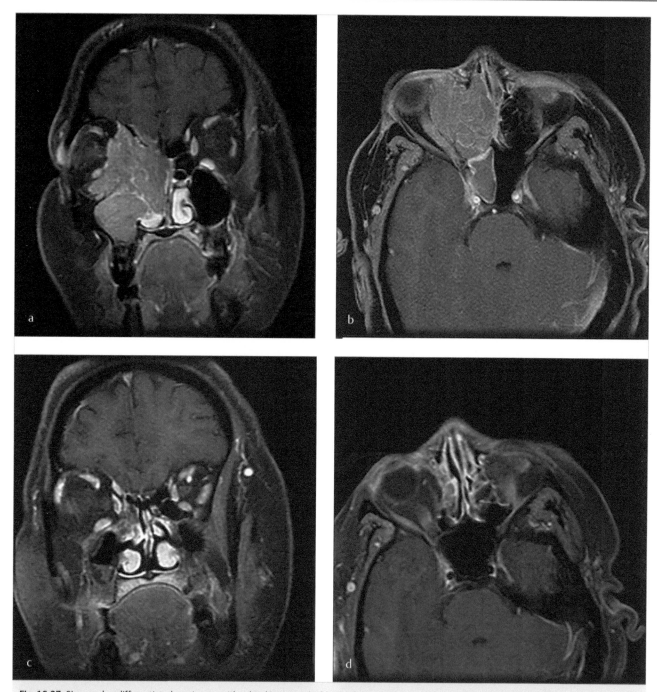

Fig. 16.37 Sinonasal undifferentiated carcinoma with orbital invasion. (a, b) MRI showing tumor of the right sinonasal region with gross invasion of the medial and inferior orbital contents. The tumor also invades the anterior skull base with limited intracranial extension. (c, d) MRI of same patient 3 years after completing treatment with induction chemotherapy followed by concurrent chemoradiation. Imaging shows no evidence of residual disease. Surgery was avoided, and the orbit was preserved.

Surgical reconstruction of palatal defects using tissue flaps has the advantage of eliminating the need for regular hygiene of the surgical cavity. However, flap reconstruction requires more extensive surgery, adds donor site morbidity, does not allow rapid dental restoration, and conceals the surgical cavity from inspection for recurrent tumor. These disadvantages make prosthetic obturators the method of choice for reconstruction of surgical defects of the palate. The use of tissue flaps is usually reserved for patients who need additional

reconstruction to the maxillary skeleton, orbital floor, or cranial base. In these cases, osseointegrated implants are used to facilitate dental restoration.

Cranial Base Reconstruction: Cranionasal Separation

Whenever the cranial and nasal cavities are joined by a surgical defect, as is the case with anterior craniofacial resection,

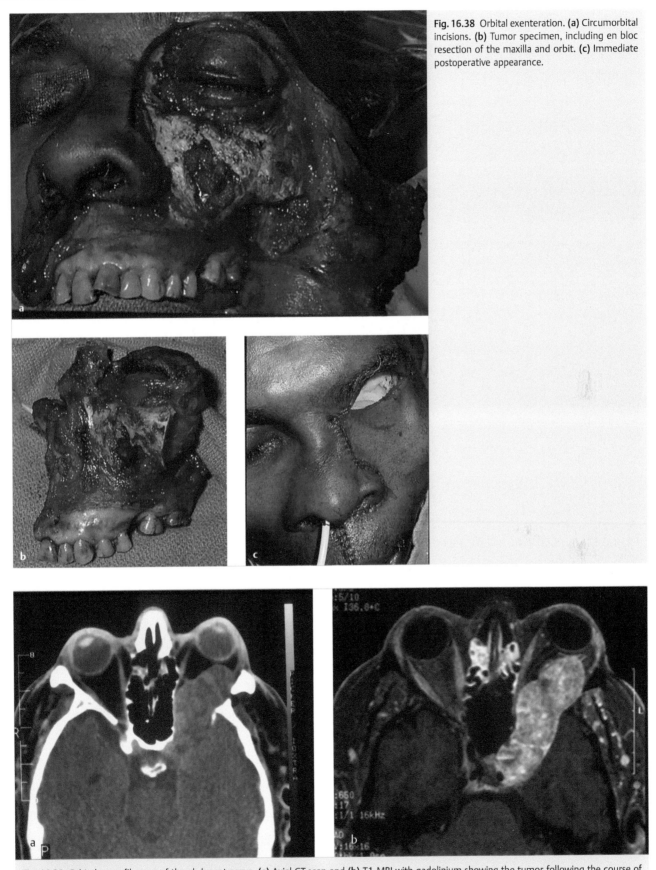

Fig. 16.38 Orbital exenteration. **(a)** Circumorbital incisions. **(b)** Tumor specimen, including en bloc resection of the maxilla and orbit. **(c)** Immediate postoperative appearance.

Fig. 16.39 Orbital neurofibroma of the abducent nerve. **(a)** Axial CT scan and **(b)** T1-MRI with gadolinium showing the tumor following the course of the abducent nerve in the lateral orbit and extending to the cavernous sinus.

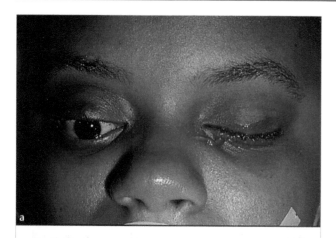

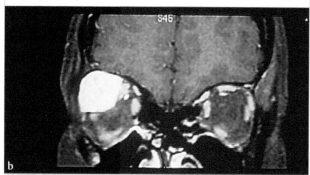

Fig. 16.40 Pleomorphic adenoma of the lacrimal gland. (a) This young woman presented with proptosis and a palpable mass in the upper lateral right orbit. (b) Coronal MRI shows the mass in the region of the right lacrimal gland. Surgical resection via a lateral orbitotomy revealed a pleomorphic adenoma.

watertight cranionasal separation is essential to reduce the risk of CSF leak, meningitis, and pneumocephalus. Meticulous closure of all dural incisions is necessary. Larger defects of the dura should be repaired using temporalis fascia, pericranium, or fascia lata grafts. Although bony reconstruction of the anterior skull base has been described using vascularized and nonvascularized bone grafts as well as bone cement, reconstruction of the bone defect is not necessary in most patients. The vascularized pericranial flap is currently the most frequently used flap for reconstructing defects of the floor of the anterior cranial fossa (▶ Fig. 16.32d). Flap handling and suturing should be meticulous to achieve a watertight seal (▶ Fig. 16.45). Fibrin glue and tissue adhesives do not compensate for an imperfect closure. Lumbar subarachnoid drainage may be used for several days postoperatively to reduce CSF pressure and the possibility of a leak. Excessive lumbar drainage, however, may encourage the development of pneumocephalus.

Occasionally more bulk is needed to reconstruct the surgical cavity and reduce dead space, such as with extensive defects of the cranial base. Regional flaps, such as the temporalis muscle, are usually adequate for this purpose. If the muscle bulk is inadequate, or if its blood supply has been sacrificed, then a microvascular free flap is used.[50] Vascularized tissue may also be needed to protect the carotid artery if it is exposed to the surgical defect. This is done to prevent desiccation

of the arterial wall and carotid artery blowout. This is particularly important if the patient received prior radiation therapy or will receive postoperative adjuvant radiation. For more detail on microvascular reconstruction, please refer to Chapter 7 of this book.

Orbitomaxillary Reconstruction: Eye and Cheek Support

The maxilla has three bony buttresses: the nasomaxillary, zygomaticomaxillary, and pterygomaxillary. In addition to a palatal defect, total maxillectomy results in resection of all three buttresses and loss of adequate skeletal support to the soft tissues of the cheek (▶ Fig. 16.29d). Loss of the zygomaticomaxillary buttress results in inferior displacement of the orbit and flattening of the malar eminence. Loss of the nasomaxillary buttress results in superior and posterior deviation of the alar base of the nose. Loss of the pterygomaxillary buttress results in superior and posterior deviation of the upper lip. Resection of the inferior orbital rim and floor leads to loss of skeletal support to the eyelid and globe. The lack of adequate orbital support leads to enophthalmos, ectropion, hypoglobus, and diplopia, resulting in unacceptable esthetic and functional outcome. The combined effects of loss of support of the eye and cheek result in the "typical" postmaxillary deformity (▶ Fig. 16.46). Although a split thickness skin graft and a palatal obturator are commonly used in reconstruction after maxillectomy, these methods of reconstruction do not provide adequate support for the cheek and eye.

Skeletal reconstruction of the maxillary and orbital defects may be done using bone grafts, most commonly autogenous calvarial grafts. Demineralized and banked bone grafts, which are available in a variety of shapes and sizes, may also be used. Alternatively, alloplastic implants may be used for reconstruction of the maxillary buttresses, orbital rim, or orbital floor. Titanium mesh, bone cement, and porous polyethylene have all been successfully used in orbital and maxillary bony reconstruction.

Whatever method is used for bone reconstruction, adequate coverage with well-vascularized soft tissue is essential to prevent resorption of bone grafts and infection or extrusion of alloplastic implants. The pedicled temporalis muscle flap, temporoparietal fascial flap, and septal mucosal flap are most commonly used for this purpose. Microvascular free flaps may be used to either provide soft tissue coverage of bone grafts or implants, or composite vascularized bone flaps may be used for full reconstruction of both soft tissue and bone defects.[50]

Primary reconstruction of defects of the maxilla and orbit at the time of maxillectomy is easier and results in better esthetic and functional outcome than delayed reconstruction does (▶ Fig. 16.47). Although secondary reconstruction after globe-sparing maxillectomy is feasible, it is often difficult, and the results are limited by excessive scarring and soft tissue contracture, especially in patients who underwent adjuvant radiation therapy. These patients may benefit more from free-tissue transfer reconstruction.[50]

Dental Restoration

Prosthetic rehabilitation using partial or full upper dentures is the easiest method of dental restoration in patients who have undergone maxillectomy (▶ Fig. 16.44). Remaining contralateral teeth facilitate retention of partial dentures. In edentulous patients, dental fixatives can be used, but denture retention is more difficult. A soft palate "band" at the posterior edge of the defect may provide enough of a ledge to retain the prosthesis. Retention of the prosthesis in edentulous patients who underwent an extended resection to include the soft palate may be extremely difficult. In such cases, the use of osteointegrated implants facilitates prosthetic dental restoration.

Another important aspect in the rehabilitation of patients after maxillectomy is the prevention of trismus. Patients who have undergone resection of the pterygoid plates or muscles of mastication are particularly prone to develop trismus that may be severe enough to interfere with inserting and wearing a denture-bearing obturator. Early postoperative jaw opening exercises using "stacked" wooden tongue blades or commercially available devices (e.g., Therabite) are extremely important in preventing or minimizing postoperative trismus.

Restoration of Facial Defects

Smaller defects of the face are optimally reconstructed using local flaps. Local skin flaps provide the best thickness and color match for facial defects. Reconstruction of more extensive facial defects may require regional or microvascular free flaps but suffer from suboptimal esthetic outcome as a result of color or thickness mismatch between donor and defect sites. Facial defects resulting from orbital exenteration or total rhinectomy are best managed using prosthetic restoration.

16.9 Outcomes and Prognosis

Much progress in prognosis of patients who have nasal and paranasal carcinoma has been made during the past 40 years (▶ Fig. 16.48), likely as a result of advances in both the evaluation and treatment of these patients. Office endoscopy and high-resolution imaging allow better assessment of the extent of disease and hence better treatment planning. Advances in cranial base surgery and microvascular reconstruction have allowed more adequate resection of advanced sinonasal cancer, even that involving the cranial base. Improvements in the delivery of radiation therapy using highly conformal radiation such as IMRT or proton therapy have allowed more targeted and homogenous dosimetry to the tumor while sparing nearby critical structures. Integration of more effective chemotherapeutic and targeted agents in the overall management of patients who have sinonasal cancer has improved local control of the disease.

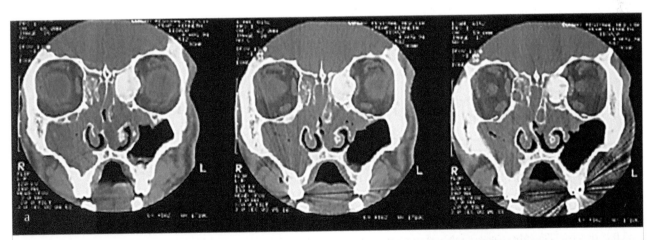

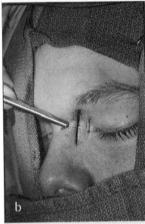
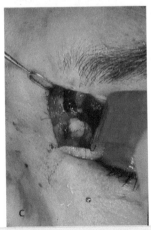
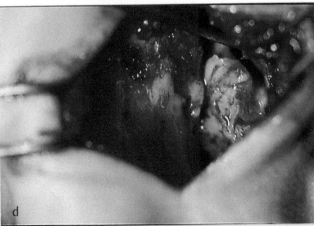

Fig. 16.41 Osteoma of the ethmoid and medial orbital wall. **(a)** Coronal CT showing an osteoma of the left ethmoid and medial orbital wall. **(b)** Lynch-type incision for an anterior ethmoidectomy. **(c)** Exposure of the tumor in the medial orbit. **(d)** Bony dissection around the tumor. *(Continued)*

(Continued)

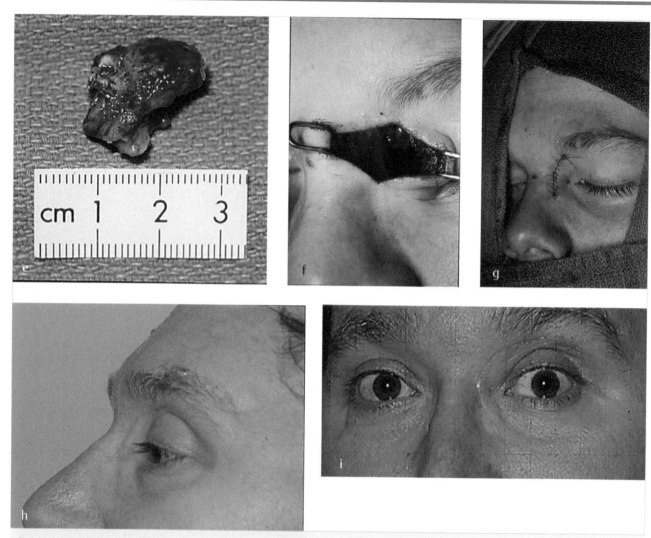

Fig. 16.41 *(Continued)* **(e)** Surgical specimen. **(f)** Surgical field showing complete resection. **(g)** Closure. **(h, i)** Postoperative appearance.

Although the literature is replete with reports describing the outcome and prognosis of patients with sinonasal cancer, several confounding factors make meaningful interpretation of the results extremely difficult, including the diversity of histological diagnoses, site of origin, extent of tumor invasion, prior therapy, extent of surgical resection, status of surgical margins, adjuvant therapy, and length of follow-up. The factor most influencing prognosis is the histopathologic type of sinonasal malignancy, which has a direct bearing on the biology and natural history of the disease and consequently on the outcome of therapy. This is highlighted in ▶ Fig. 16.49, which shows the 5-year survival rate by histology for 2,698 patients who had sinonasal cancer, seen at MD Anderson Cancer Center (MDACC) from 1944 to 2007.

The 10-year survival outcomes of patients undergoing anterior craniofacial resection for sinonasal cancer at MDACC during the past decade are shown in ▶ Fig. 16.50a. Despite these excellent outcomes, patients who have T4 tumors have a worse prognosis (▶ Fig. 16.50b). The presence of perineural invasion (▶ Fig. 16.50c) and angioinvasion (▶ Fig. 16.50d) also negatively affects survival.

Brain invasion has a particularly profound—indeed, perhaps the most dramatic—impact on survival (▶ Fig. 16.51a), likely because of the difficulty of achieving negative surgical margins, which is a major determinant of a favorable outcome in surgically treated patients (▶ Fig. 16.51b,c). It is interesting to note that the effect of method of resection (en bloc vs. piecemeal) did not affect the outcome so long as the margins were negative (▶ Fig. 16.51d). Several molecular and genetic markers of prognosis have been already discussed in their corresponding tumor-specific sections. The presence of cervical lymph node metastasis from sinonasal cancer is an uncommon event, but when it is present, survival rate is reduced by at least 50%. Finally, the presence of distant metastasis is usually an indication that the disease is incurable and that treatment strategies should focus on palliation.

The long-term oncologic results of EEA in treating malignant sinonasal tumors are still being defined. The two largest series from North America[41] and Europe[40] have demonstrated endoscopic resection to have comparable oncological results to those achieved using open surgery. Hanna et al reported on 120 patients treated at MDACC from 1992 to 2007.[41] An exclusive

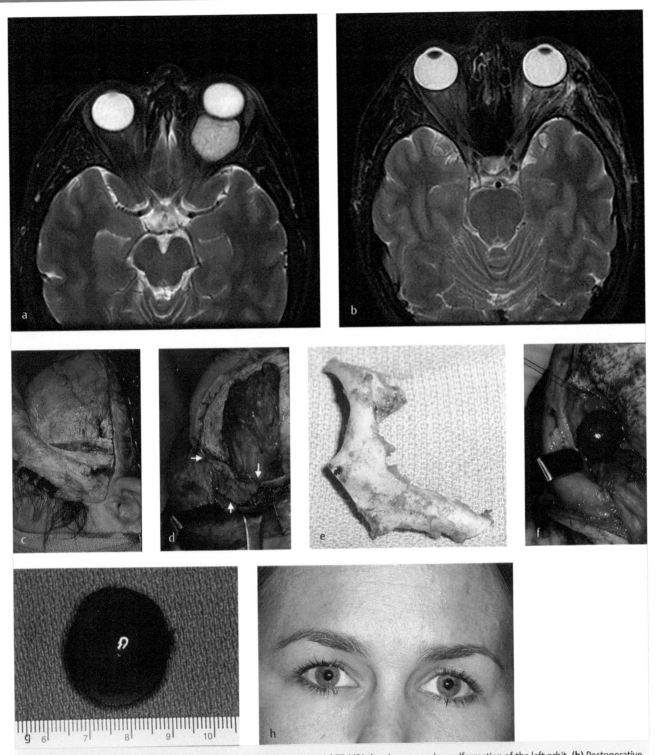

Fig. 16.42 Bicoronal approach for lateral orbitotomy. **(a)** Preoperative axial T2-MRI showing a vascular malformation of the left orbit. **(b)** Postoperative axial T2-MRI showing complete resection of the tumor. Intraoperative photographs show **(c)** bicoronal approach; **(d)** orbitozygomatic exposure and osteotomies (*arrows*), **(e)** orbitozygomatic bone segment, including the lateral orbital rim and zygomatic arch; **(f)** lateral orbitotomy providing wide exposure for tumor resection; and **(g)** tumor specimen. **(h)** Postoperative photographs showing good eye position and cosmetic result.

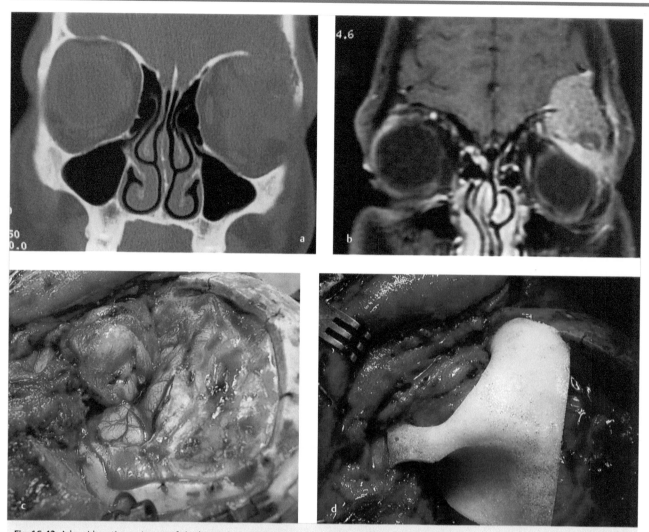

Fig. 16.43 Adenoid cystic carcinoma of the lacrimal gland. **(a)** Coronal CT and **(b)** MRI show bone destruction of the superior orbital wall and intracranial soft invasion, respectively. **(c)** The tumor was completely resected through a cranio-orbito-zygomatic approach, and **(d)** the superior lateral orbital walls were reconstructed using porous polyethylene Medpore implant.

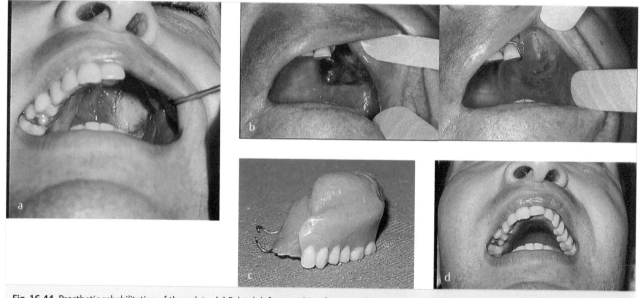

Fig. 16.44 Prosthetic rehabilitation of the palate. **(a)** Palatal defect resulting from maxillectomy, with split thickness skin graft lining the surgical cavity. **(b)** Interim obturator effectively seals the palatal defect and allows patients to resume a soft diet. **(c, d)** Permanent obturator provides excellent palatal reconstruction and dental restoration, allowing the patient to resume a normal diet.

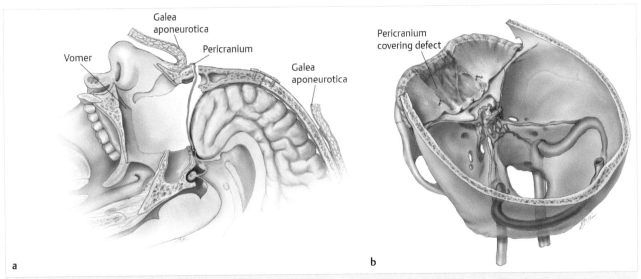

Fig. 16.45 **(a)** Sagittal and **(b)** axial views of pericranial flap reconstruction of anterior cranial base defect.

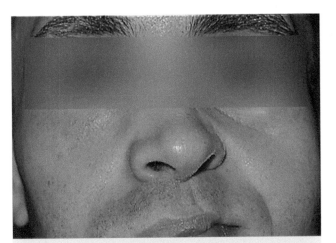

Fig. 16.46 Left total maxillectomy with no reconstruction. "Typical" postmaxillectomy deformity due to lack of support of the orbit and cheek. There is downward displacement of the orbit and medial canthus. Note the presence of enophthalmos, as evidenced by a prominent upper eyelid sulcus. There is flattening of the cheek and deviation of the nasal tip. The patient had significant diplopia. These deformities can be avoided through adequate bony reconstruction.

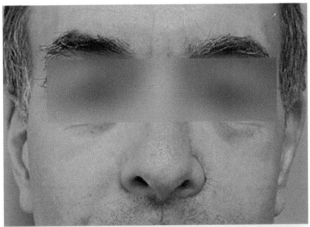

Fig. 16.47 Left total maxillectomy with orbitomaxillary reconstruction. Postoperative appearance showing good position of the eye, cheek, and nose.

endoscopic approach (EEA) was used in 77% of patients, and the cranioendoscopic approach (CEA; the transnasal endoscopic approach with the addition of a frontal or subfrontal craniotomy) was used in 23% of patients. Approximately two-thirds of patients in the EEA group had T1 to T2 tumor stage, whereas 95% of patients in the CEA group had T3 to T4 disease stage ($P < 0.01$). Positive margins were reported in 15%. Postoperative radiation therapy or chemoradiotherapy was used in 50% of patients. Mean follow-up was 37 months, with local, regional, and distant recurrences of 15%, 6%, and 5%, respectively. The 5-year and 10-year disease-specific survival (DSS) were 87% and 80%, respectively (▶ Fig. 16.52a). Disease recurrence and survival did not significantly differ between the EEA and CEA groups (▶ Fig. 16.52b).

The authors emphasized the role of appropriate adjuvant therapy and treatment by expert multidisciplinary teams in the management of sinonasal malignancies. Nicolai et al reported on 184 patients from the University of Brescia and the University of Pavia/Insubria-Varese, treated from 1996 to 2006.[40] The overall 5-year DSS was 82%. At mean follow-up of 34 months, local, regional, and distant recurrences were 15%, 1%, and 7%, respectively. Both study cohorts had similar distributions of T staging, adjuvant treatment, and proportion of EEA to CEA (▶ Table 16.4). However, compared with the MDACC group, patients in the European group were older, predominantly male, less likely to have had prior treatment (28% vs. 58%), and more likely to present with adenocarcinoma (37% vs. 14%). Irrespective of these differences, the 5-year DSS for the two series was comparable to those reported in the open anterior craniofacial resection (ACFR) cohorts. Both groups concluded that in well-selected patients, endoscopic resection of sinonasal cancers produces acceptable oncological outcomes.

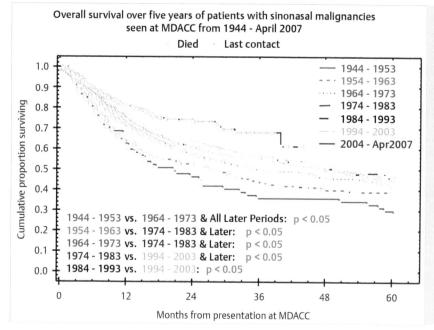

Fig. 16.48 Improvement in 5-year overall survival of patients with sinonasal malignancy. Data of 2,698 patients who had sinonasal cancer, seen at MD Anderson Cancer Center from 1944 to 2007.

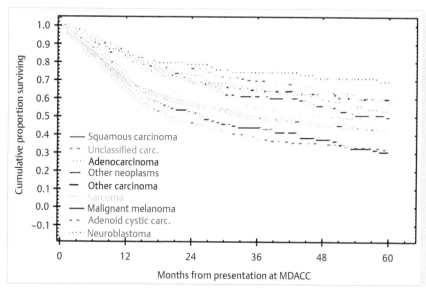

Fig. 16.49 Overall 5-year survival by histology of 2,698 patients with sinonasal cancer, seen at MD Anderson Cancer Center from 1944 to 2007.

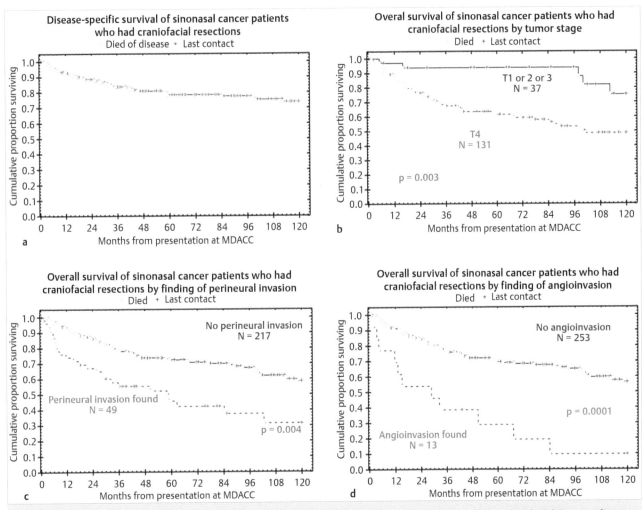

Fig. 16.50 Survival outcomes of craniofacial resection in patients treated at MD Anderson Cancer Center in the past decade. **(a)** Ten-year disease-specific survival. **(b)** Effect of stage on survival. **(c)** Effect of perineural invasion on survival. **(d)** Effect of angioinvasion on survival.

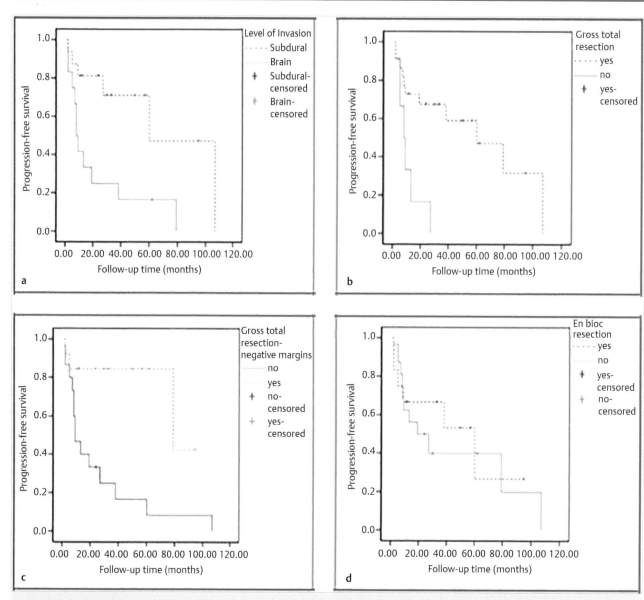

Fig. 16.51 Prognostic significance of transdural invasion of cranial base malignancies in patients undergoing craniofacial resection (per Feiz-Erfan I, Suki D, Hanna E, DeMonte F, Prognostic significance of transdural invasion of cranial base malignancies in patients undergoing craniofacial resection, Neurosurgery 2007;61[6]:1178–1185). **(a)** Brain invasion was a significant prognostic factor associated with progression-free survival (PFS; $P = 0.005$). **(b)** A significant association was found for PFS and gross total resection (GTR; $P = 0.003$). **(c)** In the cohort of patients who had GTR, the ones who had a microscopic negative surgical margin had a better PFS than those who had positive margins ($P = 0.02$). **(d)** No significant association was found for PFS between en bloc and piecemeal resection ($P = 0.64$).

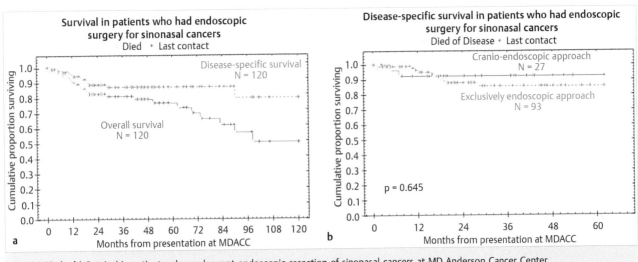

Fig. 16.52 (a, b) Survival in patients who underwent endoscopic resection of sinonasal cancers at MD Anderson Cancer Center.

Table 16.4 Comparison of results from two large studies of oncologic outcomes of endoscopic resection of sinonasal malignancy

Findings	Hanna[a]: MD Anderson Cancer Center			Nicolai[b]: U. Brescia and U. Pavia/Insubria-Varese		
Patients						
Total	120			184		
EEA	93 (77.5%)			134 (73%)		
CEA	27 (22.5%)			50 (27%)		
Mean follow-up	37 months			34 months		
Prior treatment	59%			28%		
Stage	EEA	CEA	All patients	EEA*	CEA*	All patients*
T1	32%	0%	25%	37%	6%	28%
T2	31%	5%	25%	19%	2%	14%
T3	17%	36%	21%	15%	24%	17%
T4	20%	59%	29%	16%	62%	28%
Histopathology						
Adenocarcinoma	14%			37%		
Esthesioneuroblastoma	17%			12%		
Melanoma	14%			9%		
Squamous cell carcinoma	13%			14%		
Adenoid cystic carcinoma	7%			7%		
Neuroendocrine carcinoma	4%			1%		
SNUC	2%			3%		
Sarcomas	15%			13%		
Adjuvant therapy						
None (surgery only)	50%			47%		
Radiation	37%			39%		
Chemoradiation	13%			3%		
Chemotherapy	6%			4%		
Recurrence						
Local	15%			15%		
Regional	6%			1%		
Distant	5%			7%		

(Continued)

Table 16.4 *(Continued)* Comparison of results from two large studies of oncologic outcomes of endoscopic resection of sinonasal malignancy

Findings	Hanna[a]: MD Anderson Cancer Center	Nicolai[b]: U. Brescia
5-year disease-specific survival		and U. Pavia/Insubria-Varese
Overall	87%	82%
EEA	86%	91%
CEA	92%	59%

Abbreviations: CEA, cranioendoscopic approach; EEA, endoscopic endonasal approach; SNUC, sinonasal undifferentiated carcinoma.
[a]Hanna E, DeMonte F, Ibrahim S, Roberts D, Levine N, Kupferman M. Endoscopic resection of sinonasal cancers with and without craniotomy: oncologic results. Arch Otolaryngol Head Neck Surg 2009;135(12):1219–1224.
Nicolai P, Battaglia P, Bignami M, et al. Endoscopic surgery for malignant tumors of the sinonasal tract and adjacent skull base: a 10-year experience. Am J Rhinol 2008;22(3):308–316.

16.10 Conclusion

Surgical management of tumors of the nasal cavity, paranasal sinuses, and orbit require in-depth understanding of the biologic behavior of the various tumor types originating in this region. Careful assessment of the location and extent of the tumor is crucial in planning and executing the proper surgical approach for adequate oncologic resection. Meticulous reconstruction of all surgical defects is critical in avoiding complications and maximizing functional and esthetic outcome. As for other types of cranial base tumors, multidisciplinary collaboration is essential for successful treatment of patients who have tumors of this region.

Acknowledgment

Unless otherwise credited, all figures reproduced in this chapter are courtesy of the MD Anderson Cancer Center in Houston, Texas.

References

[1] Hanna E, et al. Cancer of the nasal cavity and the paranasal sinuses. In: Myers JN, Hanna E, Myers EN, eds. Cancer of the Head and Neck. Wolters Kluwer: Philadelphia; 2017

[2] Diaz EM, Jr, Johnigan RH, III, Pero C, et al. Olfactory neuroblastoma: the 22-year experience at one comprehensive cancer center. Head Neck. 2005; 27 (2):138–149

[3] Rosenthal DI, Barker JL, Jr, El-Naggar AK, et al. Sinonasal malignancies with neuroendocrine differentiation: patterns of failure according to histologic phenotype. Cancer. 2004; 101(11):2567–2573

[4] Girod D, Hanna E, Marentette L. Esthesioneuroblastoma. Head Neck. 2001; 23 (6):500–505

[5] Lupinetti AD, Roberts DB, Williams MD, et al. Sinonasal adenoid cystic carcinoma: the M. D. Anderson Cancer Center experience. Cancer. 2007; 110(12): 2726–2731

[6] Prokopakis EP, Snyderman CH, Hanna EY, Carrau RL, Johnson JT, D'Amico F. Risk factors for local recurrence of adenoid cystic carcinoma: the role of postoperative radiation therapy. Am J Otolaryngol. 1999; 20(5):281–286

[7] Pitman KT, Prokopakis EP, Aydogan B, et al. The role of skull base surgery for the treatment of adenoid cystic carcinoma of the sinonasal tract. Head Neck. 1999; 21(5):402–407

[8] Tirado Y, Williams MD, Hanna EY, Kaye FJ, Batsakis JG, El-Naggar AK. CRTC1/MAML2 fusion transcript in high grade mucoepidermoid carcinomas of salivary and thyroid glands and Warthin's tumors: implications for histogenesis and biologic behavior. Genes Chromosomes Cancer. 2007; 46(7):708–715

[9] Hanna E, Vural E, Teo C, et al. Sinonasal tumors: the Arkansas experience. Skull Base Surg. 1998; 8 Supplement:15

[10] Hanna E, Linskey ME, Pieper D. Malignant tumors of the anterior cranial base. In: Sekhar LN, Fessler RG, eds. Atlas of Neurosurgical Techniques. New York: Thieme; 2006:588–598

[11] DeMonte F, Ginsberg LE, Clayman GL. Primary malignant tumors of the sphenoidal sinus. Neurosurgery. 2000; 46(5):1084–1091, discussion 1091–1092

[12] Hanna EY, et al. Cancer of the nasal cavity, paranasal sinuses, and orbit. In: Myers EN, ed. Cancer of the Head and Neck. 4th ed. Philadelphia: Saunders; 2003:155–206

[13] Hanna E, Vural E, Prokopakis E, Carrau R, Snyderman C, Weissman J. The sensitivity and specificity of high-resolution imaging in evaluating perineural spread of adenoid cystic carcinoma to the skull base. Arch Otolaryngol Head Neck Surg. 2007; 133(6):541–545

[14] Cohen ZR, Marmor E, Fuller GN, DeMonte F. Misdiagnosis of olfactory neuroblastoma. Neurosurg Focus. 2002; 12(5):e3

[15] Bristol IJ, Ahamad A, Garden AS, et al. Postoperative radiotherapy for maxillary sinus cancer: long-term outcomes and toxicities of treatment. Int J Radiat Oncol Biol Phys. 2007; 68(3):719–730

[16] Hanna E, DeMonte F. Comprehensive Management of Skull Base Tumors. New York: Informa; 2009

[17] Hentschel SJ, Vora Y, Suki D, Hanna EY, DeMonte F. Malignant tumors of the anterolateral skull base. Neurosurgery. 2010; 66(1):102–112, discussion 112

[18] Ganly I, Patel SG, Singh B, et al. Craniofacial resection for malignant paranasal sinus tumors: report of an international collaborative study. Head Neck. 2005; 27(7):575–584

[19] Ganly I, Patel SG, Singh B, et al. Complications of craniofacial resection for malignant tumors of the skull base: report of an international collaborative study. Head Neck. 2005; 27(6):445–451

[20] Hanasono MM, Silva A, Skoracki RJ, et al. Skull base reconstruction: an updated approach. Plast Reconstr Surg. 2011; 128(3):675–686

[21] Levine PA. Would Dr. Ogura approve of endoscopic resection of esthesioneuroblastomas? An analysis of endoscopic resection data versus that of craniofacial resection. Laryngoscope. 2009; 119(1):3–7

[22] Lund VJ, Stammberger H, Nicolai P, et al. European Rhinologic Society Advisory Board on Endoscopic Techniques in the Management of Nose, Paranasal Sinus and Skull Base Tumours. European position paper on endoscopic management of tumours of the nose, paranasal sinuses and skull base. Rhinol Suppl. 2010; 22(22):1–143

[23] Kassam A, Snyderman CH, Mintz A, Gardner P, Carrau RL. Expanded endonasal approach: the rostrocaudal axis. Part I. Crista galli to the sella turcica. Neurosurg Focus. 2005; 19(1):E3

[24] Wellman BJ, Traynelis VC, McCulloch TM, Funk GF, Menezes AH, Hoffman HT. Midline anterior craniofacial approach for malignancy: results of en bloc versus piecemeal resections. Skull Base Surg. 1999; 9(1):41–46

[25] Feiz-Erfan I, Suki D, Hanna E, DeMonte F. Prognostic significance of transdural invasion of cranial base malignancies in patients undergoing craniofacial resection. Neurosurgery. 2007; 61(6):1178–1185

[26] Su SY, Kupferman ME, DeMonte F, Levine NB, Raza SM, Hanna EY. Endoscopic resection of sinonasal cancers. Curr Oncol Rep. 2014; 16(2):369

[27] Snyderman CH, Kassam AB, Carrau R, Mintz A. Endoscopic reconstruction of cranial base defects following endonasal skull base surgery. Skull Base. 2007; 17(1):73–78

[28] Kassam A, Carrau RL, Snyderman CH, Gardner P, Mintz A. Evolution of reconstructive techniques following endoscopic expanded endonasal approaches. Neurosurg Focus. 2005; 19(1):E8

[29] Kassam AB, Thomas A, Carrau RL, et al. Endoscopic reconstruction of the cranial base using a pedicled nasoseptal flap. Neurosurgery. 2008; 63(1) Suppl 1:ONS44–ONS52, discussion ONS52–ONS53

[30] Pinheiro-Neto CD, Paluzzi A, Fernandez-Miranda JC, et al. Extended dissection of the septal flap pedicle for ipsilateral endoscopic transpterygoid approaches. Laryngoscope. 2014; 124(2):391–396

[31] Zanation AM, Snyderman CH, Carrau RL, Kassam AB, Gardner PA, Prevedello DM. Minimally invasive endoscopic pericranial flap: a new method for endonasal skull base reconstruction. Laryngoscope. 2009; 119(1):13–18

[32] Bolzoni Villaret A, Nicolai P, Schreiber A, Bizzoni A, Farina D, Tschabitscher M. The temporo-parietal fascial flap in extended transnasal endoscopic procedures: cadaver dissection and personal clinical experience. Eur Arch Otorhinolaryngol. 2013; 270(4):1473–1479

[33] Fortes FS, Carrau RL, Snyderman CH, et al. Transpterygoid transposition of a temporoparietal fascia flap: a new method for skull base reconstruction after endoscopic expanded endonasal approaches. Laryngoscope. 2007; 117(6):970–976

[34] Fortes FS, Carrau RL, Snyderman CH, et al. The posterior pedicle inferior turbinate flap: a new vascularized flap for skull base reconstruction. Laryngoscope. 2007; 117(8):1329–1332

[35] Oliver CL, Hackman TG, Carrau RL, et al. Palatal flap modifications allow pedicled reconstruction of the skull base. Laryngoscope. 2008; 118(12):2102–2106

[36] Rivera-Serrano CM, Oliver CL, Sok J, et al. Pedicled facial buccinator (FAB) flap: a new flap for reconstruction of skull base defects. Laryngoscope. 2010; 120 (10):1922–1930

[37] Rivera-Serrano CM, Snyderman CH, Carrau RL, Durmaz A, Gardner PA. Transparapharyngeal and transpterygoid transposition of a pedicled occipital galeopericranial flap: a new flap for skull base reconstruction. Laryngoscope. 2011; 121(5):914–922

[38] Gil Z, Abergel A, Leider-Trejo L, et al. A comprehensive algorithm for anterior skull base reconstruction after oncological resections. Skull Base. 2007; 17(1):25–37

[39] Villaret AB, Yakirevitch A, Bizzoni A, et al. Endoscopic transnasal craniectomy in the management of selected sinonasal malignancies. Am J Rhinol Allergy. 2010; 24(1):60–65

[40] Nicolai P, Battaglia P, Bignami M, et al. Endoscopic surgery for malignant tumors of the sinonasal tract and adjacent skull base: a 10-year experience. Am J Rhinol. 2008; 22(3):308–316

[41] Hanna E, DeMonte F, Ibrahim S, Roberts D, Levine N, Kupferman M. Endoscopic resection of sinonasal cancers with and without craniotomy: oncologic results. Arch Otolaryngol Head Neck Surg. 2009; 135(12):1219–1224

[42] Hanna EY, Holsinger C, DeMonte F, Kupferman M. Robotic endoscopic surgery of the skull base: a novel surgical approach. Arch Otolaryngol Head Neck Surg. 2007; 133(12):1209–1214

[43] Kupferman ME, Hanna E. Robotic surgery of the skull base. Otolaryngol Clin North Am. 2014; 47(3):415–423

[44] Kupferman ME, Demonte F, Levine N, Hanna E. Feasibility of a robotic surgical approach to reconstruct the skull base. Skull Base. 2011; 21(2):79–82

[45] Kupferman M, Demonte F, Holsinger FC, Hanna E, et al. Transantral robotic access to the pituitary gland. Otolaryngology–Head and Neck Surgery. 2009; 141(3):413–415

[46] Vural E, Hanna E. Extended lateral rhinotomy incision for total maxillectomy. Otolaryngol Head Neck Surg. 2000; 123(4):512–513

[47] DeMonte F, Hanna E. Transmaxillary exploration of the intracranial portion of the maxillary nerve in malignant perineural disease. Technical note. J Neurosurg. 2007; 107(3):672–677

[48] Essig GF, Newman SA, Levine PA. Sparing the eye in craniofacial surgery for superior nasal vault malignant neoplasms: analysis of benefit. Arch Facial Plast Surg. 2007; 9(6):406–411

[49] Dexter WS, Jacob RF. Prosthetic rehabilitation after maxillectomy and temporalis flap reconstruction: a clinical report. J Prosthet Dent. 2000; 83(3): 283–286

[50] Chang DW, Langstein HN, Gupta A, et al. Reconstructive management of cranial base defects after tumor ablation. Plast Reconstr Surg. 2001; 107(6): 1346–1355, discussion 1356–1357

17 Nasopharyngeal Carcinoma

Jimmy Yu Wai Chan

Summary

Nasopharyngeal carcinomas, which are among the most surgically challenging malignancies of the head and neck, commonly result in involvement of the skull base. Their deep location and the density of their intimately related critical neurovascular structures make their exposure and resection difficult. Advances in radiation therapy and especially concurrent chemoradiation have had a significantly positive effect on patient outcomes. A deep understanding of locoregional anatomy critically informs the surgical procedures needed for resection of these lesions. This chapter reviews the anatomy and comprehensively describes the maxillary swing approach, tumor resection, reconstruction, and complication avoidance and management.

Keywords: nasopharynx, maxillary swing approach, nasopharyngeal carcinoma

17.1 Introduction

Incidence of nasopharyngeal carcinoma (NPC) has distinct racial and geographic variations. The tumor is rare in most parts of the world, with incidence for either sex of less than 1 per 100,000 persons per year. However, it is endemic in the southern part of China, including Guangdong Province, where the incidence of NPC is among the highest in the world.[1]

NPC often demonstrates highly aggressive behavior, with extensive local tumor infiltration, early and multiple/bilateral lymph node metastasis, and a high chance of hematogenous metastasis to the bone, lungs, liver, and distant nodes. Local skull base erosion and intracranial extension are not uncommon. The tumor is sensitive to radiotherapy and has an overall survival of up to 90%, especially for patients who have early-stage disease[2]; treatment outcomes for late-stage tumors have also dramatically improved with use of concurrent chemoradiation.[3,4,5]

The overall rate of local tumor recurrence in the nasopharynx after primary treatment is approximately 10%.[6] Surgical salvage of recurrent tumors offers better overall survival and quality of life than re-irradiation does.[7,8,9] Conversely, surgical access to the nasopharynx is difficult because of its location[10] and its proximity to vital structures. Furthermore, complications of surgery, such as meningitis, extensive osteoradionecrosis of the skull base, and torrential bleeding from carotid artery blowout, are potentially life-threatening. Adequate preoperative assessment and meticulous intraoperative technique are essential to the success of surgery.

17.2 Surgical Anatomy

The nasopharynx is located at the posterior end of the nasal cavity. It is bounded superiorly by the floor of the sphenoid sinuses and by the clivus as the roof that slopes posteriorly and inferiorly (▶ Fig. 17.1). Inferiorly the nasopharynx is continuous with the oropharynx at the level of the soft palate. Anteriorly it is bounded in the midline by the posterior edge of the nasal septum and the vomer of the sphenoid bone. On each side, the nasopharynx is continuous with the nasal cavity via the

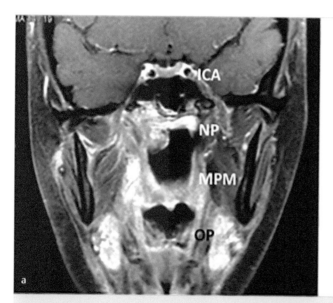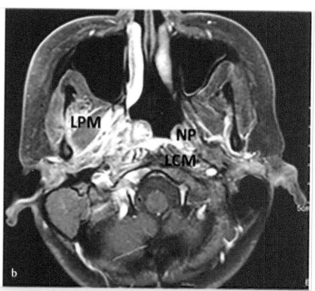

Fig. 17.1 (a) Coronal view of MRI showing the position of the internal carotid artery (ICA) in the lateral wall of the cavernous sinus. The nasopharynx (NP) is located below the floor of the sphenoid sinus, with the medial pterygoid muscle (MPM) deep to it in the parapharyngeal space. The muscle is resected en bloc with the tumor in nasopharyngectomy to ensure an adequate deep resection margin. The oropharynx (OP) is located inferior to the nasopharynx. **(b)** Axial view of MRI showing the longus capitis muscle (LCM) deep to the posterior wall of the nasopharynx. The lateral pterygoid muscle (LPM) may be infiltrated by locally advanced tumors, which may then be resected with the specimen.

choanae. Posteriorly the nasopharynx is bounded by the prevertebral muscles, the clivus, and the vertebral body of the first cervical vertebra. The lateral walls of the nasopharynx are formed by the Eustachian tube cushions on each side. The opening of the auditory tube leads to the middle ear. The auditory tube is cartilaginous in its distal third and passes into a bony canal as it traverses superiorly and laterally toward the middle ear, where it communicates on its anteroinferior wall. The levator veli palatini and the tensor veli palatini muscles are attached to the auditory tube.

The nasopharynx consists of an epithelium, deep to which is the lamina propria, followed by the superior constrictor and prevertebral muscles. The epithelium is mainly pseudostratified ciliated columnar cells, with transition to squamous cells inferiorly as it merges with the oropharynx. The lamina propria is richly filled with lymphocytes. Enveloping the nasopharynx laterally is the superior constrictor muscles. A thick fascia, the pharyngobasilar fascia, is located superior to this. This fascia lies anterior to the prevertebral muscles and its covering fascia. Laterally the pharyngobasilar fascia is continuous with the prevertebral fascia, medial to the carotid sheath, which forms the boundary of the parapharyngeal space.

Understanding of the course of the internal carotid artery is crucial to avoid inadvertent injury during nasopharyngectomy. After originating from the common carotid artery, the cervical portion of the internal carotid artery ascends about 2.5 cm posterior to the coronal plane of the pterygoid plates, lateral to the lateral pterygoid plate. It then enters the bony carotid canal of the petrous bone, where it passes medially and superiorly, making its first turn. Within this bony carotid canal, it is located posterior and medial to the auditory tube. As the internal carotid leaves the carotid canal medially, it reaches close to the lateral edge of the sphenoid sinus, where it now ascends in a medial and superior direction. Here the internal carotid artery passes posterior and above the foramen lacerum. The internal carotid artery finally enters the cranial cavity via the foramen lacerum, posterior to the anterior clinoid process. It traverses the cavernous sinus and divides into the anterior and middle cerebral arteries.

In nasopharyngectomy, depending on the extent of the tumor, the lateral resection margin often requires that the pterygoid plates be completely or partially transected. After the pterygoid plates are transected, the internal carotid artery will be in proximity. It may be identified by gently dissecting through the fibrofatty tissue in the pterygopalatine fossa and palpating for pulsation or by using intraoperative Doppler ultrasonography or MRI stereotaxy. A sheet of connective tissue, the pharyngobasilar fascia, is superficial to the internal carotid artery and must be breached before reaching the wall of the artery.

17.3 Regional Pathology and Differential Diagnosis

In endemic regions, such as South China (particularly Guangdong Province), Southeast Asia, northern circumpolar region, and the Mediterranean basin, NPC is the most common tumor arising from the nasopharynx. More than 95% of these tumors are of World Health Organization (WHO) type III (undifferentiated,

nonkeratinizing), which is associated with Epstein-Barr virus (EBV) infection. Other differential diagnosis of tumors in the region includes squamous cell carcinoma, salivary gland tumors (mucoepidermoid carcinoma, adenoid cystic carcinoma), adenocarcinoma, and sarcoma. Head and neck lymphoma may also present with tumor involving the nasopharynx.

17.4 Clinical Assessment

In endemic areas, such as South China, NPC is the most common malignancy giving rise to nasal symptoms. Symptomatology of patients suffering from NPC can be divided into four categories: (1) nasal symptoms, (2) otological symptoms, (3) cranial nerve symptoms, and (4) neck symptoms.

A patient presenting with unprovoked epistaxis on just one side should raise concern about a malignant cause. In early tumors, bleeding is usually trivial and stops spontaneously after several minutes. New-onset persistent unilateral nasal obstruction is also more worrying, as nasal obstructions that have inflammatory causes are more likely to be bilateral and episodic. NPC patients frequently experience postnasal discharge that is bloodstained. The olfaction of NPC patients, however, is rarely affected, because the nasopharynx is quite far from the cribriform plate that houses the olfaction nerves.

NPC is frequently located near the fossa of Rosenmüller, so that disturbance of Eustachian tube function is seen on one side early in the disease's progression. This disturbance causes unilateral otitis media with effusion, after which patients experience unilateral conductive hearing loss associated with low-pitch nonpulsatile tinnitus. Pasame ear. However, true otalgia and ear discharge are rare, because the tympanic membrane usually remains intact.

Neck swelling secondary to cervical lymphadenopathy is the most common presenting symptom of NPC. Up to 76% of NPC patients have enlarged cervical lymph nodes on presentation.[11] Systemic symptoms, such as anorexia and weight loss, are uncommon in NPC, and distant metastasis should be suspected if such symptoms are present.

Physical examination of the nasal cavity begins with anterior rhinoscopy by a nasal speculum, but this is usually unrevealing in NPC patients. Postnasal space mirror examination provides a satisfactory view of the region in fewer than half of patients. Otoscopy should be carried out to look for the presence of otitis media with effusion, the presence of which should warrant endoscopic examination of the nasopharynx in all adult patients. The neck should be palpated carefully to look for the presence of cervical lymphadenopathy. The most common locations of metastatic lymph nodes from NPC are level II and the apex of level V, and it is not uncommon to have bilateral nodal involvement because of the decussation of the lymphatic supply of the nasopharynx. Finally, the cranial nerves, particularly the abducent nerve and the trigeminal nerves, should be examined, as up to 20% of patients have cranial nerve palsies on presentation.[12]

In patients who have suspicious symptoms or family history of NPC, blood should be tested for EBV serology, with positive EBV serology another indication for nasal endoscopy.[13] The diagnosis of NPC is made on the basis of a positive biopsy result of the nasopharyngeal tumor visualized on nasal endoscopy.

Early tumors tend to be near the fossa of Rosenmüller, which is just medial to the Eustachian tube. In patients who have a high clinical suspicion of suffering from NPC, cross-sectional imaging such as CT or MRI of the nasopharynx should be undertaken even if initial nasal endoscopy is unrevealing, with the aim of picking up the infrequent instances of submucosal tumors in which the nasopharyngeal mucosa can remain completely smooth. A targeted deep biopsy of the submucosal tumor identified on imaging can then be done to confirm the diagnosis.

17.5 Diagnostic Imaging

MRI has taken over CT as the primary imaging tool for the staging of NPC. Tumors are isointense or hypointense on T1-weighted images (relative to muscles) and intermediate hyperintense on T2-weighted images. Modest contrast enhancement is noted, but less than that seen in normal nasopharyngeal mucosa (▶ Fig. 17.2).

Eighty-two percent of early tumors arise in the posterolateral recess of the nasopharynx, usually in the fossa of Rosenmüller.[14]

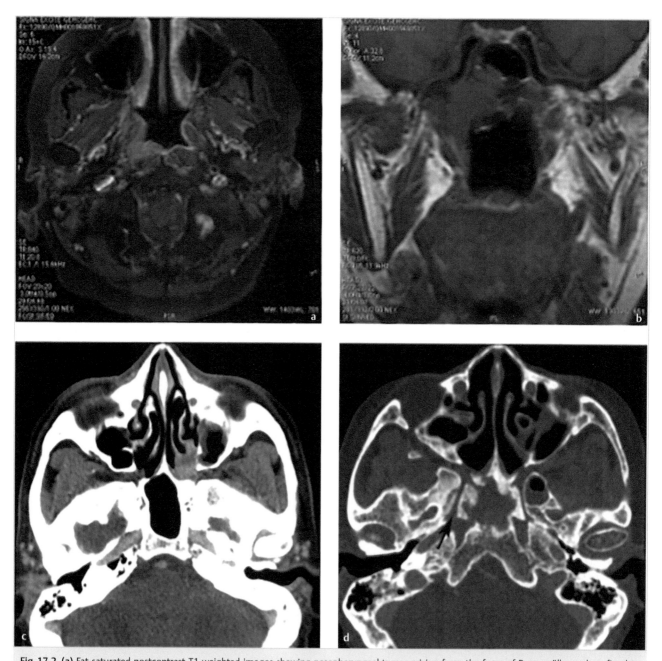

Fig. 17.2 (a) Fat-saturated postcontrast T1-weighted images showing nasopharyngeal tumor arising from the fossa of Rosenmüller and confined to the nasopharynx. (b) Tumor invading the sphenoid sinus and replacing the normal fatty marrow signal with the hypointense tumor. (c) Early tumor invasion to the left sphenopalatine foramen. (d) Tumor invasion of the right pterygopalatine fossae via the vidian canal (*arrow*) toward the foramen lacerum.

The fossa is located posterior to the torus tubarius on axial images and superior to it on the coronal images. The torus tuberous contains the cartilaginous portion of the Eustachian tube and the levator veli palatine. Anterior to the torus tubarius is the opening of Eustachian tube. Fluid collection in the middle ear cavity secondary to tumor obstruction or Eustachian tube dysfunction is commonly seen. Although ventral tumor extension to the choanal orifice is not uncommon, extensive disease extension into the nasal cavity is encountered only occasionally. Careful imaging examination of the nasal septum is essential, for tumor involving the roof of the nasopharynx may extend anteriorly to invade the septum.[15]

The retropharyngeal lymph nodes are the first echelon of nodes of lymphatic drainage of the nasopharynx. Most of them are seen at the C1/C2 level. Tumors extending posterolaterally may involve the carotid artery and the jugular and hypoglossal canal and thus affect cranial nerves IX, X, XI, and XII. Assessment of tumor involvement of the carotid is essential when planning surgery.

Locally advanced tumors have a propensity to extend superiorly and involve the base of skull. Invasion of the sphenoid sinus is common, as it is separated from the roof of the nasopharynx by only a thin plate of bone. Replacement of the normal high T1-weighted fatty marrow signal should raise suspicions of skull base involvement. The clivus, pterygoid plates, and body of the sphenoid are commonly involved (▶ Fig. 17.2). The pterygopalatine fossa can be involved with disease extension via the sphenopalatine foramen. Once the fossa is involved, disease can spread to the orbit via the inferior orbital fissure, to the infratemporal fossa via the pterygomaxillary fissure, to the middle cranial fossae via the foramen of rotundum, to the foramen of lacerum via the vidian canal, and to the oral cavity via the greater palatine foramen.

Direct invasion of the base of skull is the most common manner of intracranial tumor extension.[16] Sphenoid and the foramen of lacerum can be involved by direct tumor spread (▶ Fig. 17.3). After the foramen lacerum is involved, the tumor will be sitting next to the internal carotid artery, which runs over the superior portion of the foramen lacerum.

Cranial nerve involvement is seen in 15 to 20% of patients who have NPC.[16,17,18] Perineural spread, particularly through the mandibular division of the trigeminal nerve via the foramen ovale, has been shown to be the most common route of intracranial disease extension with the advent of MRI,[19,20] but perineural spread can also involve the maxillary division of the trigeminal nerve with tumor extending through the foramen rotundum. Perineural invasions are best seen in fat-saturated postcontrast T1-weighted MR images in the coronal plane. Cranial nerve enlargement, irregularity, excessive enhancement, and foraminal enlargement with destruction are MR features of perineural spread. Effacement of the normal intraforaminal fat signal on T1-weighted images is also suggestive of perineural tumor invasion.[21] The foramen ovale can be seen on the coronal images at and slightly ventral to the condylar head of the mandible. Dural involvement in the middle cranial fossae and involvement of the cavernous sinus and Meckel's caves should be checked as well. Tumors that invade the cavernous sinuses can lead to multiple cranial nerve palsies, including oculomotor, trochlear, and the ophthalmic and maxillary divisions of the trigeminal and the abducent nerves.

17.6 Preoperative Preparation

Before contemplating salvage nasopharyngectomy, a thorough endoscopic examination of the nasopharynx and oropharynx is important. Suspicious mucosal ulceration should be biopsied for histological confirmation of tumor recurrence. For submucosal tumors, deep biopsy is required; in some patients, biopsy under general anesthesia is indicated. Fine-needle aspiration of cervical lymph nodes is useful for nodal staging, although its

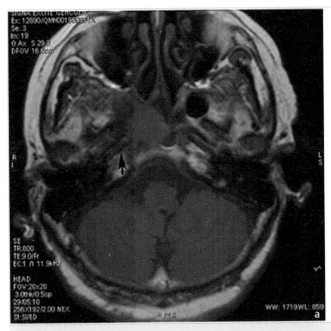 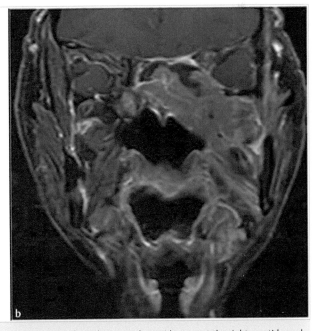

Fig. 17.3 (a) Locally advanced tumor with invasion of the right foramen lacerum. The tumor abuts the internal carotid artery at the right carotid canal (*arrow*). (b) Intracranial tumor extension via direct skull base invasion and left foramen ovale infiltration. The left cavernous sinus is involved.

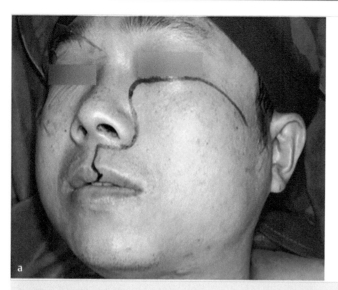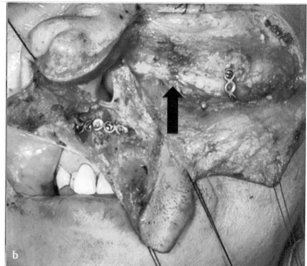

Fig. 17.4 (a) Weber-Ferguson-Longmire incision for left maxillary swing operation. **(b)** Soft tissue dissection is carried out to expose the underlying osteotomy site. The infraorbital nerve (*arrow*) is transected. The osteotomy site at the anterior wall of the maxillary antrum is defined and preplated with titanium plates and screws.

efficacy is diminished in cases of prior radiotherapy.[22] Patients are assessed for fitness of general anesthesia, with particular attention to the stability of the cervical spine in patients who have osteoradionecrosis and to the presence of hypopituitarism. The presence of trismus from previous radiotherapy, which may cause difficulty in intubation during anesthesia, should be noted. If necessary, surgeons should be available during the induction of anesthesia and should prepare for the creation of a surgical airway should intubation fail. Preoperative dental assessment is important, and an obturator should be fabricated for postoperative application.

17.7 Surgical Technique

Although early recurrent tumors in the nasopharynx can be resected using an endoscopic or transoral robotic-assisted approach, the traditional open approach offers a wide exposure that is particularly advantageous for locally advanced tumor. Among the various open approaches described, the maxillary swing approach, first described in 1991,[23] offers wide access to the ipsilateral nasopharynx and parapharyngeal space up to the infratemporal fossa. It offers access to the middle cranial base superiorly, the contralateral nasopharynx, and the oropharynx inferiorly. Exposure of the contralateral parapharyngeal space, however, is limited, so the approach is contraindicated in tumors infiltrating the contralateral parapharyngeal space.

17.8 Positioning

Patient is positioned supine, with neck extended. In general, intubation via the transnasal route is avoided to prevent trauma and bleeding from the tumor. Transoral intubation is preferred, although tracheostomy under local anesthesia should be considered in patients who have severe trismus after radiotherapy. Induction of anesthesia can subsequently be performed via the tracheostomy.

The ipsilateral eyelids are then apposed with a temporary tarsorrhaphy, with the contralateral orbital contents protected using watertight adhesives. The mid- and lower face are prepared with antiseptic solution and draped accordingly. If vastus lateralis muscle flap is indicated for reconstruction, the thigh is prepared and draped as well. The oral cavity is then cleansed with antiseptic solution.

17.9 Incision

A Weber-Ferguson-Longmire incision is placed on the side of tumor (▶ Fig. 17.4). The subciliary incision is placed 5 mm inferior to the lower lid margin. The angle between the skin incisions at the subciliary region and the nasal sidewall should not be acute, so as to avoid ischemic necrosis of the tip of the angle, which is not uncommon after previous radical radiotherapy.

A palatal incision is placed along the gingiva in a curvilinear fashion on the ipsilateral side of the hard palate. It is then gently curved behind the last molar tooth.

17.10 Soft Tissue Dissection

Soft tissue dissection after the skin incision exposes the underlying osteotomy sites. However, it is crucial not to detach soft tissues from the underlying bone/periosteum to an excessive degree, so as to maximally preserve the blood supply to the maxillary bone, thus minimizing the risk of osteonecrosis after surgery.

Soft tissue dissection starts at the upper lip. The orbicularis oris muscle is transected and the superior labial artery is ligated and divided. As the dissection is continued superiorly, part of the levator labii superioris muscle is divided. The skin at the pyriform aperture is then incised; it is important to preserve a 2- to 3-mm rim of skin from the edge of the bony aperture to allow subsequent closure. The dissection is carried out until the inferior edge of the nasal bone is exposed.

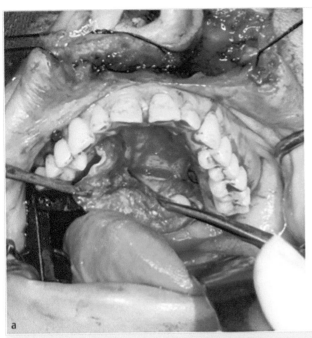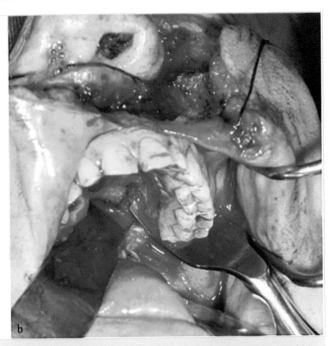

Fig. 17.5 (a) The palatal mucoperiosteal flap is prepared by making a curvilinear mucosal incision at the gingiva and performing subperiosteal dissection afterward. **(b)** The first osteotomy is performed at the pterygoid plates. The curved osteotome is placed anterior to the maxillary tuberosity, with the osteotome traveling in the cephalad direction.

The lower eyelid skin is separated from the underlying orbicularis occuli muscle by sharp dissection. The infraorbital nerve, which is located about 1 cm inferior to the infraorbital rim,[24] is identified and divided. The infraorbital foramen marks the level of the horizontal osteotomy across the maxillary bone. After defining the line of osteotomy at the body of the zygoma and the premaxillary region, the osteotomy sites are preplated at these regions using titanium miniplates, allowing restoration of the preoperative dental occlusion after the return of the maxilla on completion of surgery. The titanium plates and screws are then removed and saved for subsequent use.

At the hard palate, the curvilinear mucosal incision is made down to the underlying bone. The palatal mucosal flap is elevated at the subperiosteal plane until the midline is reached (▶ Fig. 17.5). Care must be taken, especially in patients who have torus palatinus, in whom the overlying mucosa is usually thin and thus is prone to perforation during the palatal flap dissection, increasing the risk of subsequent palatal fistula formation after surgery. The greater palatine vessels are ligated and divided to allow a complete mobilization of the palatal flap. Posterior to the last molar tooth, soft tissue is dissected until the maxillary tuberosity is exposed. The soft palate musculature is then separated from the posterior border of the ipsilateral hard palate until the midline is reached.

17.11 Bony Dissection and Osteotomies

The first osteotomy is usually performed at the pterygoid plates. A curved osteotome is placed through the mucosal incision behind the last molar tooth anterior to the maxillary tuberosity. It is important to ensure that the osteotome is

traveling horizontally in a caudal–cranial direction, lest the internal carotid artery suffer injury. In patients who have severe trismus, which prevents placement of the curved osteotome transorally, the osteotomy at the pterygoid plates must be left until the rest of the osteotomies have been performed, when a downfracture of the pterygoid plates can be performed after mobilization of the maxilla.

The second osteotomy is made just lateral to the midline at the hard palate, avoiding injury to the nasal septum. The saw blade must pass through the medial incisors, and care must be taken not to injury the dental roots. The final osteotomy is performed through the anterior wall—the body of the zygoma and the medial and lateral walls of the maxilla, at the level of the infraorbital foramen. (Bleeding can result from injury to the branches of the internal maxillary artery posteriorly.) The maxillary osteocutaneous unit is then free from bony attachment and can be swung out to expose the nasopharynx (▶ Fig. 17.6).

17.12 Tumor Resection

The tumor is exposed and its extent assessed. Nasopharyngectomy is performed with at least 1.5 cm radial margins,[25] as resection margin status is shown to be the most important independent prognostic factor in surgical outcome.[26] For small tumors arising from the fossa of Rosenmüller, the cancer is resected en bloc with the medial pterygoid muscles and the cartilaginous part of the Eustachian tube, down to the prevertebral fascia posteriorly. For tumors that have invasion of the parapharyngeal space, the surgeon must prepare wide resection of the region. All the soft tissues anteromedial to the cervical part of the internal carotid artery are resected en bloc with the tumor. To avoid injury to the internal carotid artery during tumor resection, the artery must first be identified

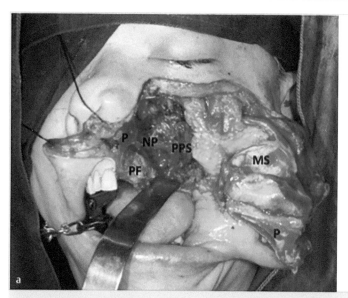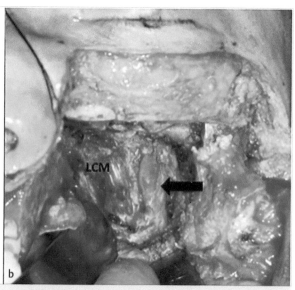

Fig. 17.6 **(a)** Left maxillary osteocutaneous unit swung out, exposing the nasopharynx (NP) and the parapharyngeal space (PPS) for tumor resection. The maxillary sinus (MS) and the bony palate (P) are shown. During osteotomy, it is important to protect the palatal mucoperiosteal flap from trauma. **(b)** For tumors that have extensive parapharyngeal invasion, the pterygoid muscles and the tumor are resected en bloc with the pharyngobasilar fascia, exposing the internal carotid artery (*arrow*) from just above the oropharynx to the skull base. The adjacent longus capitis muscle (LCM) and the clivus are often exposed after tumor extirpation.

and protected. The vessel is best identified inferiorly just above the oropharyngeal level, where there is no tumor involvement. The medial and lateral pterygoid muscles are transected until the pharyngobasilar fascia is identified and incised. The artery is located immediately underneath the fascia, where it can be identified by palpation, intraoperative Doppler ultrasound, or MRI stereotaxy. In difficult cases, it may be useful to dissect and lateralize the internal carotid artery via a transcervical route, thereby developing a plane medial to the artery and protecting it from injury during nasopharyngectomy. After identification of the artery, the dissection is performed superficial to the vessel in the cranial direction until the petrous bone is reached. For tumors close to the clivus, the surrounding bone, including the floor of the sphenoid sinuses, is resected. If necessary, the inferior portion of the bony carotid canal can be removed, exposing the petrous portion of the internal carotid artery. To avoid injury to the artery, this is usually performed under microscopic magnification.

For tumors that extend to the contralateral nasopharynx, the exposure can be improved by removing the posterior part of the nasal septum. In patients who need the nasoseptal flap for reconstruction, the flap must be prepared first and left aside for subsequent use to avoid damaging the flap during tumor exposure and resection. As already explained, the exposure of the contralateral parapharyngeal space is limited, and the contralateral internal carotid artery is at risk of injury in patients who require wide resection of tumor in the region.

17.13 Reconstruction

Soft tissue reconstruction is not necessary after nasopharyngectomy for small tumors. Reconstruction is indicated when there is exposure of the bony skull base, dura, or internal carotid

artery. For limited exposure of the clivus, the exposed bone is best resurfaced using the nasoseptal flap.[27] This a mucoperichondrial pedicled flap has blood supply based on the nasoseptal artery, a branch of the sphenopalatine artery that emerges at the sphenopalatine foramen. Horizontal incisions are made 1.5 cm inferior to the skull base and along the floor of the nasal cavity and are then joined by a vertical incision 2 cm posterior to the caudal edge of the septum. After identification of the sphenoid ostia, the mucosa is dissected from the anterior sphenoid wall while preserving its vascular pedicle to the level of the sphenopalatine foramen.

For extensive exposure of the clivus and the vertebral body of the first cervical vertebra, and for all patients who have exposure of the internal carotid artery, complete coverage of the defect is best achieved using the pedicled temporoparietal fascial flap[28] or microvascular free flaps (▶ Fig. 17.7).[29] These reconstructive strategies provide a large volume of healthy, nonirradiated tissue for secure coverage of bones, dura, cranial nerves, and blood vessels. The temporoparietal fascial flap is perfused by the anterior or posterior branch of the superficial temporal artery. The superficial soft tissue dissection is performed in the subcutaneous level immediately deep to the hair follicles. The flap passes through a tunnel that traverses the temporalis muscle, infratemporal fossa, and parapharyngeal space through a window in the posterior maxillary wall. It is important to ensure that there is no kinking or extrinsic compression on the pedicle of the flap. Microvascular free flap has the advantage of providing a large amount of healthy tissue for reconstruction, particularly after combined craniofacial resection of locally advanced tumors. It also avoids scar and depression of the temporal region of the scalp after the temporoparietal fascial flap is harvested, and the duration of the operation can be shortened by having two teams of surgeons operate simultaneously.

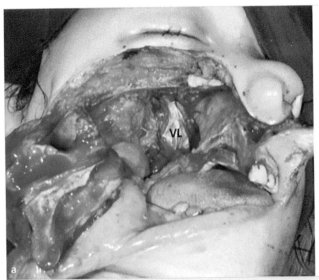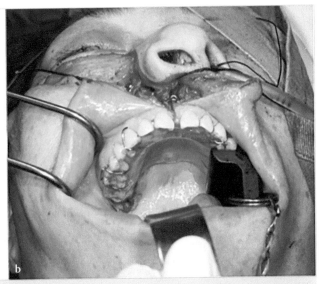

Fig. 17.7 (a) The free vastus lateralis (VL) muscle flap is used to protect the internal carotid artery and the clivus from exposure after tumor resection. Complications such as blowout bleeding and osteoradionecrosis of the skull base are prevented. (b) A prefabricated obturator is used to keep the palatal mucoperiosteal flap in situ and ensure a proper dental occlusion after surgery.

In selected patients who have tumor encasement of the cervical internal carotid artery, the ipsilateral cerebral perfusion is secured by performing an extracranial intracranial vascular bypass, using the autologous radial artery or the long saphenous vein as the vascular conduit.[30] In the neck, end-to-side anastomosis to the external carotid artery is performed, and the other end of the conduit is anastomosed in an end-to-side manner to the ipsilateral middle cerebral artery. The tumor can then be resected en bloc with the native internal carotid artery that has been invaded by the cancer.

17.14 Closure

On completion of tumor resection and reconstruction, the maxillary osteocutaneous unit is returned. A nasogastric tube is inserted. Two holes are drilled at the posterior border of the hard palate that allow the passage of stitches for fixing the soft palate to the bony hard palate. The returned maxilla is fixed with titanium plates and screws. Three-point fixation of the maxilla is achieved by adding a two-holed titanium plate at the medial anterior maxillary wall. The palatal mucoperiosteal flap is held in position by the prefabricated obturator. The facial wound is then closed in layers.

17.15 Postoperative Care

Postoperative intensive care unit admission is not necessary for the majority of patients—only those who require vascular bypass and craniofacial resection. Feeding via the nasogastric tube can commence as soon as the position of the feeding tube is confirmed. It is important to ensure the patency of the tracheostomy tube. The obturator can be removed on the first day after surgery, when the palatal mucoperiosteal flap has already adhered to the underlying hard palate. The patient receives regular chest physiotherapy and is advised to be ambulatory during the early postoperative period. The tracheostomy and

nasogastric tube can usually be weaned 5 to 6 days after surgery, and nasal douching with warm normal saline solution is started. The nasopharyngeal wound is examined endoscopically before discharge.

After extracranial intracranial vascular bypass, regular monitoring of the patency of the bypass graft is necessary. Antiplatelet agent is commenced after surgery and is maintained for 6 months afterward, although the exact duration is controversial.

17.16 Complications and Their Avoidance

Complications of maxillary swing nasopharyngectomy[31] may adversely affect quality of life after surgery.[32] Some of the complications are potentially life-threatening and should be prevented proactively during surgery.

17.16.1 Complications during the Operation

Venous Bleeding

Venous bleeding from the pterygoid plexus can be significant during the dissection of the pterygoid muscle. The pterygoid plates should be removed with diathermy and the pterygoid muscles, then plicated with sutures. Without removing the bone, stitching and applying pressure is difficult. In general, venous bleeding stops on appropriate application of adequate pressure. The returned maxilla bone, with a properly applied nasal pack, provides enough pressure to achieve venous hemostasis.

Arterial Bleeding

During dissection of tumor or lymph node in the paranasopharyngeal space, the internal carotid artery might be injured, leading to severe arterial bleeding. Pressure should be applied below the bleeding point; with wide exposure, the bleeding site might be controllable using a nonabsorbable stitch. Injury to the internal carotid artery could be avoided when the dissection is inside the tough pharyngobasilar fascia. It is advisable to perform the dissection using scissors rather than diathermy, as the injury to the vessel is usually less extensive with the former.

17.16.2 Postoperative Complications

Osteoradionecrosis

This could present as a range of problems, depending on the amount of necrotic bone (▶ Fig. 17.8), with one or more of the following potentially taking place:

- The patient might have a small amount of necrotic bone around the screws used to fix the titanium plate over the zygoma. This could be managed with removal of the screw and the titanium plate. The wound ordinarily heals with conservative treatment.
- The bone over the maxillary tuberosity is slightly removed from the anterior cheek flap and thus has less blood supply. When osteoradionecrosis took place, the patient developed a fistula between the posterior nasal cavity and the oral cavity. Because it is not along the main pathway of food ingestion, swallowing is only partly affected. Wearing a dental plate to cover the fistula will help swallowing. This fistula can be closed later using local tissue.
- When the maxillary swing procedure was initially reported, the split of the mucoperiosteum over the hard palate and the osteotomy over the hard plate was in the same plane.[23] As a result, approximately 20% of patients developed palatal fistula that affected swallowing, especially of fluids. Wearing a dental plate can significantly help oral intake, and a palatal fistula can be closed using the palatal flap based on the greater palatine vessel from the contralateral side of the swung maxilla. With the modification of the incision over the palate and the elevation of the palatal flap, the incision of the mucoperiosteum over the hard palate and the osteotomy of the hard palate are no longer in the same plane, so that this complication of palatal fistula can be avoided in nearly all patients.[33]

- A few patients may develop an extensive area of osteoradionecrosis at the skull base, and with infection this might extend intracranially, leading to meningitis. Early recognition of the problem, together with adequate debridement of necrotic tissue followed by reconstruction of the defect using a microvascular free flap, is essential for salvage. To avoid osteoradionecrosis, all exposed bone should be covered by soft tissue at the completion of operation. The mucosa of the inferior turbinate is used as a new graft to cover the exposed bone resulting from tumor resection and is usually adequate for this purpose. Occasionally, after extensive resection involving exposed bone and the internal carotid artery, a microvascular free flap, preferably a free muscle flap, should be done before the maxilla is returned.

Trismus

Another frequently encountered problem is trismus, which is more often encountered in patients who have had previous radiotherapy. It is mostly related to the contracture of, and scar formation around, the pterygoid muscles. Even with the division of the temporalis muscle insertion on the coronoid process of the mandible during the maxillary swing procedure, a degree of trismus can remain. Trismus responds to passive mechanical stretching; when the interalveolar distance reaches 2 cm, normal oral feeding is usually possible.

Facial Scar Contracture

Occasionally a patient may develop ectropion and thus also conjunctivitis when contracture of the scar along the lower eyelid pulls down the eyelid. Revision of this scar, together with the placement of a small piece of full-thickness skin graft to allow the lower eyelid to return, will solve the problem. Scar contraction in the midline over the lip leads to contraction of the lip and exposure of the upper incisors.

Epiphora

Some patients develop epiphora in the early postoperative period as a result of the transection of the lacrimal duct within the maxilla bone during the osteotomy of the medial wall of

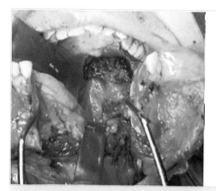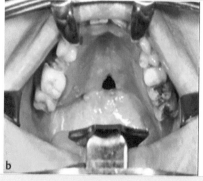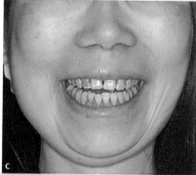

Fig. 17.8 (a) Patient with extensive exposure and necrosis of the clivus and the body of the first cervical vertebra, presenting with meningitis and blowout bleeding from the left internal carotid artery. **(b)** Long-term result after ischemic necrosis of the palatal flap showing scar contracture and the formation of oronasal fistula. **(c)** Severe trismus after nasopharyngectomy, which is particularly common in patients who require extensive dissection of the parapharyngeal space. Early jaw mobilization exercise is effective in the prevention of trismus after surgery.

the maxilla while carrying out the maxillary swing. Because the lacrimal duct is adherent to the bony canal wall, stenosis is uncommon. When the edema at the divided lacrimal duct has subsided, the epiphora decreases; in most patients the symptoms become less noticeable after 6 months.

Serous Otitis Media

When the resection of the primary pathology must include the cartilaginous orifice of the auditory tympanic tube, such as in cases of recurrent or persistent NPC, the patient will develop serous otitis media. The patient will then experience decreased hearing acuity because of the accumulation of fluid in the middle ear on the side of the swing. Myringotomy and insertion of ventilation tube will release the fluid and restore hearing. Patients who have had previous radiotherapy might have increased incidence of perforated tympanic membrane, persistent otorrhea, and later decrease in hearing acuity.[34] In these patients, if serous otitis media is left undisturbed, the patient can still use a hearing aid. In the unlikely event that the patient develops otalgia, a myringotomy is indicated.[35] More recently, internal stenting of the Eustachian tube[36] is used to prevent the development of middle ear effusion and has been shown to be effective in alleviating the symptoms of aural fullness and conductive hearing loss after maxillary swing nasopharyngectomy.

17.17 Follow-up and Rehabilitation

Patients are followed up regularly and indefinitely after salvage surgery for recurrent NPC. After discharge from the hospital, patients attend frequent training sessions with the physiotherapist and speech therapist. Jaw-opening exercise is commenced early, and trismus is preventable in most patients. Swallowing exercises improve swallowing and prevent aspiration of food into the trachea, which may occasionally develop in some patients during the early postoperative period.

Patients are followed up for detection of tumor recurrence or development of second malignancy, including squamous cell carcinoma or sarcoma. Regular endoscopic examination and biopsy of suspicious lesions, plasma EBV DNA, and contrast MRI of the skull base down to the neck region are useful.

17.18 Conclusion

Surgical access to the nasopharynx is challenging because of the deep-seated location and complicated anatomy of the region. Surgeons must understand the anatomy and choose the best surgical approach for individual patients. The maxillary swing approach offers a wide exposure that is advantageous for the management of locally advanced tumor in the region.

References

[1] Luo J, Chia KS, Chia SE, Reilly M, Tan CS, Ye W. Secular trends of nasopharyngeal carcinoma incidence in Singapore, Hong Kong and Los Angeles Chinese populations, 1973–1997. Eur J Epidemiol. 2007; 22(8):513–521

[2] Lee AW, Sze WM, Au JS, et al. Treatment results for nasopharyngeal carcinoma in the modern era: the Hong Kong experience. Int J Radiat Oncol Biol Phys. 2005; 61(4):1107–1116

[3] Al-Sarraf M, LeBlanc M, Giri PG, et al. Chemoradiotherapy versus radiotherapy in patients with advanced nasopharyngeal cancer: phase III randomized Intergroup study 0099. J Clin Oncol. 1998; 16(4):1310–1317

[4] Lee AW, Lau WH, Tung SY, et al. Hong Kong Nasopharyngeal Cancer Study Group. Preliminary results of a randomized study on therapeutic gain by concurrent chemotherapy for regionally-advanced nasopharyngeal carcinoma: NPC-9901 Trial by the Hong Kong Nasopharyngeal Cancer Study Group. J Clin Oncol. 2005; 23(28):6966–6975

[5] Lee AW, Tung SY, Chan AT, et al. Preliminary results of a randomized study (NPC-9902 Trial) on therapeutic gain by concurrent chemotherapy and/or accelerated fractionation for locally advanced nasopharyngeal carcinoma. Int J Radiat Oncol Biol Phys. 2006; 66(1):142–151

[6] Yu KH, Leung SF, Tung SY, et al. Hong Kong Nasopharyngeal Carcinoma Study Group. Survival outcome of patients with nasopharyngeal carcinoma with first local failure: a study by the Hong Kong Nasopharyngeal Carcinoma Study Group. Head Neck. 2005; 27(5):397–405

[7] You R, Zou X, Hua YJ, et al. Salvage endoscopic nasopharyngectomy is superior to intensity-modulated radiation therapy for local recurrence of selected T1-T3 nasopharyngeal carcinoma—a case-matched comparison. Radiother Oncol. 2015; 115(3):399–406

[8] Fee WE, Jr, Moir MS, Choi EC, Goffinet D. Nasopharyngectomy for recurrent nasopharyngeal cancer: a 2- to 17-year follow-up. Arch Otolaryngol Head Neck Surg. 2002; 128(3):280–284

[9] Chang KP, Hao SP, Tsang NM, Ueng SH. Salvage surgery for locally recurrent nasopharyngeal carcinoma—a 10-year experience. Otolaryngol Head Neck Surg. 2004; 131(4):497–502

[10] Wilson CP. The approach to the nasopharynx. Proc R Soc Med. 1951; 44(5):353–358

[11] Wei WI, Sham JST. Nasopharyngeal carcinoma. Lancet. 2005; 365(9476):2041–2054

[12] Lee AW, Foo W, Law SC, et al. Nasopharyngeal carcinoma: presenting symptoms and duration before diagnosis. Hong Kong Med J. 1997; 3(4):355–361

[13] Wei WI, Kwong DLW. Current management strategy of nasopharyngeal carcinoma. Clin Exp Otorhinolaryngol. 2010; 3(1):1–12

[14] Slootweg PJ, Richardson M. Squamous cell carcinoma of the upper aerodigestive system. In: Gnepp DR, ed. Diagnostic Surgical Pathology of the Head and Neck. Philadelphia: Saunders; 2001:19–29

[15] King AD, Bhatia KS. Magnetic resonance imaging staging of nasopharyngeal carcinoma in the head and neck. World J Radiol. 2010; 2(5):159–165

[16] Sham JS, Cheung YK, Choy D, Chan FL, Leong L. Cranial nerve involvement and base of the skull erosion in nasopharyngeal carcinoma. Cancer. 1991; 68(2):422–426

[17] King AD, Leung SF, Teo P, Lam WW, Chan YL, Metreweli C. Hypoglossal nerve palsy in nasopharyngeal carcinoma. Head Neck. 1999; 21(7):614–619

[18] Mineura K, Kowada M, Tomura N. Perineural extension of nasopharyngeal carcinoma into the posterior cranial fossa detected by magnetic resonance imaging. Clin Imaging. 1991; 15(3):172–175

[19] Chong VF, Fan YF, Khoo JB. Nasopharyngeal carcinoma with intracranial spread: CT and MR characteristics. J Comput Assist Tomogr. 1996; 20(4):563–569

[20] Su CY, Lui CC. Perineural invasion of the trigeminal nerve in patients with nasopharyngeal carcinoma. Imaging and clinical correlations. Cancer. 1996; 78(10):2063–2069

[21] Gandhi D, Gujar S, Mukherji SK. Magnetic resonance imaging of perineural spread of head and neck malignancies. Top Magn Reson Imaging. 2004; 15(2):79–85

[22] Chan YW, Lee VH, Chow VL, To VS, Wei WI. Extracapsular lymph node spread in recurrent nasopharyngeal carcinoma. Laryngoscope. 2011; 121(12):2576–2580

[23] Wei WI, Lam KH, Sham JS. New approach to the nasopharynx: the maxillary swing approach. Head Neck. 1991; 13(3):200–207

[24] Liu HL, Chan YW, Ng RWM, Wei WI. The clinical landmark of infraorbital foramen in Chinese population: a prospective measurement study. Eur J Plast Surg. 2014; 37(10):517–522

[25] Chan JY, Wong ST, Wei WI. Whole-organ histopathological study of recurrent nasopharyngeal carcinoma. Laryngoscope. 2014; 124(2):446–450

[26] Chan JY, Wei WI. Impact of resection margin status on outcome after salvage nasopharyngectomy for recurrent nasopharyngeal carcinoma. Head Neck. 2016; 38 Suppl 1:E594–E599

[27] El-Sayed IH, Roediger FC, Goldberg AN, Parsa AT, McDermott MW. Endoscopic reconstruction of skull base defects with the nasal septal flap. Skull Base. 2008; 18(6):385–394

[28] Veyrat M, Verillaud B, Herman P, Bresson D. How I do it: the pedicled temporoparietal fascia flap for skull base reconstruction after endonasal endoscopic approaches. Acta Neurochir (Wien). 2016; 158(12):2291–2294

[29] Chan JY, Chow VL, Tsang R, Wei WI. Nasopharyngectomy for locally advanced recurrent nasopharyngeal carcinoma: exploring the limits. Head Neck. 2012; 34(7):923–928

[30] Chan JY, Wong ST, Chan RC, Wei WI. Extracranial/intracranial vascular bypass and craniofacial resection: new hope for patients with locally advanced recurrent nasopharyngeal carcinoma. Head Neck. 2016; 38 Suppl 1:E1404–E1412

[31] Chan JY, Tsang RK, Wei WI. Morbidities after maxillary swing nasopharyngectomy for recurrent nasopharyngeal carcinoma. Head Neck. 2015; 37(4): 487–492

[32] Chan YW, Chow VL, Wei WI. Quality of life of patients after salvage nasopharyngectomy for recurrent nasopharyngeal carcinoma. Cancer. 2012; 118(15): 3710–3718

[33] Ng RW, Wei WI. Elimination of palatal fistula after the maxillary swing procedure. Head Neck. 2005; 27(7):608–612

[34] Wei WI, Engzell UC, Lam KH, Lau SK. The efficacy of myringotomy and ventilation tube insertion in middle-ear effusions in patients with nasopharyngeal carcinoma. Laryngoscope. 1987; 97(11):1295–1298

[35] Ho AC, Chan JY, Ng RW, Ho WK, Wei WI. The role of myringotomy and ventilation tube insertion in maxillary swing approach nasopharyngectomy: review of our 10-year experience. Laryngoscope. 2013; 123(2): 376–380

[36] Ho AC, Chan JY, Ng RW, Ho WK, Wei WI. Stenting of the Eustachian tube to prevent otitis media with effusion after maxillary swing approach nasopharyngectomy. Laryngoscope. 2014; 124(1):139–144

18 Clival Tumors

Franco DeMonte, Shaan M. Raza, Michael E. Kupferman, Shirley Su, Marc-Elie Nader, Paul W. Gidley, and Ehab Y. Hanna

Summary

Clival tumors are among the most challenging of all neoplasms affecting the skull base. Their deep central location and the density of their intimately related critical neurovascular structures make their exposure and resection difficult. Advances in visualization technology and endoscopic microinstrumentation have significantly changed the surgical approaches to these tumors. Approaches that translocate or remove craniofacial structures are no longer used, having been supplanted by endonasal endoscopic approaches. At times these anterior approaches need to be supplemented by lateral or posterolateral approaches to achieve maximal resection, which is the most critical predictor of patient outcome. This chapter reviews regional surgical anatomy and surgical approaches to the clivus, with particular attention to the endonasal endoscopic approaches and the transcondylar approaches.

Keywords: clivus, chordoma, endonasal endoscopic transclival and transpterygoid approaches, anterior and posterior transcondylar approaches

18.1 Introduction

This chapter focuses on the surgical treatment of clival tumors. Because clival chordoma is the archetypal tumor in this location, specific comments regarding this tumor type will be made. Irrespective of the pathology, the bone of the clivus may be infiltrated by tumor and require resection beyond the grossly visible tumor margin. The majority of tumors in this location are large at diagnosis and extend to the anterior cranial fossa or parasellar region; ventrally into the nasal cavity, paranasal sinuses, or nasopharynx; or to the middle fossa.

18.2 Surgical Anatomy

The clivus is formed from the part of the basilar occipital bone that extends anteriorly and superiorly from the foramen magnum and from the body of the sphenoid bone. These two bones articulate at the spheno-occipital synchondrosis. The clivus thus extends from the dorsum sella and the posterior clinoid processes to the foramen magnum. At its superior aspect the clivus is bordered laterally by the petroclival fissure synchondrosis) and the petrous temporal bone. The petroclival fissure terminates in the jugular foramen posterolaterally. The pharyngeal tubercle located on the anterior and inferior surface of the clivus is the site of attachment of the pharyngeal raphe and the anterior longitudinal ligament. Laterally, the supracondylar groove marks the location of the underlying hypoglossal canal. A rich venous plexus exists between the periosteal and meningeal layers of the clival dura. The inferior petrosal sinus runs along the petroclival fissure and connects the clival venous plexus and the posterior cavernous sinus to the jugular bulb. The abducens nerve penetrates the inferior petrosal sinus at Dorello's canal, at the lateral limits of the midclivus, and courses

superiorly medial to the petrous apex to enter the posterior cavernous sinus. The foramen lacerum and the internal carotid artery are at the level of the floor of the sphenoid sinus and are identified surgically by following the vidian canal superiorly and laterally. Mobilization of the Eustachian tube allows access to the inferoventral clivus and petroclival fissure to the jugular foramen. The medulla, pons, and midbrain and the vertebrobasilar arterial tree lie directly behind the clivus. The posterolateral aspects of the basiocciput form the occipital condyles and transmit the hypoglossal nerves.[1,12,13,18]

18.3 Diagnostic Imaging, Regional Pathology, and Differential Diagnosis

High-resolution CT scanning allows the accurate assessment of bony destruction by the tumor, which is universally present in chordomas (▶ Fig. 18.1).[40] Integrity of the optic and carotid canals can be best assessed in this way. Tumoral calcification is well seen if present. If there is a question of occipitocervical instability, plain X-ray films of the cervical spine, both in flexion and extension, are performed.

Multiplanar MRI with and without contrast enhancement best demonstrates the extent of the tumor and best identifies important adjacent neurovascular structures, such as brainstem, optic nerves and chiasm, and internal carotid and basilar

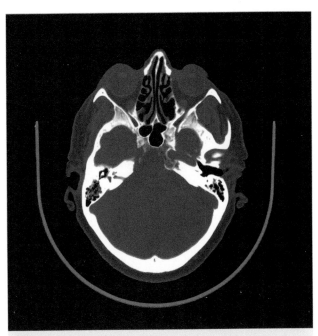

Fig. 18.1 Axial CT scan with bone windowing in a patient who has clival chordoma. Note the destruction of the central portion of the clivus with a loss of the cortical bone and islands of calcification within the tumor. (Courtesy of the Department of Neurosurgery, MD Anderson Cancer Center.)

arteries. Fat-suppression techniques highlight tumoral contrast enhancement within or adjacent to fatty areas such as the orbits and bone marrow.[39,40]

CT angiography is very valuable in the assessment and surgical management of clival tumors. It accurately visualizes the relationships of the internal carotid artery (ICA) to the tumor and the tumor-infiltrated bone of the clivus. Along with pre-operative volumetric MRI, it is typically coregistered and imported into intraoperative navigational devices so as to aid anatomic navigation of the central skull base.

Cerebral angiography is not typically necessary for the diagnosis of clival tumors; it is used when a detailed view of the head and neck and intracranial vasculature is desired. Important anatomic variations are noted, such as the pattern of venous drainage or the integrity of the circle of Willis. Vascular distortion and narrowing are well identified. Preoperative temporary balloon occlusion testing of the ICA may be performed if ICA occlusion or sacrifice is planned or if risk of arterial injury is deemed high. One or more complementary investigations of cerebrovascular reserve, such as transcranial Doppler, cerebral blood flow, or single-photon emission CT, may be used in conjunction with the temporary balloon occlusion test.

The differential diagnosis of an invasive clival mass includes chordoma, chondrosarcoma (although these tumors are usually found in a paramedian location), pituitary adenoma, metastasis, meningioma, nasopharyngeal carcinoma, plasmacytoma, and primary sphenoid sinus malignancy.

On conventional spin echo T1-weighted MRI, chordoma produces an intermediate to low signal intensity and is easily recognized amid the high signal intensity of the fat within the marrow of the clivus. Occasionally small foci of hyperintensity may be seen within the tumor on T1-weighted sequences. This finding may represent either intratumoral hemorrhage or mucin production by the tumor. T2-weighted MRI usually demonstrates high signal as a result of the high fluid content of the vacuolated cellular components. Areas within the tumor containing calcium, hemorrhage, or densely proteinaceous mucus will most often produce T2 hypointensity. Interlaced low-intensity septations separating high-signal intensity lobules are commonly visualized

and correspond to the multilobular gross morphology of the tumor. Contrast enhancement is seen in the majority of chordomas and ranges from moderate to marked. The enhancement pattern of the tumor is often described as a "honeycomb" appearance that is created by intratumoral areas of low signal intensity (▶ Fig. 18.2). Fat-suppressed images are useful for differentiating enhanced tumor margins from adjacent bright fatty bone marrow.[39,40]

As opposed to intracranial chordomas, which have a predilection for the midline of the skull base, the majority of chondrosarcomas are located more laterally along the petroclival fissure. Chondrosarcomas may, however, have a midline origin that makes preoperative differentiation from chordoma more challenging, as both have similar signal intensity on T1- and T2-weighted MR images (▶ Fig. 18.3). Chondrosarcoma can sometimes be distinguished by the presence of linear, globular, or arclike matrix calcifications best identified on CT imaging.

Clival meningiomas represent another small subset of the pathologies encountered in this area. On MRI they appear as a well-circumscribed avidly and homogeneously contrast-enhancing mass with a dural attachment. They do not have the bony destruction associated with chordomas but may be associated with hyperostosis.

Nasopharyngeal cancers, including nasopharyngeal carcinoma, lymphoma and plasmacytomas, must always be considered in the differential for clival chordoma. They usually extend more anteriorly and may be associated with head and neck lymphadenopathy. These masses may produce lytic destruction of the skull base as well, which when centrally located may produce imaging that exactly mimics clival chordoma. Most of these tumors tend to be of low to intermediate signal intensity on T2-weighted imaging.

Pituitary macroadenomas may at times appear to involve and/or originate from the clivus. The inability to identify the pituitary gland in the presence of a large clival mass should raise the possibility of pituitary macroadenoma. A markedly elevated serum prolactin level may obviate the need for biopsy or resection.

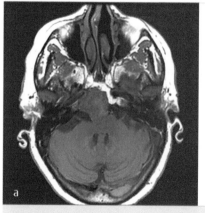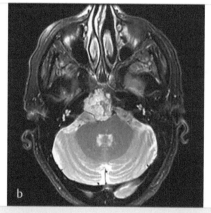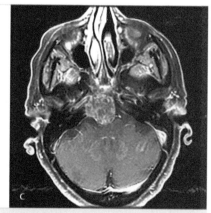

Fig. 18.2 **(a)** Axial T1-weighted MRI. **(b)** Axial T2-weighted MRI. **(c)** Axial T1-weighted postcontrast MRI of the skull base in a patient who has a left lower clival chordoma with extension to the cervicomedullary junction. On precontrast T1-weighted imaging, note the loss of the marrow fat signal in the lower left clivus. The tumor is isointense to brain on T1-weighted imaging. On T2-weighted imaging the tumor is bright, but there are areas of heterogeneity within the tumor that are of lesser signal intensity. After contrast administration, only mild contrast enhancement is identified. (Courtesy of the Department of Neurosurgery, MD Anderson Cancer Center.)

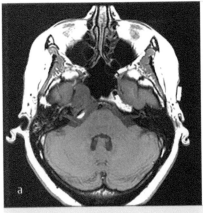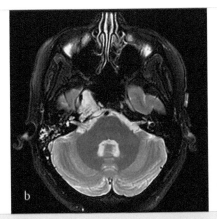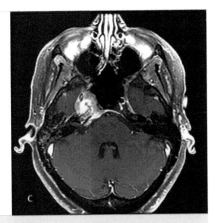

Fig. 18.3 **(a)** Axial T1-weighted MRI. **(b)** Axial T2-weighted MRI. **(c)** Postcontrast T1-weighted MRI of a patient who has a right skull base chondrosarcoma. On T1-weighted imaging the tumor is of decreased signal intensity. Note the loss of marrow fat in the right petrous apex. On T2-weighted imaging the lesion is homogenously of high signal—slightly unusual for chondrosarcoma, which tends to have more of a heterogenous T2-signal, similar to chordoma. There is moderate to marked homogenous enhancement after contrast administration. (Courtesy of the Department of Neurosurgery, MD Anderson Cancer Center.)

Table 18.1 Symptoms of clival tumors based on site of origin

Upper clivus	Pituitary endocrinopathy, visual loss, chiasmal syndrome, cavernous sinus syndrome
Midclivus	Nasopharyngeal mass, abducens nerve palsy, multiple cranial neuropathies, brainstem syndrome, hydrocephalus, cerebellopontine angle syndrome
Lower clivus	Hypoglossal nerve palsy, foramen magnum syndrome

Rhabdomyosarcoma represents another pathology that in children may develop in the clival region. This lesion takes origin in the nasopharynx and manifests as a large, bulky intra- and extracranial tumor with associated lytic osseous destruction of the skull base.

18.4 Clinical Assessment

All patients have a complete history and physical examination, including a neuro-ophthalmologic evaluation, which assesses visual acuity and fields, pupillary function, and ocular motility. Less than a third of these patients have a normal neuro-ophthalmological exam. Patients who have upper clival tumors undergo a complete endocrinologic assessment to identify evidence of pituitary or hypothalamic dysfunction. Patients who have mid- to lower clival tumors are assessed by an otolaryngologist with specific attention to hearing and lower cranial nerve (CN) function. An audiogram and direct laryngoscopy are usually performed.

The symptoms resulting from clival tumors depend on the specific sites of their extension (▶ Table 18.1). The most common manifestation is a headache in the occipital or occipito-cervical area, which may be aggravated by changes in neck position. Diplopia, the initial symptom experienced by most patients, is almost always the result of abducens neuropathy. Larger tumors may produce additional CN palsies manifesting as decreased visual acuity, facial weakness or numbness, hearing loss, dysphagia, and dysphonia. When tumors enlarge and produce brainstem or cerebellar compression, patients may develop ataxia, dysmetria, and motor weakness. When tumor

extends into the retropharyngeal space or the nasal cavity, symptoms such as nasal obstruction, epistaxis, and throat fullness may develop.

18.5 Surgical Management

Numerous surgical approaches have been used to access the clivus. The choice of one approach over another should factor in the parameters of tumor location, size, and extension; unique patient anatomy and functional requirements; and the experience, expertise, and preferences of the surgical team. Small, midline upper clival tumors without lateral extension, for example, are probably best removed through an endoscopic transsphenoidal approach, whereas large tumors having lateral and intradural extensions may require both an endoscopic and an intracranial approach for adequate tumor removal. The advent of high-resolution cameras and the development of appropriate endoscopic microsurgical tools has supplanted the need for many of the open approaches traditionally used to access the central skull base. We no longer perform transfacial approaches and craniofacial translocations simply for tumor access but rather do so only when tumor resection requires the removal of tissues along these corridors. ▶ Table 18.2 lists the various surgical approaches traditionally used for clival tumor resection as well as the approaches currently used by our surgical team. The endonasal endoscopic approach to the clivus, and the transcondylar approaches, will be dealt with in detail.

18.6 Transsphenoidal (Microscopic) Approach

The transsphenoidal approach works well for smaller tumors located in the upper and middle clivus. Excellent exposure of the sphenoid sinus, sella turcica, and upper and middle clivus is possible.[37] It has the disadvantages of limited inferior and lateral exposure, although the lateral exposure can be improved by entry into the medial maxillary sinus and removal of the pterygoid plate. The surgical field is typically deep and narrow,

Table 18.2 Surgical approaches to the clivus

Historical	Current
Transsphenoidal (microscopic)	Endonasal, endoscopic, transclival, and transpterygoid
Transsphenoethmoidal	
Transmaxillary	
Transoral/transpalatal	
Transmandibular	
Transbasal (biorbital frontal)	
Transtemporal—anterior (Kawase's)	Transtemporal—anterior (Kawase's)
Transtemporal—posterior (petrosal)	Transtemporal—posterior (petrosal)
Transcondylar—anterior	Transcondylar—anterior
Transcondylar—posterior	Transcondylar—posterior

so there is little room available for aggressive bone resection.[35] This approach has essentially been replaced by the endoscopic endonasal transsphenoidal approach, which offers greatly improved visualization, ease of expansion, and freedom of surgical movement.

18.7 Transsphenoethmoidal Approach

To expand the exposure offered by the microscopic transsphenoidal approach, an external ethmoidectomy with or without a medial maxillectomy was employed. Lalwani et al found this approach to be "adequate for the majority of tumors and disease processes present in the sphenoid sinus and clivus."[33] Addition of medial maxillectomy in instances of a narrow ethmoid sinus or inferiorly extending tumor allows improved access. Disadvantages include the necessity for facial incision and the limited exposure. The inferior limits can be extended by a medial maxillectomy as already described, but lateral reach is limited to approximately 2 cm from the midline.

18.8 Transoral–Transpalatal

After placement of an appropriate oral retractor system, the posterior pharyngeal wall and soft palate are divided to expose the clivus and upper cervical spine. Relatively limited exposure is obtained using this approach, which is most commonly employed for odontoidectomy.[15] It is adequate for tumor biopsy or in the case of small lower clival tumors, but repair of intraoperative cerebrospinal fluid (CSF) leakage is problematic. Although fat and/or fascial tissue can be placed posterior to the pharyngeal wall, the pharyngeal wall rarely approximates well, and gaps are common, thus increasing the risk of CSF leakage. The transoral–transpalatal approach should not be the primary approach to intradural lesions at the foramen magnum unless other approaches prove ineffective.[38]

18.9 Transmaxillary Approaches

The transmaxillary approaches may prove useful for clival tumors that extend into the nasopharynx or craniocervical junction with minimal lateral extension. Numerous variations of this approach have been described. Most are based on a Le Fort I osteotomy with or without midline splitting of the hard and soft palates or a unilateral maxillotomy with median or paramedian splitting of the hard and soft palates.[5,11,27,50] In the past, we preferred to avoid displacing or sectioning the palate and alveolar arch.[13,14,41,42] Access to the maxilla was obtained via a facial degloving approach or through a lateral rhinotomy with lip split.[13,49] Lateral exposure is limited by the pterygoid plates, the ICA at the level of the foramen lacerum and cavernous sinus, the hypoglossal canal, and the jugular foramen. Removal of the pterygoid plates allows access to the infratemporal fossa (ITF).[17,43]

Disadvantages of the transmaxillary approaches include the risk of ischemic osteonecrosis with multisegment osteotomies. This risk can be minimized by subtotally splitting the soft palate if palatal osteotomies are necessary and by leaving wide soft tissue attachments to freed maxillary compartments during swing procedures, or it can be avoided entirely by using transantral approaches. The principal disadvantage of the transmaxillary approach, however, is the inability to reliably stop CSF leakage. Direct repair of the dura is rarely possible and must rely on packing with fat, fascia, and fibrin glue without firm tissue available as a support to hold the repair in place. Elevation and use of vascularized mucosal flaps (septal, nasal, or turbinate) helps with healing and reduces CSF leak rate. Currently our only indication for this approach is the need to surgically resect the maxillary sinus in the presence of malignancy.

18.10 Transmandibular, Circumglossal, Retropharyngeal, Transpalatal Approach to Clivus and Upper Cervical Spine

Initially described by Biller et al and popularized by Krespi, and later by Ammirati, the transmandibular approach to the skull base provides simultaneous exposure of the middle and lateral compartments of the skull base, allows excellent vascular control and access to CNs IX to XII, and by straightforward expansion allows exposure that extends from the ipsilateral ITF to the contralateral medial pterygoid plate, from the anterior cranial fossa to the lower clivus and the anterior cervical spine down to C7 (▶ Fig. 18.4).[2,3,6, 16,30,31,32] The main indications for this approach are large tumors involving both the middle and lateral compartments and tumors of the craniocervical junction and upper cervical spine, where wide resection of soft tissue and bone is required.

A good deal of anatomic dissection is required for this approach, which results in predictable morbidity. A temporary tracheostomy is required. Conductive hearing loss and serous otitis media result from section of the Eustachian tube. Temporary swallowing difficulties induced by the circumglossal and palatal incisions, the extensive retropharyngeal dissection, and the section of the tensor and levator pallatini muscles occasionally necessitate the insertion of a gastrostomy. Preoperative consultation with dentistry should be obtained to fashion a palatal stent with which to support the palatal mucosa after closure. This stent allows for improved apposition of the mucosa against the residual hard palate, helping prevent acute mucosal loss.

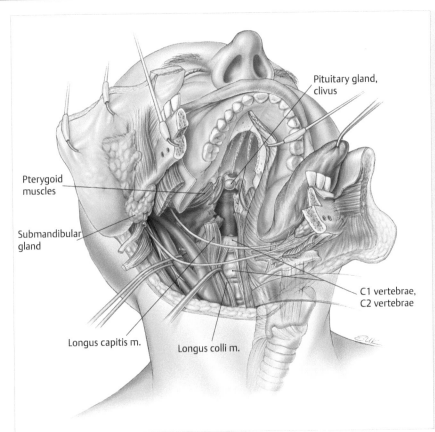

Pituitary gland, clivus

Pterygoid muscles

Submandibular gland

C1 vertebrae, C2 vertebrae

Longus capitis m.

Longus colli m.

Fig. 18.4 Artist's representation of the transmandibular approach to the clivus after clivectomy. The bone has been removed from the sella and the undersides of the optic nerves. Bone removal can continue inferiorly down to the foramen magnum. At this point it can be extended laterally to the hypoglossal canals bilaterally. (Courtesy of the Department of Neurosurgery, MD Anderson Cancer Center.)

Because of this inherent morbidity, long and careful consideration should be given to the use of this approach, which should be reserved for instances in which surgical cure or significant palliation are likely.[16] As noted, this approach is no longer used as a means of access to the clivus: the endoscopic approaches, at times in combination with posterolateral approaches, have obviated the need for this extensive operation (▶ Fig. 18.5).

18.11 Extended Transbasal Approach

Developed by Tessier and Derome, the transbasal approach to the clivus was subsequently modified to incorporate orbital osteotomies in an effort to reduce frontal lobe retraction and to allow exposure of more posteriorly and laterally related structures such as the medial walls of the cavernous sinus and the hypoglossal canals.[5,19,20,21,28,44,48] The approach consists of bifrontal craniotomy, bilateral orbital osteotomy (removal of supraorbital bar), ethmoidectomy, sphenoidectomy, and the extradural resection of the clivus. The limits of exposure are the foramen magnum inferiorly and the hypoglossal canals inferolaterally; the intracavernous carotid arteries form the superolateral limits. The posterior clinoids, dorsum sella, and the region behind and above the pituitary gland are obscured by the gland, making this a blind area when using the extended transbasal approach. The endoscopic approaches to the clivus have eliminated the use of this approach by offering improved visualization and access to the entire clivus without the need to manipulate the frontal lobes of the brain.

18.12 Transpetrous Approaches

In the presence of clival tumors with lateral extensions beyond the ICA or jugular foramen, adequate access for tumor resection may necessitate the use of a variety of transpetrous approaches. The amount of petrous bone resection is tailored to the location of the tumor. Anterior, posterior, or, rarely, total petrosectomy may be necessary.

An anterior petrosectomy will access tumor extensions in and around the petroclival synchondrosis, the posterior cavernous sinus, and the prepontine and cerebellopontine cisterns. The limits of bone removal include the carotid canal laterally, the superior petrosal sinus medially, the inferior petrosal sinus inferiorly, and the internal auditory canal and cochlea posteriorly.[29] Sacrifice of the mandibular nerve and anterolateral displacement of the ICA allows further inferior exposure of the clivus.[26,47] Although a few appropriately located small tumors can be resected through this surgical corridor, an anterior-based approach is typically required as a second stage for tumor extensions superolateral to the internal carotid artery.

Of the posterior transpetrous approaches, the petrosal or subtemporal–retrolabyrinthine approach is best suited for large posterolateral intradural tumor extensions, whereas the ITF approach can be used for both extra and intradural tumor extensions (▶ Fig. 18.6).[7,35] In the latter approach the structures of the jugular foramen can be identified and skeletonized using a high-speed drill. The extradural removal of tumors from around the exiting lower CNs can result in neurological improvement. The approach can be extended inferiorly by the posterior mobilization of the vertebral artery from the foramina transversaria of C1 and C2. In

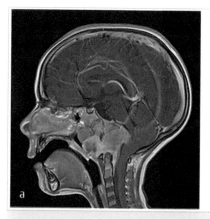
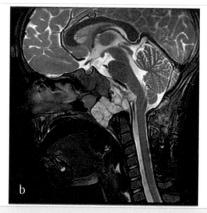
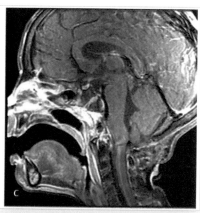

Fig. 18.5 Sagittal postcontrast T1-weighted MRI of a patient who has a large and complex clival chordoma. **(a)** The tumor prior to any surgical intervention. **(b)** Residual tumor after first-stage transcondylar resection of the portion of the tumor that was causing marked neural compression. **(c)** The final appearance after transmandibular circumglossal retropharyngeal resection of the anterior components of the tumor. Complex tumors such as this may require extensive and multistaged procedures to maximize resection. (Courtesy of the Department of Neurosurgery, MD Anderson Cancer Center.)

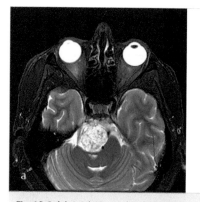
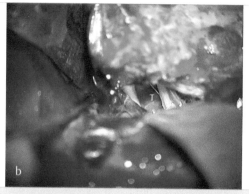
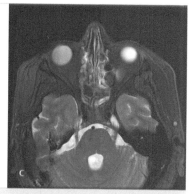

Fig. 18.6 **(a)** Axial T2-weighted MRI reveals a large intradural laterally extending chordoma. The trigeminal nerve is displaced laterally. **(b)** Intraoperative photograph following completion of the petrosal exposure. The petrosal vein, trigeminal nerve and VII–VIII nerve bundle are well identified, as are the anteroinferior cerebellar artery and the tumor between the VII–VIII nerve complex and the trigeminal nerve. **(c)** Axial T2-weighted image following resection via the petrosal approach of this large intradural extension of chordoma. A secondary transmaxillary approach completed the resection in this patient. (Courtesy of the Department of Neurosurgery, MD Anderson Cancer Center.)

this way, the region of the odontoid process and arch of C1 can be exposed.[10,23,24,25] Craniospinal fixation may be necessary.

Total petrosectomy allows access from the sphenoid sinus to the foramen magnum and from the upper cervical spine to the intradural structures of the middle and posterior fossae. Destruction of the inner ear and complete mobilization of the facial nerve, with their attendant morbidities, are consequences of this approach. The problem of limited midline access remains.

18.13 Endonasal Endoscopic Transclival/Transpterygoid Approach

Taking advantage of the nasopharynx as a corridor, the endoscopic endonasal approaches provide direct access to the clivus with the theoretical benefit of reductions to both neurovascular manipulation and soft tissue morbidity. Particularly for clival malignancies, such as chordomas, the endoscopic transclival approach is now the preferred initial strategy of choice (▶ Fig. 18.7). From the endoscopic standpoint, the clivus is divided into thirds in the craniocaudal direction, with clear anatomic considerations associated with each third. The lateral limits of the endoscopic transclival approach for each third of the clivus are the CNs of the cavernous sinus (upper third), the paraclival carotid arteries (middle third), and the Eustachian tubes (lower third). Within the subarachnoid space of the posterior fossa, the transclival approach provides the ability to manage disease along the ventral brainstem and vertebrobasilar system using standard microsurgical techniques; however, disease extension lateral to the abducens nerve is a clear limit of this approach. In this section, we will cover strategies for maximizing the endoscopic transclival approach for each third of the clivus to access disease within not only the clivus but also adjacent bony and soft tissue compartments.

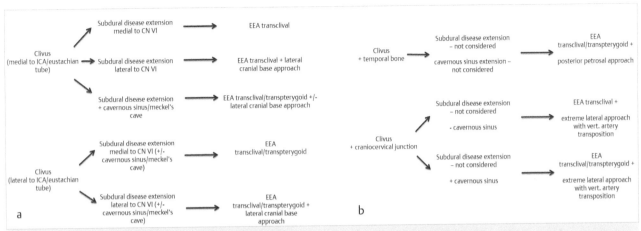

Fig. 18.7 (a, b) Decision-making algorithm regarding indications for endoscopic and open cranial base approaches for clival chordomas based on anatomic extensions. (Courtesy of Dr. Shaan Raza, University of Texas, MD Anderson Cancer Center.)

18.13.1 Positioning/Preprocedure Planning

Preoperative imaging necessary for planning consists of a MRI and CT–angiogram (CT-A) to assess the need for access to soft tissue and bony compartments (e.g., disease extension lateral to the petroclival synchondrosis, occipital condyles). Vascular imaging, in the form of a CT-A, additionally provides information regarding the bony anatomy around the carotid arteries (e.g., intact or dehiscent bony canal) while allowing assessment of the completeness of the circle of Willis in case of intraoperative injury to the carotid artery. For anticipated high-flow CSF leaks, the procedure commences with placement of a lumbar subarachnoid drain, which is left clamped during the procedure but employed for postoperative CSF diversion. The patient is placed into rigid fixation with an approximate angulation of 30°. The nostrils are decongested using topically placed patties.

18.13.2 Sinonasal Dissection

The first step of sinonasal dissection is the harvesting of a nasoseptal flap pedicled on the sphenopalatine artery. To ensure adequate coverage of not only the anticipated defect but also the exposed internal carotid arteries and bony skull base, the flap length and width are maximized by extending relevant incisions anteriorly toward the columella and laterally along the nasal floor toward the inferior turbinate, respectively. The flap is typically stored within the maxillary sinus. If an extremely large holoclival defect is anticipated, then bilateral nasoseptal flaps are harvested.

The paranasal sinuses are then opened selectively to provide sufficient access. At the very least, this consists of performing bilateral posterior ethmoidectomies and a wide sphenoidotomy with a view to identifying landmarks such as the orbital apex, opticocarotid recesses, and paraclival carotid arteries. For midclival access, to ensure sufficient lateral access to the internal carotid arteries, bilateral maxillary antrostomies may be performed along and the sphenopalatine foramina and the medial aspect of the pterygopalatine fossae opened. With subsequent transposition of the nasoseptal flap–sphenopalatine

artery–pterygopalatine fossa complex, the vidian neurovascular bundle can be identified and sectioned. This maneuver can enhance the transpterygoid approach by avoiding the sacrifice of any intranasal flaps. To access the lower clival region, a U-shaped incision is made in the mucosa of the posterior nasopharynx. The underlying longus capitis muscle is dissected (or resected if there is tumor invasion) and reflected separately. After this initial approach, the sphenoid sinus floor is resected to the clivus and laterally to the vidian canals.

18.13.3 Clival Window/Resection

The extent of clival resection is tailored to the extension of the tumor and ultimately to which components of the posterior fossa need to be accessed. Providing access to the interpeduncular cistern posteriorly and cavernous sinuses laterally, an upper clival approach requires bony removal in such a manner that the ventral surface and floor of the sella are removed along with exposure of the medial aspect of the cavernous carotid arteries bilaterally (▶ Fig. 18.8). The posterior clinoids can be removed via an extradural approach, working inferior and posterior to the gland, or via a transcavernous approach with pituitary transposition. Any tumor extension into the lateral cavernous sinus can be resected endoscopically by performing a dural incision lateral to the carotid artery, which can be extended posteriorly along the floor of the cavernous sinus and inferiorly into Meckel's cave (▶ Fig. 18.9). For lateral cavernous sinus resections, the abducens nerve is typically at greatest risk and can be electrically monitored.

A midclival approach should take into consideration tumor extension not only into the prepontine cistern but also laterally into the petrous apex (▶ Fig. 18.10). Lateral petrous apical extension typically requires the addition of a transpterygoid approach. This requires additional work within the sinonasal cavity to facilitate lateral exposure. A medial maxillectomy is performed with resection of the ipsilateral middle turbinate and the inferior turbinate (if needed for access to the jugular foramen). The contents of the pterygopalatine fossa are subsequently dissected in order to gain access to the medial infratemporal fossa. After skeletonizing and mobilizing the

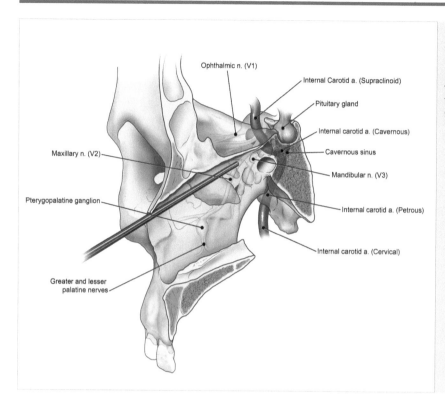

Fig. 18.8 The endonasal endoscopic approach to the upper clivus. The internal carotid artery and the divisions of the trigeminal nerve that are located laterally require exposure to adequately visualize lateral extensions of tumor posterior to the artery. (Courtesy of Dr. Shaan Raza, University of Texas, MD Anderson Cancer Center.)

descending palatine nerve, V2 at foramen rotundum is identified at the superiormost aspect of the pterygoid plates. The inferior head of the lateral pterygoid muscle is detached and the pterygoid plates isolated medially and laterally, then drilled away in their entirety. Of note, the medial pterygoid muscle attachment to the lateral aspect of the medial pterygoid plate marks the posterior endpoint of the bony resection. The middle fossa floor is subsequently resected exposing the dura over Meckel's cave, circumferentially exposing V3 and the foramen ovale and stopping medial to foramen spinosum.

The paraclival and laceral segments of the carotid artery are circumferentially skeletonized along with V3 as a marker of the horizontal petrous segment of the carotid artery. In this process, the thin bony plate between the carotid artery and superior surface of the Eustachian tube is resected and the fibrocartilaginous tissue along the inferior half of foramen lacerum exposed and sharply transected.

The Eustachian tube is subsequently exposed by detaching the superior half of the medial pterygoid muscle. The tensor veli palatini muscle is detached from the lateral surface of the Eustachian tube, and the levator veli palatini is now exposed inferiorly and is similarly detached to complete exposure of the cartilaginous portion of the Eustachian tube. To further mobilize the Eustachian tube, the fibrocartilaginous tissue at the foramen is sharply incised from medial to lateral while mobilizing the internal carotid artery superiorly. At this point the decision is made of whether the Eustachian tube is mobilized purely for lateral petrous apex access or whether resection of its medial component is required. This decision ultimately depends on the target pathology and the goals of surgery. An incision through the lateralmost aspect of the exposed Eustachian tube is subsequently made to remove this structure and gain access to the lateral clivus, petrous apex, and medial jugular foramen.

Working further inferiorly, considerations pertinent to a low clival approach are management of the occipital condyles and resection of bony disease extending lateral to the occipital condyles. When viewed in the axial plane, the occipital condyles lie in the ten o'clock and two o'clock positions along the ventral aspect of the foramen magnum. When using an endonasal approach, resection of the medial aspect of one or both occipital condyles may be necessary in order to widen access to intradural disease extension. A limitation of the endonasal transclival approach is management of disease extending lateral to the condyles. In such a situation, either the use of an endoscopic transpterygoid approach with Eustachian tube mobilization/resection or an extreme/far lateral craniotomy is needed.

18.13.4 Reconstruction

Dural reconstruction is performed in a multilayered fashion. It is important to note that beyond prevention of a CSF fistula, vascularized reconstruction is necessary for carotid artery coverage and promotion of skull base healing prior to initiation of adjuvant therapy (if indicated). For large defects when the entire bony clivus has been resected, supplementary flaps (i.e., the inferior turbinate, pericranial, and temporoparietal fascia) beyond the traditional nasal septal flap are needed to ensure sufficient vascularized coverage.

18.14 Transcondylar Approach

Tumors of the lower clivus that have lateral extension to the atlanto-occipital joint, jugular foramen, or upper cervical spine are well addressed via this approach.[4,8,9,22,34,45,46] Important advantages of the transcondylar approach include a short and wide surgical field, vascular control of the vertebral artery,

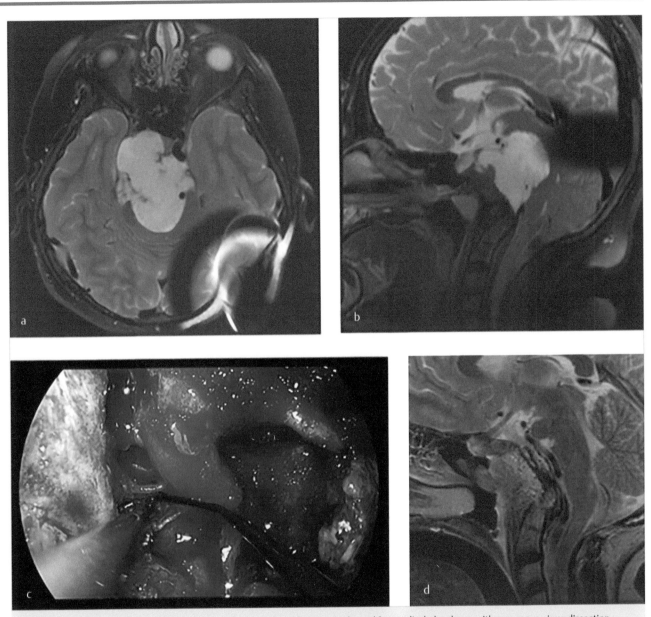

Fig. 18.9 Expanded endoscopic endonasal transclival resection of upper, mid-, and lower clival chordoma with cavernous sinus dissection. **(a, b)** Preoperative T1-weighted MRI with contrast. **(c)** Intraoperative view during lateral cavernous sinus dissection along the right cavernous sinus. **(d)** Postoperative MRI scan demonstrating gross total resection with pedicled flap reconstruction. (Courtesy of Dr. Shaan Raza, University of Texas, MD Anderson Cancer Center.)

and an uncontaminated surgical field. The direct lateral exposure of the craniocervical junction afforded by this approach allows for a direct line of sight to the structures ventral to the cervicomedullary junction and upper cervical cord.[51] This is an excellent approach for large lower clival chordomas. Neural decompression can be directly confirmed and craniocervical fixation performed if necessary. This typically removes the patient from immediate danger and allows time for a staged anterior approach, which in most cases is required for maximal tumor removal. The region of the occipital condyle may be accessed from a posterolateral or anterolateral approach.[10,25] The posterolateral approach affords excellent anterior intradural midline access but does not permit a surgical corridor to the anterior extradural region. It is an excellent approach for

clival tumors that penetrate the dura and extend posteriorly to compress the cervicomedullary region and is typically used as a staged procedure, with a secondary anterior endoscopic approach. The posterior midline access it affords allows immediate craniocervical stabilization if necessary.

18.15 Anterolateral Transcondylar Approach

18.15.1 Positioning and Incision

The patient is positioned in the supine position with the head slightly elevated and turned to the opposite side or in the direct

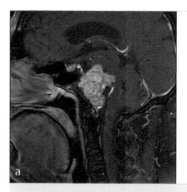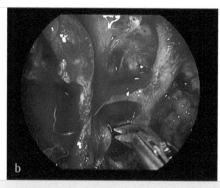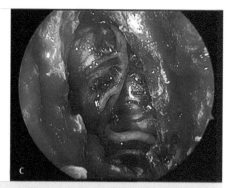

Fig. 18.10 Expanded endoscopic endonasal transclival resection of upper, mid-, and lower clival chordoma with intradural extension and brainstem compression. (a) Preoperative T1-weighted MRI with contrast demonstrating extent of involvement. (b) Intraoperative view demonstrating sharp dissection off basilar artery and duplicated left anteroinferior cerebellar artery segments. (c) Intraoperative view at the completion of the tumor resection, with entire vertebrobasilar system exposed. (Courtesy of Dr. Shaan Raza, University of Texas, MD Anderson Cancer Center.)

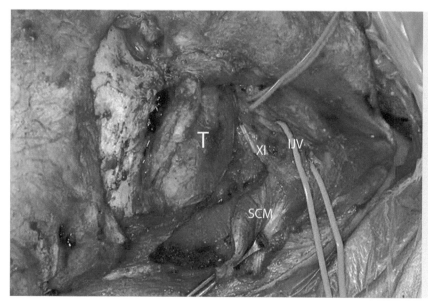

Fig. 18.11 Intraoperative photograph of a patient operated on via the anterolateral approach. The sternocleidomastoid muscle (SCM) is reflected posteriorly. The accessory nerve is protected and the jugular vein is controlled in the vascular loop. The tumor is identified just below the tip of the mastoid overlaying the region of the condyle and vertebral artery. (Courtesy of the Department of Neurosurgery, MD Anderson Cancer Center.)

lateral position. There are several options for the incision. We have used a large retroauricular C-shaped incision, although an incision that begins along the upper anterior border of the sternomastoid muscle, curves across the mastoid process, and then travels along the occipital crest to the external occipital protuberance can also be used. The exact choice of skin incision will depend on the extensions of the tumor, the need to combine this approach with another approach for resection, and the presence of concurrent occipitocervical fusion.

18.15.2 Soft Tissue Dissection

After the flap is elevated, the sternomastoid muscle is dissected along its anterior border to identify the jugular vein. The dissection continues superiorly, with the sternomastoid muscle detached from the mastoid tip and reflected posterolaterally (▶ Fig. 18.11). The accessory nerve is identified in relation to the jugular vein and dissected superiorly as far as possible toward the skull base. Its distal portion, just prior to its penetration of the sternomastoid, is also freed so as to mobilize the

nerve inferiorly. The fatty tissue around the midportion of the nerve is left undisturbed to serve as a protective cushion around the nerve. The transverse process of the atlas is palpated just below and anterior to the tip of the mastoid process. The rectus minor, superior and inferior obliques, and levator scapulae muscles are detached from the transverse process while attending to the vertebral artery, which lays immediately deep to these muscles. As described by George, the vertebral artery is first exposed inferiorly between the transverse processes of C1 and C2. Here it is crossed anteriorly by the anterior branch of the C2 nerve root. The vertebral artery is then exposed above C1 and dissection carried posteriorly along the arch of C1 in a subperiosteal plane. The foramen transversarium of C1 is opened and the vertebral artery dissected free and translocated posteriorly. The C1 transverse process is resected, and then the anterior arch of C1 is exposed and cleared off subperiosteally. Finally, the vertebral artery in its periosteal sheath is separated from the atlanto-occipital membrane and capsule of the C1–C2 joint, fully exposing the lateral foramen magnum.

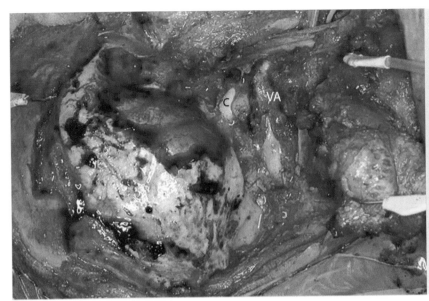

Fig. 18.12 This intraoperative photograph was taken after resection of the tumor identified in ▶ Fig. 18.11. The vertebral artery is entirely skeletonized, and the capsule of the atlantoaxial joint has been removed completely to identify the occipital condyle. A mastoidectomy and retrosigmoid craniectomy has been performed to achieve total tumor removal, in this case of radiation-associated osteogenic sarcoma. (Courtesy of the Department of Neurosurgery, MD Anderson Cancer Center.)

18.15.3 Bony Dissection and Osteotomies

A standard mastoidectomy is performed; bone should be removed to unroof the lower half of the sigmoid sinus and jugular bulb. The superior extent of exposure is the jugular foramen. Tumor extensions above this level will require the addition of a transpetrous approach. A retromastoid craniotomy may be added if needed (▶ Fig. 18.12). The extent of condylar resection depends on the extent of the tumor. Care must be taken in identifying the hypoglossal nerve, which passes through the midportion of the condyle. Resection of greater than 50% of the condyle typically necessitates occipitocervical fixation. This can be performed as part of the same operation or in a secondary procedure, with the patient maintained in a rigid collar in the interim.

18.15.4 Tumor Resection

The tumor is resected using standard intralesional ultrasonic aspiration or suction and bipolar cautery. When significant encasement of the lower CNs and the vertebral artery exists, CN monitoring serves as a useful adjunct. The dissection plane should proceed from normal to abnormal anatomy, especially when prior surgery and treatment have created distorted anatomy and scar tissue.

18.15.5 Reconstruction and Closure

Standard techniques for dural closure, including primary dural closure and patch duraplasty, are used to facilitate watertight dural closure so as to prevent CSF leak.

18.16 Posterolateral Transcondylar Approach

18.16.1 Positioning and Incision

The patient is positioned in the lateral position, tumor side up. The back of the operating room bed is elevated. The incision is marked with the patient's head in the neutral position. The head is then rigidly fixated and laterally flexed downward but not rotated. A hockey stick–type incision is made that extends from above the ear to the posterior midline of the neck. This will give the needed access for craniocervical fixation should it be required (▶ Fig. 18.13).

18.16.2 Soft Tissue Dissection

The suboccipital musculature is elevated en bloc from the occipital bone. The soft tissue elevation continues laterally to expose the mastoid and the digastric groove. Beginning at the coronal plane of the digastric groove, dissection of the fibroadipose tissue, found below the groove, from the occipital bone should be done without electrocautery to avoid vertebral artery injury (▶ Fig. 18.14).

The posterior cervical musculature is elevated off the arch of C1 and the spinous process and lamina of C2 to its lateral mass. Sharp dissection of the soft tissue between C1 and the occipital bone exposes the V3 portion of the vertebral artery in the sulcus arteriosus of the arch of C1. Laterally, the upper V2 segment of the vertebral artery is identified between the foramina transversaria of C1 and C2, where it is crossed posteriorly by the C2 nerve root.

18.16.3 Bony Dissection and Osteotomies

A suboccipital craniotomy is performed to expose the inferior sigmoid sinus as it turns anteriorly to the jugular bulb. Bone removal continues anteriorly to the jugular fossa, removing the jugular tubercle (supracondylar drilling). The V3 portion of the vertebral artery is freed subperiosteally from the arch of C1 and the arch removed to the lateral mass just posterior and medial to the foramina transversaria. Inferior reflection of the vertebral artery allows access to the occipital condyle, but full exposure of the occipitoatlantal joint requires posteromedial transposition of the vertebral artery. The vertebral is freed from the foramina transversaria of C1. Usually the C2 nerve root needs to be

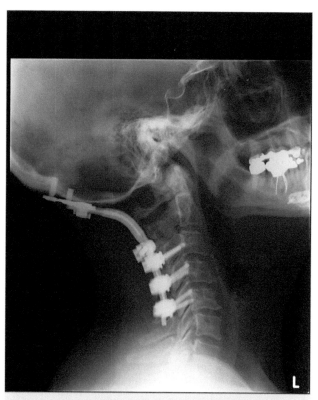

Fig. 18.13 Lateral radiograph of the spine after occipital–cervical fusion in a patient who underwent complete condylar resection for removal of a clival chordoma. (Courtesy of the Department of Neurosurgery, MD Anderson Cancer Center.)

divided to fully allow the posteromedial transposition of the V2/V3 segment of the vertebral. With the vertebral artery transposed and protected, the occipital and atlantal condyles can be removed using the drill. Typically chordoma is accompanied by condylar involvement, which is immediately accessed at this time.

The hypoglossal canal runs through the junction of the posterior and middle thirds of the occipital condyle from posteromedial to anterolateral and is directed forward and laterally at a 45° angle to the sagittal plane.

18.16.4 Tumor Resection

Tumor removal begins extradurally with protection of the vertebral artery, hypoglossal nerve and lower CNs, and jugular venous system anteriorly. The rectus capitus lateralis muscle separates the vertebral artery from the jugular vein and jugular fossa anteriorly. After extradural tumor removal, the dura is opened posterior to the vertebral artery and extended superiorly and inferiorly as needed. The upper dentate ligaments are sectioned to allow greater freedom of movement and dissection. The C1 and C2 nerve roots can also be sectioned if needed. The rootlets of the spinal accessory nerve are dissected free to allow anterior or posterior transposition of the accessory nerve. The dissection continues from normal to abnormal anatomy, carefully following the vertebral artery to its junction with the basilar artery. The rootlets of CNs IX, X, and XI are consistently posterior to the vertebral artery, whereas the hypoglossal

rootlets may be split by the vertebral artery. If necessary, the dural incisions can be extended around the vertebral artery dural entry to allow access anterior to the vertebral artery.

18.16.5 Reconstruction and Closure

A watertight primary dural closure is usually possible, but there should be no hesitation over using a dural patch to achieve this. If circumvertebral dural incisions have been made or dura resected anterior to the vertebral artery, then primary dural closure is unlikely and a multilayered reconstruction is necessary. We use a soft, commercially available dural substitute both intra- and extradurally. This is reinforced with commercially available tissue adhesives and subcutaneous fat. The occipital bone flap is replaced and plated. The cervical and suboccipital musculature is carefully approximated.

If craniocervical instability is likely, then the patient is carefully repositioned into the prone position and alignment is checked with fluoroscopy. An occipital cervical fusion is then performed. An alternative would be to manage the patient in a stiff collar and perform occipital cervical fusion as a second stage, depending on the likelihood and degree of craniospinal instability.

18.16.6 Postoperative Care and Follow-up

The most important aspect of the patient's postoperative care is the identification and aggressive management of lower cranial neuropathy. All patients are evaluated by speech pathology in the immediate postoperative period and a swallowing evaluation is performed. A modified barium swallow or direct laryngoscopy may be recommended. Only when deemed safe is oral intake allowed.

CSF leakage may occur after endoscopic clival resection for myriad reasons, including technical errors in reconstruction, graft migration, and presence of unrecognized hydrocephalus (including temporarily secondary to "posterior fossa syndrome"). Among all skull base sites, endoscopic reconstruction of transclival defects can be uniquely challenging because of anatomic factors such as the extensive size of the defects, long exposed segments of the internal carotid arteries bilaterally, and potential space within the clival recess. Patient-specific factors such as an elevated body mass index also need to be considered. For leak management, it is necessary to differentiate between a "low-flow" and "high-flow" leak based on clinical examination and CT imaging, assessing for pneumocephalus. Low-flow leaks can commonly be managed via 5 days of CSF diversion via a lumbar drain; leaks recurring after this initial trial drainage are treated with venticuloperitoneal (VP) shunt placement on the assumption that a underlying pressure-related issue is involved. High-flow leaks (usually associated with significant pneumocephalus on CT) warrant immediate surgical exploration of the reconstruction to determine the cause of failure. At this point, the entire reconstruction is performed again, with secondary vascularized flaps (i.e., the pericranial and temporoparietal fascial flaps) potentially necessary depending on the viability of the original flaps. Prolonged CSF diversion is also undertaken. If a leak recurs after this revision,

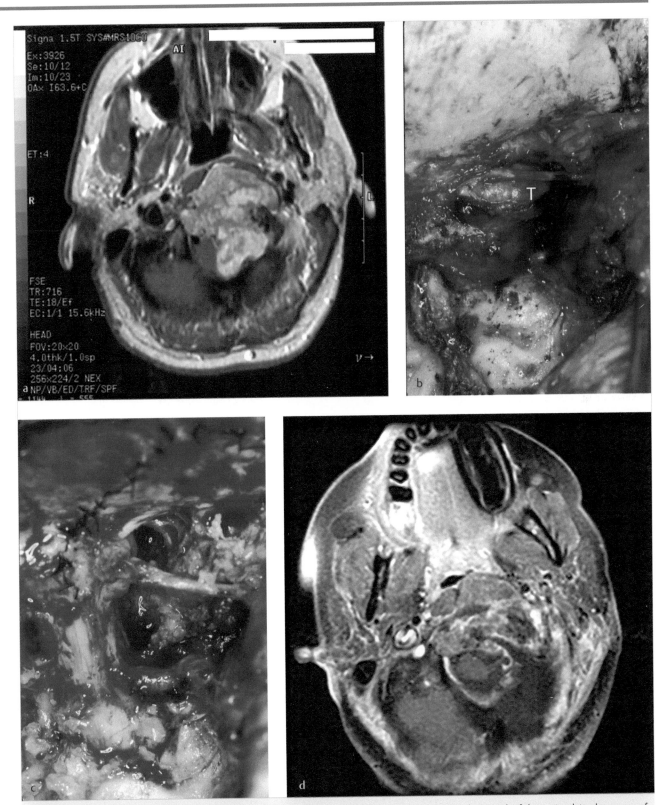

Fig. 18.14 (a) Axial postcontrast MRI revealing a large intra- and extradural chordoma. (b) Intraoperative photograph of the posterolateral exposure of the condyle. The tumor is well identified, as is the overlying hypoplastic vertebral artery. (c) Intraoperative photograph after resection and direct and complete decompression of the cervicomedullary junction. (d) Postoperative contrast-enhanced axial MRI confirms neural decompression and removal of the posterolateral component of the tumor. A secondary transmandibular approach accessed and resected the remaining anterior disease. (Courtesy of the Department of Neurosurgery, MD Anderson Cancer Center.)

then a repeat intraoperative evaluation of the reconstruction, along with VP shunt placement, is often necessary.

Disturbances of ocular movement are managed initially by patching and subsequently by prisms and extraocular muscle surgery under the supervision of an ophthalmologist.

A noncontrast CT of the brain is done on the first postoperative day to identify any subclinical complications. A baseline postoperative MRI is done within 48 hours of surgery. If clinically indicated, dynamic imaging of the craniocervical junction with flexion extension radiographs is obtained.

Close follow-up with clinical evaluation and imaging is essential, the frequency of which depends on the tumor pathology. For patients who have chordoma or chondrosarcoma, if no tumor is visualized on baseline postoperative imaging, additional imaging is obtained at 3-month intervals for the first year, at 6-month intervals for the next 2 years, and yearly thereafter. When residual disease is identified, the patient should be referred to a specialized radiation treatment facility, ideally one that has proton beam capability as well as radiation oncologists who are familiar with the treatment of disease processes that affect the clivus. Referral to medical oncology may also be necessary.

Management algorithms for residual or recurrent local disease is complex and beyond the scope of this chapter. Multiple variables should be analyzed, including the clinical condition of the patient, the size and location of the recurrence, the tumor histology at the initial operation, the extent of the previous resection, and the dose, field, and fractionation scheme of prior radiation therapy.

References

[1] Alfieri A, Jho HD. Endoscopic endonasal cavernous sinus surgery: an anatomic study. Neurosurgery. 2001; 48(4):827–836, discussion 836–837

[2] Ammirati M, Bernardo A. Analytical evaluation of complex anterior approaches to the cranial base: an anatomic study. Neurosurgery. 1998; 43(6): 1398–1407, discussion 1407–1408

[3] Ammirati M, Ma J, Cheatham ML, Mei ZT, Bloch J, Becker DP. The mandibular swing-transcervical approach to the skull base: anatomical study [technical note]. J Neurosurg. 1993; 78(4):673–681

[4] Babu RP, Sekhar LN, Wright DC. Extreme lateral transcondylar approach: technical improvements and lessons learned. J Neurosurg. 1994; 81(1):49–59

[5] Beals SP, Joganic EF, Hamilton MG, Spetzler RF. Posterior skull base transfacial approaches. Clin Plast Surg. 1995; 22(3):491–511

[6] Biller HF, Shugar JM, Krespi YP. A new technique for wide-field exposure of the base of the skull. Arch Otolaryngol. 1981; 107(11):698–702

[7] Blevins NH, Jackler RK, Kaplan MJ, Gutin PH. Combined transpetrosal-subtemporal craniotomy for clival tumors with extension into the posterior fossa. Laryngoscope. 1995; 105(9 Pt 1):975–982

[8] Borba LA, Al-Mefty O. Skull-base chordomas. Contemp Neurosurg. 1998; 20: 1–6

[9] Canalis RF, Martin N, Black K, et al. Lateral approach to tumors of the craniovertebral junction. Laryngoscope. 1993; 103(3):343–349

[10] Carpentier A, Blanquet A, George B. Suboccipital and cervical chordomas: radical resection with vertebral artery control. Neurosurg Focus. 2001; 10(3):E4

[11] Catalano PJ, Biller HF. Extended osteoplastic maxillotomy: a versatile new procedure for wide access to the central skull base and infratemporal fossa. Arch Otolaryngol Head Neck Surg. 1993; 119(4):394–400

[12] Cavallo LM, Messina A, Cappabianca P, et al. Endoscopic endonasal surgery of the midline skull base: anatomical study and clinical considerations. Neurosurg Focus. 2005; 19(1):E2

[13] Cavallo LM, Messina A, Gardner P, et al. Extended endoscopic endonasal approach to the pterygopalatine fossa: anatomical study and clinical considerations. Neurosurg Focus. 2005; 19(1):E5

[14] Couldwell WT, Sabit I, Weiss MH, Giannotta SL, Rice D. Transmaxillary approach to the anterior cavernous sinus: a microanatomic study. Neurosurgery. 1997; 40(6):1307–1311

[15] Crockard HA, Sen CN. The transoral approach for the management of intradural lesions at the craniovertebral junction: review of 7 cases. Neurosurgery. 1991; 28(1):88–97, discussion 97–98

[16] DeMonte F, Diaz E, Jr, Callender D, Suk I. Transmandibular, circumglossal, retropharyngeal approach for chordomas of the clivus and upper cervical spine [technical note]. Neurosurg Focus. 2001; 10(3):E10

[17] DeMonte F, Hanna E. Transmaxillary exploration of the intracranial portion of the maxillary nerve in malignant perineural disease [technical note]. J Neurosurg. 2007; 107(3):672–677

[18] de Oliveira E, Rhoton AL, Jr, Peace D. Microsurgical anatomy of the region of the foramen magnum. Surg Neurol. 1985; 24(3):293–352

[19] Feiz-Erfan I, Spetzler RF, Horn EM, et al. Proposed classification for the transbasal approach and its modifications. Skull Base. 2008; 18(1):29–47

[20] Fujitsu K, Saijoh M, Aoki F, et al. Telecanthal approach for meningiomas in the ethmoid and sphenoid sinuses. Neurosurgery. 1991; 28(5):714–719, discussion 719–720

[21] Gay E, Sekhar LN, Rubinstein E, et al. Chordomas and chondrosarcomas of the cranial base: results and follow-up of 60 patients. Neurosurgery. 1995; 36(5): 887–896, discussion 896–897

[22] George B, Archilli M, Cornelius JF. Bone tumors at the cranio-cervical junction. Surgical management and results from a series of 41 cases. Acta Neurochir (Wien). 2006; 148(7):741–749- (Wien)

[23] George B, Dematons C, Cophignon J. Lateral approach to the anterior portion of the foramen magnum: application to surgical removal of 14 benign tumors [technical note]. Surg Neurol. 1988; 29(6):484–490

[24] George B, Laurian C. Surgical approach to the whole length of the vertebral artery with special reference to the third portion. Acta Neurochir (Wien). 1980; 51(3–4):259–272

[25] George B, Lot G. Anterolateral and posterolateral approaches to the foramen magnum: technical description and experience from 97 cases. Skull Base Surg. 1995; 5(1):9–19

[26] Harsh GR, IV, Sekhar LN. The subtemporal, transcavernous, anterior transpetrosal approach to the upper brain stem and clivus. J Neurosurg. 1992; 77(5): 709–717

[27] James D, Crockard HA. Surgical access to the base of skull and upper cervical spine by extended maxillotomy. Neurosurgery. 1991; 29(3):411–416

[28] Kawakami K, Yamanouchi Y, Kawamura Y, Matsumura H. Operative approach to the frontal skull base: extensive transbasal approach. Neurosurgery. 1991; 28(5):720–724, discussion 724–725

[29] Kawase T, Shiobara R, Toya S. Anterior transpetrosal-transtentorial approach for sphenopetroclival meningiomas: surgical method and results in 10 patients. Neurosurgery. 1991; 28(6):869–875, discussion 875–876

[30] Krespi YP, Har-El G. Surgery of the clivus and anterior cervical spine. Arch Otolaryngol Head Neck Surg. 1988; 114(1):73–78

[31] Krespi YP, Sisson GA. Skull base surgery in composite resection. Arch Otolaryngol. 1982; 108(11):681–684

[32] Krespi YP, Sisson GA. Transmandibular exposure of the skull base. Am J Surg. 1984; 148(4):534–538

[33] Lalwani AK, Kaplan MJ, Gutin PH. The transsphenoethmoid approach to the sphenoid sinus and clivus. Neurosurgery. 1992; 31(6):1008–1014, discussion 1014

[34] Lang DA, Neil-Dwyer G, Iannotti F. The suboccipital transcondylar approach to the clivus and cranio-cervical junction for ventrally placed pathology at and above the foramen magnum. Acta Neurochir (Wien). 1993; 125(1–4): 132–137 (Wien)

[35] Laws ER, Jr. Transsphenoidal surgery for tumors of the clivus. Otolaryngol Head Neck Surg. 1984; 92(1):100–101

[36] Leonetti JP, Reichman OH, al-Mefty O, Li J, Smith PG. Neurotologic considerations in the treatment of advanced clival tumors. Otolaryngol Head Neck Surg. 1992; 107(1):49–56

[37] Maira G, Pallini R, Anile C, et al. Surgical treatment of clival chordomas: the transsphenoidal approach revisited. J Neurosurg. 1996; 85(5):784–792

[38] Menezes AH, VanGilder JC. Transoral-transpharyngeal approach to the anterior craniocervical junction: ten-year experience with 72 patients. J Neurosurg. 1988; 69(6):895–903

[39] Meyers SP, Hirsch WL, Jr, Curtin HD, Barnes L, Sekhar LN, Sen C. Chordomas of the skull base: MR features. AJNR Am J Neuroradiol. 1992; 13(6):1627–1636

[40] Oot RF, Melville GE, New PF, et al. The role of MR and CT in evaluating clival chordomas and chondrosarcomas. AJR Am J Roentgenol. 1988; 151(3):567–575

[41] Rabadán A, Conesa H. Transmaxillary-transnasal approach to the anterior clivus: a microsurgical anatomical model. Neurosurgery. 1992; 30(4):473–481, discussion 482

[42] Sabit I, Schaefer SD, Couldwell WT. Extradural extranasal combined transmaxillary transsphenoidal approach to the cavernous sinus: a minimally invasive microsurgical model. Laryngoscope. 2000; 110(2 Pt 1):286–291

[43] Sabit I, Schaefer SD, Couldwell WT. Modified infratemporal fossa approach via lateral transantral maxillotomy: a microsurgical model. Surg Neurol. 2002; 58(1):21–31

[44] Sekhar LN, Nanda A, Sen CN, Snyderman CN, Janecka IP. The extended frontal approach to tumors of the anterior, middle, and posterior skull base. J Neurosurg. 1992; 76(2):198–206

[45] Sen CN, Sekhar LN. An extreme lateral approach to intradural lesions of the cervical spine and foramen magnum. Neurosurgery. 1990; 27(2):197–204

[46] Sen CN, Sekhar LN. Surgical management of anteriorly placed lesions at the craniocervical junction—an alternative approach. Acta Neurochir (Wien). 1991; 108(1–2):70–77

[47] Sen CN, Sekhar LN. The subtemporal and preauricular infratemporal approach to intradural structures ventral to the brain stem. J Neurosurg. 1990; 73(3):345–354

[48] Terasaka S, Day JD, Fukushima T. Extended transbasal approach: anatomy, technique, and indications. Skull Base Surg. 1999; 9(3):177–184

[49] Uttley D, Moore A, Archer DJ. Surgical management of midline skull-base tumors: a new approach. J Neurosurg. 1989; 71(5 Pt 1):705–710

[50] Wei WI, Lam KH, Sham JS. New approach to the nasopharynx: the maxillary swing approach. Head Neck. 1991; 13(3):200–207

[51] Wen HT, Rhoton AL, Jr, Katsuta T, de Oliveira E. Microsurgical anatomy of the transcondylar, supracondylar, and paracondylar extensions of the far-lateral approach. J Neurosurg. 1997; 87(4):555–585

19 Tumors of the Infratemporal Fossa

Mathieu Forgues, Rahul Mehta, and Daniel W. Nuss

Summary

This chapter reviews the anatomy, pathology, and clinical evaluation of the infratemporal fossa and describes the surgical
management of this complex structural space. Because of its proximity to critical neurovascular structures, resection of tumors in
this space requires precise surgical planning. Historically, many
open approaches have been available to the surgeon, which can
be tailored to the extent and behavior of the tumor. Beginning in
the 1980s, advances in endoscopic endonasal techniques have cat-
alyzed efforts to minimize surgical morbidity. A multidisciplinary
team should be assembled to perform a comprehensive evaluation
of the patient and establish a coordinated treatment plan.

Keywords: infratemporal fossa, tumor, endoscopic endonasal,
facial translocation, multidisciplinary

19.1 Introduction

Tumors of the infratemporal fossa (ITF) can arise primarily or
can invade by direct extension from surrounding structures,
such as the parotid gland, upper aerodigestive tract, nasopharynx, paranasal sinuses, temporal bone, pterygopalatine fossa
(PPF), and parapharyngeal space (PPS). Many of these tumors
require surgery, which can carry significant risk to the critical
neurovascular structures contained within this space. Proper
evaluation requires intimate knowledge of the anatomy and a
multidisciplinary approach to treatment planning. Management decisions should ensure both effective eradication of
disease and acceptable function and cosmesis.

19.2 Surgical Anatomy

The ITF, located medial to the vertical ramus of the mandible
and zygomatic arch and lateral to pharynx, is not lined by a
single consistent fascia and lacks rigid borders. Anteriorly, it is
limited by the posterior surface of the maxilla, and its posterior
border is the mastoid and tympanic temporal bone. Its superior
border is the inferior surface of the greater wing of the sphenoid, through which communication with the middle cranial
fossa occurs through the foramina ovale and spinosum.

Its medial and inferior borders have varying definitions. Medial limits may be defined by the bony landmarks of the lateral
pterygoid plate, the lateral portion of the clivus, the first cervical vertebra, and the inferior surface of the petrous temporal
bone. Soft tissues can also delineate the medial border: the
superior pharyngeal constrictor and tensor and levator veli
palatini. Inferior limits are variably defined in some descriptions; some sources consider the lateral inferior insertion of the
medial pterygoid muscle or the posterior belly of the digastric
muscle as the inferior boundary of the ITF.[1]

The ITF communicates with the orbit through the inferior
orbital fissure and with the PPF through the pterygomaxillary
fissure. Tumors can spread to and from surrounding spaces
through these openings or along venous connections. Careful
attention must be paid to these potential corridors of spread,
which are often best evaluated using MRI.

The contents of the ITF include the medial and lateral pterygoid, masseter, and temporalis muscles, the deep lobe of the
parotid gland, and neurovascular elements: the mandibular
division of the trigeminal nerve (V3), chorda tympani branch
of the facial nerve, otic ganglion, jugular vein, internal carotid
artery (ICA), internal maxillary artery, and pterygoid venous
plexus.

19.3 Regional Pathology and Differential Diagnosis

Because the contents of the ITF include multiple tissue types, a
variety of tumors can occur there. Common benign neoplasms
of the ITF include schwannomas, pleomorphic adenomas, vascular lesions (arteriovenous malformations, paragangliomas),
and meningiomas. Less commonly, deep lipomas and inflammatory pseudotumor may also arise in the ITF.

Malignant primary tumors of the ITF include rhabdomyosarcoma, osteosarcoma, fibrosarcoma, and malignant hemangiopericytoma. The ITF can also be involved by spread of tumors
from adjacent spaces. Malignant salivary tumors can originate
from the aerodigestive tract, parotid gland, or microscopic
minor salivary rests. Locally aggressive mucosal cancers can
extend from the oral cavity, sinuses, and nasopharynx. Hematologic proliferative disorders, such as lymphoma, plasmacytoma,
or histiocytosis X, may also present in the ITF.[2] Occasionally,
distant metastases may appear in the ITF, such as from the kidney, thyroid, and adrenal glands.[3]

19.4 Clinical Assessment

The interview with the patient should address any history of
previous cancers or tumors in the head and neck or other locations, particularly details of management, including prior head
and neck surgery or radiation. The patient's medical health,
functional status, alcohol and tobacco use are also important.
The history of present illness should include a thorough investigation of any neurologic complaints, with an emphasis on
any cranial nerve (CN) dysfunction, which can sometimes be
quite subtle and easily missed unless careful examination is
performed.

Dysfunction of the trigeminal nerve is common with tumors
of the ITF. This may present as localized numbness or dysesthe-
sia in the distribution of the trigeminal nerve, especially V2 and
V3. Malocclusion, deviation of the jaw, or other dysfunction of
mastication may be present due to mass effect or denervation
atrophy of the masticator muscles. Trismus suggests possible
spread of tumor into the pterygoid musculature or the temporomandibular joint (TMJ).[4]

Facial weakness suggests tumor involvement either by nerve
compression or direct invasion. A detailed assessment of the
function of all facial nerve (VII) branches should be carefully

documented in the medical record, both to assess initial status and to serve as a baseline for comparison in the case of postoperative dysfunction. Tumors approaching the jugular foramen may cause deficits of CNs IX through XII.[5] Any complaints of dysphagia, cough, choking episodes, or aspiration should be thoroughly investigated. Any of these deficits warrant further evaluation by a speech-language pathologist, often in conjunction with a videoradiographic examination of swallowing. Again, surgery or radiation may worsen these problems, highlighting the importance of precise documentation of pretreatment status. The presence of dysarthria or tongue atrophy, indicating CN XII dysfunction, is significant for both treatment planning and postoperative rehabilitation.

A detailed otologic history and exam should be conducted, including audiogram and vestibular testing as indicated. Eustachian tube (ET) compression by tumor can lead to middle ear effusion and conductive hearing loss. Invasion of the temporal bone and middle or posterior cranial fossa can lead to conductive or sensorineural hearing loss and vestibular dysfunction.

The ITF is relatively inaccessible to direct inspection and palpation, but indirect or secondary signs can be appreciated on careful physical exam. Subtle swelling of the temporal area above the zygomatic arch may be noted. Visual changes such as proptosis, diplopia, and blurring may indicate orbital or cavernous sinus involvement by tumor. Ophthalmologic history should be taken, and visual acuity and visual fields should be assessed. Any deficits should trigger a referral to an ophthalmologist.

Finally, the patient's airway must be thoughtfully assessed. Flexible fiberoptic rhinoscopy and laryngoscopy will offer the most thorough visual examination of the upper airway. Patients who have significant trismus may require fiberoptic intubation or even a tracheostomy if a major resection and reconstruction are planned. If the management plan includes endoscopic surgery, nasal endoscopy is helpful to assess the adequacy of the intended surgical corridor.

19.5 Diagnostic Imaging

Because accessibility for direct physical examination of the ITF is limited, radiographic imaging is essential in determining precise tumor location and extent. Bony changes are best seen on CT. Frank bone erosion, especially if mottled or irregular, indicates aggressive behavior and suggests malignancy, whereas remodeled bone with smooth or tapered borders may be a sign of slow compression from benign tumor growth. Widening of cranial foramina is best seen on CT. MRI is best for evaluation of soft tissue planes and identifying neural invasion, tumor extension into the orbit, and involvement of adjacent dura. It is important to obtain fat-suppressed T1-weighted contrast-enhanced MRI. These images will more accurately display tumor-related contrast enhancement and reduce potential confusion due to high signal from surrounding adipose tissue and fat-containing bone marrow of the skull base.

Evaluation of the ICA is always important; ITF tumors located lateral to the ICA at the carotid foramen will require an external or combined approach. If there is any concern for ICA involvement following initial imaging, a CT angiogram (CTA), MR angiogram (MRA), or formal angiogram is indicated. Preoperative evaluation of collateral cerebral blood flow with a balloon occlusion test

should be considered if intraoperative manipulation of the ICA is likely. Consultation with a neurovascular surgeon is warranted if intraoperative vascular bypass is a possibility.

19.6 Preoperative Preparation

Tissue biopsy to determine the precise pathologic diagnosis and help predict likely biologic behavior is necessary before considering a treatment plan for ITF tumors, with very few exceptions. This information is critical. Although management of many tumors will require surgical resection, others (e.g., lymphoma, plasmacytoma) will best be treated with other modalities.

An image-guided fine-needle aspiration biopsy is preferable for the majority of tumors of the ITF, having lower risk and morbidity than an open biopsy. Transnasal endoscopic biopsy is possible for tumors of the medial ITF, which can usually be accessed well through either the maxillary sinus or the nasopharynx. Highly vascular lesions such as glomus tumors, when suspected on imaging, should usually not be biopsied if they fit classic radiographic criteria for diagnosis. When necessary, such as when a fine needle aspiration (FNA) has been inconclusive, open biopsies (through the upper neck or temporal region) are sometimes justified. Open biopsies of the ITF through the mouth are generally discouraged due to their potential for hemorrhage and contamination.

A multidisciplinary tumor board should evaluate each case and assist in deciding optimal treatment plans, taking into consideration the patient's overall health and fitness for surgery. When applicable, alternate treatment plans can be considered, such as when patients have unacceptably high risk for surgery or when a patient will not accept the risk of certain treatments (e.g., sacrifice of facial nerve or carotid artery). Reconstructive needs and options are assessed preoperatively, and reconstructive surgeons are engaged as needed. In most cases, reconstruction is performed immediately after the surgical resection, although occasionally it may be electively delayed for a second-stage surgery if there is uncertainty about tumor margins.

Preoperative counseling should inform the patient that intact preoperative CN function is no assurance of functional preservation. In addition to injury to CNs, other operative risks include cerebrospinal fluid (CSF) leak, injury to the orbit, injury to adjacent brain, and vascular injury, including ICA injury, with risks of resultant cerebrovascular accident or death.

Facial nerve monitoring is helpful in cases in which the facial nerve may be at risk. Select CN monitoring, such as of the vagus nerve via electromyographic endotracheal tube or of the spinal accessory nerve via the trapezius, is indicated in some cases.[6] If neurophysiologic monitoring is performed, paralytic agents should be avoided by the anesthesia team.

Antibiotic prophylaxis should provide coverage against flora of the skin and upper aerodigestive tract. If imaging reveals skull base or intracranial invasion, neurosurgical consultation is essential. If intracranial surgery is anticipated, the use of an antibiotic that exhibits good penetration of the blood–brain barrier should be considered. A lumbar drain should be considered if significant intradural dissection with risk of postoperative CSF leak is anticipated. Tumor involvement of the ICA with failed balloon occlusion test is generally a contraindication for surgery, as is extensive invasion of brain parenchyma by a malignancy.

19.7 Surgical Technique

The precise location and extent of the tumor, along with its histology and vascularity, will dictate the optimal surgical approach. The most commonly used approaches to the ITF include the *preauricular, postauricular, transtemporal, facial translocation*, and *endoscopic endonasal* approaches. Each has its own advantages and limitations, discussed hereafter.

Many tumors of the ITF can be accessed through a *preauricular approach*[7] (▶ Fig. 19.1), including tumors that arise in the deep lobe of the parotid gland, the mandible, the TMJ, the greater wing of the sphenoid, or the anterior temporal bone. (Note: This approach does not allow safe resection of the entire temporal bone or control of the infratemporal facial nerve or jugular bulb.) A *postauricular approach*[7] (▶ Fig. 19.2) is well suited for tumors originating within, or substantially involving, the temporal bone. Common indications include meningiomas, facial schwannomas, arteriovenous malformations (AVMs), smaller glomus tumors, and certain malignancies of the temporal bone that extend downward into the ITF.

The *lateral infratemporal approaches* (▶ Fig. 19.3) described and popularized by Ugo Fisch[8] are appropriate for a wide variety of ITF tumors, including large glomus tumors and other tumors that extend from the mastoid and middle ear to the infratemporal skull base, and those that involve the carotid artery or carotid canal. Surgery for such tumors may require rerouting of the facial nerve, which can be readily achieved with these approaches. Prof. Fisch described a system of transtemporal (otologic) approaches, called types A, B, and C, with progressively more exposure for each type (later a more limited type D was also described). These approaches are thus quite adaptable for many different lesions that extend into the ITF, ranging from tumors of the ear canal to those of the nasopharynx and clivus.

The *facial translocation approach* (▶ Fig. 19.4) described by Ivo Janecka[9] was developed as an alternative to address very extensive lesions of the ITF, central skull base, masticator space, pterygomaxillary fossa, and paraclival region as well as certain tumors of the nasopharynx extending into the ITF. The chief advantage of this approach is that it allows direct, open-field access in three dimensions for maximal external access to tumor and critical structures.

The introduction of *endoscopic endonasal approaches* (▶ Fig. 19.5) has offered a "minimally invasive" alternative to open surgery for ITF tumors. Not long after endoscopic sinus surgery was introduced, it became clear that the endoscope could often be helpful for diagnostic biopsy of tumors in the medial ITF. With introduction of more sophisticated tools (e.g., high-definition video images, image-guided intraoperative CT- and MRI-navigation, and improved methods of endohemostasis), the use of the endoscopic technique has expanded to include totally endoscopic tumor resections. At first this was applied to tumors within just the medial ITF, but endoscopic techniques are now used to resect many tumors deep in the ITF, including jugular foramen and even extension into the PPS.[10] With endoscopic resections, as opposed to open craniofacial resections, significant decreases in operative time, hospital stay, and blood loss have been reported.[11,12] It has also been argued, based on studies of CT images, that open approaches do not afford a substantially larger working space or visual field.[13] In properly selected patients, endoscopic approaches can be quite effective.

19.7.1 Positioning

For open procedures, the patient is placed supine on the operating table and the head is turned to the side contralateral to the lesion. When intracranial neurovascular work is anticipated, the head may be fixed in a Mayfield headrest or in fixation pins. The patient's body is secured with straps and carefully cushioned to avoid pressure points; this facilitates rotation of the entire table to enhance visualization. Hair is parted, clipped or shaved along the path of the planned incision, and the face, scalp and neck are prepped in sterile fashion.

For endoscopic approaches, the patient is positioned supine in the operating table with the head in neutral position. The head of the table is raised, in a reverse Trendelenburg position, to decrease central venous pressure. The nasal cavity is prepared with pledgets bearing topical decongestant. The eyes are lubricated but kept accessible for intraoperative monitoring of the pupils and globes. A 3D stereotactic navigation system, though not absolutely necessary, can aid in confirmation of landmarks and locations of structures at the skull base and can be helpful in defining trajectory and assessing completeness of resection. Navigation should be based on thin-cut CT images obtained immediately prior to surgery. The system is set up prior to the start of the case and calibrated using reliable external surface anatomy.

19.7.2 Incision

In the *preauricular approach*, a hemicoronal or bicoronal incision is made in the coronal plane of the scalp and extended inferiorly in front of the ear, usually following the preauricular skin crease, down to the lobule of the ear (▶ Fig. 19.1a). Additional extension into a neck skin crease is sometimes also required, depending on how low the tumor extends and on whether the mandible needs to be displaced forward. The contralateral extent of the scalp incision can be extended as needed for broader rotation of the flap.

The *postauricular approach* begins with a generous C-shaped postauricular incision extending approximately 4 to 5 cm behind the postauricular sulcus, from superior and posterior to the root of the helix down to the mastoid tip (▶ Fig. 19.2). This incision is further extended inferiorly into a natural crease in the midneck to provide access to the great vessels and lower CNs, as described hereafter.

Incisions for the Fisch[8] transtemporal approaches usually include a generous postauricular incision with variable extension into the scalp and neck, as required by the extent of the disease (▶ Fig. 19.3).

Incisions for the *facial translocation approach* are more complex. First, a modified Weber-Fergusson incision is made and extended down to nasal and maxillary periosteum, with an optional lip-split for additional access (▶ Fig. 19.4). The Weber-Fergusson incision is then joined to a transmucosal, subconjunctival lower-eyelid horizontal incision that begins by going through the medial canthus, then into an inferior-fornix incision in the palpebral conjunctiva as far as the lateral canthus. This oculoplastic technique allows release of the

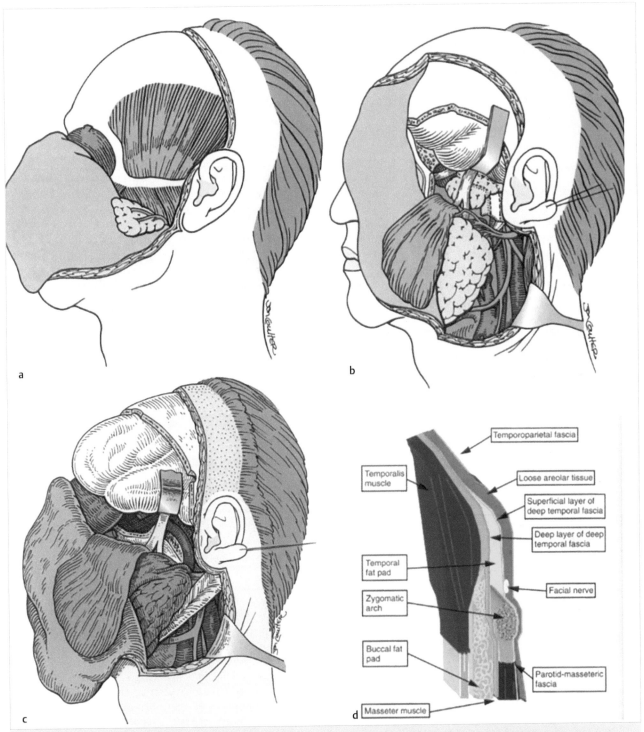

Fig. 19.1 Preauricular subtemporal–infratemporal approach. **(a)** Bicoronal incision extended preauricularly reveals temporalis muscle and orbitozygomatic bone. The facial nerve can be identified entering parotid tissue using a standard parotidectomy technique. **(b)** Reflection of temporalis muscle anteriorly, removal of orbitozygomatic bone, and temporal craniotomy enhances superior access, whereas extension of the incision into the midneck allows dissection to reach the internal jugular vein, hypoglossal nerve, and internal carotid artery. Under the brain retractor, a beige tumor is seen deep to V3. **(c)** Further dissection reveals the petrous carotid (visualized just left of the auricle from this perspective) passing behind V3. **(d)** Coronal cut-through view of the temporal region illustrating that the temporal fat pad lies between the two layers of the deep temporal fascia. Note the temporal branch of the facial nerve, which lies in the superficial layer of the deep temporal fascia. (Reproduced with permission from Carrau R, Vescan A, Snyderman C, Kassam A, Surgical approaches to the infratemporal fossa, in: Eugene Myers, ed., Operative Otolaryngology/Head and Neck Surgery, 2nd ed., Saunders Elsevier Figs. 101–6, 101–20, 101–21, 101–5.)

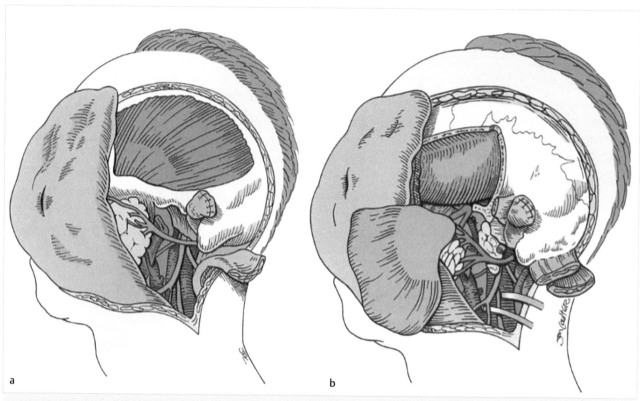

Fig. 19.2 (a, b) Postauricular approach to allow temporal bone dissection. **(a)** The cervicofacial flap has been reflected forward to expose temporalis muscle, orbitozygomatic bone, closed-off external auditory canal, main trunk of facial nerve entering parotid gland, hypoglossal nerve, and great vessels deep. **(b)** Temporalis muscle has been reflected forward and orbitozygomatic bone removed, and temporal bone craniotomy reveals extent of approach to the infratemporal fossa. (Reproduced with permission from Carrau R, Vescan A, Snyderman C, Kassam A, Surgical approaches to the infratemporal fossa, in: Eugene Myers, ed., Operative Otolaryngology/Head and Neck Surgery, 2nd ed., Saunders Elsevier Figs. 101–33, 101–35.)

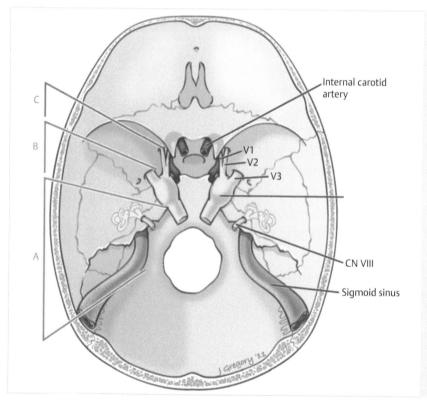

Fig. 19.3 Transtemporal–infratemporal approaches of Fisch (see text for details): types A, B, and C. (Reproduced with permission from Persky M, Manolidis S, Vascular tumors of the head and neck, in: Johnson J, Rosen C, eds., Bailey's Head and Neck Surgery—Otolaryngology, 5th ed., Wolters Kluwer Fig. 127.12.)

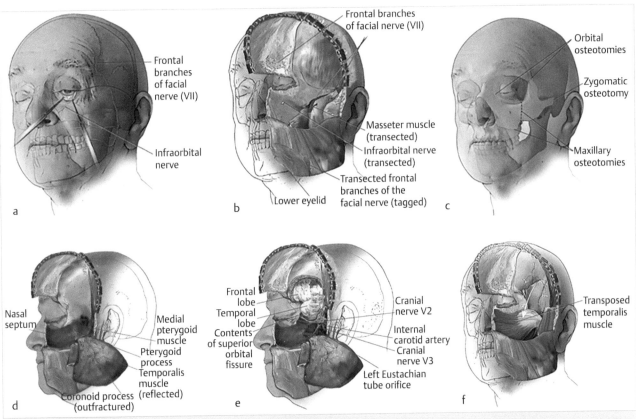

Fig. 19.4 Facial translocation approach to ITF and adjacent cranial base. **(a)** Incisions: Note that the frontalis branches of facial nerve are electively transected and tagged for neural repair at the end of the surgery. The infraorbital nerve is likewise electively transected at its foramen and repaired at the end of the surgery. **(b)** Skeletal exposure after transposition of skin flaps from face and frontotemporal area. **(c)** Osteotomies for removal of orbital–zygomatic–maxillary (OZM) bone segment, which includes anterior maxilla, portions of nasal bone and orbital floor, lateral orbital wall and rim, and zygoma. **(d)** Exposure of the ITF after the OZM segment has been removed. **(e)** Addition of frontotemporal craniotomy provides access to distal ICA, orbital fissures, cavernous sinus, and adjacent brain. **(f)** The temporalis muscle flap is one option for reconstruction of defects left after removal of ITF tumors. (Reproduced with permission from Nuss D, Facial translocation approach to the central cranial base, in: Snyderman C, Gardner P, eds., Master Techniques in Otolaryngology–Head and Neck Surgery: Skull Base Surgery, Wolters Kluwer Figs. 20.5, 20.6, 20.10, 20.12, 20.13, 20.14.)

lower eyelid yet does not leave any visible external eyelid scar on the skin of the face. (The cornea is protected with a shield once this has been accomplished.) Next is a hemicoronal incision, taken down to the subgaleal plane. Finally, the facial incisions are united with the hemicoronal incision by making a horizontal temporal incision, which is parallel to the zygomatic arch. This connecting incision allows maximal exposure of the facial skeleton, permitting extensive osteotomies when needed.[14]

This horizontal temporal incision will require transection of frontal branches of the facial nerve, which should be identified as they cross the zygoma and tagged for reapproximation at the end of the case. EMG stimulation and loupe magnification are essential in this endeavor. Inferior reflection of the medial–inferior facial flap then requires transection of the infraorbital nerve (V2). If uninvolved by tumor, V2 can be reapproximated at the end of the case.

19.7.3 Soft Tissue Dissection

In the *preauricular approach*, deeper dissection begins by raising the frontotemporal scalp flap and rotating it anteriorly. This flap is supplied by the anterior branches of the superficial temporal artery, which are preserved. The scalp is rotated forward in the subgaleal plane until the temporal fat pad is visible as a yellow color showing through the pink–gray deep temporal fascia. At this point, the plane of dissection must be deepened so as to avoid injury to the frontalis branches of the facial nerve (▶ Fig. 19.6a,b,c).

An incision through the deep temporal fascia (the *interfascial* incision) deepens the plane of dissection enough to lift the fat pad upward and off the temporalis muscle, thus ensuring that the facial nerve branches are also liberated and protected. (A good topographical approximation for the location of this interfascial incision is to draw a line from the midforehead, roughly 1 cm above the brow, to the tragus.) Further anterior–inferior dissection must remain deep to this adipose tissue pad to protect the frontal branches of the facial nerve, which run in the superficial layer of the deep temporal fascia. Once the fat pad is elevated from its fossa, a subperiosteal exposure of the entire zygoma, lateral orbital rim, and malar region is possible (▶ Fig. 19.6d), allowing for a variety of midface osteotomies specific to the needs of the patient.

In many cases, especially when the pathology is located low in the ITF, the preauricular incision should be extended around the earlobe, gently curving upward across the mastoid, and

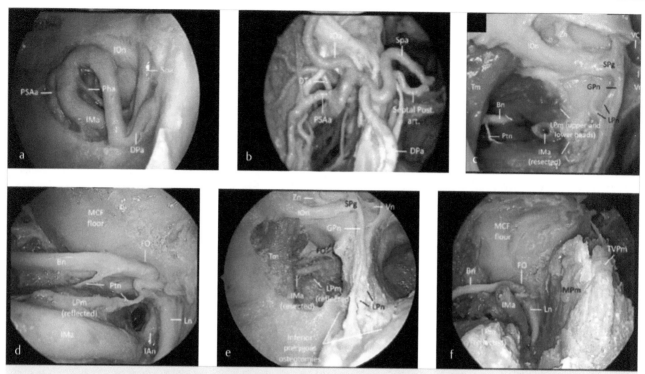

Fig. 19.5 Endoscopic endonasal approach to the infratemporal fossa (right side). **(a)** After wide antrostomy and removal of posterior wall of maxillary sinus, the pterygopalatine fossa is viewed with prominent blood vessels. **(b)** View of distal third of internal maxillary artery branches seen after further removal of bone and fat. **(c)** Right infratemporal fossa seen with transected internal maxillary artery as well as upper and lower heads of lateral pterygoid muscles. **(d)** V3 is seen exiting from foramen ovale and dividing into lingual nerve, inferior alveolar nerve, buccal nerve, and lateral pterygoid nerves. Internal maxillary artery is seen prominently. **(e)** View from the nasal cavity into the ITF is enhanced with removal of the pterygoid plates and reflection of the lateral pterygoid muscles. **(f)** Perspective with endoscope in ITF showing transected internal maxillary artery and V3 exiting foramen ovale with early branching of buccal nerve and lingual nerve. Medial pterygoid muscles and tensor veli palatine muscle reflected. (Reproduced with permission from Falcon RT, Rivera-Serrano CM, Miranda JF, Prevedello DM, Snyderman CH, Kassam AB, Carrau RL, Endoscopic endonasal dissection of the infratemporal fossa: anatomical relationships and importance of Eustachian tube in the endoscopic skull base surgery, The Laryngoscope 2011;121:31–41, Figs. 4A, 4B, 7A, 7B, 8A, 8B.)

then turning to align with a prominent skin crease in the midneck. The neck skin flap will be initially elevated in a subplatysmal plane, taking care to look for and protect the cervical and marginal mandibular branches of the facial nerve. The addition of the neck incision allows access for dealing with the extratemporal facial nerve, the internal jugular vein (IJV), the internal and external carotid artery (ICA and ECA), and CNs IX to XII.

The *postauricular approach* requires anterior reflection of the auricle (▶ Fig. 19.2). Once the generous **C**-shaped incision has been done and the postauricular scalp has been elevated in the subgaleal plane, circumferential conchal incisions are made, avoiding incisions deep within the external auditory canal (EAC) that risk canal stenosis. Portions of the pinna can be included in the resection if involved by malignancy. If pathology dictates sacrifice of the middle ear and there is a risk of CSF leak, the EAC must be transected and carefully sewn together in layers. Then the scalp flap and the entire external ear can be rotated forward to expose the preauricular structures (face, parotid, mandible, etc.).

For both the preauricular and the postauricular approaches, at this point, dissection proceeds anteriorly until the orbitozygomatic (OZ) complex is exposed. Further soft tissue dissection and scalp rotation are performed as needed, remaining in a subplatysmal plane in the cervical area, superficial to the superficial muscular aponeurotic system (SMAS) over the parotid, and along the deep layer of the deep temporal fascia over the cranium.

A standard parotidectomy technique is then used to identify and preserve the main trunk of the facial nerve. It is extremely important to minimize traction on VII, and the nerve should only be exposed as much as necessary to reach the target. The most proximal trunk of the nerve can be tagged with a vessel loop for identification as the dissection proceeds (▶ Fig. 19.7). (The senior author finds this very helpful as a constant visual marker of the position of the facial nerve trunk, which becomes vulnerable when the much deeper ITF dissection commences.) Access to the ITF, jugular bulb, and lower CNs may require further mobilization of the nerve with a mastoidectomy and distal dissection of the infratemporal portion of the nerve.

Once the facial nerve is protected, further exposure can be achieved by detaching soft tissue structures anterior to the temporal bone, most notably the digastric, stylohyoid, and styloglossus muscles and the stylomandibular and sphenomandibular ligaments. The styloid process is then removed. (Kerrison rongeurs are helpful for this maneuver.) Releasing these structures provides significantly better access to the distal ICA and proximal IJV and CN IX to XII at the skull base, which are exposed one by one in a manner similar to that used for a neck dissection.

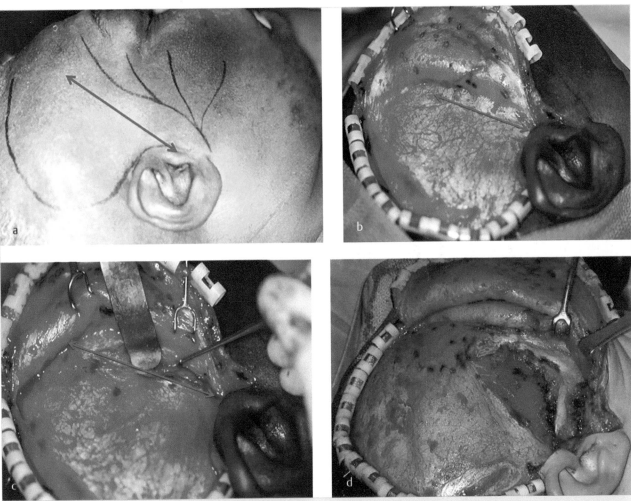

Fig. 19.6 Operative views from two different patients, showing a method for preserving the frontalis branches of the facial nerve by elevating scalp flap for exposure of ITF. *Arrows* mark the transition zone from a single thick layer of deep temporal fascia superiorly to the separation of layers (superficial and deep) that envelope the temporal fat pad. It is along this line that the "interfascial incision" is made. **(a)** Intraoperative photo showing topographical markings for anticipated course of frontalis nerve branches (see text for detail) as well as planned hemicoronal incision with preauricular extension. **(b)** With the scalp flap elevated in the subgaleal plane, the transition zone appears along the expected oblique line. In most cases, this is easily recognizable because of the yellow color of the fat pad just beneath the fascia. **(c)** The interfascial incision has been made, elevating the fat pad and exposing the muscle fibers of temporalis. Facial nerve branches are in the superficial layer now and can be safely mobilized with the scalp flap. **(d)** When the fat pad has been lifted from the temporalis, subperiosteal dissection along the zygoma, lateral orbital rim, and malar region provides ample access for desired osteotomies.

The temporalis muscle is then elevated out of its temporal fossa and reflected inferiorly. Its blood supply comes from the deep temporal artery branches of the internal maxillary artery, near the attachment to the coronoid process of the mandible. The muscle is left attached at this location to preserve the vascular pedicle. Superiorly, a cuff of fascia can be preserved on the cranium for suturing the muscle at its superior attachment during closure.

Endoscopic Endonasal Approach

The endoscopic procedure (▶ Fig. 19.5) is begun with bilateral diagnostic endoscopy. Lidocaine with epinephrine is injected to minimize bleeding. A septoplasty is performed if a septal deviation obstructs surgical access. A wide maxillary antrostomy is created and can be extended anteriorly to involve the nasolacrimal duct in order to increase lateral access. Achieving wider

superolateral access may require disruption of the nasolacrimal sac, necessitating an endoscopic dacryocystorhinostomy for repair. Extending the dissection further anteriorly, an endoscopic Denker maxillotomy can be performed by drilling the entire medial buttress.[15] Even further exposure can be provided laterally by a traditional sublabial Caldwell-Luc antrostomy or by using a posterior septectomy to allow transseptal surgical access. Improved medial exposure can be obtained by removal of the posterior portion of the inferior turbinate.

The medial maxillectomy should be taken down flush to the nasal floor with a drill so as to allow free movement of the instruments. Continuing to the posterior wall of the maxillary sinus, the crista ethmoidalis is identified and guides the surgeon to the sphenopalatine artery, which is ligated with a vascular clip or bipolar cautery. The posterior wall of the maxillary sinus is then gently removed to reveal the PPF. The internal

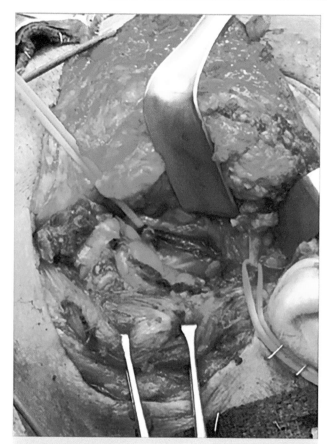

Fig. 19.7 Intraoperative photo of preauricular–infratemporal approach to a distal internal carotid lesion, illustrating that the facial nerve trunk has been exposed for approximately 2 cm of its course to mobilize the parotid. Before deeper work in the ITF proceeds, a vessel loop is placed around the facial nerve, with no tension, and is then secured behind the ear. This keeps the position of the VII trunk clearly identifiable while the surgeon's attention is focused on the deeper spaces.

maxillary artery is identified and ligated. At this point drilling can proceed through the medial and lateral pterygoid plates, with resection of portions of the pterygoid muscles as needed. V3 is identified and is followed to the foramen ovale. V2 can be found traversing the PPF to the foramen rotundum, where it enters the middle cranial fossa. The vidian canal is identified posteriorly at the level of the sphenoid sinus floor. The ET is located posterior to the medial pterygoid plate; both vidian and ET are important landmarks in identifying the petrous ICA.[12,16] After the ICA has been identified, tumor resection can safely commence.

19.7.4 Bony Dissection and Osteotomies

Preauricular and postauricular approaches (▶ Fig. 19.1; ▶ Fig. 19.2): For access to structures deep to the OZ complex, the periosteum is elevated off both sides of the zygoma and the periorbita is elevated from the lateral orbit, exposing the area from the orbital roof to the inferior orbital fissure. A reciprocating saw is used to make beveled cuts at the root of the zygoma, zygomaticofrontal suture, and zygomaticomaxillary

buttress. Similar technique is used in the Fisch approaches. During these maneuvers, a malleable retractor protects the periorbita inside the orbit. In a *facial translocation approach*, unilateral maxillary Le Fort I or II osteotomies are performed along with OZ osteotomies to free the anterior face of the maxilla with the OZ complex (▶ Fig. 19.4). The free bone segment is then saved in saline for later reattachment. Prebending plates and drilling screw holes prior to detachment will facilitate precise replacement at the end of the procedure.

Various osteotomies of the mandible can lend significant additional exposure to the ITF. A limited osteotomy of the coronoid process can increase the temporalis flap's downward arc of rotation, providing more space through which to access the ITF from above; care should be taken to protect the nearby deep temporal arteries. If access to the petrous portion of the ICA is required, the glenoid fossa must be exposed, usually by dislocating (but sometimes by resecting) the condyle of the mandible. A temporal craniotomy may be required for exposure of the superior aspect of the glenoid fossa and, further medially, exposure of foramina. Removing the pterygoid plates will provide further access medially or to the nasopharynx. An "angular osteotomy" limited to the mandibular angle can provide additional working space from below without the need for disrupting mandibular continuity. Finally, a complete through-and-through osteotomy of the ramus or condyle of the mandible, or even midline as part of a mandibular swing approach,[17] well described elsewhere, can allow even greater access to the ITF but comes with the disadvantages of potential injury to the inferior alveolar nerve and the need to restore dental occlusion, usually using a combination of mandibulomaxillary dental fixation and mandibular plates. These latter steps are not usually necessary unless the mandible is directly involved in tumor or the tumor is so large that no other approach will suffice. In such cases, appropriate oral–maxillofacial consultation is helpful.

Cranial considerations: To enhance middle fossa dural exposure or provide intracranial access, multiple transtemporal approaches were described by Fisch, predicated on temporal bone drilling and rerouting of the intratemporal facial nerve.[8] Detailed descriptions of these microsurgical procedures are found in otologic texts. Briefly, *Fisch Type A* can be used for glomus jugulare surgery or tumors that are limited to the middle ear cleft. The facial nerve is transposed along with the tail of the parotid and periosteum of the stylomastoid foramen. *Type B* is used to achieve complete exposure of the ICA and foramen ovale. The zygomatic arch and temporalis muscle are reflected inferiorly, a subtotal petrosectomy is performed, and the TMJ is disarticulated. *Type C*, by further resection of the pterygoid plates, provides access to the ET orifice, nasopharynx, and posterior maxillary sinus.[18]

19.7.5 Tumor Resection

Once the ITF is adequately exposed from the appropriate direction, tumor resection can proceed. If the surgery is done for malignancy, complete resection with negative margins is the goal even if en bloc resection is not possible. Malignancies involving the temporal bone may necessitate a lateral temporal bone resection for clear margins.

Decisions about whether to sacrifice various structures of the ITF are driven by the goals of the surgery. Unilateral loss of the muscles of mastication will lead to mandibular drift on mouth-opening but usually will not have debilitating effects on diet or nutrition. However, if the *sensory* branches of V3 are also lost, the dietary and nutritional impact is much more significant and sometimes severe. Similarly, loss of V2 can lead to unpleasant numbness of the face and palate, sometimes accompanied by troublesome neuralgia that can be difficult to treat.

Representative margins should be sent for frozen section pathological analysis. Clear communication with nursing staff and the pathologist is critical considering the complex and easily confused 3D anatomy of the surgical field. For the purposes of postoperative tumor board discussions, it is helpful to use specimen names that are anatomically as objective, specific, and detailed as possible in case of any questionable or positive margins.

19.7.6 Reconstruction

Any large tissue defect must be obliterated with vascularized soft tissue, either by rotation of a local flap or by free tissue transfer with microvascular anastomosis. The decision to reconstruct defects using local flap or free tissue transfer will depend on defect size, location, and complexity; availability of expertise; and other patient factors, such as history of or plan for radiation therapy. Options for local flaps include the temporalis muscle flap, the temporoparietal fascia flap, and the galeal–pericranial flap.

Many reconstructive surgeons believe that free tissue transfer reconstruction provides better functional and cosmetic results.[3] Additionally, in large skull base resections with resultant dural defects, free tissue is more reliable in providing support to the brain and orbit and separating the central nervous system from the aerodigestive tract.[19] Commonly used free tissue donor sites for ITF defects include rectus abdominis, anterolateral thigh, latissimus dorsi, and radial forearm.

In endoscopic resections, some defects can be managed without formal reconstruction if there is no exposed major vessel or dura. If such defects are adjacent to the maxillary sinus and accessible for endoscopic debridement, they may eventually mucosalize and become fairly maintenance-free. However, the bigger the cavity, the more prolonged and difficult the healing.

Reconstruction of endoscopic defects can also be performed using free grafts such as buccal mucosa, mucoperichondrium, mucoperiosteum, fascia, fat, and noncellular grafts. Although these are useful for small defects, pedicled vascularized flaps offer more robust reconstructive options for larger defects. Radiation therapy may increase the risk of reconstructive failure[20] and should be considered when planning the repair. Vascularized pedicled flaps available for endoscopic repair include the nasoseptal flap, middle and inferior turbinate flaps, endoscopic-assisted pericranial flap, and tunneled temporoparietal fascia flap.[21]

19.7.7 Closure

Closure is predicated on obliterating dead space and ensuring that there is no communication between the intracranial compartments and the aerodigestive tract. Otherwise, standard soft tissue closure is performed, restoring uninvolved tissues to their anatomical places of origin. A suction drain is left under the scalp flap unless dura has been opened. Fixation with craniofacial plates and screws proceeds according to standard principles of bony reconstruction.

If the lacrimal system was transected, the lacrimal canaliculi should be stented with silicone stents secured in the nasal cavity. When the eyelid has been released as part of the approach, a temporary tarsorrhaphy may be placed for 10 to 14 days to prevent lower-lid ectropion.

19.8 Postoperative Care

Monitoring in an intensive care unit is recommended for at least one night after ITF surgery owing to the proximity of dissection to the skull base and neurovascular structures. Opening of the dura, or dissection in proximity to it, places the patient at risk of CSF leak. Early recognition is important, and lumbar drainage or reoperation may be indicated if it occurs. In most cases, noncontrast CT is done immediately after, or at least early the morning after, ITF surgery. This is primarily to look for any hemorrhage, vascular injury, or brain swelling and to confirm the adequacy of resection and reconstruction.

Postoperative surveillance of facial nerve function is essential. Incomplete eye closure carries the highest risk during the immediate postoperative period, for it may lead to keratoconjunctivitis and even blindness. Prevention of these sequelae involves moisturization techniques such as lubrication, humidity chambers, and taping of the eyelid. Tarsorrhaphy, tarsoconjunctival flap, or gold/platinum weight placement may also be considered in these patients to prevent chronic exposure keratopathy.

Patients who have undergone endoscopic approaches may develop epistaxis. Nasal bleeding may occur from the internal maxillary artery or its branches or even from the ICA. The nasal cavity should be packed for 3 to 7 days to reduce the risk of epistaxis and to support any endoscopically placed tissue grafts or flaps if used. If carotid arterial bleed is suspected after endoscopic surgery, urgent arteriography will determine the best method of management—most often endovascular occlusion.

Antibiotics are usually discontinued after 48 to 72 hours unless there is retained nasal packing or an indwelling lumbar drain. Nutrition is allowed as early as possible. If patients are expected to have significant dysphagia or are unable to eat or drink, nasogastric feedings should be considered. If lower CN deficits are known to be severe postoperatively, gastrostomy should be initiated early. Airway edema or trismus, or injury or sacrifice of the vagus nerve, may require some patients to undergo tracheotomy until improvement can be achieved.

19.9 Complications and Their Avoidance

Facial nerve injury can be due to transection or excessive traction during the standard parotidectomy, during retraction of the mandible, during intratemporal drilling, or when elevating the frontotemporal flap, as already discussed. Sacrifice of V2 and/or V3 may be required for tumor resection, and the resultant facial anesthesia can put the patient at risk for self-injury, such as when chewing food or shaving. Loss of V3 motor function will lead to masticator atrophy, malocclusion and mandibular drift, and sometimes nutritional deficits.

Vascular complications are a serious risk following dissection along the ICA or IJV; bleeding can be severe and challenging to control and can lead to ischemic brain injury. Significant bleeding can also occur from the internal maxillary artery. Delicate exposure and protection of the ICA and any other major arteries during surgery are paramount to avoid vascular injury. Compatible blood products should be available intraoperatively.

Injury to the orbit is a risk in all ITF approaches but is a special concern during endoscopic endonasal approaches. The eyes should be taped shut during most open approaches but are best left accessible for evaluation during endoscopic endonasal surgery. Intraoperative disruption of the lamina papyracea and endonasal exposure of orbital fat should lead to heightened caution and frequent careful evaluation of the globe for the duration of the surgery and also postoperatively. Retrobulbar bleeding can occur from injury to the anterior ethmoidal artery and can be recognized by a proptotic globe with a fixed, dilated pupil. Urgent decompression must then be performed, whether endoscopic or by means of a lateral canthotomy and cantholysis.

Finally, cosmetic deformities may arise even with careful planning of incisions and meticulous reconstruction. Transposition or sacrifice of the temporalis muscle leads to a pronounced concavity in the temporal fossa, which can be reconstructed with a free fat graft or implant at the time of surgery or at a later date. Accordingly, any unused portion of the temporalis should be placed in this anterior defect intraoperatively to preserve cosmesis.

19.10 Follow-up and Rehabilitation

Patients treated for malignant tumors in our practice are seen monthly for the first few months, then every 2 months during the first year after treatment, and should undergo posttreatment imaging at 3 months (ideally with a PET-CT) for evaluation of recurrent disease. Patients should be seen 1 week after an endoscopic endonasal approach for removal of any packing material. After this, the patient is instructed on frequent nasal saline irrigations. Regular in-office debridement may be required until mucosal healing is complete.

Trismus can occur both in the immediate postoperative period, due to pain, and chronically, due to scarring and fibrosis of the pterygoid musculature. This is even more likely if radiation is part of the treatment plan. Jaw-opening exercises should be performed early and regularly to prevent permanent trismus.

19.11 Conclusion

Due to the complex anatomy and high potential for morbidity and complications, tumors of the ITF require a comprehensive evaluation by a multidisciplinary team to form an individualized treatment plan. It is imperative to obtain detailed imaging and (with few exceptions) a biopsy-proven diagnosis, as the biologic behavior and extent of the tumor will determine the most appropriate management. When surgery is indicated, a wealth of approaches are available to achieve ideal exposure, including traditional open techniques and rapidly evolving endoscopic endonasal techniques.

Acknowledgments

The authors gratefully acknowledge the assistance and contributions to this chapter of each of the following colleagues: Neal Jackson MD, Meghan Wilson MD, Moises Arriaga MD, Frank Culicchia MD, Anna Pou MD, Michael DiLeo MD, Rohan Walvekar MD, Laura Hetzler MD, and, especially, Annette Barnes, RN, coordinator of cranial base surgery at Louisiana State University Health Sciences Center.

References

[1] Arya S, Pawan R, D'Cruz A. Infratemporal fossa, masticator space and parapharyngeal space: can the radiologist and surgeon speak the same language? Int J Otorhinolaryngol Clin. 2012; 4(3):125–135

[2] Tiwari R, Quak J, Egeler S, et al. Tumors of the infratemporal fossa. Skull Base Surg. 2000; 10(1):1–9

[3] Givi B, Liu J, Bilsky M, et al. Outcome of resection of infratemporal fossa tumors. Head Neck. 2013; 35(11):1567–1572

[4] Jackson NM, Wilson MN, Nuss DW. Surgical approaches to the infratemporal fossa. In: Myers EN, Snyderman CH, eds. Operative Otolaryngology: Head and Neck Surgery. 3rd ed. Philadelphia: Elsevier; 2018:809–819

[5] Burke E, Nuss D. Schwannomas of the skull base. In: Hanna EY, Demonte F, eds. Comprehensive Management of Skull Base Tumors. New York: Informa Healthcare; 2008:513–538

[6] Netterville JL, Groom K. Function-sparing intracapsular enucleation of cervical schwannomas. Curr Opin Otolaryngol Head Neck Surg. 2015; 23(2): 176–179

[7] Sen CN, Sekhar LN. The subtemporal and preauricular infratemporal approach to intradural structures ventral to the brain stem. J Neurosurg. 1990; 73(3):345–354

[8] Fisch U, Pillsbury HC. Infratemporal fossa approach to lesions in the temporal bone and base of the skull. Arch Otolaryngol. 1979; 105(2):99–107

[9] Janecka IP, Sen CN, Sekhar LN, Arriaga M. Facial translocation: a new approach to the cranial base. Otolaryngol Head Neck Surg. 1990; 103(3):413–419

[10] Vaz-Guimaraes F, Nakassa ACI, Gardner PA, Wang EW, Snyderman CH, Fernandez-Miranda JC. Endoscopic endonasal approach to the ventral jugular foramen: anatomical basis, technical considerations, and clinical series. Oper Neurosurg (Hagerstown). 2017; 13(4):482–491

[11] Eloy JA, Vivero RJ, Hoang K, et al. Comparison of transnasal endoscopic and open craniofacial resection for malignant tumors of the anterior skull base. Laryngoscope. 2009; 119(5):834–840

[12] Oakley GM, Harvey RJ. Endoscopic resection of pterygopalatine fossa and infratemporal fossa malignancies. Otolaryngol Clin North Am. 2017; 50(2): 301–313

[13] Fahmy CE, Carrau R, Kirsch C, et al. Volumetric analysis of endoscopic and traditional surgical approaches to the infratemporal fossa. Laryngoscope. 2014; 124(5):1090–1096

[14] Nuss D. Facial translocation approach to the central cranial base. In: Snyderman C, Gardner P, eds. Master Techniques in Otolaryngology–Head and Neck Surgery: Skull Base Surgery. Philadelphia: Wolters Kluwer; 2015

[15] Upadhyay S, Dolci RL, Buohliqah L, et al. Effect of incremental endoscopic maxillectomy on surgical exposure of the pterygopalatine and infratemporal fossae. J Neurol Surg B Skull Base. 2016; 77(1):66–74

[16] Rivera-Serrano CM, Terre-Falcon R, Fernandez-Miranda J, et al. Endoscopic endonasal dissection of the pterygopalatine fossa, infratemporal fossa, and post-styloid compartment: anatomical relationships and importance of Eustachian tube in the endoscopic skull base surgery. Laryngoscope. 2010; 120 Suppl 4:S244

[17] Krespi YP, Sisson GA. Transmandibular exposure of the skull base. Am J Surg. 1984; 148(4):534–538

[18] Carrau RL, Kassam AB, Arriaga MA. Anterior and subtemporal approaches to the infratemporal fossa. In: Brackmann DE, Shelton C, Arriaga MA, eds. Otologic Surgery. 3rd ed. Philadelphia: Elsevier; 2009:649–665

[19] Pusic AL, Chen CM, Patel S, Cordeiro PG, Shah JP. Microvascular reconstruction of the skull base: a clinical approach to surgical defect classification and flap selection. Skull Base. 2007; 17(1):5–15

[20] Zanation AM, Carrau RL, Snyderman CH, et al. Nasoseptal flap reconstruction of high flow intraoperative cerebral spinal fluid leaks during endoscopic skull base surgery. Am J Rhinol Allergy. 2009; 23(5):518–521

[21] Thorp BD, Sreenath SB, Ebert CS, Zanation AM. Endoscopic skull base reconstruction: a review and clinical case series of 152 vascularized flaps used for surgical skull base defects in the setting of intraoperative cerebrospinal fluid leak. Neurosurg Focus. 2014; 37(4):E4

20 Tumors of the Parapharyngeal Space

Daniel L. Price, Eric J. Moore, and Kerry D. Olsen

Summary

The parapharyngeal space is deep compartment medial to the mandible and is often challenging and foreign to inexperienced surgeons. Tumors in this location are most commonly benign deep-lobe parotid tumors, but up to a third of tumors here will be malignant, and the number of pathologies encountered here is dizzying. This chapter discusses the anatomy, pathology, and work-up of tumors of the parapharyngeal space, describing in detail the surgical approaches and postoperative care of patients who have parapharyngeal tumors.

Keywords: parapharynx, parotid, deep lobe, facial nerve, mandibulotomy, pleomorphic adenoma, salivary gland, salivary tumors, deep-lobe tumors, prestyloid, poststyloid, carotid space, adenoid cystic carcinoma, mucoepidermoid carcinoma

20.1 Surgical Anatomy

The anatomy of the parapharyngeal space is either wonderfully intricate or frighteningly complicated, depending on the operator's level of experience. Failure to appreciate the anatomic relationships can lead to selection of an incorrect surgical approach. The result may be inadequate access, difficult tumor removal, damage to vital structures, or tumor spillage and thus recurrence of neoplasms.

The parapharyngeal space is often described as an inverted pyramid with its base at the skull and apex at the greater cornu of the hyoid bone (▶ Fig. 20.1). The parapharyngeal space is further compartmentalized by thick fascial layers that direct tumor growth. Prior descriptions of these fascial layers have varied.[1]

The superior border of the parapharyngeal space is a small portion of the temporal bone (▶ Fig. 20.2). The superomedial wall is enclosed by a fascial connection from the medial pterygoid plate to the spine of the sphenoid. This fascia passes lateral to the foramen ovale and the foramen spinosum. These foramina are not included in the superior limits of the parapharyngeal space but rather are in the infratemporal fossa. The inferior boundary of the parapharyngeal space ends at the junction of the posterior belly of the digastric muscle and the greater cornu of the hyoid bone. The firm fascial attachments in this area limit parapharyngeal space extension inferior to the hyoid bone. This fascia, however, can be weak and may be an ineffective barrier to the spread of infection.

The posterior border of the parapharyngeal space is formed by the fascia over the vertebral column and paravertebral muscles. The anterior limit is composed of the pterygomandibular raphe and medial pterygoid fascia.

The medial wall of the parapharyngeal space is made up of the fascia overlying the medial pterygoid muscle and the ramus of the mandible. The fascia of the medial pterygoid muscle superiorly incorporates the sphenomandibular ligament that extends from the spine of the sphenoid to the lingula of the mandible. This dense fascia then continues to the skull base and separates the parapharyngeal space from the inferior alveolar

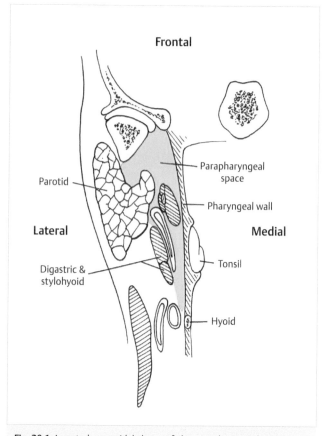

Fig. 20.1 Inverted pyramidal shape of the parapharyngeal space.

nerve, the lateral pterygoid muscle, and the condyle of the mandible. The retromandibular portion of the deep lobe of the parotid gland also forms a small portion of the lateral border, as does a portion of the posterior belly of the digastric muscle.

Superiorly, the medial border is formed by the approximation of the fascia from the tensor veli palatini muscle to the medial pterygoid muscle. The pharyngobasilar fascia forms the posteromedial border of the poststyloid space near the levator palatini muscle. Inferiorly, the medial border is contiguous with the fascia over the superior constrictor muscle and contains attachments of the stylopharyngeal aponeurosis. The inferomedial wall continues with fascia that joins the styloglossus and stylopharyngeus muscles.

The parapharyngeal space is divided into a prestyloid and a poststyloid compartment (▶ Fig. 20.2) by fascia that extends from the styloid process to the tensor veli palatini muscle. Posteriorly, this fascial plane blends with the styloid muscles. The prestyloid space extends superiorly into a blind pouch formed by the joining of the medial pterygoid fascia to the tensor veli palatini fascia. This space contains a variable portion of the retromandibular deep lobe of the parotid gland. In addition, a small branch of cranial nerve V crosses this area to reach the tensor veli palatini muscle. Most of the prestyloid parapharyngeal space is composed of fat. As a result, tumors in this area are

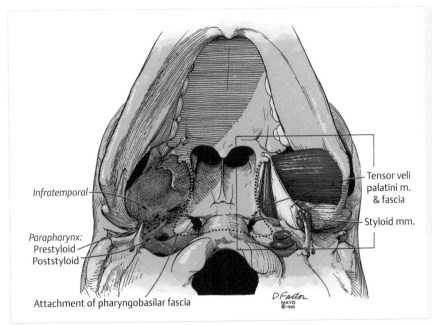

Fig. 20.2 The superior border of the parapharyngeal space is formed by the base of skull. Note the tensor veli palatine fascia, which separates the parapharyngeal space into a prestyloid and poststyloid compartment.

Labels in figure:
Infratemporal
Parapharynx:
Prestyloid
Poststyloid
Attachment of pharyngobasilar fascia
Tensor veli palatini m. & fascia
Styloid mm.
D.Factor MAYO ©1992

Table 20.1 Contents of prestyloid and poststyloid compartments of the parapharyngeal space

Structure	Prestyloid compartment	Poststyloid compartment
Vessels	Internal maxillary artery	Internal carotid artery
	Ascending pharyngeal artery	Internal jugular vein
Nerve	Auriculotemporal nerve	Cranial nerves IX, X, XI, and XII; cervical sympathetic chain
Other	Lymph nodes	Lymph nodes
	Deep-lobe parotid gland	Glomus bodies
	Ectopic salivary rests	

generally limited to salivary lesions, lipomas, and rare neurogenic tumors (▶ Table 20.1).

The poststyloid compartment contains the carotid artery and jugular vein located posterolateral to the artery at the skull base. Cranial nerves IX through XII accompany these vessels, with X occupying a position between the artery and the vein. Cranial nerve XI crosses the vein anteriorly or posteriorly, and IX crosses the carotid artery laterally. This compartment also contains the sympathetic chain, lymph nodes, and glomus tissue. The retropharyngeal space is separated from the poststyloid space by a thin fascial layer that is a minimal barrier to the spread of tumor or infection.

The stylomandibular ligament is fascia that unites the styloid process to the mandibular ramus and forms one of the boundaries of the stylomandibular tunnel.[2] The remaining borders include the skull base and ascending ramus of the mandible. Extension of tumors through the rigid opening of the stylomandibular tunnel will often be noted as a result of constricted tumor growth in this narrow area.

The parapharyngeal space has numerous lymphatics that drain the paranasal sinuses, the oropharynx, the oral cavity, and a portion of the thyroid gland. These nodes are connected superiorly to the node of Rouvière, situated in the retropharyngeal space, which drains the nasopharynx, upper oropharynx, and sinuses.

20.2 Regional Pathology and Differential Diagnosis

Tumors of the parapharyngeal space include primary neoplasms, direct extension from adjacent regions, and metastatic disease (▶ Table 20.2). The majority of neoplasms in this area are of salivary gland origin, followed in order of frequency neurogenic, lymphatic, and metastatic lesions.[3,4,5] Malignant tumors can invade the parapharyngeal space from the nasopharynx, oropharynx, mandible, maxilla, oral cavity, or parotid gland. Primary parapharyngeal tumors can extend intracranially through the jugular foramen or into the retropharyngeal space.

20.2.1 Salivary Gland Neoplasms

Pleomorphic adenoma is the most common parapharyngeal space tumor and generally originates from the deep lobe of the parotid gland but also can occur from extraparotid salivary tissue. A deep-lobe parotid tumor may have an external component palpable anterior to the tragus and may have a pharyngeal component that extends through the stylomandibular tunnel into the parapharyngeal space. This "dumbbell" tumor may have a variable portion of the mass in the parapharyngeal space.[6]

Pleomorphic adenomas can also arise from the retromandibular portion of the parotid gland. Medial extension occurs where the external carotid pierces the parotid fascia inferior to the stylomandibular ligament. The tumor expands into the parapharyngeal space and displaces the tonsil and palate. They do not expand laterally to present as a pretragal mass, as do dumbbell tumors, but may become palpable below the angle of the jaw.[7]

A final origin of parotid parapharyngeal space tumors is the tail of the inferior deep portion of the gland. These tumors can form round lesions that grow medially and cranially to present as a parapharyngeal space mass. The pharyngeal component is

Table 20.2 Neoplasms of the parapharyngeal space

	Benign	Malignant
Salivary gland	Pleomorphic adenoma	Adenoid cystic carcinoma
	Warthin's tumor	Acinic cell carcinoma
	Oncocytoma	Adenocarcinoma
	Benign lymphoepithelial lesion	Mucoepidermoid carcinoma
		Carcinoma ex pleomorphic adenoma
Neurogenic	Neurilemmoma	Neurofibrosarcoma
	Neurofibroma	
	Vagal paraganglioma	
	Carotid body tumor	
Other	Lymphatic malformation	Lymphoma
	Hemangioma	Rhabdomyosarcoma
	Vascular malformation	Plasmacytoma
	Dermoid tumor	Chordoma
	Meningioma	Fibrosarcoma
	Rhabdomyoma	Fibrous histiocytoma
	Teratoma	Hemangiopericytoma
	Lipoma	Liposarcoma
	Branchial cleft cyst	
	Hibernoma	
	Leiomyoma	
	Hemangioepithelioma	
Metastatic		Squamous cell carcinoma
		Thyroid carcinoma

generally the largest, but the tumors also have an external palpable component situated posterior and inferior to the angle of the jaw.

Extraparotid salivary tissue is also a source of parapharyngeal space neoplasms and is usually pleomorphic adenoma. They may arise in ectopic salivary rests in lymph nodes or from ectopic salivary gland lateral to the superior pharyngeal constrictor muscle.[8]

The ratio of malignant parapharyngeal salivary tumors to benign salivary tumors is approximately 1:3.[5] The spectrum of malignant and benign salivary tumors largely reflects that of the parotid gland and is listed in ▶ Table 20.2.

20.2.2 Neurogenic Tumors

The most common neurogenic neoplasm found in the parapharyngeal space is the neurilemmoma (schwannoma), followed by paraganglioma and neurofibroma. The site of origin is generally the vagus nerve or sympathetic chain. The vagus nerve has been reported to be the nerve of origin in 50% of parapharyngeal neurilemmomas.[9,10] The most common tumor of the vagus nerve, however, is a paraganglioma. Cranial nerves IX through XII and the sympathetic chain are all encased in Schwann cells and can give rise to neurilemmomas.

The cervical sympathetic chain is the second most common nerve of origin of the parapharyngeal space. The glossopharyngeal nerve and hypoglossal nerve are rarely the source of parapharyngeal neurogenic tumors. When large parapharyngeal neurilemmomas involve adjacent nerves, determining the true nerve of origin can be difficult.

Neurilemmomas of the parapharyngeal space are generally benign and slow-growing neoplasms. They rarely cause neuropathy of their nerve of origin. They frequently present as neck masses or incidentally noted lesions on imaging. Removal of large neurilemmomas can rarely be accomplished with preservation of the nerve of origin and potential return of function.

Paragangliomas that involve the parapharyngeal space originate from the vagal or carotid bodies. Glomic tissue of neural-crest origin has been found around the surface of the nodose ganglion, and vagal paragangliomas are most commonly found in the parapharyngeal space.

Carotid body tumors that extend into the parapharyngeal space are rarer. They can present as a painless mass below the angle of the jaw that extends above the posterior belly of the digastric muscle into the parapharyngeal space. Paragangliomas can be multicentric 10% of the time, and bilateral imaging of the parapharyngeal space is indicated. Patients who have multiple paragangliomas or a family history of paraganglioma have, by definition, the familial form of paraganglioma. The gene for paraganglioma has been identified as a mutation in the succinate dehydrogenase (SDH) D, B, and C genes.[11] Many times, the multiple tumors are occult and screening and imaging is necessary for detection.

Neurofibromas generally occur as multiple lesions—they intimately involve the nerve, and removal of tumor with preservation of the nerve is not possible. Cranial nerve deficits occur with neurofibromas more often than with schwannomas.

Several malignant nerve tumors, such as malignant paragangliomas and schwannosarcomas, occur in the parapharyngeal space. Malignant neuroblastoma has been reported, as has malignant solitary schwannoma.[12]

20.2.3 Miscellaneous Tumors

Other rare tumors that have been found in the parapharyngeal space are listed in ▶ Table 20.2.

20.3 Clinical Assessment

Tumors of the parapharyngeal space most often present as an asymptomatic mass in the neck or oropharynx. They are often discovered on routine physical examination. Their presence should be suspected when a subtle fullness is noted in the soft palate or tonsillar region or when there is mild fullness near the angle of the jaw. The tumors often must grow to 3 cm before they can be palpated.

Small tumors in the parapharynx cause few symptoms. As the tumors enlarge and extend superiorly, they may cause symptoms related to the Eustachian tube. As tumors expand medially, voice change, nasal obstruction, aspiration, and dyspnea may occur. Rarely, tumors have been found that require immediate tracheotomy for relief of upper airway obstruction. As tumors enlarge, they may compress cranial nerves IX, X, XI, or XII, causing hoarseness, dysphagia, and dysarthria. Horner's syndrome may also be produced by tumor pressure on the superior cervical ganglion. For a benign tumor to cause significant nerve deficits, it must enlarge to a considerable degree. Pain, trismus, or cranial nerve palsy often suggests malignancy.

Malignant tumors of the parapharyngeal space can cause carotid sinus hypersensitivity and glossopharyngeal neuralgia. Asystole, bradycardia, and hypertension have been reported.[13]

Tumors of the parapharyngeal space are often misdiagnosed as infections or tonsil tumors. Patients often complain of a mild sore throat or globus sensation, and sometimes they complain of dysphagia. The swelling in the tonsillar and soft palatal region maybe misdiagnosed as a peritonsillar abscess.

Delays in diagnosis have also occurred because patients were being treated for presumed nasal obstruction, Eustachian tube dysfunction, or serous otitis media. Patients have been known to be misdiagnosed with temporomandibular joint pathology when they actually had a parapharyngeal space lesion.

A complete head and neck examination is an essential part of the evaluation of parapharyngeal space tumors. However, the anatomic location of the parapharyngeal space makes it difficult to accurately assess tumor presence and size. Bimanual palpation with one finger in the patient's mouth and the other hand on the patient's neck assesses mobility, pulsation, and tumor extent. The finding of a pulsatile mass is generally not a helpful differentiating sign, as many of the tumors will transmit carotid pulsations. If a preauricular mass is noted at physical examination in addition to a lateral pharyngeal mass, this indicates a parotid tumor extending through the stylomandibular tunnel. The presence of cervical lymphadenopathy may indicate malignancy. Cranial nerve function should be noted.

Flexible nasal endoscopy can help determine the inferior extent of tumor, and it can also offer information about the function of cranial nerves IX and X. The status of the patient's airway should be assessed and the expected difficulty of orotracheal intubation determined.

20.4 Diagnostic Imaging

Radiographic study of all parapharyngeal space tumors is essential. CT scan with and without contrast medium or a MRI study with gadolinium should be performed in all cases. Angiographic procedures may also be necessary in select cases. The results of these studies aid significantly in diagnosis and treatment planning.

CT imaging is capable of displaying the soft tissues of the parapharyngeal space extremely well. One of the most important features in radiographic evaluation of parapharyngeal space lesions is to assess whether they lie anterior or posterior to a plane from the styloid process to the medial pterygoid plate. This is the plane of the fascia of the tensor veli palatini muscle, which divides the parapharyngeal space into a prestyloid and poststyloid compartment. A lesion in the prestyloid compartment will be anterior to the carotid artery and posterior to the medial pterygoid muscle (▶ Fig. 20.3).[14] Prestyloid tumors are usually salivary gland neoplasms that displace the carotid sheath contents posteriorly. Poststyloid tumors are normally of neurogenic or vascular origin. Poststyloid tumors displace the internal carotid artery in an anteromedial direction.

The exception to this rule is schwannomas, which can displace the carotid artery in different directions because of the unpredictable tumor position between the great vessels and the site of origin of the tumor. Vessel displacement depends on the nerve of origin and on whether the tumor arises near the

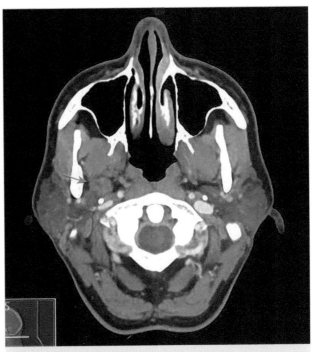

Fig. 20.3 Axial CT scan of patient who has right parapharyngeal pleomorphic adenoma. Note that lesion is anterior to the internal carotid artery and posterior to the medial pterygoid muscle.

base of the skull or in the inferior portion of the parapharyngeal space. A recent review found that neurogenic tumors that splayed the internal carotid artery and internal jugular vein with medial displacement of the carotid carried an 86% probability of vagal nerve origin, whereas the absence of vessel splaying and lateral carotid displacement had a 91% chance of sympathetic chain origin.[15]

CT scans may be helpful in separating prestyloid deep-lobe parotid tumors from extraparotid salivary neoplasms. The best way to distinguish between these two lesions is the finding of a fat plane between the deep lobe of the parotid gland and the posterolateral aspect of a mass. When seen, the tumor is extraparotid. Unfortunately, for lesions larger than 4 cm, the fat plane is obliterated.

It is important to look for evidence of skull base or cervical vertebral erosion and extension through the jugular foramen into the cranial cavity as well. Benign prestyloid tumors can cause erosion of the pterygoid plate, a finding that is not pathognomonic for malignant lesions. Radiographically, low-grade malignancies are difficult to distinguish from benign parapharyngeal space tumors.

Large pleomorphic adenomas have a less homogeneous appearance on CT and contain irregular areas of minimal enhancement, which can give them an appearance similar to that of many neuromas. Neurilemmomas also often have areas of hemorrhage, cystic necrosis, and fatty deposition.[16] Lesions that show enhancement on CT with contrast include paragangliomas, hemangiomas, hemangiopericytomas, aneurysms, and neurilemmomas.

Irregular tumor margins, spread into surrounding tissues and fat planes on CT, and evidence of enlarged necrotic cervical or retropharyngeal nodes indicate malignancy.

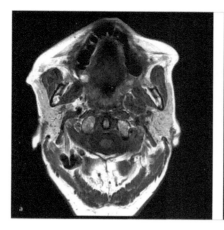
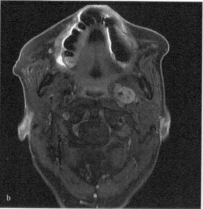

Fig. 20.4 **(a)** Axial T1-weighted and **(b)** T1 post-gadolinium fat-suppressed MRIs demonstrating left parapharyngeal pleomorphic adenoma.

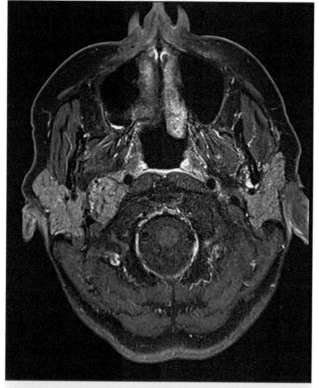

Fig. 20.5 Axial T1 fat-suppressed MRI with gadolinium of patient who has a vagal paraganglioma. The carotid artery is pushed anterior and medial and the jugular vein posterior and lateral, suggesting vagal origin.

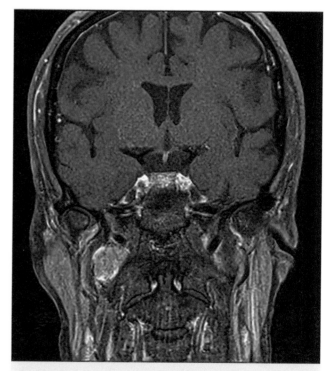

Fig. 20.6 Coronal T1 fat-suppressed MRI with gadolinium of the same patient. Note flow voids within the tumor.

The capability of MRI to image the coronal and sagittal planes directly through MR scan is a significant advantage over CT. MRI also has the ability to distinguish lesions based on their signaling and enhancement. Pleomorphic adenomas, for instance, have low signal on T1-weighted images and bright signal on T2-weighted images, and paragangliomas often demonstrate flow voids within areas of high vascularity (▶ Fig. 20.4; ▶ Fig. 20.5; ▶ Fig. 20.6). The presence of flow voids on imaging of a poststyloid lesion can suggest paraganglioma over less vascular schwannomas.

Distinguishing between malignant and benign parapharyngeal lesions based on images is difficult, but some findings may suggest malignancy. Irregular borders and obliteration of fat

planes, particularly around nerves, can suggest malignancy. Invasion of the skull base and dura is often an indicator of malignancy, as is the presence of lymphadenopathy.

If a paraganglioma is suspected, then patients should undergo angiography. Angiography can help confirm the diagnosis and allow identification of feeding vessels for which simultaneous embolization can be performed. Embolization is used by the authors for extensive paragangliomas extending to the skull base and for some carotid body tumors. If embolization is planned, it should be performed within 24 hours of the definitive operative therapy to prevent revascularization and inflammatory reaction from complicating tumor removal. It may also be necessary to perform a carotid occlusion study during the angiogram. This must be done when a malignant tumor involves the poststyloid portion of the parapharyngeal space or for extensive vascular tumors that surround the carotid artery at the base of skull.

Ultrasound is rarely indicated for assessment of tumors of the parapharyngeal space, with the exception of possible use to aid in fine-needle aspiration (FNA) biopsy. PET may be useful in assessment of malignant tumors in some circumstances.

20.5 Preoperative Preparation

Biopsy of tumors of the parapharyngeal space is rarely necessary after careful history, physical examination, and imaging. Transoral biopsy is contraindicated, for it causes the pharyngeal mucosa to adhere to the tumor capsule and can lead to tumor spillage and other untoward complications. If needed, FNA can be performed either directed by palpation or with the assistance of ultrasound or CT guidance. Fine-needle biopsy may be useful in confirmation of malignancy to help with treatment planning and patient counseling. FNA is generally accurate in diagnosis of pleomorphic adenoma and other tumors of salivary origin, but it may be less useful in neurogenic tumors, which often yield a hypocellular aspirate.

Not every tumor of the parapharyngeal space deserves surgical extirpation. Removal of paraganglioma of neural origin is nearly always associated with permanent disability of the involved nerve. Some authors have questioned the benefit of removal of paragangliomas of the base of skull.[17] Similarly, removal of neurilemmomas can result in morbidity such as dysphagia and dysphonia. These neural tumors often grow slowly, and some reports demonstrate good growth control using nonoperative therapy such as external beam irradiation.[18] In general, we recommend operative therapy of prestyloid parapharyngeal space lesions. These tumors often arise from salivary gland, and the morbidity associated with their removal is usually low. The benefit of definitive diagnosis and avoidance of long-term morbidity associated with growth and malignant potential outweighs potential complications in most of these patients. Counseling regarding removal of paragangliomas and parapharyngeal space schwannomas is heavily influenced by patient age. Patients younger than 70 years who are acceptable surgical candidates based on other comorbidities are usually offered surgery. Patients older than 70 years are commonly counseled regarding serial imaging and selection for removal based on location and evidence of growth, malignant potential, and morbidity of observation.

If a paraganglioma is suspected, the patient should undergo testing for possible catecholamine secretion. Labile hypertension, tremulousness, headache, palpitations, and sweating may indicate catecholamine secretion. Urine should be collected to asses for the presence of vanillylmandelic acid, metanephrines, dopamine, epinephrine, and norepinephrine. Serum catecholamines should be quantitated. Failure to discover a secreting tumor preoperatively can have dire consequences during surgical removal of the tumor. If a secreting tumor is found, preoperative blockade with propranolol and phenoxybenzamine may help control intraoperative arrhythmias and hypertension.

Following the complete evaluation, the surgeon should thoroughly discuss with the patient the assessment, treatment plan, and goals of surgery. Even in the setting of FNA diagnosis, the surgeon should prepare the patient for an alteration of the diagnosis based on intraoperative findings and frozen section analysis. The treatment plan must be designed around safe and complete tumor extirpation, avoidance of piecemeal removal, appropriate management of cervical lymphatics, nerve preservation if oncologically sound, and appropriate rehabilitation measures as necessary. All patients undergoing parapharyngeal surgery should be counseled regarding incisional placement; expected cosmetic defect; expected postoperative function and time to full recovery; possibility of need for additional therapy as indicated by tumor type; and postoperative sequelae, such as paresthesia, dysphagia, dysphonia, and first-bite pain.

20.6 Surgical Technique

The vast majority of tumors in this area can be treated by the cervical–parotid approach with or without minor variations. The four most commonly applied operations are (1) the cervical, (2) the cervical–parotid, (3) the cervical–parotid with a lateral or midline mandibulotomy, and (4) the transoral. The transoral approach has been reported to be effective for removing select benign, minor salivary tumors that originate high in the parapharyngeal space.[19] However, this approach gives poor exposure, lack of access to regional vessels and nerves, and high risk of tumor spillage with possible recurrence. The transoral robotic approach has gained momentary popularity in the literature. We do not favor this approach, noting that more than a quarter of patients in published reports had tumor fragmentation.[20] Tumor recurrence in the parapharynx is often an incurable problem, and an incorrect approach can result in significant morbidity and mortality.

Our most commonly used surgical approaches for parapharyngeal lesions are the cervical–parotid approach and the cervical–parotid approach with midline mandibulotomy. The cervical–parotid approach is used for deep-lobe parotid neoplasms, extraparotid salivary tumors, and most neurogenic tumors. This approach can be combined with a craniotomy for tumors that extend intracranially at the same operation. The cervical approach with midline mandibulotomy is used for highly vascular tumors that extend into the superior parapharyngeal space and for tumors confined to the superior parapharyngeal region—that is, the Eustachian tube and skull base. This procedure is indicated for tumors that have invaded the skull base or vertebral bodies. In these cases, and in cases involving obvious intracranial extension, the operation is performed in conjunction with a neurosurgeon.

20.6.1 Positioning

Before entering the operating theater, the surgeon should arrange for the availability of a pathologist to provide reliable frozen section review of the tissue. Patients who have paragangliomas should have type and cross-matched blood available. Antibiotics are not routinely administered. Intraoperative electroencephalographic (EEG) monitoring or cranial nerve monitoring is performed for carotid body tumors and skull base paragangliomas. The operation is performed under general anesthesia with the nasotracheal tube in the nostril opposite the lesion, which significantly improves mandibular distraction and tumor exposure. The patient is placed in a 45° reverse Trendelenburg position so that the head is higher than the heart. The head is turned to the opposite side of the lesion, and the neck is extended by placement of a rolled sheet under the shoulders. The patient is then prepared by sterile scrub and draped so that the ear, lateral corner of the ipsilateral eye, ipsilateral oral commissure, and entire ipsilateral neck are visible in the field. The surgeon stands on the side of the patient ipsilateral to the gland to be dissected, the assistant stands at the head and opposite the surgeon, and the scrub tech stands on the side of the surgeon.

20.6.2 Incision

The incision begins in the preauricular crease at the superior root of the helix, descends in a preauricular crease, curves gently below the lobule, and then turns anteriorly to run horizontally in a skin crease approximately two fingerwidths below the angle of the mandible. This limb of the incision should be oriented so that it could be extended into an incision able to accommodate dissection of the neck or could be extended up through the submental and lip area to incorporate mandibulotomy. The incision should not extend far posteriorly into the thin skin below the lobule over the mastoid tip. This skin will become ischemic in patients who have tobacco abuse or diabetes, risking skin flap loss. The skin incision can be combined with a postauricular incision to perform mastoidectomy or craniotomy for tumors that extend intracranially, via the jugular foramen.

20.6.3 Soft Tissue Dissection

The incision is brought through the superficial musculoaponeurotic system (SMAS) and the flap raised immediately over the parotid fascia. The neck flap is dissected in the subplatysmal plane to expose the sternocleidomastoid muscle, submandibular gland, and anterior and inferior neck. The inferior portion of the parotid gland is separated sharply from the sternocleidomastoid muscle, the posterior belly of the digastric muscle, and cartilaginous ear canal. The main trunk of the facial nerve is identified. A superficial parotidectomy is often performed if the patient has a bilobe deep-lobe parotid tumor. For extraparotid tumors, the facial nerve trunk and inferior division are isolated and retracted gently superiorly (▶ Fig. 20.7). The sternocleidomastoid muscle is retracted laterally, and the accessory nerve can be identified. The posterior belly of the digastric muscle is isolated completely down to its insertion on the hyoid bone. The dense stylomandibular fascia between the inferior parotid gland and the submandibular gland is divided so that the submandibular gland can easily be retracted medially for exposure. The posterior bellies of the digastric muscle and the stylohyoid muscle are separated from their attachments at the mastoid tip and from the styloid process and are retracted medially to give further superior exposure of the internal carotid artery, jugular vein, and adjacent nerves.

The external and internal carotid arteries, common carotid artery, and internal jugular vein are isolated, and vessel loops are placed around the internal and external carotid arteries for security. Upper jugular nodes may be removed to aid in exposure, and cranial nerves X and XII are isolated.

The external carotid artery is now easily seen passing into parotid tissue in front of the styloglossus muscle. This artery

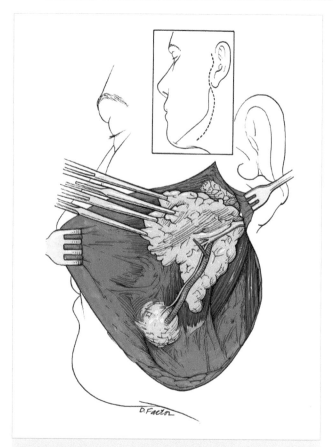

Fig. 20.7 Exposure and mobilization of the inferior division and trunk of the facial nerve.

and its corresponding vein are divided. The angle of the mandible is retracted anteriorly if necessary for exposure—paralysis of the patient may help at this point. This stretches the stylomandibular ligament so that it can easily be palpated and divided. Dividing the ligament creates a wide opening into the parapharyngeal space (▶ Fig. 20.8). The tumor may be able to be visualized and palpated at this point.

20.6.4 Bony Dissection and Osteotomies

Although rarely necessary for parapharyngeal tumors, the cervical approach with midline mandibulotomy can be used for the removal of highly vascular or malignant tumors that extend to the superior portion of the parapharyngeal space. Tumors that are confined solely to the superior parapharynx are also approached in this way. The procedure is also indicated for tumors that have invaded the skull base or vertebral bodies. Mandibulotomy should be included in the informed consent discussion with any patient who has a parapharyngeal tumor that extends to the skull base or in whom bleeding and/or poor exposure are anticipated.

A tracheostomy is performed first, because subsequent edema can compromise the airway. The incision is the same as for the cervical parotid approach, and it is extended up through the submental incision, through or around the mentum, and into the midline lower lip (▶ Fig. 20.9). The digastric

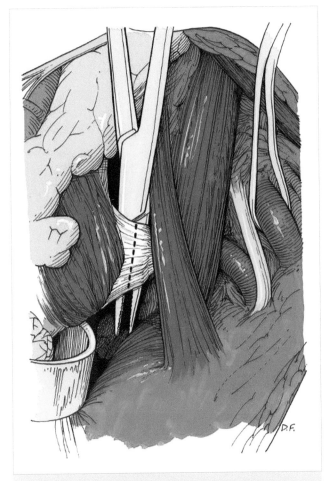

Fig. 20.8 Division of the stylomandibular fascia to open the parapharyngeal space.

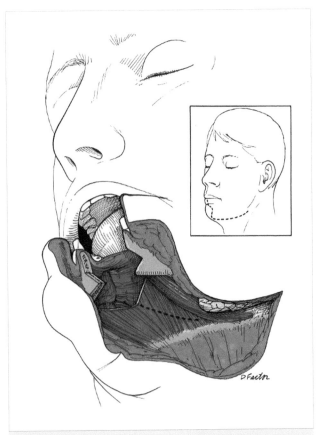

Fig. 20.9 Splitting the submental skin and lip and dividing the mylohyoid muscle.

muscle is freed from the hyoid bone, and the digastric tendon and anterior belly are retracted superiorly with the submandibular gland. A plating system with an inferior border plate and a smaller upper plate is bent, applied, drilled, and then set aside for subsequent closure. The mandible is then divided with a sagittal saw in a stair-step manner in the midline, preserving the incisor teeth if good dentition is present. An incision is made intraorally along the floor of the mouth extending this behind the anterior tonsillar pillar and onto the hard palate. The submandibular duct is included with the soft tissue of the mandible, and the lingual nerve is preserved as it stretches across the operative field. The hypoglossal nerve is followed to its entrance into the tongue and forms the lower border for division of the musculature of the tongue (▶ Fig. 20.10).

The supporting musculature of the floor of the mouth is divided, as are the styloglossus and stylopharyngeus muscles where they enter the pharynx and tongue. A plane is then established lateral to the constrictor muscles, and the parapharyngeal space is widely exposed (▶ Fig. 20.11). If the tumor involves the region of the nasopharynx, the muscles of the Eustachian tube can be divided. The retropharyngeal space is entered and the contents of the nasopharynx can be retracted medially. Tumor removal can safely be done by following the carotid intracranially if necessary.

20.6.5 Tumor Resection

Deep-lobe parotid tumors can usually be palpated and removed using blunt and digital dissection. It is not necessary to perform a superficial or total parotidectomy for most deep-lobe parotid tumors. In our experience, most deep-lobe parotid tumors are not the dumbbell type but rather are rounded and originate from the retromandibular portion of the deep lobe of the parotid gland. There often is a narrow attachment of parotid tissue to the tumor that can be separated easily under direct vision and included with the specimen. For deep-lobe tumors that extend through the stylomandibular tunnel into the parapharyngeal space, an initial superficial parotidectomy can be performed. Care should be taken not to compress the tumor against the styloid process, mastoid tip, or pterygoid plates, as this may cause rupture of the tumor and spillage of tumor into the wound. This can lead to increased risk of recurrence. The styloid process or portion of the mastoid tip can be removed to aid in tumor exposure and removal.

For malignant tumors of the parapharyngeal space, a total parotidectomy is performed both for complete tumor removal and for adequacy of lymphadenectomy. The superficial and deep portions of the parotid gland both contain lymph nodes that may be involved by malignant salivary tumors of metastatic tumors to the parapharyngeal nodes.

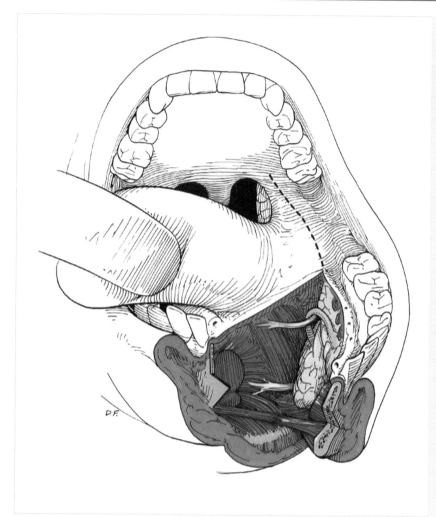

Fig. 20.10 Retraction of the mandible and incision of the anterior tonsillar pillar.

Removal of poststyloid tumors of the parapharyngeal space is performed through similar exposure, but removal of the parotid gland is not usually necessary. Only after adequate exposure of the cranial nerves and vessels above and below the tumor should the surgeon begin tumor removal. The surgeon should achieve exposure and vessel security between the tumor and the skull base if possible. The uninvolved cranial nerves are isolated from the tumor completely for preservation. After isolation of the cranial nerves, the great vessels are freed from the tumor. For carotid body tumors, the dissection proceeds in the subadventitial plane of the common carotid artery. The external carotid artery may be preserved, but in many cases division of the external carotid artery aids in mobilization of the tumor and isolation of the common and internal carotid arteries. Dissection proceeds with a combination of bipolar cautery and sharp and blunt dissection until the tumor is totally mobilized and removed.

In select cases of neurilemmoma, the tumor may be able to be dissected away from a portion of the involved nerve. If the nerve can be preserved, then functional recovery may occur. For paragangliomas and neurofibromas, complete resection of the tumor requires division of the nerve above and below the tumor and preservation of function is not possible except with the possibility of nerve grafting. Tumor margins should be checked by frozen section at the proximal and distal ends of division.

20.6.6 Closure

After tumor removal is completed and the margins are confirmed with frozen section analysis, the wound is prepared for closure. Inspection for bleeding points and correction with suture ligation and bipolar cautery is meticulously performed. The wound is irrigated with saline. If mandibulotomy has been performed, then the mandible is fixated internally with the previously drilled and contoured miniplates placed across the stair-step mandibulotomy. The intraoral incisions are closed with absorbable sutures, and a suction drain is placed in the parapharyngeal space. The skin and subcutaneous layers are closed with absorbable sutures. If a tracheostomy tube has been placed, then it is sutured into position to the skin to prevent accidental decannulation.

The transoral approach must be mentioned, although its use should be very rare. Several series in the literature use a pure transoral approach with or without robotic assistance or combined transoral and transcervical approaches, but patients must be very carefully selected for this approach. The surgeon should have significant robotic experience and open parapharyngeal

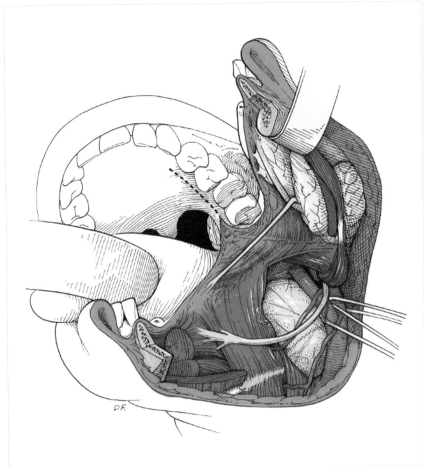

Fig. 20.11 Exposure of the tumor by mandibulotomy.

experience prior to embarking. In the largest series, 24% of pleomorphic adenomas were violated or spilled.[20] Management of recurrence from this approach is incredibly difficult.

20.7 Postoperative Care

Removal of large parapharyngeal tumors by the cervical–parotic approach leaves significant dead space that is prone to hematoma formation and infection. A broad-spectrum antibiotic is used for several days postoperatively. If the intraoral mucosa has been violated, metronidazole is also used. It is essential to maintain constant suction drainage to collapse the cavity left by the tumor. The drain is removed when the 24-hour collection value is negligible. Antibiotics are continued until the drain is removed.

Patients who have removal of high vagal lesions may have significant dysphagia after the operation. The challenges associated with dysphagia increase with additional injury to cranial nerves IX and XII. A feeding tube and swallowing therapy may be necessary in some patients. The possibility for aspiration is high, and precautions with positioning during feeding and thickening of liquids may be necessary. In our experience, younger patients and those who have isolated vagal injuries recover the ability to swallow early. Older patients and those who have multiple cranial neuropathies may have significantly longer periods of trouble swallowing or may even have permanent dysphagia.

If a tracheotomy has been placed for airway precautions, it is removed only when the patient can tolerate occlusion of the tracheostomy during sleep and the airway is well visualized on endoscopy.

20.8 Complications and Avoidance

Complications of surgical approaches in the parapharyngeal space have been reported in a few large series in the literature.[21,22] Surgical complications can result in expected sequelae from resection of cranial nerves as a planned part of tumor resection. This can occur frequently in operations of parapharyngeal space masses and can result in both temporary and permanent morbidity. The most frequently reported unexpected complications of surgery in the parapharyngeal space include tumor spillage (20%), first-bite pain (12%), trismus and jaw pain (4%), temporary facial paresis (4%), palatal weakness (2.7%), and cerebrospinal fluid leak (2.0%).[22] Wound infection, orocutaneous fistula, hemorrhage, compromised airway, surgical incision morbidity, and complications of catecholamine-secreting tumors are rare.

Fortunately, most operations in the parapharyngeal space are for primary benign neoplasms and have low expected morbidity. In contrast, cancers that extend into the parapharyngeal space or into the infratemporal fossa are associated with significantly higher levels of morbidity after attempts at removal. Reported complications have included major vessel injury,

Table 20.3 Complications of surgery in the parapharyngeal space

Complication	Sequelae
Recurrent tumor	Additional treatment/death
Cranial nerve injury: VII, IX, X, XII	Aspiration
	Dysphonia
Greater auricular nerve	Dysarthria
Inferior alveolar nerve	Velopharyngeal insufficiency
Cervical sympathetic chain	Horner's syndrome
	Facial paralysis
	Facial numbness
	Shoulder dysfunction
Vessel injury: carotid artery, jugular vein	Hemorrhage
	Stroke
	Death
Airway compromise	Emergency tracheotomy/death
Mandibular osteotomy	Tooth loss
	Malunion
	Nonunion
Catecholamine-secreting tumor	Hypertensive crisis
Parotid gland complications	Frey's syndrome
	Soft tissue depression
	Salivary fistula
	"First-bite pain"
Cerebrospinal fluid leakage	Rhinorrhea
	Wound drainage
	Meningitis
Infection	Delayed wound healing
	Abscess
	Fistula
Other	Seroma
	Scar
	Thrombophlebitis
	Pneumonia
	Pulmonary embolism
	Myocardial infarction

stroke, and death. ▶ Table 20.3 lists the reported complications and sequelae of surgery in the parapharyngeal space.[23]

Avoidance of complications involves two important steps: (1) adequate and accurate preoperative assessment and (2) excellent surgical exposure. Accurate preoperative imaging is essential to avoid complications. Both CT and MRI scans help determine the extent of the lesion and the possibility of intracranial extension while delineating vascular and nonvascular masses. Displacement of the carotid vessels (anteriorly by neurogenic tumors, posteriorly by salivary tumors) can give clues to the origin of the tumor. Angiography can define vascular tumors and give information about carotid blood flow. FNA can provide helpful information about parapharyngeal tumors and can be performed safely. Cranial nerve monitoring can decrease the incidence of nerve injury in tumors that extend intracranially.

Intimate knowledge of anatomy and good meticulous surgical exposure can lead to low parapharyngeal surgical complications. A well-prepared and experienced surgeon can expect to operate in the parapharyngeal space with minimal morbidity and excellent outcomes as long as complications are anticipated and appropriate steps taken for prevention.

20.9 Follow-up and Rehabilitation

Timely institution of speech and swallowing rehabilitation can facilitate recovery in patients after resection of neurogenic tumors.[24] Laryngoplasty with injectable material or framework medialization can improve dysphonia and aspiration in selected patients with vocal cord paralysis. Unilateral palatal adhesion has been shown to improve velopharyngeal competence and speech in patients who have glossopharyngeal nerve sacrifice.[25] We usually assess for the need of these procedures several weeks to months after resection to allow for recovery and stability of the patients. In this way, a more specific and efficient intervention can be planned.

The patient should be scheduled for regular follow-up physical examinations that include nasopharyngeal endoscopy to assess for both the recovery and the possibility of recurrent tumor. Serial imaging may be obtained to help in detection of recurrent tumor. The schedule and type of these examinations are tailored to the location and type of the tumor and the likelihood of regrowth or metastasis.

In general, patients who have parapharyngeal tumors recover and achieve an excellent quality of life when they have excellent preoperative, operative, and postoperative care. Most patients achieve a high level of functional and cosmetic recovery. For those patients in whom this cannot be expected based on preoperative assessment, the benefits of surgery should be heavily contemplated by the surgeon and patient before proceeding to the operating room.

References

[1] Work WP, Hybels RL. A study of tumors of the parapharyngeal space. Laryngoscope. 1974; 84(10):1748–1755

[2] Patey DH, Thackray AC. The pathological anatomy and treatment of parotid tumours with retropharyngeal extension (dumb-bell tumours); with a report of 4 personal cases. Br J Surg. 1957–1957; 44(186):352–358

[3] Robbins KT, Woodson GE. Thyroid carcinoma presenting as a parapharyngeal mass. Head Neck Surg. 1985; 7(5):434–436

[4] Stell PM, Mansfield AO, Stoney PJ. Surgical approaches to tumors of the parapharyngeal space. Am J Otolaryngol. 1985; 6(2):92–97

[5] Olsen KD. Tumors and surgery of the parapharyngeal space. Laryngoscope. 1994; 104(5 Pt 2) Suppl 63:1–28

[6] Chu W, Strawitz JG. Parapharyngeal growth of parotid tumors: report of two cases. Arch Surg. 1977;112(6):709–711

[7] Carr RJ, Bowerman JE. A review of tumours of the deep lobe of the parotid salivary gland. Br J Oral Maxillofac Surg. 1986; 24(3):155–168

[8] Warrington G, Emery PJ, Gregory MM, Harrison DF. Pleomorphic salivary gland adenomas of the parapharyngeal space: review of nine cases. J Laryngol Otol. 1981; 95(2):205–218

[9] Chu W, Strawitz JG. Parapharyngeal growth of parotid tumors: report of two cases. Arch Surg. 1977; 112(6):709–711

[10] Green JD, Jr, Olsen KD, DeSanto LW, Scheithauer BW. Neoplasms of the vagus nerve. Laryngoscope. 1988; 98(6 Pt 1):648–654

[11] Baysal BE, Ferrell RE, Willett-Brozick JE, et al. Mutations in SDHD, a mitochondrial complex II gene, in hereditary paraganglioma. Science. 2000; 287 (5454):848–851

[12] Ferlito A, Pesavento G, Recher G, Nicolai P, Narne S, Polidoro F. Assessment and treatment of neurogenic and non-neurogenic tumors of the parapharyngeal space. Head Neck Surg. 1984; 7(1):32–43

[13] Sobol SM, Wood BG, Conoyer JM. Glossopharyngeal neuralgia-asystole syndrome secondary to parapharyngeal space lesions. Otolaryngol Head Neck Surg. 1982; 90(1):16–19

[14] Myers EN, Johnson JT, Curtin HD. Tumors of the parapharyngeal space. In: Myers EN, Smith MR, Myers J, Hanna EY (eds). Cancer of the Head and Neck, 4th ed. Saunders, 2003

[15] Graffeo CS, Van Abel KM, Morris JM, et al. Preoperative diagnosis of vagal and sympathetic cervical schwannomas based on radiographic findings. J Neurosurg. 2017; 126(3):690–697

[16] Whyte AM, Hourihan MD. The diagnosis of tumours involving the parapharyngeal space by computed tomography. Br J Radiol. 1989; 62(738):526–531

[17] van der Mey AG, Frijns JH, Cornelisse CJ, et al. Does intervention improve the natural course of glomus tumors? A series of 108 patients seen in a 32-year period. Ann Otol Rhinol Laryngol. 1992; 101(8):635–642

[18] Evenson LJ, Mendenhall WM, Parsons JT, Cassisi NJ. Radiotherapy in the management of chemodectomas of the carotid body and glomus vagale. Head Neck. 1998; 20(7):609–613

[19] Ducic Y, Oxford L, Pontius AT. Transoral approach to the superomedial parapharyngeal space. Otolaryngol Head Neck Surg. 2006; 134(3):466–470

[20] Chan JYK, Tsang RK, Eisele DW, Richmon JD. Transoral robotic surgery of the parapharyngeal space: a case series and systematic review. Head Neck. 2015; 37(2):293–298

[21] Carrau RL, Myers EN, Johnson JT. Management of tumors arising in the parapharyngeal space. Laryngoscope. 1990; 100(6):583–589

[22] Hughes KV, III, Olsen KD, McCaffrey TV. Parapharyngeal space neoplasms. Head Neck. 1995; 17(2):124–130

[23] Moore EJ, Olsen KD. Complications of surgery of the parapharyngeal space. In: Eisele DW, ed. Complications of Head and Neck Surgery. 2nd edition. Mosby, 2008

[24] Netterville JL, Civantos FJ. Rehabilitation of cranial nerve deficits after neurotologic skull base surgery. Laryngoscope. 1993; 103(11 Pt 2) Suppl 60:45–54

[25] Netterville JL, Vrabec JT. Palatal adhesions. Arch Otolaryngol Head Neck Surg. 1994; 120:218–221

21 Tumors of the Temporal Bone

Paul W. Gidley

Summary

This chapter discusses the evaluation and management of benign and malignant tumors of the temporal bone. The primary benign tumors of the temporal bone are paragangliomas, meningiomas, and schwannomas. Temporal bone cancer is mainly squamous cell carcinoma, but basal cell carcinoma, ceruminous adenoid cystic carcinoma, ceruminous adenocarcinoma, endolymphatic sac tumors, melanoma, and neuroendocrine carcinomas are also seen. Primary temporal bone cancers are rare. The temporal bone is more commonly invaded by tumors from the external ear, periauricular skin, or parotid gland. A comprehensive approach for diagnosis and management is presented. The surgical techniques for resecting these tumors is described. The possible postoperative complications for these procedures, and tips to avoid them, are outlined.

Keywords: paraganglioma, meningioma, schwannoma, squamous cell carcinoma, basal cell carcinoma, ceruminous adenoid cystic carcinoma, ceruminous adenocarcinoma, temporal bone cancer, external auditory canal cancer, endolymphatic sac tumors, middle ear adenocarcinoma, neuroendocrine carcinoma, lateral temporal bone resection, subtotal temporal bone resection, total temporal bone resection

21.1 Introduction

A large variety of benign and malignant tumors affect the temporal bone. Benign tumors are far and away more common than malignant tumors. Excluding cholesteatoma, the most common benign tumors that affect the temporal bone are schwannomas (trigeminal, facial, vestibular, vagal), paragangliomas, and meningiomas. Entire textbooks are dedicated to the evaluation and management of these tumors. Additionally, because tumors of the petrous apex, cerebellopontine angle, and jugular foramen are covered in other chapters, this chapter concentrates on tumors of the temporal bone.

This chapter will discuss the evaluation and management of benign and malignant tumors of the temporal bone. The primary benign tumors of the temporal bone are paragangliomas, meningiomas, and schwannomas. Temporal bone cancer is mainly squamous cell carcinoma (SCC). Primary temporal bone cancers are rare. However, given the temporal bone's anatomical relationship to the parotid and sun-exposed skin of the ear and face, it is frequently involved by primary tumors from these locations. Primary temporal bone tumors make up about 2% of all head and neck cancers. Primary temporal bone cancers occur at a rate of 1/1,000,000 persons per year. SCC accounts for more than 60% of primary temporal bone cancers. The remainder are primary ear canal cancers (ceruminous adenoid cystic carcinoma, ceruminous adenocarcinoma), middle ear cancers (middle ear adenocarcinoma, neuroendocrine carcinoma), and primary temporal bone tumors (chondrosarcoma, osteosarcoma, rhabdomyosarcoma).

Emphasis is placed on the surgical management of these tumors, but properly speaking, these tumors demand multidisciplinary care. Postoperative radiotherapy (PORT) is given for malignant tumors stage T2 or higher on the Pittsburgh scale. Chemotherapy has emerged as an important treatment for T4 tumors. Several recent reports have demonstrated the efficacy of chemotherapy—usually a taxane, a platinum compound, and 5-FU—and radiotherapy for these large unresectable tumors.

21.2 Surgical Anatomy

The temporal bone is situated in the center of the skull base and is roughly pyramidal. It has six bony processes: zygomatic, mastoid, styloid, tympanic, squamous, and petrous (▶ Fig. 21.1). It articulates with the sphenoid bone, along its squamous and petrous portion; with the maxilla, along its zygomatic process; with the occipital bone posteriorly; and with the clivus medially. Extracranially, the squamosal portion is covered by the temporalis muscle. The sternocleidomastoid muscle attaches at the mastoid tip. The digastric muscle attaches at the digastric grove, medial to the mastoid tip. The medial surface communicates with the infratemporal fossa. The mandible articulates at the glenoid fossa, which is on the anteroinferior surface.

Intracranially, the temporal bone has two surfaces: a superior surface that makes up the majority of the middle cranial fossa and a posterior surface that makes up part of the posterior cranial fossa (▶ Fig. 21.2). Accordingly, the temporal bone is closely related to the temporal lobe on its superior surface and to the cerebellum on its posterior surface.

The bony ear canal (external auditory canal) is made up the tympanic portion anteriorly and inferiorly. This bony process joins with the squamous portion superiorly (tympanosquamous suture line) and mastoid portion posteriorly (tympanomastoid suture line). The bony ear canal is covered with thin skin (0.2 mm average thickness) and does not contain hair follicles or cerumen glands. The ear canal ends at the tympanic membrane. The cartilaginous canal makes up a third to half of the length of the ear canal and is covered with thicker skin containing hair follicles and cerumen glands.

The internal auditory canal (IAC) is located at the medial petrous portion of the posterior surface of temporal bone. The facial nerve (and its nervus intermedius) and cochleovestibular nerve enter through the IAC. The cochlear portion occupies the anteroinferior quadrant of the IAC and terminates at the perforated area of the cochlea. The vestibular nerve occupies the posterior half of the IAC and divides into a superior and an inferior branch to terminate in the vestibular organs.

The facial nerve is located in the anterosuperior quadrant of the IAC and has a long and complicated course through the temporal bone. It emerges out of the IAC and travels anteriorly through a short labyrinthine segment to reach the geniculate ganglion. The greater superficial petrosal nerve (GSPN) branches from the geniculate ganglion to supply preganglionic parasympathetic axons to the pterygopalatine (also called sphenopalatine) ganglion. The facial nerve continues posteriorly,

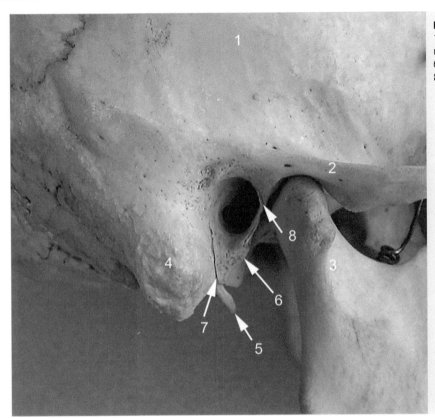

Fig. 21.1 Lateral surface of the temporal bone. 1, squamosal process; 2, zygomatic process; 3, mandible; 4, mastoid process; 5, styloid process; 6, tympanic process; 7, tympanomastoid suture; 8, tympanosquamous suture.

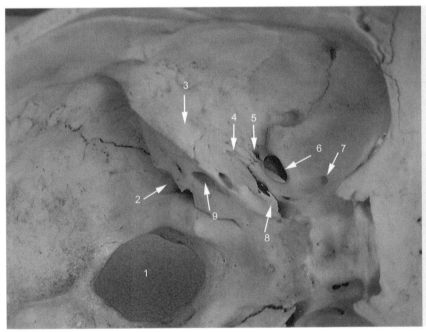

Fig. 21.2 Middle and posterior fossae. 1, foramen magnum; 2, groove for sigmoid sinus; 3, arcuate eminence; 4, hiatus for greater superficial petrosal nerve; 5, foramen spinosum; 6, foramen ovale; 7, foramen rotundum; 8, foramen lacerum; 9, internal auditory canal.

superior to the cochleariform process (tendon of the tensor tympani muscle), and continues as the tympanic portion inferior to the horizontal semicircular canal and superior to the oval window and stapes. The nerve makes a gentle turn inferiorly (the second genu) to continue in its mastoid portion; here the nerve gives off a small branch to the stapedius muscle and a larger branch, the chorda tympani nerve, which contains special sensory afferents for taste on the anterior two-thirds of the tongue and preganglionic parasympathetic fibers for the submandibular ganglion. From there, the nerve exits the temporal bone at the stylomastoid foramen and continues its extratemporal course to the muscles of facial expression.

The petrous portion of the temporal bone contains the cochlea and vestibular organs. This portion of the temporal bone is quite dense. The otic capsule is surrounded by aerated bone. This aeration is highly variable.

The internal carotid artery enters the temporal bone medial to the tympanic process. It has a short intratemporal vertical segment that closely approximates the cochlea, after which it turns anteromedially underneath the Eustachian tube. The carotid continues in its horizontal petrous portion, which is closely marked by the GSPN, until it reaches the cavernous sinus.

The sigmoid sinus is the continuation of the transverse sinus and is the major venous outflow from the brain. This sinus lies in a deep grove along posterior portion of the temporal bone. Its serpentine tract continues underneath the temporal bone to exit at the jugular foramen (pars vasculosa). Cranial nerves IX, X, and XI exit the skull base in the anteromedial portion of the jugular foramen (pars nervosa).

Cranial nerves V and VI are closely related to the petrous apex. The trigeminal nerve is bounded by Meckel's cave at the petrous apex. This nerve passes over the most medial aspect of the petrous apex and its divisions pass through their respective foramina of the sphenoid bone: V_1 (ophthalmic) through the superior orbital fissure, V_2 (maxillary) through the foramen rotundum, and V_3 (mandibular) through the foramen ovale. Located close to the foramen ovale is the foramen spinosum, which is in the temporal bone and admits the middle meningeal artery from the internal

maxillary artery. Cranial nerve VI passes through a meningeal tunnel, Dorello's canal, which is also closely applied to the petrous apex.

21.3 Regional Pathology and Differential Diagnosis

A wide range of benign and malignant tumors affect the temporal bone. Entire textbooks are dedicated to the evaluation and management of these tumors. Additionally, because tumors of the petrous apex, cerebellopontine angle, and jugular foramen are covered in other chapters, this chapter concentrates on primary cancers of the temporal bone.

Half the tumors that involve the temporal bone arise from sites outside the temporal bone. Parotid gland and periauricular skin account for 25% apiece of tumors that invade the temporal bone.[1] Periauricular skin cancers are particularly bad players, because they tend to follow along embryologic fusion and often invade the temporal bone. Large neglected external ear cancers can grow into the ear canal (▶ Fig. 21.3). Ear canal, middle ear and mastoid, and temporal bone tumors are rare. Finally, tumors from the temporomandibular joint can grow into the ear canal (▶ Fig. 21.4).

SCC is by far the most common tumor type seen in the ear canal and temporal bone. Basal cell carcinoma, adenoid cystic carcinoma, adenocarcinoma, and melanoma are the next most common tumors of the ear canal. In the middle ear and mastoid, adenocarcinoma and neuroendocrine carcinoma are the next most common tumors in that location. Excluding SCC, most common temporal bone primary tumors include endolymphatic sac tumors (ELSTs) and adenocarcinomas. Unusual tumors that occur within the temporal bone include plasmacytoma and metastatic tumors. Tumors that grow from the temporomandibular joint to involve the ear canal and middle

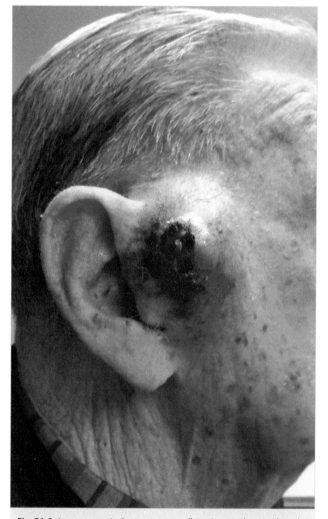

Fig. 21.3 Large preauricular squamous cell carcinoma that involves the ear canal.

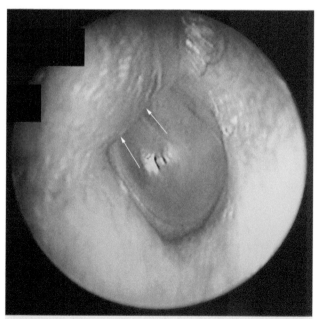

Fig. 21.4 Chondrosarcoma of the temporomandibular joint bulging (*arrows*) into the ear canal.

ear include giant cell tumor, chondrosarcoma, and pigmented villonodular synovitis.

Tumors of the ear canal and temporal bone generally present with ear blockage, pain, or drainage. These tumors are nonspecific and often occur with chronic otitis externa or chronic otitis media. Because chronic ear infections are so common and temporal bone cancers so rare, many patients are treated for infection (sometimes for months or years) before a definitive diagnosis of cancer is made.

Any unusual tissue in the ear canal that does not respond within a few weeks to standard treatment for otitis externa (ear cleaning and antibiotics drops) should be biopsied.

21.4 Clinical Assessment

The clinical assessment of the patients who have skull base tumors is covered in detail in Chapter 4 of this book. Some of these tumors have typical appearances that help in formulating the diagnosis (▶ Fig. 21.5). Because benign ear canal tumors arise from cerumen glands, these tumors are usually subcutaneous and present as an external auditory meatus obstruction. Benign tumors, such as paragangliomas, are easily seen as a retrotympanic mass or as vascular engorgement of ear canal vessels. SCC of the ear canal appears as a reddish, friable tissue that can be confused for granulation tissue and often obscures the view of the tympanic membrane. Basal cell carcinoma appears as a raised ulcerated lesion. Adenoid cystic carcinoma is frequently subcutaneous.

Tumors of the ear canal are examined under the operative microscope. Care is taken to note the extent of disease with respect to the bony–cartilaginous junction. Tumors solely within the cartilaginous canal can be excised with wide local excision. Tumors that involve the bony canal are removed with a lateral temporal bone resection (LTBR).

All patients who undergo temporal bone surgery undergo an audiogram. This test measures the preoperative hearing level. Occasionally, the tumor is in the better (or only) hearing ear. These patients need appropriate counseling about hearing outcomes and rehabilitation. Patients who have significant preoperative hearing loss should have appropriate amplification for the uninvolved ear, for surgery will produce at least a maximum conductive hearing loss.

Patients who have T2 or higher-staged SCC, recurrent tumors, and tumors that have cervical lymph node involvement or perineural spread are referred to radiation oncology for a preoperative evaluation.[2,3]

Late-stage SCC, T3 and T4, are referred to medical oncology for consideration of preoperative or neoadjuvant chemotherapy.[4,5,6,7,8,9] Patients who respond to therapy are then considered for surgical resection. Patients who do not respond to therapy can still undergo surgery, but long-term results for these patients are very poor.

21.5 Diagnostic Imaging

Cross-sectional imaging is needed to understand the extent of temporal bone disease. CT is used as the primary technique for imaging, because it offers excellent soft tissue and bony definition. CT will generally demonstrate aggressive bony erosion with cancers of the ear canal and mastoid (▶ Fig. 21.6a,b). Soft

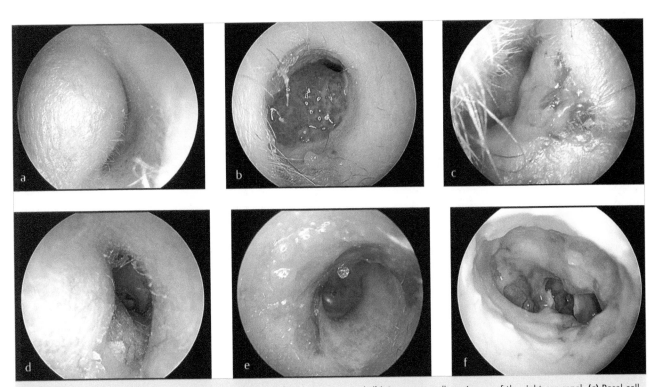

Fig. 21.5 Various tumors of the ear canal. (a) Benign tumor of the right ear canal. (b) Squamous cell carcinoma of the right ear canal. (c) Basal cell carcinoma of the left ear canal. (d) Adenoid cystic carcinoma of the left ear canal. (e) Melanoma of the left ear canal. (f) Squamous cell carcinoma of left middle ear and mastoid.

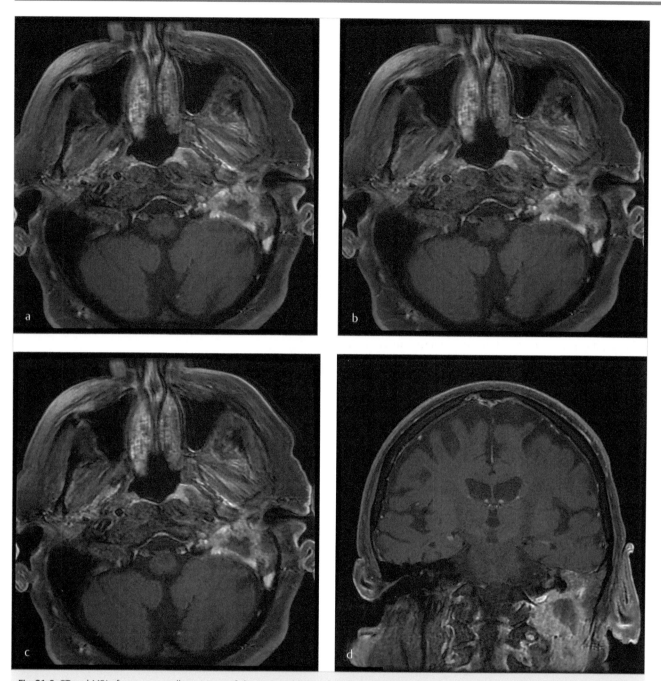

Fig. 21.6 CT and MRI of squamous cell carcinoma of the temporal bone of the patient depicted in Fig. 21.5f. **(a)** Axial soft tissue windows. **(b)** Axial bone windows. Note the loss of the bone of the posterior fossa (*arrows*). **(c)** Axial contrast-enhanced T1 MRI. **(d)** Coronal contrast-enhanced T1 MRI.

tissue invasion and lymph node metastasis are also well defined on CT. MRI adds improved resolution when the dura is involved or for perineural invasion (▶ Fig. 21.6c,d).

The differential diagnosis of ear canal and temporal bone lesions is long and includes benign and malignant processes.[10,11,12] Benign processes include skull base osteomyelitis, histiocytosis, tuberculosis, Wegener's granulomatosis, osteoradionecrosis, paragangliomas, and ELSTs. SCC is the most common malignant process, but other cancers in the temporal bone include basal cell carcinoma, adenoid cystic carcinoma, adenocarcinoma, melanoma, lymphoma, myeloma, chondrosarcoma, osteosarcoma, and metastatic lesions (▶ Table 21.1).

Arriaga et al examined CT scans systematically in patients who had temporal bone cancer.[13] They identified 12 important areas to evaluate for extent of disease: the four quadrants of the ear canal, middle ear, otic capsule, mastoid, jugular fossa, carotid canal, tegmen for middle fossa, posterior fossa, and infratemporal fossa. In comparing the CT findings to histopathologic slides, they concluded that CT accurately diagnosed the extent of disease.

Leonetti et al retrospectively reviewed stage III and IV SCC cases and compared intraoperative findings with radiographic analysis.[14] They identified five invasion patterns: superiorly through the tegmen, anteriorly through the glenoid fossa and

Table 21.1 Differential diagnosis of malignant ear canal, middle ear, and temporal bone tumors

Ear canal	Squamous cell carcinoma
	Basal cell carcinoma
	Ceruminous adenoid cystic carcinoma
	Ceruminous adenocarcinoma
	Melanoma
Middle ear	Squamous cell carcinoma
	Neuroendocrine carcinoma
	Middle ear adenocarcinoma
Temporal bone	Squamous cell carcinoma
	Endolymphatic sac tumor
	Neuroendocrine carcinoma
	Adenocarcinoma
	Plasmacytoma
	Sarcomas (chondrosarcoma, neurofibrosarcoma, osteosarcoma, rhabdomyosarcoma, leiomyosarcoma, pleomorphic sarcoma)

Table 21.2 Pittsburgh 2000 staging system

Staging system	Description
T classification	
T1	Limited to the EAC without bony erosion or evidence of soft tissue involvement
T2	Limited to the EAC with bone erosion (not full thickness) or limited soft tissue involvement (<0.5 cm)
T3	Erosion through the osseous EAC (full thickness) with limited soft tissue involvement (<0.5 cm), or tumor involvement in the middle ear and/or mastoid
T4	Erosion of the cochlea, petrous apex, medial wall of the middle ear, carotid canal, jugular foramen, or dura with extensive soft tissue involvement (>0.5 cm, such as involvement of the TMJ or styloid process) or evidence of facial paresis
N classification	
N0	No regional nodes involved
N1	Single metastatic regional node <3 cm in size
N2	
N2a	Single ipsilateral metastatic node 3–6 cm in size
N2b	Multiple ipsilateral metastatic lymph nodes
N2c	Contralateral metastatic lymph node
N3	Metastatic lymph node >6 cm in size
Overall stage	
I	T1N0
II	T2N0
III	T3N0
IV	T4N0 and T1–4N1–3

Abbreviations: EAC, external auditory canal; TMJ, temporomandibular joint.

infratemporal fossa, inferiorly through the hypotympanum and jugular foramen, posteriorly though the mastoid air cells, and medially though the middle ear and carotid canal. They found that CT and MRI underestimated disease in the tegmen tympani, middle fossa dura, and intradural extension of disease.

Accurate assessment of imaging is required for staging of these tumors. A number of staging systems have been proposed for SCC.[15,16,17,18,19,20] Although there is not an American Joint Committee on Cancer (AJCC) approved staging system, the Pittsburgh staging system has been widely used in the literature (▶ Table 21.2).[21,22]

21.6 Preoperative Preparation

Patients who have temporal bone cancer are thoroughly questioned about their underlying medical history and carefully examined. Because temporal bone surgery usually requires several hours under general anesthetic, these patients must be of good general health. All underlying medical illnesses must be identified and optimized to minimize the chance of postoperative complications. When patients have multiple medical problems, a consultation with an internist is indicated to help manage these issues.

21.7 Surgical Technique: Benign Tumors

The most common benign tumor affecting the temporal bone is paraganglioma. Small paragangliomas that are found only within the middle ear (so-called glomus tympanicum) are easily excised via a transcanal approach (▶ Fig. 21.7). A postauricular incision is made, and the ear canal is entered medially to the bony–cartilaginous junction. An incision is made anteriorly, and a large tympanomeatal flap is elevated to expose the inferior tympanic ring. The drill can be used to remove the inferior tympanic ring to expose the inferior extent of the tumor, if necessary. The tumor is carefully dissected away from the ossicular

chain and out of the Eustachian tube. Bipolar cautery or CO_2 laser is used to coagulate the feeding vessels into the tumor. The tumor is then removed. Bleeding is easily controlled using absorbable gelatin sponge and thrombin solution. The tympanomeatal flap is repositioned and the ear canal filled with packing material. The postauricular wound is closed in layers.

Larger tumors that extend beyond the tympanic ring will require either a tympanomastoid approach or an infratemporal fossa approach (Fisch type C).[23] For the tympanomastoid approach, a postauricular incision is made and a complete mastoidectomy performed. A tympanomeatal flap, as already described, is elevated to expose the tumor in the middle ear. Standard techniques are used to identify the facial nerve. The fallopian canal can be skeletonized to create an "intact fallopian bridge" (▶ Fig. 21.8).[24] Tumor resection is performed by working through both the middle ear and mastoid. Hemostasis is achieved using gelatin packing and thrombin. The tympanomeatal flap is replaced and the ear canal is packed. The postauricular wound is closed in layers.

Larger tumors that invade the jugular bulb require an infratemporal fossa approach. These larger tumors are evaluated with angiography preoperatively. Feeding vessels are embolized or coiled to help reduce blood loss. Because these patients are at high risk of developing lower cranial nerve deficits, all patients are evaluated preoperatively by a speech and swallowing

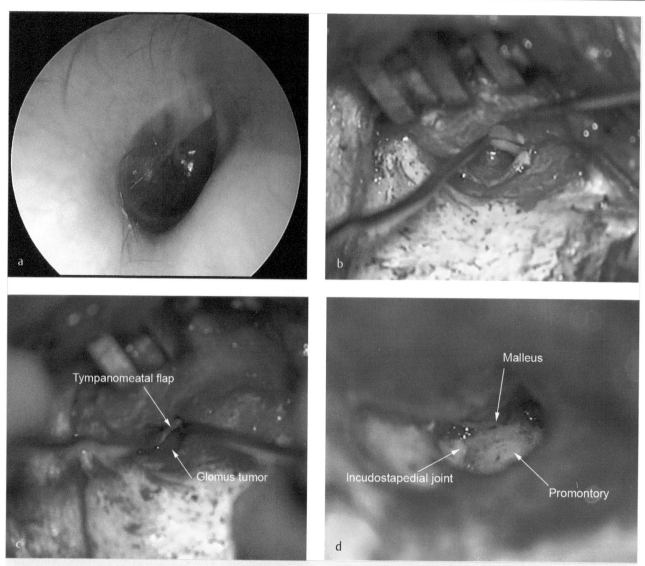

Fig. 21.7 Glomus tympanicum. **(a)** Otoendoscopic photograph of glomus tympanicum. **(b)** Postauricular approach with anterior canal incision. **(c)** Flap elevation exposing tumor in middle ear. **(d)** Tumor resection completed.

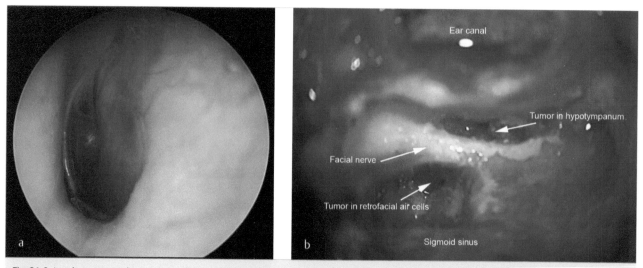

Fig. 21.8 Jugulotympanic glomus tumor, left ear. **(a)** Otoendoscopic photograph. **(b)** Intact fallopian bridge being developed.

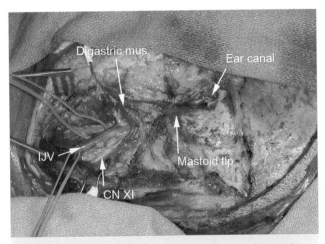

Fig. 21.9 Neck exposure for glomus jugulare. The internal carotid artery is looped with a red vessel loop and is not seen. IJV, internal jugular vein.

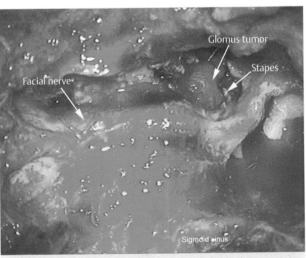

Fig. 21.10 Facial nerve fully decompressed. Labyrinthectomy has been performed. Sigmoid sinus is being compressed with retractor.

therapist. Intraoperative nerve monitoring is employed for the facial and vagus nerves.

This approach requires removal of the ear canal and overclosure of the external auditory meatus. As a result, conductive hearing loss is an expected outcome. Furthermore, the facial nerve is elevated out of its canal, and temporary facial weakness is common.

A large postauricular C-shaped incision is made and elevated over the temporalis muscle, sternocleidomastoid muscle, and parotid gland. A palva flap is elevated, and the ear canal is divided medial to the bony–cartilaginous junction. After the canal is divided, the skin flap can be elevated over the parotid gland and held with a fishhook retractor. The skin of the external auditory meatus is undermined, everted, and sewn shut. The palva flap is sewn to the undersurface of the ear as a second layer.

Neck dissection is performed to identify the lower cranial nerves (IX–XII), the internal carotid artery, and the internal jugular vein. Vascular loops are placed around the great vessels (▶ Fig. 21.9).

The skin of the bony canal, tympanic membrane, incus, and malleus are removed. A radical mastoidectomy is performed. The sigmoid sinus is skeletonized and 1 to 2 cm of retrosigmoid dura is exposed. The mastoid tip is removed, unifying the temporal bone with the neck. The facial nerve is skeletonized for 270° of its circumference from the second genu to the stylomastoid foramen (▶ Fig. 21.10). Fisch instruments are used to remove the last thin shell of bone on the nerve and to open the periosteal cuff at the stylomastoid foramen. Blunt dissection along the nerve with a fine hemostat and sharp dissection with a no. 12 blade are used to dissect the extratemporal portion of the nerve until the pes anserinus is reached. The nerve is then gently elevated out of its canal. The digastric muscle is divided and grasped to avoid injuring the nerve, and the nerve is sewn up to the parotid gland.

Bone over the jugular bulb is then removed to expose the entire tumor. The styloid process and its muscular attachments are removed. The digastric is reflected anteriorly. Resection of the tumor requires ligation of the sigmoid. Suture ligatures are placed around the sigmoid and the sinus

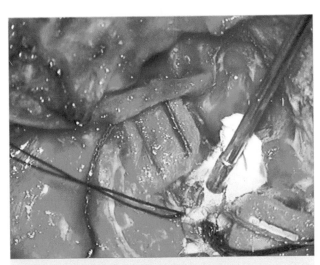

Fig. 21.11 Sigmoid sinus is doubly ligated and divided.

is divided (▶ Fig. 21.11). The jugular vein is then ligated and divided in the neck. Tumor removal is then performed. Bleeding from the petrosal sinuses is controlled with packing.

Once the tumor is removed, reconstruction begins by harvesting an abdominal fat graft to fill in the mastoid defect. The dura can be repaired with a temporalis fascia graft, and strips of fat are packed on top of this.

21.8 Surgical Technique: Malignant Tumors

Malignant tumors that are confined to the external auditory meatus are excised via an endaural incision. The tumor is excised with 4 mm margins. The underlying cartilage is removed with the overlying skin. Orienting marks or sutures are placed for the pathologist, and the margins are checked with frozen section. If the margins are all clear, then reconstruction is performed with a split thickness skin graft. If the medial or bony

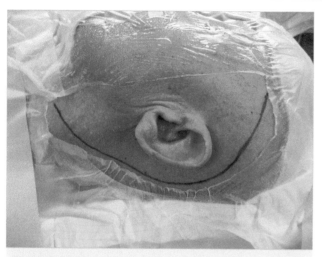

Fig. 21.12 C-shaped postauricular incision for resection of malignant ear canal tumor.

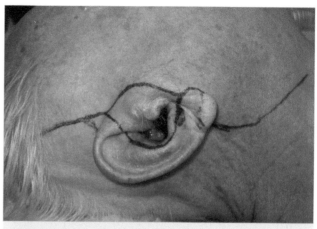

Fig. 21.13 Preauricular incision for recurrent squamous cell carcinoma of the ear canal.

canal margin is positive, then LTBR is performed as described hereafter.

The following sections will describe the techniques for LTBR and for subtotal (STBR) and total (TTBR) temporal bone resection.

21.8.1 Operative Preparation and Positioning

These procedures are performed under general anesthetic. The patient is positioned supine, padded, and strapped to the operating table, which is turned 180° so that the anesthesia stand is at the patient's feet. The head can be positioned in a Mayfield head holder when an image guidance system is used, but these procedures do not require this technique except in cases of STBR or TTBR.

The hair is clipped around the ear. The head, neck, and thighs are prepared in a sterile manner, because anterolateral thigh is the most common donor site for reconstruction.

Electrodes for facial nerve monitoring are placed. Monitoring is performed for all patients with facial function; this modality is not performed for patients who have facial paralysis. A temporary tarsorrhaphy stitch is often placed to protect the eye.

21.8.2 Incisions

A variety of incisions can be used for these procedures. The choice of incision depends on the presence of previous scars and the location and extent of the primary tumor. Tumors that are confined to the ear canal can be excised using a large postauricular C-shaped incision (▶ Fig. 21.12). The incision is designed to permit neck dissection for level 2. The skin flap is elevated over the temporalis muscle and mastoid periosteum. The ear canal is divided at the external auditory meatus, and the outer ear and surround skin are elevated as a large visor flap over the parotid gland and upper neck.

Alternatively, a preauricular modified Blair incision can be used (▶ Fig. 21.13). This incision is extended superiorly to

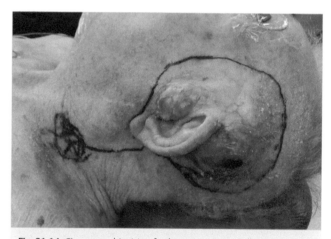

Fig. 21.14 Circumaural incision for large squamous cell carcinoma of periauricular skin.

ellipse the ear canal and is further extended superiorly into the temporal scalp. The advantage of this incision is that the external ear is elevated with a broad blood supply and is especially useful when either a prior parotidectomy has been performed or the patient has received prior radiotherapy.

Finally, a large circumaural incision is used when the primary involves the majority of the outer ear (▶ Fig. 21.14). In this case, a margin of 1 to 2 cm is drawn around the tumor, and the skin is incised down to the temporal bone and sternocleidomastoid muscle and parotid gland.

Regardless of the incision that is used, margins from the surrounding normal skin are sent for frozen section.

21.8.3 Bony Dissection and Osteotomies

Temporal bone dissection is performed in a stepwise fashion prior to parotidectomy and neck dissection. This order is preferred because the facial nerve can be identified in the mastoid and followed into the parotid.

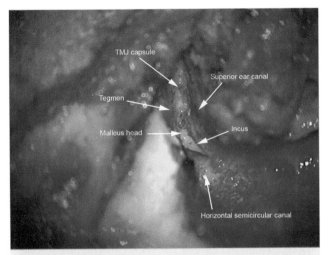

Fig. 21.15 Lateral temporal bone resection, with exposure of the joint capsule.

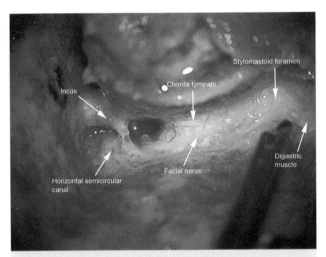

Fig. 21.16 Facial nerve to stylomastoid foramen.

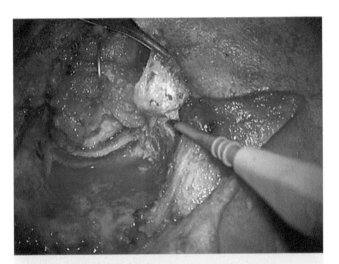

Fig. 21.17 Mastoid tip is freed.

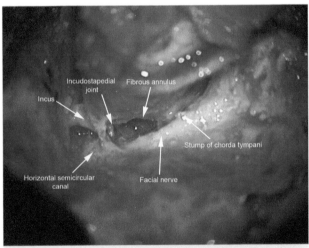

Fig. 21.18 Extended facial recess and opening hypotympanic air cells.

LTBR is usually a required first step prior to STBR or TTBR. The goal of LTBR is en bloc resection of the ear canal. LTBR can be combined with parotidectomy, neck dissection, partial mandibulectomy, or resection of the zygoma, infratemporal fossa, or middle fossa dura depending on the extent of the disease.

A complete mastoidectomy is performed, identifying the mastoid tegmen, sigmoid sinus, and digastric ridge. The operating microscope is brought into place and used for the remaining procedure. The antrum is opened, allowing identification of the horizontal semicircular canal. The antrum is widened until the incus and malleus head are exposed. The root of the zygoma is drilled away until the capsule of the temporomandibular joint is exposed. Bone lateral to the ossicular chain is removed, following the bone of the ear canal and tegmen. Exposure of the joint capsule superior to the ear canal marks the anterior superior extent of the dissection (▶ Fig. 21.15).

The facial recess is opened and the middle ear examined. If the middle ear is normal, LTBR can continue. If the middle ear contains tumor, then STBR is necessary. The tympanic portion of the facial nerve is identified and is followed to the second genu of the facial nerve. The mastoid portion of the facial nerve is followed to the stylomastoid foramen (▶ Fig. 21.16).

The stylomastoid foramen is widened, and the digastric muscle is exposed. A bone cut is made lateral to the facial nerve and inferior to the ear canal. The mastoid tip is mobilized and is freed from its muscular attachments (▶ Fig. 21.17). This move unifies the temporal bone with the neck and permits tracing the facial nerve from the mastoid into the parotid gland.

The facial recess is extended and widened so that the fibrous annulus is identified. Drilling is performed between the facial nerve and the annulus to open the hypotympanic air cells (▶ Fig. 21.18). In the process, the chorda tympani nerve is sacrificed.

The inferior tympanic ring bone is drilled away until soft tissue is reached. These two bony cuts are joined together to complete the inferior canal cut. Care is taken to avoid injury to the carotid artery, which can lie at the level of the annulus.

Thumb pressure on the canal fractures the ear canal at the level of the annulus. A Freer elevator can be used to elevate the ear canal and ear drum. Care is taken to avoid using either

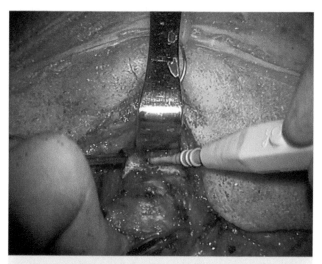

Fig. 21.19 Dissection anterior to the ear canal to separate the canal from the surrounding soft tissues. The ear canal is being retracted posteriorly.

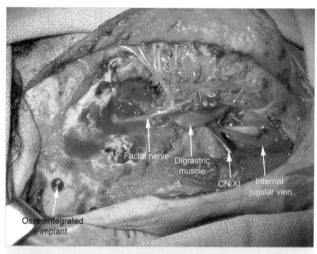

Fig. 21.20 Osseointegrated implant placed at the time of oncologic resection. In this example, parotidectomy and neck dissection were performed along with lateral temporal bone resection.

the dura or the facial nerve as a fulcrum for the Freer. The ear canal is attached only by soft tissue anteriorly. If parotidectomy and neck dissection are not planned, then the attached soft tissues can be divided following the bloodless plane along the cartilage and bone of the ear canal (▶ Fig. 21.19).

If parotidectomy is performed, then the ear canal and overlying soft tissues are left intact to be removed with the parotid. When parotidectomy is planned, facial nerve decompression is performed. Bone covering the mastoid portion of the facial nerve is thinned using diamond burs. The last thin shell of bone is removed using Fisch instruments. At the stylomastoid foramen, the periosteal cuff is opened using Fisch instruments and the facial nerve is dissected from the surrounding soft tissues using a fine Jacobsen hemostat, bipolar electrocautery, and a no. 12 blade.

When the face is paralyzed preoperatively, facial nerve sacrifice is required. In this circumstance, the facial nerve is divided proximal to the sight of involvement and a nerve segment is sent for frozen section.

The decision to sacrifice a normally functioning facial nerve is usually very difficult. Occasionally, abnormal tissue around the facial nerve can be biopsied to confirm malignant invasion of the nerve.

STBR implies that the middle ear is involved. To achieve a negative margin, the labyrinth and cochlea are removed. In these late stage 3 and 4 tumors, facial nerve sacrifice is often required. The carotid canal is skeletonized. Tumor within the middle ear, mastoid, and inner ear is removed piecemeal.

TTBR implies that the petrous apex is involved. This deepens the surgical defect from STBR to include the petrous apex and IAC.

Often such advanced stage tumors involve the dura. If the dura is involved, a craniotomy is performed to allow resection and repair of the dura.

21.8.4 Soft Tissue Dissection

After the temporal bone work has been completed and the facial nerve decompressed, parotidectomy and neck dissection are performed. For SCC of the ear canal, parotidectomy is performed, because the tumor can directly involve the parotid gland through the fissures of Santorini or the gland can be involved indirectly with intraparotid metastases. Level 2 lymph nodes are removed for ear canal and temporal bone cancers. If level 2 nodes are involved, then levels 3 and 4 are removed.

The branches of the facial nerve are individually followed so that the superficial lobe of the gland is removed.

21.8.5 Reconstruction

The rate of facial nerve sacrifice approaches 45% in patients who have temporal bone malignancies.[12] Facial nerve reconstruction is performed using the greater auricular nerve, the sural nerve, or a donor nerve from the free flap site (lateral cutaneous thigh nerve). Good outcomes can be achieved even when the proximal margin of the facial nerve is positive for tumor and when PORT is given.[25,26]

Eyelid loading with either a gold weight or platinum chain and static slings can be placed at the time of oncologic resection when the facial nerve is sacrificed. Additional surgery to rehabilitate the paralyzed face, such as brow lift or tarsorrhaphy, is generally performed at a later time.

Osseointegrated implants can be placed at the time of oncologic resection for attachment of a bone-conducting hearing aid and auricular prosthesis (▶ Fig. 21.20). These implants have better osseointegration and lower rates of extrusion if they are placed prior to radiation.[27]

Historically, lateral temporal bone defects were left open; however, this lack of reconstruction led to a high rate of osteoradionecrosis.[28] As a result, these defects are always closed off. The choice of reconstruction technique depends on the final defect and any prior treatment (e.g., radiotherapy). LTBR defects can be repaired using either a temporalis flap and split-thickness skin graft or a microvascular flap. Temporalis muscle flap is chosen when the soft tissue defect is small and when the blood supply to the muscle has not been disturbed.

Larger defects, especially defects that include mandibulectomy or dural resection, are closed using a microvascular free flap. Patients who have previously been irradiated are also reconstructed using a free flap, regardless of the size of the defect. A number of different flaps have been used for reconstruction, but the anterolateral thigh flap has been a reliable donor site having enough bulk for closure of even very large defects (defect diameter up to 15 cm).[29]

Whether temporalis muscle flap or microvascular free flap is performed, closed suction wound drains are placed to minimize hematoma formation.

21.8.6 Postoperative Care

Perioperative antibiotics are used for just 24 hours. Because patients' average age exceeds 65 years, many have underlying medical problems that require appropriate medical management. Patients who have facial weakness or paralysis are started on eyedrops and moisturizing ointment to prevent exposure keratopathy.

Patients who undergo LTBR and temporalis muscle flap are usually observed for two nights before being discharged home. The main complication in this circumstance has been hematoma formation.

Patients who undergo microvascular free flap reconstruction are usually observed in the hospital for 5 to 7 days. Close monitoring of the flap is essential to identify signs of early flap failure and to instigate salvage of the flap when it appears to be in trouble.

Jugular foramen tumor patients are at high risk for developing aspiration. These patients are evaluated by a speech and swallowing therapist before starting an oral diet. Those patients who have trouble protecting the airway are fed by alternate means (either a nasogastric or a percutaneous gastrostomy tube).

21.8.7 Complications and Their Avoidance

Facial weakness or paralysis is a common outcome from this surgery. Despite careful surgical technique, patients who undergo temporal bone resection and parotidectomy have a high incidence of temporary facial weakness. Eye care is mandatory for these patients to prevent exposure keratopathy. If the nerve is intact, facial function will return with time. To encourage nerve regeneration, facial nerve exercises are started before discharge from hospital.

Cerebrospinal fluid (CSF) leak can occur in patients who have had dural resection. Watertight closure of the dura is the goal, but this can be difficult to achieve medially along the floor of the middle fossa. Reinforcing the dural repair with a free flap can help prevent CSF from leaking through the wound or the Eustachian tube. In the MD Anderson series, fewer than 1% of patients developed a CSF leak that required either lumbar drainage or reoperation.

Wound infection occurs in about 5 to 10% of temporal bone resections. Ulcerated necrotic tumors, prior radiation, obesity, and diabetes are risk factors for postoperative wound infection.

21.8.8 Follow-up and Rehabilitation

These patients are seen for suture removal about 10 days to 2 weeks after surgery. The results of the final pathology report are discussed with the patient, and a decision about postoperative radiotherapy is made.

Perineural invasion, lymph node involvement, bone invasion, positive margin, and recurrent tumors are all indications for PORT, which is usually started about 4 to 6 weeks after surgery. The decision about radiation modality is left to the radiotherapist. The patient is seen halfway during radiotherapy and at the conclusion of therapy. A follow-up CT scan is performed about 6 weeks after radiotherapy, with imaging repeated every 3 months for the first 2 years, then every 6 months until the 5-year mark.

If radiotherapy is not necessary, then the patient is seen every 3 months and so on, as already described.

Hearing rehabilitation is important for patients who lose the sound-conducting mechanism of the ear. For this reason, osseointegrated implants are placed in almost all patients at the time of the oncologic resection. If radiotherapy is not required, then a second-stage procedure to place the transcutaneous abutment is performed about 3 months postoperatively. The postoperative CT scan can help in locating the implant, whose small, flat head can be difficult to palpate when the skin thickness is greater than 10 mm.

If radiotherapy was administered, then second-stage abutment procedure is delayed for at least 6 months to allow for adequate osseointegration.[27] Frequently, such patients have received a microvascular free flap, and flap revision is performed at the same setting.

Rehabilitation of the paralyzed face is beyond the scope of this chapter. Eyelid loading, brow lift, static slings, and occasionally powered gracilis muscle transfer each have their role in helping these patients.

Lower cranial nerve deficits are particularly difficulty to manage. Preoperative evaluation with a speech and swallowing therapist helps in identifying patients who are at risk, and corrective therapies can be started. Modified barium swallows are helpful postoperatively to identify patients who have aspiration. Vocal fold augmentation and thyroplasty can help with voice and swallowing. Unfortunately, many of these patients have a high vagal injury, and sensory afferents have been destroyed. Gastrostomy tube is required for patients who aspirate.

21.9 Conclusion

Temporal bone tumors are rare. Benign tumors, such as schwannomas, paragangliomas, and meningiomas, are more common than malignant tumors. SCC is the most common malignant tumor in the temporal bone. Most of these tumors are managed using surgical resection primarily. The surgical procedures for these lateral skull base tumors has been discussed. Postoperative complications and their management have been outlined.

References

[1] Gidley PW, DeMonte F. Temporal bone malignancies. Neurosurg Clin N Am. 2013; 24(1):97–110
[2] Moffat DA, Wagstaff SA, Hardy DG. The outcome of radical surgery and postoperative radiotherapy for squamous carcinoma of the temporal bone. Laryngoscope. 2005; 115(2):341–347

[3] Gidley PW, Roberts DB, Sturgis EM. Squamous cell carcinoma of the temporal bone. Laryngoscope. 2010; 120(6):1144–1151

[4] Nishimura Y. Rationale for chemoradiotherapy. Int J Clin Oncol. 2004; 9(6): 414–420

[5] Nakagawa T, Kumamoto Y, Natori Y, et al. Squamous cell carcinoma of the external auditory canal and middle ear: an operation combined with preoperative chemoradiotherapy and a free surgical margin. Otol Neurotol. 2006; 27 (2):242–248, discussion 249

[6] Shiga K, Ogawa T, Maki A, Amano M, Kobayashi T. Concomitant chemoradiotherapy as a standard treatment for squamous cell carcinoma of the temporal bone. Skull Base. 2011; 21(3):153–158

[7] Shinomiya H, Hasegawa S, Yamashita D, et al. Concomitant chemoradiotherapy for advanced squamous cell carcinoma of the temporal bone. Head Neck. 2015

[8] Kitani Y, Kubota A, Furukawa M, et al. Primary definitive radiotherapy with or without chemotherapy for squamous cell carcinoma of the temporal bone. Eur Arch Otorhinolaryngol. 2015

[9] Morita S, Homma A, Nakamaru Y, et al. The outcomes of surgery and chemoradiotherapy for temporal bone cancer. Otol Neurotol. 2016; 37(8):1174–1182

[10] Juliano AF, Ginat DT, Moonis G. Imaging review of the temporal bone: part I. Anatomy and inflammatory and neoplastic processes. Radiology. 2013; 269 (1):17–33

[11] Ahmed S, Gupta N, Hamilton JD, Garden AS, Gidley PW, Ginsberg LE. CT findings in temporal bone osteoradionecrosis. J Comput Assist Tomogr. 2014; 38 (5):662–666

[12] Gidley PW, Thompson CR, Roberts DB, DeMonte F, Hanna EY. The oncology of otology. Laryngoscope. 2012; 122(2):393–400

[13] Arriaga M, Curtin HD, Takahashi H, Kamerer DB. The role of preoperative CT scans in staging external auditory meatus carcinoma: radiologic-pathologic correlation study. Otolaryngology–Head and Neck Surgery. 1991; 105(1):6–11

[14] Leonetti JP, Smith PG, Kletzker GR, Izquierdo R. Invasion patterns of advanced temporal bone malignancies. Am J Otol. 1996; 17(3):438–442

[15] Goodwin WJ, Jesse RH. Malignant neoplasms of the external auditory canal and temporal bone. Arch Otolaryngol. 1980; 106(11):675–679

[16] Stell PM, McCormick MS. Carcinoma of the external auditory meatus and middle ear. Prognostic factors and a suggested staging system. J Laryngol Otol. 1985; 99(9):847–850

[17] Shih L, Crabtree JA. Carcinoma of the external auditory canal: an update. Laryngoscope. 1990; 100(11):1215–1218

[18] Austin JR, Stewart KL, Fawzi N. Squamous cell carcinoma of the external auditory canal: therapeutic prognosis based on a proposed staging system. Arch Otolaryngol Head Neck Surg. 1994; 120(11):1228–1232

[19] Pensak ML, Gleich LL, Gluckman JL, Shumrick KA. Temporal bone carcinoma: contemporary perspectives in the skull base surgical era. Laryngoscope. 1996; 106(10):1234–1237

[20] Manolidis S, Pappas D, Jr, Von Doersten P, Jackson CG, Glasscock ME, III. Temporal bone and lateral skull base malignancy: experience and results with 81 patients. Am J Otol. 1998; 19(6) Suppl:S1–S15

[21] Arriaga M, Curtin H, Takahashi H, Hirsch BE, Kamerer DB. Staging proposal for external auditory meatus carcinoma based on preoperative clinical examination and computed tomography findings. Ann Otol Rhinol Laryngol. 1990; 99(9 Pt 1):714–721

[22] Moody SA, Hirsch BE, Myers EN. Squamous cell carcinoma of the external auditory canal: an evaluation of a staging system. Am J Otol. 2000; 21(4): 582–588

[23] Fisch U. Infratemporal fossa approach for glomus tumors of the temporal bone. Ann Otol Rhinol Laryngol. 1982; 91(5 Pt 1):474–479

[24] Pensak ML, Jackler RK. Removal of jugular foramen tumors: the fallopian bridge technique. Otolaryngol Head Neck Surg. 1997; 117(6):586–591

[25] Gidley PW, Herrera SJ, Hanasono MM, et al. The impact of radiotherapy on facial nerve repair. Laryngoscope. 2010; 120(10):1985–1989

[26] Wax MK, Kaylie DM. Does a positive neural margin affect outcome in facial nerve grafting? Head Neck. 2007; 29(6):546–549

[27] Nader ME, Beadle BM, Roberts DB, Gidley PW. Outcomes and complications of osseointegrated hearing aids in irradiated temporal bones. Laryngoscope. 2015

[28] Nadol JB, Jr, Schuknecht HF. Obliteration of the mastoid in the treatment of tumors of the temporal bone. Ann Otol Rhinol Laryngol. 1984; 93(1 Pt 1): 6–12

[29] Hanasono MM, Silva AK, Yu P, Skoracki RJ, Sturgis EM, Gidley PW. Comprehensive management of temporal bone defects after oncologic resection. Laryngoscope. 2012; 122(12):2663–2669

22 The Evaluation and Management of Sellar Tumors

Tony R. Wang and John A. Jane Jr.

Summary

Sellar region tumors, though diverse in pathology, most frequently present as tumors of adenohypophyseal origin. Detailed history, physical examination, and biochemical and radiographic work-up are necessary to confirm diagnosis. Although various surgical approaches can be used to access the sella, the endoscopic endonasal transsphenoidal approach has gained significant popularity within the past two decades, starting in the 1990s. Here we detail the technical nuances and anatomical knowledge necessary for complication avoidance and successful surgery.

Keywords: sellar tumor, pituitary, transsphenoidal, endoscopic, technique, complication

22.1 Introduction

The sella turcica is a small saddle-shaped indentation in the posterior aspect of the sphenoid bone that houses the pituitary gland. Sellar tumors of both pituitary and nonpituitary origin may cause endocrinopathy and/or neurologic deficit secondary to mass effect. Although initial attempts at sellar tumor surgery in the late 1800s were via transcranial approaches, luminaries in neurosurgery such as Cushing[1] and Hardy[2] adopted the transsphenoidal approach at the beginning of the 20th century. After being abandoned in the 1920s, the approach became popular again in the 1970s and again recently in the 1990s with the introduction of endoscopic endonasal transsphenoidal (EETS) approaches.[3]

22.2 Surgical Anatomy

Sellar tumors are most often accessed via a transsphenoidal approach. Accordingly, knowledge of extracranial structures such as the nasal cavity and sphenoid sinus, as well as of the sellar and parasellar regions, is essential for successful surgery.

22.2.1 Nasal Cavity

In the sagittal orientation, the nasal septum, which comprises the perpendicular plate of the ethmoid along with the vomer, divides the nasal cavity in half. From the lateral walls of the nasal cavity arise the superior, middle, and inferior turbinates. At the posterior end of the nasal cavity, the inferior turbinate marks the location of the choana, an aperture that demarcates the transition from nasal cavity to nasopharynx. Approximately 1.5 cm superior to the choana, at the level of the inferior third of the superior turbinate within the sphenoethmoidal recess, is the sphenoid os, the passageway from the nasal cavity to the sphenoid sinus.

22.2.2 Sphenoid Sinus

The sphenoid sinus can be classified into one of three classes based on the degree of pneumatization: conchal, presellar, and sellar. Conchal sphenoid sinuses, though rare in the adult

population, are the most common type in the pediatric population and are characterized by lack of pneumatization—that is, a solid block of bone. Approximately 25% of adult sphenoid sinuses are presellar, the other 75% sellar. Presellar sphenoid sinuses denote a sinus in which the air cavity does not extend beyond the anterior border of the sellar wall. Sellar sphenoid sinuses have air that extends below the sella and as far back as the clivus.[4]

Knowledge of the sphenoid type allows the surgeon to anticipate what degree of bony removal is necessary for the anterior sphenoidotomy. After this, the sphenoid septae should be visible. Although the major sphenoid septum may occasionally mark midline, studies have shown that it more often does not and can be up to 8 mm off midline.[4] A more consistent marker of midline is the sphenoidal rostrum. Other bony landmarks that can orient the surgeon to midline include the carotid protuberances and the opticocarotid recesses. The lateral opticocarotid recesses represents the space between the carotid and optic protuberances. These protuberances mark the location of the cavernous internal carotid artery (ICA) and optic nerves. The midpoint between either the carotid protuberances or opticocarotid recesses will also serve as a marker of midline. Structures inferior to the sella include the clivus and clival recess; superior to the anterior wall of the sella are the tuberculum sellae and planum sphenoidale (▶ Fig. 22.1).

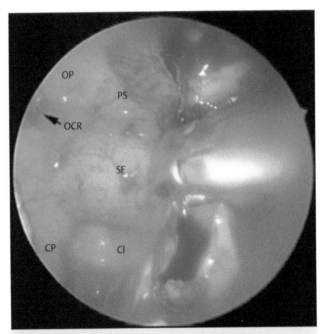

Fig. 22.1 Endoscopic view within sphenoid sinus during removal of sphenoid septae. Here the sellar floor (SL), clival recess (CI), and planum sphenoidale (PS) can be appreciated in the middle. On the left the optic and carotid processes (OP, CP) and opticocarotid recess are seen. (Reproduced with permission from Jane JA Jr, Han J, Prevedello DM, et al, Perspectives on endoscopic transsphenoidal surgery, Neurosurg Focus 2005;19:E2.)

22.2.3 Sellar and Parasellar Regions

Anterior to the sella are the tuberculum sella and the chiasmatic groove. The posterior limits of the sella are demarcated by the dorsum sellae, which transitions laterally into the posterior clinoid processes and posteriorly as the clivus. The sella itself contains the pituitary gland, whose anterior and posterior lobe correspond to the adenohypophysis and neurohypophysis, respectively. The pituitary stalk descends from the hypothalamus to the pituitary through a small opening in the diaphragma, a small dural fold that serves as the roof of the sella. Lateral to the sella is the cavernous sinus, within which runs the cavernous ICA. Here the ICA gives off the meningohypophyseal trunk and capsular artery of McConnell, which supply the neurohypophysis (via a branch off the meningohypophyseal trunk, the inferior hypophyseal artery) along with the capsule of the pituitary and dura of the anterior wall and floor of the sella. The adenohypophysis derives its blood supply from the hypophyseal portal system, a plexus of capillaries that ultimately derives its origin from the superior hypophyseal artery, a branch off the ICA after it leaves the cavernous sinus. The cavernous sinus also contains the oculomotor nerve, the trochlear nerve, the ophthalmic and maxillary divisions of the trigeminal nerve, and the abducens nerve. The abducens nerve, unlike the other nerves, is not within the lateral wall but rather is in close association with the cavernous ICA.

Superior to the sella are the suprasellar cistern. The suprasellar cistern contains the optic chiasm along with additional structures which we list. Superior to the optic chiasm lie the anterior cerebral arteries, anterior communicating artery, lamina terminalis, and third ventricle. Sellar tumors that have significant suprasellar extension, in addition to causing visual disturbances secondary to optic chiasm compression, may encase the anterior cerebral arteries or cause hydrocephalus if sufficient tumor invades the third ventricle.

22.3 Regional Pathology and Differential Diagnosis

22.3.1 Tumors of Pituitary Origin

Pituitary adenomas comprise an estimated 14% of all brain tumors and trail only meningioma and glioma in prevalence[5]; they can be classified as either nonfunctioning or functioning adenomas. Nonfunctioning adenomas are the most common, comprising just over a third of pituitary adenomas.[6] Although not themselves hormonally active, nonfunctional adenomas, particularly large macroadenomas, can compress normal pituitary tissue, leading to hormonal hyposecretion and hypopituitarism. Compressive effects on the pituitary stalk may also cause endocrinopathy in the form of hyperprolactinemia. Hormonally active adenomas, in order of prevalence, include prolactinoma, growth hormone (GH) adenoma, adrenocorticotropic hormone (ACTH) adenoma, postadrenalectomy ACTH adenoma, and thyroid stimulating hormone (TSH) adenoma. Gonadotropin adenomas, conversely, are typically hormonally silent, albeit very rarely hormonally active[7]; nonfunctioning adenomas frequently arise from gonadotrophs.

Pituitary carcinoma, unlike nonfunctional and functional adenomas, is a malignant process having a poor prognosis. Fortunately, pituitary carcinoma is rare, accounting for 0.1 to 0.2% of all pituitary tumors.[8] Hallmarks of pituitary carcinoma include spread throughout the central nervous system (CNS) as well as sites external to the CNS, such as the liver, ovaries, and bone. Most pituitary carcinomas are hormonally active, producing either ACTH or prolactin.

Neurohypophyseal tumors are also quite rare and can include granular cell tumors or gliomas. Granular cell tumors typically afflict women in the fourth or fifth decade of life but are neurochemically silent and rarely grow large enough to exert mass effect.[9] Interspersed among the axons of the neurohypophysis are glial cells, referred to as pituicytes. Tumors of the pituicytes, known as pituicytomas, typically present with mass effect.[10]

22.3.2 Tumors of Nonpituitary Origin

Craniopharyngioma is a frequently cystic and locally aggressive lesion thought to arise from the rests of squamous epithelium from the embryological remnant of the craniopharyngeal duct.[11] Among children who have sellar masses, craniopharyngioma is the most common diagnosis, accounting for 1.2 to 4% of all brain tumors.[12] Although craniopharyngiomas may present at any age, they classically have a bimodal distribution, with a predilection for pediatric patients aged 5 to 14 years and adults aged 50 to 74 years.[13] Among the two histological types of craniopharyngioma, the adamantinomatous type follows a bimodal distribution, whereas the papillary type is almost exclusively found in adults.[14] Craniopharyngiomas have a propensity for suprasellar extension, with a majority of tumors (75%) having suprasellar origin alone with invasion of the third ventricle.[15] Additional sellar tumors of nonpituitary origin can include germ cell tumors, gliomas of the optic apparatus or hypothalamus with inferior extension, meningioma, and chordoma.

22.3.3 Cyst, Hamartomas, and Malformations of the Sellar Region

Rathke's cleft cysts are thought to arise from the embryologic remnant of Rathke's pouch[11] and classically have been thought to represent a separate entity from craniopharyngioma. Some have challenged this distinction, as multiple accounts of cystic tumors of indeterminate radiographic and histological features have been reported. These practitioners have advocated that Rathke's cleft cyst and craniopharyngioma represent two spectrums of the same disease process.[11] Nevertheless, recent studies have identified genetic mutations that are specific to papillary (BRAF V600E) and adamantinomatous (CTNNB1 encoding beta-catenin) craniopharyngiomas, supporting an immunohistochemical distinction between craniopharyngiomas and Rathke's cleft cysts.[16] Other cystic sellar lesions include arachnoid, epidermoid, and dermoid cysts. Epidermoid and dermoid cysts are composed of abnormal rests of surface ectoderm, with epidermoid cysts comprising epithelial cell debris, keratin and dermoid cysts of dermal elements such as hair follicles, and glands.

22.4 Clinical Assessment

Patients who have sellar tumors can present with endocrinopathy secondary to pituitary hypersecretion, hypopituitarism, or neurologic symptoms secondary to mass effect. Careful history and physical examination often strongly suggests a diagnosis, particularly in cases of endocrinopathy, in which many syndromes have classic clinical features. Nevertheless, laboratory and radiographic work-up help further establish diagnosis.

22.4.1 Pituitary Hypersecretion

Functioning adenomas include prolactinoma, GH adenoma, ACTH adenoma, and TSH adenoma. Each of these conditions will present with their own respective clinical symptoms—namely, galactorrhea/amenorrhea, acromegaly, or gigantism; Cushing's disease; or secondary hyperthyroidism. Initial laboratory work-up for any of these conditions includes baseline measures of prolactin, GH, ACTH, luteinizing hormone, follicle stimulating hormone, TSH, free-T4, α-subunit, cortisol, IGF-1, testosterone, and estradiol. Aberrations in any of these tests may subsequently trigger provocative tests that stress the hypothalamic–pituitary–end organ axes.[6]

Prolactinoma

Classic manifestations of prolactinoma include galactorrhea and hypogonadism. Women, who present three times more often than men,[17] typically present earlier in life with endocrinopathy. Men generally present later in life with symptoms attributable to mass effect.[18] Prolactin levels > 200 ng/mL coupled with a pituitary adenoma confirmed on MRI establish a diagnosis of prolactinoma.[18] Patients who have signs and symptoms of prolactinemia and who display lower-than-expected prolactin levels may suffer from the hook effect, in which excessively elevated levels of prolactin oversaturate the antibodies used in prolactin assays, leading to an artificially low result. For suspected cases of hook effect, a 1:100 sample dilution will lead to accurate results.[19] Hyperprolactinemia is not exclusive to cases of prolactinoma, however. Sellar masses, regardless of hormonal function, can compress the pituitary stalk and release lactotrophs from tonic dopaminergic inhibition in what is termed the stalk effect. Hyperprolactinemia secondary to stalk effect, however, is generally mild to moderate, with levels < 94 ng/mL.[20]

GH Adenoma

Symptoms of GH adenoma depend on age of presentation. Prior to closure of the epiphyseal plate, GH adenomas present with gigantism, whereas after the closure of the epiphyseal plate, acromegaly prevails. Although signs of gigantism are often obvious at ultimate presentation, the progression of acromegaly is insidious, with an average time from symptom onset to diagnosis of 7 years.[21] Symptoms can include coarsening of facial features, acral enlargement, headaches, carpal tunnel syndrome, hypertension, sleep apnea, cardiovascular disease, and diabetes.[21] Although historical diagnostic metrics have relied on GH levels for diagnosis, recent guidelines do not support this. Rather, diagnosis of acromegaly rests on elevated levels of IGF-1 along with lack of GH suppression to < 0.4 μg/L after an oral glucose tolerance test.[22]

ACTH Adenoma

Hypersecretion from an ACTH adenoma leads to overproduction of cortisol from the adrenal glands and a clinical diagnosis of Cushing's disease. Signs of Cushing's disease can include central obesity, diabetes, hypertension, plethora, abdominal striae, osteoporosis, myopathy, and neuropsychiatric disturbances. Diagnosis of Cushing's disease must first exclude hypercortisolemic states such as iatrogenic causes, ectopic ACTH lesions, and ACTH-independent lesions. First hypercortisolemia must be established, which can be done by measuring free cortisol in a 24-hour urine sample. With hypercortisolemia confirmed, serum ACTH level should be analyzed to distinguish between ACTH-dependent and ACTH-independent cases of hypercortisolemia. ACTH-dependent cases display elevated levels of ACTH, whereas ACTH-independent cases (e.g., an adrenal adenoma) in which cortisol is directly secreted would be expected to have low levels of ACTH secondary to feedback inhibition. The final step in diagnosis, distinguishing Cushing's disease from ectopic ACTH conditions, remains perhaps the most challenging step. Provocative tests such as high-dose dexamethasone and corticotropin-releasing hormone stimulation tests can be performed to aid diagnosis. If testing remains inconclusive or conflicting, inferior petrosal sinus sampling (IPSS)[23] can be pursued.

22.4.2 Hypopituitarism

Hypopituitarism may occur when a sellar mass compresses the anterior pituitary, leading to its impairment. The hormones of the anterior pituitary have differing susceptibilities to hyposecretion, with gonadotropins being the most sensitive, followed by TSH, GH, and ACTH.[15] Consequently, hypopituitarism may present with diminished libido, infertility, fatigue, and/or hypothyroidism. Pituitary apoplexy due to hemorrhagic necrosis of a pituitary adenoma may present with acute features of hypopituitarism along with sudden-onset headache, meningismus, visual decline, and ophthalmoplegia.

22.4.3 Neurologic Symptoms Secondary to Mass Effect

Bitemporal hemianopsia may occur secondary to suprasellar extension of a sellar mass, leading to optic chiasm compression. Moreover, patients may also experience declines in acuity and, more rarely, ptosis and ophthalmoplegia secondary to lateral extension into the cavernous sinus. Baseline ophthalmologic evaluation, including assessment of acuity and fields, is recommended for patients who have preoperative visual complaints and/or chiasmal compression, as they may portend prognostic recovery of visual complaints after surgery while documenting any postoperative change.[24] Beyond visual symptoms, suprasellar extension of sellar masses, particularly craniopharyngioma, may encroach on the hypothalamus and third ventricle, causing neurologic disturbance and hydrocephalus. Giant pituitary adenomas with lateral extension into the temporal lobes may additionally present with seizures.[6]

22.5 Diagnostic Imaging

Imaging of suspected sellar pathology begins with MRI unless contraindicated. Attention should be paid to the coronal and sagittal images, because the sella is best delineated in these planes. Basic work-up includes T1 pre- and postcontrast images along with T2 images. Further sequences can be performed, depending on the suspected pathology.

Pituitary adenomas are often slightly hypointense compared with the normal pituitary, which is isointense. Moreover, adenomas have delayed enhancement relative to the normal gland, which avidly enhances in a homogenous manner.[25] Special consideration should be given to cases of suspected Cushing's disease. Spoiled gradient recalled acquisition in the steady state sequences should be obtained in the work-up of Cushing's disease due to its superior characterization of soft tissue contrasting and improved sensitivity compared with standard T1 postcontrast spin echo images, which may miss up to 40% of cases (▶ Fig. 22.2).[26] For macroadenomas, the cavernous sinuses should also be examined, because these tumors are frequently locally invasive. In such cases, the Knosp score, which is determined based on the macroadenoma's relationship to the cavernous and supracavernous ICA, can be highly predictive of cavernous sinus invasion (▶ Fig. 22.3).[27]

Other sellar tumors may have common imaging characteristics that can help narrow the differential diagnoses. Examples include sellar/parasellar meningioma (homogenous enhancement, dural tail, possible calcification), craniopharyngioma (solid/cystic components with calcification), Rathke's cleft cyst (cystic structure with possible fluid/debris level), and arachnoid cyst (cystic mass with signal comparable to CSF without fluid restriction on diffusion weighted imaging).[25]

22.6 Preoperative Preparation

Any comorbid conditions, such as diabetes, hypertension, and cardiovascular disease, should be optimized prior to surgery. Attention should be paid to cases of Cushing's disease and acromegaly, as the aforementioned conditions are frequently present. In patients who have hypopituitarism, proper hormonal replacement should be instituted prior to surgery. This is of utmost importance for hypocortisolemia, which if left untreated could result in an Addisonian crisis brought on by surgery.

22.7 Surgical Technique

Because our experience and expertise lie with the EETS approach, our discussion focuses on this approach (**Video 22.1**). Details regarding microscopic sublabial, microscopic endonasal, and transcranial approaches can be found elsewhere.[28]

22.7.1 Positioning

Patients are placed in a semirecumbent position with their right shoulder at the right upper corner of the operating table with the right arm tucked. A horseshoe headrest supports the head; we do not routinely use rigid fixation. The horseshoe headrest is then shifted left, moving the patient's left ear toward the left shoulder. The operating table is then turned until the patient's ears are parallel to the operating room walls. This moves the patient's body and allows the surgeon to be positioned directly in front of the surgical field. The head of bed is then elevated to approximately 20° so that the nose bridge is parallel to the floor. Positioning the head in such a manner improves venous outflow and thereby decreases cavernous sinus bleeding. The bed height should be appropriately lowered to allow the surgeon to comfortably operate with elbows at 90° (▶ Fig. 22.4).[29]

22.7.2 Nasal Preparation

We administer nasal oxymetazoline prior to induction and then again following induction and prior to positioning. After the patient is prepped, each nare is packed with three half-by-three patties soaked with oxymetazoline and left in place for 5 to 10 minutes. During this period, the patient is draped in the usual sterile manner. We customarily additionally prep and drape the abdomen for possible abdominal fat graft for sellar floor reconstruction. Patties are then removed from the nares, and the middle turbinates, nasal septum, and rostrum are instilled with 0.2% ropivacaine with 1:200,000 epinephrine, under direct visualization.

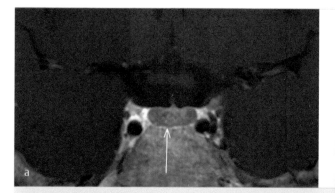
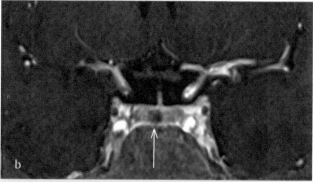

Fig. 22.2 Coronal T1 postcontrast images of the sella for a case of suspected Cushing's syndrome. **(a)** Standard T1 postcontrast spin echo image shows no obvious pathology; note the homogenous enhancement of the pituitary. **(b)** Postcontrast spoiled gradient recalled acquisition in the steady state shows an area of hypoenhancement suggestive of adenoma.

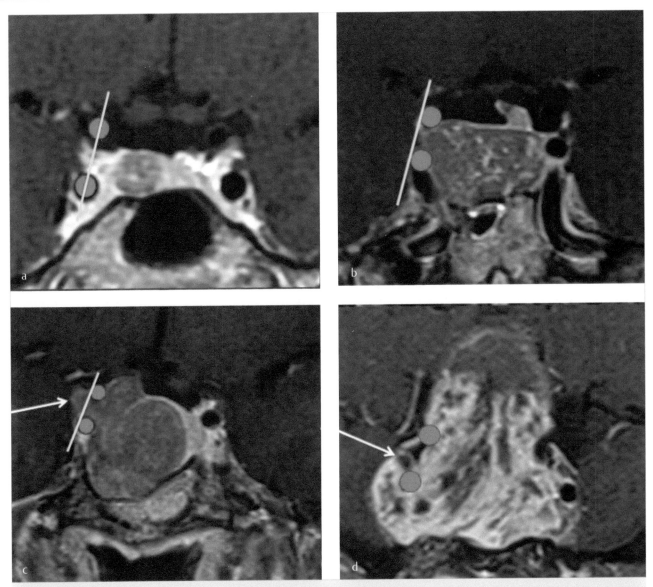

Fig. 22.3 Coronal T1 postcontrast images of the sella, cavernous internal carotid artery (ICA) denoted by white circles. **(a)** Knosp grade I adenoma does not extend past the midline of the cavernous ICA. **(b)** Knosp grade II adenoma extends to the lateral tangential line of the cavernous ICA, but not past. **(c)** Knosp grade III adenoma extends past the lateral tangential line of the cavernous ICA. **(d)** Knosp grade IV adenoma completely surrounds the cavernous ICA.

22.7.3 Soft Tissue Dissection

The 0° endoscope is used to inspect each nare; we prefer to pick the nare with more space for initial approach. If each nare is approximately equal, the right side is selected by convention. The inferior and middle turbinates are identified and then lateralized in succession with a Cottle instrument. With the turbinates lateralized, the inferior third to half of the superior turbinate is removed using a straight Thru-Cut sinus forceps. This maneuver should then allow identification of the sphenoid os. Once identified, the sphenoid os is enlarged superiorly and laterally. At the level of the sphenoid os, a rectangular incision is then made on the septal mucosa and using a soft tissue shaver the posterior 1.0 to 1.5 cm of the nasal septum is removed to complete the posterior septectomy. The same procedure is then performed in the other nare. Up until the posterior septectomy, the

procedure is performed in a two-handed mononarial fashion. The posterior septectomy allows additional instruments to pass into the sphenoid sinus, transitioning the procedure to a three-handed binarial technique.

22.7.4 Sphenoidotomy and Sellar Entry

The sphenoidotomy is enlarged lateral to the sphenoid ostia to ensure adequate exposure. This can be accomplished using Kerrison punches, a soft-tissue shaver, or a drill. While drilling down the sphenoid rostrum, care must be taken to not injure the sphenopalatine artery, which is typically found in the mucosa of the infero-lateral rostrum. Accordingly, mucosa from the inferior portion of the rostrum is carefully separated from the bone prior to its removal, after which the mucosa—along with the sphenopalatine

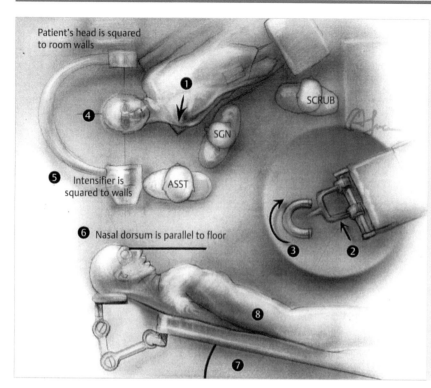

Patient's head is squared to room walls

SCRUB

SGN

Intensifier is squared to walls

ASST

Nasal dorsum is parallel to floor

Fig. 22.4 Patient positioning. (1) Right shoulder moved to top right corner of operating table. (2) Headrest frame moved to the left. (3) Horse-shoe headrest angled so that the patient's left ear moves toward the left shoulder. (4,5) Operating table oriented such that the patient's ears are parallel to the walls of the operating room. (6) Head positioned such that the nasal dorsum is parallel to the floor. (7) Head of Bed (HOB) raised approximately 20°, the height of the bed can be adjusted to allow the surgeon to operate with his or her elbows at 90°. (8) The right arm is tucked. (Reproduced with permission from Jane JA Jr, Thapar K, Kaptain GJ, Maartens N, Laws ER Jr, Pituitary surgery: transsphenoidal approach, Neurosurgery 2002;51(2):435–442.)

artery—is preserved. Damage to the sphenopalatine artery may result in postoperative epistaxis. The sphenoidotomy should continue until certain structures become visible: the optic protuberances, opticocarotid recesses, the sellar floor, clival recess, and planum sphenoidale. Identification of these structures, and particularly of the optic protuberances and opticocarotid recesses, will help establish the midline. Image guidance may also be used to establish midline, but we reserve its use for repeat surgeries in which anatomical landmarks may not be easily identifiable as well as cases involving presellar or conchal sphenoid sinuses. Some sellar tumors may erode through the floor of the sella itself or leave the floor thin enough to flake off with a blunt hook. In other cases, a small chisel or a high-speed drill may be used to open the sellar floor. With the floor opened, a Kerrison punch is used to widen the opening to the medial border of the cavernous sinuses. A small lip of bone is left in place to help facilitate sellar floor reconstruction at the conclusion of the case.

22.7.5 Tumor Removal

The dura is first opened using a 15-blade scalpel, avoiding entry into the pituitary capsule or tumor. A plane is then developed between the dura and the tumor/pituitary. Removal of macroadenomas may be performed in two basic manners: traditional piecemeal removal or resection using the pseudocapsule[30] as a plane of dissection. It is our practice to initially attempt to identify a pseudocapsule over the anterior face of the tumor in all cases. However, this is not always possible, in which case a piecemeal removal is pursued.

For piecemeal removal, the tumor is removed in a sequential fashion, first along the floor of the sella, until the posterior aspect of the tumor is identified. At times a pseudocapsule may be identified posteriorly at this point and allow a pseudocapsular dissection to proceed. If a pseudocapsule is not identified, a

plane posterior to the tumor is developed with ringed curettes and tumor is then progressively removed from posterior to anterior until the inferior half of the cavernous sinus walls are identified. Care should be taken to not remove the superior portions of the tumor prematurely lest the diaphragma descend and obstruct the view of the remaining tumor. Tumor removal proceeds progressively until the diaphragma sella is identified and freed of tumor. Although techniques such as instillation of air or fluid via a lumbar drain placed preoperatively will help deliver suprasellar tumor into the operative field, we find that use of controlled hypercapnia and a Valsalva maneuver applied by the anesthesia team provides adequate delivery of suprasellar tumor. The entire surgical bed should be inspected, especially the cavernous sinus walls and superolateral margins at the junction of the cavernous sinus walls and the diaphragma, for tumor remnants. This can be accomplished using a 30° endoscope.

When a pseudocapsule can be identified in patients who have macroadenomas, the pseudocapsule is used as a plane of dissection. Even with presence of macroadenomas, patients may still have an identifiable pituitary capsule and thin rim of gland anterior to the tumor pseudocapsule. The pseudocapsule can be identified by careful scoring of the pituitary capsule and gland, followed by careful blunt dissection until the pseudocapsule is identified. If identified, the pseudocapsular plane is dissected superiorly and laterally until it is clearly established. For larger macroadenomas, the tumor will need to be internally debulked to allow progressive dissection of the pseudocapsule. The removal proceeds with progressive internal debulking followed by delivery of the pseudocapsule until a circumferential removal has been achieved.

Surgical resection of microadenomas is slightly more nuanced. Unlike in cases of macroadenomas, microadenomas pose a distinct challenge, because after the dura is opened, the

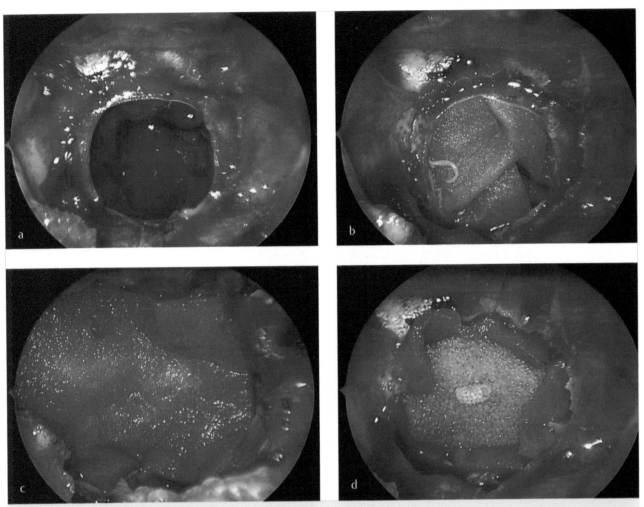

Fig. 22.5 Gasket seal repair for cerebrospinal fluid leak. **(a)** Defect in the anterior cranial base after use of the endoscopic endonasal transsphenoidal approach. **(b)** Dural substitute is placed within the sella. **(c)** Dural substitute (larger than the size of the defect) is centered on the defect. **(d)** Autologous bone or artificial plate is the tucked underneath the bony edges with redundant dural graft draped over the bone or artificial plate.

surgeon is often confronted with normal-appearing pituitary gland. In patients who have Cushing's disease, a vertical incision is made in the gland overlying the location of the tumor based on the preoperative imaging. This incision is then carried posteriorly until the pseudocapsule is identified, after which circumferential dissection proceeds until the tumor is removed. In cases of MRI-negative Cushing's disease in which IPSS was performed, the initial incision is made on the side of lateralization. If tumor is not identified, the gland is explored using serial vertical incisions. If tumor is still not identified, we consider removal of the lateral wings and inferior central portion of the gland, preserving the central wedge attached to the pituitary stalk.

22.7.6 Reconstruction and Closure

Closure techniques depend on whether a CSF leak has been encountered. A useful way to discuss intraoperative CSF leaks was described by Kelly and colleagues.[31] In cases without CSF leak, (grade 0), Gelfoam and/or a dural substitute may be packed into the sella to close off dead space. For cases of a weeping-type

(grade I) CSF leak, either abdominal fat or a dural substitute may be placed within the sella. Either autologous bone (often harvested during the posterior septectomy) or an artificial plate can then be tucked under the bony margins to complete sellar reconstruction. When an overt hole in the diaphragma is nonetheless too small to permit placement of instruments in the supradiaphragmatic space (grade II), a dural substitute is first placed against the diaphragma and held in place with either fat or a rolled dural substitute that approximates the size of the sella. The anterior dura is then reconstructed using a dural substitute and either septal bone or an artificial plate in a gasket-seal manner, as described by the Cornell group (► Fig. 22.5).[32]

For large diaphragmatic defects (grade III), this same technique is used, but a nasoseptal flap is also used to augment the repair. Lumbar drainage may also be used, but its utility has not been clearly established. After sellar reconstruction, the nasal cavity and sphenoid are irrigated. The turbinates are then medialized back to their anatomical position. The oropharynx and stomach are then suctioned free of blood. If an abdominal fat graft has been harvested, this is closed in a layered manner using absorbable sutures.

22.8 Postoperative Care

Postoperatively, patients are admitted to a general ward and are placed on intravenous antibiotics (cefazolin 1gm Q8 H x 24 hours) for surgical infection prophylaxis; if a lumbar drain has been placed, antibiotics continue while the drain is in place. Patients are mobilized ad lib except for cases of CSF leak. For cases involving grade II or III CSF leak without use of postoperative lumbar drainage, patients are placed on bedrest until postoperative day 1. For cases of CSF leak involving use of postoperative lumbar drainage, patients may be placed on 2 to 3 days of bedrest with the head of bed (HOB) at 30 to 45°. In cases of prolonged bed rest, we obtain a lower-extremity ultrasound to screen for deep vein thrombosis prior to mobilization.

All patients will have sodium and cortisol checked immediately postoperatively and every morning while hospitalized. The patient's fluid status and urine specific gravity are closely monitored for signs of diabetes insipidus (DI). Although postoperative diuresis is not uncommon, we do not routinely use desmopressin unless a patient is not able to keep up with fluid loses orally and sodium levels are increasing. Daily cortisols are obtained, with physiologic steroid replacement not given unless levels are less than 8 µg/dL. For Cushing's disease, however, we check cortisol every 6 hours postoperatively and do not initiate exogenous steroid replacement until cortisol levels are less than 1 µg/dL.

22.9 Complications and Their Avoidance

Although the EETS approach has proven to be efficacious, it is not without complication. The existing literature for pituitary adenomas reports complication rates of 10 to 26.3%, with an intraoperative mortality rate of 0 to 0.68%.[33,34,35,36,37] EETS resection of craniopharyngioma has higher complication rates, with reports ranging up to 48.1%.[38,39] Complications can be grouped into the following categories: sinonasal, neurologic, endocrinopathy, vascular, CSF leak, and infectious.

22.9.1 Sinonasal Complications

Although rarely life-threatening, sinonasal complications are frequently annoying to the patient and lead to a lower quality of life.[40] Failure to achieve hemostasis may result in postoperative epistaxis, which in severe cases may require reoperation. Other complications, such as impaired mucociliary clearance leading to sinusitis, can occur secondary to obstruction of the osteomeatal complex if the turbinates are not adequately medialized at the conclusion of the case. Caution should be exercised in not overmedializing the turbinates, as this may cause synechiae between the turbinates and the nasal septum. Nasal mucosa disruption, especially during the removal of the superior turbinate and septectomy, may lead to postoperative anosmia.

22.9.2 Neurologic Complications

Neurologic complications may encompass a wide array of conditions, including hypothalamic injury, visual decline, and cranial nerve injury. Hypothalamic injury after EETS surgery for pituitary adenomas is somewhat rare but is a well-recognized complication of EETS surgery for craniopharyngiomas, which commonly have suprasellar and hypothalamic extension.[12] Signs of hypothalamic injury could include DI, memory disturbance, hypothalamic obesity, and disturbances in temperature regulation. Careful surgical technique minimizing tumor retraction and pituitary stalk manipulation will help avoid these complications. For tumors—i.e., craniopharyngiomas—having direct hypothalamic involvement, subtotal resection followed by local radiation may be advocated to avoid hypothalamic injury.[41]

Postoperative visual decline after EETS surgery is frequently secondary to chiasmal and/or optic nerve manipulation during surgery.[42] Careful dissection of the tumor off the chiasm, along with preservation of blood supply to the chiasm, will help mitigate these concerns. Rarely, postoperative hematoma may cause visual deficits secondary to chiasmal compression. Similarly, overpacking of the sella during reconstruction may also lead to chiasmal compression. Visualization of brain pulsations after graft placement helps ensure that undue pressure has not been transmitted to the chiasm.

As pituitary adenomas frequently invade the cavernous sinus, entry into the cavernous sinus is at times inevitable, bringing the risk of neurologic injury, which can present as ophthalmoplegia or facial numbness in the V_1 and V_2 distributions. Ophthalmoplegia most often presents as abduction deficit, for the abducens nerve is the most medial nerve in the cavernous sinus and thus is the most susceptible to injury. Such injury may occur with cavernous sinus bleeding when the sinus is overpacked with hemostatic material. Careful surgical technique and visualization of neural structures may decrease the likelihood of these complications.

22.9.3 Endocrine-Related Complications

New onset anterior pituitary dysfunction is a well-known complication after EETS surgery, with a reported incidence of 3 to 14%. This hypopituitarism, however, is short-lived: most patients can discontinue exogenous hormonal replacement within 2 to 6 months of surgery.[43] In addition to anterior pituitary dysfunction, posterior pituitary dysfunction in the form of DI may also occur after EETS surgery, particularly in cases of nonadenomatous pathology[44,45] and cases involving CSF leak.[46] Although postoperative DI may be seen in up to 18.3%[45] of patients, it is often transient, with only 1 to 5% of patients necessitating permanent treatment.[43] Postoperative derangements in sodium may also take the form of syndrome of inappropriate antidiuretic hormone secretion (SIADH), which has an incidence of 1.1 to 7%.[37] This typically presents approximately 1 week after surgery and often can be managed by outpatient fluid restriction provided the patient is not overly symptomatic or hyponatremic.

22.9.4 Vascular Complications

The cavernous ICA is most susceptible to injury and can be damaged during cavernous sinus exploration or during dural opening. Loss of midline orientation during the surgical approach may lead to the inadvertent opening of the dura over the cavernous ICA, resulting in its laceration. Scrutiny of pre-operative imaging and maintaining midline orientation are crucial in order to avoid this complication. In cases involving unclear anatomy, techniques that can be used to avoid injury to the ICA include navigation, micro-Doppler, or even puncture of the dura with a 25-gauge needle prior to dural opening.[29]

22.9.5 Cerebrospinal Fluid Leak

CSF leak after EETS surgery has an incidence of 2 to 16%[43] and results from damage to the diaphragma, to which sellar tumors are frequently adherent. Careful dissection and avoidance of tugging at the tumor will minimize damage to the diaphragma. In some instances, tumor may invade and disrupt the diaphragma, leading to inevitable intraoperative CSF leak. For such cases—and all cases in which CSF is visualized intraoperatively—prevention of postoperative CSF leak rests on the integrity of sellar reconstruction. Our technique for sellar reconstruction has already been detailed. Although lumbar drainage may be used when an intraoperative CSF leak is identified, we often advocate for surgical reexploration, leak identification, and repair if any CSF rhinorrhea occurs early postoperatively.

22.9.6 Infectious Complications

Limiting sinonasal complications and CSF leak may subsequently decrease the likelihood of infection, because infection is often a sequela of these complications. Sinonasal complications such as obstruction leading to impaired mucociliary clearance may predispose patients to sinusitis. Similarly, prolonged postoperative CSF rhinorrhea may increase the likelihood of meningitis. Moreover, repeated reoperation for CSF leak repair and protracted use of lumbar drainage with persistent leakage further increases the risk of meningitis.[46]

22.10 Follow-up and Rehabilitation

Barring complication, patients are typically discharged to home on postoperative day 2. A sodium level is drawn at 1 week postoperatively to screen for delayed-onset SIADH. If patients are not sent home on steroid replacement, then a morning cortisol is also drawn. Patients are then seen in our neuroendocrine clinic at 2 to 3 months postoperatively for endocrine testing, with exogenous hormonal replacement initiated as indicated. Neuro-ophthalmological examination is also performed for those who have preoperative visual deficits or who developed them postoperatively. An MRI with and without contrast is also obtained at the initial follow-up visit, with additional imaging performed yearly.

22.11 Conclusion

The introduction of EETS surgery has revolutionized the field of sellar surgery. Although sellar surgery has classically been associated with pituitary adenomas, adenomas represent just one of the many possible lesions that can be found in the sellar region.

Knowledge of this, local anatomy, and proper surgical technique will ultimately help avoid complications and lead to a successful surgery.

References

[1] Cushing H. Partial hypophysectomy for acromegaly: with remarks on the function of the hypophysis. Ann Surg. 1909; 50(6):1002–1017

[2] Hardy J. Transphenoidal microsurgery of the normal and pathological pituitary. Clin Neurosurg. 1969; 16:185–217

[3] Jho HD, Carrau RL. Endoscopic endonasal transsphenoidal surgery: experience with 50 patients. J Neurosurg. 1997; 87(1):44–51

[4] Renn WH, Rhoton AL, Jr. Microsurgical anatomy of the sellar region. J Neurosurg. 1975; 43(3):288–298

[5] Dolecek TA, Propp JM, Stroup NE, Kruchko C. CBTRUS statistical report: primary brain and central nervous system tumors diagnosed in the United States in 2005–2009. Neuro-oncol. 2012; 14 Suppl 5:v1–v49

[6] Jane JA, Jr, Laws ER, Jr. The surgical management of pituitary adenomas in a series of 3,093 patients. J Am Coll Surg. 2001; 193(6):651–659

[7] Cote DJ, Smith TR, Sandler CN, et al. Functional gonadotroph adenomas: case series and report of literature. Neurosurgery. 2016; 79(6):823–831

[8] Ragel BT, Couldwell WT. Pituitary carcinoma: a review of the literature. Neurosurg Focus. 2004; 16(4):E7

[9] Gagliardi F, Spina A, Barzaghi LR, et al. Suprasellar granular cell tumor of the neurohypophysis: surgical outcome of a very rare tumor. Pituitary. 2016; 19 (3):277–285

[10] Pirayesh Islamian A, Buslei R, Saeger W, Fahlbusch R. Pituicytoma: overview of treatment strategies and outcome. Pituitary. 2012; 15(2):227–236

[11] Zada G, Lin N, Ojerholm E, Ramkissoon S, Laws ER. Craniopharyngioma and other cystic epithelial lesions of the sellar region: a review of clinical, imaging, and histopathological relationships. Neurosurg Focus. 2010; 28(4):E4

[12] Sterkenburg AS, Hoffmann A, Gebhardt U, Warmuth-Metz M, Daubenbüchel AM, Müller HL. Survival, hypothalamic obesity, and neuropsychological/psychosocial status after childhood-onset craniopharyngioma: newly reported long-term outcomes. Neuro-oncol. 2015; 17(7):1029–1038

[13] Bunin GR, Surawicz TS, Witman PA, Preston-Martin S, Davis F, Bruner JM. The descriptive epidemiology of craniopharyngioma. J Neurosurg. 1998; 89(4): 547–551

[14] Rao YJ, Hassanzadeh C, Fischer-Valuck B, et al. Patterns of care and treatment outcomes of patients with craniopharyngioma in the National Cancer Database. J Neurooncol. 2017; 132(1):109–117

[15] Jane JA, Jr, Laws ER. Craniopharyngioma. Pituitary. 2006; 9(4):323–326

[16] Brastianos PK, Taylor-Weiner A, Manley PE, et al. Exome sequencing identifies BRAF mutations in papillary craniopharyngiomas. Nat Genet. 2014; 46(2): 161–165

[17] Agustsson TT, Baldvinsdottir T, Jonasson JG, et al. The epidemiology of pituitary adenomas in Iceland, 1955–2012: a nationwide population-based study. Eur J Endocrinol. 2015; 173(5):655–664

[18] Carter JN, Tyson JE, Tolis G, Van Vliet S, Faiman C, Friesen HG. Prolactin-screening tumors and hypogonadism in 22 men. N Engl J Med. 1978; 299 (16):847–852

[19] Melmed S, Casanueva FF, Hoffman AR, et al. Endocrine Society. Diagnosis and treatment of hyperprolactinemia: an Endocrine Society clinical practice guideline. J Clin Endocrinol Metab. 2011; 96(2):273–288

[20] Karavitaki N, Thanabalasingham G, Shore HCA, et al. Do the limits of serum prolactin in disconnection hyperprolactinaemia need re-definition? A study of 226 patients with histologically verified non-functioning pituitary macroadenoma. Clin Endocrinol (Oxf). 2006; 65(4):524–529

[21] Rajasoorya C, Holdaway IM, Wrightson P, Scott DJ, Ibbertson HK. Determinants of clinical outcome and survival in acromegaly. Clin Endocrinol (Oxf). 1994; 41(1):95–102

[22] Katznelson L, Laws ER, Jr, Melmed S, et al. Endocrine Society. Acromegaly: an endocrine society clinical practice guideline. J Clin Endocrinol Metab. 2014; 99(11):3933–3951

[23] Oldfield EH, Doppman JL, Nieman LK, et al. Petrosal sinus sampling with and without corticotropin-releasing hormone for the differential diagnosis of Cushing's syndrome. N Engl J Med. 1991; 325(13):897–905

[24] Newman SA, Turbin RE, Bodach ME, et al. Congress of Neurological Surgeons systematic review and evidence-based guideline on pretreatment ophthalmology evaluation in patients with suspected nonfunctioning pituitary adenomas. Neurosurgery. 2016; 79(4):E530–E532

[25] Go JL, Rajamohan AG. Imaging of the sella and parasellar region. Radiol Clin North Am. 2017; 55(1):83–101

[26] Patronas N, Bulakbasi N, Stratakis CA, et al. Spoiled gradient recalled acquisition in the steady state technique is superior to conventional postcontrast spin echo technique for magnetic resonance imaging detection of adrenocorticotropin-secreting pituitary tumors. J Clin Endocrinol Metab. 2003; 88(4): 1565–1569

[27] Knosp E, Steiner E, Kitz K, Matula C. Pituitary adenomas with invasion of the cavernous sinus space: a magnetic resonance imaging classification compared with surgical findings. Neurosurgery. 1993; 33(4):610–617, discussion 617–618

[28] Rhoton AL, Jr. The sellar region. Neurosurgery. 2002; 51(4) Suppl:S335–S374

[29] Jane JA, Jr, Thapar K, Kaptain GJ, Maartens N, Laws ER, Jr. Pituitary surgery: transsphenoidal approach. Neurosurgery. 2002; 51(2):435–442, discussion 442–444

[30] Oldfield EH, Vortmeyer AO. Development of a histological pseudocapsule and its use as a surgical capsule in the excision of pituitary tumors. J Neurosurg. 2006; 104(1):7–19

[31] Esposito F, Dusick JR, Fatemi N, Kelly DF. Graded repair of cranial base defects and cerebrospinal fluid leaks in transsphenoidal surgery. Oper Neurosurg (Hagerstown). 2007; 60(4) Suppl 2:295–303, discussion 303–304

[32] Leng LZ, Brown S, Anand VK, Schwartz TH. "Gasket-seal" watertight closure in minimal-access endoscopic cranial base surgery. Neurosurgery. 2008; 62(5 Suppl 2):ONSE342–342

[33] Cappabianca P, Cavallo LM, Colao A, de Divitiis E. Surgical complications associated with the endoscopic endonasal transsphenoidal approach for pituitary adenomas. J Neurosurg. 2002; 97(2):293–298

[34] Frank G, Pasquini E, Farneti G, et al. The endoscopic versus the traditional approach in pituitary surgery. Neuroendocrinology. 2006; 83(3–4):240–248

[35] Dehdashti AR, Ganna A, Karabatsou K, Gentili F. Pure endoscopic endonasal approach for pituitary adenomas: early surgical results in 200 patients and comparison with previous microsurgical series. Neurosurgery. 2008; 62(5): 1006–1015, discussion 1015–1017

[36] Gondim JA, Almeida JP, Albuquerque LA, et al. Endoscopic endonasal approach for pituitary adenoma: surgical complications in 301 patients. Pituitary. 2011; 14(2):174–183

[37] Berker M, Hazer DB, Yücel T, et al. Complications of endoscopic surgery of the pituitary adenomas: analysis of 570 patients and review of the literature. Pituitary. 2012; 15(3):288–300

[38] Moussazadeh N, Prabhu V, Bander ED, et al. Endoscopic endonasal versus open transcranial resection of craniopharyngiomas: a case-matched single-institution analysis. Neurosurg Focus. 2016; 41(6):E7

[39] Cavallo LM, Frank G, Cappabianca P, et al. The endoscopic endonasal approach for the management of craniopharyngiomas: a series of 103 patients. J Neurosurg. 2014; 121(1):100–113

[40] Little AS, Kelly D, Milligan J, et al. Predictors of sinonasal quality of life and nasal morbidity after fully endoscopic transsphenoidal surgery. J Neurosurg. 2015; 122(6):1458–1465

[41] Müller HL, Gebhardt U, Teske C, et al. Study Committee of KRANIOPHARYNG-EOM 2000. Post-operative hypothalamic lesions and obesity in childhood craniopharyngioma: results of the multinational prospective trial KRANIOPHARYNGEOM 2000 after 3-year follow-up. Eur J Endocrinol. 2011; 165(1):17–24

[42] Halvorsen H, Ramm-Pettersen J, Josefsen R, et al. Surgical complications after transsphenoidal microscopic and endoscopic surgery for pituitary adenoma: a consecutive series of 506 procedures. Acta Neurochir (Wien). 2014; 156(3): 441–449

[43] Dallapiazza RF, Jane JA, Jr. Outcomes of endoscopic transsphenoidal pituitary surgery. Endocrinol Metab Clin North Am. 2015; 44(1):105–115

[44] Schreckinger M, Walker B, Knepper J, et al. Post-operative diabetes insipidus after endoscopic transsphenoidal surgery. Pituitary. 2013; 16(4):445–451

[45] Nemergut EC, Zuo Z, Jane JA, Jr, Laws ER, Jr. Predictors of diabetes insipidus after transsphenoidal surgery: a review of 881 patients. J Neurosurg. 2005; 103(3):448–454

[46] Ivan ME, Iorgulescu JB, El-Sayed I, et al. Risk factors for postoperative cerebrospinal fluid leak and meningitis after expanded endoscopic endonasal surgery. J Clin Neurosci. 2015; 22(1):48–54

23 Tumors of the Cavernous Sinus and Parasellar Space

Ramsey Ashour, Siviero Agazzi, and Harry R. van Loveren

Summary

This chapter focuses on a region having a history of innovation, from Oscar Batson's description of a no man's land in the 1920s to Dwight Parkinson's description of an anatomical jewel box in the 1970s to Vinko Dolenc's pioneering work that created the foundation of skull base surgery in the 1980s. Today's neurosurgeons find a refined strategy for their cavernous sinus armamentarium using traditional surgical approaches with skull base modifications (when needed) as well as increasing roles for endoscopic surgery and radiosurgery. The authors provide a nuanced guide for evaluating the lesions of this region, performing clinical assessment and diagnostic imaging, and using a building block concept for treatment approach. Success in complex cranial surgery depends on factors such as individual/team competencies, tumor characteristics, and patient characteristics. This chapter highlights some basic strategies as a guide to avoid complications and failures that often result from noncompliance with these concepts. Given the breadth of this subject with its exhaustive list of anatomical structures, surgical steps, and tumor names, interspersed within this chapter are specific topics from the authors' lectures and hands-on courses on the cavernous sinus and parasellar space that illuminate the most critical issues for the skull base surgeon.

Keywords: cavernous sinus, middle fossa, parasellar, sellar, skull base surgery

23.1 History

In the late 1920s, anatomist Oscar Batson at the University of Cincinnati created plastic casts of the venous anatomy of the cavernous sinuses (similar to those of the lumbar plexus) that would eventually bear his name. Passed down from Batson to our neuroanatomical mentor and partner Dr. Jeffrey Keller, they are a physical reminder of Dr. Batson's admonition that the cavernous sinus was truly a "no-man's land" for neurosurgeons, with exsanguination the expected outcome of the folly of surgical exploration (▶ Fig. 23.1).

In 1973, Dwight Parkinson described the surgical opening of the lateral wall of the cavernous sinus, including insertion of pieces of muscle to obliterate cavernous sinus fistulas. This seminal publication transformed what was fiction to become the reality of Dwight Parkinson's "Anatomical Jewel Box," the cavernous sinus.[1] Fast-forward 20 years and 5,000 miles to Yugoslavia (now Slovenia), where Vinko Dolenc's[2,3] pioneering work defined a comprehensive surgical approach to the cavernous sinus. In proving its feasibility and utility in hundreds of cases worldwide, Dolenc established cavernous sinus surgery as the centerpiece for the development of skull base surgery and sparked a renaissance of descriptive neuroanatomy.

As with any new technique or novel idea, adoption is met with skepticism and then embraced with fanaticism before finally finding its proper place in the world—in this case, the neurosurgical armamentarium. After many years of pursuing the aggressive surgical cure of cavernous sinus meningiomas, we witnessed the collision of this concept with a counterrevolution fueled by the combination of failure of cure, persistent cranial nerve morbidities, and gradual acceptance of a rational role for radiosurgery in the treatment of these tumors. Eventually we moved toward a more balanced two-part approach that included, first, retention of portions of tumor that encased the cavernous carotid artery and, second, radiosurgery as an adjunctive treatment for select cases and circumstances.

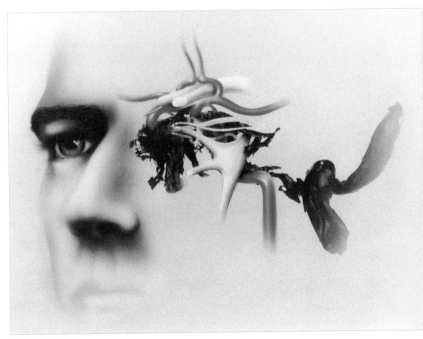

Fig. 23.1 Artist's enhancement of Dr. Oscar Batson's original cast of the cavernous sinus, made at the University of Cincinnati in the 1920s. (Reproduced with permission from J Neurosurg 74:837–844, 1991.)

In recent years, a new set of pioneers have defined and promoted a surgical approach to the medial cavernous sinus that uses a transnasal route and an endoscopic technique. Once again, the idea was met with skepticism and then embraced with fanaticism before only now beginning to find its role in the neurosurgical armamentarium.

23.2 Surgical Anatomy

Key anatomical structures for the surgical approach to the cavernous sinus are discussed in the appendix. Briefly, topics include the anterior clinoid process (ACP), whose removal typically unlocks the anterior compartment of the cavernous sinus, and the major landmarks of the foramen lacerum and lacerum segment of the internal carotid artery (ICA), greater superficial petrosal nerve (GSPN), and vidian nerve, among others.[4,5,6]

The ACP overlies the clinoid segment of the ICA and is almost invariably removed to unlock the anterior part of the cavernous sinus. The ACP has three points of insertion to the skull base: the optic strut (also known as lateral opticocarotid recess from a transnasal endoscopic view), roof of the optic canal, and lesser wing of the sphenoid (part of the superior orbital fissure). Removal of the ACP extradurally exposes the clinoidal space (or anteromedial triangle in Dolenc's description) and the anterior loop of the ICA. Its removal is essential if the distal dural ring of the ICA is to be sectioned and/or mobilized.

The foramen lacerum and lacerum segment of the ICA are major landmarks used to navigate the exposure of the cavernous sinus from an endonasal approach. From a transcranial perspective, the foramen lacerum and lacerum segment of the ICA are never really exposed; they are situated just underneath (deep to) the root of the trigeminal nerve and covered by the petrolingual ligament.

The term *paraclival ICA* is often used in the endoscopic literature but does not have an exact correlate in the currently accepted ICA nomenclature. The endoscopic paraclival ICA corresponds to the lacerum (C3) segment and vertical portion of the cavernous (C4) segment of the ICA (the C1–C7 segments per Bouthillier et al).[4,5]

The GSPN remains a classic landmark for transcranial surgery of the middle fossa and parasellar space. Fortuitously, then, its anatomical continuation, the vidian nerve, has become a classic landmark for the transnasal approach to the same region. Both the GSPN and vidian nerve serve as reliable landmarks for the location of the ICA. During a transcranial approach, the GSPN must be carefully dissected from the temporal lobe dura to provide the lateral limit of Kawase's quadrangle. During anterior petrosectomy, the GSPN that overlies the petrous ICA defines the lateral extent of the drilling. This nerve also serves as one of the landmarks of the internal auditory canal (IAC) during the middle fossa approach to vestibular schwannomas. During an expanded transnasal approach, the vidian canal and vidian nerve are identified in the pterygopalatine fossa and carefully followed back along the floor of the sphenoid sinus to the anterior skull base for safe exposure of the lacerum segment of the ICA.[5,6]

23.3 Regional Pathology and Differential Diagnosis

Various lesions originate in, grow contiguously into, or metastasize to the middle cranial fossa and parasellar space. Meningiomas, schwannomas, and chondrosarcomas are the most frequently encountered tumors in the parasellar space. Pituitary adenomas, craniopharyngiomas, and chordomas are parasellar tumors that can extend into the cavernous sinus. Cholesterol granulomas are nonneoplastic lesions often found in the petrous apex that should also be included in the differential diagnosis of parasellar lesions. Rare are the tumors that can affect the middle cranial fossa and parasellar space, including metastases, epidermoid tumors, cavernous sinus hemangioma, lymphoma, osteosarcoma, angiofibroma, nasopharyngeal carcinoma, and rhabdomyosarcoma.

23.3.1 Meningioma

Meningiomas of the parasellar space also involve the sphenoid wing and have been classified historically among medial, middle, and lateral sphenoid wing types. Clinoidal meningiomas are medial sphenoid wing meningiomas that have been classified separately on the basis of their relationship to the ACP.[7] Along with tuberculum meningiomas, clinoidal meningiomas tend to present early with ophthalmologic disturbances secondary to optic nerve involvement. In contrast, middle sphenoid wing meningiomas often grow slowly and silently from the temporal fossa floor. They tend to present later, sometimes growing large enough to cause seizures from mass effect on the temporal lobe. Sphenocavernous meningiomas may present with signs and symptoms referable to cavernous sinus involvement, including eye movement problems (III, IV, VI), facial sensory disturbance (V), headaches (dura), or orbital venous congestion (venous obstruction).

For purposes of surgical planning, we group the middle fossa and parasellar meningiomas into clinoidal, sphenocavernous, and sphenoid wing types (▶ Fig. 23.2). Sphenoid wing meningiomas are converted to convexity meningiomas once the wing is removed, allowing for complete resection of the tumor and its dural attachment. Although this is possible for clinoidal meningiomas, opening of the optic canal for removal of en plaque canalicular extension is generally required. Depending on the tumor's consistency and adherence at surgery, leaving residual tumor is sometimes necessary to protect the optic nerve or surrounding vasculature or both. Complete resection of sphenocavernous meningiomas is limited to a small subset of tumors that superficially involve the lateral wall without significant cavernous sinus invasion (e.g., carotid encasement). For those that truly invade the sinus and are deemed to need treatment, in light of unacceptably high rates of neurological morbidity associated with intracavernous sinus surgery, we routinely remove the extracavernous tumor if it is large and symptomatic and radiate the intracavernous portion.[8,9] If the tumor's size is acceptable and the extracavernous portion is asymptomatic, we opt to radiate the entire tumor when treatment is necessary. Given the classic appearance of cavernous sinus meningiomas on imaging, radiosurgery or radiotherapy can usually be undertaken without biopsy confirmation.

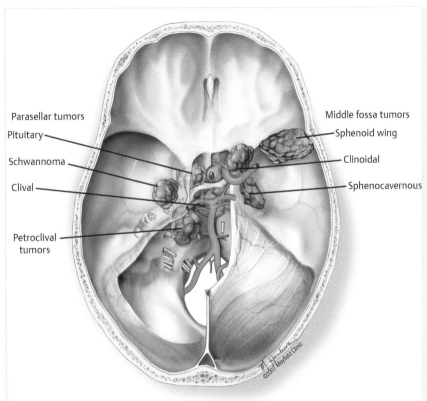

Fig. 23.2 Lesions that can originate in, grow contiguously into, or metastasize to the cavernous sinus include middle fossa tumors, parasellar tumors, and petroclival tumors. (Courtesy of the Mayfield Clinic.)

Parasellar tumors
Pituitary
Schwannoma
Clival
Petroclival tumors

Middle fossa tumors
Sphenoid wing
Clinoidal
Sphenocavernous

Petroclival meningiomas are posterior fossa tumors that can grow into the cavernous sinus or middle fossa. Because of their deep location and association with multiple critical neurovascular structures, they remain one of the most challenging skull base tumors to treat surgically and thus require a command of the gamut of skull base approaches.[10,11,12] When petroclival meningiomas extend anteriorly to involve the cavernous sinus or superolaterally toward the middle fossa, an anterior petrosal approach can deal with those tumor components and provide a window from the middle to the posterior fossa. Conversely, a retrosigmoid intradural suprameatal approach[13] provides a window from the posterior to the middle fossa, allowing for removal of the middle fossa extension of a petroclival meningioma from below. Over time, as with cavernous sinus meningiomas, our strategy for managing petroclival meningiomas has evolved, reflecting our greater willingness to leave residual tumor behind, the better to preserve neurologic function, and radiate the residual as needed.

23.3.2 Trigeminal Schwannoma

Trigeminal schwannomas are benign tumors that arise from Schwann cells of the trigeminal nerve. Although rare—accounting for only < 0.4% of all intracranial tumors—they are the second most common intracranial schwannoma, after vestibular schwannoma. Trigeminal schwannomas may be situated anywhere along the course of the trigeminal nerve, from its root in the prepontine cistern and ganglion in Meckel's cave to major divisions in the middle fossa interdural space and extracranial locations (e.g., infratemporal fossa, pterygopalatine fossa, orbit). The numerous classifications

with which to characterize trigeminal schwannomas anatomically all reflect the potential for involvement in the posterior or middle fossa, or both to varying extent.[14,15,16] Common presenting symptoms include facial pain and numbness, headache, diplopia (cavernous sinus involvement), and signs of brainstem compression.

Typically, small or asymptomatic lesions are observed or radiated, whereas larger, symptomatic lesions undergo surgery, especially in young patients.[17] At surgery, trigeminal schwannomas are typically soft and avascular, displacing (rather than encasing) surrounding nerves and vessels. Cystic changes, found in up to 7% of cases,[18] can make the tumor more adherent to surrounding neurovascular structures and thus more difficult to resect.

Any approach should account for the almost universal finding that trigeminal schwannomas have a Meckel's cave component. Accordingly, even with significant encroachment into the posterior fossa, our approach typically begins in the middle cranial fossa and includes opening Meckel's cave. Overall, the surgical strategy should focus on radical resection of the tumor with preservation of neurological function. More recently, transnasal endoscopic approaches have achieved success in resecting these tumors and are becoming an important strategy in the management of trigeminal schwannomas.[19]

23.4 Clinical Assessment

Signs and symptoms of parasellar tumors depend on the lesion's type, site of origin, size, morphology, growth rate, and involvement of surrounding anatomical structures. Benign, slow-growing lesions tend to gradually develop an onset of symptoms.

Malignant lesions or infectious processes manifest a more rapid clinical course. Furthermore, a lesion that arises from or in proximity to a cranial nerve may produce symptoms referable to the nerve, facilitating diagnosis earlier than for a similar lesion located elsewhere (e.g., clinoidal versus middle sphenoid wing meningioma).

23.5 Diagnostic Imaging

Although the imaging characteristics of common skull base lesions are well described in an earlier chapter, certain observations deserve emphasis. For example, cavernous sinus tumors that track along nerves are more likely malignant than benign. Carotid encasement is a typical feature of meningiomas. Bony lesions, such as chondrosarcoma, will instead displace the vascular structures. Most of the parasellar cavernous sinus tumors are vascularized by branches of the ICA or ophthalmic artery that cannot be embolized or by branches of the middle meningeal artery that can be controlled early in the operation. Catheter angiography is not routinely necessary when managing these tumors; it should only be requested in specific situations, such as for the study of collaterals when carotid sacrifice is contemplated.

23.6 Preoperative Preparation

Success in complex cranial surgery depends on many factors, including individual and team competencies, tumor characteristics (e.g., softness, "suckability," adherence), and patient characteristics. Complications and failures often result from noncompliance with just a handful of simple strategic concepts. The night before a complex surgery, we review our checklist, such as this example for cavernous sinus/parasellar and middle fossa pathologies for goal of surgery, extent of resection, neurological deficits, relation of tumor to ICA, anatomical variations, prevention of cerebrospinal fluid (CSF) leak, imaging, special equipment, and communications with the anesthesiologist.

Our checklist guides us in defining the goal of the surgery and implications if we fail to reach that goal. For example, will the surgical strategy change significantly based on intraoperative biopsy, and if so, can that change be accommodated in the same setting? Other important questions include the following: Will we conduct a complete resection, or a partial one? How aggressive should resection be? Should we check the extent of resection using intraoperative MRI or rely on intraoperative visual assessment and MRI on postoperative day 1? What are the implications if the goal is not achieved?

Any neurological deficit and deficits that we or the patients are willing to accept are carefully evaluated. For instance, damaging the oculomotor nerve in a blind eye is probably acceptable, but causing a permanent ptosis in a seeing eye will make that eye functionally blind.

Assessment includes the relationship of the carotid artery to the tumor and the extent of collateral circulation in case of carotid injury. If the cavernous ICA is narrowed (as is often the case in cavernous sinus meningiomas), one should expect that tumor is tightly adherent to the ICA and will be difficult to separate from the vessel, because the adventitia can be invaded by the tumor. What are the criteria for stopping? Are we prepared to do a bypass procedure if necessary? When the ICA is displaced laterally (as is often the case for chondrosarcomas), is an expanded transnasal approach preferred to a transcranial approach? Do we have the right team for such an approach?

Anatomical variations to consider include degree of pneumatization of the optic strut and the presence of a middle clinoid process, interosseous bridge, or bony carotid ring. An unrecognized pneumatization of the optic strut during a transcranial anterior clinoidectomy will result in a profuse CSF leak on the patient's arrival in the recovery room. An unrecognized carotid ring could turn a routine clinoidectomy into a life-threatening vascular complication. With today's availability of high-quality CTs and MRIs, basing our surgical strategy on the described frequency of such anatomical variations no longer makes sense. Rather, we ascertain the exact anatomical situation of each patient before surgery using dedicated imaging and design an "individualized" surgical plan accordingly.

The best time to think about the closure is before the opening. Preserving a vascularized pericranial flap is the most basic step in anterior cranial base surgery. However, in some instances, avoiding a postoperative CSF leak will require the planned involvement of a plastic surgery team to supplement the closure with a free tissue transfer graft.

Once again we cannot stress enough the importance of preoperative studies in complex skull base cases. **Are all radiographic studies/ancillary investigations completed, reviewed, and, if necessary, uploaded into the operating room navigation system?** Not only should they be ordered, but the surgeon is responsible to ensure their proper format. Aside from their anatomical accuracy, these studies must be compatible with the hospital's navigation system and in the proper format for uploading to the navigation system. Finally, if fusion of other image sets or postprocessing sets (e.g., fiber tractography) is necessary, complete those steps before the day of surgery.

Complex skull base procedures often require special equipment. For example, have the pieces of equipment needed for the case arrived and been cleared by the hospital's biomedical department? The surgeon is responsible to know what equipment is available "off the shelf" and what must be specifically ordered. It is far more efficient to notify the operating room well in advance and to follow up on the request before surgery than to either postpone the case or scramble to have a piece of equipment brought in emergently.

Keeping the anesthesiologist in the loop is mandatory. Aside from routine cases, close communication with the anesthesia team before a complex case significantly affects the flow of the case and shortens the time to incision on the morning of the surgery.

23.7 Surgical Technique

The workhorse approach for the transcranial exposure of the cavernous sinus and parasellar space is the FTOZ (frontotemporal orbitozygomatic osteotomy), sometimes referred to as the COZ (cranio-orbito-zygomatic). A full FTOZ with orbital and zygomatic osteotomy always achieves a wide, generous approach to this region. It should be the default approach for large tumors or when the exact degree of necessary exposure is unclear from preoperative imaging. With greater experience and detailed understanding of the exposure added by each of those osteotomies, a more limited and tailored approach can be designed.

Exposure of the middle fossa is typically via a standard temporal craniotomy. A zygomatic osteotomy can bring the exposure flush with or even through the middle fossa floor. Anterior petrosectomy will allow resection of tumors that extend deep into the petrous apex or into the posterior fossa.

23.7.1 Surface Landmarks

The McCarty bur hole, a key step in the one-piece FTOZ craniotomy, is drilled over the frontosphenoidal suture 1 cm behind the frontozygomatic junction, between the frontal process of the zygomatic bone and zygomatic process of the frontal bone; its upper half exposes the frontal lobe dura and its lower half the periorbita. Note that the McCarty bur hole is usually located 5 to 10 mm below the standard keyhole bur hole.

Two surface landmarks are important for surgical exposures of the middle fossa. First, the external auditory canal (EAC) nearly perfectly aligns with the IAC in both the coronal and the axial planes. The geniculate ganglion is also found in the same coronal plane as the EAC and IAC. Second, the root of the zygoma is the external landmark for the middle fossa floor. The root has both a vertically oriented component, which is lateral, and a horizontal component, which is medial and connected to the squamous temporal bone. A coronal cut through the center of this root also runs through the foramen ovale, whereas a coronal cut through the posterior aspect of the zygomatic root runs through the foramen spinosum. The depression that overlies the lesser wing of the sphenoid marks the sylvian fissure and the anterior wall of the middle cranial fossa. The root of the zygoma marks the middle fossa floor near its junction with the petrous bone. These external landmarks and their reference to internal structures facilitate proper positioning of the craniotomy and help orient the surgeon during extradural exposure of the middle fossa.

23.7.2 Selection of the Approach: Building Block Concept

In designing our approaches from simple to complex, we ensure that every building block is justified and necessary to achieve the surgical goal. The core surgical approach starts with a pterional (frontotemporal) craniotomy in the parasellar space and with a temporal craniotomy in the middle fossa (▶ Fig. 23.3).

The need for a zygomatic osteotomy is determined more by trajectory of view and working angle than by tumor location. Indeed, a front-to-back working trajectory (e.g., resection of a sphenocavernous meningioma) benefits from a zygomatic osteotomy, because it allows downward retraction of the temporalis muscle and a craniotomy flush with the tip of the middle fossa. Conversely, in a posterior-to-anterior working trajectory (e.g., Meckel's cave tumor), a zygomatic osteotomy would be superfluous, because the zygomatic root is already flush with the middle fossa floor and the temporalis muscle can be retracted anteriorly.

Addition of an orbital rim osteotomy to a pterional craniotomy increases the viewing angle under the frontal lobe and decreases the depth of the surgical field. Removal of the zygomatic arch or the orbital rim can be done either in one piece with the frontotemporal bone flap or as separate osteotomies. We usually keep the orbital rim with the frontotemporal flap (one piece) but downfracture the zygomatic arch as a separate step from the craniotomy; this keeps it attached to the masseter muscle and decreases the incidence of postoperative temporomandibular joint dysfunction.

With completion of the superficial working window, the tumor often dictates the need to further enlarge the deep working window. In the parasellar space and middle fossa, this is accomplished most often by adding an anterior petrosectomy to the FTOZ craniotomy. The anterior petrosectomy (Kawase approach) lowers the medial petrous apex to the level of the IAC and creates a window between the middle and posterior fossae.

The exposure provided by an anterior petrosectomy is constant and predictable from preoperative imaging studies. The floor of the viewing trajectory through the anterior petrosectomy is the IAC and cisternal course of the cranial nerve VII to VIII complex. In this approach, the scope of view progressively constricts from top to bottom. When normal anatomy is relatively well preserved, the exposure is limited laterally by the IAC and medially by the inferior petrosal sinus, which is traversed by the abducens nerve. A tumor, however, can expand the anterior petrosectomy approach by naturally eroding the petrous apex. Such lesions can often be radically resected through a middle fossa approach even when their caudal extent reaches as low as the jugular foramen.

In planning for large tumors, the combination of all the building blocks described can obtain a complete exposure of the parasellar space, cavernous sinus, middle fossa, petrous apex, and upper posterior fossa.

23.7.3 Positioning

For a parasellar/cavernous sinus exposure, the patient's head is rotated 20 to 30° toward the contralateral side and tilted back to bring the zygoma to the apex of the field. This brings the sylvian fissure to nearly vertical, allowing it to open "like a book" after its dissection. The greater the extension into the middle fossa, the more the tumor will need a subtemporal exposure and the more the patient's head should be turned to the contralateral side. For a pure middle fossa/subtemporal approach, we position the head with the zygomatic arch parallel to the floor with use of a lumbar drain.

In fact, we always use a drain for the middle fossa approach. We believe that draining CSF facilitates safe retraction of the brain and lessens the potential for temporal lobe injury. After drainage of CSF in 20-mL aliquots as necessary, the drain is removed at the end of surgery.

23.7.4 Execution of the Approach

Skin Incision

The standard incision is a frontotemporal incision behind the hairline. If an orbital osteotomy will be added, the incision should extend past the midline to allow proper skin retraction. Conversely, if the tumor is exclusively located in the middle fossa, a 5-cm straight incision often suffices. Combined approaches

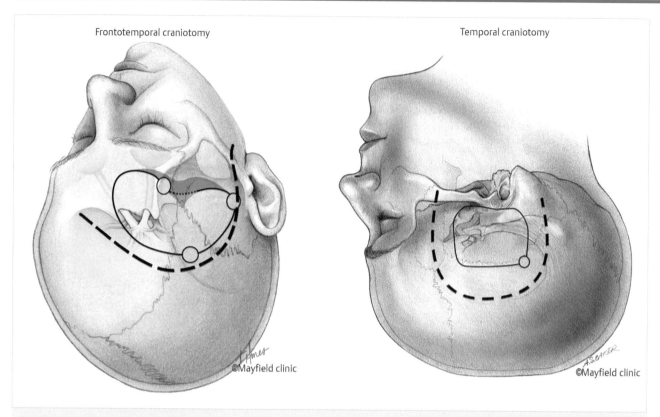

Fig. 23.3 The frontotemporal (pterional) and temporal craniotomies are the building blocks for all approaches to the parasellar and middle fossa regions. Additions of zygomatic osteotomy, orbital rim osteotomy, and anterior petrosectomy are customized to expose the lesion. (Courtesy of the Mayfield Clinic.)

(in particular posterior petrosal approaches) necessitate combination of skin incisions.

Soft Tissue Dissection

The temporalis muscle stretches from the back of the orbit to the pinna of the ear. Its thickness, which varies by patient, must be considered when designing the approach. For most pterional and all full FTOZ craniotomies, the temporalis muscle is reflected inferiorly while the skin is reflected anteriorly. This opens up the anterolateral corridor along the lesser wing of the sphenoid. To separate the skin from the temporalis muscle and avoid damage to the frontal branch of the facial nerve, either a subfascial or interfascial dissection can be used depending on the surgeon's preference. For a temporal craniotomy and middle fossa approach, the temporalis muscle can be retracted anteriorly while still allowing access to the floor of the middle fossa.

Craniotomy

The bony cuts of an FTOZ craniotomy are illustrated in ▶ Fig. 23.4. Some variations of the FTOZ include an orbital variant (orbital osteotomy only) of sufficient exposure for parasellar tumors having little to no middle fossa extension. Similarly, a temporal variant (zygomatic osteotomy only) would be sufficient to expose parasellar tumor having little subfrontal extension. A pterional craniotomy combined with a posterior orbitotomy would appropriately expose small tumors of the anterior cavernous sinus.

Because of concerns with temporomandibular joint pain and chewing difficulties, our strategy is to preserve the patient's masseter insertion on the zygomatic arch. For a full FTOZ, we first cut and down fracture the zygomatic arch (i.e., keeping it attached to the masseter muscle) and then proceed with the cuts. Plating the zygomatic arch before cutting it is routine and ensures exact repositioning at the end of the case.

The temporal part of the craniotomy should be flush with the middle fossa floor—a critical step that is often ignored. If the lesion extends to or arises from the infratemporal fossa, the middle fossa floor should be removed.

Anterior Clinoidectomy

Proper exposure of the ACP requires that the meningo-orbital band be fully severed all the way to the superior orbital fissure. The meningo-orbital band is a dural reflection lateral to the ACP that extends all the way to the medial end of the superior orbital fissure. A small branch of the middle meningeal artery, the meningo-orbital branch, runs in this dural fold and should be coagulated. This fold is surprisingly wide and must be completely divided for good visualization of the ACP. Good microscopic magnification and hemostasis help in identifying the lateral extent of the fold and the beginning of the superior orbital fissure.

Once the band is severed, the three roots of the ACP can be drilled out sequentially. Generally, start with a posterior orbitotomy and unroof the superior orbital fissure (sever the lateral

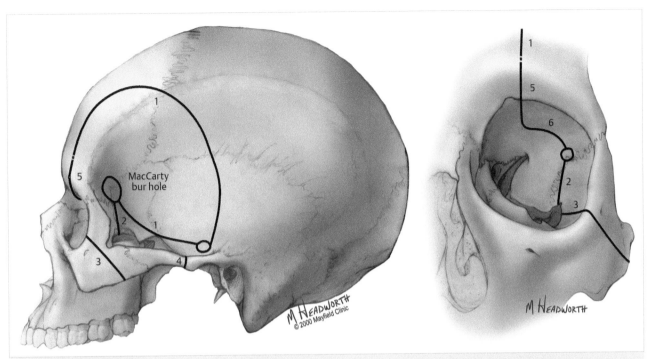

Fig. 23.4 Illustrations depicting the location of the bur holes (MacCarty keyhole, temporal keyhole) and all bony cuts in sequence for a total one-piece FTOZ. First cut (1) extends from the temporal bur hole superiorly, then anteriorly, to a point just lateral to the supraorbital notch at the supraorbital ridge. Returning to the temporal bur hole, the cut is extended anteriorly along the squamous temporal bone toward the frontal component of the MacCarty keyhole bur hole. The sphenoid ridge is thinned to a point that allows it to be cracked safely. Second cut (2), made in the lateral wall of the orbit with the B1 footplate, extends from the orbital component of the MacCarty keyhole to the anterolateral portion of the inferior orbital fissure. Third cut (3) is made just above the zygomaticofacial foramen across the body of the zygoma, starting at the lateral orbital edge and cutting across the zygoma to the anterolateral edge of the inferior orbital fissure. Fourth cut (4) is made across the posterior end of the zygomatic root of the temporal bone. Fifth cut (5) extends from the first cut through the supraorbital ridge just lateral to the supraorbital notch. Sixth cut (6) is made from inside the orbit with a small chisel across the orbital roof to the orbital component of the MacCarty keyhole bur hole. Intraorbital view shows the fifth and sixth cuts made lateral to the supraorbital notch, across the orbital roof, and extending to the orbital portion of the MacCarty keyhole bur hole. (Courtesy of the Mayfield Clinic.)

root/sphenoid wing), then unroof the optic canal (sever the medial/planum sphenoidale root), and finally drill the optic strut that sits just inferior (underneath) the optic nerve. As the optic strut is drilled, gentle traction on the clinoid allows the surgeon to feel when the ACP is free. It can then be removed by rotating it, which detaches it from the surrounding connective tissue. Bleeding from the anteromedial triangle of the cavernous sinus (around the clinoidal segment of the ICA) is common and can be effectively controlled with gentle packing.

Dissection of the Cavernous Sinus

The cavernous sinus is exposed by peeling away the dura covering the medial aspect of the temporal lobe, which covers the parasellar compartment and its contents. This area of dura is often called "the lateral wall of the cavernous sinus," although no such specific structure actually exists. Mobilization of this lateral wall is done mostly extradurally with just one intradural cut along the oculomotor nerve. The lateral wall almost "peels itself off," without requiring major effort, provided three meningeal bands are sharply severed: First and most important is the meningo-orbital band already described. Two other areas requiring sharp dissections are the second and third divisions of the trigeminal nerve (V_2 and V_3) as they exit the middle

cranial fossa through the foramen rotundum and ovale. These two nerves take with them a sleeve of dura, which must be cut sharply to allow further dissection of the lateral cavernous sinus wall.

After the superior orbital fissure, V_2, and V_3 have been uncovered by dissection away from the temporal lobe dura, we often shift our dissection more laterally and posteriorly.

From a subtemporal approach, we identify the foramen spinosum, section the middle meningeal artery, and look for the greater superficial petrosal nerve (GSPN). We dissect the temporal lobe dura from posterior to anterior because it has proved the most reliable way to preserve the GSPN, which courses along the middle fossa floor after exiting the facial hiatus. Elevation of the dura then continues medially to expose the "true" edge of the petrous ridge, which is slightly posterior to the "false" edge created by the groove for the superior petrosal sinus. Every effort should be made to essentially "hook" the blades of the retractors behind the true edge of the petrous ridge rather than just have them press on the temporal dura and underlying temporal lobe.

Before cutting the structure that runs through it, be certain that it is the foramen spinosum. The best way to confirm this is to go back to the dura, find the middle meningeal artery, and follow it. Next, identify the larger foramen (foramen ovale) just anterior and slightly medial to it. Finally, if you already started cutting or dissecting across the foramen without first coagulating it and it did not bleed, it is likely not the foramen spinosum.

When disoriented, go to the foramen rotundum. In the middle fossa, we call the foramen rotundum "home," because it represents a very reliable and easily identifiable landmark. When dissecting the dura anteriorly until the rise of the greater sphenoid wing is encountered, you will always see the maxillary division (V_2) in the dural sleeve entering the foramen rotundum. Once the foramen rotundum is identified, the foramen ovale can be localized posteriorly and slightly lateral to it. The foramen spinosum will be posterior and lateral to the foramen ovale. This path from anterior to posterior facilitates reorientation at the expense of causing some venous bleeding.

Use of a nerve stimulator can help in finding the GSPN. Indeed, the first nerve that is found during elevation of the middle fossa dura will be the lesser superficial petrosal nerve (LSPN), which runs parallel and lateral to the GSPN. The GSPN, which does not look like a nerve, exits the facial hiatus and imitates the periosteum (which did not elevate with the rest of the dura); it will stimulate the facial nerve retrograde. The LSPN conveys presynaptic parasympathetic fibers from the glossopharyngeal nerve (IX) to the otic ganglion, where, after synapsing, it provides secretory fibers to the parotid gland. If what at first appears to be the GSPN does not stimulate, then it is likely the LSPN. The LSPN will not stimulate the facial nerve, whereas stimulation of the GSPN will result in positive contraction signal on neuromonitoring.

Importantly, the GSPN should not be cut, preventing traction injury to the facial nerve. Indeed, the absence of lacrimation from the ipsilateral eye is bothersome only when isolated. However, it could prove to be a very significant complication if during tumor resection injury to the ophthalmic (V_1) division of the trigeminal nerve adds corneal numbness to the dry eye caused by GSPN sectioning (▶ Fig. 23.5).

Drilling of the Petrous Apex (Anterior Petrosectomy)

The first step is to define the borders of Kawase's triangle (or quadrangle, if geometrical accuracy is desired), including the petrous ridge, arcuate eminence, GSPN, and mandibular (V_3) division of the trigeminal nerve. To maximize the anterior petrosectomy, the petrous ICA can be exposed by drilling

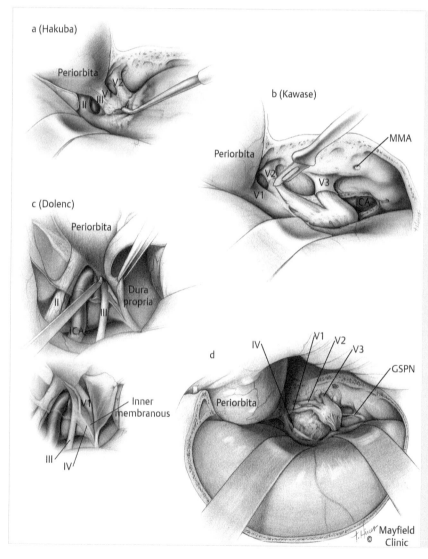

Fig. 23.5 Three techniques for mobilization of the lateral wall of the cavernous sinus. **(a)** Hakuba technique: from an extradural approach, the outer layer of the lateral wall of the cavernous sinus is cut sharply from its attachments at the superior orbital fissure and swept anterolaterally to posteromedially. **(b)** Kawase technique: from an extradural approach, the middle meningeal artery is sacrificed. Outer layer of the lateral wall of the cavernous sinus is then cut sharply from its attachments at the foramen rotundum and foramen ovale and swept laterally to medially, thereby exposing the trigeminal ganglion. **(c)** Dolenc technique: from an intradural approach, outer layer (dura propria) of the lateral wall of the cavernous sinus is first incised along the oculomotor nerve and then stripped from the underlying inner membranous layer in a medial-to-lateral fashion. **(d)** Surgical exposure of a parasellar cavernous chordoma using the Hakuba and Kawase techniques to mobilize the lateral wall of the cavernous sinus. Note the well-defined nature of the tumor from the cavernous sinus structures. (Courtesy of the Mayfield Clinic.)

under irrigation just medial to the GSPN. Drilling can be more aggressive in the anteromedial "safe zone" of Kawase's triangle but should be more careful posterolaterally when approaching the IAC. Drilling the anteromedial safe zone leads to the posterior fossa dura, which serves as a roadmap.

Drilling stops when the inferior petrosal sinus is reached in the depth of the dissection. Intentional sacrifice of the inferior petrosal sinus should be avoided because of the high risk of abducens nerve injury. Drilling near the posterior aspect of Kawase's triangle will eventually lead to dura within the petrous bone. That dura localizes the IAC and is the roadmap for removing further bone laterally. Medial-to-lateral IAC exposure is preferred, because the nerves are more vulnerable laterally toward the fundus of the meatus. A small arch of hard cortical bone is preserved in the angle between the GSPN and the IAC, which contains the cochlea. We estimate the location of the cochlea without fully exposing it; to date this has been effective in preserving it (▶ Fig. 23.6).

Dural Opening

The dural opening for a cavernous sinus meningioma is unique and purposeful. Just as the dural base of a convexity meningioma is often resected, so also with cavernous meningiomas. However, the dura removed is the lateral wall of the cavernous sinus—or, stated more clearly, a large area of the deep temporal dura. If the dura is opened in a conventional fashion along the line of craniotomy and the deep dura resected, you may risk losing the entire dural flap and require a larger-than-necessary dural reconstruction.

The first line of dural incision follows the sylvian fissure (from lateral to medial) to reach deep, nearly to the clinoidal space (created by your earlier clinoidectomy). The second dural cut turns medially under the deep frontal lobe, leaving just 5 mm of dural edge along the falciform ligament and anterior fossa floor for partial suture closure. The third dural cut turns laterally across the anterior pole of the temporal lobe. We refer to

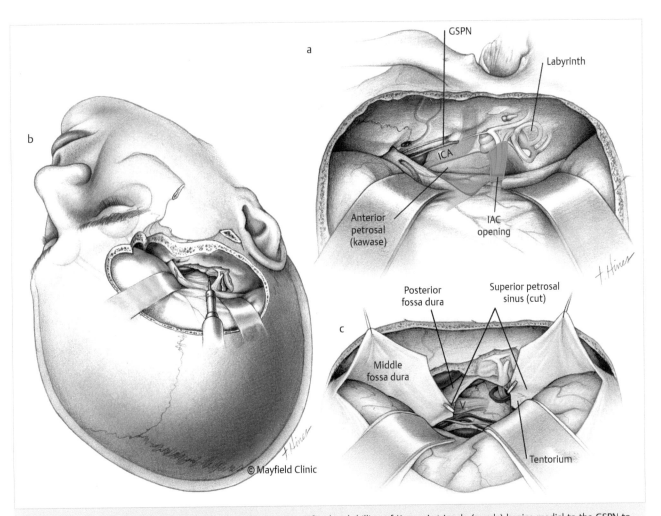

Fig. 23.6 Anterior petrosectomy. **(a)** Middle meningeal artery is sacrificed and drilling of Kawase's triangle (purple) begins medial to the GSPN to unroof the petrous ICA. **(b)** Overview of the craniotomy, placement of the retractors, and anterior petrosectomy drill-out. **(c)** Remaining bone of Kawase's triangle is removed. After dura is opened along the inferior temporal lobe and reflected inferiorly, the dural flap is split in midsection to the level of the superior petrosal sinus. Clips are placed across the superior petrosal sinus and the tentorium is incised toward a point posterior to the trochlear nerve. Dura is then further split down exposing the upper posterior fossa. (Courtesy of the Mayfield Clinic.)

this particular method of dural opening as the "Dolenc technique." Not only did Vinko Dolenc show us how to do it, but he also modeled meticulous patience in suturing the dura "nearly" closed. We usually place a small fat graft at the clinoidal space, where the dura is impossible to suture watertight, and then seal the suture line with a dural sealant. A large sphenocavernous meningioma will dictate that the cuts are made more superficially, along the edge of tumor, with a small margin.

The next step is to debulk the tumor directly to gain exposure of critical structures. We use whatever tools (e.g., ultrasonic aspiration, cutting loops, or just forceps and scalpel) will achieve the most rapid decompression given the texture of the tumor. The best structure to identify first is the optic nerve at its optic canal and then the subjacent carotid artery. With proper debulking of tumor, begin to incise the deep dura around the base of the tumor across the optic canal region and medial anterior fossa floor. You may have to open the optic sheath and remove tumor from the canal.

Next, focus on the dura at the superior orbital fissure area. Identify the deep edge and use a Penfield dissector no. 1 or 4 to literally push the dura, or lateral wall of the cavernous sinus. It dissects rather easily from the cavernous sinus, leaving the nerves down with the inner membranous layer or embedded in residual meningioma within this sinus. Use caution in cauterizing bleeding from small areas of cavernous sinus: you might be cauterizing directly over the cranial nerves.

Next, cut the deep temporal lobe dura near the foramen rotundum and foramen ovale. Grab the free deep edge of dura and again dissect it off maxillary and mandibular nerves from the bottom up. Continue dissection of the dura off Meckel's cave. "Encourage" the dural sleeves of the mandibular and maxillary nerves a bit with a no. 15 blade. Those cuts are difficult to explain: just do it, and don't be afraid.

Make your way to the upper medial aspect of the tumor. Find the oculomotor nerve in the pontine cistern and track its path until you can identify the oculomotor foramen. Make an incision in the dura along the course of the oculomotor nerve to release the upper aspect of the "lateral wall." You should already know that the trochlear nerve will cross the oculomotor nerve in the anterior cavernous sinus—if not, you are not ready for this operation.

The tumor and its dural base are now nearly completely detached. Ready for that moment of awe and wonder, lift the remaining tumor en bloc out of the head except for one last dural incision. The last dural cut crosses behind the tumor from the area of the mandibular nerve upward toward the oculomotor. This cut requires a bit of blind faith, in the most literal sense. Holding the tumor up with a forceps, we typically cut blindly across the dura behind it, knowing that no critical structures will pull up with the tumor. Using this method, you have figuratively (if not literally) converted a cavernous sinus or sphenocavernous meningioma into a convexity meningioma.

Some tumors confined solely to the middle fossa have little or no cavernous sinus involvement. Simply opening the dura parallel to the middle fossa floor is usually sufficient to gain appropriate exposure. If an anterior petrosectomy is performed, then the goal of the dural opening is to eliminate any boundary between the middle and posterior fossae (▶ Fig. 23.7).

Achieving this goal requires cutting of the superior petrosal sinus and tentorium. In its anterior third, the root of the trigeminal nerve, crosses the petrous apex en route to the Gasserian ganglion. The nerve is in danger of being cut accidentally, because posterior fossa tumors compress it against the tentorium and superior petrosal sinus. At this step in the exposure, the dura and superior petrosal sinus are fairly tight. Accordingly, the safest way to avoid injuring the trigeminal nerve is to section the superior petrosal sinus with a sharp blade, millimeter by millimeter, under good illumination and high magnification. This technique enables identification of the fibers of the trigeminal nerve root that are compressed against the inferior aspect of the superior petrosal sinus wall. The sinus should be interrupted and cut between two vascular ligaclips or coagulated using a bipolar cautery. When sectioning the tentorium and reaching its free edge, the trochlear nerve (IV) must be identified and protected before the final cut into the incisura is made.

Preservation of the trochlear nerve is feasible. This nerve enters the tentorium fairly anteriorly and is usually not directly threatened during dural opening. In the posterior part of its trajectory, the trochlear nerve is protected by a layer of arachnoid that separates it from the tentorial edge. Look either above or below the tentorium to identify the nerve before making the final cut through the incisura.

Avoid bleeding when cutting the tentorium by refining your cutting trajectory. Venous lakes present in the tentorium should be coagulated before each cut is made. Nevertheless, bleeding may be excessive when the tentorium is cut too far anteriorly, near the origins of the petrosal sinuses and their connections to the cavernous sinus. When excessive bleeding occurs, redirecting the cutting trajectory more posteriorly usually helps. Conversely, if the cutting trajectory is too posterior, follow the rise of the tentorium behind rather than through the incisura. To avoid these aberrant trajectories, it is best to visualize the incisura before cutting the tentorium.

23.8 Tumor Resection

The most important concept in safe and effective tumor resection is the preoperative establishment of reasonable goals that keep in mind the patient's age and physiologic status and the predicted natural history of the lesion. This assessment results in a set of decisions regarding partial versus total resection and the validity or nonvalidity of intentionally producing neurologic deficits to achieve a radical resection.

The existence of a dissection plane between tumor and brain can be occasionally predicted by the presence of a subarachnoid plane on MRI; similarly, the softness can be indirectly inferred from the brightness of the lesion on T2 sequences. However, many important factors that determine the resectability of a given tumor (i.e., consistency, vascularity, invasiveness, adherence to surrounding structures) are unknown until the operation.

23.9 Closure

Watertight dural closure is never achieved in cavernous sinus or middle fossa exposures, especially when an anterior petrosectomy is also performed. Important steps to help prevent CSF leak consist of careful waxing of exposed air cells, in particular around the IAC ostium, placement of a fat graft in the

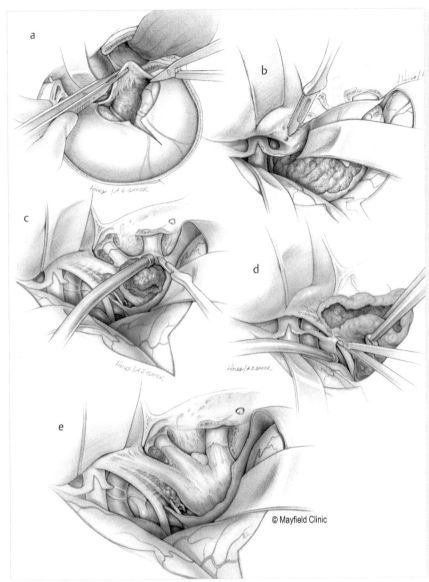

Fig. 23.7 Steps of tumor removal. **(a)** After the dura has been opened along the sylvian fissure and underneath the frontal and temporal lobe, the tumor is debulked. **(b)** Once the residual tumor mass is small enough to be easily manipulated, the capsule is further peeled off the superior orbital fissure/anterior cavernous sinus and **(c)** from the V_2–V_3 branches/lateral cavernous sinus. Often this dissection needs to be "encouraged" with a no. 15 blade, around the dural sleeves of V_2 and V_3. **(d)** The final dural cut is done along cranial nerve III as it enters the roof of the cavernous sinus, carefully avoiding the trochlear nerve that crosses the oculomotor nerve on its way into the superior orbital fissure. **(e)** Residual tumor encasing the trochlear nerve and meningohypophyseal trunk is avoided to prevent neurovascular injury. (Courtesy of the Mayfield Clinic.)

petrosectomy defect, and use of a dural sealant to keep the fat in place.

Although we typically use a lumbar drain in a purely subtemporal surgical approach to gain exposure, it is usually not required for cavernous sinus approaches. Because patients after subtemporal surgery are at risk for temporal lobe swelling, we discontinue the lumbar drain at the conclusion of surgery. The lumbar drain is probably unnecessary to prevent postoperative leak; it may be additionally harmful by adding multiple days of bed rest and producing headache.

23.10 Postoperative Care

With the combination of the delicacy of the temporal lobe and the small working space, temporal lobe swelling is not uncommon. Swelling can result in severe consequences, including uncal herniation, if not recognized and managed aggressively. If the vein of Labbé is injured, more severe temporal lobe swelling should be anticipated, with worse clinical consequences if the

dominant hemisphere is injured. We typically obtain a postoperative head CT on the day of the procedure, administer intravenous antibiotics for 24 hours after surgery, taper steroids to discontinue within 1 week, and continue anticonvulsant medications for 3 months. The lumbar drain is discontinued in the operating room after surgery. Most patients are observed in the intensive care unit for 24 to 48 hours and undergo hourly neurological checks intended to detect any clinical deterioration at an early stage.

23.11 Complications and Their Avoidance

Complications are defined by three necessary characteristics: they are events that are simultaneously undesirable, unintended, and uncommon. They can be minimized, though not always avoided, by adequate planning before surgery and meticulous execution during surgery. We believe that staging lengthy procedures helps reduce time-dependent complications, such as deep venous thrombosis, infection, pneumonia, and pressure ulcers. A willingness to leave behind residual tumor, particularly the cavernous sinus component, has also reduced neurological complications after middle fossa surgery. We have highlighted the anatomical knowledge and pointed out many surgical techniques required to operate safely in the middle cranial fossa. Developing and maintaining an appropriate skill set for this kind of surgery depends on a steady volume of cases and the availability of a cadaveric dissection laboratory for study and practice.

23.12 Follow-up and Rehabilitation

Follow-up should be based on the prediction of time to recurrence, which is based on an understanding of the natural history of the specific tumor histology, resection achieved, and impact of surgical resection on that histology. These factors help guide the timing of surveillance imaging or adjuvant treatment. A multidisciplinary skull base team (e.g., otolaryngologists, ophthalmologists, radiation oncologists, pathologists, radiologists, physical therapists) facilitates the identification and management of important specialty-specific patient care issues after surgery.

23.13 Conclusion

The cavernous sinus, parasellar space, and middle fossa constitute an important landscape in the realm of skull base surgery. Contemporary treatment strategies for tumors in these locations combine traditional surgical approaches with skull base modifications where needed. Continually increasing roles for endoscopic surgery and radiosurgery are expected in the future. Successful management of tumors in this region requires a multidisciplinary approach and a thorough understanding of the wide range of concepts highlighted in this review.

References

[1] Parkinson D. Carotid cavernous fistula: direct repair with preservation of the carotid artery. Technical note. J Neurosurg. 1973; 38(1):99–106

[2] Dolenc V. Direct microsurgical repair of intracavernous vascular lesions. J Neurosurg. 1983; 58(6):824–831

[3] Dolenc V. Anatomy and Surgery of the Cavernous Sinus. Wien: Springer-Verlag; 1989

[4] Bouthillier A, van Loveren HR, Keller JT. Segments of the internal carotid artery: a new classification. Neurosurgery. 1996; 38(3):425–432, discussion 432–433

[5] Alikhani P, Sivakanthan S, van Loveren H, Agazzi S. Paraclival or cavernous internal carotid artery: One segment but two names. J Neurol Surg B Skull Base. 2016; 77(4):304–307

[6] Kasemsiri P, Solares CA, Carrau RL, et al. Endoscopic endonasal transpterygoid approaches: anatomical landmarks for planning the surgical corridor. Laryngoscope. 2013; 123(4):811–815

[7] Al-Mefty O. Clinoidal meningiomas. J Neurosurg. 1990; 73(6):840–849

[8] Abdel-Aziz KM, Froelich SC, Dagnew E, et al. Large sphenoid wing meningiomas involving the cavernous sinus: conservative surgical strategies for better functional outcomes. Neurosurgery. 2004; 54(6):1375–1383, discussion 1383–1384

[9] O'Sullivan MG, van Loveren HR, Tew JM, Jr. The surgical resectability of meningiomas of the cavernous sinus. Neurosurgery. 1997; 40(2):238–244, discussion 245–247

[10] Erkmen K, Pravdenkova S, Al-Mefty O. Surgical management of petroclival meningiomas: factors determining the choice of approach. Neurosurg Focus. 2005; 19(2):E7

[11] Little KM, Friedman AH, Sampson JH, Wanibuchi M, Fukushima T. Surgical management of petroclival meningiomas: defining resection goals based on risk of neurological morbidity and tumor recurrence rates in 137 patients. Neurosurgery. 2005; 56(3):546–559

[12] Miller CG, van Loveren HR, Keller JT, Pensak M, el-Kalliny M, Tew JM, Jr. Transpetrosal approach: surgical anatomy and technique. Neurosurgery. 1993; 33(3):461–469

[13] Samii M, Tatagiba M, Carvalho GA. Retrosigmoid intradural suprameatal approach to Meckel's cave and the middle fossa: surgical technique and outcome. J Neurosurg. 2000; 92(2):235–241

[14] Samii M, Migliori MM, Tatagiba M, Babu R. Surgical treatment of trigeminal schwannomas. J Neurosurg. 1995; 82(5):711–718

[15] Jefferson G. The trigeminal neurinomas with some remarks on malignant invasion of the gasserian ganglion. Clin Neurosurg. 1953; 1:11–54

[16] Yoshida K, Kawase T. Trigeminal neurinomas extending into multiple fossae: surgical methods and review of the literature. J Neurosurg. 1999; 91(2):202–211

[17] Niranjan A, Barnett S, Anand V, Agazzi S. Multimodality management of trigeminal schwannomas. J Neurol Surg B Skull Base. 2016; 77(4):371–378

[18] Wanibuchi M, Fukushima T, Zomordi AR, Nonaka Y, Friedman AH. Trigeminal schwannomas: skull base approaches and operative results in 105 patients. Neurosurgery. 2012; 70(1 Suppl Operative):132–143; discussion 143–144

[19] Raza SM, Donaldson AM, Mehta A, Tsiouris AJ, Anand VK, Schwartz TH. Surgical management of trigeminal schwannomas: defining the role for endoscopic endonasal approaches. Neurosurg Focus. 2014; 37(4):E17

24 Tumors of the Petrous Apex

Ricardo Ramina, Maurício Coelho Neto, Gustavo Nogueira, and Erasmo Barros da Silva Jr.

Summary

The petrous apex and petroclival junction are difficult areas to access. Conceptually the region can be divided into areas inferomedial and superolateral to the petrous carotid artery. Endonasal approaches are favored for inferomedially located pathology, whereas approaches through the temporal bone are preferred for pathologies superior and lateral to the internal carotid artery. This chapter discusses the common lesions in this region and their surgical management.

Keywords: petrous apex, petroclival, temporal bone, cholesterol granuloma, trigeminal schwannoma, middle fossa, suprameatal triangle

24.1 Introduction

The petrous apex (PA) is defined as the pyramidal, medial projection of the petrous portion of the temporal bone lying anteromedial to the inner ear, between the sphenoid bone anteriorly and the occipital bone posteriorly, with the apex at the foramen lacerum.[1,2] It is located in the center of the skull base and is surrounding by critical structures. The PA is pneumatized in approximately 33% of people.[3] Pneumatization may be variably and asymmetrical in 4 to 7% of cases.[4] Neoplastic and inflammatory processes are the most common lesions in the PA. These lesions may originate within the PA as primary lesions (e.g., chondrosarcomas, congenital cholesteatomas, cholesterol granuloma) or may arise from structures related to the PA, as secondary lesions (e.g., petroclival meningiomas, trigeminal schwannomas, chordomas). Neoplastic lesions produce symptoms through invasion and mass effect. Surgery is the treatment of choice for most PA lesions, with the exception of petrous apicitis and osteomyelitis. Surgical difficulties are related to the involvement of the internal carotid artery (ICA) and the basilar arteries and their branches, as well as to brain retraction, tumor extension to the cavernous sinus and brainstem, preservation of the vein of Labbé and other temporal lobe veins, and surgical defect after extensive drilling of skull base bone. Careful preoperative clinical and radiological evaluation is very important to select the surgical approach and minimize intra- and postoperative complications.

Several surgical approaches have been used to resect these lesions. In the last two decades endonasal endoscopic approaches have been used as a single approach or in association with microsurgery. Factors influencing the choice of approach include the nature, location, and extension of the lesion; status of hearing and vestibular function; preoperative facial nerve function; presence of infection; and experience level of the surgical team. If the tumor has relationship with the sphenoid sinus or is located medial to the ICA, the endoscopic approach is favored. Continuous developments in surgical techniques, improvements in imaging studies, neuroanesthesia, intraoperative monitoring, antimicrobials, and postoperative care have made possible the radical removal of many PA lesions with preservation of cranial nerves and vessels while avoiding postoperative cerebrospinal fluid (CSF) leak and infection.

24.2 Surgical Anatomy

The temporal bone has four parts: petrous, squamous, tympanic, and mastoid. The PA is formed by the medial portions of the temporal bone. This pyramid-shaped structure has its apex pointing anteromedially and its base located posterolaterally. Its limits are medially the petro-occipital fissure, anteriorly the petrosphenoidal fissure, posteriorly the posterior fossa, and laterally the inner ear structures. The PA has three surfaces between the middle and the posterior fossae (▶ Fig. 24.1)[5]: An anterior surface (temporal), a posterior surface (posterior fossa) and an inferior surface (occipital). The anterosuperior portion of the PA forms the middle fossa floor. The main anatomical structures related to this portion are the great superficial petrosal nerve, which runs posterior to the mandibular branch of the trigeminal nerve; the arcuate eminence; the Eustachian tube; the ICA; and the gasserian and geniculate gangliae.[6]

The posterior surface of the PA is the anterolateral wall of the posterior cranial fossa and extends medially from the posterior semicircular canal and the endolymphatic sac to the petroclinoid ligament and the canal for the abducens nerve (Dorello's canal). This surface extends from the petro-occipital suture line inferiorly to the superior petrosal sinus superiorly. Inferiorly, the petrous pyramid is bounded by the jugular bulb and the inferior petrosal sinus. The inferior surface has also a foramen for the entry of the ICA. Medial to the jugular fossa is a depression that is associated with the cochlear aqueduct (perilymphatic duct). The petrous bone articulates with the greater wing of the sphenoid anteriorly. The foramen lacerum is found between the apex of the petrous bone and the sphenoid bone and contains but does not transmit the ICA. The ICA penetrates the skull through the carotid canal of the temporal bone, then makes a curve medially to form the horizontal portion over the lacerum foramen penetrating the cavernous sinus (▶ Fig. 24.2).

The relationship of PA tumors with the ICA is of critical importance for endoscopic endonasal approaches. The vidian canal is used as a landmark to expose the petrous portion of the ICA.[7] The segment of facial nerve mainly related (3–5 mm) to the PA is the labyrinthine portion (▶ Fig. 24.3).[8] The geniculate ganglion is anterior and medial to the arcuate eminence. In about 15% of cases the temporal bone is dehiscent over the geniculate ganglion.[9] The internal auditory canal divides the PA into an anterior portion and a smaller posterior portion.[10] In children, the PA is usually filled with fat but becomes pneumatized with age, as the mastoids do. Embryologically its ossification is endochondral from mesenchymal tissue present in this region. The PA may be pneumatic (20% of the population), sclerotic, or diploic. The anterior portion of the PA is filled with marrow in approximately 60% of temporal bones. Pneumatization is relatively symmetric between right and left side, and asymmetric pneumatization may be mistaken for tumor.[11]

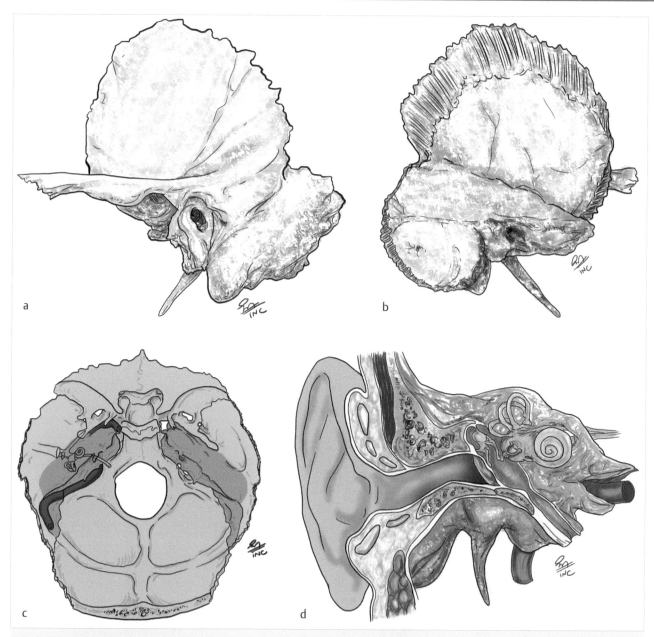

Fig. 24.1 **(a)** Temporal bone, lateral view. **(b, c)** Petrous apex (*arrows*). **(d)** Inner ear and anatomical structures of temporal bone.

There is no nervous or vascular structure within the PA, but it is surrounded by vital structures. These important vessels, nerves, and brainstem may be embedded or related to tumors arising in this region. Most surgical approaches require identification and dissection of these structures from the tumor capsule.[12]

24.2.1 Regional Pathology and Differential Diagnosis

Various pathologies may arise within the PA. The differential diagnosis includes infection, benign tumors, malignant tumors, congenital entities (cholesteatomas, asymmetric fatty marrow), obstructive processes (cholesterol granulomas), vascular (ICA aneurysms), and miscellaneous lesions (Paget's disease, fibrous

dysplasia).[2,13,14,15,16,17] Embryologically the PA has a mesodermic origin and is formed by osseous and fat tissue. It is closely related to the clivus and the spheno-occipital and sphenopetrous synchondroses, which have rests of notochordal and cartilaginous matrix. The temporal bone has pneumatized cells filled with mucosa of ectodermic origin. The cranial nerves related to this region also have an ectodermic origin. Lesions of the PA may be classified on the basis of their etiology as inflammatory lesions, developmental lesions, benign and malignant tumors, vascular lesions, and osseous dysplasias. PA tumors are divided into two groups by site of origin: primary, originating within the PA, and secondary, originating from neighboring structures with secondary involvement of the PA. PA destruction is most frequently caused by a

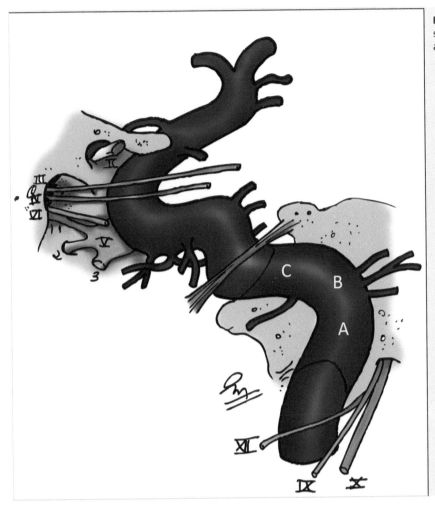

Fig. 24.2 The three portions of the petrous segment of the internal carotid artery: A, ascending (vertical); B, genu; C, horizontal.

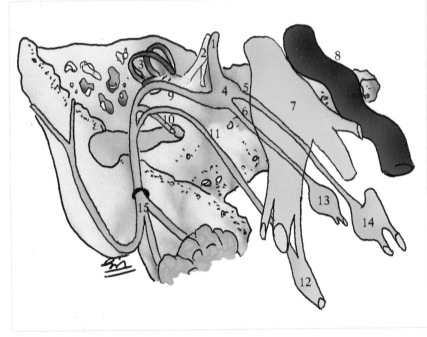

Fig. 24.3 Facial nerve anatomy. 1, intracanalicular portion; 2, cochlear nerve; 4, geniculate ganglion; 7, gasserian ganglion; 9, labyrinthic and mastoid portions; 15, extratemporal portion.

secondary process from either contiguous lesions or metastasis. The most frequent primary PA lesions are as follows:

- Mesenchymal origin:
  - Squamous cell carcinoma
  - Rhabdomyosarcoma
  - Chondrosarcoma
  - Aneurysmal bone cyst
  - Cholesteatoma
  - Cholesterol granuloma
  - Meningioma
  - Facial nerve schwannoma
  - Trigeminal nerve schwannoma
- Ectodermic origin:
  - Epidermoid cyst
  - Chordoma
  - Neurofibroma
  - Mucocele
- Mesenchymal/ectodermic origin:
  - Multiple myeloma
  - Lymphoma
  - Metastasis

The most frequent secondary PA lesions are as follows:
- Neoplastic:
  - Adenoid cystic carcinomas
  - Juvenile angiofibromas
  - Vestibular nerve schwannomas
  - Nasopharyngeal carcinoma
  - Chondrosarcoma
  - Meningiomas
  - Jugular foramen paragangliomas
  - Chordoma
  - Metastasis
- Nonneoplastic:
  - Epidermoid cyst
  - Arachnoid cyst

- Fibrous dysplasia
- Intrapetrous carotid artery aneurysm
- Petrous apicitis
- Mucocele

24.2.2 The Most Frequent Petrous Apex Lesions

Chondrosarcomas

Chondrosarcomas arise from mesenchymal cells in the embryonic cartilaginous matrix of the cranium, generally with an epicenter in the petroclival synchondrosis. They typically grow by infiltrating the bone, replacing the normal bone marrow with chondroid tissue, and spreading through Harver's canals.[18] Although similar in clinical and radiological presentation, chordomas and chondrosarcomas have very different patterns on immunohistology. Unlike chordoma (even chondroid), chondrosarcomas are nonreactive for cytokeratin and brachyury. They share reactivity to vimentin and S-100. Most chordomas are positive for epithelial membrane antigen, but a few chondrosarcomas are positive for it.[19,20,21]

Another marker in the last 10 years identified as an important tool in this differential is the presence of IDH1 mutation, which is associated with chondrosarcomas rather than chordoma and had a sensitivity of 71.4% and specificity of 100% in one series, although this association had no impact on prognosis.[20] Prognosis of PA chondrosarcomas is related to histological grade. Grade I tumors present a 5-year survival rate of 90%, grade II 81%, and grade III 43%. Facial nerve palsy, vertigo, diplopia (cranial nerve VI dysfunction), and pulsatile tinnitus are the most frequent complaints.[22] Surgical approach depends on extension of the tumor. The middle fossa approach has been used in our clinic to remove PA chondrosarcomas that extended lateral to the ICA (▶ Fig. 24.4). Tumors with extensions medial to the ICA are approached thorough a transnasal endoscopic

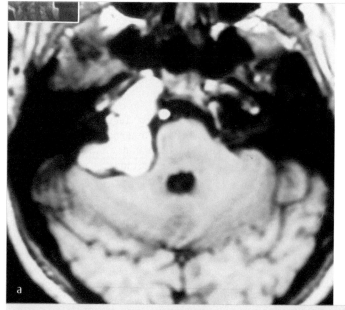
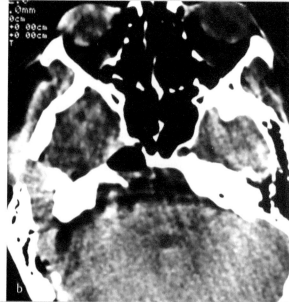

Fig. 24.4 **(a)** T1-weighted MRI showing a petrous apex chondrosarcoma. **(b)** CT scan after removal of the tumor.

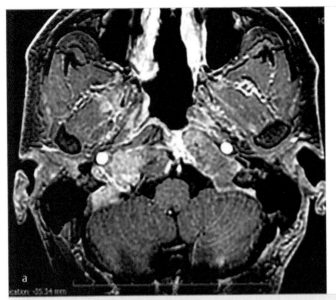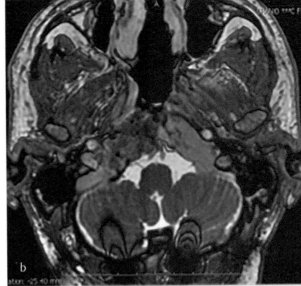

Fig. 24.5 (a, b) Recurrent petrous apex chondrosarcoma. Surgical approach: transnasal endoscopic.

approach (▶ Fig. 24.5). Radical resection is difficult in large and infiltrative tumors, and postoperative radiosurgery is performed in high-grade tumors.

Chordomas

Chordomas correspond to 1 to 4% of all bone malignancies and 0.2 to 0.4% of all intracranial tumors, with higher incidence in men, mainly between 20 and 40 years of age. Fewer than 5% of these tumors occur in children and adolescents. The annual incidence is 0.089/100.000 in the United States.[13,19,23] These slow-growing tumors arise from notochordal remnants and originate from the clivus and PA (▶ Fig. 24.6).[6] Chordomas are usually not related to any syndrome, but some reports of familial cases do exist. Duplication of a region in 6q27 plays a role in susceptibility to hereditary chordomas. This genetic abnormality is related to the brachyury gene.[21,24] Recurrence after surgical removal is frequent, and radiotherapy/radiosurgery (proton beam) is indicated as adjuvant therapy.[25] Proton therapy presents a 5-year estimate for local control of 69.6% and overall survival of 81.4%.[26]

Carbon ion particle therapy is increasingly being used to treat chordomas and chondrosarcomas. The Heidelberg Group has published a series of 54 cases of chondrosarcomas treated using carbon ions, for a tumor control rate of 89% and overall survival of 98% in 5 years.[27] Uhl et al reported a series of chondrosarcomas treated using carbon ion therapy, for 90% local control rates in 5 years and 88% in 10 years.[28] Results of carbon ion therapy for chordomas present 72 to 85% of local control and 85 to 88% of overall survival in 5 years.[29]

Chondromas

Chondromas arise at the base of the skull from residual rests of primordial cartilage in basilar synchondrosis entrapped during endochondral ossification.[30,31] Usually they are located at the sphenoethmoidal, sphenopetrosal, petro-occipital, and spheno-occipital synchondroses.[31,32] Another possible origin of chondromas is from metaplasia of meningeal fibroblasts or perivascular mesenchymal tissue, which would explain their presence in other locations, such as cerebral parenchyma, dura, and different bone sites.[33] They may occur alone or as part of Ollier's disease or Mafucci's syndrome.[34,35] These tumors are rare and benign and may be cured by radical resection (▶ Fig. 24.7).

Meningiomas

Most meningiomas involving the PA originate from the petroclival region, the cerebellopontine angle, or the sphenoid ridge.[36] True PA meningiomas are rare (▶ Fig. 24.8). Involvement of the trigeminal nerve and Meckel's cave causes often intractable trigeminal neuralgia. Meningiomas may cause hyperostosis of the PA, and in MRI studies they are hypointense on T1 and iso- to hyperintense on T2. They enhance with gadolinium, and a "dural tail" may be observed.

Schwannomas

Schwannomas affecting the PA most frequently originate from the trigeminal and facial nerves. Trigeminal nerve schwannomas (TSs) are the second most common type of intracranial schwannoma (▶ Fig. 24.9).[37] These tumors are benign in the majority of the cases and have their highest incidence between 38 and 40 years of age. They are more common in middle-aged women.[37,38] Facial pain, hypesthesia, headaches, and diplopia are the most common symptoms. Usually trigeminal schwannomas are slow-growing tumors and when the patient presents with clinical symptoms the lesion has already reached a large size. Radical resection is curative in the majority of cases. The main challenge of surgical removal is preservation of nonaffected fibers of the trigeminal nerve. Facial nerve schwannomas are uncommon tumors that are extremely slow-growing, that are benign in the majority of cases, and that frequently present

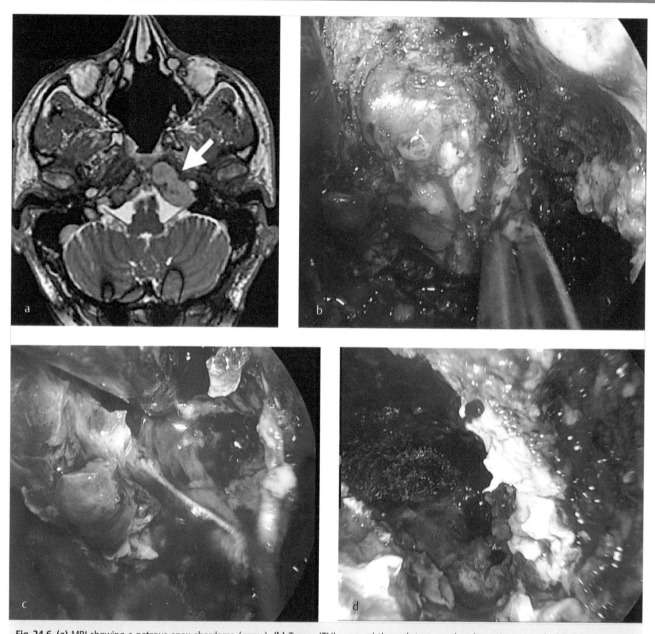

Fig. 24.6 **(a)** MRI showing a petrous apex chordoma (*arrow*). **(b)** Tumor (TU) exposed through transnasal endoscopic approach. **(c)** Tumor removal (TU). **(d)** After tumor removal. Surgicel covering the jugular foramen (JF).

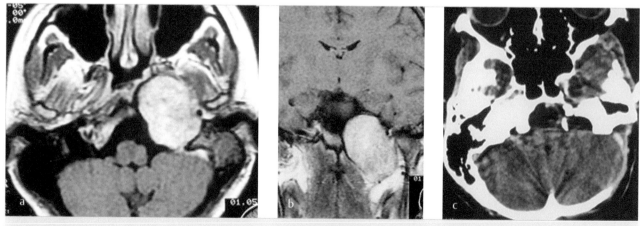

Fig. 24.7 **(a, b)** Large petrous apex chondroma. **(c)** CT scan after total removal of the tumor.

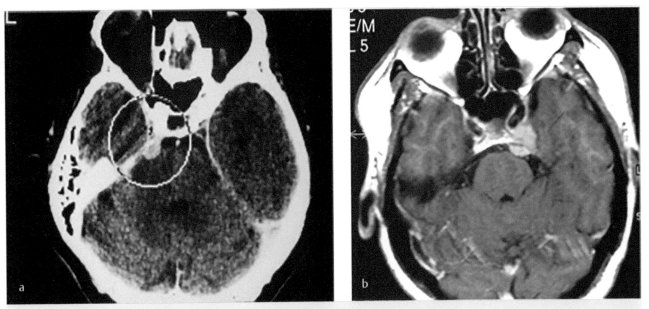

Fig. 24.8 (a) CT scan showing a small petrous apex meningioma. (b) MRI of a petrous apex meningioma.

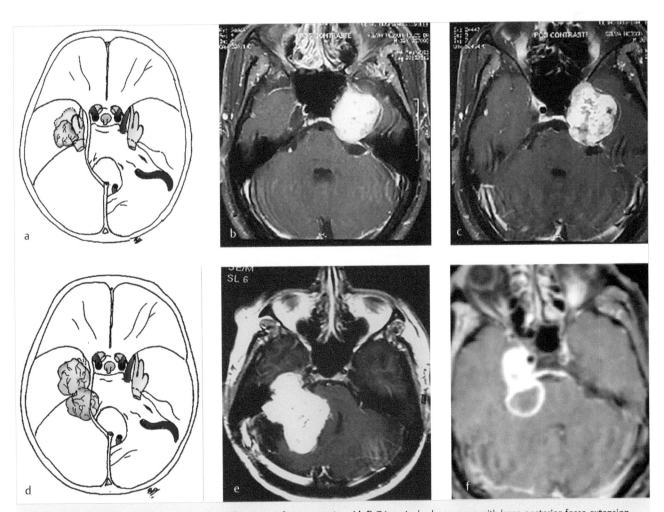

Fig. 24.9 (a–c) Trigeminal schwannoma with small posterior fossa extension. (d–f) Trigeminal schwannoma with large posterior fossa extension.

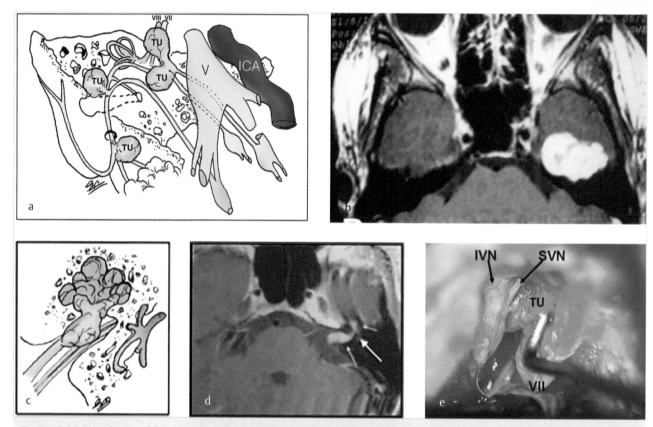

Fig. 24.10 (a) Sites of origin of facial nerve schwannomas. (b) Geniculate ganglion facial nerve schwannoma involving the petrous apex. (c–e) Intrameatal facial nerve schwannoma (TU). IVN, inferior vestibular nerve; SVN, superior vestibular nerve.

without facial dysfunction. They can be mistaken for vestibular schwannomas. The most common origin sites of these tumors are the geniculate ganglion and internal auditory canal (▶ Fig. 24.10).

Indication for surgical removal and choice of surgical approach of facial nerve schwannomas depends on tumor extension, grade of facial nerve palsy, hearing function, and surgical experience. The best postoperative function of facial nerve after tumor resection and nerve reconstruction is a House-Brackmann grade III palsy. Patients who have preoperative facial palsy grade III or higher or those who have large tumors compressing the brainstem are the best candidates for surgery.

Metastasis

The PA is the most common site for metastases in the temporal bone. The most frequent metastases from the following tumors have been found in the PA: breast, lung, kidney, prostate, and gastrointestinal. The petrous bone may be involved by metastatic disease through hematogenous spread or leptomeningeal extension from distant neoplasms or by direct extension of an extra or intracranial tumor. Treatment and prognosis depend on extension of the disease.

Cholesterol Granulomas

Cholesterol granuloma is the most common PA lesion. The granuloma contains cholesterol crystals, granulation tissue, and blood breakdown products. It may be a sequela of chronic otitis

media. The cyst has a fibrous capsule without a true epithelial lining. The most common symptoms are hearing loss, tinnitus, and headache. MRI shows a hyperintense, non-enhancing lesion on T1- and T2-weighted sequences. CT scans demonstrate a well-defined PA lesion with no cortical destruction (▶ Fig. 24.11).

Cholesteatomas

PA cholesteatomas are uncommon and may be congenital or acquired (▶ Fig. 24.12). They constitute 4 to 9% of all PA lesions.[39] Congenital lesions are rare, arise from aberrant ectoderm that is trapped during embryogenesis, and develop behind the tympanic membrane.[22] Headaches, hearing loss, and facial nerve palsy are the most frequent symptoms. Large lesions may produce symptoms of other cranial nerves. Persistent otorrhea after previous mastoid surgery is an indication of an acquired cholesteatoma. A high recurrence rate is associated with difficulty clearing all the disease at primary surgery, and long-term follow-up is required.

24.3 Clinical Assessment

The presenting symptoms of PA lesions may be vague and nonspecific. They may remain undetected for long periods, and some lesions are incidentally diagnosed on imaging studies for nonrelated symptoms. Progressive and long-standing symptoms suggest benign tumors. Pain, multiple cranial nerve

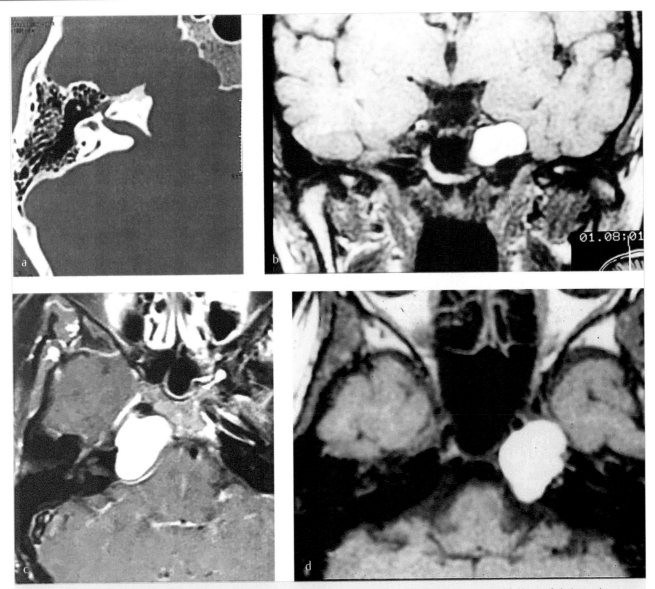

Fig. 24.11 Petrous apex cholesterol cyst. **(a)** CT scan demonstrating petrous apex erosion. **(b–d)** MRIs show typical findings of cholesterol cysts.

deficits, and short history are more frequently encountered with malignant lesions. Clinical symptoms are attributable to mass effect of an expansile lesion or infiltration of anatomical structures within or adjacent to the apex. The presenting signs and symptoms of PA tumors may be specific (related to the structures of this region) or nonspecific. The most common presenting symptoms are headache, visual symptoms, and hearing loss.[40] Retroauricular pain and headache (retro-orbital and at the vertex) may occur with malignant or aggressive lesions from infiltration of the dura. Facial pain, hypoesthesia, and paresthesia are observed with involvement of the trigeminal nerve at Meckel's cave. Diplopia due to compression or invasion of cranial nerve VI is observed in chondrosarcomas. The facial nerve may be affected anywhere along its course in the temporal bone. Tinnitus, vertigo, and hearing loss occur due to Eustachian tube dysfunction, involvement of the bony labyrinth and the vestibulocochlear nerve, erosion of the ossicular chain, and compression of the cerebellum and brainstem. Other cranial nerves from II through XII may be affected. Involvement of the ICA may produce pain (invasion of the adventitia), syncope, amaurosis fugax, and stroke.

24.3.1 Diagnostic Imaging

The differential diagnosis for PA lesions is extensive. Evaluation of the temporal bone with standard radiography includes Towne's and Stenver's views and polytomography. However, accurate diagnosis is possible only using imaging studies, such as CT scanning and MRI; usually both studies are required for elucidation of a more definitive diagnosis.[41] CT scanning with contrast enhancement, thin slices, and 3D reconstruction is useful to evaluate the extension of the lesion and erosion of the cranial base bone and in planning the surgical approach. Bone erosion with smooth or scalloped margins suggests a slow-growing benign lesion (cholesterol granuloma, meningocele, mucocele, schwannoma). Infections and aggressive tumors may present

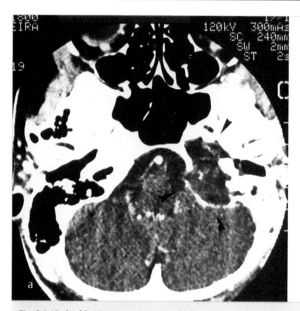
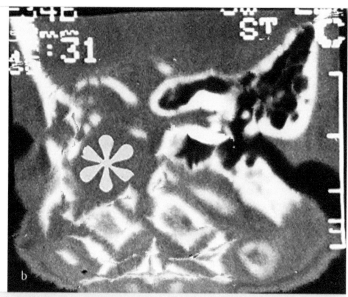

Fig. 24.12 (a, b) CT scans presenting large petrous apex erosion by a cholesteatoma (*asterisk*).

Table 24.1 Petrous apex lesions on CT scanning

Lesion	Bone erosion	Eroded margin	Contrala-teral apex	Contrast enhance-ment
Cholesterol granuloma	+	Smooth	Highly pneuma-tized	–
Cholestea-toma	+	Smooth	Often not pneuma-tized	–
Petrous apicitis	+	Irregular	Variable	–
Effusion	–	–	Usually pneuma-tized	–
Bone mar-row asym-metry	–	–	Variable	–
Carotid aneurysm	+	Smooth	Variable	+
Neoplasia	+	Variable	Variable	+

Source: Adapted with permission from Jackler RK, Parker D, The radiographic differential diagnosis of petrous apex lesions, Am J Otol 1992;13:561–574.

on CT as osteolytic lesions with ill-defined margins and a moth-eaten pattern. CT scanning is helpful in the differential diagnosis of lesions in this region (▶ Table 24.1).[42]

Tumors such as fibrous dysplasia, multiple myeloma, and calcified chondrosarcomas can be well demonstrated using CT examination.[43,44] about the nature and extension of the lesion and involvement of other structures, such as vessels, nerves, and the brainstem (▶ Table 24.2).[10,42]

Inflammatory diseases (e.g., petrositis, osteomyelitis) and epidermoid cyst have characteristic findings on MRI. Petrous carotid and cavernous carotid aneurysms as well as venous sinus variations are well demonstrated using MR angiography and

venography. Special sequences are helpful to visualize cranial nerves and relations of the tumor with the brainstem. Digital angiography is performed when an aneurysm is suspected, when a balloon occlusion test is needed, and for preoperative embolization (e.g., paragangliomas and other highly vascularized tumors).

24.3.2 Preoperative Preparation

Careful preoperative evaluation is critical in minimizing intraoperative and postoperative complications. Preoperative preparation involves evaluation of the patient's clinical condition. Because PA tumors occur commonly in elderly patients, adequate evaluation of clinical condition and associated comorbidities is mandatory (▶ Table 24.3).

Management of PA pathologies poses a challenge. A correct preoperative diagnosis is needed to define treatment modality and surgical approach. The central location in the skull base, with adjacent critical neurovascular structures, makes diagnostic biopsy difficult and hazardous. Preoperative imaging studies may define the exact size and location of the lesion. If the tumor has extension into the sphenoid sinus, then an endoscopic biopsy may be performed. Careful evaluation of the involved cranial nerves is needed to define the best form of treatment. Facial nerve function and the quality of preoperative hearing are important factors in choosing the surgical approach. Removal of the labyrinth should be avoided in patients who have good hearing. Patients who have associated infection, such as otitis, require antibiotic treatment. Radiosurgery may be an option in some cases.

24.3.3 Surgical Approaches

Different surgical approaches to this region have been described, each of which has its advantages and disadvantages. Choice of surgical approach depends on the clinical status of the patient, etiology of the lesion, extent of the tumor, involvement

Table 24.2 Petrous apex lesion on MRI scanning

Lesion	T1 images	T2 images	T1 gadolinium enhancement	Tumor margins	Other characteristics
Chondrosarcoma	↓ (B)	↑ ↑ ↑ (B)	Heterogenous	Irregular invasive	Chondroid matrix
Chordoma	↓ or ↔ (B)	↑ ↑ ↑ ↑ (B)	Heterogenous	Irregular invasive	Bone "islands" midline
Cholesteatoma	↔ (L)	↔ (L)	No enhancement	Regular expansive	Prussak spaces
Epidermoid cyst	↓ ↓ (L)	↑ ↑ or ↔ (L)	No enhancement	Regular expansive	↑ ↑ ↑ Diffusion
Cholesterol granuloma	↑ ↑ ↑ ↑ (L)	↑ ↑ ↑ ↑ (L)	No enhancement	Regular expansive	Confined petrous apex
Meningioma	↔ (B)	↔ (B)	Homogeneous intense	Regular	Calcifications "Dural tail"
Schwannoma	↔ (B)	↑ ↑ (B)	Homogeneous intense	Regular	"Ice-cream cone sign" cysts
Carcinoma	↔ (M)	↔ (M)	Heterogeneous	Irregular destructive	Extracranial extension
Metastasis	↔ (M)	↔ (M)	Heterogeneous	Irregular destructive	Primary tumor
Plasmocytoma	↓ or ↔	↓ or ↓ ↓ or ↔	Homogeneous moderate	Irregular	Middle clivus

Abbreviations: ↓, hypointense; ↑, hyperintense; ↔, isointense; B, brain; L, CSF; M, muscle.

Table 24.3 Preoperative preparation in petrous apex tumors

General evaluation	Routine preoperative examination for a major surgery Evaluation of comorbidities: heart, lung, kidneys, liver, diabetes, infection, and more History of thromboembolism, bleeding, and use of drugs
Specific evaluation	CT with 3D reconstruction MRI, MRA Angiography (embolization) Audiometry, BAER, facial and trigeminal nerve functional testing
Preoperative anesthetic care	Adequate venous access for blood transfusion Monitoring of invasive BP, CVP, O_2, CO_2 Monitoring of cranial nerves III, IV, VI, VII, VIII, IX, X, and XI (jugular foramen lesions) Careful head rotation, avoiding jugular vein and vertebral artery compression

of ICA and cavernous sinus, presence of facial nerve paralysis, quality of preoperative hearing, vestibular function, presence of infection, and experience level of the surgeon.[5,45] Skull morphology may also be a factor, for the distance between the external cortical table of the skull and the PA varies with skull types.[5] In selected cases the endoscopic endonasal approach offers advantages over transcranial approaches by avoiding risks to the facial nerve and hearing.

24.4 Translabyrinthine Approach

24.4.1 Indications

The main indications for this approach are PA cholesteatomas, facial nerve schwannomas, and malignant lesions involving the temporal bone and the PA.[46] This approach should be avoided in patients who have preserved preoperative hearing. Many authors use the translabyrinthine approach to resect vestibular schwannomas and labyrinthectomy in cases of intractable vertigo. We prefer the retrosigmoid approach for treatment of vestibular schwannomas.

24.4.2 Surgical Technique

In supine position with head turned toward the opposite side, a retroauricular skin incision is made 2 cm posterior to the postauricular sulcus. The mastoid cortex is exposed after periosteal incisions and an extended mastoidectomy with removal of bone over the sigmoid sinus and the middle cranial fossa is performed (▶ Fig. 24.13).

Removal of bone over the sigmoid sinus must be done carefully. The middle fossa dura is dissected, the antrum is opened, and the lateral semicircular canal is identified. The short process of the incus and the semicircular canal are landmarks for the horizontal segment of the facial nerve. After identification of facial nerve a complete labyrinthectomy is performed. If infection is present (PA cholesteatoma with secondary infection), marsupialization of the cavity and a wide meatoplasty using a skin flap are carried out to allow postoperative care of the cavity. Management of the facial nerve depends on the preoperative facial nerve function, presence of infection, and whether the proximal and distal stumps of the nerve can be identified. If the facial nerve is involved by the tumor but not infiltrated and its function is normal, the nerve is dissected from the lesion, preserving the perineural tissues (neurolysis). If the nerve is infiltrated by the tumor and there is infection, reconstruction of cranial nerve VII should be postponed. If there is no infection, the affected portion of the nerve is resected and an end-to-end reconstruction or interposition nerve graft (sural nerve or great auricular nerve) is performed. When identification of the proximal stump of the facial nerve is possible only at the brainstem,

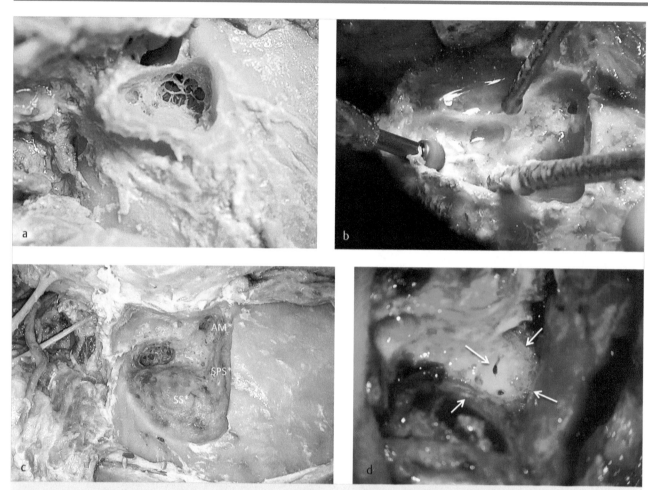

Fig. 24.13 **(a)** Anatomical specimen showing mastoidectomy with exposure of the mastoid antrum. **(b)** Surgical specimen. **(c)** Anatomical specimen. AM, mastoid antrum; SPS, superior petrous sinus; SS, sigmoid sinus. **(d)** Labyrinthine block and semicircular canals (*arrows*).

a sural graft is sutured with 10–0 nylon or glued with fibrin glue at the brainstem and at the stylomastoid foramen (▶ Fig. 24.14).

When direct reconstruction of the facial nerve by direct suture or grafting is not possible, a facial–hypoglossal anastomosis is carried out. In such cases we prefer to perform an end-to-side anastomosis to avoid atrophy of the tongue. In our experience the postoperative results with this technique are similar to an end-to-end VII–XII anastomosis. After tumor removal and reconstruction of the facial nerve, the dural opening and the mastoid cavity are obliterated with fat tissue and fibrin glue to avoid CSF leak. The wound is closed using vascularized muscle–periosteal flaps.

24.5 Middle Fossa Approach

24.5.1 Indications

The most frequent pathologies treated by this approach are petroclival meningioma with its main portion in the middle fossa, facial and trigeminal schwannomas, small vestibular schwannomas, cholesteatomas, cholesterol granulomas, chondrosarcomas, teratomas, CSF fistulas, and facial nerve lesions at or medial to the geniculate ganglion. This approach exposes

the PA intradurally and extradurally and allows dissection of the second and third divisions of the trigeminal nerve, the gasserian ganglion, the petrosal portion of the ICA, and the meatal and petrosal portions of the facial nerve.[47] Both damage of the temporal lobe with excessive retraction and injury to the temporal lobe draining veins can be avoided by using adequate anesthetic and microsurgical techniques.

24.5.2 Surgical Technique

Under general anesthesia, and with head rotated to the opposite side, a semicircular or straight skin incision is cut, beginning at the tragus and extending anteriorly to the frontal region. A temporalis muscle fascia flap is dissected, exposing the temporalis muscle, the zygomatic arch, and the upper portion of the external auditory canal. The temporal muscle is cut and the bone of the temporal bone exposed. If exposure of the infratemporal fossa is needed, the temporal muscle is rotated down, the zygomatic arch is temporarily removed, and in some selected cases opening of the glenoid fossa or resection of the mandibular condyle is performed. A craniotomy flap is cut, exposing the basal portion of the temporal fossa from the middle portion of the zygomatic arch to the transverse sinus (▶ Fig. 24.15).

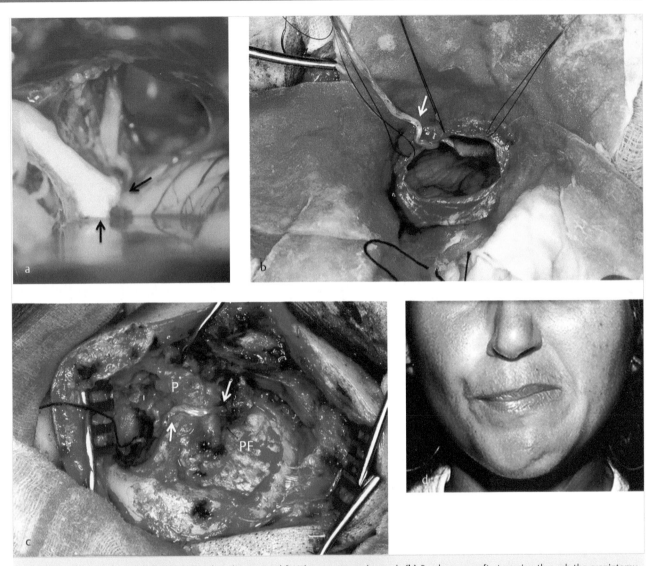

Fig. 24.14 (a) Sural nerve graft (SNG) sutured at the proximal facial nerve stump (*arrows*). **(b)** Sural nerve graft at passing through the craniotomy border (*arrow*). **(c)** Sural nerve anastomosed at the distal facial nerve stump (*arrow*). **(d)** House-Brackmann grade III 2 years after surgery.

Temporal lobe retraction is reduced by this basal approach, assisted by the infusion of mannitol and lumbar CSF drainage. The extradural approach to the PA is carried out by elevating the dura mater of the middle fossa so as to expose the middle meningeal artery, the greater superficial petrosal nerve, and the second and third divisions of the trigeminal nerve. The middle meningeal artery is coagulated and cut. The greater superficial petrosal nerve is carefully dissected from the dura up to its exit at the facial nerve hiatus. The arcuate eminence (superior semicircular canal) is identified. This extradural approach allows exposure of the PA, internal auditory canal, labyrinthine and tympanic portions of the facial nerve, and petrosal and horizontal portions of the ICA by drilling the bone medial to the Eustachian tube. To intradurally expose the PA region, the dura is incised parallel to the sylvian fissure. The temporal lobe is carefully retracted, avoiding damage to the draining veins—especially the vein of Labbé. The free border of the tentorium is dissected; the fourth cranial nerve is identified at the margin of the tentorium and the oculomotor nerve, medial to the troclear nerve. Splitting the tentorial border allows exposure of the posterior fossa and cranial nerves V, VI, VII, and VIII (▶ Fig. 24.16).

The posterior communicating artery and its branches, as well as the posterior cerebral and superior cerebellar arteries, are identified. All these anatomical structures may be displaced or embedded in the lesion and must be preserved. The posterior clinoid process and bone between the trigeminal nerve and the internal auditory meatus may be removed using a high-speed drill to enlarge the exposure of the middle line. In cases of petroclival meningiomas, perforating branches from the basilar artery may be embedded in the tumor so that complete removal may be impossible. After tumor removal, watertight dura closure is performed. All opened mastoid cells are closed using temporal muscle graft or wax. The temporalis fascial flap is rotated to cover the dural opening and the craniotomy flap is replaced.

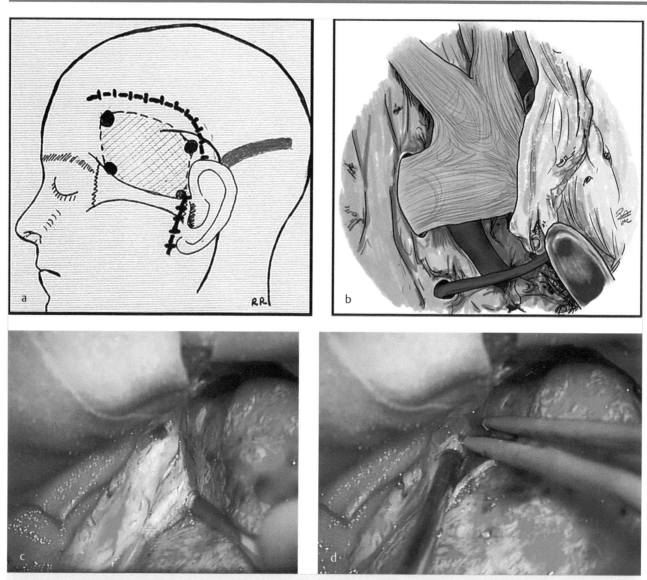

Fig. 24.15 (a) Drawing of middle fossa approach (skin incision 7 craniotomy). **(b)** Extradural middle fossa approach showing the trigeminal nerve and the middle meningeal and internal carotid arteries. **(c)** Surgical view of middle fossa extradural approach. **(d)** Coagulation of the middle meningeal artery.

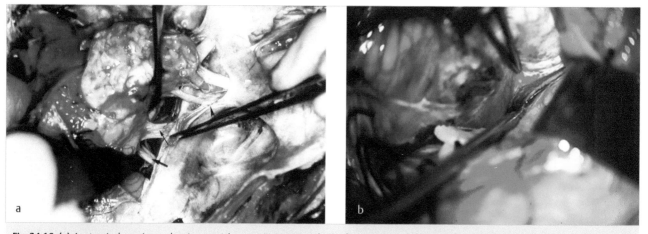

Fig. 24.16 (a) Anatomical specimen showing cranial nerves III, V, VII, and VIII after opening of the tentorium. **(b)** Tentorium border and cranial nerve IV.

24.6 Endoscopic Endonasal Approach

24.6.1 Indications

The endoscopic endonasal approach is indicated for midline and paramedian lesions extending or invading the sphenoid sinus lying medial to the ICA.[48] Cholesterol granulomas, cholesteatomas, chordomas, and chondrosarcomas are the most common lesions treated by this approach (▶ Fig. 24.17). The advantages of this route are avoidance of a lateral temporal craniotomy, unlikeliness of facial weakness (temporary or permanent) and hearing–vestibular loss, and shorter hospitalization.

24.6.2 Surgical Technique

Zanation et al described the endoscopic approaches to the PA as medial approach, medial approach with ICA lateralization, and transpterygoid infrapetrous approach according to the relationship of the lesion to the ICA (medial or inferior), degree of medial expansion, and pathology.[49] The head is fixed in a Mayfield skull clamp and the nasal cavity is prepared by injection with epinephrine. A nasoseptal flap is elevated when CSF leak is anticipated. The middle turbinate and the posterior nasal septum are removed using a 0° endoscope. The sphenoid ostium is identified and the anterior sphenoid sinus wall removed. A wide bilateral sphenoidotomy allows four-hands surgery. After removal of the sphenoid sinus septations, both carotid and optic protuberances are visualized (▶ Fig. 24.18).

The ICA may be surrounded by the lesion, and a micro-Doppler probe is used to identify this vessel. Lesions extending to the sphenoid sinus are approached by drilling the bone medial to the ICA with diamond burs. A larger medial window is obtained by additional bone removal and decompression and lateral displacement of the ICA. For more lateral lesions, a transpterygoid infrapetrous approach may be required. Following

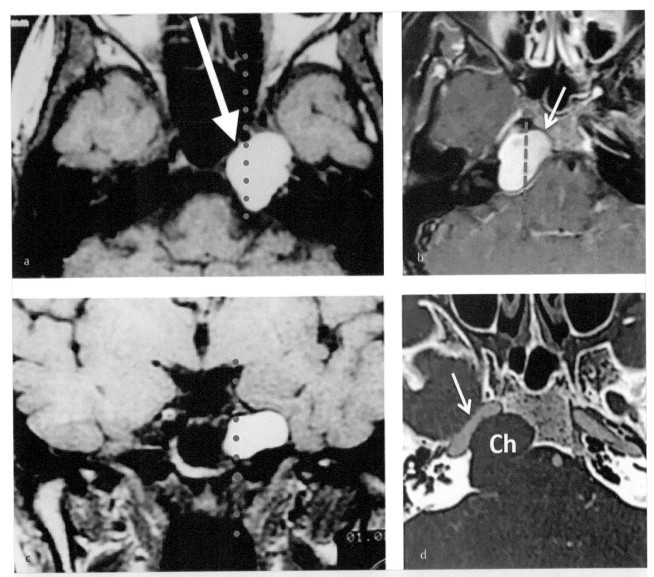

Fig. 24.17 (a–c) MRIs show cholesterol cysts with extension medial to the internal carotid artery (*arrow*). (d) CT scan of a cholesterol cyst (Ch) medial to the internal carotid artery (*arrow*).

the vidian canal, by drilling the bone between the horizontal segment of the petrous ICA and the Eustachian tube, medial to the third division of the trigeminal nerve, the PA is exposed (▶ Fig. 24.19).

In cases of cholesterol granuloma, complete removal of the cyst wall versus only marsupialization, with or without placement of a stent, remains a matter of controversy, and recurrences may occur irrespective of the approach used.[50,51,52,53] After draining the cholesterol granuloma, we avoid stenosis or closure of the stoma by rotation of a vascularized mucosal flap into the cavity.[54,55] In our experience this pedicle vascularized flap maintains the drainage to the sphenoid sinus, reducing risk of recurrence (▶ Fig. 24.20).

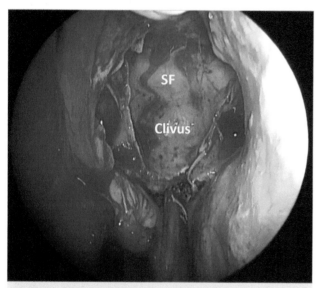

Fig. 24.18 Endoscopic view of the sella floor (SF) and clivus.

24.7 Retrosigmoid Approach

24.7.1 Indications

This approach is used to remove vestibular schwannomas, meningiomas of the cerebellopontine angle, and petroclival meningiomas with the main portion beneath the tentorium, trigeminal schwannomas, and epidermoid cysts (▶ Fig. 24.21).[56] It permits a wide exposition of the posterior fossa structures and the tentorial margin.

24.7.2 Surgical Technique

The patient may be placed in supine decubitus "mastoid position" (our preference), semisitting position, or "park-bench position" (▶ Fig. 24.22). The supine position makes air embolism, arterial hypotension, and postoperative venous bleeding unlikely and is more comfortable for the surgeon during more prolonged surgeries. The head is rotated about 30° to the opposite side, with light lateral extension. A pillow is placed under the ipsilateral shoulder to avoid excessive rotation of the head and compression of vertebral artery at the craniocervical junction (▶ Fig. 24.22).

The opposite internal jugular vein (IJV) must be checked to ensure that it is not compressed. Neurophysiological monitoring of cranial nerves V, VI, VII, VIII, IX, X, XI, and XII is performed. A retroauricular skin incision (straight or slightly curved) starts in the retromastoid region about 5 cm behind the external auditory canal and extends 2 cm behind the mastoid tip, ending in the upper neck. Fascia and muscles are cut straight down, exposing the occipital bone, the asterium, and the retromastoid region, and are held with a self-retaining retractor. A small bur hole is drilled in the asterium region, identifying the junction of the transverse and sigmoid sinuses. A 5-cm diameter craniotomy is cut (▶ Fig. 24.23).

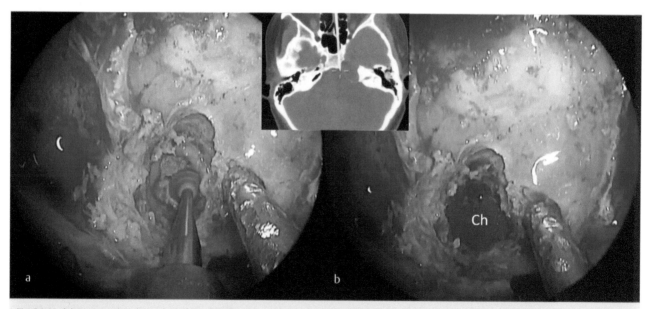

Fig. 24.19 (a) Transnasal endoscopic drilling of the petrous apex. **(b)** Drainage of a petrous apex cholesterol granuloma (Ch).

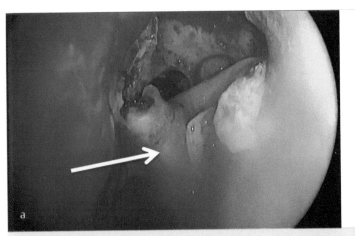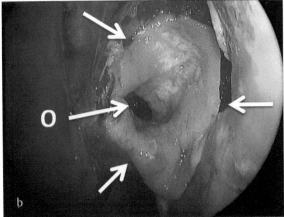

Fig. 24.20 **(a)** Nasoseptal flap being rotated inside the petrous apex cavity (*arrow*). **(b)** Final aspect of the nasoseptal flap and the ostium (O) of the petrous apex cavity.

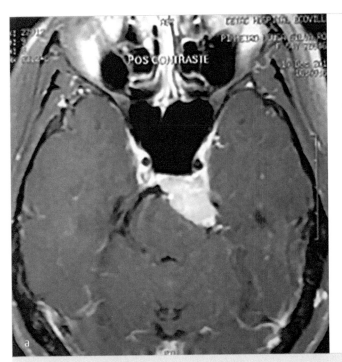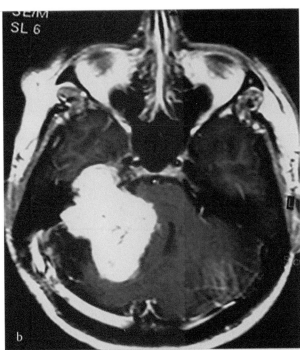

Fig. 24.21 **(a)** Petrous apex meningioma. **(b)** Large trigeminal schwannoma in the posterior fossa.

Its superior limit is the transverse sinus, and the anterior limit is the sigmoid sinus. The mastoid emissary vein is coagulated and cut. Jugular vein compression in the neck or use of the Valsalva maneuver helps identify venous bleeding. Small sigmoid sinus lacerations are repaired using either sutures or small pieces of muscle, fascia, and fibrin glue. Care should be taken to avoid occluding the sinus, including by packing lacerations with hemostatic material or muscle. The opened mastoid cells are packed with bone wax or muscle pieces and fibrin glue to avoid postoperative CSF fistula. Under the surgical microscope the dura mater is incised parallel to the sigmoid and transverse sinuses. The cerebellomedullary cistern is opened, exposing the lower cranial nerves; the facial, cochlear and trigeminal nerves; and the tentorium (▶ Fig. 24.24).

In cases of petroclival meningiomas, these nerves are dislocated posteriorly. Intracapsular tumor removal facilitates dissection of the cranial nerves from the tumor capsule. Tumor removal exposes the prepontine region and the PA. Infiltrated dura mater and bone are removed to avoid recurrence. Opening of the tentorium and removal of the supra-meatal tubercle allows a better approach to the middle fossa (▶ Fig. 24.25).

The use of the endoscope is helpful to dissect the tumor from cranial nerves. After tumor removal, watertight continuous suture of dura mater is performed. The bone flap is replaced and fixed with miniplates, or cranioplasty with methyl methacrylate is performed. The wound is sutured in the usual fashion, and no drain is used.

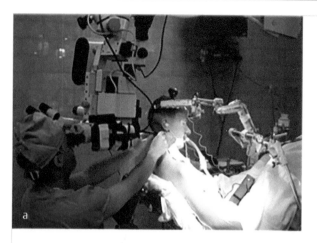
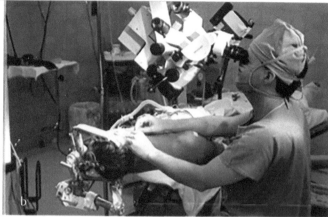
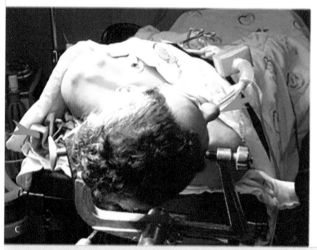
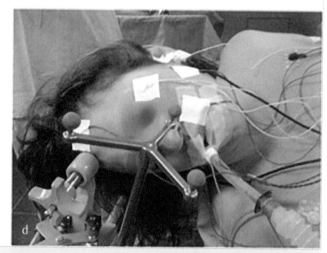

Fig. 24.22 Retrosigmoid approach. **(a)** Semisitting position. **(b)** Supine ("mastoid") position. **(c)** Supine position: rotation of the head (*arrow*) and pillow under the shoulder (*arrowhead*). **(d)** Intraoperative monitoring of cranial nerves.

24.8 Presigmoid (Retrolabyrinthine) Approach

24.8.1 Indications

The presigmoid approach allows wide exposure of the middle fossa, posterior fossa (up to the internal auditory canal), and clivus. It is used for tumors that have extension into the middle and posterior fossae (e.g., large petroclival meningiomas and trigeminal schwannomas).[57] Removal of the semicircular canals or labyrinth is not performed if the patient has good preoperative hearing.

24.8.2 Surgical Technique

Surgery is performed with the patient in supine decubitus and the head rotated to the opposite side. A semicircular skin incision from the temporal region—4 cm above the zygomatic arch, passing 3 cm behind the ear, extending 2 cm behind the mastoid tip—is performed (▶ Fig. 24.26).

The skin and subcutaneous flap is folded anteriorly, exposing the temporalis muscle and the craniocervical fasciae. To avoid postoperative CSF leak, a skull base reconstruction technique using fascia/muscle flaps was developed. The temporalis muscle fascia is cut and dissected with the mastoid periosteum, the craniocervical fascia, and the sternocleidomastoid muscle (SCM) that is detached from its insertion. These structures form a large vascularized muscle/fascia flap that is rotated back at the end of surgery to cover the entire surgical field. The temporal muscle is dissected in an anterior direction and is used to cover the dura mater as a vascularized muscle flap at the end of the surgery. The cortical bone of the mastoid is drilled exposing the antrum, tegmen mastoid, and sinus plate. The labyrinthine block and the facial nerve canal are identified. These canals are not opened. Two bur holes above the sigmoid sinus and two below are placed, and a craniotomy exposing the middle fossa and the posterior fossa (retrosigmoid) is cut (▶ Fig. 24.27). The superior petrosal, the sigmoid, and the transverse sinuses are identified. The retrofacial mastoid cells down to the jugular bulb are removed. The dura mater anterior to the sigmoid sinus is exposed. The zygomatic and supra labyrinthine cells are removed, maintaining the semicircular canals and middle ear intact. The superior petrosal sinus is coagulated and ligated between two stitches. The dura mater is incised parallel to the middle fossa floor and in front of the sigmoid sinus (▶ Fig. 24.27).

The superior petrosal sinus is ligated and sectioned and the tentorium is opened, exposing the PA region. The tentorium is

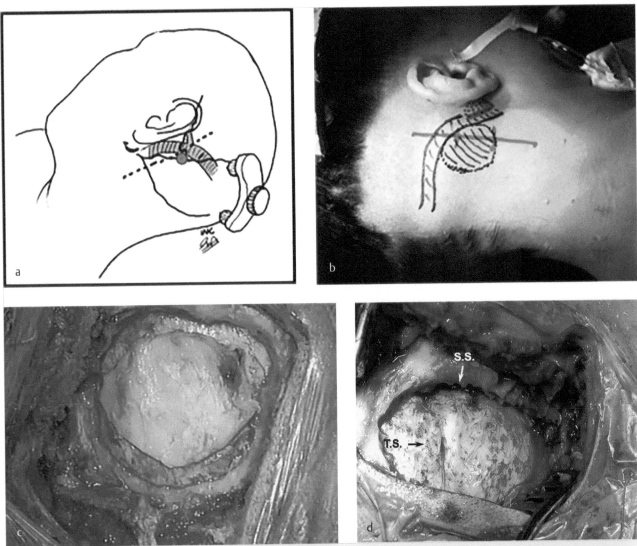

Fig. 24.23 **(a, b)** Retrosigmoid approach: skin incision. **(c)** Craniotomy flap. **(d)** Sigmoid (SS) and transverse sinus (TS) are the limits of craniotomy.

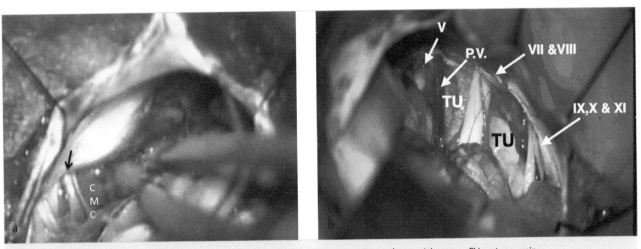

Fig. 24.24 **(a)** Cerebellopontine angle cistern (CMC) opening. **(b)** Tumor (TU) anterior to the cranial nerves. PV, petrous vein.

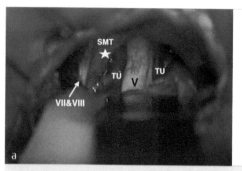
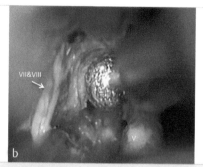
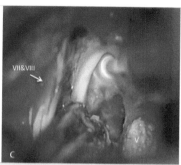

Fig. 24.25 (a) Petrous apex meningioma (TU). (b, c) Drilling of the suprameatal tubercle. SMT, suprameatal tubercle.

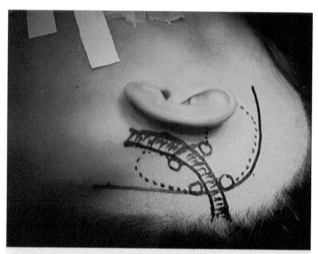

Fig. 24.26 Presigmoid approach: skin incision and planned craniotomy.

severed initially perpendicular to the superior petrosal sinus for a distance of 2 or 3 cm and then medially, parallel to the transverse sinus, for an additional 3 cm. The tentorial incision is continued up to the incisura, where cranial nerve IV is exposed and preserved. This maneuver allows a wide exposure of the cerebellum, separating it from the posterior aspect of temporal lobe like "opening a book" (▶ Fig. 24.28).

Care should be taken to preserve the vein of Labbé, which has a variable anatomy and usually enters the transverse sinus 10 mm before its junction with the sigmoid sinus. Temporal lobe retraction is minimal to avoid postoperative temporal lobe edema. Cranial nerves V, VII, and VIII are identified in the posterior fossa. In meningiomas, the devascularization of feeding vessels is performed before intracapsular tumor removal is started. After reduction of the size of the lesion, the tumor capsule is dissected from cranial nerves, vessels, and the brainstem. Some meningiomas invade the pia mater, and total removal may result in damage to the brainstem. In such cases, a small portion of the capsule is not removed. The infiltrated dura

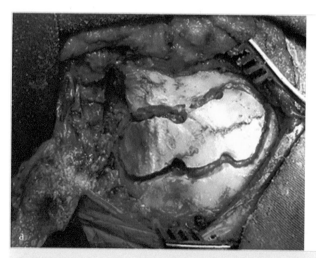
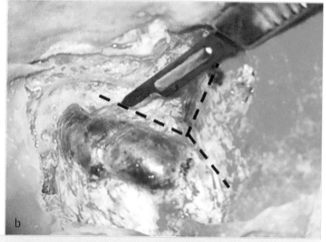

Fig. 24.27 (a) Presigmoid craniotomy: two bur holes above the sinuses and two below. (b) Opening of the dura.

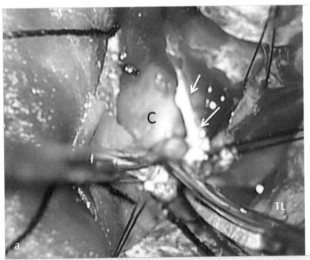
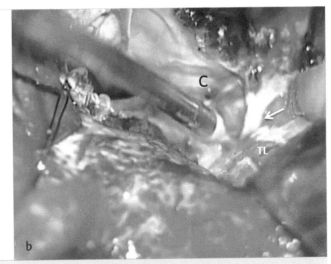

Fig. 24.28 (a) Initial opening of tentorium (*arrows*). (b) Tentorium opening to expose the incisura. C, cerebellum; TL, temporal lobe.

mater and bone should be resected. After tumor removal, the dura mater is closed in a watertight fashion or with fascia graft and fibrin glue. The aditus and antrum are closed using muscle plugs, and the temporalis muscle flap is rotated to cover the entire exposed dura mater. All opened mastoid cells and pneumatized bone are covered with muscle graft and fibrin glue. The fascia–muscle flap (temporalis, cranial–cervical fasciae, and SCM) is sutured in its original position and the skin is closed.

24.9 Craniocervical Approach

24.9.1 Indications

This approach is mainly used for resection of jugular foramen tumors with extension to the PA and cervical region (e.g., paragangliomas, schwannomas, meningiomas).[45,58,59,60,61]

24.9.2 Surgical Technique

Intermittent compression of the lower limbs to prevent deep vein thrombosis is used for patients who are at risk of this complication. A nasoenteral tube is inserted. The patient is placed in supine position with the head fixed in a cranial clamp (Mayfield), slightly extended and rotated 30 to 45° to the contralateral side. The ipsilateral shoulder is elevated, and the opposite IJV must be free (▶ Fig. 24.29).

All body contact areas must be checked due to the long duration of the surgery. Electrophysiological monitoring of cranial nerves V, VI, VII, VIII, IX, X, XI, and XII, as well as bilateral somatosensory evoked responses (SAEPs), are performed depending on the extension of the tumor. All parameters for neuronavigation are checked. A C-shaped skin incision starts in the temporal region, about 5 cm superior to the zygomatic arch, circumscribes the ear and the mandibular angle, and continues in a cervical fold over the border of the SCM, reaching the midline (▶ Fig. 24.30).

The great auricular nerve is identified and dissected. This nerve may be used as a graft for reconstruction of the facial

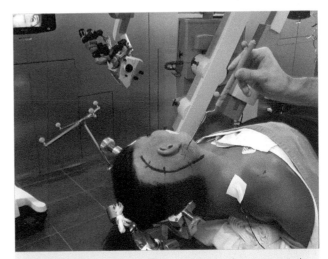

Fig. 24.29 Patient's position and skin incision for the craniocervical approach.

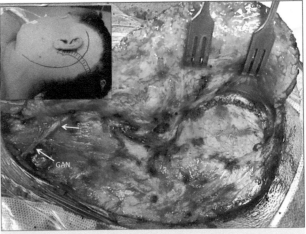

Fig. 24.30 Craniocervical approach: rotation of skin flap exposing the great auricular nerve (GAN).

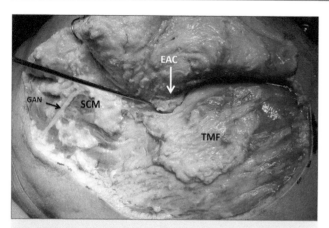

Fig. 24.31 Anatomical specimen showing the external auditory canal (EAC), temporal muscle fascia (TMF), sternocleidomastoid muscle (SCM), and great auricular nerve (GAN).

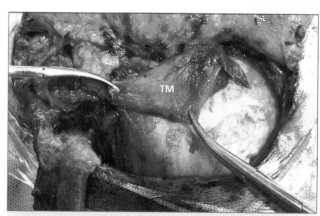

Fig. 24.32 Skull base reconstruction: the temporal muscle (TM) is rotated over the surgical defect.

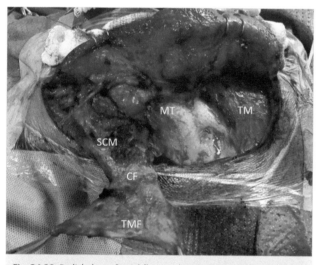

Fig. 24.33 Pedicled myofascial flap used to reconstruct the skull base. CF, cervical fascia; MT, mastoid tip; SCM, sternocleidomastoid muscle; TM, temporal muscle; TMF, temporal muscle fascia.

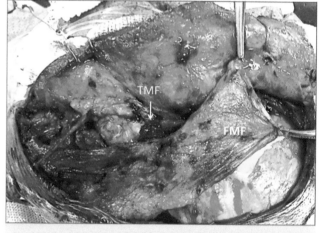

Fig. 24.34 Final aspect of skull base reconstruction technique using the temporal muscle (TM) and the fascia–muscle flap (FMF).

nerve when cranial nerve VII is infiltrated by the tumor and must be resected. The skin flap is rotated anteriorly, exposing the temporal muscle fascia, the external auditory canal, the mastoid tip, and the anterior border of the SCM muscle. If the tumor invades the middle ear, destroying the ossicular chain extending to the external auditory canal, the canal is cut at the osseocartilaginous junction (▶ Fig. 24.31).

To avoid postoperative CSF leak, the external auditory meatus is sutured in two layers. A special surgical technique of skull base reconstruction using vascularized flaps was developed.[61] This technique reconstructs the surgical defect in three layers, reduces CSF leak, and promotes a very good cosmetic result. The first reconstruction layer is a watertight dura closure. If the dura mater is infiltrated by the tumor and was removed, a temporalis muscle fascia graft and fibrin glue are used to cover the defect. The second reconstruction layer is formed by the posterior third of the temporalis muscle, which is rotated down to cover the dura and the mastoid cavity while remaining attached to its insertion (▶ Fig. 24.32).

We avoid the use of abdominal fat grafts, because they require an abdominal skin incision and may thus increase the risk of infection. The third reconstruction layer is formed by the temporalis muscle fascia, the cervical fasciae, and the SCM. The temporalis muscle fascia is elevated and dissected with the cervical fascia that is incised close to the external auditory canal and mastoid tip and over the SCM (▶ Fig. 24.33).

These fasciae remain attached to the SCM, which is dissected in the neck and removed from its insertion at the mastoid. At the end of surgery, this large vascularized muscle–fasciae flap will be rotated back, over the temporalis muscle flap (▶ Fig. 24.34). The contour of the SCM is preserved, and the cosmetic results are excellent (▶ Fig. 24.35).

After these flaps are prepared, the next surgical step is neck dissection. The greater auricular nerve is dissected and the external jugular vein and common facial vein are ligated with suture/ligature and cut. The digastric muscle, a key landmark for neck dissection, is identified (▶ Fig. 24.36).

The facial nerve runs at its superior border and the hypoglossal nerve at its posteroinferior border. The posterior belly of the digastric muscle, the superior belly of the omohyoid muscle,

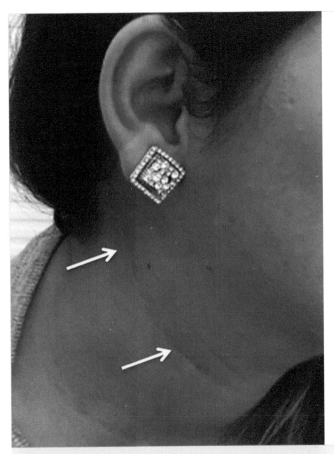
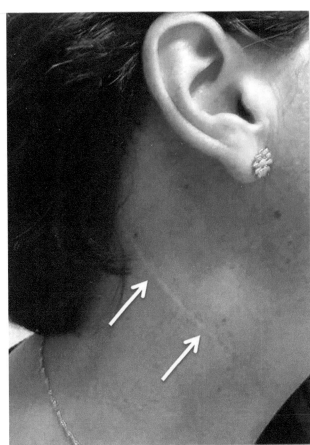

Fig. 24.35 Cosmetic results using the skull base reconstruction technique. *Arrows*, skin incision.

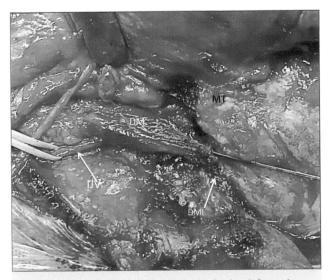

Fig. 24.36 The digastric muscle (DM) is a key landmark for neck dissection. DMI, digastric muscle incisure in the mastoid; IJV, internal jugular vein.

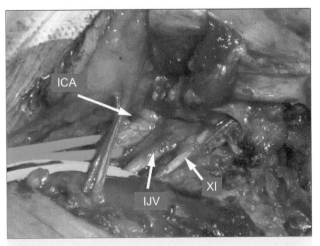

Fig. 24.37 Neck dissection. ICA, internal carotid artery; IJV, internal jugular vein; XI, accessory nerve.

and the anterior margin of the SCM delimit the carotid triangle. This triangle contains the carotid sheath, the IJV, and deep cervical lymph nodes. The major vessels of the neck (common CA, ICA, external CA and its branches, and IJV) are identified (▶ Fig. 24.37).

The digastric muscle is removed from its insertion in the mastoid groove and rotated down. Cranial nerve XII passes to the submandibular region, where the ansa cervicalis is identified and reaches the tongue. This nerve crosses the external carotid artery. The vagal nerve and the sympathetic trunk are lateral and inferior to the common carotid artery. The occipital artery is coagulated and cut. The transverse process of the C1

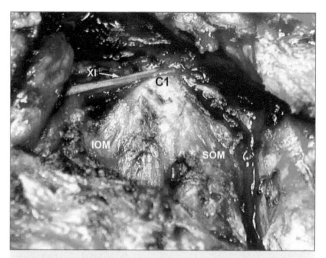

Fig. 24.38 The transverse process of C1 (C1) and the superior (SOM) and inferior (IOM) obliquus capitis muscles are landmarks for dissection of the vertebral artery.

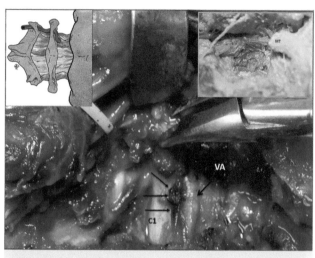

Fig. 24.39 The vertebral artery is identified (VA) and may be removed from the transverse foramen of C1.

vertebra is identified; cranial nerve XI runs inferior to the transverse process of C1, in most cases lateral to the IJV, entering the SCM. The transverse process of C1 is a "key point" to dissect the accessory nerve and the vertebral artery (▶ Fig. 24.38).

The superior and inferior capitis oblique muscle's insertion at the transverse process of C1 is cut and the groove of the vertebral artery in the C1 lamina is identified. The transverse process of C1 is removed using a rongeur. The vertebral artery may be removed from the transverse foramen and rotated posteriorly (▶ Fig. 24.39).

This maneuver associated with removal of the transverse process of C1 vertebra enlarges the approach to the jugular foramen. The glossopharyngeal nerve leaves the cranium through the jugular foramen and runs down anterolateral to the ICA. The IJV is dissected up to the jugular foramen. The ICA is also dissected upward to the skull base. Very often tumor is compressing or involving this vessel. Careful dissection under the operation microscope is recommended. If vasospasm occurs as a result of the dissection, cotton soaked with papaverine is placed around the ICA. The facial nerve is identified at its exit from the stylomastoid foramen. The following anatomical landmarks are helpful for dissecting cranial nerve VII: the mastoid tip, the posterior belly of the digastric muscle, the "tragal pointer," and the tympanomastoid suture (▶ Fig. 24.40).[14,19,38]

If the nerve is not infiltrated by the tumor, then it remains in the fallopian canal. Rerouting of the nerve is avoided, because most patients develop temporarily facial paresis. After transposition of the facial nerve in 18 patients, 10 (56%) developed facial paralysis (House-Brackmann grade V or VI) as assessed 1 month after surgery. At 1 year after surgery, six patients recovered to a grade of III or IV weakness (60%).[62] If the nerve is infiltrated (most commonly infiltration occurs with paragangliomas and meningiomas), the nerve is resected and grafted with the greater auricular nerve or a sural nerve graft. Radical mastoidectomy and antrostomy are performed exposing the mastoid antrum, ossicular chain, sigmoid sinus, superior petrosal sinus, the labyrinth, and the sinodural angle. The lateral semicircular canal and the short process of the incus are anatomical land-

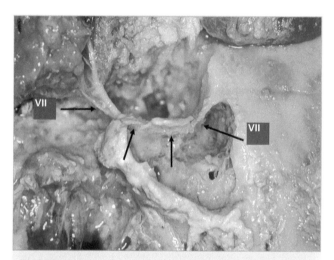

Fig. 24.40 Anatomical specimen showing the course of the facial nerve (cranial nerve VII) at the stylomastoid foramen and mastoid.

marks for identifying the facial nerve. In the mastoid the facial nerve is exposed by drilling the bone over and parallel to the nerve using a diamond bur larger than its diameter. A fine curette is used to remove small bone fragments close to the nerve. The retrofacial mastoid cells are removed. The sigmoid sinus and the jugular bulb are completely skeletonized. The posterior and anterior walls of the external auditory meatus are drilled when the tumor extends to the ear canal. Jugular foramen paragangliomas usually invade the middle and external ear through the hypotympanum. Tumor extensions within the ear, Eustachian tube, and mastoid cells are resected after removal of the tympanic membrane. The ICA travels through the temporal bone. It is anterior to the jugular foramen and medial to the Eustachian tube. The ICA can be dissected by removal of the tympanic bone (distal control of the ICA; ▶ Fig. 24.41).

The carotid–tympanic branches of the ICA are feeding vessels to paragangliomas and meningiomas. A bur hole is placed behind the sigmoid sinus and a craniectomy 3 cm in diameter is performed (▶ Fig. 24.42).

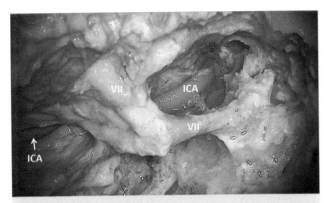

Fig. 24.41 Anatomical specimen. Internal carotid artery (ICA) in the neck and in the ear, after removal of the tympanic membrane and tympanic bone. VII, facial nerve.

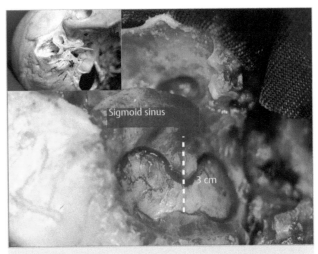

Fig. 24.42 Craniectomy exposing the sigmoid sinus and jugular foramen.

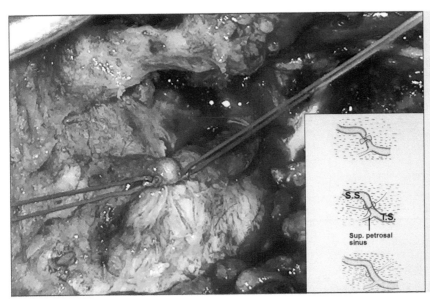

Fig. 24.43 Sigmoid sinus ligation below the exit of the superior petrosal sinus.

The retrosigmoid dura mater is exposed and the emissary mastoid vein is coagulated; the bone over the sigmoid sinus is removed using diamond bur and curettes, and the sinus is followed down to the jugular bulb. A diamond bur is used to remove bone at the mastoid tip, behind the facial nerve. The posterior portion of the jugular fossa is widely opened using Kerrison rongeurs, communicating the jugular bulb with the IJV. The dura mater anterior to the sigmoid sinus is dissected. If the jugular bulb is occluded by the tumor (mainly in paragangliomas and meningioma cases), the sigmoid sinus is ligated. Small dural openings in front and behind the sigmoid sinus, below the superior petrous sinus, are made, and the IJV is double-ligated using two nonabsorbable sutures and is cut (▶ Fig. 24.43).[61] The posterior wall of the sigmoid sinus is incised, exposing the tumor within the sinus and jugular bulb. Removal of the portion of the lesion inside the jugular vein is accomplished with the ligation of the IJV. Bleeding from the inferior petrous sinus (within the jugular bulb) is controlled using Surgicel or Gelfoam. The caudal cranial nerves are located anterior to the venous lumen, and there is a thin membrane between these two structures.

Some tumors may have anterior extensions to the hypoglossal canal and following the ICA. In such cases the ICA is dissected from the ear until its entrance at skull base. If the carotid wall is infiltrated by the tumor, the following strategies are employed:

- If the patient tolerates a balloon occlusion test, the ICA may be sacrificed.
- If the patient does not tolerate the balloon occlusion test:
  a) In elderly patients, radical resection of the lesion is not possible for malignant tumors. Tumors around the ICA are left behind and postoperative radiotherapy or radiosurgery is indicated.
  b) In young patients, benign tumor and total removal are possible. A high-flow bypass between the external or internal carotid artery and the middle cerebral artery is performed. Patency of the bypass is checked and the ICA is ligated below the posterior communicating artery and in the neck. The infiltrated vessel is removed with the tumor.

c) Alternatively, the insertion of a covered stent may be used. The patient is placed under aspirin for 3 months until reepithelialization inside the stent occurs. After this time the tumor can be dissected from the carotid wall with protection of the stent.

After removal of the extradural portion of the tumor, the dura mater is opened. The cerebellomedullary cistern is drained, and minimal retraction of the cerebellum is needed to expose the intradural posterior fossa structures. Tumor within the jugular foramen around the lower cranial nerves is identified. Cranial nerves VII and VIII, the vertebral artery, the posterior inferior cerebral artery (PICA), and brainstem are exposed. When the intradural tumor extension is small, the lower cranial nerves are easily identified at the brainstem and preserved. Intra- and extradural dissection of these nerves from tumor capsule, under electrophysiological monitoring, is important to preserve the caudal cranial nerves anatomically and functionally. Some fascicles may be infiltrated or embedded by benign tumors such as paragangliomas and meningiomas.[12,13] If fascicles of cranial nerves IX and X are infiltrated and the patient has no deficits from these nerves, subtotal removal is preferred. Total removal will only be attempted if there are preoperative lower cranial nerve deficits. Identification of the lower cranial nerves is difficult in cases of large intradural extensions, because these structures are embedded in the lesion. Bipolar coagulation of the tumor capsule and intracapsular tumor removal under monitoring of the cranial nerves will allow identification of the nerves, first at brainstem and then at the jugular foramen. Dissection of tumor capsule is easier with schwannomas than with paragangliomas and meningiomas. Closure of the wound is performed using the reconstruction technique already described. Postoperative lumbar drainage is used only in cases involving very large skull base and dural defects that could not be closed in a watertight fashion.

24.10 Temporal Bone Resection

24.10.1 Indications

This surgical procedure is indicated when a tumor involving the petrous bone can be totally resected based on preoperative radiological studies. For benign tumors this surgery may be curative.[38] For low-grade malignancies, surgery followed by radiation therapy is indicated. High-grade tumors are usually treated using adjuvant therapy, and surgical indication depends on extension of the lesion. In our institution, high-grade malignancies with tumor spread into the cavernous sinus, infratemporal fossa, and upper cervical soft tissue and medial to the petrous ICA are not surgically treated because of the expected failure of this treatment modality and postoperative morbidity.

24.10.2 Surgical Technique

A **C**-shaped incision starting from the frontotemporal region to the neck is performed. Tumors infiltrating the skin or the presence of infection may need a modified incision (▶ Fig. 24.44).

The external auditory canal is transected at its osteocartilaginous junction, sutured, and covered with a fascia flap to prevent CSF leak. The vessels (carotid artery and jugular vein) and cranial nerves are exposed in the neck. The facial nerve is dissected at the stylomastoid foramen. The temporal muscle is elevated from the middle fossa and a craniotomy is performed. The zygomatic arch, the squamous portion of the temporal bone, the condyle, and the neck of the mandible are cut with a drill. A mastoidectomy with skeletonization of the sigmoid and transverse sinuses is carried out. A suboccipital craniotomy is performed. Extradural dissection of the temporal fossa exposes the greater superficial petrosal nerve and middle meningeal artery, which is coagulated and cut. The third division of the trigeminal nerve is identified and the petrous carotid unroofed with

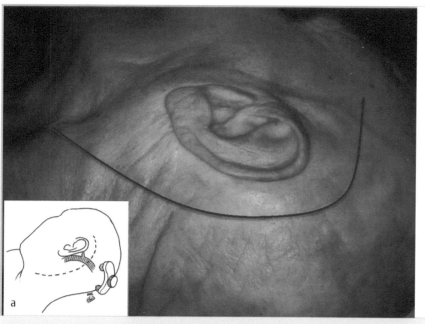
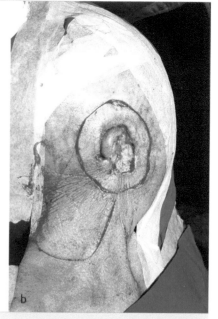

Fig. 24.44 (a) Skin incisions for temporal bone resection. (b) Tumor infiltration in the ear and skin.

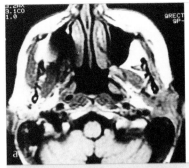
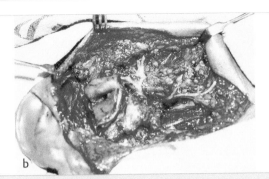
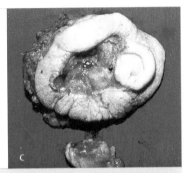

Fig. 24.45 **(a)** MRI showing squamous cell carcinoma with petrous apex infiltration. **(b,c)** Temporal bone dissection: en bloc resection of infiltrative squamous cell carcinoma.

diamond burs. The opened Eustachian tube is packed with pieces of temporal muscle to avoid CSF fistula. If the sigmoid sinus is infiltrated, then it is ligated with a double ligature and divided. The IJV is ligated and transected. The PA and bone in clivus region are removed with a drill. The dura is incised in the middle fossa across Meckel's cave, superior petrosal sinus, tentorium, and posterior fossa behind the sigmoid sinus. The facial and vestibulocochlear nerves are transected at the internal auditory canal and the dura medial to these nerves is incised. Malignant tumors are resected en bloc (▶ Fig. 24.45).

Careful bipolar coagulation and Surgicel are used for hemostasis. Reconstruction of the facial nerve is performed using a sural nerve graft. The dural defect is closed using pericranium or bovine pericardium flap and fibrin glue. The temporalis muscle is rotated to cover the surgical field and sutured to the SCM. Large defects are closed with rotation of trapezius or pectoralis rotation flap. Tarsorrhaphy is done to protect the eye and a lumbar CSF drain is inserted to reduce risk of CSF leak. Excessive CSF drainage should be avoided.

24.10.3 Postoperative Care

Patients are monitored in an intensive care unit (ICU) setting, as for all major intracranial surgeries. Usually patients do not complain of postoperative pain and regular analgesics or diclofenac are sufficient. Additional analgesia can be achieved by morphine infusion. Nausea and vomiting are controlled with ondansetron. Intravenous access is maintained for drug and fluid replacement. In cases of large jugular foramen tumors, patients remain intubated in the ICU until adequate evaluation of the lower cranial nerves is feasible with strict blood pressure control. The function of these nerves should be carefully evaluated before extubation and continued for some days after surgery. Postoperative dysfunction of cranial nerves IX and X causing dysphagia with bronchial aspiration and pneumonia may be a severe or even fatal complication. Patients who have involvement of these nerves should be extubated only when they are awake and after careful evaluation of the function of the caudal cranial nerves. The nasoenteral tube for feeding is kept in place and eventually a percutaneous endoscopic gastrostomy must be performed.

Tracheostomy and gastrostomy are performed without any delay in patients who have severe dysphasia and vocal cord palsy. In moderate cases of caudal cranial nerve dysfunction,

grade of reflux is evaluated using endoscopy and video fluoroscopy. These cases are usually managed using a nasoenteral tube and phonorehabilitation. Procedures for vocal cord medialization may be helpful when these measures fail. When a lumbar drain has been placed, the drain is maintained for 48 to 72 hours. The drain is clamped for 24 hours, after which it is removed if there is no CSF leak or swelling of the wound. Prophylactic antibiotics are continued for 24 hours. Thromboembolism prophylaxis is initiated early, especially in elderly patients. A CT scan examination is performed in the first 24 hours and a MRI before discharge from the hospital. Skin sutures are removed from the scalp after 8 days.

Functional evaluation of the cranial nerves is performed as soon as possible. Facial nerve palsy, especially when associated with palsy of the first trigeminal nerve division, requires care of the eye to avoid lesion to the cornea. When the facial nerve is sectioned, it is preferentially reconstructed using an end-to-end suture or a graft from the greater auricular nerve or from the sural nerve. An anastomosis between cranial nerves VII and XII is usually performed 2 weeks after surgery if a VII–VII reconstruction was not possible. A tarsorrhaphy is carried out as soon as possible in cases of complete facial nerve lesion.

24.10.4 Complications and Avoidance

CSF fistula is a common complication after intradural surgeries involving the mastoid and the temporal bone (▶ Table 24.4). The described myofascial vascularized flaps were developed in our department to close a large surgical defect while avoiding CSF fistula. The cosmetic results using this reconstruction technique are excellent. Postoperative infection may occur as a result of intraoperative contamination or preexisting ear and/or

Table 24.4 Cerebrospinal fluid fistula in temporal bone surgery

Fistula types	Prevention and management
Through mastoid cells	Prevention: Watertight dura mater closure. All opened pneumatized cells are closed with muscle graft, fibrin glue, and bone wax. Management: Lumbar drainage, acetazolamide for 3 days. In case of failure, reoperation.
Subcutaneous	Prevention: Watertight dura mater closure. Vascularized myofascial flap rotation. Management: Compressive dressing and lumbar drainage. In case of failure, reoperation.

mastoid infection. Careful otoscopy and endoscopic evaluation of mastoid cells and paranasal sinuses is mandatory to diagnose infection in these regions. Damage to the greater superficial petrosal nerve will produce "dry eye." The petrous portion of the ICA may be dehiscent, and careful drilling of the PA bone is needed to avoid damage to this vessel. Drilling the petrous bone may damage the arcuate eminence (superior semicircular canal), the geniculate ganglion, and the cochlea. Injury to cranial nerves within the jugular foramen may occur in tumors of the posterior portion of the temporal bone. Excessive temporal lobe retraction will produce venous compression—postoperative edema that may cause hemiplegia, aphasia, and even death.

This complication may be avoided by using a basal approach with drilling of the temporal bone, good anesthesia, and adequate microsurgical technique and, in some cases, lumbar drainage for brain relaxation. Identification and dissection of the vein of Labbé is very important to avoid venous infarction of the temporal lobe. Aspiration pneumonia resulting from palsy of the lower cranial nerves is one of the most dangerous complications in patients undergoing surgical resection of jugular foramen tumors.

References

[1] Curtin HD, Som PM. The petrous apex. Otolaryngol Clin North Am. 1995; 28 (3):473–496

[2] Larson TL. Petrous apex and cavernous sinus: anatomy and pathology. Semin Ultrasound CT MR. 1993; 14(3):232–246

[3] Virapongse C, Sarwar M, Bhimani S, Sasaki C, Shapiro R. Computed tomography of temporal bone pneumatization: 1. Normal pattern and morphology. AJR Am J Roentgenol. 1985; 145(3):473–481

[4] Moore KR, Harnsberger HR, Shelton C, Davidson HC. "Leave me alone" lesions of the petrous apex. AJNR Am J Neuroradiol. 1998; 19(4):733–738

[5] Meneses MS, Moreira AL, Bordignon KC, Pedrozo AA, Ramina R, Nikoski JG. Surgical approaches to the petrous apex: distances and relations with cranial morphology. Skull Base. 2004; 14(1):9–19, discussion 19–20

[6] Gudmundsson K, Rhoton AL, Jr, Rushton JG. Detailed anatomy of the intracranial portion of the trigeminal nerve. J Neurosurg. 1971; 35(5):592–600

[7] Kassam AB, Vescan AD, Carrau RL, et al. Expanded endonasal approach: vidian canal as a landmark to the petrous internal carotid artery. J Neurosurg. 2008; 108(1):177–183

[8] Pait TG, Harris FS, Paullus WS, Rhoton AL, Jr. Microsurgical anatomy and dissection of the temporal bone. Surg Neurol. 1977; 8(5):363–391

[9] Rhoton AL, Jr, Pulec JL, Hall GM, Boyd AS, Jr. Absence of bone over the geniculate ganglion. J Neurosurg. 1968; 28(1):48–53

[10] Schmalfuss IM. Petrous apex. Neuroimaging Clin N Am. 2009; 19(3):367–391

[11] Roland PS, Meyerhoff WL, Judge LO, Mickey BE. Asymmetric pneumatization of the petrous apex. Otolaryngol Head Neck Surg. 1990; 103(1):80–88

[12] Fournier HD, Mercier P, Velut S, Reigner B, Cronier P, Pillet J. Surgical anatomy and dissection of the petrous and peripetrous area. Anatomic basis of the lateral approaches to the skull base. Surg Radiol Anat. 1994; 16(2):143–148

[13] Chambers KJ, Lin DT, Meier J, Remenschneider A, Herr M, Gray ST. Incidence and survival patterns of cranial chordoma in the United States. Laryngoscope. 2014; 124(5):1097–1102

[14] Franklin DJ, Jenkins HA, Horowitz BL, Coker NJ. Management of petrous apex lesions. Arch Otolaryngol Head Neck Surg. 1989; 115(9):1121–1125

[15] Jackler RK, Parker DA. Radiographic differential diagnosis of petrous apex lesions. Am J Otol. 1992; 13(6):561–574

[16] Kveton JF, Brackmann DE, Glasscock ME, III, House WF, Hitselberger WE. Chondrosarcoma of the skull base. Otolaryngol Head Neck Surg. 1986; 94(1):23–32

[17] Muckle RP, De la Cruz A, Lo WM. Petrous apex lesions. Am J Otol. 1998; 19 (2):219–225

[18] Bloch OG, Jian BJ, Yang I, et al. A systematic review of intracranial chondrosarcoma and survival. J Clin Neurosci. 2009; 16(12):1547–1551

[19] George B, Bresson D, Herman P, Froelich S. Chordomas: A Review. Neurosurg Clin N Am. 2015; 26(3):437–452

[20] Kanamori H, Kitamura Y, Kimura T, Yoshida K, Sasaki H. Genetic characterization of skull base chondrosarcomas. J Neurosurg. 2015; 123(4):1036–1041

[21] Van Gompel JJ, Janus JR. Chordoma and chondrosarcoma. Otolaryngol Clin North Am. 2015; 48(3):501–514

[22] Glasscock ME, III, Woods CI, III, Poe DS, Patterson AK, Welling DB. Petrous apex cholesteatoma. Otolaryngol Clin North Am. 1989; 22(5):981–1002

[23] Koutourousiou M, Snyderman CH, Fernandez-Miranda J, Gardner PA. Skull base chordomas. Otolaryngol Clin North Am. 2011; 44(5):1155–1171

[24] Gulluoglu S, Turksoy O, Kuskucu A, Ture U, Bayrak OF. The molecular aspects of chordoma. Neurosurg Rev. 2016; 39(2):185–196, discussion 196

[25] Tzortzidis F, Elahi F, Wright D, Natarajan SK, Sekhar LN. Patient outcome at long-term follow-up after aggressive microsurgical resection of cranial base chordomas. Neurosurgery. 2006; 59(2):230–237, discussion 230–237

[26] McDonald MW, Linton OR, Moore MG, Ting JY, Cohen-Gadol AA, Shah MV. Influence of Residual Tumor Volume and Radiation Dose Coverage in Outcomes for Clival Chordoma. Int J Radiat Oncol Biol Phys. 2016; 95(1):304–311

[27] Schulz-Ertner D, Nikoghosyan A, Hof H, et al. Carbon ion radiotherapy of skull base chondrosarcomas. Int J Radiat Oncol Biol Phys. 2007; 67(1):171–177

[28] Uhl M, Mattke M, Welzel T, et al. High control rate in patients with chondrosarcoma of the skull base after carbon ion therapy: first report of long-term results. Cancer. 2014; 120(10):1579–1585

[29] Uhl M, Mattke M, Welzel T, et al. Highly effective treatment of skull base chordoma with carbon ion irradiation using a raster scan technique in 155 patients: first long-term results. Cancer. 2014; 120(21):3410–3417

[30] Mariniello G, Cappabianca P, Stella L, Del Basso De Caro ML, Buonamassa S, de Divitiis E. Chondroma of the petrous apex. Clin Neurol Neurosurg. 2003; 105 (2):135–139

[31] Sarwar M, Swischuk LE, Schecter MM. Intracranial chondromas. AJR Am J Roentgenol. 1976; 127(6):973–977

[32] Komisar A, Som PM, Shugar JM, Sacher M, Parisier SC. Benign chondroma of the petrous apex. J Comput Assist Tomogr. 1981; 5(1):116–118

[33] Fountas KN, Stamatiou S, Barbanis S, Kourtopoulos H. Intracranial falx chondroma: literature review and a case report. Clin Neurol Neurosurg. 2008; 110 (1):8–13

[34] Nakase H, Nagata K, Yonezawa T, Morimoto T, Sakaki T. Extensive parasellar chondroma with Ollier's disease. Acta Neurochir (Wien). 1998; 140(1):100–101

[35] Ramina R, Coelho Neto M, Meneses MS, Pedrozo AA. Maffucci's syndrome associated with a cranial base chondrosarcoma: case report and literature review. Neurosurgery. 1997; 41(1):269–272

[36] Ichimura S, Kawase T, Onozuka S, Yoshida K, Ohira T. Four subtypes of petroclival meningiomas: differences in symptoms and operative findings using the anterior transpetrosal approach. Acta Neurochir (Wien). 2008; 150(7):637–645

[37] Pollack IF, Sekhar LN, Jannetta PJ, Janecka IP. Neurilemomas of the trigeminal nerve. J Neurosurg. 1989; 70(5):737–745

[38] Ramina R, Mattei TA, Sória MG, et al. Surgical management of trigeminal schwannomas. Neurosurg Focus. 2008; 25(6):E6–, discussion E6

[39] Sanna M, Zini C, Gamoletti R, et al. Petrous bone cholesteatoma. Skull Base Surg. 1993; 3(4):201–213

[40] Goyal N, Liu J, Kanekar SG, Ghossaini S. Symptoms of Petrous Apex Lesions. J Neurol Surg B Skull Base. 2012; 73(S 01):A:292

[41] Struffert T, Grunwald IQ, Papanagiotou P, Politi M, Roth C, Reith W. [Imaging of the temporal bone. An overview]. Radiologe. 2005; 45(9):816–827

[42] Greess H, Baum U, Römer W, Tomandl B, Bautz W. [CT and MRI of the petrous bone]. HNO. 2002; 50(10):906–919

[43] Brown RV, Sage MR, Brophy BPCT. CT and MR findings in patients with chordomas of the petrous apex. AJNR Am J Neuroradiol. 1990; 11(1):121–124

[44] Razek AA, Huang BY. Lesions of the petrous apex: classification and findings at CT and MR imaging. Radiographics. 2012; 32(1):151–173

[45] Samii A, Gerganov V, Herold C, Gharabaghi A, Hayashi N, Samii M. Surgical treatment of skull base chondrosarcomas. Neurosurg Rev. 2009; 32(1):67–75, discussion 75

[46] Brackmann DE, Toh EH. Surgical management of petrous apex cholesterol granulomas. Otol Neurotol. 2002; 23(4):529–533

[47] Youssef S, Kim EY, Aziz KM, Hemida S, Keller JT, van Loveren HR. The subtemporal interdural approach to dumbbell-shaped trigeminal schwannomas: cadaveric prosection. Neurosurgery. 2006; 59(4) Suppl 2:ONS270–ONS277, discussion ONS277–ONS278

[48] Patel SJ, Sekhar LN, Cass SP, Hirsch BE. Combined approaches for resection of extensive glomus jugulare tumors. A review of 12 cases. J Neurosurg. 1994; 80(6):1026–1038

[49] Zanation AM, Snyderman CH, Carrau RL, Gardner PA, Prevedello DM, Kassam AB. Endoscopic endonasal surgery for petrous apex lesions. Laryngoscope. 2009; 119(1):19–25

[50] Eisenberg MB, Haddad G, Al-Mefty O. Petrous apex cholesterol granulomas: evolution and management. J Neurosurg. 1997; 86(5):822–829

[51] Hoa M, House JW, Linthicum FH, Jr. Petrous apex cholesterol granuloma: maintenance of drainage pathway, the histopathology of surgical management and histopathologic evidence for the exposed marrow theory. Otol Neurotol. 2012; 33(6):1059–1065

[52] Paluzzi A, Gardner P, Fernandez-Miranda JC, et al. Endoscopic endonasal approach to cholesterol granulomas of the petrous apex: a series of 17 patients: clinical article. J Neurosurg. 2012; 116(4):792–798

[53] Sanna M, Dispenza F, Mathur N, De Stefano A, De Donato G. Otoneurological management of petrous apex cholesterol granuloma. Am J Otolaryngol. 2009; 30(6):407–414

[54] Ishi Y, Kobayashi H, Motegi H, et al. Endoscopic transsphenoidal surgery using pedicle vascularized nasoseptal flap for cholesterol granuloma in petrous apex: A technical note. Neurol Neurochir Pol. 2016; 50(6):504–510

[55] Karligkiotis A, Bignami M, Terranova P, et al. Use of the pedicled nasoseptal flap in the endoscopic management of cholesterol granulomas of the petrous apex. Int Forum Allergy Rhinol. 2015; 5(8):747–753

[56] Samii M, Tatagiba M, Carvalho GA. Retrosigmoid intradural suprameatal approach to Meckel's cave and the middle fossa: surgical technique and outcome. J Neurosurg. 2000; 92(2):235–241

[57] Samii M, Tatagiba M. Experience with 36 surgical cases of petroclival meningiomas. Acta Neurochir (Wien). 1992; 118(1–2):27–32

[58] Ramina R, Maniglia JJ, Fernandes YB, et al. Jugular foramen tumors: diagnosis and treatment. Neurosurg Focus. 2004; 17(2):E5

[59] Ramina R, Maniglia JJ, Fernandes YB, Paschoal JR, Pfeilsticker LN, Coelho Neto M. Tumors of the jugular foramen: diagnosis and management. Neurosurgery. 2005; 57(1) Suppl:59–68, discussion 59–68

[60] Ramina R, Neto MC, Fernandes YB, Aguiar PH, de Meneses MS, Torres LF. Meningiomas of the jugular foramen. Neurosurg Rev. 2006; 29(1):55–60

[61] Ramina R, Maniglia JJ, Paschoal JR, Fernandes YB, Neto MC, Honorato DC. Reconstruction of the cranial base in surgery for jugular foramen tumors. Neurosurgery. 2005; 56(2) Suppl:337–343, discussion 337–343

[62] Huy PT, Kania R, Duet M, Dessard-Diana B, Mazeron JJ, Benhamed R. Evolving concepts in the management of jugular paraganglioma: a comparison of radiotherapy and surgery in 88 cases. Skull Base. 2009; 19(1):83–91

25 Tumors of the Cerebellopontine Angle

Joshua W. Lucas, Alexandra Kammen, Rick A. Friedman, and Steven L. Giannotta

Summary

This chapter describes the clinical presentation and imaging of the three most common tumors occurring in the cerebellopontine angle: acoustic neuroma, meningioma, and epidermoid tumor. A general management scheme is proposed for all three that includes surveillance imaging and clinical follow-up. In preparation for a discussion of surgical options, the relevant surgical anatomy is presented. Using the acoustic neuroma as a template, details of the retrosigmoid, middle fossa, and translabyrinthine approaches as well as their potential complications are presented.

Keywords: acoustic neuroma, cerebellopontine angle, cerebrospinal fluid (CSF) leakepidermoid tumor, facial nerve, meningioma, middle fossa approach, retrosigmoid approach, stereotactic radiosurgery, translabyrinthine approach, vestibular schwannoma, vestibulocochlear nerves

25.1 Introduction

Acoustic neuromas, or vestibular schwannomas, are the most common masses found in the cerebellopontine angle (CPA), accounting for approximately 75% of lesions in this location and about 6% of all intracranial tumors combined. Meningiomas and epidermoid tumors are the next most common masses found in the CP angle and must be considered in the differential diagnosis of a newly discovered CP angle mass.[1]

Symptoms of patients who have acoustic neuromas closely correlate with the size of the tumor. The three most common presenting symptoms are hearing loss, tinnitus, and disequilibrium.[2] Larger tumors may produce facial numbness, weakness, or twitching. If tumors become very large, then compression of the brainstem is possible, which can cause weakness or sensory changes of the extremities or hydrocephalus from compression of the fourth ventricle.

In a series of 131 patients, 66% had no abnormal physical findings except for hearing loss on the ipsilateral side of the acoustic neuroma.[2] Patients will often complain of inability to use the telephone in the affected ear. Lateralization of Weber's test to the normal ear and normal or indeterminate Rinne's tests can be used to confirm sensorineural hearing loss. Facial nerve function should be graded on the House-Brackmann scale.[3] Excluding hearing loss, the next three most common abnormal signs in patients who have acoustic neuromas are abnormal corneal reflex, nystagmus, and facial hypoesthesia.[2]

A pure tone audiogram is often the first screening test for patients when the diagnosis of acoustic neuroma is suspected. High-frequency hearing loss is the most common abnormality seen on pure tone audiometry in patients who have these lesions.[4] Care must be taken in interpretation of pure tone audiogram results, however, as this is also the most common type of hearing loss with age and from noise exposure. In general, a hearing difference of greater than 10 to 15 dB from one ear to the other warrants further investigation. Notably, Johnson et al found that the likelihood of abnormal audiometry correlates with acoustic neuroma size.[4]

Another important aspect of the pure tone audiogram and clinical assessment is speech discrimination, which is not always related to the degree of pure tone hearing loss. Some patients may have exceptionally poor speech discrimination despite near-normal pure tone audiometry.[5] Speech discrimination is an integral part of the clinical decision-making process, especially when determining the optimal surgical approach. When hearing in the contralateral ear is normal, residual hearing on the operated side is socially useful only if speech discrimination is good and the pure tone audiogram is within 30 dB of the normal side.[5]

MRI has been used to characterize the natural history of acoustic neuromas. In a series of patients treated conservatively and followed with serial scans, the average rate of tumor growth was 0.91 mm per year.[6] Of these patients, 42% experienced no growth or reduction in tumor size. Overall postoperative growth rate for patients who underwent a subtotal resection was 0.35 mm per year; 68.5% of these patients demonstrated no growth or reduction in tumor size.[6]

25.2 Imaging

Tremendous improvements in both the quality and sensitivity of diagnostic imaging for acoustic neuromas have been made over the past several decades. Imaging techniques have evolved from plain films to CT scans. Currently, MRI is the imaging investigation of choice when evaluating and monitoring tumors of the CP angle. The increased sensitivity for detecting CP angle tumors is affecting the pattern of patient presentation and will likely influence management strategies and outcomes.[5]

25.2.1 Computed Tomography

Prior to MRI, CT was the primary imaging modality for the diagnosis of acoustic neuromas. Contrast-enhanced CT scans, with 5 mm axial slices through the cranial base, are generally sensitive enough to detect even small tumors.[7] Although MRI is now the gold standard for diagnosis of acoustic neuromas, patients will occasionally be diagnosed after undergoing a CT scan for other reasons. The classic CT appearance of an acoustic neuroma is an iso- or hypodense lesion centered on the internal auditory meatus, with homogeneous enhancement after intravenous contrast.

CT imaging remains the best modality available for delineating bony anatomy, which may help in establishing the diagnosis and aid in surgical planning. The size and location of perimeatal and labyrinthine air cells can be visualized on thinly cut scans. If a high-resolution CT scan is performed, the anatomical relationship between the semicircular canals, the vestibule, and the internal auditory meatus can also be appreciated. Bony erosion by tumor in the region of the jugular bulb may also be apparent.[5] Finally, in cases of cerebrospinal fluid (CSF) leak postoperatively, thin-cut CT scans (cisternogram) can aid in identifying the area of leakage for repair.

25.2.2 Magnetic Resonance Imaging

MRI has become the best imaging modality for acoustic neuroma diagnosis and management. Most acoustic neuromas are hypo- or isointense on T1-weighted images (T1WI) when compared with normal brain parenchyma. These tumors demonstrate marked enhancement after administration of intravenous gadolinium (▶ Fig. 25.1). On T2-weighted images (T2WI), acoustic neuromas are usually hyperintense when compared with normal brain. Large tumors may demonstrate a component of cystic degeneration (▶ Fig. 25.2). Fluid attenuated inversion recovery sequences (FLAIR) may demonstrate peritumoral edema from tumor compression or transependymal edema suggestive of hydrocephalus. Compared with CT imaging, MRI offers superior resolution, a lack of beam-hardening artifacts, the ability to image the tumor in multiple planes, and the ability to identify adjacent vascular structures and possible vascular displacement or encasement.[5]

25.3 Surgical Anatomy

The anatomy of the CP angle was described in great detail several years ago by Rhoton.[8] Briefly, the CP angle cistern is bound

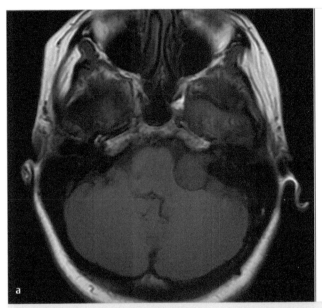
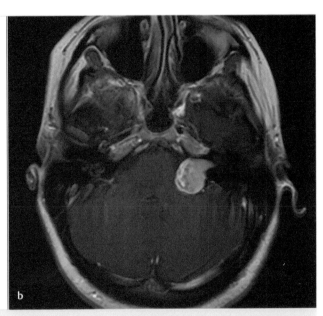

Fig. 25.1 (a) Precontrast and (b) postcontrast T1-weighted images of a left acoustic neuroma demonstrating avid enhancement with gadolinium contrast.

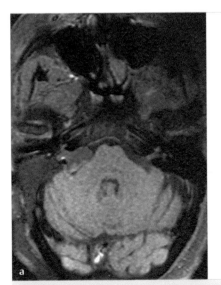
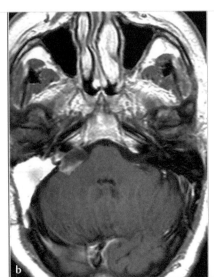
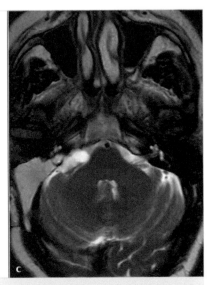

Fig. 25.2 A right-sided cystic acoustic neuroma. (a) T1-weighted noncontrast image, (b) T1-weighted postcontrast image, (c) T2-weighted image showing a small cyst in the anterior aspect of the tumor.

laterally by the petrous face, medially by the pons, and superiorly by the tentorium cerebelli.[5] The cerebellopontine fissure opens medially and has superior and inferior limbs that meet at a lateral apex. Cranial nerves (CNs) IV through XI are located within the CP angle.[8] The superior cerebellar artery and anteroinferior cerebellar artery (AICA) both arise medially from the basilar artery and course through the CP angle cistern.[1] Veins from the pons, middle cerebellar peduncle, and cerebellopontine fissure unite near the trigeminal nerve and form the superior petrosal venous complex.[9]

The trochlear and trigeminal nerves are located in the superior CP angle, whereas the glossopharyngeal, vagus, and accessory nerves are located in the inferior CP angle. The abducens nerve is located near the base of the fissure.[8] Although the facial and vestibulocochlear nerves may appear to pass as a single bundle from the pontomedullary junction to the internal auditory meatus, they are separate and distinct. Within the vestibulocochlear nerve complex, the superior and inferior vestibular nerves lie posteriorly and superiorly, whereas the cochlear nerve lies posteriorly and inferiorly. A shallow groove marks the boundary between them. The facial nerve normally lies anteriorly and slightly superiorly, separated from the vestibular nerves by the labyrinthine artery.[5] Specific anatomical relationships, however, are often distorted in larger tumors.

The internal auditory meatus houses the facial, cochlear, and inferior and superior vestibular nerves. The lateral portion of the meatus is divided into a superior and an inferior portion by a horizontal ridge called the transverse or falciform crest. The facial and the superior vestibular nerves are superior to the crest. The facial nerve is anterior to the superior vestibular nerve and is separated from it at the lateral end of the meatus by a vertical ridge of bone, called the vertical crest (Bill's bar, named after William House).[10] The cochlear and inferior vestibular nerves run below the transverse crest, with the cochlear nerve located anteriorly.

A consistent set of anatomical relationships at the brainstem facilitates the identification of the CNs on the medial side of an acoustic neuroma.[11] The facial and vestibulocochlear nerves arise from the brainstem near the lateral end of the pontomedullary sulcus, anterosuperior to the choroid plexus protruding from the foramen of Luschka.[8] In most cases, the AICA passes below the facial and vestibulocochlear nerves and would be displaced inferiorly by an acoustic neuroma. The labyrinthine, recurrent perforating, and subarcuate branches arising from the AICA are frequently stretched around a large acoustic neuroma.[8] Venous structures that have a predictable relationship to the facial and vestibulocochlear nerves are the vein of the pontomedullary sulcus and the veins of the cerebellomedullary fissure, middle cerebellar peduncle, and cerebellopontine fissure.[12] Identification of any of these veins during the tumor removal allows for easier identification of the CNs leaving the brainstem.

25.4 Treatment Considerations

Careful preoperative preparation and evaluation of a patient who has an acoustic neuroma incorporates clinical symptoms and signs, pure tone audiogram and speech discrimination testing results, and diagnostic imaging. Treatment options include observation, surgical intervention, and stereotactic radiosurgery. Surgical options consist of the hearing-preserving approaches of the retrosigmoid craniotomy and the middle fossa craniotomy as well as the hearing-sacrificing approach of the translabyrinthine craniotomy. A substantial amount of literature exists regarding diverse treatment paradigms of patients with acoustic neuromas.[13,14,15]

The general management scheme at our center has been refined over several decades.[16] Patient age factors heavily into the decision-making process. Young patients (those 40 years old or younger) are generally advised to undergo surgical intervention with the goal of total excision. Middle-aged patients (those aged 41–70) in otherwise good health are typically offered surgery, although stereotactic radiosurgery is a viable option, especially in the case of small tumors with few symptoms. Gross total resection of the acoustic neuroma in these patients is the goal, but it is pursued less aggressively than in younger patients. In older patients (those older than 70 years of age), small tumors are generally followed using serial MRIs and treated using stereotactic radiosurgery if there is evidence of tumor growth. Older patients who have symptomatic, large tumors are offered surgery for tumor debulking followed by stereotactic radiosurgery.

The retrosigmoid approach is the workhorse of acoustic neuroma surgery. This hearing-preserving approach is selected for patients who have small tumors (< 2.5 cm) and good hearing (< 50 dB on pure tone average [PTA] and > 50% speech discrimination), as well as for patients who have large tumors (> 2.5 cm) on the side of their only hearing ear. Additional considerations are the amount of tumor within the CP angle and the amount of intracanalicular tumor (▶ Fig. 25.3; ▶ Fig. 25.4).

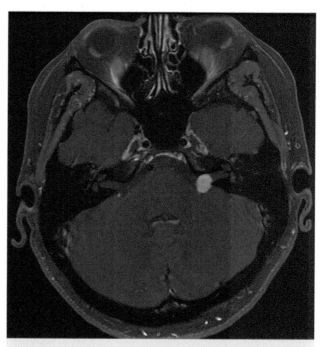

Fig. 25.3 A left acoustic neuroma with the majority of the tumor in the CP angle and a small intracanalicular component. This tumor was approached via a retrosigmoid craniotomy.

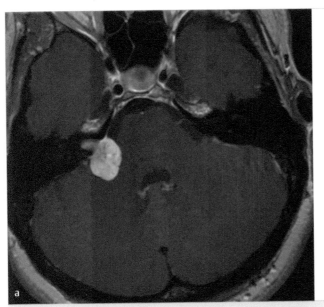
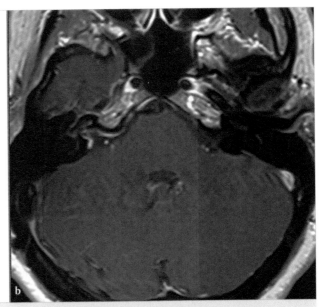

Fig. 25.4 A right acoustic neuroma resected via a retrosigmoid approach: preoperative **(a)** and postoperative **(b)** images.

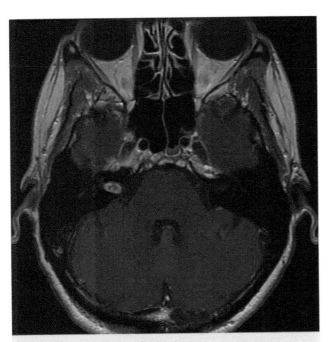

Fig. 25.5 A small right-sided intracanalicular acoustic neuroma resected via a middle fossa craniotomy.

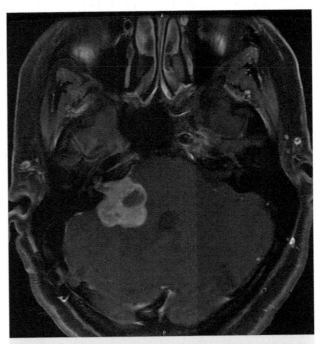

Fig. 25.6 A large right acoustic neuroma with significant cerebellopontine angle and intracanalicular components, resected via a translabyrinthine approach in a patient who had nonserviceable hearing in the right ear.

In cases of tumor extension far laterally into the internal auditory canal, a large amount of drilling into the petrous temporal bone is required via a retrosigmoid approach, which increases the risk of injury to labyrinthine structures. For small tumors confined to the internal auditory canal that have no discernable CP angle component, a middle fossa craniotomy is the preferred hearing-preserving approach (▶ Fig. 25.5). The translabyrinthine approach is a hearing-sacrificing approach that is preferred in patients who have poor hearing (>50 dB on PTA and <50% speech discrimination) and large tumors, especially when the tumor has a large canalicular component as well as a large CP angle component (▶ Fig. 25.6; ▶ Fig. 25.7).

During the operation, constant facial nerve electromyography (EMG) is used to detect facial nerve irritation/injury and provide the ability to directly stimulate the facial nerve so as to test for function and aid in localization. Brainstem auditory evoked responses (BAERs) are also used to assess the function of the cochlear nerve. Early warning of prolongation of BAERs can alert the surgeon of overzealous cerebellar retraction and allow for correction prior to permanent cochlear nerve damage. Selective somatosensory evoked potentials (SSEPs) and motor evoked potentials (MEPs) are also used to monitor brainstem function.

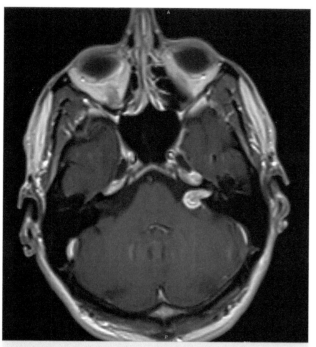

Fig. 25.7 A left acoustic neuroma resected via a translabyrinthine approach in a patient who had nonserviceable hearing in the left ear.

25.5 Approaches

25.5.1 Retrosigmoid Approach

Positioning

The semisitting, prone, supine–oblique, lateral decubitus, and park bench positions have all been used for suboccipital retrosigmoid removal of acoustic neuromas.[17,18] For a right-handed surgeon at our center, a right retrosigmoid approach is done in the left lateral decubitus position, whereas a left retrosigmoid approach is done supine with the patient's head turned to the right; this is reversed for a left-handed surgeon. The goal of this positioning scheme is to prevent the ipsilateral shoulder from obstructing the surgeon's primary operating hand during the case. The patient's head is held in place using a Mayfield three-point fixation device.

Incision and Soft Tissue Dissection

A "question-mark" shaped incision centered 2 to 3 cm posterior to the mastoid process is made (▶ Fig. 25.8). Scalp flaps are then developed using monopolar electrocautery and elevated using fishhooks and rubber bands. The suboccipital fascia and muscles are incised in a hockey-stick fashion and carefully separated from their attachments to the bone using subperiosteal dissection and monopolar electrocautery and then are reflected with fishhooks. This two-layer opening facilitates better closure and may have a role in decreasing incidence of postoperative CSF leaks. Brisk bleeding from an emissary, which can be expected in the dissection just medial to the mastoid process, should be stopped with bone wax.

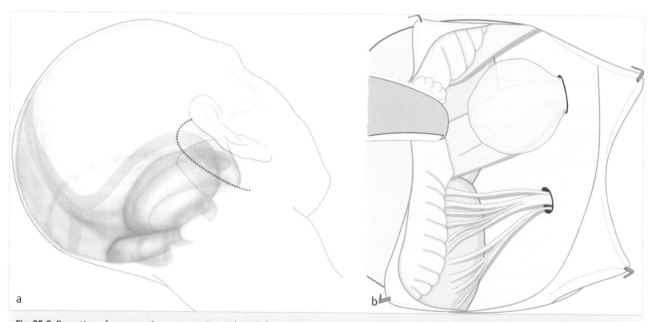

Fig. 25.8 Resection of an acoustic neuroma via a right-sided retrosigmoid approach. **(a)** Retrosigmoid craniotomy scalp incision (*dotted line*) and craniotomy (*green shaded region*). **(b)** Dural opening. The acoustic neuroma can be seen in the center of the field, with arachnoid adhesions between the tumor capsule and the petrous dura. The vestibulocochlear nerve can be seen splayed over the posteroinferior surface of the tumor.

Bony Dissection

A standard suboccipital craniotomy is performed by placing a bur hole behind the mastoid and using a combination of a diamond-bur drill and Kerrison rongeurs to enlarge the craniotomy. The craniotomy is widened to the edge of the transverse sinus superiorly and the sigmoid sinus anteriorly (▶ Fig. 25.8a). Exposure sometimes requires a partial mastoidectomy, during which the mastoid air cells may be opened. Repair involves sealing the opened air cells using bone max or a muscle graft.

Tumor Resection

When the dura is adequately relaxed, it is opened under the microscope in a curvilinear fashion and reflected anteriorly (▶ Fig. 25.8b). A Fujita snake retractor is then used to gently retract the cerebellum until the arachnoid of the cisterna magna is identified. The cisterna magna is sharply opened, which leads to brisk CSF drainage and, invariably, recession of the cerebellum from the posterior surface of the petrous bone.[19] At this point, careful dissection of remaining arachnoid adhesions will reveal the CNs and the acoustic neuroma within the CP angle. In many cases, the vestibulocochlear nerve can be identified splayed out into the medial–caudal aspect of the tumor. The cochlear nerve can be significantly attenuated in patients who have large tumors and may be unrecognizable even under high magnification. The origin of the facial nerve almost always remains hidden by the overlying CN VIII and tumor.

After the tumor is identified, attention is turned to internally decompressing it. The posterior aspect of the tumor is queried with the stimulating probe to ensure that the facial nerve has not been displaced posteriorly. Microscissors are used to sharply open the tumor capsule, and ultrasonic aspiration is used to internally debulk the acoustic neuroma. When it is clear that the tumor is originating from the superior vestibular nerve, this nerve can be divided. As the tumor is decompressed, the cochlear nerve usually becomes increasingly apparent to the point that a plane may be visualized between the cochlear nerve and the tumor capsule. The cochlear nerve dissection is followed toward the porus acusticus.

The dura overlying the porus acusticus is then stripped off, and a diamond bur is used to drill a small trough in the petrous temporal bone so as to expose the dura of the internal auditory canal and the lateral extent of tumor. Excessive drilling may result in inadvertent opening of the posterior semicircular canal or endolymphatic duct and compromise hearing. The cochlear and facial nerves are identified within the internal auditory canal. The tumor is then carefully dissected from the nerves and removed piecemeal. The entire operative field is then inspected for residual tumor. Bleeding should be addressed, but bipolar cauterization should be used sparingly to prevent interruption of blood supply to the facial and cochlear nerves.

Closure

Once hemostasis is achieved, the dura is closed in watertight fashion using a small piece of suturable Duragen (Integra LifeSciences) as an inlay graft. This closure is then reinforced with fibrin glue. The cranial defect is repaired using a titanium mesh plate. The wound is then thoroughly irrigated and closed in a multilayer fashion.

25.5.2 Translabyrinthine Approach

Positioning

The patient is placed supine on the operating table, with the head resting on a doughnut. The head is turned as far as possible away from the side of the tumor.

Incision and Soft Tissue Dissection

A curvilinear incision is made, starting from just below the tip of the mastoid process, running upward over the lateral surface of the mastoid and just behind the root of the pinna, to a point about 2 cm above the tip of the pinna. Scalp flaps are developed using monopolar electrocautery and elevated using fishhooks and rubber bands. A hockey-stick incision is then made with the monopolar cautery in the temporalis fascia and muscle. The muscle and fascia are separated off the bone using subperiosteal dissection and monopolar electrocautery. The fascia and muscle are then elevated using fishhooks and rubber bands.

Bony Dissection

A high-speed drill with a cutting bur is used to begin the bony dissection. Anteriorly, the posterior wall of the external meatus is thinned. Superiorly, the dissection should expose the edge of the middle fossa dura and superior petrosal sinus. The sigmoid sinus is exposed posteriorly. Inferiorly, the mastoid process is hollowed out. It is important to remove sufficient bone posteriorly and superiorly to allow for significant dural retraction.[5]

With the aid of the operating microscope, the dissection is then deepened in the space between the middle fossa dura and superior margin of the meatus to open the mastoid antrum and aditus. After exposure of the incus and the head of the malleus, the incus is removed. The lateral semicircular canal is then identified on the medial wall of the epitympanic recess (▶ Fig. 25.9).

Dense bone marks the otic capsule surrounding the semicircular canals. The lateral semicircular canal is removed first. The superior canal is then drilled until the identification of the common crus, which can then be used to find the posterior canal. After completion of the labyrinthectomy, the bone covering the internal auditory canal is completely skeletonized. The bone over the porus acusticus is then removed. The cavity resulting from this dissection is roughly pyramidal in shape, with its base at the cortical opening of the mastoid (▶ Fig. 25.9b). The dura of the posterior fossa lies posteriorly. Dura of the middle fossa lies above, and the petrous bone, middle ear cavity, and descending facial nerve lie anteriorly.

Tumor Resection

The dura of the meatus and posterior fossa is subsequently opened to expose the full extent of the acoustic neuroma (▶ Fig. 25.9b,c). In all but the smallest tumors, internal decompression of both the cisternal and the intracanalicular portions of the mass is emphasized before any attempt at identification of the facial nerve is carried out. Internal debulking allows the dissection to be extended under direct vision around the far side of the tumor, where the arteries, CNs, and brainstem lie. As

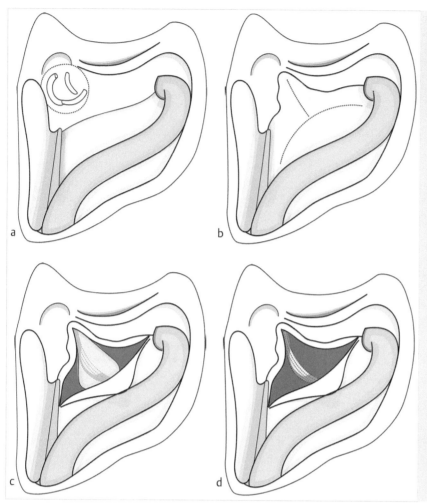

Fig. 25.9 Translabyrinthine craniotomy. **(a)** Location of the semicircular canals in relation to the facial nerve. **(b)** The internal auditory canal (IAC) after bony removal, with dural incision represented by the dotted line. **(c)** Tumor exposure. **(d)** View of the facial nerve after tumor removal.

the tumor is reduced in size, dissection proceeds along its upper, lower, anterior, and posterior poles.

As the residual cisternal portion of the mass becomes more mobile, CN VIII is definitively identified at its junction with the tumor and divided. A stimulator is used to define the facial nerve exit zone as distinct from the vestibulocochlear nerve. Dissection of the plane between the facial nerve and tumor is carried out in a medial to lateral direction to avoid traction injury. Traction on the facial nerve is further avoided by leaving a small dural attachment adherent to the bulk of the tumor until most of the mass has been reduced. Attention is then turned to the lateral end of the internal auditory canal, where Bill's bar is identified, facial nerve position is confirmed, and any further tumor is removed (▶ Fig. 25.9d).

Closure

The edges of the dural opening into the posterior fossa are approximated, as watertight closure is essentially impossible. An abdominal fat graft is harvested and placed in the surgical corridor to seal off the middle ear from CSF communication. A piece of titanium mesh is then fashioned to cover the cranial defect. The wound is then irrigated and closed in a multilayered fashion.

25.5.3 Middle Fossa Approach

Positioning

Much as in the translabyrinthine approach, the patient's head is placed on a soft doughnut and turned as far as possible from the side of the acoustic neuroma.

Incision and Soft Tissue Dissection

The incision is made starting just anterior to the tragus, coursing around and over the pinna to a point several centimeters behind the external auditory canal, where it turns superiorly for approximately 6 cm and then turns anteriorly to the hairline. The temporalis muscle is incised using monopolar electrocautery, and the entire musculocutaneous flap is reflected anteriorly and held in place with retention sutures.

Bony Dissection

A 5 × 5 cm craniotomy is performed, with approximately a third of the craniotomy anterior to the external auditory canal and approximately two-thirds posterior to it. The temporal squamous bone is drilled down to the middle fossa floor to allow the following of an appropriate trajectory to the petrous apex. Under the operative microscope, the dura is elevated from the petrous ridge in a posterior to anterior direction until the greater superficial petrosal nerve is identified. A House-Urban retractor system is used to retract the temporal lobe superiorly. The superior semicircular canal is identified, and bone is drilled anterior and medial to this structure so as to expose the dura around the porus acusticus. Bone is subsequently removed from medial to lateral to expose Bill's bar and the entirety of the internal auditory canal.

Tumor Resection

The dura of the internal auditory canal is opened sharply, and tumor is usually readily identified within the canal. The facial nerve is stimulated to confirm its location. If the tumor is sufficiently large, then primary internal decompression may be required to reduce manipulation of the surrounding nerves. The tumor is dissected from the facial and cochlear nerves and removed.

Closure

After meticulous hemostasis has been achieved, a small abdominal fat graft is placed within the defect to reduce the incidence of postoperative CSF rhinorrhea. The temporal lobe retractor is removed, and the wound is closed in a multilayered fashion.

25.6 Complication Avoidance

Postoperative CSF leak is the most common complication of acoustic neuroma surgery, regardless of approach. It has been reported with a frequency of 2 to 25%.[20,21,22] CSF leak may present as rhinorrhea or leakage from the wound. Although it is most commonly evident within a few days of surgery, it may also present in a delayed fashion. A thin-cut CT scan through the temporal bone can often demonstrate the area of leakage (▶ Fig. 25.10). In most cases, lumbar drainage for several days allows the site of CSF egress to heal, but if the leak continues, then surgery for reexploration and graft repacking may be necessary.

Facial nerve dysfunction is another common complication of acoustic neuroma surgery. Should facial paralysis be noted, care of the affected eye becomes paramount, especially if facial analgesia is present and the corneal reflex is absent. The patient should have Lacrilube ointment and artificial tears regularly applied to the affected eye and should wear an optically clear eye chamber while sleeping, for further eye protection. During follow-up, the patient is specifically examined for corneal ulcerations. Early ophthalmology consultation is warranted. Sampath et al[22] have summarized the results of facial nerve function from several large series of acoustic neuroma patients. The House-Brackmann facial nerve grading system is the standard system used to record facial nerve function.[3] When facial paralysis does not recover, the patient may need to undergo a hypoglossal–facial anastomosis. Additionally, tarsorrhaphy and/or gold weight placement in the upper eyelid might be needed.

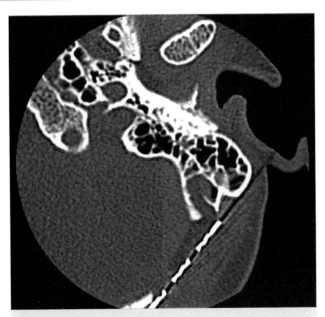

Fig. 25.10 A CT scan of the left temporal bone after a left retrosigmoid craniotomy in a patient who experienced postoperative cerebrospinal fluid rhinorrhea. A defect in the mastoid air cells can be seen just medial to the anterior surface of the plate. This patient required reoperation for closure of the air cell.

Other less common complications include postoperative hematoma, aseptic or bacterial meningitis, hydrocephalus, and wound infection. These complications are rare but must be managed expeditiously and appropriately when they occur.

References

[1] Osborn AG, Rauschning W. Brain tumors and tumorlike masses: classification and differential diagnosis. In: Osborn AG, ed. Diagnostic Neuroradiology. 1st ed. St. Louis: Mosby; 1994:401–528

[2] Harner SG, Laws ER, Jr. Clinical findings in patients with acoustic neurinoma. Mayo Clin Proc. 1983; 58(11):721–728

[3] House JW, Brackmann DE. Facial nerve grading system. Otolaryngol Head Neck Surg. 1985; 93(2):146–147

[4] Johnson EW. Auditory test results in 500 cases of acoustic neuroma. Arch Otolaryngol. 1977; 103(3):152–158

[5] Kaye AH, Briggs RJS. Acoustic neuroma (vestibular schwannoma). In: Kaye AH, Laws ER, eds. Brain Tumors. 2nd ed. London: Churchill Livingstone; 2001:619–669

[6] Rosenberg SI. Natural history of acoustic neuromas. Laryngoscope. 2000; 110 (4):497–508

[7] Harner SG, Reese DF. Roentgenographic diagnosis of acoustic neurinoma. Laryngoscope. 1984; 94(3):306–309

[8] Rhoton AL, Jr. The cerebellopontine angle and posterior fossa cranial nerves by the retrosigmoid approach. Neurosurgery. 2000; 47(3) Suppl:S93–S129

[9] Matsuno H, Rhoton AL, Jr, Peace D. Microsurgical anatomy of the posterior fossa cisterns. Neurosurgery. 1988; 23(1):58–80

[10] House WF. Translabyrinthine approach. In: House WF, Luetje CM, eds. Acoustic Tumors: II–Management. Baltimore: University Park Press; 1979:43–87

[11] Rhoton AL, Jr. Microsurgical anatomy of the brainstem surface facing an acoustic neuroma. Surg Neurol. 1986; 25(4):326–339

[12] Matsushima T, Rhoton AL, Jr, de Oliveira E, Peace D. Microsurgical anatomy of the veins of the posterior fossa. J Neurosurg. 1983; 59(1):63–105

[13] Rutherford SA, King AT. Vestibular schwannoma management: What is the "best" option? Br J Neurosurg. 2005; 19(4):309–316

[14] Kondziolka D, Lunsford LD, Flickinger JC. Acoustic tumors: operation versus radiation—making sense of opposing viewpoints. Part II. Acoustic neuromas: sorting out management options. Clin Neurosurg. 2003; 50:313–328

[15] Mangham CA, Jr. Retrosigmoid versus middle fossa surgery for small vestibular schwannomas. Laryngoscope. 2004; 114(8):1455–1461

[16] Chakrabarti I, Apuzzo MLJ, Giannota SL. Acoustic tumors: operation versus radiation—making sense of opposing viewpoints. Part I. Acoustic neuroma: decision making with all the tools. Clin Neurosurg. 2003; 50: 293–312

[17] Ojemann RG. Suboccipital transmeatal approaches to vestibular schwannomas. In: Schmidek HH, Sweet, WH, eds. Operative Neurosurgical Techniques. Philadelphia: W.B. Saunders Company; 1995:829–841

[18] Tew JM, Scodary DJ. Neoplastic disorders—surgical positioning. In: Apuzzo MLJ, ed. Brain Surgery Complication Avoidance and Management. New York: Churchill Livingstone; 1993:1609–1620

[19] Ciric I, Zhao JC, Rosenblatt S, Wiet R, O'Shaughnessy B. Suboccipital retrosigmoid approach for removal of vestibular schwannomas: facial nerve function and hearing preservation. Neurosurgery. 2005; 56(3):560–570

[20] Gjurić M, Wigand ME, Wolf SR. Enlarged middle fossa vestibular schwannoma surgery: experience with 735 cases. Otol Neurotol. 2001; 22(2):223–230, discussion 230–231

[21] Gormley WB, Sekhar LN, Wright DC, Kamerer D, Schessel D. Acoustic neuromas: results of current surgical management. Neurosurgery. 1997; 41(1): 50–58, discussion 58–60

[22] Sampath P, Rini D, Long DM. Microanatomical variations in the cerebellopontine angle associated with vestibular schwannomas (acoustic neuromas): a retrospective study of 1006 consecutive cases. J Neurosurg. 2000; 92(1):70–78

26 Tumors of the Jugular Foramen

Samer Ayoubi, Badih Adada, Marcio S. Rassi, Luis A. B. Borba, and Ossama Al-Mefty

Summary

Tumors in the jugular foramen frequently present a great challenge to the neurosurgeon because of its intimate relationship with the facial and lower cranial nerves as well as the internal carotid artery. The high morbidity associated with damage to these structures requires extensive laboratory training and deep knowledge of local anatomy.

Keywords: jugular foramen, glomus jugulare, paraganglioma, schwannoma, meningioma

26.1 Anatomical Background

The jugular foramen is an opening in the skull connecting the posterior cranial fossa and the jugular fossa.[1] It is located between the temporal and occipital bones, around the sigmoid and inferior petrosal sinuses, extending in a posterolateral to anteromedial direction. The foramen houses two venous compartments: the sigmoid part, which receives flow from the sigmoid sinus, and the petrosal part, which receives drainage from the inferior petrosal sinus. A fibro-osseous diaphragm separates these two vascular channels, and the lower cranial nerves lie on either side of this partition at the site of the intrajugular processes of the temporal and occipital bones (▶ Fig. 26.1a).[2,3,4]

The jugular fossa is a deep depression at the inferior surface of the petrous portion of the temporal bone that communicates with the posterior cranial fossa via the jugular foramen. It hosts the jugular bulb, which continues as the jugular vein inferiorly (▶ Fig. 26.1b). Cranial nerves IX, X, and XI enter the dura on the medial side of the intrajugular process. The entrance orifice of the glossopharyngeal nerve is separated from the entrance of

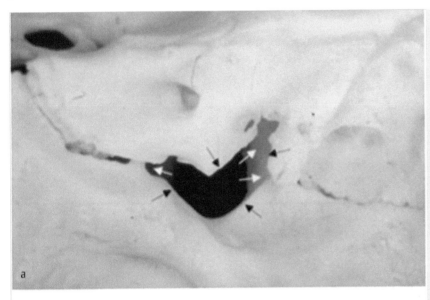

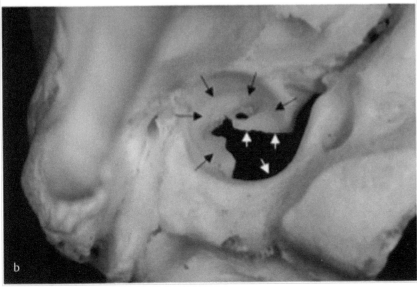

Fig. 26.1 Photographs of dry anatomical specimens from the right side. **(a)** Anterior perspective, in which the view extends from the outside to the inside, delineating the jugular foramen (*white arrows*) and jugular fossa (*black arrows*). **(b)** Posterior perspective, in which the view extends from the inside to the outside, delineating the jugular foramen (*black arrows*) and jugular fossa (*white arrows*). Note the difference between the two perspectives. (Reproduced with permission from Arnautovic KI, Al-Mefty O, Primary meningiomas of the jugular fossa, J Neurosurg 2002;97(1):12–20.)

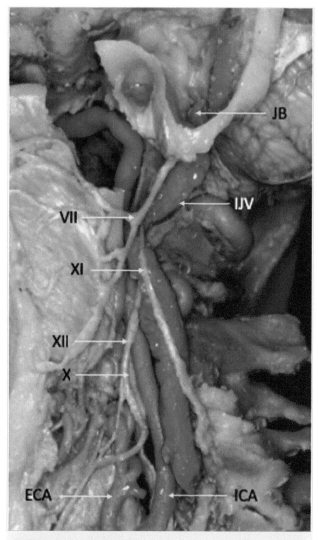

Fig. 26.2 Anatomical dissection demonstrating the relationship of the jugular bulb to the carotid artery and cranial nerves VII, X, XI, and XII. ECA, external carotid artery; ICA, internal carotid artery; IJV, internal jugular vein; JV, jugular bulb.

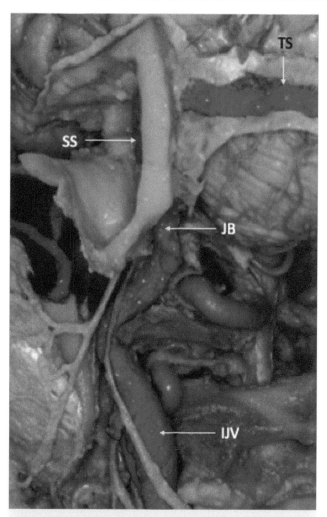

Fig. 26.3 Anatomical dissection demonstrating the course of the sigmoid sinus from the transverse sinus, into the temporal bone and down the neck. IJV, internal jugular vein; JB, jugular bulb; SS, sigmoid sinus; TS, transverse sinus.

the vagus and accessory nerves by a dural crest in the jugular fossa.[5] The glossopharyngeal nerve (▶ Fig. 26.2) passes forward, coursing through the jugular fossa, and exits on the lateral surface of the internal carotid artery deep to the styloid process. The vagus nerve exits the fossa vertically, in intimate relation with the accessory nerve behind the glossopharyngeal nerve on the posteromedial wall of the internal jugular vein.[4] The accessory nerve descends laterally between the carotid artery and the internal jugular vein and then backward across the lateral surface of the vein to the sternomastoid and trapezius muscles. The hypoglossal nerve passes through the hypoglossal canal and does not traverse the jugular foramen. It passes adjacent to the vagus nerve and descends between the internal carotid artery and the jugular vein. Then it turns abruptly forward toward the tongue. Lesions located lateral to the fibro-osseous diaphragm frequently displace the nerves medially, favoring their preservation during tumor removal. By contrast, medially positioned tumors displace the cranial nerves onto the lateral tumor

surface, where they interpose between the surgeon and the tumor—an unfavorable location.[3]

The carotid artery passes anteromedial to the internal jugular vein to reach the carotid canal. At the level of the skull base, this artery runs anterior to the vein and is separated from it by the carotid ridge. It ascends a short distance in the canal (the vertical segment), then turns at a right angle anteromedially toward the petrous apex (the horizontal segment). Three branches of the external carotid artery—the ascending pharyngeal, occipital, and posterior auricular arteries—can contribute significant blood supply to lesions of the jugular fossa. The sigmoid sinus (▶ Fig. 26.3) courses down the sigmoid sulcus, turning anteriorly toward the jugular foramen and crossing it into the jugular bulb. It then flows downward behind the carotid canal into the internal jugular vein. The inferior petrosal sinus courses on the surface of the petroclival fissure, forming a plexiform confluence as it enters the petrosal part of the jugular fossa. Because the position of the lower cranial nerves with respect to the inferior petrosal sinus varies, overpacking or cautery over the sinus can injure these nerves.[6]

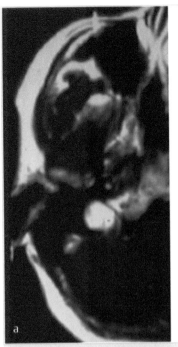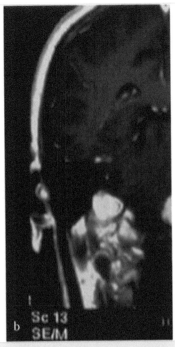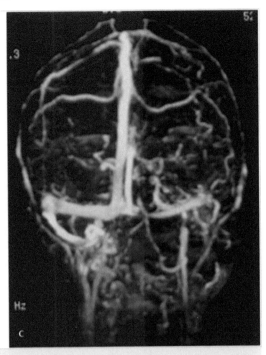

Fig. 26.4 Example of a high jugular bulb that may be mistaken for a glomus jugulare tumor. T1-weighted postcontrast MRI, **(a)** axial and **(b)** coronal. **(c)** MR venography.

26.2 Regional Pathology and Differential Diagnosis

Several lesions can arise within the structures of the jugular foramen and fossa or from contiguous structures. Nevertheless, the surgeon must be able to recognize anatomical variations of the jugular bulb, particularly a high jugular bulb or turbulent flow within the bulb, so as not to misdiagnose them as disease (▶ Fig. 26.4). Though rare, the three most common tumors within the jugular foramen are paragangliomas, schwannomas, and meningiomas.[3,7,8,9] Precise preoperative diagnosis of these lesions, though not always possible, is crucial, because each has different surgical considerations, such as the need for preoperative embolization with glomus jugulare tumors or the removal of a certain amount of bone with meningiomas. MRI complemented by thin-cut bony window CT facilitates differentiation between these tumors (▶ Table 26.1).

Differential diagnoses to be considered are acoustic schwannomas and lesions such as chordomas and chondrosarcomas, malignant tumors (carcinomas), metastases, peripheral primitive neuroectodermal tumors, cholesteatomas, chondromas, lymphangiomas, choroid plexus papillomas, salivary gland tumors, lipomas, aneurysmal bone cysts, hemangiopericytomas, plasmacytomas and inflammatory granulomas, pseudomasses such as normal vascular asymmetry, a high jugular bulb or jugular diverticulum, and aneurysms of the petrous carotid artery.[7,9,10,11,12,13,14,15,16] A jugular foramen abscess has also been reported.[17]

Table 26.1 Imaging differences according to type of tumor

Tumor	CT	MRI
Glomus jugulare	Erosion and destruction of the jugular spine and carotid crest Moth-eaten pattern	Salt-and-pepper appearance Nonhomogeneous enhancement
Schwannoma	Enlarged fossa with smooth, distinct, sclerotic margin	Low to isointense on T1 and high signal on T2 May be cystic Often dumbbell-shaped Moderate to marked enhancement
Meningioma	Hyperostosis and bone thickening without erosion	Dural tail Extensive enhancement

26.3 Glomus Jugulare Tumors

26.3.1 Pathology

Benign paragangliomas originating within the jugular foramen are known as glomus jugulare tumors.[18] These tumors grow along the path of least resistance and can gain access to the subarachnoid space by penetrating the dura of the posterior fossa, growing along cranial nerves, or, less commonly, penetrating the dura of the middle fossa.[19] Glomus jugulare tumors are uncommon tumors of the head and neck, accounting for only 0.03% of all neoplasms and 0.6% of head and neck tumors.[20] Nonetheless, they are the most common neoplasms of the middle ear and are the most common tumor involving the temporal bone, after only vestibular schwannomas. Glomus tumors have no clear racial predilection, but they seem to be more common among Caucasians. There is a marked predominance among females; women are affected three to six times more than men, with a peak incidence during the fifth decade of life. Multiple paragangliomas are reported in more than 10% of cases. Familial cases, most of which involve fathers and daughters, have a much higher rate of multicentricity, up to 55%. Evidence supports an autosomal dominant inheritance pattern consistent with genomic imprinting and an association with the haplotype at chromosome band 11q23. Most multicentric tumors are carotid body tumors. Only a few cases of bilateral glomus jugulare tumors associated with carotid body tumors have been reported.[21] The two established classifications of these tumors, those of Fisch and Jackson, are based mainly on tumor size, with special emphasis on intracranial extension as a decisive factor for resectability.[22,23] A subgroup of glomus jugulare tumors is rarely encountered but presents a formidable challenge for treatment. Al-Mefty and colleagues used the following criteria to describe this group[24]:

- Giant size (▶ Fig. 26.5)
- Multiple paragangliomas (bilateral or ipsilateral) (▶ Fig. 26.6)
- Malignancy (▶ Fig. 26.7)
- Catecholamine secretion
- Association with other lesions, such as a dural arteriovenous malformation or an adrenal tumor, or previous treatment that produced an adverse outcome that makes surgical intervention a much greater risk, such as sacrifice of the carotid artery, radiation therapy, or postoperative deficits or adverse effects from embolization

26.3.2 Clinical Presentation

Frequently reported symptoms of glomus tumors include pulsatile tinnitus, hearing loss, and cranial nerve palsies.[23] Lower cranial nerve deficits are the prominent feature in patients who have symptomatic jugular tumors (▶ Fig. 26.8).[24] Conductive hearing loss is the result of mechanical obstruction of the ossicular mechanism by the tumor, whereas sensorineural hearing loss is a result of the involvement of the labyrinth. Patients may also present signs of elevated catecholamine production such as palpitations, excessive sweating, and headache, which must be investigated in all patients who have a glomus jugulare tumor. Eventually, large tumors can cause obstructive hydrocephalus and intracranial hypertension.

26.3.3 Appearance on Diagnostic Imaging

Bony-window CT scans show skull base infiltration with erosion and enlargement of the jugular foramen, characterized by an irregular "moth-eaten" pattern (▶ Fig. 26.9).[25,26] MRI shows an enhancing tumor with flow voids and a "salt-and-pepper" appearance on T2-weighted sequences (▶ Fig. 26.10) and also discloses the presence of multiple tumors. MRI of the neck is done to exclude associated paragangliomas. The arteriographic findings of glomus jugulare tumors are typically a hypervascular mass with an intense characteristic tumor "blush." Large feeding vessels and early draining veins are commonly encountered, suggesting early arteriovenous shunting. Like other tumors in this region, glomus jugulare tumors are predominantly supplied by the external carotid artery system, mainly the ascending pharyngeal artery (▶ Fig. 26.11).[25] Angiographic studies are critical for assessing the appropriateness of preoperative

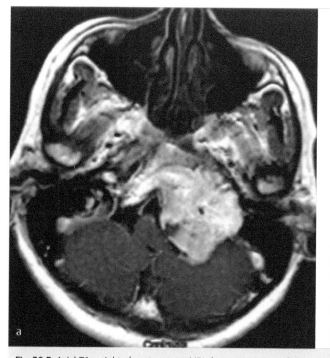
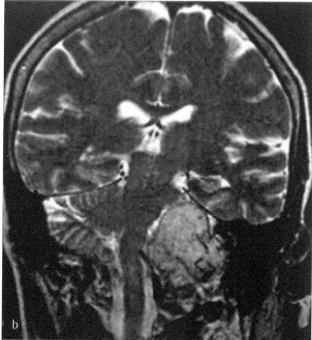

Fig. 26.5 Axial T1-weighted postcontrast MRI depicting a giant glomus jugulare tumor: **(a)** axial and **(b)** coronal.

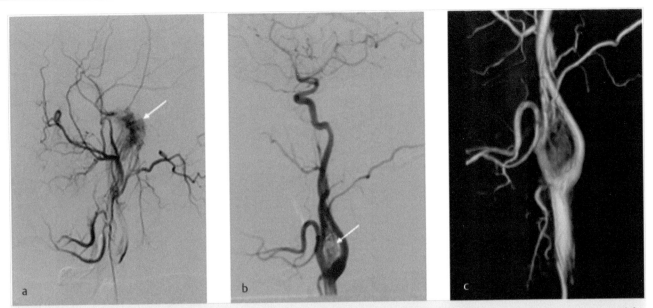

Fig. 26.6 Angiogram of a patient with multiple paragangliomas. (a) Left external carotid artery injection, lateral view, demonstrating a recurrent left glomus jugulare tumor (arrow). (b) Right common carotid artery injection, lateral view, demonstrating a right carotid body tumor. (c) Three-dimensional reconstruction of the right common carotid artery injection demonstrating the carotid body tumor.

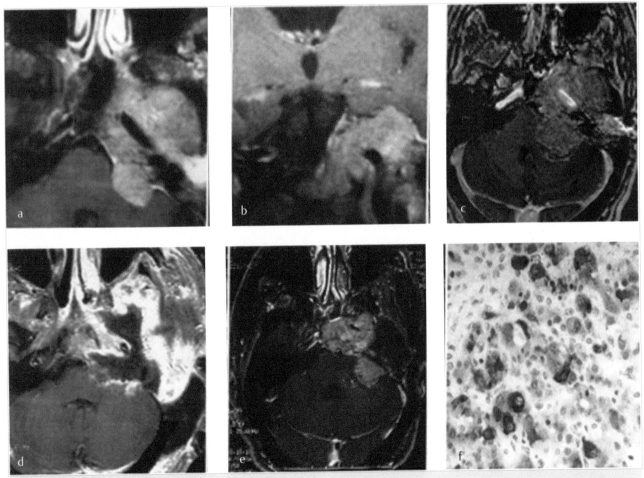

Fig. 26.7 Examples of malignant paraganglioma. (a,b) MRI after previous treatment with surgery and radiotherapy. (c) MRI showing marked growth a year later. (d) MRI after resection. (e) MRI showing rapid growth after 4 months. (f) Immunochemical staining for chromogranin. Note the brown granules in the cytoplasm. (Reproduced with permission from Al-Mefty O, Teixeira A, Complex tumors of the glomus jugulare: criteria, treatment, and outcome, J Neurosurg 2002;97(6):1356–1366.)

embolization after the tumor's blood supply has been delineated. The most critical aspect of angiographic evaluation in patients who have undergone previous embolization or carotid occlusion is the identification of new feeding vessels from the internal carotid artery and the vertebrobasilar circulation (▶ Fig. 26.12).[24]

26.3.4 Preoperative Preparation

With some modifications, the same preoperative protocol is used for all lesions of the jugular foramen. Audiologic and otolaryngologic evaluations are carried out, and speech evaluations and swallowing studies are conducted before surgery.

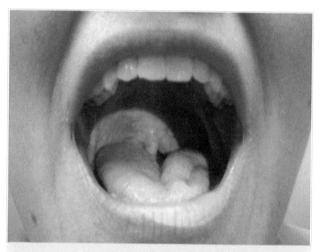

Fig. 26.8 Deviation of the soft palate with atrophy of the tongue as presenting symptoms in a patient who had a jugular foramen lesion.

Hormonal Studies

Paragangliomas have the potential to secrete a wide variety of neuropeptide hormones, including adrenocortical hormones, serotonin, catecholamines, and dopamine.[24,27] Patients who have hypersecreting tumors (catecholamine levels at least four times higher than normal) require preparation with combined alpha- and beta-blocker medication before surgery, angiography, or embolization. Beta-blockers should not be given before or without alpha-blockers. Screening for excess catecholamines is necessary in all patients who have a glomus jugulare tumor, and the actual treatment and duration of prophylaxis depend on the level of catecholamine secretion and its source. Patients who have these tumors might also harbor adrenal norepinephrine-secreting tumors. Accordingly, adrenal imaging is part of our work-up and is particularly important for patients who have hypersecreting tumors.

Diagnostic Imaging

MRI scans with and without contrast injection, angiography, and thin-cut bony-window CT scans constitute the radiologic workup needed to explore the anatomy of each patient's jugular fossa, temporal bone, and condyles, as well as the nature of the tumor (cystic or solid) and its extensions (intracranial, extracranial, or dumbbell) and bone involvement (the presence of sclerosis and enlargement of the canal). The dominant vertebral artery and the characteristics of the vertebrobasilar system are also studied. Special attention is paid to the venous phase with a view to determining the size, dominance, and tributaries (superior petrosal, inferior petrosal, and vein of Labbé) of the transverse and sigmoid sinuses as well as the position and size of the jugular bulb.

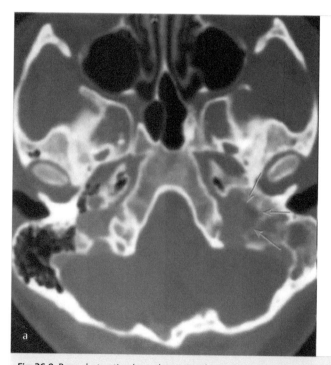
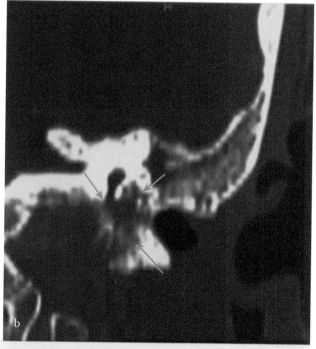

Fig. 26.9 Bone destruction by a glomus jugulare tumor, as seen on the bone window of a CT scan: **(a)** axial and **(b)** coronal.

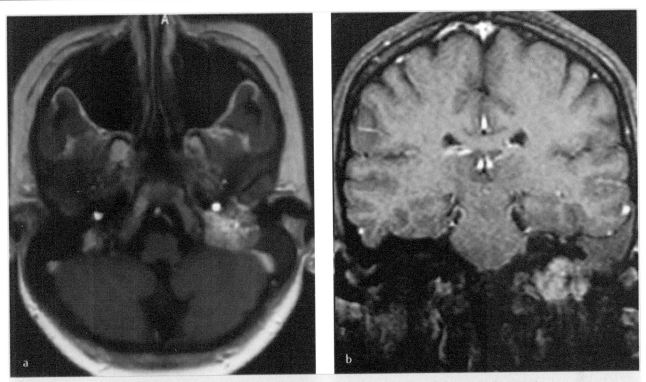

Fig. 26.10 Axial T1-weighted postcontrast MRI depicting the typical salt-and-pepper enhancement: **(a)** axial and **(b)** coronal.

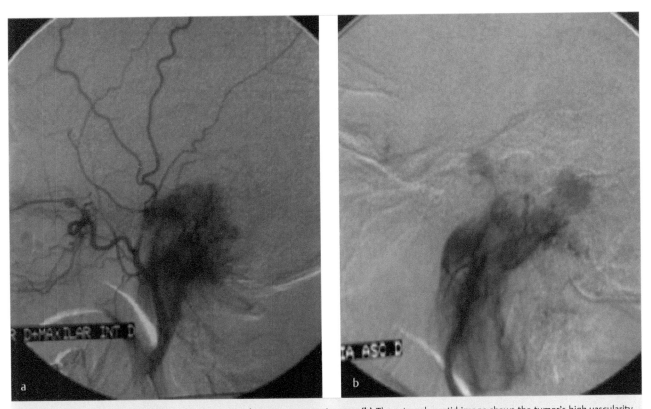

Fig. 26.11 **(a)** The typical appearance of a glomus jugulare tumor on angiogram. **(b)** The external carotid image shows the tumor's high vascularity, venous shunting, and blood supply through the ascending pharyngeal artery.

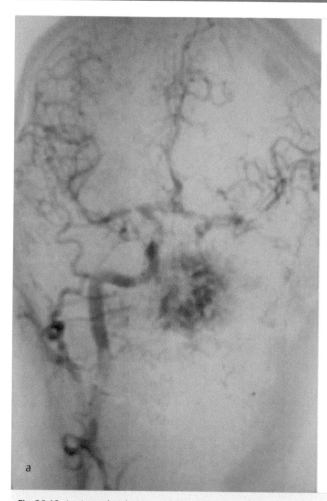
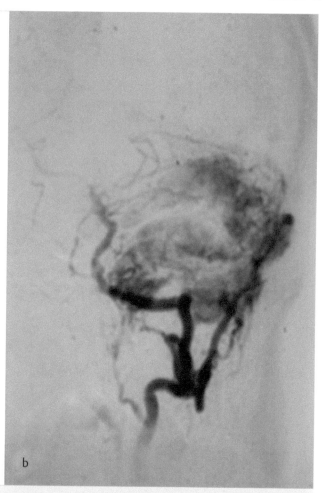

Fig. 26.12 Angiographic depiction of a new blood supply through the contralateral internal carotid artery and the vertebrobasilar system in a patient who had prior treatment with embolization and carotid occlusion. **(a)** Contralateral carotid injection. **(b)** Vertebral injection.

Embolization

Embolization is indicated for patients who have paragangliomas and other highly vascular lesions.[7,13,28] Surgery is more challenging when the patient has undergone prior embolization or carotid artery occlusion that was followed by development of new feeding vessels from the internal carotid and vertebrobasilar circulation.[24] Current techniques are successful for embolizing the tumor bed and reducing blood loss (▶ Fig. 26.13).

The thoroughness of embolization is critical, but partial embolization of the external carotid feeder augments the internal carotid feeders. Furthermore, embolization has accompanying risks and complications, including reflux cerebral emboli in the internal carotid artery, cranial nerve deficits from a "dangerous anastomosis," and tumor hemorrhage. Carrier and colleagues reported that preoperative embolization of the inferior petrosal sinus, the anterior condylar vein complex, and the posterior condylar vein reduced preoperative bleeding considerably.[29] Because of the absence of shift at the rigid structures of the jugular foramen, intraoperative image-guided frameless navigation is particularly useful during the surgical procedure.

Intraoperative Neurophysiological Monitoring

Cranial nerve X is monitored intraoperatively using an electromyographic endotracheal tube. Electromyographic needles are inserted into the facial musculature, the sternocleidomastoid muscle, and the tongue to monitor cranial nerves VII, XI, and XII, respectively. Auditory evoked potentials are obtained if hearing is present and no plan is made for closing the ear canal or resecting tumor from the middle ear. The external auditory speaker is placed under sterile conditions after the ear is prepared. Multiple paragangliomas present the greatest challenge to treating complex paragangliomas, because the treatment decision is based not on a single tumor but rather on the quality and length of the patient's life. Whether to treat, when to treat, and which tumors to treat, as well as with which modality (surgery or radiation) and in what sequence, are all questions that must be addressed at the first evaluation and thoroughly considered throughout the patient's follow-up. The surgeon must try to prevent the consequences of multiple bilateral cranial nerve deficits.[24]

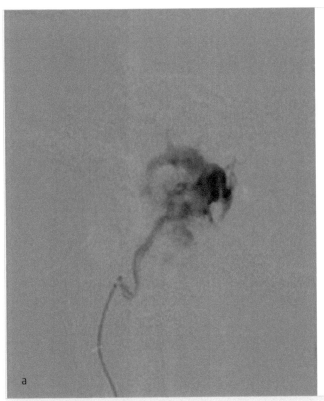
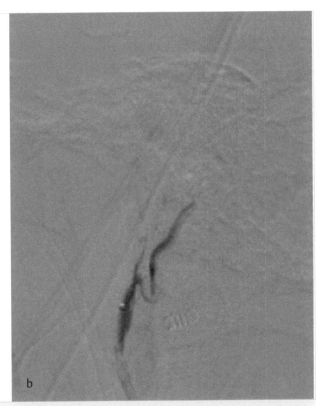

Fig. 26.13 Preoperative embolization is of great value in decreasing the tumor's blood supply, particularly from the external carotid artery. **(a)** Preembolization angiogram. **(b)** Postembolization angiogram.

26.3.5 Surgical Approach

The surgical approach is tailored in each patient to the findings of preoperative imaging, the local anatomy, and the tumor's characteristics and extension. Jugular foramen tumors that have an intracranial extension should be carefully evaluated with regard to size, position, infiltrative potential, and vascularization. On the basis of these data, the surgeon can then settle on the most appropriate approach.[30] Possible approaches include the infratemporal, combined infratemporal–posterior fossa, and combined approaches with a total petrosectomy.[24]

Patient Position

The patient is placed supine with the head elevated, turned away from the side of the lesion, and fixed in the three-point head frame (▶ Fig. 26.14). The abdomen and thigh are prepared for removal of fat and fascia lata grafts.

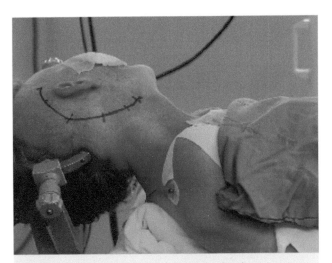

Fig. 26.14 Skin incision and patient positioning for glomus tumor surgery.

Incision and Soft Tissue Dissection

An open C-shaped incision is made behind the ear and extended up to the temporal area and down transversely along the natural skin crease in the neck. In selected patients in whom the middle ear is involved, the external ear canal is transected at the bony cartilaginous junction. The skin of the external ear canal is everted and closed as a blind sac. A small periosteal flap is kept attached to the skin flap and closed over the ear canal. The skin flap, including the auricle, is reflected anteriorly, and the sternomastoid muscle is detached from its insertion in the mastoid process. The neurovascular structures in the neck are dissected and exposed; these include the common carotid artery, internal carotid artery, external carotid artery, jugular vein, and cranial nerves IX–XII.

Bone Removal

The mastoidectomy is done using a high-speed drill, and bleeding is anticipated during drilling of the bone. The eardrum is removed, and the tumor is located in the middle ear. The semicircular canals are exposed, and the facial canal is located caudal to the lateral semicircular canal. The facial nerve is skeletonized from the stylomastoid foramen to the geniculate ganglion.

We have abandoned the practice of routine transposition of the facial nerve; after its skeletonization, we keep it in a tiny protective bony canal.[10] If the nerve needs to be transposed, it is moved out of the fallopian canal and secured anteriorly. A radical mastoidectomy exposes the sigmoid sinus down to the jugular bulb and in cases of intradural extension is followed by a lateral and low posterior fossa craniectomy.

Tumor Isolation

To isolate the tumor, the internal carotid artery and the jugular vein are followed upward toward the base of the skull. To expose the tumor, the posterior belly of the digastric muscle and the styloid musculature is transected and the styloid process is removed. The ascending mandibular ramus is dislocated anteriorly if necessary. The sigmoid sinus is then ligated distal to the tumor's extension and proximal to the mastoid emissary vein. If the tumor extends into the middle ear or along the petrous carotid artery, the remnant of skin in the external ear canal is removed with the tympanic membrane. The internal carotid artery is exposed in the petrous canal by drilling the bone, if not already destroyed by the tumor, over the carotid canal. The Eustachian tube is obliterated using a piece of muscle. The anterior pole of the tumor is then dissected from the internal carotid artery, and the small feeding arteries are coagulated with bipolar electrocautery. At this stage, the extradural tumor is completely exposed.

If the tumor does not extend into the middle ear, the approach should be modified to preserve both the middle and the inner ear, so that the tumor is exposed in the infralabyrinthine space. The superior pole of the tumor is freed from the infratemporal fossa. The inferior pole is removed by dissecting and elevating the jugular vein after it is ligated, to prevent early venous drainage. The lower cranial nerves are preserved as they emerge from the jugular foramen. Intrabulbar dissection, a maneuver described by Al-Mefty and Teixeira, helps preserve the lower cranial nerves.[24] This maneuver can be used for any tumor so long as the tumor itself has not penetrated the wall of the jugular bulb or actually infiltrated the cranial nerves. The outer wall of the lower sigmoid sinus is incised along the jugular bulb into the jugular vein. The tumor is then removed from inside the jugular bulb and the sigmoid sinus, and the tail end of the jugular vein is separated from the lower cranial nerves. The innermost venous wall separating the tumor from the nerves is left in situ to minimize dissection, trauma, manipulation, and devascularization of the lower cranial nerves.

Using this technique helps preserve the immediate postoperative function of the lower cranial nerves for patients in whom the tumor does not transgress the venous wall at the jugular foramen. When the tumor does transgress the venous wall, the cranial nerves can be infiltrated on a microanatomical level despite having normal function. In such situations, total resection may not be possible without sacrificing these nerves. Profuse bleeding from the inferior petrosal artery is controlled through gentle and judicious packing with appropriate hemostatic materials.

Intradural Tumor Removal

To remove the intradural portion of the tumor, the dura mater is incised posterior to the sigmoid sinus and carried forward, and the intradural extension of the tumor is exposed. The cranial nerves (VIII–XII) are meticulously dissected from the tumor and kept intact. Tumor encroachment on the medulla is removed through microdissection, and the basilar artery, the anteroinferior cerebellar artery (AICA), and the posteroinferior cerebellar artery (PICA) are dissected from the tumor and preserved. Any tumor extension into the foramen magnum is followed and removed after it is freed from the lateral and anterior surfaces of the medulla and the vertebrobasilar junction. When it is giant, the tumor should be isolated for safe surgical removal. This is best done in one stage through the combined posterior fossa and infratemporal approach described earlier.[31] This approach allows the tumor to be devascularized from the intrapetrous carotid artery. It is also used to separate the tumor from the posterior fossa and to dissect the lower portion from the nerves with minimal blood loss while preserving the vessels.

Resecting tumors of the glomus jugulare requires special techniques in the handling of both arterial and venous dissection. Although paragangliomas engulf, adhere to, and receive blood from the internal carotid artery, with the aid of the operating microscope, a plane of dissection can be identified to separate the tumor from the carotid. Thus the carotid artery does not need to be sacrificed or reconstructed. Because exposing tumors of the glomus jugulare requires neck dissection, associated tumors of the carotid body can be removed at the same time without additional morbidity or undue lengthening of the operating time. Glomus jugulare tumors often shunt blood with high venous outflow. Accordingly, they should be handled as arteriovenous malformations. Thus venous drainage from the tumor should be preserved and the proximal end of the jugular vein should not be ligated until the tumor is isolated and its arterial supply is devascularized.

Closure

After total removal of the tumor is assured, the Eustachian tube (if exposed) is covered with a small piece of muscle and fascia. The dura mater is repaired with a graft of fascia lata, and the cavity is obliterated with fat. The temporal muscle is swung inferiorly and sutured to the sternomastoid muscle, and the skin is closed in two layers.

26.3.6 Postoperative Care

The patient's ability to swallow is tested postoperatively, and oral intake is allowed only if these studies show satisfactory results, which ensure that the function of the lower cranial nerves can protect the airway. Otherwise, the patient is kept on transpyloric feeding by Dobhoff tube until swallowing recovers. Adaptations are made for satisfactory airway protection, and other appropriate precautions are taken.

A CT scan is obtained during the early postoperative period to check for hemorrhage, hydrocephalus, edema, and infarction. Any residual tumor is better assessed on later contrast-enhanced and fat-suppression MRIs.

26.3.7 Reconstruction

Large surgical defects must be repaired using vascularized flaps (temporalis fascia, cervical fascia, sternocleidomastoid muscle, and temporalis muscle). Reconstruction of the carotid artery as a graft bypass to the middle cerebral artery may be necessary if the carotid is injured beyond repair. Facial nerve reconstruction with the greater auricular nerve, the sural nerve, or a 12/7 anastomosis might be needed if the facial nerve was transected.

26.3.8 Results

The results of surgical treatment of glomus jugulare tumors have improved drastically with advances in skull base surgery. Surgical resection with long-term follow-up shows the effectiveness of total removal in achieving a cure (▶ Fig. 26.15).[21,23,32] Even the most formidable tumors have been successfully resected with no mortality and low morbidity.[24,33] Deficits of the lower cranial nerves are the main surgical complications. However, the success in maintaining function has alleviated many of these concerns, and vigilant pulmonary toilet postoperatively has minimized pulmonary complications from aspiration until the patient adapts or vocal cord medialization is done. Thus total resection is indicated and successful in treating complex glomus jugulare tumors despite the challenge encountered.[24] The rarely encountered malignant type, however, carries a poor prognosis.[24,34]

26.3.9 Other Treatments

Radiation therapy has long been used to treat glomus tumors, particularly those that are only partially removed or that have recurred. However, glomus tumors are known to be radioresistant, and radiation often induces fibrosis, mainly along the vessels supplying the tumor. Furthermore, persistent viable tumors are often present long after the patient undergoes radiation therapy. Radiation therapy has also been associated with long-term side effects that include osteonecrosis of the temporal bone, development of a new malignancy, and demyelination. Radiosurgery appears to provide control if the target size is within the optimal size for treatment, and the preliminary results of this treatment suggest a symptomatic improvement of cranial nerve function, but the long-term recurrence rate is still unknown.[35]

26.3.10 Complications

In patients who have glomus jugulare tumors, mortality is around 1%. Leaks of cerebrospinal fluid (CSF) occur in 8% of patients. Other complications include aspiration, wound infection, pneumonia, and meningitis.[35] Postoperative CSF leakage is one of the most important complications in the surgery of jugular fossa tumors. A CSF leak can occur either from the skin or, more often, in the form of rhinorrhea. Meticulous closure is very important in preventing the leak. If a leak does occur, spinal drainage is carried out for 72 hours. If the leak continues, the wound is reexplored. If meningitis occurs as a result of a CSF leak, it is treated with antibiotics and spinal drainage.

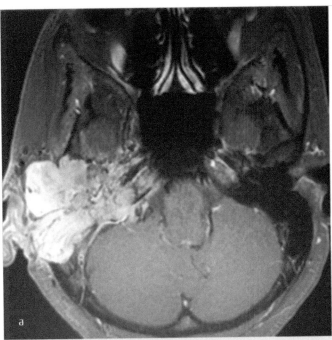 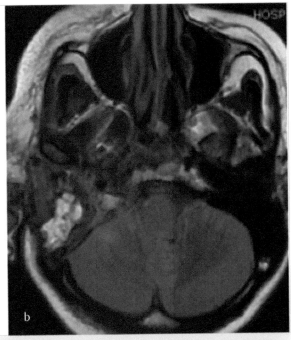

Fig. 26.15 Complete surgical resection is successful in the overwhelming number of patients who have large or giant glomus tumors and provides the prospect of cure. (a) Preoperative MRI depicting a giant glomus tumor. (b) Postoperative MRI demonstrating complete resection; note the hyperintensity of the fat graft used for reconstruction.

26.3.11 Follow-up and Rehabilitation

After surgery, each patient is followed up with MRI images at 3 months, 6 months, and then annually to detect any recurrence. Dysphonic symptoms are treated with medialization of the vocal cords. Most patients adapt to unilateral deficits of the lower cranial nerves, but the older the patient, the longer the recovery. Hence aspiration must be avoided and tube feeding is needed in the early stages, or a jejunostomy is done if aspiration persists for prolonged periods of time. Eye weights or tarsorrhaphy may be necessary if facial weakness is present.

26.4 Schwannomas

26.4.1 Pathology

Jugular foramen schwannomas are a rare pathological condition comprising 2 to 4% of intracranial schwannomas, with approximately 100 cases reported in the literature.[7,36] Schwannomas located at the jugular foramen may arise from the glossopharyngeal, vagus, or accessory nerves.[7,36,37] The proximity and clinical manifestation of schwannomas originating from the hypoglossal nerve have led some authors to classify these tumors with jugular foramen schwannomas. These tumors can originate from the cisternal portion of the nerve and present with major intracranial growth, or from the foraminal portion expanding the bone, or from the distal portion and present with extracranial growth. Some appear with both extra- and intracranial growth through an enlarged jugular foramen.[7] Pellet and colleagues have classified jugular foramen schwannomas into four types[38]:

- Type A: primarily intracranial, minimal extension into the jugular foramen
- Type B: primarily intraosseous, with or without an intracranial extension
- Type C: primarily extracranial, minimal extension into the jugular foramen
- Type D: saddlebag- or dumbbell-shaped intra- and extracranial extensions

26.4.2 Clinical Presentation

The primary symptoms of a jugular foramen schwannoma include dizziness, hearing loss, dysphagia, diplopia, tongue paresis, and hoarseness.[37] Preoperative findings include mainly audiovestibular (hearing loss, tinnitus, and dizziness) and lower cranial nerve signs (dysphagia, hoarseness, weakness of the shoulder, and tongue paresis).[36,37] Almost all patients who have dumbbell-shaped schwannomas also have glossopharyngeal and vagal deficits. Hypoglossal and accessory nerve deficits appear in most patients, but hearing loss is less common.[7] In cases of large tumors, the abducens and facial nerves can be affected and patients may develop cerebellar signs or hydrocephalus. Careful evaluation of the lower cranial nerves is particularly important in jugular foramen schwannomas, because they are the source of most life-threatening postoperative complications.

26.4.3 Appearance on Diagnostic Imaging

An enlarged jugular foramen having well-delineated sclerotic margins is seen on thin-cut CT scans with bone algorithms.[7,25,39] Schwannomas usually expand the foramen without eroding it and have a low to isointense signal on T1-weighted images and a high signal on T2-weighted images.[40] The tumor shows moderate to marked enhancement after the injection of gadolinium.[7,25,37,39,41] Cystic degeneration can occur and is well delineated on MRIs (▶ Fig. 26.16).[37,42] On conventional or MR angiography, schwannomas are avascular.[7]

26.4.4 Preoperative Preparation

Diagnostic imaging and intraoperative neurophysiological monitoring are done in the same way as for patients with glomus tumors. Hormonal studies and embolization are not needed.

26.4.5 Surgical Approach

The real challenge in neurosurgical treatment of these tumors is to preserve the function of the lower cranial nerves while achieving radical resection and decreasing the risk of recurrence. A repeated operation drastically increases the chance of injury to the lower cranial nerves. These challenges are found especially in patients who have dumbbell-shaped tumors, in which the nerves are at risk during resection of the intracranial, intraforaminal, and extracranial sections. Schwannomas differ from glomus tumors and meningiomas within the jugular foramen and fossa because they compress rather than invade the jugular bulb—and the nerves of origin are positioned anterior to this structure. The labyrinth is also preserved, as hearing might occasionally improve after removal of the tumor. Because schwannomas within the jugular foramen tend to displace the jugular bulb posteriorly, the suprajugular approach allows the surgeon to remove the tumor without opening the wall of the bulb. Even if preoperative studies reveal an absence of flow into the jugular bulb, the transjugular approach is not used, because the sinus usually recovers its patency after decompression. The suprajugular approach is essentially a presigmoid infralabyrinthine route.

The suprajugular approach is used if the tumor extends anteriorly to the jugular bulb. A postauricular incision is made, and the internal carotid artery, external carotid artery, and internal jugular vein, as well as cranial nerves IX to XII, are identified in the cervical region. The sternomastoid muscle is dissected, mobilized, and reflected inferiorly. A mastoidectomy is followed by complete skeletonization of the sigmoid sinus, jugular bulb, and jugular vein. The presigmoid, infralabyrinthine space is exposed and the dura mater is identified superior to the patent jugular bulb and inferior to the labyrinth. After the cerebellomedullary cistern is opened, releasing CSF, the tumor is exposed and debulked. The lower cranial nerves (IX–XII), the PICA, the AICA, and the vertebral artery are dissected away from the tumor through the arachnoid plane, and the lesion is radically removed. The removal of a schwannoma is accomplished without sectioning the ear canal, entering the middle ear, or transposing the facial nerve. Some surgeons transpose the facial nerve for

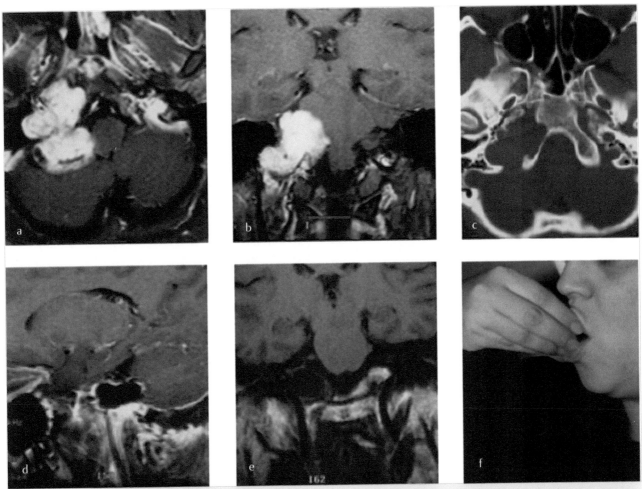

Fig. 26.16 Jugular foramen schwannoma. T1-weighted **(a)** axial and **(b)** coronal MRI with gadolinium demonstrating an enhancing lesion extending through the jugular foramen into the high cervical region. **(c)** Preoperative CT scan demonstrating the scalloping of the bone at the jugular foramen, classically associated with underlying schwannoma. Postoperative MRI scan, **(d)** coronal and **(e)** sagittal planes, demonstrating complete resection. **(f)** Postoperative photograph demonstrating intact swallowing function.

selective circumstances, such as when scar tissue from a previous operation impedes control of the carotid artery and safe removal, the tumor has a large extension anteriorly to the petrous apex, or the middle ear is extensively involved.[36,43]

Because schwannomas are avascular and are largely soft and amenable to suction decompression, we have not found a need to transpose the facial nerve. Dumbbell-shaped jugular foramen schwannomas present a special challenge, with a risk of injury to the lower cranial nerves intracranially, intraforaminally, and extracranially.[7] However, these tumors can be removed without creating additional neurological deficits. Furthermore, the patient can be expected to recover function in the affected cranial nerves.[7]

26.4.6 Postoperative Course

In these patients, the acute development of postoperative deficits before the development of compensatory mechanisms requires careful attention. Speech pathology and otolaryngological evaluations with pre- and postoperative swallowing studies are obtained. Oral intake is withheld and parenteral nutrition is administered. Swallowing exercises and soft mechanical diets

with swallowing precautions are prescribed if the patient exhibits a risk of aspiration. Vocal cord medialization is done if there is persistent dysphasia or aspiration.

26.4.7 Results

Complete excision is achieved in the majority of patients who have a schwannoma.[7,37,42,44] Preoperative palsy of cranial nerves V, VI, VII, IX, X, and XII can improve after the removal of a jugular foramen schwannoma.[7,37] Hearing can also improve.[7,42]

26.4.8 Other Treatments

Stereotactic radiosurgery can be offered to patients who have small tumors or intact lower cranial nerve function and to those who have declined surgery. It is also considered for patients who have residual or recurrent tumors after microsurgical resection.[45] However, experience with this modality is limited due to the rarity of these tumors. We prefer to reserve radiosurgery treatment for the rare patient in whom the venous anatomy presents a considerable risk, such as when the patient has a single functioning ipsilateral sigmoid sinus and jugular bulb (► Fig. 26.17).

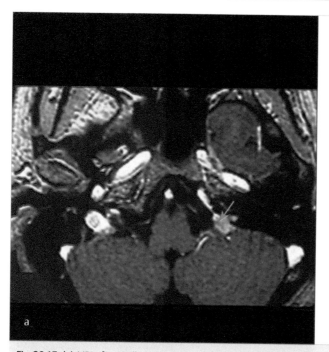
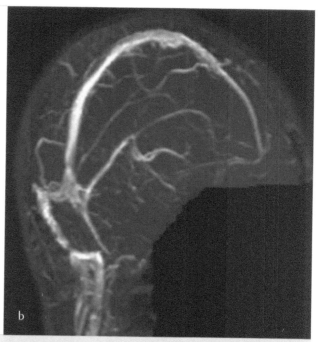

Fig. 26.17 (a) MRI of a small intraforaminal schwannoma. (b) MR venography image showing a single and dominant drainage through the corresponding jugular bulb. Radiosurgery might be preferable because of the increased risks presented by the venous configuration.

26.5 Meningiomas

26.5.1 Pathology

Primary jugular fossa meningiomas are one of the rarest subgroups of meningioma, with fewer than 40 cases reported in the literature.[1,46] They constitute 9% of jugular fossa tumors.[47] These meningiomas presumably arise from arachnoid cells lining the jugular bulb in the jugular fossa.[1] Women are affected more than men.[1] The transitional type of meningioma is most commonly found, closely followed by the meningotheliomatous type and then by the less common psammomatous meningioma.[48] Their intimate relationship with the lower cranial nerves and jugular bulb, their involvement of the temporal bone, and their tendency to extend intracranially and extracranially have traditionally made their removal fraught with difficulty.[1] As a result, the surgeon should tailor the approach to the local anatomy (the tumor–neurovascular relationship).

26.5.2 Clinical Presentation

The symptoms of a jugular foramen meningioma are similar to those of a schwannoma, with signs of lower cranial nerve deficits and altered hearing.[1]

26.5.3 Appearance on Diagnostic Imaging

A meningioma of the jugular foramen permeates and shows sclerotic changes on bone algorithm CT studies (▶ Fig. 26.18).

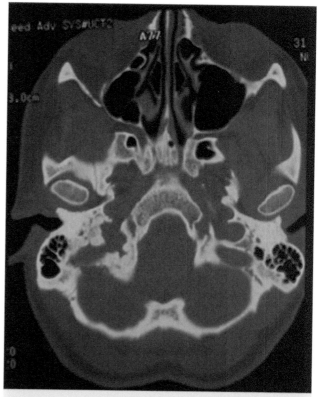

Fig. 26.18 CT scan of a jugular foramen meningioma showing bone invasion with hyperostotic features, which is characteristic of meningiomas.

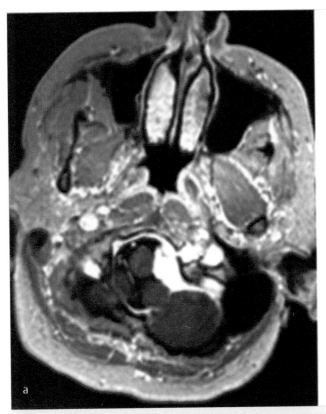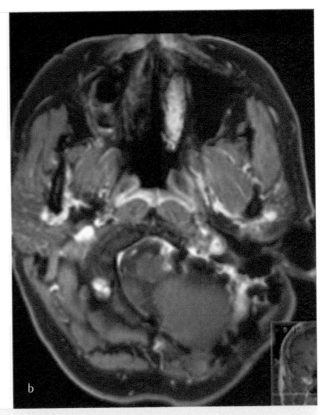

Fig. 26.19 Axial T1-weighted postcontrast MRI of a jugular foramen meningioma showing intense homogeneous enhancement and the typical dural tail. **(a)** Preoperative image. **(b)** Postoperative image.

These lesions are most often isointense or of low signal on T1-weighted MRI and of intermediate signal intensity on T2-weighted images. They also show avid, homogeneous enhancement on contrast MRIs, as well as a dural tail (▶ Fig. 26.19). Meningiomas of the jugular foramen may demonstrate a relatively more aggressive appearance than similar intracranial lesions but most often retain their CSF/vascular cleft against the brain parenchyma intracranially. Angiography shows avid arterial blushing and prolonged contrast retention into the venous phase.[37] MRAs have mostly replaced conventional angiography as a preoperative evaluation.

26.5.4 Preoperative Preparation

The steps to prepare the patient for surgery are similar to those for patients who have glomus tumors and schwannomas. Particular emphasis is given to the position, patency, and size of the jugular bulb as seen on MRA performed during both arterial and venous phases.

26.5.5 Surgical Approach

For patients who have meningiomas, the involved dura mater and the bone of the jugular fossa should be resected to minimize the chance of tumor recurrence.[1] The surgical approach is tailored to the local anatomy of the tumor and its relation to the neurovascular structures. Three different routes can be used. The suprajugular approach, a presigmoid, infralabyrinthine route, is chosen if the jugular bulb is patent and the tumor extends

primarily anteriorly. The retrojugular approach, a transcondylar, transtubercle, retrosigmoid route, is chosen if the jugular bulb is patent and the tumor extends primarily posteriorly.

The transjugular approach, an infratemporal route, is chosen for patients in whom the jugular bulb is totally occluded by the tumor. The position, incision, and soft tissue dissection for each approach are similar to those used for schwannomas.

The Suprajugular Approach

In the suprajugular approach, a total mastoidectomy is done with complete skeletonization of the sigmoid sinus, jugular bulb, and jugular vein. The jugular fossa is accessed in the presigmoid infralabyrinthine space. The dura mater located superior to the patent jugular bulb and inferior to the labyrinth is opened. CSF is released from the cerebellomedullary cistern, and the tumor is dissected away from the lower cranial nerves (IX–XI), the PICA, the AICA, and the vertebral artery while preserving the arachnoidal surgical dissection planes. The tumor is debulked with suction and bipolar coagulation or with an ultrasonic aspirator. The procedure is completed with microsurgical radical resection of the tumor.

The Retrojugular Approach

In the retrojugular approach, the suboccipital bone is exposed and a small, inferior, lateral suboccipital craniotomy is performed, followed by a mastoidectomy and complete skeletonization of the sigmoid sinus, jugular bulb, and jugular vein. Drilling approximately a third of the condyle usually suffices for exposure; postoperative stabilization is not necessary. Attention is then turned to the jugular tubercle, which is completely drilled away to facilitate opening of the jugular fossa, which lodges the jugular bulb. With the aid of an operating microscope, the dura mater is incised along the posterior border of the sigmoid sinus. The tumor is carefully separated from the medulla oblongata, lower cranial nerves, vertebral artery, and PICA along arachnoidal planes and is followed toward the jugular fossa. Careful, meticulous dissection of the tumor from the jugular bulb and the wall of the jugular vein is important. Ultrasonic aspiration or suction and bipolar coagulation are used to debulk the tumor.

The Transjugular Approach

For patients in whom the meningioma has invaded the sinus and occupied the jugular bulb, a transjugular approach similar to that for a glomus tumor is used (▶ Fig. 26.20). The neurovascular structures in the neck (cranial nerves IX–XII, jugular vein, and carotid artery) are dissected and exposed. A radical mastoidectomy exposes the sigmoid sinus down to the jugular bulb and is followed by a posterior fossa craniotomy. The jugular vein is followed superiorly to the jugular bulb. To enlarge the exposure, the posterior belly of the digastric muscle and the styloid musculature are transected and the styloid process is removed. The sigmoid sinus and jugular vein are ligated at a location proximal to the mastoid emissary vein and distal to the tumor obstruction. The inferior pole of the tumor is then dissected off the internal carotid artery and the jugular vein. The extradural tumor is thus completely exposed.

Bleeding from the inferior petrosal sinus may be profuse and is controlled by packing with Gelfoam. With the aid of the microscope, the dura mater is opened posterior to the sigmoid

sinus and carried forward. The intradural tumor extension is then exposed. Meticulous intradural dissection of the tumor, performed while maintaining the arachnoidal dissection planes, helps preserve the function of the lower cranial nerves and the vertebral artery, the PICA, and the AICA at the anterolateral surface of the medulla oblongata.

26.5.6 Results

Radical tumor removal can be achieved in 83 to 100% of patients who have jugular fossa meningiomas.[1,46,47] The most common complications are transient deficits of the lower cranial nerves, which resolve or are compensated for in all patients within 1 month.[1,47] Accordingly, jugular fossa meningiomas can be radically resected with the expectation of a good outcome provided that extensive evaluation and appropriate tailoring of the operative approach are done.

26.5.7 Other Treatments

As in the case of schwannomas, experience with radiosurgery is limited because of the rarity of these tumors. The results, however, are expected to be the same as those of radiosurgery for basal meningiomas when it is used for residual or recurrent tumors or as the primary treatment. Recent literature is expanding the data on the efficacy, technique, control rates, risks, and complications of this treatment. The goal of radiosurgery, however, is "control," and long-term results are not yet available. The average follow-up for the usual reported radiosurgery series is too short to ascertain significant control of this slow-growing tumor. The risks and complications of radiosurgery are not negligible and include seizures, brain edema, neurological

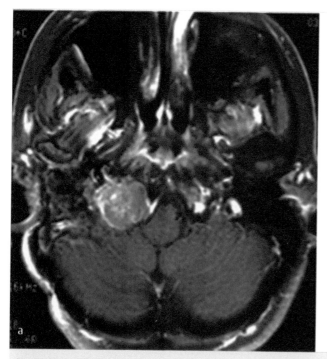
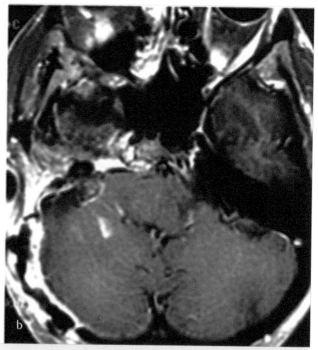

Fig. 26.20 Axial T1-weighted postcontrast MRI of a patient who had a jugular foramen meningioma that involved and occupied the jugular bulb. This lesion was targeted through the transjugular approach. (a) Preoperative image. (b) Postoperative image.

deficits, cranial nerve deficits, and the potential for radiation-induced tumors or a new malignant progression. Some authors have reported a pattern of aggressive recurrence after years of control using radiosurgery.[49] For tumors of the jugular foramen, we prefer to reserve radiosurgery for the rare patient in whom the venous anatomy presents a considerable risk, such as a patient having a single functioning ipsilateral sigmoid sinus and jugular bulb or a recurrent tumor, or for patients who are unsuitable for or decline surgery.

References

[1] Arnautović KI, Al-Mefty O. Primary meningiomas of the jugular fossa. J Neurosurg. 2002; 97(1):12–20

[2] Katsuta T, Rhoton AL, Jr, Matsushima T. The jugular foramen: microsurgical anatomy and operative approaches. Neurosurgery. 1997; 41(1):149–201; discussion 2

[3] Lustig LR, Jackler RK. The variable relationship between the lower cranial nerves and jugular foramen tumors: implications for neural preservation. Am J Otol. 1996; 17(4):658–668

[4] Rhoton AL, Jr. Jugular foramen. Neurosurgery. 2000; 47(3) Suppl:S267–S285

[5] Ozveren MF, Türe U. The microsurgical anatomy of the glossopharyngeal nerve with respect to the jugular foramen lesions. Neurosurg Focus. 2004; 17(2):E3

[6] Inserra MM, Pfister M, Jackler RK. Anatomy involved in the jugular foramen approach for jugulotympanic paraganglioma resection. Neurosurg Focus. 2004; 17(2):E6

[7] Kadri PA, Al-Mefty O. Surgical treatment of dumbbell-shaped jugular foramen schwannomas. Neurosurg Focus. 2004; 17(2):E9

[8] Lee YB, Kim SH, Kim HT, Kim JH, Kim MH, Ko Y. Jugular foramen neurilemmoma mimicking an intra-axial brainstem tumor—a case report. J Korean Med Sci. 1996; 11(3):282–284

[9] Tekdemir I, Tuccar E, Aslan A, Elhan A, Ersoy M, Deda H. Comprehensive microsurgical anatomy of the jugular foramen and review of terminology. J Clin Neurosci. 2001; 8(4):351–356

[10] Borba LA, Ale-Bark S, London C. Surgical treatment of glomus jugulare tumors without rerouting of the facial nerve: an infralabyrinthine approach. Neurosurg Focus. 2004; 17(2):E8

[11] Chao CK, Sheen TS, Lien HC, Hsu MM. Metastatic carcinoma to the jugular foramen. Otolaryngol Head Neck Surg. 2000; 122(6):922–923

[12] Harvey SA, Wiet RJ, Kazan R. Chondrosarcoma of the jugular foramen. Am J Otol. 1994; 15(2):257–263

[13] Ramina R, Maniglia JJ, Fernandes YB, Paschoal JR, Pfeilsticker LN, Coelho Neto M. Tumors of the jugular foramen: diagnosis and management. Neurosurgery. 2005; 57(1) Suppl:59–68

[14] Iwasaki S, Ito K, Takai Y, Morita A, Murofushi T. Chondroid chordoma at the jugular foramen causing retrolabyrinthine lesions in both the cochlear and vestibular branches of the eighth cranial nerve. Ann Otol Rhinol Laryngol. 2004; 113(1):82–86

[15] Prasanna AV, Muzumdar DP, Goel A. Lipoma in the region of the jugular foramen. Neurol India. 2003; 51(1):77–78

[16] Yamazaki T, Kuroki T, Katsume K, Kameda N. Peripheral primitive neuroectodermal tumor of the jugular foramen: case report. Neurosurgery. 2002; 51(5):1286–1289

[17] Mirza S, Dutt SN, Irving RM. Jugular foramen abscess. Otol Neurotol. 2001; 22(6):973–974

[18] Rosenwasser H. Carotid body tumor of the middle ear and mastoid. Arch Otolaryngol. 1945; 41:64–67

[19] Jackson CG, Kaylie DM, Coppit G, Gardner EK. Glomus jugulare tumors with intracranial extension. Neurosurg Focus. 2004; 17(2):E7

[20] Batsakis J. Paraganglioma of the head and neck. In: Batsakis J, ed. Tumors of the Head and Neck: Clinical and Pathological Considerations. Baltimore: Williams and Wilkins; 1979:369–380

[21] Borba LA, Al-Mefty O. Paragangliomas of the skull base. Neurosurg Q. 1995; 5(4):255–277

[22] Fisch U. Infratemporal fossa approach for lesions in the temporal bone and base of the skull. Adv Otorhinolaryngol. 1984; 34:254–266

[23] Jackson CG. Basic surgical principles of neurotologic skull base surgery. Laryngoscope. 1993; 103(11 Pt 2) Suppl 60:29–44

[24] Al-Mefty O, Teixeira A. Complex tumors of the glomus jugulare: criteria, treatment, and outcome. J Neurosurg. 2002; 97(6):1356–1366

[25] Löwenheim H, Koerbel A, Ebner FH, Kumagami H, Ernemann U, Tatagiba M. Differentiating imaging findings in primary and secondary tumors of the jugular foramen. Neurosurg Rev. 2006; 29(1):1–11, discussion 12–13

[26] Oghalai JS, Leung MK, Jackler RK, McDermott MW. Transjugular craniotomy for the management of jugular foramen tumors with intracranial extension. Otol Neurotol. 2004; 25(4):570–579

[27] Borba LA, Al-Mefty O. Intravagal paragangliomas: report of four cases. Neurosurgery. 1996; 38(3):569–575

[28] Kinney SE. Glomus jugulare tumors with intracranial extension. Am J Otol. 1979; 1(2):67–71

[29] Carrier DA, Arriaga MA, Gorum MJ, Dahlen RT, Johnson SP. Preoperative embolization of anastomoses of the jugular bulb: an adjuvant in jugular foramen surgery. AJNR Am J Neuroradiol. 1997; 18(7):1252–1256

[30] Fisch U.. Intracranial extension of jugular foramen tumors. Otol Neurotol. 2004; 25(6):1041, author reply 2

[31] Al-Mefty O, Fox JL, Rifai A, Smith RR. A combined infratemporal and posterior fossa approach for the removal of giant glomus tumors and chondrosarcomas. Surg Neurol. 1987; 28(6):423–431

[32] Michael LM, II, Robertson JH. Glomus jugulare tumors: historical overview of the management of this disease. Neurosurg Focus. 2004; 17(2):E1

[33] Borba LA, Araújo JC, de Oliveira JG, et al. Surgical management of glomus jugulare tumors: a proposal for approach selection based on tumor relationships with the facial nerve. J Neurosurg. 2010; 112(1):88–98

[34] Bojrab DI, Bhansali SA, Glasscock ME, III. Metastatic glomus jugulare: long-term followup. Otolaryngol Head Neck Surg. 1991; 104(2):261–264

[35] Gottfried ON, Liu JK, Couldwell WT. Comparison of radiosurgery and conventional surgery for the treatment of glomus jugulare tumors. Neurosurg Focus. 2004; 17(2):E4

[36] Cokkeser Y, Brackmann DE, Fayad JN. Conservative facial nerve management in jugular foramen schwannomas. Am J Otol. 2000; 21(2):270–274

[37] Wilson MA, Hillman TA, Wiggins RH, Shelton C. Jugular foramen schwannomas: diagnosis, management, and outcomes. Laryngoscope. 2005; 115(8):1486–1492

[38] Pellet W, Cannoni M, Pech A. The widened transcochlear approach to jugular foramen tumors. J Neurosurg. 1988; 69(6):887–894

[39] Eldevik OP, Gabrielsen TO, Jacobsen EA. Imaging findings in schwannomas of the jugular foramen. AJNR Am J Neuroradiol. 2000; 21(6):1139–1144

[40] Flint D, Fagan P, Sheehy J. An intracranial vagal schwannoma without jugular foramen erosion or vagal dysfunction. Otolaryngol Head Neck Surg. 2005; 132(3):507–508

[41] Valvassori G, Palacios E. Schwannoma of the jugular foramen. Ear Nose Throat J. 1998; 77(9):732

[42] Carvalho GA, Tatagiba M, Samii M. Cystic schwannomas of the jugular foramen: clinical and surgical remarks. Neurosurgery. 2000; 46(3):560–566

[43] Al-Mefty O. Atlas of Meningiomas. New York: Lippincott-Raven Press, 1997

[44] Ramina R, Maniglia JJ, Fernandes YB, et al. Jugular foramen tumors: diagnosis and treatment. Neurosurg Focus. 2004; 17(2):E5

[45] Muthukumar N, Kondziolka D, Lunsford LD, Flickinger JC. Stereotactic radiosurgery for jugular foramen schwannomas. Surg Neurol. 1999; 52(2):172–179

[46] Gilbert ME, Shelton C, McDonald A, et al. Meningioma of the jugular foramen: glomus jugulare mimic and surgical challenge. Laryngoscope. 2004; 114(1):25–32

[47] Ramina R, Neto MC, Fernandes YB, Aguiar PH, de Meneses MS, Torres LF. Meningiomas of the jugular foramen. Neurosurg Rev. 2006; 29(1):55–60

[48] Molony TB, Brackmann DE, Lo WW. Meningiomas of the jugular foramen. Otolaryngol Head Neck Surg. 1992; 106(2):128–136

[49] Couldwell WT, Cole CD, Al-Mefty O. Patterns of skull base meningioma progression after failed radiosurgery. J Neurosurg. 2007; 106(1):30–35

27 Tumors of the Craniovertebral Junction

Karolyn Au, Michael Paci, Michael Wang, and Jacques Morcos

Summary

The complex anatomy of the craniovertebral junction is critical both to allow necessary movement of the head and to prevent excess motion that would injure the neurologic and vascular structures at the cervicomedullary junction. Pathology in this area may disrupt the stability of the craniovertebral junction or require surgical intervention that introduces instability. Surgical approaches have been developed to access the region from any direction. Thorough knowledge of the regional anatomy, surgical approaches and their variants, and stabilization techniques is critical to safely manage tumors in this location. This chapter reviews the relevant osseoligamentous, vascular, and neurologic structures; describes investigations and selection of surgical approach; and discusses potential pitfalls of carrying out surgery in this location.

Keywords: craniocervical junction, cervicomedullary junction, clivus, foramen magnum, atlanto-occipital, atlantoaxial

27.1 Introduction

Management of tumors that arise at the craniovertebral junction (CVJ) is made challenging by the complex osseoligamentous, vascular, and neural anatomy of the region as well as the need to balance dynamic function with mechanical stability. Both erosive neoplasms and extensive operative approaches can destroy bone, joints, and ligaments, resulting in excess movement that encroaches on the traversing neurovascular elements. Tumor compression or invasion, surgical manipulation, or ischemia can compromise the cervicomedullary junction, which contains critical autonomous neurologic functions, the motor decussation, and multiple cranial nerve nuclei, as well as the cranial nerves themselves. A number of surgical approaches have been developed to access the CVJ from all directions, using corridors from different trajectories to decrease morbidity on neighboring structures. This chapter describes the basic anatomy of the CVJ, outlines the primary surgical approaches for gaining access to the region, and discusses considerations for stabilization.

27.2 Surgical Anatomy

The CVJ, which comprises the occiput, atlas, and axis and their associated joints and ligaments, surrounds vital neural and vascular structures that represent the transition between the brain and spinal cord. The majority of the rotation, flexion, and extension of the head relative to the spine occurs at the CVJ, yet a high degree of stability is critical to the integrity of the neurovascular components.

The occipital bone forms the clivus, which leads caudally to the basion at the anterior aspect of the foramen magnum. The dorsal surface of the clivus is concave, the extent of which can affect the exposure achieved from posterolateral surgical approaches. Flanking the anterior half of the foramen magnum are the occipital condyles, which extend in an inferomedial-to-superolateral orientation from anterior to posterior. Immediately rostral to the condyle lies the hypoglossal canal, opening medially one-third of the distance from the posterior edge of the condyle and exiting extracranially one-third of the distance behind its anterior edge. The squamous occipital bone completes the dorsal ring of the foramen magnum, a thickened keel arising in the midline to the inion. Projecting laterally from the posterior aspect of the condyle is the jugular process, which bears on its anterior surface a notch that forms the posterior portion of the jugular foramen.

The articular surface of the condyle is convex and is received by the concave superior articular surface of the lateral mass of the atlas. The lateral masses are joined by an anterior and posterior arch, the latter of which in particular may contain a developmental defect.[1] The posterior arch also bears on its rostral surface the groove of the sulcus arteriosus, over which courses the vertebral artery (VA). The transverse processes and transverse foramina of the atlas extend farther laterally than at the levels below. The inferior articular surface of the lateral mass meets the superior articular process of the axis in a biconvex configuration, allowing for extensive movement at the atlantoaxial segment. At a third interface, the ventral aspect of the dens apposes the dorsal surface of the anterior atlas arch. The pars interarticularis, lamina, and prominent bifid spinous process complete the dorsal ring of the axis.

Much of the stability of the craniocervical junction is provided by ligamentous structures, which can be disrupted by both pathology and surgical dissection. The transverse ligament of the cruciate complex is the strongest ligament of the spine and thus is a critical source of stability for the CVJ.[2] It inserts on the medial aspect of each lateral mass of the atlas, arching dorsal to the dens and holding it against the anterior arch while permitting rotation at the atlantoaxial joint. The other major stabilizers of the CVJ are the paired alar ligaments, which extend from the upper dens to the region of the medial occipital condyle and anterolateral foramen magnum.[3] Each alar ligament limits contralateral axial rotation and lateral flexion. They are second in tensile strength only to the transverse ligament and in the setting of disruption of the latter are responsible for preventing atlantal subluxation.[4] Additional structures, including the vertical part of the cruciate ligament, which inserts on the clivus rostrally and posterior axis body caudally, and the apical ligament, which extends from the tip of the dens to the basion, are consistently identified but contribute little to CVJ stability.

The tectorial membrane sits posterior to the cruciate ligament, blending with dura rostrally at the spheno-occipital synchondrosis and attaching caudally to the posterior axis body. It helps prevent posterior impingement of the odontoid process during flexion and demarcates the posterior border of the supraodontoid space.[5] The anterior border of this space is formed by the anterior atlanto-occipital membrane, a thin structure attached to the anterior atlas arch and foramen magnum rim that lies immediately posterior to the prevertebral muscles. The posterior atlanto-occipital membrane attaches the posterior foramen magnum to the atlas arch and is related to the posterior atlantoaxial membrane caudally, the dura ventrally, and the rectus capitis posterior minor muscle dorsally.

The dorsal myoligamentous complex, which includes the interspinous ligament, nuchal ligament, rectus capitis posterior minor and major muscles, and obliquus capitis superior and inferior muscles, supports the stability of the CVJ.[6] The latter three muscles form the suboccipital triangle, the deepest layer of musculature in the posterior neck. The rectus capitis posterior major takes its origin from the spinous process of the axis and inserts on the occipital bone to form the medial border of the triangle. The obliquus capitis superior also inserts on the occipital bone after arising from the transverse process of the atlas, and the obliquus capitis inferior arises from the spinous process of the axis and inserts on the transverse process of the atlas, respectively forming the superior and inferior borders of the triangle. They are covered by the semispinalis capitis and splenius capitis muscles, which are in turned overlaid by the trapezius and sternocleidomastoid (SCM) muscle. Lateral to the occipital condyle, the rectus capitis lateralis arises from the transverse process of the atlas and inserts onto the jugular process. From the anterior aspect of the atlas lateral mass arises the rectus capitis anterior, which inserts onto the occipital bone anterior to the condyle and is covered anteriorly by the longus capitis. In the midline roughly 1 cm anterior to the foramen magnum, the pharyngeal tubercle provides the point of attachment for the fibrous raphe of the superior pharyngeal constrictor.

The predominant movements at the atlanto-occipital joint are flexion and extension, contributing 23 to 24.5° of the range of the skull on the spine.[7] Other movements are limited, as the cupped configuration of the condyles in the lateral masses provide stability to this segment. In contrast, the atlantoaxial joint allows for a wide range of motion, adding 10.1 to 22.4° of flexion/extension and providing 25 to 30° of axial rotation.[8] The basion and dens act as a central pillar around which the occiput and atlas rotate, and overrotation is prevented by the ligaments and joint capsules. Less than 10° of lateral bending occurs, and translation, distraction, and compression are minimal at the CVJ.

Although the VA takes a roughly vertical course as it ascends the subaxial spine, movement at the CVJ requires greater mobility and redundancy of the vessel. Above the transverse foramen of the axis, the VA travels laterally to pass through the transverse foramen of the atlas, then turns posteromedially behind the lateral mass. It crosses over the sulcus arteriosus in the depths of the suboccipital triangle, passing under the inferior border of the posterior atlanto-occipital membrane, and finally turns anteriorly to penetrate the dura. The artery is surrounded by a rich venous plexus, which can cause brisk bleeding during surgical dissection. Although the intradural course of each VA can be highly variable, they typically give rise to the posteroinferior cerebellar arteries (PICAs), ascend ventral to the hypoglossal nerves, and join to form the basilar artery at the pontomedullary junction.

The jugular foramen is situated between the occipital and petrous temporal bones, its intracranial opening superolateral to that of the hypoglossal canal and its extracranial opening lateral to the anterior occipital condyle. The glossopharyngeal, vagus, and accessory nerves exit in the anteromedial portion of the foramen, whereas the jugular bulb transitions to the internal jugular vein (IJV) and exits the posterolateral portion anterior to

the rectus capitis lateralis, posteromedial to the styloid process and posterolateral to the opening of the carotid canal. Ascending within the carotid sheath, the internal carotid artery lies anterior to the transverse processes of the axis and atlas and the longus capitis.

27.3 Regional Pathology and Differential Diagnosis

Neoplasms of the CVJ may arise from neural elements or from the surrounding osseous or soft tissue structures. As with other parts of the skull base, intradural lesions such as meningiomas, schwannomas, neurofibromas, epidermoids, and paragangliomas occur in this region, as do extradural lesions such as metastases, plasmacytomas, and giant cell tumors. More specific to the CVJ are chordomas and chondrosarcomas and extensions of pituitary tumors, craniopharyngiomas, and nasopharyngeal malignancies. Lesions that should be distinguished from skull base neoplasms include exophytic intra-axial tumors, rheumatoid pannus, fibrous dysplasia, and congenital segmentation abnormalities.

27.4 Clinical Assessment

Because the cross-sectional area of the foramen magnum and spinal canal at the CVJ is much larger than that of the traversing neurovascular structures, by the time symptoms are apparent a slow-growing lesion may have attained a large size. Clinical presentation may follow a pattern in keeping with posterior fossa pathology, abnormality of the cervicomedullary junction, or high myelopathy and may additionally manifest hydrocephalus, syringohydromyelia, or vascular compromise. The most common initial symptom is pain in the suboccipital region, referred to the C2 dermatome, that is aggravated by head and neck motion.[9] The head is held flexed, and torticollis may be apparent. In contrast, bone erosion and mechanical instability can result in nondermatomal pain. Such nonspecific complaints may lead to delay in diagnosis, sometimes for years, until other findings develop.

Cranial neuropathies may arise due to involvement of brainstem nuclei, subarachnoid space segments, or intraforaminal nerves. The glossopharyngeal, vagus, and hypoglossal nerves are most commonly affected, manifesting as dysarthria, dysphagia, or repeated aspiration, with secondary pneumonia and weight loss. Involvement of the accessory nerve may result in SCM and trapezius weakness and atrophy. Abnormal or diminished pain, temperature, and deep pressure sensation in the face may result from compression of the caudal extent of the spinal trigeminal nucleus. Compression or traction of the vestibulocochlear nerve may result in vertigo, tinnitus, or hearing loss.

Effects on the ascending long tracts may produce a variety of sensory deficits. Paresthesias or dysesthesias are common, often in a suspended pattern affecting the hands first. Although typically suggestive of intramedullary disease, a dissociated pattern of decreased pain and temperature sensation with preserved joint position and vibration sensation can be seen with extradural lesions.

Weakness and clumsiness associated with spasticity is a common motor finding, although atrophy of intrinsic hand muscles may also be seen. A pattern of weakness beginning in the ipsilateral upper extremity, progressing to the ipsilateral lower extremity and then the contralateral lower extremity, and finally affecting the contralateral upper extremity, is a classic syndrome associated with pathology of the lateral craniocervical junction.[10] The syndrome of cruciate paralysis, with upper extremity weakness and preserved lower extremity power, has been described in tumors of the CVJ.

Vascular compromise can result in a variety of vertebrobasilar syndromes. Ataxia, nystagmus, vertigo, dysarthria, dysphagia, diplopia, hemiparesis, or paraparesis may occur, transiently or progressively. Venous obstruction may cause spinal cord edema, with findings of myelopathy. Hydrocephalus may result from obstruction of cerebrospinal fluid (CSF) flow or absorption.

27.5 Diagnostic Imaging

CT is often the first imaging obtained when pathology of the CVJ is suspected, and it is invaluable for delineating osseous anatomy and involvement. Planning of surgical approach and targeting extent of bone removal is facilitated by multiplanar thin-slice CT studies. Patterns of hyperostosis, erosion, lysis, and sclerosis help in narrowing the differential diagnosis. CT venography and angiography can be used to evaluate the caliber, course, dominance, and compromise of adjacent vessels and potential segments at risk during surgical resection. Particularly in older patients, the course of the vertebral and carotid arteries may become tortuous as they approach the skull base, and imaging studies should be reviewed to anticipate any anomalies.

MRI can distinguish tumors of the CVJ from intramedullary and nonneoplastic lesions that present in similar fashion. Patterns of enhancement with gadolinium contrast, as well as patterns on susceptibility-weighted imaging, diffusion-weighted imaging, and steady-state sequences, can further narrow the differential diagnosis, identify the likely anatomical site of origin, and provide detailed information about the location of neighboring vascular and neural structures. Fluid-attenuated inversion recovery sequences can reveal the presence of edema within the brainstem or spinal cord. MR venography and angiography can also be obtained in the same session.

Digital subtraction angiography may be needed for dynamic evaluation of collateral circulation and to assess whether a patient will tolerate vascular occlusion. Highly vascular tumors such as paragangliomas may benefit from preoperative embolization of feeding arteries.

Additional imaging can identify instances in which the tumor has caused destruction of the bony and ligamentous structures that provide stability at the CVJ. Surgical stabilization should be considered when patients are found to have instability before resection—that is, instability caused by the tumor itself. Such instability can be identified using both static and dynamic X-rays. Static X-rays of the CVJ allow many widely used parameters to be drawn and measured. These measurements, such as the Chamberlain and McRae lines and the basion–dens and basion–atlanto intervals, can help distinguish whether instability is present.[11] Dynamic X-rays, such as flexion–extension X-rays, allow for identification of translation, which is also indicative of instability.

27.6 Preoperative Preparation

In patients who have decreased hearing on presentation, formal evaluation using an audiogram will determine baseline function and may identify those at greatest risk of complete hearing loss. Patients who have glossopharyngeal, vagal, and/or hypoglossal nerve palsies may require tracheostomy and gastrostomy. Long-standing dysphagia may have resulted in malnourishment, and nutritional support may be required preoperatively to lessen problems of wound healing. The patient should be examined for development of neurological symptoms with the head in rotation or flexion to ensure that they will tolerate surgical positioning. Prior to transnasal or transoral approaches, examination for and treatment of infections that may lead to contamination of the surgical field should be undertaken.

Even in the absence of preoperative mechanical instability, disruption of the CVJ caused by the surgical approach warrants stabilization. The posterior midline approach can cause instability by disrupting the posterior tension band, as well as if the bony resection is taken laterally to involve the condyle. Lateral approaches involve drilling of the condyle, with stabilization often performed if more than 70% of the condyle is drilled.[12] The anterolateral approach can require drilling of the lateral mass of the atlas, as well as the atlanto-occipital and atlantoaxial joints. This bony removal can also lead to instability. Finally, the transoral route may lead to resection of a significant portion of the bony and ligamentous complex that unites the clivus, atlas, and dens. This results in instability in the majority of patients who undergo this approach.[13] The extent of bone removal may be determined intraoperatively, but if the approach may be destabilizing, a plan should be in place to perform surgical stabilization at the same session or to maintain alignment until stabilization is carried out at later session.

The anesthesiologist should be made aware of patients who have CVJ instability or cervicomedullary compression and should modify the intubation technique accordingly. Standard protocols to facilitate brain relaxation are employed, including mild hyperventilation, mannitol administration, and head elevation. A ventriculostomy may be considered in patients who have obstructive hydrocephalus. Electrophysiologic monitoring of somatosensory, motor and brainstem–auditory evoked potentials can provide early warning of neurologic compression, retraction, or ischemic injury. Electromyographic monitoring of cranial nerve function may also be useful, particularly when the tumor has caused displacement of normal structures.

27.7 Surgical Technique

Numerous surgical approaches have been developed to access the CVJ, allowing for circumferential access to the region. In selecting a technique, factors for consideration include (1) likely histology and possibility of complete resection, (2) site of origin and direction of growth and neurovascular compression/displacement, (3) pathological or surgical breach of dura and need for CSF containment, and (4) mechanical craniospinal stability. Slow-growing tumors have often pushed away the neurovascular structures, creating working space and allowing for reduced surgical manipulation.

The available corridors can be considered in four categories: posterior midline, far lateral, anterolateral, and anterior transoral–transpharyngeal. For dorsal and paramedian tumors, the posterior midline suboccipital craniotomy is a routine and familiar approach and is often combined with C1 and C2 laminectomy. It allows for bony decompression of the foramen magnum, provides wide access to the CVJ on both sides of midline, and is essentially unlimited in potential rostrocaudal extension. It can be used for intradural pathology, as the dura is easily repaired, and dorsal instrumentation and fusion can be performed in the same exposure. For lateral or anterolateral tumors, a posterolateral trajectory is needed, which can be achieved using a far lateral approach (▶ Fig. 27.1).

Further ventral exposure is gained with drilling of the occipital condyle, C1 lateral mass, or jugular tubercle, although extensive removal of the O–C1 joint may cause instability requiring fusion,[14] and the dorsal jugular bulb can be accessed with removal of the jugular process. Because the dura is also readily closed, intradural pathology to and past the ventral midline can be treated using this approach. Anterior and anterolateral tumors can be directly accessed by an anterolateral approach, also called extreme lateral—a useful technique, particularly for extradural tumors or dumbbell lesions having a large extradural component and when a posterolateral approach has previously been performed.[15] If the prevertebral region anterior to the CVJ is exposed, this approach carries risk of pharyngeal dysfunction as well as injury to the extracranial segments of the hypoglossal nerves. As in any setting of extensive O–C1 or C1–C2 joint removal, stabilization may be required. For primarily extradural ventral pathology, the transoral–transpharyngeal approach is direct and relatively simple, avoiding manipulation of the cervicomedullary junction,

cranial nerves, and VA. However, morbidity of the approach includes postoperative tube feeding while the pharynx heals as well as potential long-term velopharyngeal insufficiency. Endoscopic endonasal approaches have become increasingly applied to directly ventral pathology, as they may result in less pharyngeal morbidity. Detailed discussions of endoscopic techniques are provided elsewhere in this volume.

27.7.1 Posterior Midline Approach

Positioning

The patient is placed in the Concorde position, with the head fixed in flexion at the atlanto-occipital segment to increase working space at the posterior CVJ, taking care to avoid obstruction of cerebral venous outflow. The upper chest and pelvis are supported, allowing free movement of the chest and abdominal wall, and the operating table is placed in the reverse Trendelenburg position to reduce cerebral venous congestion.

Incision

The incision is placed in the midline, from 2 cm above the inion to the spinous process of C2. The pericranial layer above the superior nuchal line is preserved.

Soft Tissue Dissection

The avascular midline aponeurosis is opened to expose the occipital bone, and the superficial muscles are reflected inferolaterally, maintaining a cuff along the superior nuchal line on each side to facilitate tight closure and decrease risk of CSF leak. As the subperiosteal muscle elevation proceeds caudally,

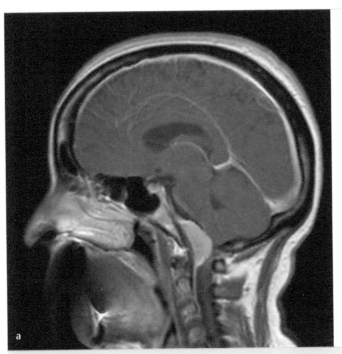
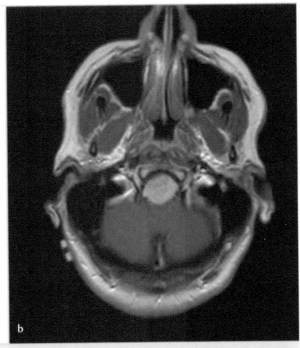

Fig. 27.1 A 38-year-old woman presents with several months of difficulty swallowing and neck pain. Her physical examination reveals a mildly hoarse voice and severe hyperreflexia. MRI T1 sequences with contrast of the craniovertebral junction on **(a)** sagittal and **(b)** axial cuts demonstrate a midline, anteriorly arising foramen magnum meningioma. A far lateral approach was selected for this tumor.

an instrument is used to palpate for the rim of foramen magnum, which is identified in the midline. The posterior arch of the atlas can then be palpated in the midline and the fibrous attachments freed from the posterior tubercle to expose the subperiosteal surface of the lamina. Developmental defects in the posterior arch should be identified on preoperative imaging. The lamina is further exposed using a gauze to sweep the soft tissues laterally, to the beginning of the sulcus arteriosus. Depending on the caudal extent of the tumor, the spinous process and lamina of the axis may need to be exposed. Where possible, the inferior muscle attachments are preserved to help maintain stability. Hooked retractors on elastics reduce the muscle bulk better than hinged self-retaining retractors do.

Bony Dissection and Osteotomies

The suboccipital craniotomy extends superiorly to encompass the pathology and inferiorly across the foramen magnum. The opening crosses the midline but may extend further laterally on one side if the lesion is asymmetric. Laminectomy of the atlas may also be wider on one side. Removal of bone of the axis is determined by the caudal extent of the tumor, allowing for sufficient room to close the durotomy.

Tumor Resection

The dura is opened in the midline dorsal to cisterna magna to allow for CSF egress, although this may be modified if the tumor is present there. The opening is extended superolaterally, on either side of a potential occipital sinus, and inferiorly below the extent of the tumor. Because a dorsally located tumor will be encountered first, it may require internal debulking before its interface with ventral neurovascular structures can be dissected. Involved dura may need to be excised.

Reconstruction

The edges of the dura should be sutured, primarily or with a graft particularly if dura has been excised. A large craniotomy flap may be replaced to minimize the superior bone defect.

Closure

The deep muscle layers may be sutured to reduce the potential space for hematoma formation, taking care to avoid muscle strangulation. The midline raphe is closed tightly, and the superior edge of cut muscle is reattached to the cuff at the superior nuchal line.

27.7.2 Far Lateral Approach

Positioning

The patient is placed in the three-quarters prone position, which allows gravity to draw away the cerebellar hemisphere and has a lower risk of venous air embolism than the sitting position does. A gel roll supports the chest, and the dependent arm is suspended in a sling beyond the end of the operating table. Head positioning incorporates four movements: (1) anteroposterior flexion to open the suboccipital region and rostral

clivus, (2) contralateral flexion to increase room for the surgeon beside the ipsilateral shoulder, (3) contralateral rotation to place the suboccipital surface highest in the surgical field, and (4) vertical translation to partially sublux the ipsilateral O–C1 joint and facilitate condylar drilling (▶ Fig. 27.2). The ipsilateral shoulder is pulled toward the feet, taking care to avoid excessive traction on the brachial plexus.

Incision

The incision begins in the midline and extends from the spinous process of C2 to 2 cm above the inion, continues laterally on the side of the lesion to a point level with the mastoid process, and then turns inferiorly to end at the mastoid tip. Retromastoid incisions direct the exposure through the musculature to reduce its bulk, but these approaches increase muscle trauma and place the VA at greater risk of injury.

Soft Tissue Dissection

The midline raphe is opened, decreasing muscle trauma and allowing for identification of the atlas in the midline, away from the VA. On the side of the lesion, a muscle cuff along the superior nuchal line is preserved for closure, and the muscles are reflected laterally from the occipital bone to expose the mastoid process and digastric groove. As the subperiosteal dissection proceeds caudally, electrocautery should be avoided to prevent inadvertent thermal injury to the VA. The foramen magnum is identified in the midline and the rim freed of soft tissue to the occipital condyle. The posterior tubercle of the atlas is palpated and cleared of soft tissue, and a gauze used to sweep the soft tissue laterally. When the sulcus arteriosus is identified, dissection in the subperiosteal plane from the inferior toward the superior aspect of the posterior atlas arch preserves the venous plexus surrounding the VA, which reduces troublesome bleeding.

If access to the atlanto-occipital joint is required, then the muscle attachments on the C1 transverse process are divided and reflected medially. If the posterior aspect of the jugular bulb is to be exposed, the rectus capitis lateralis is detached from the jugular process and reflected inferiorly.

Bony Dissection and Osteotomies

An ipsilateral hemilaminectomy of the atlas is performed, from just beyond midline on the opposite side to the ipsilateral lateral mass. A suboccipital craniotomy extends superiorly to the rostral extent of pathology, laterally to the sigmoid sinus, and inferiorly across the foramen magnum at the midline. The rim of foramen magnum is further removed to the occipital condyle, facilitated by use of a high-speed drill while an assistant retracts and protects the VA with its venous plexus. Bleeding may be encountered from the posterior condylar emissary vein in the condylar canal, which lies in the condylar fossa at the base of the condyle. This lateral exposure is key to the far lateral approach, creating an inferolateral corridor to the anterior brainstem without retraction (▶ Fig. 27.3).[16]

Additional access to the anterior medulla may be gained by drilling the jugular tubercle intradurally with direct visualization of the lower cranial nerves, or to the lower clivus by drilling the occipital condyle in part or whole.[17] Removal of

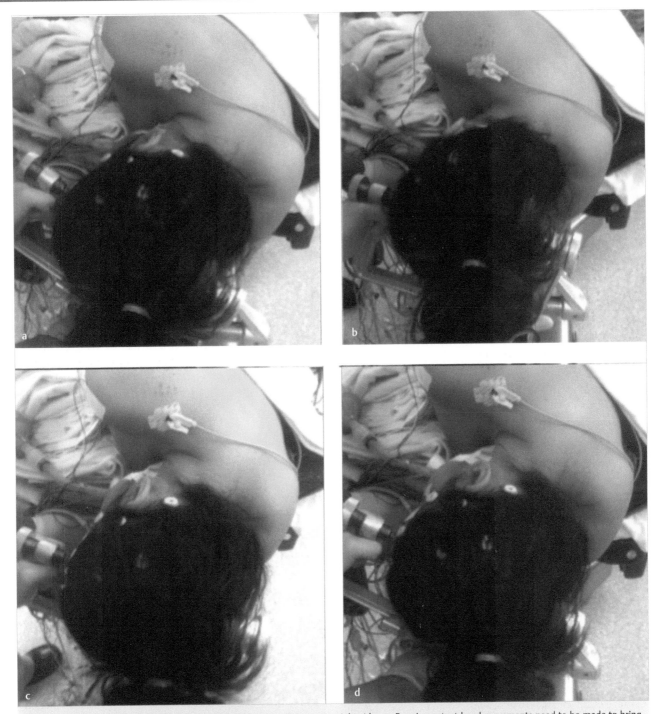

Fig. 27.2 Positioning for right far lateral approach is three-quarters prone, right side up. Four important head movements need to be made to bring the craniovertebral junction in the best exposure: **(a)** flexion, **(b)** contralateral rotation, **(c)** lateral bending, and **(d)** upward translocation.

the posterior third of the condyle is demarcated by encountering the cortex of the hypoglossal canal medially, at its intracranial opening. Further condylar resection can be performed, although instability of the atlanto-occipital joint may result and require fixation. Access to the O–C1 articular pillar requires mobilization of the VA, which runs dorsal to the joint before crossing the C1 lamina. The C1 transverse foramen is opened posteriorly and the VA freed from surrounding connective tissue between the C1 and C2 transverse foramina and displaced inferomedially. The far lateral approach can

also be extended laterally to expose the posterior aspect of the jugular bulb by removing the jugular process and opening the jugular foramen dorsally.

Tumor Resection

One limb of the paramedian dural opening extends across the foramen magnum, and the other reaches the superolateral corner of the exposure; the flap is retracted laterally (▶ Fig. 27.4). A transdural PICA or posterior spinal artery incorporated into

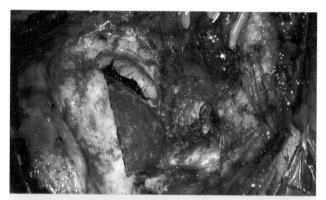

Fig. 27.3 After a hockey stick incision, a suboccipital craniotomy, a C1 hemilaminectomy, and a thorough drilling of the juxtacondylar bone, the craniovertebral angle is flattened maximally at the foramen magnum and the dura is ready to be opened.

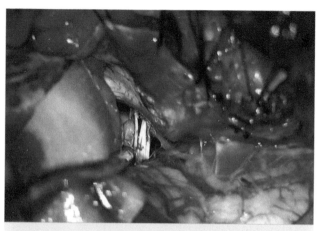

Fig. 27.4 After the dural opening, the advantages of a thorough drilling are appreciated: flat unobstructed view of the jugular foramen and lateral cervical canal wall.

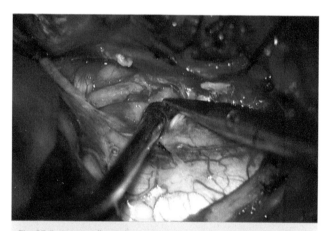

Fig. 27.5 Gravity allows the compressed cervicomedullary junction to fall away from the tumor. The tumor is seen here after the dentate ligament has been divided. The V4 segment of the vertebral artery is seen partially engulfed by the tumor. The hypoglossal rootlets are also seen stretched posteriorly.

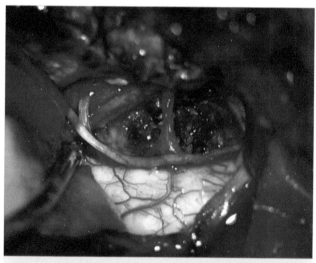

Fig. 27.6 The lower pole of the tumor has been debulked. The C1 nerve root was not sacrificed, because it carried a radicular artery contributing blood supply to the dorsal arterial network of the cervical cord.

the fibrous ring surrounding the VA at its dural penetration must be recognized and preserved. The first two dentate ligaments are divided to access and mobilize the pathology (▶ Fig. 27.5). Lower cranial nerves may be displaced, splayed, or encased by tumor, and intraoperative electromyographic stimulation can assist in identifying them (▶ Fig. 27.6). Tumor resection is necessarily piecemeal, as dissection is carried out through multiple small windows between neurovascular structures (▶ Fig. 27.7).

Reconstruction

The dura should be sutured to reduce likelihood of CSF leak. Air cells encountered during the exposure must be completely occluded with bone wax. The suboccipital bone flap can be replaced so as not to leave a large defect.

Closure

The muscle flap is closed at the midline and reattached to the cuff along the superior nuchal line (▶ Fig. 27.8).

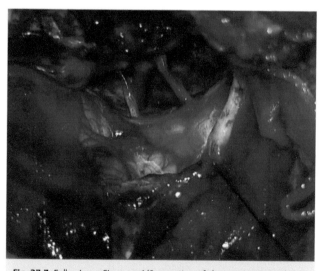

Fig. 27.7 Following a Simpson 1/2 resection of the meningioma, the space created ventral to the medulla and cervical cord is well appreciated.

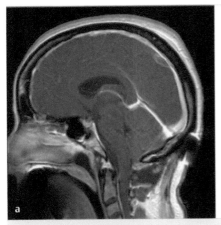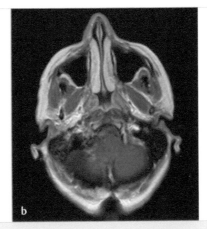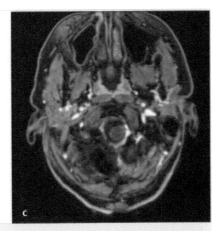

Fig. 27.8 A T1-weighted MRIs with contrast, in (**a**) sagittal and (**b, c**) axial views, done on postoperative day 2, show complete resection of the anterior lesions from a posterolateral approach.

27.7.3 Anterolateral Approach

Positioning

The patient is positioned supine, with the head extended and rotated contralaterally: ~ 15° for access to the anterior CVJ or 30° or more to expose the posterior atlas.

Incision

The incision begins at the medial border of the SCM, 6 cm below the mastoid tip. It extends superiorly along the muscle border over the mastoid tip to the level of the external auditory meatus, then curves medially along the superior nuchal line.

Soft Tissue Dissection

The SCM, splenius capitis, and longissimus capitis are detached from the mastoid and occipital bones with preservation of a cuff for closure. Dissection is carried along the medial aspect of the SCM, separating it from the lateral border of the IJV. The sole nerve crossing the surgical field, the spinal accessory, is found 3 to 4 cm below the mastoid tip. It is identified most readily along the SCM border but should be freed as proximally as possible toward the skull base to allow safe mobilization. The fatty and lymphatic tissue through which the nerve runs should be freed and used to cushion its retraction caudally. The transverse process of the atlas can be palpated 10 to 15 mm anterior and inferior to the mastoid tip. The C1 transverse process is the lateral apex of the suboccipital triangle, which is located in the depth of the space bordered by the mastoid process rostrally, IJV medially, spinal accessory nerve caudally, and SCM laterally.[18] Separation of the small muscle attachments exposes the C1 transverse process.

The VA is first exposed between the C1 and C2 transverse foramina, being mindful of the increased relative anterior position of the C1 lateral mass on C2 with greater contralateral head rotation. The anterior ramus of the C2 nerve root crosses the VA and needs to be divided for mobilization of the artery. The horizontal portion of the VA is then freed, beginning at the inferior edge of the C1 posterior arch and working to the superior aspect. Attachments near the occipital condyle may need to be sharply divided. Subperiosteal dissection preserves the periarterial venous plexus and reduces bleeding, and this plane is finally followed into the transverse foramen.

Bony Dissection and Osteotomies

The C1 transverse foramen is opened and enlarged enough to completely transpose the VA and mobilize it dorsally. Drilling of the lateral mass of the atlas brings the anterior thecal sac and lateral dens into view. The C1 posterior arch, C2 lamina, atlanto-occipital joint, atlantoaxial joint, C1 anterior arch, and C2 vertebral body and dens are exposed and can also be removed if needed, according to the extent of pathology.[19] If a posterior fossa component is present, a retrosigmoid craniotomy can be performed and the foramen magnum rim removed, including a partial condylectomy if needed.

Tumor Resection

As tumor is removed, the medial aspect of the opposite lateral mass may come into view. If access to intradural tumor is required, the dura is opened linearly. Tumor is debulked internally before the capsule is dissected from the neurovascular structures. As tumor is removed, the nerve roots of the contralateral side may be visualized.

Reconstruction

A sutured closure of the dura is ideal. A piece of subcutaneous fat obtained from a separate abdominal incision may be placed in the epidural space to reinforce the dural repair.

Closure

The muscles are reapproximated to the cuffs left on the bone.

27.7.4 Transoral Approach

Positioning

The patient is positioned supine with the head in extension. The orotracheal tube is retracted out of view of the surgical approach. A self-retaining oral retractor is used to keep the mouth open and to retract the tongue. To reduce velopharyngeal morbidity caused by splitting the palate, the uvula is retracted into the nasopharynx by securing it to a soft rubber catheter that is passed out the nares.

Incision

The anterior tubercle of the atlas and the body of the axis are palpable at the posterior oropharynx. A midline incision is made from the lower clivus to the lower body of C2. Frameless stereotaxy or lateral fluoroscopy can help determine the required exposure.

Soft Tissue Dissection

The pharyngeal mucosa and pharyngeal constrictors are elevated as a single layer, incorporating the longus capitis and longus colli as the dissection is carried laterally. The underlying anterior atlanto-occipital membrane and anterior longitudinal ligament are dissected using electrocautery to expose the inferior clivus, anterior arch of C1, and anterior body of C2. The exposure can be extended to the body of C3 if needed. The myomucosal flaps are incorporated in the self-retaining retractor system.

Bony Dissection and Osteotomies

The extent of bone removal depends on the histology and extent of tumor to be removed. Benign and nonaggressive lesions can be removed piecemeal, whereas primary bone tumors may require en bloc resection with more extensive bone removal. An exposure of 10 mm on each side of midline can be gained, with further lateral exposure limited by the opening of the Eustachian tube, hypoglossal nerve, vidian nerve, and VA segment at C1–C2; caution during resection must be exercised if the pathology extends laterally to involve these structures. The anterior arch of C1 is drilled to create a trough 15 to 20 mm wide, which is maintained as exposure is extended rostrocaudally. Removal of the dens is performed by first detaching it from its associated ligaments, then drilling it from within to leave an "eggshell" rim posteriorly that can be removed using curettes. The inferior clivus rostrally and cervical vertebrae caudally can be removed as far as the transoral exposure allows. The cruciate ligament and tectorial membrane are further removed if exposure of the dura is needed.

Tumor Resection

Intraosseous pathology may be encountered upon elevation of the prevertebral musculature and tumor resected as the bone exposure is carried out.

Reconstruction

Although intradural pathology can be directly accessed using the transoral approach, this technique is infrequently used, because closure without CSF leak is challenging. Dural closure is performed using an inlay graft of dural substitute and a patch placed on the extradural surface. These can be affixed with fibrin glue. Fat graft obtained from a separate abdominal incision is placed in the defect left from bone removal, with further

application of fibrin glue. In cases of dural opening, a lumbar drain is left open for several days postoperatively to decrease CSF pressure on the repair.

Closure

The pharyngeal musculature and mucosa are closed as separate layers with absorbable suture. An orogastric tube is placed during anesthesia, for oral intake will not be possible while the soft tissues of the pharynx heal. Tracheal intubation is left in place for at least the first 24 hours after surgery, until airway swelling has adequately subsided.

27.7.5 Surgical Stabilization

Current methods of occipitocervical stabilization involve rigid internal instrumentation. The types of hardware used include plates, screws, and rods. Although constructs can vary, most involve an occipital plate that is connected through rods to screws in the cervical spine. The types of occipital plates may differ, but these are usually secured to the bone through bicortical screws at the inion as well as extra screws laterally.[11] Screws can be placed in the atlantoaxial complex by numerous techniques, including C1 lateral mass and C2 pars screws (Harms technique), C1–C2 transarticular screws (Magerl technique), and C2 translaminar screws. Additional fixation points can be obtained through lateral mass screws in the subaxial cervical spine. Controversy remains over how many levels of fixation are necessary to achieve satisfactory stabilization for fusion (▶ Fig. 27.9).

Instrumentation techniques including sublaminar wires, hooks, and clamps were developed in the early- and mid-20th century, and have generally been supplanted by screw fixation. Nevertheless, these strategies may be necessary when anatomic or technical factors render the more modern techniques impossible to carry out.

27.8 Postoperative Care

Patients should be monitored in an ICU during the early postoperative period, particularly if prolonged anesthetic times and new or worsened lower cranial nerve deficits place them at risk for aspiration and airway compromise.

27.9 Complications and Their Avoidance

In all posterior and posterolateral approaches, the horizontal segment of the VA between the C1 transverse foramen and its dural entry is particularly vulnerable to injury. An aberrant or tortuous loop of the VA toward the occipital bone should be recognized on preoperative imaging. Electrocautery should also be avoided in this area, because an inadvertent sharp arteriotomy is more readily repaired than a thermal injury. The VA may be avulsed or compressed against an ossified posterior atlanto-occipital ligament arch, which effectively turns the groove of the sulcus arteriosus into a bony canal. Other variants may also occur, such as an extradural origin of the PICA or posterior spinal artery.[20] The VA may also have a tortuous course between the transverse foramina of C2 and C1 and be susceptible to

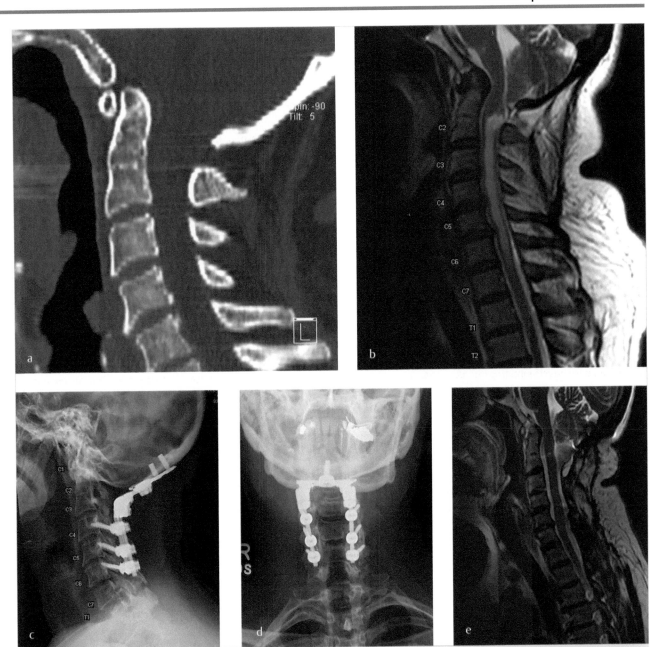

Fig. 27.9 A patient presenting with myelopathy due to basilar invagination demonstrates the use of surgical stabilization of the craniovertebral junction following decompression. **(a)** Sagittal CT showed the diagnosis of basilar invagination. **(b)** Sagittal T2-weighted MRI demonstrated marked signal hyperintensity in the spinal cord. Surgical intervention included posterior decompression and spinal realignment with a construct extending from the occiput to C5 on **(c)** lateral and **(d)** AP X-ray. **(e)** Postoperative sagittal MRI demonstrated satisfactory decompression with improvement in T2-weighted spinal cord signal hyperintensity.

injury during lateral approaches. The carotid artery typically veers laterally before its penetration of the skull base, but ectatic loops may bring it close to the midline; these must be recognized prior to performing the anterior transoral approach.

Particularly when tight dural closure is difficult, CSF leak with subsequent meningitis is a potential source of major morbidity. Whenever possible, a sutured closure should be performed, using a patch graft as necessary. Fat grafts and fibrin glue sealants can additionally be helpful to reinforce the closure. Continuous lumbar drainage in the first several days is helpful to facilitate healing.

27.10 Follow-up and Rehabilitation

Evaluation of the extent of tumor resection and need for adjuvant treatment such as radiotherapy is based on postoperative contrast-enhanced MRI imaging. X-ray and CT are useful to assess mechanical stability, fixation constructs, and progression of bone fusion.

Patients may require hearing assessment, swallowing assessment, and physical therapy depending on the extent of postoperative deficit. Prolonged lower cranial nerve palsy and dysphagia may require consideration of tracheostomy and/or percutaneous gastrostomy for nutrition.

The overall outcomes of CVJ stabilization are good.[21,22,23] Complications can be a result of injury to neurovascular structures during instrumentation, hardware problems postoperatively, or perioperative issues such as infection. Bhatia et al reported that of 100 patients who underwent occipitocervical instrumentation, 5 suffered from hardware breakage or failure, 5 developed a surgical site infection, 1 had a VA injury, and 1 died perioperatively.[21] For a series of 49 patients who underwent occipito-cervical fusion, Kukreja et al reported 2 cases of infection, 2 cases of nonunion, and 4 perioperative mortalities.[22] Nockels et al presented a series of 69 patients who underwent occipitocervical fusion who were followed for a mean time of 37 months: none suffered pseudarthrosis, and there were no perioperative deaths.[23]

Neurological recovery after occipitocervical fusion in the context of CVJ tumor resection depends on preoperative neurological status, the type and location of tumor encountered, and the resection performed.[24] The main goal of stabilization is to prevent further neurological deterioration after the tumor has been satisfactorily resected. However, surgeons should clearly counsel patients on the potential for lost neck motion as well as the possibility of fusion's placing the neck into a position that affects horizontal gaze permanently.

27.11 Conclusion

The numerous techniques that have been developed to access the CVJ reflect the complexity of anatomy in the region and the myriad tumors that may arise. The principal tenet of removing bone to avoid retraction on neural structures is applied, but the need for surgical stabilization must also be considered. Selection of the appropriate surgical strategy must be individualized for each patient, depending on clinical symptoms, tumor histology, and the goals of the operation.

References

[1] Gehweiler JA, Jr, Daffner RH, Roberts L, Jr. Malformations of the atlas vertebra simulating the Jefferson fracture. AJR Am J Roentgenol. 1983; 140(6): 1083–1086

[2] Dickman CA, Mamourian A, Sonntag VK, Drayer BP. Magnetic resonance imaging of the transverse atlantal ligament for the evaluation of atlantoaxial instability. J Neurosurg. 1991; 75(2):221–227

[3] Tubbs RS, Hallock JD, Radcliff V, et al. Ligaments of the craniocervical junction. J Neurosurg Spine. 2011; 14(6):697–709

[4] Dvorak J, Schneider E, Saldinger P, Rahn B. Biomechanics of the craniocervical region: the alar and transverse ligaments. J Orthop Res. 1988; 6(3): 452–461

[5] Tubbs RS, Kelly DR, Humphrey ER, et al. The tectorial membrane: anatomical, biomechanical, and histological analysis. Clin Anat. 2007; 20(4):382–386

[6] Offiah CE, Day E. The craniocervical junction: embryology, anatomy, biomechanics and imaging in blunt trauma. Insights Imaging. 2017; 8(1):29–47

[7] Panjabi M, Dvorak J, Duranceau J, et al. Three-dimensional movements of the upper cervical spine. Spine. 1988; 13(7):726–730

[8] Lopez AJ, Scheer JK, Leibl KE, Smith ZA, Dlouhy BJ, Dahdaleh NS. Anatomy and biomechanics of the craniovertebral junction. Neurosurg Focus. 2015; 38(4):E2

[9] Benglis D, Levi AD. Neurologic findings of craniovertebral junction disease. Neurosurgery. 2010; 66(3) Suppl:13–21

[10] Meyer FB, Ebersold MJ, Reese DF. Benign tumors of the foramen magnum. J Neurosurg. 1984; 61(1):136–142

[11] Benke M, Yu WD, Peden SC, O'Brien JR. Occipitocervical junction: imaging, pathology, instrumentation. Am J Orthop. 2011; 40(10):E205–E215

[12] Bejjani GK, Sekhar LN, Riedel CJ. Occipitocervical fusion following the extreme lateral transcondylar approach. Surg Neurol. 2000; 54(2):109–115, discussion 115–116

[13] Dickman CA, Locantro J, Fessler RG. The influence of transoral odontoid resection on stability of the craniovertebral junction. J Neurosurg. 1992; 77(4): 525–530

[14] Vishteh AG, Crawford NR, Melton MS, Spetzler RF, Sonntag VK, Dickman CA. Stability of the craniovertebral junction after unilateral occipital condyle resection: a biomechanical study. J Neurosurg. 1999; 90(1) Suppl: 91–98

[15] Sen CN, Sekhar LN. An extreme lateral approach to intradural lesions of the cervical spine and foramen magnum. Neurosurgery. 1990; 27(2):197–204

[16] Heros RC. Lateral suboccipital approach for vertebral and vertebrobasilar artery lesions. J Neurosurg. 1986; 64(4):559–562

[17] Spektor S, Anderson GJ, McMenomey SO, Horgan MA, Kellogg JX, Delashaw JB, Jr. Quantitative description of the far-lateral transcondylar transtubercular approach to the foramen magnum and clivus. J Neurosurg. 2000; 92 (5):824–831

[18] Bruneau M, Cornelius JF, George B. Antero-lateral approach to the V3 segment of the vertebral artery. Neurosurgery. 2006; 58(1) Suppl:ONS29–ONS35

[19] George B, Lot G. Anterolateral and posterolateral approaches to the foramen magnum: technical description and experience from 97 cases. Skull Base Surg. 1995; 5(1):9–19

[20] Fine AD, Cardoso A, Rhoton AL, Jr. Microsurgical anatomy of the extracranial-extradural origin of the posterior inferior cerebellar artery. J Neurosurg. 1999; 91(4):645–652

[21] Bhatia R, Desouza RM, Bull J, Casey AT. Rigid occipitocervical fixation: indications, outcomes, and complications in the modern era. J Neurosurg Spine. 2013; 18(4):333–339

[22] Kukreja S, Ambekar S, Sin AH, Nanda A. Occipitocervical fusion surgery: review of operative techniques and results. J Neurol Surg B Skull Base. 2015; 76 (5):331–339

[23] Nockels RP, Shaffrey CI, Kanter AS, Azeem S, York JE. Occipitocervical fusion with rigid internal fixation: long-term follow-up data in 69 patients. J Neurosurg Spine. 2007; 7(2):117–123

[24] Jiang H, He J, Zhan X, He M, Zong S, Xiao Z. Occipito-cervical fusion following gross total resection for the treatment of spinal extramedullary tumors in craniocervical junction: a retrospective case series. World J Surg Oncol. 2015; 13:279

28 Tumors of the Orbit

Alan Siu, Jurij Bilyk, Kelsey Moody, Ashley Maglione, Marc Rosen, and James J. Evans

Summary

The clinical and surgical management of tumors that invade the orbit can be quite complex but is greatly facilitated by a comprehensive understanding of the orbital anatomy. The orbit can be separated into compartments and can be associated with specific clinical findings. The subsequent clinical work-up and diagnosis can be guided by the clinical findings. Pathologies within the orbit are typically described relative to the orbital cone and in relation to the rectus musculature. Accordingly, the surgical approach is selected that optimizes the opportunity for a complete surgical resection while respecting the orbital anatomy.

Keywords: orbital tumor, orbit, orbital anatomy, orbitotomy

28.1 Introduction

Clinical familiarity with the orbit is important for the comprehensive care of skull base lesions. Pathologies can originate within the orbit and extend into the skull base or, conversely, can invade the orbit from surrounding structures. The complexity of orbital anatomy requires a thorough understanding for determination of the optimal surgical approach for improving outcomes and minimizing complications. Depending on the location of the lesion, surgical approaches may also be performed in conjunction with other surgical services, including ophthalmology and otolaryngology. We present a review of the anatomy, differential diagnosis, and surgical approaches for orbital pathology.

28.2 Osteology

The orbit is a complex bony structure that houses the globe and ocular adnexal tissue (▶ Fig. 28.1). The shape of the orbit can be described in a simplified manner as a pyramid with its apex pointing posteriorly.[1] The four sides of the pyramid represent the roof, medial and lateral walls, and floor of the orbit, each having unique landmarks and clinical significance. The anterior face subsumes a roughly rectangular shape formed by the orbital rim (arcus marginalis), which is discontinuous medially to accommodate the lacrimal sac.[1,2] The periosteum of the face turns roughly 90° to enter the orbit as periorbita and is tightly tethered to the orbital rim.

The orbital roof is formed largely by the frontal bone, with a small contribution made posteriorly by the sphenoid bone. The frontal bone thickens and protrudes anteriorly to form the orbital rim so as to accommodate the frontal sinus. At the superior orbital rim, the supraorbital notch and trochlear foramen allow for passage of the supraorbital and trochlear branches of the frontal division (V_1) of the trigeminal nerve, providing sensory innervation to the upper face.[3] Laterally, a concave fossa is found just posterior to the orbital rim that accommodates the lacrimal gland. Medially, the fibrocartilaginous trochlea is found 3 to 5 mm posterior to the orbital rim and acts as a pulley for the superior oblique muscle (SOM); careful disinsertion of the trochlea at its osseous insertion (rather than the SOM from the trochlea) is important to prevent injury to the muscle and postoperative diplopia.

The lateral orbital wall is formed by the zygomatic bone anteriorly and the greater wing of the sphenoid posteriorly. Two foramina are also found within the zygomatic bone, the zygomaticofacial and zygomaticotemporal, through which the respective nerves, arteries, and veins pass to provide sensory innervation and vascular supply to the midface. On axial radiographic images, the lateral wall subsumes an appearance of two triangles with their apices meeting at the sphenozygomatic suture; this anatomical landmark is important surgically, as it provides an

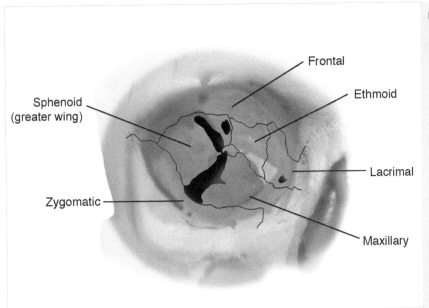

Fig. 28.1 Bony orbital anatomy.

Frontal

Ethmoid

Sphenoid (greater wing)

Lacrimal

Zygomatic

Maxillary

area of weakness that can be exploited when fashioning a bone flap during lateral orbitotomy. An arterial anastomosis between the middle meningeal and ophthalmic artery is present in about 40% of patients along the frontosphenoidal suture line (foramen meningo-orbitale); control of this artery is important during orbitotomy to prevent vessel retraction and intracranial bleeding.[1]

The medial wall of the orbit is formed by multiple contributing bones. Most anteriorly, the frontal process of the maxilla forms the orbital rim and the anterior lacrimal crest. The maxilla also contributes to the inferomedial portion of the medial wall, extending toward the orbital apex as a thickening often referred to as the "maxillary strut." The lacrimal bone is found just posterior to the frontal process, forming the bulk of the lacrimal sac fossa and the posterior lacrimal crest. The lacrimal sac sits within the fossa, whereas the anterior and especially the posterior lacrimal crests provide anchorage points for the medial canthal tendon. The majority of the medial orbital wall is made up of the ethmoid bone, abutting the ethmoid and sphenoid sinuses. This portion of the medial wall is the thinnest of the orbit (lamina papyracea) but might not be the weakest because of the trestlelike support of the underlying ethmoidal air cell septations.[4]

The anterior and posterior ethmoidal arteries pass through the anterior and posterior canals, respectively. The anterior ethmoidal artery is usually located at the level of the frontoethmoidal suture and the posterior ethmoidal artery at the sphenoethmoidal recess, and in many patients the canals define the level of the skull base (fovea ethmoidalis and cribriform plate). Not only do the locations of ethmoidal canals delimit endonasal landmarks, but they can also be used to define regions of the orbit.[5] The bulbar part of the orbit is ventral to the anterior ethmoidals, followed by the retrobulbar portion between the anterior and posterior ethmoidal arteries, and the orbital apex is posterior to the posterior ethmoidal arteries. The medial orbital wall ends at the optic canal, comprising the body and lesser wing of the sphenoid bone, and is typically found 42 mm (range 32–53 mm) posterior to the anterior lacrimal crest.[6] As a general rule we use the pneumonic "24, 12, 6": the anterior ethmoidal artery is 24 mm posterior to the orbital rim, the posterior ethmoidal artery 12 mm behind the anterior ethmoidal, and the optic canal 6 mm posterior to the posterior ethmoidal.

Finally, the majority of the orbital floor is composed of the maxillary bone medially and the zygoma laterally, with a small contribution posteriorly by the orbital process of the palatine bone. The orbital floor is sloped upward by about 20° from anterior to posterior, an important consideration during fracture repair.[1] The inferior orbital fissure (IOF) travels anteriorly at the junction of the inferior and lateral orbital walls and carries the zygomatic branch of V_2, the infraorbital branch of V_2, the infraorbital artery (a branch of the internal maxillary artery) and vein, and the parasympathetic postganglionic branches from the pterygopalatine ganglion that travel to the lacrimal gland. The IOF ends approximately 24 mm (range 17–29 mm) posterior to the orbital rim and communicates posteriorly with the foramen rotundum.[1] The IOF is an important surgical landmark for many endoscopic procedures. In addition, because the IOF neighbors the superior orbital fissure and pterygopalatine fossa, spread of pathology can readily occur in these regions.[7] The

orbital floor is the most deformable wall when exposed to static loading, which explains the high frequency of fractures.[4] When attempting to access the orbital apex surgically, it is important to remember that the floor does not extend to the apex but rather ends at the pterygopalatine fossa.

On imaging, axial view of the midorbit will reveal relatively straightforward normal relationships between the orbital walls; any variation should alert the clinician of possible pathology. The medial orbital walls maintain a roughly parallel configuration. The lateral and medial orbital walls meet at a 45° angle, whereas the lateral orbital walls are roughly 90° apart.[1]

The superior orbital fissure (SOF) lies at the apex of the orbit and is formed by the lesser and greater wings of the sphenoid, separating the orbital roof from the lateral orbital wall and forming a rough **V**-shape as it joins the more anteriorly oriented IOF. It provides an opening for many important anatomical structures to pass from the cranium into the orbit. It can be divided into two regions by a ring of fibrous tissue, known as the annulus of Zinn, which envelops structures within the superior orbital fissure as well as the optic nerve and ophthalmic artery, which traverse the optic canal. The four rectus muscles arise from the annulus of Zinn and travel anteriorly to form the intraconal and extraconal spaces of the orbit. The nasociliary, oculomotor, and abducens nerves pass within the annulus of Zinn. The frontal, lacrimal, and trochlear nerves as well as the superior and inferior ophthalmic veins pass outside the annulus of Zinn in the superior orbital fissure.

The optic canal exits the orbit superomedially along the apex of the orbital roof, traveling medially and superiorly at about a 35° angle toward the optic chiasm. The canal is 8 to 12 mm long and abuts the posterior ethmoid and/or sphenoid sinuses, depending on individual anatomy. Notably, in about 40% of individuals, the optic canal may bulge into the adjacent sinus, occasionally surrounded by a pneumatized sinus.[8,9] A detailed review of all aspects of orbital anatomy can be found in Dutton's highly regarded atlas on the subject.[1]

28.3 Regional Pathology and Differential Diagnosis

The differential diagnosis of orbital pathology is broad but can be concisely established based on the location of the pathology within the orbit and structures involved.[10] It is important to keep in mind the variability of clinical manifestations depending on the location of the lesion. Rhoton et al described the division of the regional pathologies into three anteroposterior compartments delimited by the anterior and posterior ethmoidal arteries.[5] A fourth region where pathology can lie is posterior to the orbit in the region of the optic nerves.

1. The most anterior compartment is the **bulbar region**, which contains the globe. Pathologies in this region can originate in the retina, choroid, sclera, and vitreous body but most frequently arise from the lacrimal gland through posterior spread of eyelid processes. The most common pediatric and adult intraocular malignancies are retinoblastoma and choroidal melanoma, respectively. A variant of idiopathic orbital inflammatory syndrome (IOIS) known as posterior scleritis affects the bulbar region and frequently spills posteriorly into the intraconal orbital fat. Various forms of inflammation

(e.g., sarcoidosis, granulomatosis with polyangiitis, IgG4-related orbitopathy) may affect the peribulbar tissue, also extending posteriorly into orbital fat.

2. The middle compartment, or **retrobulbar region**, can be further divided into the intraconal and extraconal space. The cone is defined by the rectus muscles. Common intraconal pathologies (▶ Fig. 28.2a,b) include cavernous hemangioma, IOIS, schwannomas, non-Hodgkin's lymphomas (NHL), solitary fibrous tumors, and metastases (usually breast, prostate, or lung carcinoma), among others. The conal space (essentially the rectus muscles) is often affected by thyroid eye disease, IOIS, and NHL. Extraconal lesions are located external to the rectus muscles and can be further distinguished by their location relative to the periorbita. Lesions deep to the periorbita are considered "intradural" (▶ Fig. 28.2c), and lesions outside the periorbita are extradural (▶ Fig. 28.2d). Common extraconal lesions are dermoid cysts and benign or malignant lacrimal gland masses (e.g., pleomorphic adenoma, adenoid cystic carcinoma, NHL) that mimic salivary gland pathology. Common extradural lesions include mucoceles and subperiosteal abscesses from adjacent paranasal sinuses, as well as bony lesions such as osteomas, fibrous dysplasia, and hyperostotic sphenoid wing meningiomas.

3. The posterior compartment is the **orbital apex**. Pathologies affecting the orbital apex include parasellar or sphenoid wing meningiomas, schwannomas, and cavernous hemangiomas.

4. The optic nerve and its surrounding meningeal sheath may harbor a variety of neoplastic and inflammatory processes, including optic nerve glioma in children and optic nerve sheath meningioma in adults, as well as sarcoidal or lymphomatous infiltration, infection (Lyme's disease), and demyelinating disease (optic neuritis with or without multiple sclerosis).

Other pathologies can originate from adjacent structures and grow to invade the orbit. Sinonasal malignancies are the most common lesions to secondarily involve the orbit. Tumors originating from the adjacent sphenoid wing include spheno-orbital meningiomas, metastases (especially from the prostate), lymphoproliferative disease (plasmacytoma, multiple myeloma), and histiocytosis X (especially eosinophilic granuloma in adults). The skin may also serve as the origin of subsequent orbital pathology; perineural spread of cutaneous squamous cell carcinoma into the orbit and skull base is an often overlooked condition and a leading cause of orbital exenteration.[11,12]

28.4 Clinical Assessment

Orbital pathology can present with a host of symptoms that vary in severity and duration. In general, pain is associated with infection, inflammation, or malignancy (especially with perineural invasion). Globe dystopia, either axially (exophthalmos) or nonaxially (e.g., hypoglobus, hyperglobus), may be noted. Diplopia may occur but is often absent, especially in slowly progressive, noninflamed, well-tolerated processes such as cavernous hemangioma, sphenoid wing meningioma, and NHL. Likewise, visual loss may be profound secondary to rapidly expansile or compressive lesions (orbital hemorrhage, subperiosteal abscess) or subtle in cases of slowly progressive

processes (thyroid eye disease, cavernous hemangioma, sphenoid wing meningioma).

Clinical assessment begins with evaluation of the afferent system for signs of optic nerve dysfunction.[13] Visual acuity with the Snellen chart and pupillary reaction to light are two methods of determining function of the afferent system. Confrontation fields can also be performed monocularly in all four peripheral and central quadrants with finger counting. Note that not all afferent visual parameters need be abnormal. As an example, a patient may have 20/20 central acuity and still harbor a significant optic neuropathy.

The efferent system should also be evaluated. A cardinal rule to remember when evaluating the efferent system is that pupils, extraocular motility, and eyelid position are related: when one is abnormal, it is extremely important to carefully check the other two. Anisocoria may be either physiologic or nonphysiologic. Physiologic anisocoria can be seen in up to 20% of normal individuals but is typically mild and seen in dim light.[13] Nonphysiologic anisocoria may result from abnormalities of the sympathetic and parasympathetic innervation to the iris musculature but may also occur following intraocular surgery (e.g., cataract extraction).

Extraocular motility testing should be performed to look for full and smooth pursuits (slow, tracking movements) and saccades (rapid movements toward an eccentric target) in the four principle gazes, as well as oblique gazes.[14] If either eye has a limitation of gaze, then forced duction and force generation testing with forceps should be performed to evaluate for a restrictive or paretic process, respectively. If the patient complains of diplopia, it is of paramount importance to ascertain whether the diplopia is monocular or binocular.[13] Monocular diplopia is rarely caused by neurologic disease and typically connotes an abnormality of the eye (corneal or lens aberration, macular abnormality, etc.), whereas binocular diplopia points to an ocular misalignment.

The third parameter for evaluation of the efferent system is eyelid position. Palpebral apertures size should be measured as well for any signs of ptosis or eyelid retraction. Of note, in addition to the upper eyelid ptosis, patients who have Horner's syndrome may also have asymmetry of lower eyelid position, with the affected lower eyelid positioned higher than the unaffected side in what is called "reverse ptosis."

Slit lamp examination may reveal signs of conjunctival chemosis or hyperemia, indicating a possible orbital process. Arterialization of the conjunctival veins suggests an arteriovenous malformation of the orbit or skull base; this finding is most frequently encountered in a carotid–cavernous fistula.

Dilated funduscopic examination should be performed to evaluate the optic nerve, retina, and retinal vascular tree. Unilateral optic disc swelling suggests a localized orbital or optic nerve process, whereas bilateral disc swelling often indicates increased intracranial pressure and requires urgent neuroimaging.[13,14] Optic disc pallor may be present in a variety of pathologies but usually indicates that the process is at least 4 weeks old. Chorioretinal folds are highly suggestive of an orbital (usually intraconal) process.

One additional useful technology for orbital and skull base disease is optical coherence tomography (OCT), which provides detailed information on the topography of the optic nerve and macula, supplying the clinician with objective measurements of

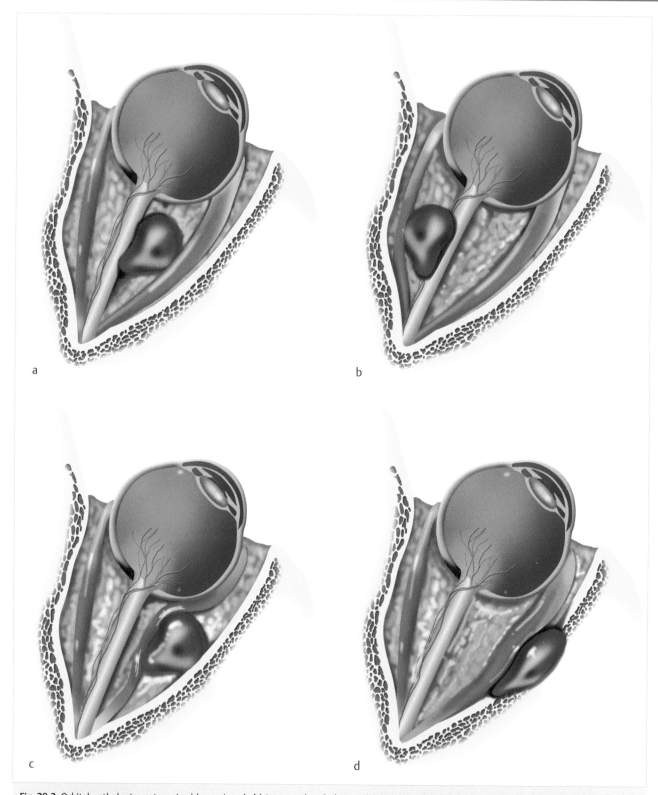

Fig. 28.2 Orbital pathologies categorized by region: **(a,b)** intraconal pathologies, **(c)** "intradural" pathologies within the periorbita, and **(d)** "extradural" pathologies outside the periorbita.

a variety of parameters, including nerve fiber layer thickness. In addition, preoperative OCT has been shown to have prognostic implication in patients who have preoperative visual loss and who are undergoing transnasal hypophysectomy.[15,16]

In general, lesions closer to the orbital apex wreak greater havoc on the afferent and efferent visual system than those found in the anterior orbit. Optic neuropathy and concomitant multiple sensory and motor cranial neuropathies are seen frequently with lesions of the orbital apex, cavernous sinus, and adjacent areas of the skull base.

28.5 Diagnostic Imaging

The two imaging modalities that are critical for evaluation of orbital pathology are CT and MRI studies of the orbits. Sequences used for routine imaging of the brain do not provide the same detail as dedicated orbital studies.[17] Multidetector CT is a rapid, readily available study that is highly useful in emergency or posttraumatic situations and when bony detail is necessary. CT of the orbit has distinct advantages over that of the brain, mainly because the fat in the orbit is relatively radiolucent on CT, providing excellent detail of nonlipomatous normal anatomy and pathologic processes. However, this detail diminishes significantly at the orbital apex and skull base.[14] When possible, intravenous contrast should be used, although this is unnecessary in cases of orbital trauma or in thyroid eye disease.

Contrast-enhanced MRI with fat saturation (fat suppression) is critical in providing the soft tissue definition necessary to delineate the location and extent of an orbital lesion, especially at the orbital apex and skull base.[14,17] Lack of fat saturation and contrast greatly diminish the efficacy of orbital MRI, mainly because in contradistinction to CT, the hyperintensity of the fat on T1-weighted images overwhelms normal anatomy and pathologic processes.

CT and MR angiography play an important role in certain orbital pathologies when there is a suspicion of abnormal vasculature. The three most common clinical situations include Horner's syndrome (possible internal carotid artery dissection), oculomotor nerve palsy (posterior communicating artery aneurysm), and suspected carotid cavernous fistula (admittedly, CT angiography and MR angiography may not visualize small caliber vascular abnormalities). Color Doppler ultrasonography is useful in a variety of suspected embolic or vascular processes of the orbit, including evaluation for a carotid–cavernous fistula. Finally, four-vessel cerebral angiography remains the gold standard in the work-up of neuro-orbital vascular disease. Although the cerebral angiogram may be more invasive, it also allows the possibility of concurrent endovascular intervention.

28.6 Preoperative Preparation

The goal of surgery should be clearly delineated, especially when a pathology involves the orbital apex or skull base. Because of the density and complexity of important efferent and afferent neural structures in this area, significant potential risks exist, and these should be reviewed with the patient in detail. Any patient undergoing orbitotomy must be warned about the possibility of partial or complete iatrogenic visual loss, most of which has no effective treatment. Visual loss in orbital surgery is unpredictable and may occur secondary to intraoperative manipulation or compression of the globe and/or optic nerve, vasospasm of the ophthalmic and/or central retinal arteries, or laceration of the globe and/or optic nerve. The risk of visual loss is higher with surgery in the orbital apex.[18,19] External ophthalmoplegia with symptomatic diplopia and ptosis is a common sequela of orbital surgery and is almost guaranteed following orbital apical surgery.

Much or all of the external ophthalmoplegia will resolve spontaneously over weeks to months, but the patient is often quite symptomatic in the interim. Pupillary abnormalities are less common and less symptomatic, but the patient should be warned about this possibility.

28.7 Surgical Technique

The location of the lesion will dictate the surgical approach. Additional considerations are the surgical goals with biopsy, decompression, or resection. The surgical approaches to the orbit can be broadly divided into two categories: transcranial extraorbital and transorbital extracranial. In general, the transcranial route is indicated for posteriorly placed lesions in the orbit (orbital apex and optic canal) or if there is infiltration into the skull base. Tumors in the anterior orbit that are superficial can often be reached extracranially. Each of the approaches is described in more detail hereafter.

28.7.1 Extraorbital Transcranial Approaches

The transcranial surgical approaches to the orbit may be arbitrarily divided into two types based on whether the superior orbital rim is removed when exposing the orbital lesion. Early approaches involved removal of a frontal or frontotemporal bone flap, with preservation of the supraorbital rim, and opening of the orbit behind the rim.[10,16,17,18,19,20,21,22] The transcranial approaches to the orbit use exposures of the orbital roof and lateral wall that are very common to neurosurgeons. We offer a brief description of these approaches within the context of treating lesions of the orbit.

A standard frontotemporal craniotomy can provide optimal access to the optic canal and orbital apex through the orbital roof, as well as the SOF and IOF and the cavernous sinus. It is important to drill and flatten the sphenoid wing so as to facilitate access to the anterior cranial fossa floor, which corresponds to the superior border of the orbit. The meningo-orbital band is incised to relax the frontal and temporal dura and to minimize retraction. The floor of the anterior fossa can then be drilled with a diamond bit. Care must be taken to maintain the periorbital plane. The periorbita is then opened in a semilunar fashion. At this point, three routes can be taken to access the lesion relative to the optic nerve. The medial route is between the SOM and the superior rectus/levator complex. The central route requires splitting of the superior rectus/levator complex. The lateral route is directed between the superior rectus/levator complex and the lateral rectus muscle. Blunt dissection with cotton-tipped applicators and neurosurgical cottonoids is used to access the specific route. The motor nerves (III, IV, and VI) are often encountered via the superior approach and should be gently reflected to minimize iatrogenic injury. The oculomotor nerve branches are typically robust and easily identified and lie within the intraconal space. In contrast, the trochlear nerve travels from the superior orbital fissure in the extraconal space and is the smallest cranial nerve; it is frequently injured during orbital dissection, especially with the superomedial approach.

The borders of the lesion are defined circumferentially, and the tumor is either excised en bloc or decompressed internally.

If possible, the tumor is carefully dissected off the surrounding structures and removed. The extraocular muscles are often bluntly retracted during tumor dissection, which must be done with care in the orbital apex, because the motor nerves innervate each rectus muscle on its internal aspect at the junction of the posterior third and anterior two-thirds of the muscle. The orbital roof is reconstructed with a collagen sponge and a malleable titanium plate, taking care to avoid iatrogenic compression of the orbital apex and trapping of the muscles. The supraorbital osteotomy via an eyelid or eyebrow incision offers a less invasive approach to access the floor of the anterior cranial fossa, and specifically the retrobulbar area and orbital apex. The contralateral optic nerve and canal are more difficult to visualize. The size of the frontal sinus must also be considered, as a large and more lateral sinus extension may be better suited for a frontotemporal craniotomy to facilitate access for frontal sinus reconstruction or cranialization. An incision along the inferior or superior border of the eyebrow may also be used and is extended medially up to the supraorbital notch.

The periorbita is cut with a 15-blade or Bovie cautery along the orbital roof, and this dissection proceeds posteriorly and subperiosteally along the orbital roof, laterally to the zygoma, medially to the supraorbital notch, and superiorly along the frontal bone. The temporalis is dissected to expose the keyhole. The soft tissue is retracted with fish hooks. For the eyelid and eyebrow approaches, a bur hole is placed at the keyhole to expose the frontal dura and periorbita. A frontal craniotomy with orbital osteotomy is performed from this bur hole, starting superiorly over the frontal bone medial to the supraorbital notch. Next the orbital roof is drilled from the bur hole while protecting the periorbita. Finally the zygoma is detached inferior to the frontozygomatic suture. The anterior fossa floor can then be thinned to permit access to the superior orbit. These approaches permit access to the superior and lateral orbit from the retrobulbar region to the orbital apex, optic canal, and superior orbital fissure. The periorbita is opened with a no. 12 Bard-Parker sickle blade. Blunt dissection allows for identification of the lateral rectus and superior rectus/levator complex. The tumor can then be resected using microsurgical techniques. The orbital wall is reconstructed with a malleable titanium plate. The frontal sinus can be packed with iodine-soaked Gelfoam if the opening is small; otherwise it will need to be cranialized and obliterated with pericranium. The craniotomy bone is then reapproximated with low-profile titanium plates at the bur hole, zygoma, and frontal areas. The galea and skin are closed with 2–0 Vicryl and 4–0 Monocryl subcuticular sutures, respectively.

A subfrontal craniotomy provides circumferential access to the orbit from medial to superior to lateral walls, from bilateral retrobulbar areas to orbital apex. Possible modifications include an extended subfrontal craniotomy, which includes a bilateral orbital osteotomy where the bilateral keyholes are connected to transect the superior orbital rims along with the roofs of the orbits.

28.7.2 Extracranial Transorbital Approaches

The transorbital approaches are categorized based on the anatomy of the orbital pyramid. The specific surgical approach for the management of orbital pathology is dependent on multiple variables, including location in the orbit (anterior, midorbit, orbital apex, intraconal, extraconal, etc.), nature of the pathology (neoplasm, infection, fracture, etc.), goal of the surgery (placement of implant for reconstruction, drainage of abscess, biopsy of tumor, complete tumor excision), and availability of specialized equipment and personnel (intraoperative image guidance, endoscopes, skull base team).[20] It is important to remember that for any given clinical situation, multiple approaches may be acceptable (▶ Fig. 28.4).

Superior Orbitotomy

Superior orbitotomy can be performed in either a limited or an extended fashion and combined with a lateral or medial orbitotomy for access to the entire superior half of the orbit. An extended superior orbitotomy with removal of the superior orbital rim provides limited access to the anterior cranial vault and may also be used to facilitate removal or debulking of superiorly located orbital apical lesions.[21] A more limited superomedial approach provides access to the frontal sinus and the superior ophthalmic vein for cannulization in transorbital, transvenous closure of carotid cavernous fistulas (CCFs) and is one surgical option for optic nerve sheath decompression.[22,23,24,25]

Incision and Soft Tissue Dissection

The lid crease is marked and infiltrated with local anesthetic with epinephrine after placement of a scleral shell over the eye. An incision is made in the medial half of the lid crease and can be extended as laterally as needed for exposure. A suborbicularis oculi muscle plane is dissected. One of two options can be used, depending on the location of the pathology and goal of the surgery. A dissection can be made to the superior orbital rim, with an incision created through the periosteum, staying lateral to the supraorbital notch. A subperiosteal dissection proceeds as described in the previous section. The second option allows for immediate entry into the intraconal space and is useful for anteriorly located lesions, cannulation of the superior ophthalmic vein, or optic nerve sheath decompression. The orbital septum is identified medially by gently pushing on the globe. This forces the medial and preaponeurotic fat to prolapse forward beneath the orbital septum. The septum is incised using Westcott scissors, resulting in immediate prolapse of the fat pads. The levator aponeurosis can be identified just beneath the preaponeurotic fat centrally. The skin/muscle flap is reflected superiorly using a Desmarres retractor, and two cotton-tipped applicators are used to create a dissection plane between the medial and preaponeurotic fat pads into the orbit.

After blunt separation of medial and preaponeurotic fat pads, blunt dissection with cotton-tipped applicators, neurosurgical cottonoids, and thin malleable (ribbon) retractors proceeds either between the SOM and medial rectus muscle (MRM), for medially located lesions, or between the SOM and superior rectus/levator complex (SRLC), for superolaterally located pathology. Anteriorly, the superior ophthalmic vein is identified coursing through the fat between the SOM and SRLC. More posteriorly, numerous short posterior ciliary arteries are encountered coursing over the surface of the optic nerve sheath. If optic nerve sheath decompression is the goal of the procedure, this is completed with a vitrectomy blade, and either slitlike fenestrations or a window are created in the optic nerve sheath. Cerebrospinal fluid is encountered during the initial nerve sheath incision, and the sheath will be seen to collapse as the subarachnoid space drains. If tumor excision is needed, then blunt dissection proceeds as previously described. If wider exposure is needed, the trochlea may be detached from the underlying periosteum sharply using a Freer elevator. Reattachment of the trochlea is usually unnecessary—it will simply reattach at or near its initial insertion.

Closure

For a limited, soft tissue medial orbitotomy, a drain may be placed if needed. Only skin closure is needed, usually in a running fashion. Deeper closure of the orbital septum should be avoided, as this may result in tethering of the eyelid and postoperative lagophthalmos. If a brow incision was made, then a two-layered closure of soft tissue should be used.

Lateral Orbitotomy

Lateral orbitotomy provides excellent exposure to the lateral extraconal and intraconal spaces, the orbital apex, and much of the inferior and superior orbit.[20,26,27,28] A limited lateral orbitotomy also provides access to the frontozygomatic suture area for repair of zygomatic complex fractures.

Incision and Soft Tissue Dissection

The upper eyelid crease incision provides excellent access to the lateral and superior orbit.[29] A lateral canthal incision with a swinging eyelid approach (i.e., with a lateral canthotomy and inferior cantholysis) is also popular because it affords facile dissection and excellent exposure to the lateral and inferior orbit.[20] A limited, inferior brow incision along its lateral 1 cm is often used for access to frontozygomatic fractures when plating is necessary.

For an eyelid crease approach, the upper lid is gently elevated at the eyelid margin, revealing the individual patient's natural crease. The incision may be extended in a curvilinear fashion 3 to 4 mm above the lateral canthal angle toward the lateral orbital rim but should not extend past this point to minimize scarring. Deeper dissection proceeds as previously described.

For a lateral canthal, eyelid-swinging approach, a lateral canthotomy is performed as described for an inferior orbitotomy. The canthotomy may be extended for up to 2 cm to provide increased exposure, although a longer incision will result in a more visible scar. An inferior and superior cantholysis is performed using Westcott scissors. The soft tissues are retracted using rake retractors and a coated malleable retractor, providing direct exposure to the lateral orbital rim, the periosteum of which is incised as heretofore described.

Once the orbital rim periosteum is incised, it is elevated using Cottle and Freer elevators. The zygomaticotemporal and zygomaticofacial neurovascular bundles will be encountered and are sacrificed using bipolar cautery. This will result in hypesthesia over a small area of temporal skin, which is usually well tolerated by patients. The recurrent meningeal artery, an anastomosis between the orbital and cerebral vessels, may be encountered along the orbital roof and should be carefully isolated, cauterized, and cut to ensure that no intracranial retraction occurs. Subperiosteal dissection proceeds posteriorly as far as needed for the particular pathology. Traction sutures may be passed through the cut edge of periosteum to reflect orbital soft tissue inferiorly and medially.

Osteotomy

If a bone flap is needed to improve visualization, it is performed after the lateral subperiosteal dissection has been completed. The osteotomies are extended posteriorly to the sphenozygomatic suture. The lateral orbital wall is grasped using an Allis clamp and bent outward, creating a fracture across the sphenozygomatic suture and completing the osteotomies.

If a deep lateral decompression of the orbital apex is needed (most commonly for compressive optic neuropathy from thyroid eye disease), the greater wing of the sphenoid is removed, using either a drill or an ultrasonic bone aspirator, to the level of the superior orbital fissure.[20,30,31] Thinning of the greater sphenoid wing may also facilitate intraconal dissection for orbital apical masses.

Additional Soft Tissue Dissection

Once the periorbita has been elevated (with or without a bone flap), a periorbital window is created by incising in the quadrant of the pathology using a no. 12 Bard Parker sickle blade parallel to the long axis of the rectus muscles. The periorbital window is usually created in an oblique quadrant either above or below the lateral rectus muscle. Intraconal dissection is carried out as previously described, using blunt technique with cotton-tipped applicators, neurosurgical cottonoids, malleable retractors, and a Freer elevator. The lateral rectus muscle and SRLC are frequently encountered and may be gently retracted with neurosurgical cottonoids or malleable retractors. Dissection in the intraconal space proceeds using a blunt technique. Prolapsing orbital fat may be retracted using either malleable retractors or neurosurgical cottonoids. Care should be taken during dissection of the orbital apex. The motor nerves exiting the superior orbital fissure are often encountered during deeper dissection and should be gently reflected. The abducens nerve is especially vulnerable to injury. In addition, the ciliary ganglion may be encountered during dissection along the lateral aspect of the optic nerve. Manipulation of the ciliary ganglion often results in pupillary dilation intraoperatively; injury may result in a postoperative tonic (Adie's) pupil.

Closure

After the tumor has been biopsied or excised, there is no need to repair the periorbita. It is important to avoid packing the deep orbit with a sterile compressed sponge (Gelfoam) or hemostatic matrix, as these products may expand in the orbital apex and result in compressive optic neuropathy. If any blood oozing is seen, a quarter-inch Penrose drain may be placed along the lateral wall and exteriorized at the lateral edge of the incision; it should be tacked to eyelid skin loosely with a suture to prevent accidental removal of the drain. The drain is typically removed 24 to 48 hours postoperatively, depending on the patient's postoperative course. The bone flap is secured back into position using curved miniplates and screws.

Medial Orbitotomy

Medial orbitotomy provides excellent exposure of the entire lamina papyracea to the optic canal. The medial orbitotomy is used for medial wall orbital decompressions, repair of medial fractures, drainage of medial and superomedial orbital abscesses, and biopsy or excision of tumors located in the medial extraconal and intraconal spaces.[32,33,34,35,36] The procedure can be performed transcutaneously through a classic Lynch or medial canthal incision but has been performed almost exclusively via a transcaruncular (transconjunctival) approach (▶ Fig. 28.3).[33,37] The transnasal, endoscopic approach is also a popular alternative (▶ Fig. 28.4).

Incision and Approach

For the transconjunctival approach a lid speculum is placed to retract the eyelids. An incision is made midway between the caruncle and the plica semiluminaris of the bulbar conjunctiva, and Tenon's capsule is also incised. A 4–0 silk traction suture is passed through the lateral aspect of the incised tissue and reflected laterally. This provides an abducting force on the globe as well as some lubrication for the cornea. A blunt-tipped curved Stevens scissors is then inserted at an approximately 45° angle in the direction of the posterior lacrimal crest. The key in this step is to avoid injury to the lacrimal sac medially and the MRM laterally. The lamina papyracea is then palpated

with the tips of the scissors as blunt spreading of orbital soft tissue occurs, resulting in prolapse of orbital fat. A thin malleable retractor is then inserted along the dissection plane to reflect and protect orbital fat, MRM, and globe. The periorbital of the lamina papyracea is identified and incised using either a Beaver or a no. 15 Bard Parker blade. The periorbita is then elevated using a Freer elevator and malleable retractor in a hand-over-hand technique, entering the subperiosteal space. The anterior and posterior ethmoidal foramina with their vessels and nerves are identified superiorly, roughly delineating the level of the skull base. The vessels and nerves can either be bluntly reflected or cauterized and divided, if additional visualization is required.

Intraconal dissection proceeds bluntly either superiorly (between the MRM and SOM) or inferiorly (between the medial and inferior rectus muscles). The MRM is often substantially retracted during medial orbitotomy, which can result in injury to either the muscle or the attendant motor nerve. Care should be taken to avoid pressure on the inner aspect of the posterior third of the MRM with a malleable retractor to minimize injury to the motor supply. The optic nerve is encountered at the orbital apex as it travels superomedially to the optic canal. Because of tight tethering at the annulus of Zinn, traction on the apical optic nerve should be avoided to minimize iatrogenic injury.

For the endoscopic endonasal approach, a 0° endoscope is introduced into the ipsilateral nostril (▶ Fig. 28.3). The middle turbinate is medialized to visualize the uncinate process and

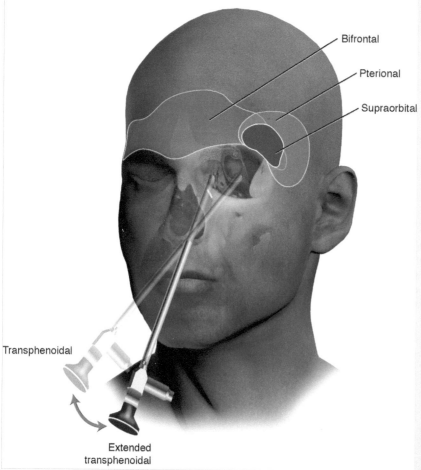

Transphenoidal

Extended transphenoidal

Bifrontal

Pterional

Supraorbital

Fig. 28.3 Transorbital approaches to orbital pathologies.

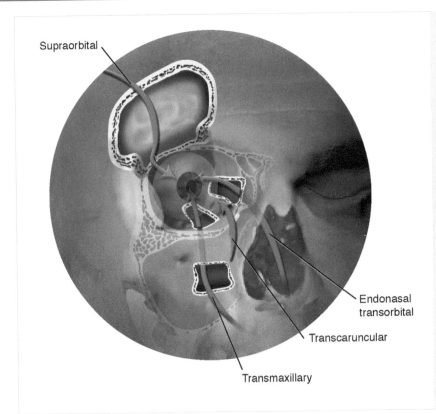

Supraorbital

Endonasal
transorbital

Transcaruncular

Transmaxillary

Fig. 28.4 Endoscopic endonasal approaches to orbital pathologies.

ethmoid bulla. The medial orbital wall is exposed. First the middle turbinate is medialized, followed by an uncinectomy and opening of the ethmoid bulla. The anterior ethmoidal cells are resected to the lateral orbital wall, which is the lamina papyracea. The basal lamella of the middle turbinate is resected to enter the posterior ethmoidal cells, which are resected up to the sphenoid sinus. In the posteroanterior approach, the sphenoid sinus is opened to provide a corridor for dissection anteriorly. The optic protuberance can be identified within the posterior sphenoid wall. Next, the posterior ethmoidal cells can be resected anteriorly until the lamina papyracea is exposed.

Orbital Decompression and Tumor Resection

The lamina papyracea is in-fractured into the nasal cavity and removed. The degree of lamina papyracea removal depends on the amount of preoperative exophthalmos and optic neuropathy. In cases of compressive optic neuropathy, removal of the apical medial orbital wall is essential for adequate decompression. Once the bony decompression has been completed, the periorbita is incised with a sickle blade along its entire length, resulting in prolapse of orbital fat and the MRM into the nasal cavity. If additional visualization and access are required, then a lateral orbitotomy may be performed in conjunction with a transcaruncular medial approach to reflect the globe and orbital soft tissue laterally.

Reconstruction

For repair of a medial orbital wall fracture, the same technique described for orbital floor fracture repair is followed (see hereafter), with one caveat: a medial orbitotomy provides direct access to the optic canal, and care should be taken to avoid direct injury to the optic nerve either during soft tissue dissection or by impingement from the orbital implant.

Inferior Orbitotomy

Inferior orbitotomy is most frequently used for repair of orbital floor fractures and for inferior orbital decompression. Inferior lesions in the anterior and midorbit may also be managed using this approach. The orbital floor, however, ends at the pterygopalatine fossa, and orbital apical lesions are thus inaccessible inferiorly.

The preseptal approach begins with a subconjunctival injection of local anesthetic with epinephrine for hemostasis.[38,39] A 4–0 silk suture is then passed through the lower eyelid margin centrally and the eyelid is everted on a Desmarres (vein) retractor. If a large dissection is planned or if inferomedial orbital exploration is needed, an inferior cantholysis should be performed. An incision is made beginning at the lateral canthal angle and extended for about 1 cm with a mild inferior angle. The lateral canthotomy is completed using Westcott scissors across the full thickness of the eyelid along the length of the skin incision. The cut end of the lower eyelid is grasped with toothed forceps and retracted superiorly while the Westcott scissors are aimed inferomedially toward the tip of the nose and all subcutaneous tissue, including the conjunctiva, is cut to complete the inferior cantholysis. If only limited access is needed (e.g., small orbital floor fracture repair, orbital floor decompression), then lateral canthotomy and inferior cantholysis are unnecessary. Care should be taken medially to avoid injury to the canaliculus; this is most easily done by extending the cautery line away from the tarsal plate, toward the caruncle. The conjunctiva is then grasped just below the cautery line with toothed forceps and the conjunctiva is incised along the cautery line using Westcott scissors. A natural plane is then easily developed and the conjunctival flap along with adherent lower lid retractors is reflected toward the eye. The Desmarres retractor is then repositioned to retract the skin and orbicularis, creating a natural preseptal plane. If orbital fat is seen, then the orbital septum has been violated.

The preseptal dissection toward the inferior rim is performed bluntly using either blunt Stevens scissors or cotton-tipped applicators. A coated malleable retractor is then placed over the conjunctival flap at the inferior orbital rim, accentuating the rim and protecting the globe and orbital soft tissue from injury while the skin and orbicularis are reflected inferiorly using the Desmarres retractor. Bovie cautery is then used to incise soft tissue and periosteum just anterior to the arcus marginalis (orbital rim) along its entire length. Periorbita is then elevated around the orbital rim into the orbit using the malleable retractor and an elevator. Once around the orbital rim, a subperiosteal dissection is easily performed using the malleable retractor and a Freer elevator. The entire orbit is easily degloved of the loosely adherent periorbita except laterally in the area of the UIOF. Care should be taken in this area to avoid elevation of the adherent periorbita to avoid laceration of the infraorbital artery. Once the orbit and periorbita are removed, a multitude of implants can be placed to fill the space to maintain cosmesis. Options include vascularized flaps with fat (i.e., radial or anterolateral thigh grafts) or prosthetic eyes.

Closure

The surgical field should remain dry, and the lids and orbit should be soft to palpation. All traction sutures are removed. Although a layered closure is advocated by some surgeons, the authors typically use no closure and simply realign the edges of the conjunctiva using forceps.[38,40] This minimizes the risk of adhesions and lid retraction and does not result in an increased risk of implant extrusion or fistula formation. If the surgeon is more comfortable performing a sutured incision, then an absorbable suture along the conjunctival incision may be performed in a running fashion, avoiding any deeper tissue. Orbital septum should never be sutured, as doing so increases the risk of lower eyelid tethering.

28.8 Postoperative Care

Postoperative care will depend on the approach and the extent of orbital dissection. Patients undergoing a craniotomy require the usual postoperative care in the form of close observation with serial neurologic and ophthalmologic assessments. We prefer to wrap the head so as to minimize postoperative swelling. Postoperative imaging can be delayed unless there are concerns. The patient's visual function should be assessed as soon as the patient is awake enough to cooperate for the exam. Patching of the orbit should be avoided, as this puts pressure on the orbit and does not allow for adequate visual and pupillary assessment. Serial examinations during the first 24 hours postoperatively are recommended to check for orbital compartment syndrome (OCS). Intravenous corticosteroids for 24 to 48 hours

may decrease orbital soft tissue edema. Diplopia is common after orbital surgery and can be managed by patching of one eye after the patient is discharged home.

Follow-up care is usually with neurosurgery, ophthalmology, and, when taking an endonasal approach, also otolaryngology.

28.9 Complications and Their Avoidance

From the orbital standpoint, the greatest surgical risk is visual loss. This possibility is minimized with judicious intraoperative manipulation of the optic nerve, avoidance of surgical packing of the orbital apex, and careful postoperative assessment and monitoring of the visual and pupillary function. If postoperative hemorrhage results in OCS, a bedside canthotomy and inferior cantholysis (as previously described) and intravenous mannitol may be necessary to reverse compressive optic neuropathy. Diplopia and ptosis may occur even with careful surgical dissection. Both should be followed conservatively for at least 6 months postoperatively before considering strabismus or eyelid surgery, because these findings frequently resolve or improve without intervention. Symptomatic diplopia is managed temporarily with patching of one eye.

28.10 Conclusion

A thorough understanding of the complex orbital anatomy is necessary to achieve a successful operation with minimal complications. The clinical examination and work-up are important to document baseline visual function and to assess the urgency of surgical intervention. Careful review of the orbital and cranial base imaging will delineate the location of the pathology and the differential diagnosis while helping determine the best surgical approach. Numerous transorbital, transcranial, and endonasal surgical approaches can be used alone or in combination depending on the location and extent of the pathology. Recent refinement of these techniques and the cooperation of multispecialty surgical teams have improved outcomes.

References

[1] Dutton J. Atlas of Clinical and Surgical Anatomy. 2nd ed. Philadelphia: Elsevier Saunders; 2011:262

[2] Nitek S, Wysocki J, Reymond J, Piasecki K. Correlations between selected parameters of the human skull and orbit. Med Sci Monit. 2009; 15(12): BR370–BR377

[3] Webster RC, Gaunt JM, Hamdan US, Fuleihan NS, Giandello PR, Smith RC. Supraorbital and supratrochlear notches and foramina: anatomical variations and surgical relevance. Laryngoscope. 1986; 96(3):311–315

[4] Jo A, Rizen V, Nikolić V, Banović B. The role of orbital wall morphological properties and their supporting structures in the etiology of "blow-out" fractures. Surg Radiol Anat. 1989; 11(3):241–248

[5] Martins C, Costa E Silva IE, Campero A, et al. Microsurgical anatomy of the orbit: the rule of seven. Anat Res Int. 2011; 2011:468727

[6] McQueen CT, DiRuggiero DC, Campbell JP, Shockley WW. Orbital osteology: a study of the surgical landmarks. Laryngoscope. 1995; 105(8 Pt 1): 783–788

[7] De Battista JC, Zimmer LA, Theodosopoulos PV, Froelich SC, Keller JT. Anatomy of the inferior orbital fissure: implications for endoscopic cranial base surgery. J Neurol Surg B Skull Base. 2012; 73(2):132–138

[8] Goodyear HM. Ophthalmic conditions referable to diseases of the paranasal sinuses. Arch Otolaryngol. 1948; 48(2):202–208

[9] Van Alyea OE. Sphenoid sinus: Anatomic study with considerations of the clinical significance of the structural characteristics of the sphenoid bone. JAMA Arch Otolaryngol. 1941;34:225–253

[10] Dolman PJ, Goold LA. Clinical evaluation and disease patterns. In: Dolman PJ, Faye A, eds. Diseases of the Orbit and Ocular Adnexa. Edinburgh: Elsevier; 2017:35–56

[11] Heffelfinger R, Murchison AP, Parkes W, et al. Microvascular free flap reconstruction of orbitocraniofacial defects. Orbit. 2013; 32(2):95–101

[12] Hanasono MM, Lee JC, Yang JS, Skoracki RJ, Reece GP, Esmaeli B. An algorithmic approach to reconstructive surgery and prosthetic rehabilitation after orbital exenteration. Plast Reconstr Surg. 2009; 123(1):98–105

[13] Miller NR, et al. Walsh and Hoyt's Clinical Neuro-Ophthalmology: The Essentials. 2nd ed. Philadelphia: Wolters Kluwer Lippincott; 2008:539

[14] Pane A, Burdon M, Miller NR. The Neuro-ophthalmology Survival Guide. Edinburgh: Mosby Elsevier; 2006:415

[15] Danesh-Meyer HV, Papchenko T, Savino PJ, Law A, Evans J, Gamble GD. In vivo retinal nerve fiber layer thickness measured by optical coherence tomography predicts visual recovery after surgery for parachiasmal tumors. Invest Ophthalmol Vis Sci. 2008; 49(5):1879–1885

[16] Lin A, Foroozan R, Danesh-Meyer HV, De Salvo G, Savino PJ, Sergott RC. Occurrence of cerebral venous sinus thrombosis in patients with presumed idiopathic intracranial hypertension. Ophthalmology. 2006; 113(12):2281–2284

[17] Lee AG, Johnson MC, Policeni BA, Smoker WR. Imaging for neuro-ophthalmic and orbital disease: a review. Clin Exp Ophthalmol. 2009; 37(1):30–53

[18] Cristante L. Surgical treatment of meningiomas of the orbit and optic canal: a retrospective study with particular attention to the visual outcome. Acta Neurochir (Wien). 1994; 126(1):27–32

[19] McCord CD, Jr. Current trends in orbital decompression. Ophthalmology. 1985; 92(1):21–33

[20] Rootman J. Orbital Surgery: A Conceptual Approach. 2nd ed. Philadelphia: Wolters Kluwer; 2014:419

[21] Shanno G, Maus M, Bilyk J, et al. Image-guided transorbital roof craniotomy via a suprabrow approach: a surgical series of 72 patients. Neurosurgery. 2001; 48(3):559–567, discussion 567–568

[22] Pelton RW, Patel BC. Superomedial lid crease approach to the medial intraconal space: a new technique for access to the optic nerve and central space. Ophthal Plast Reconstr Surg. 2001; 17(4):241–253

[23] Hanneken AM, Miller NR, Debrun GM, Nauta HJ. Treatment of carotid-cavernous sinus fistulas using a detachable balloon catheter through the superior ophthalmic vein. Arch Ophthalmol. 1989; 107(1):87–92

[24] Miller NR, Monsein LH, Debrun GM, Tamargo RJ, Nauta HJ. Treatment of carotid-cavernous sinus fistulas using a superior ophthalmic vein approach. J Neurosurg. 1995; 83(5):838–842

[25] Bilyk JR. The superior ophthalmic vein approach for carotid cavernous fistulas. In: Gonzalez LF, Albuquerque FC, McDougall C, eds. Neurointerventional Surgery: Tricks of the Trade. New York: Thieme; 2014:165–169

[26] McNab AA, Wright JE. Lateral orbitotomy—a review. Aust N Z J Ophthalmol. 1990; 18(3):281–286

[27] Wirtschafter JD, Chu AE. Lateral orbitotomy without removal of the lateral orbital rim. Arch Ophthalmol. 1988; 106(10):1463–1468

[28] Viale GL, Pau A. A plea for postero-lateral orbitotomy for microsurgical removal of tumours of the orbital apex. Acta Neurochir (Wien). 1988; 90(3–4):124–126

[29] Harris GJ, Logani SC. Eyelid crease incision for lateral orbitotomy. Ophthal Plast Reconstr Surg. 1999; 15(1):9–16, discussion 16–18

[30] Iacoangeli M, Di Rienzo A, Nocchi N, et al. Piezosurgery as a further technical adjunct in minimally invasive supraorbital keyhole approach and lateral orbitotomy. J Neurol Surg A Cent Eur Neurosurg. 2015; 76(2):112–118

[31] Goldberg RA, Kim AJ, Kerivan KM. The lacrimal keyhole, orbital door jamb, and basin of the inferior orbital fissure. Three areas of deep bone in the lateral orbit. Arch Ophthalmol. 1998; 116(12):1618–1624

[32] Lee CS, Yoon JS, Lee SY. Combined transconjunctival and transcaruncular approach for repair of large medial orbital wall fractures. Arch Ophthalmol. 2009; 127(3):291–296

[33] Shorr N, Baylis HI, Goldberg RA, Perry JD. Transcaruncular approach to the medial orbit and orbital apex. Ophthalmology. 2000; 107(8):1459–1463

[34] Kim S, Helen Lew M, Chung SH, Kook K, Juan Y, Lee S. Repair of medial orbital wall fracture: transcaruncular approach. Orbit. 2005; 24(1):1–9

[35] Garcia GH, Goldberg RA, Shorr N. The transcaruncular approach in repair of orbital fractures: a retrospective study. J Craniomaxillofac Trauma. 1998; 4(1):7–12

[36] Nguyen DC, Shahzad F, Snyder-Warwick A, Patel KB, Woo AS. Transcaruncular approach for treatment of medial wall and large orbital blowout fractures. Craniomaxillofac Trauma Reconstr. 2016; 9(1):46–54

[37] Graham SM, Thomas RD, Carter KD, Nerad JA. The transcaruncular approach to the medial orbital wall. Laryngoscope. 2002; 112(6):986–989

[38] Lane KA, Bilyk JR, Taub D, Pribitkin EA. "Sutureless" repair of orbital floor and rim fractures. Ophthalmology. 2009; 116(1):135–138.e2

[39] Schmäl F, Basel T, Grenzebach UH, Thiede O, Stoll W. Preseptal transconjunctival approach for orbital floor fracture repair: ophthalmologic results in 209 patients. Acta Otolaryngol. 2006; 126(4):381–389

[40] Ho VH, Rowland JP, Jr, Linder JS, Fleming JC. Sutureless transconjunctival repair of orbital blowout fractures. Ophthal Plast Reconstr Surg. 2004; 20(6):458–460

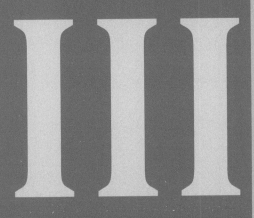

III

29 Squamous Cell Carcinoma of the Nasal Cavity and Paranasal Sinuses

Ehab Y. Hanna, Shaan M. Raza, Shirley Su, Michael E. Kupferman, and Franco DeMonte

Summary

Sinonasal squamous cell carcinoma (SNSCC) is the most common malignant tumor of the sinonasal region. Much progress has been made in the treatment of SNSCC including endoscopic endonasal resection, conformal radiation therapy such as intensity modulated radiation therapy and proton therapy, as well as the use of neoadjuvant and adjuvant chemotherapy. These advancements have improved the outcome of patients with SNSCC. Understanding of the molecular biology of SNSCC will further enhance the treatment of patients with SNSCC including developments of effective targeted therapy and immunotherapy.

Keywords: squamous cell carcinoma, sinonasal cancer, endoscopic sinus surgery, proton therapy, intensity modulated radiation therapy, neoadjuvant therapy of sinonasal cancer, cancer of the nasal cavity, cancer of the paranasal sinuses

29.1 Epidemiology

Sinonasal squamous cell carcinoma (SNSCC) is the most common histologic subtype of sinonasal cancers and accounts for almost half of all cancer in the sinonasal region. Of the 2,698 patients who had sinonasal cancers treated at MD Anderson Cancer Center, 45% had SNSCC (▶ Fig. 29.1). A recent comprehensive analysis using the U.S. National Cancer Institute's Surveillance, Epidemiology, and End Results (SEER) database registry reported the trends in the epidemiology of SNSCC.[1] A total of 4,994 cases of SNSCC were identified, composed of 65% males and 35% females, for a 1.81:1 male:female prevalence ratio. The majority of SNSCC tends to occur in people 55 years old or older, with 3,954 (79%) cases reported in patients within this age group. Dividing the data by race showed that 4,120 (82.50%) patients were white, 438 (8.77%) were black, and 436 (8.73%) were "others." The majority of cases reported the paranasal sinuses (2,693 cases, 53.92%) as the primary sites, with the remainder of cases being in the nasal cavity (2,301 cases, 46.08%). Incidence trend analysis revealed a significant decrease in yearly rates from 1973 to 2009 for the overall population, females, whites, blacks, and "others" ($P < .05$). This decrease may be partially attributable to decreased exposure to textile dust and heightened awareness and better regulation of the exposure to the carcinogenic effect of industrial substances. Another variable that may have contributed to the decrease in overall incidence of SNSCC is the decline in tobacco smoking.[1]

29.2 Histopathology

The majority of squamous cell carcinoma (SCC) of the paranasal sinuses is keratinizing but tends to be only moderately differentiated. Nonkeratinizing and poorly differentiated carcinomas are less common, and the latter show a more rapid course of growth. Variants of SCC make up 15% of all cases of SCC of the upper aerodigestive tract. There are five main histologic variants of SCC in the head and neck region: verrucous (VSCC), papillary (PSCC), spindle cell (sarcomatoid; SCSC), basaloid (BSCC), and adenosquamous (ASC). Conventional sinonasal SCC has been studied extensively, but far less is known about its major variants. In a recent SEER database analysis, a total of 4,382 cases of conventional sinonasal SCC and 328 cases of its major variants were found.[2] Sinonasal BSCC was diagnosed at a significantly lower mean age than sinonasal SCC. Sinonasal SCSC significantly affected the maxillary sinus more commonly than SCC. In the setting of advanced stage disease, sinonasal VSCC, PSCC, and BSCC appear to be associated with a better prognosis than conventional sinonasal SCC, whereas the impact of

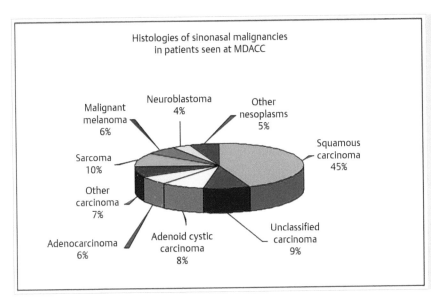

Fig. 29.1 Histopathology of patients who had sinonasal cancer seen at MD Anderson Cancer Center between 1944 and April 2007 (*N* = 2,698 patients).

histologic subtype on prognosis in early stage disease appears to be more limited. Survival for SCSC and ASC, both regarded as more lethal variants, was statistically similar to conventional SCC. This study highlights the importance of distinguishing between conventional sinonasal SCC and its major histologic variants, because histologic subtype appears to carry important prognostic implications.[2]

Another distinct entity is Schneiderian carcinoma, which commonly represents malignant transformation in a preexisting Schneiderian papilloma (SP). Carcinomas arising from SP are rare, with more carcinomas identified in the inverted type and oncocytic types but only isolated reports describing carcinomas arising from the exophytic type. Carcinoma ex-SP ranges from 2 to 27% in the literature, but based on a recent systematic review conducted in 2014, without referral or academic institution bias, the 1.9% rate might be more accurate.[3] In general, the male:female ratio of patients who have Schneiderian carcinoma ranges from 1.2:1 to 6.7:1, for an overall average of about 3.4:1. Patients range in age from 32 to 86 years, with overall mean around 61 years. Most patients experienced a mixed anatomical site presentation: nasal cavity combined with maxillary, ethmoid, sphenoid, and/or frontal sinus, with possible involvement of the nasopharynx and ear. The role of human papillomavirus (HPV) in the oncogenesis of SP and malignant transformation remains to be defined, but some studies have demonstrated that high-risk HPV is more prevalent in dysplastic SP and in those who have malignant transformation.[4,5] The majority of Schneiderian carcinomas are synchronous (carcinoma present at primary presentation of SP), with 36% metachronous (carcinoma developing after initial treatment of SP). This highlights the importance of complete excision and careful histopathologic assessment of all SP, which minimizes the risk of recurrence and allows comprehensive evaluation of the specimen for the presence of any coexisting malignancy.[6] The recurrence rates of SP quoted in the literature vary from less than 5% to as high as 75% and may depend on the surgical approach and the completeness of the surgical excision. Although multicentricity of the tumor has been suggested to be responsible for the high rate of recurrence, inadequate removal of the tumor during the initial resection seems to be the most important predictive factor of local recurrence. This was well demonstrated by Myers et al, who reported less than 5% recurrence rate of adequately resected SP.[7]

29.3 Disease Spread

29.3.1 Local Spread

The most common route of local spread of cancer of the sinonasal tract is through direct extension. Because most sinonasal cancers are relatively asymptomatic when small, local spread often prompts patients to seek medical attention. In the maxillary sinus, direct extension may occur anteriorly into the soft tissues of the cheek, superiorly into the orbit with resultant proptosis and diplopia, inferiorly into the oral cavity, or posteriorly into the pterygomaxillary space, where it may spread along the branches of the maxillary division of the trigeminal nerve (V_2). Cancer of the frontal sinus is quite rare, but the most significant direct extension is posteriorly to the frontal lobes. Cancer of the ethmoid sinus often presents with medial extension

to the orbit, superior extension to the cribriform plate, and posterior extension into the sphenoid sinus and nasopharynx. Cancers involving the sphenoid sinus may quickly become problematic because of proximity to the optic nerves, the cavernous sinus, and the pituitary fossa.

In addition to direct local extension, cancer of the paranasal sinuses can spread to nearby structures via the many fissures and foramina located in this region. Cancer of the maxillary sinus frequently erodes posteriorly into the pterygopalatine fossa (PPF). Once in the PPF, the tumor may extend laterally through the pterygomaxillary fissure into the infratemporal fossa; superiorly into the orbit via the inferior orbital fissure or into the middle cranial fossa through the foramen rotundum; posteriorly into the vidian canal, with extension to the petrous portion of the temporal bone; or inferiorly into the oral cavity by way of the palatine canal or the sphenopalatine foramen.

From the frontal sinus, cancer may extend into the nasal cavity through the nasofrontal duct. Cancer of the ethmoidal sinuses may also extend into the nasal cavity through the middle meatus and the sphenoethmoidal recess, posteriorly into the nasopharynx and along the Eustachian tube, or inferiorly along the nasolacrimal duct.

29.3.2 Perineural Spread

The dissemination of cancer cells along nerves is a frequent pathologic finding among a variety of cancers, including head and neck, upper gastrointestinal, pancreatic, and prostate carcinomas. Tumors that have a considerable propensity to disseminate along nerves are known as *neurotropic cancers*. In the head and neck, the most common tumors having a predilection to invade nerves are adenoid cystic carcinomas (ACCs), followed by SCCs.[8,9] Tumors of the paranasal sinus that exhibit perineural invasion may use this route to spread in a retrograde fashion to the skull base and even progress intracranially. Alternatively, they may spread in an antegrade fashion and along the involved nerve and its terminal branches. In either case, this neural spread makes surgical resection more complicated and makes achieving negative surgical margins less certain. Imaging, particularly MRI, is critical in determining the extent of neural spread of sinonasal cancers, as is discussed later in this chapter, under the section on imaging.[10]

Ziv et al reported the incidence and pattern of neural invasion (NI) in 208 patients who had cancers of the paranasal sinuses and anterior skull base.[11] Forty-one specimens (20%) had evidence of NI. Sinonasal undifferentiated, adenoid cystic, and SCC had a high propensity for NI, whereas melanoma and sarcoma rarely invaded nerves. Intraneural invasion was found in 32% of these cases, and 34% invaded more than 1 cm distal to the tumor. NI was associated with a high rate of positive margins, maxillary origin, and previous surgical treatment ($P < 0.04$) but not with stage, orbital invasion, or dural invasion. Patients who had NI were more likely to undergo adjuvant radiotherapy ($P = 0.003$), which significantly improved survival in patients who had minor salivary gland carcinomas ($P = 0.04$).

29.3.3 Regional Metastases

The lymphatic drainage of the posterior nasal cavities and paranasal sinuses is primarily to the retropharyngeal and lateral pharyngeal nodes at the base of the skull, then to the upper jugular lymph nodes. Cancer of the anterior nasal cavity and those that erode through the maxilla into the soft tissues of the face spread to the submandibular and upper jugular lymph nodes.

Regional metastases from paranasal sinus cancer are relatively uncommon and have been characterized to a greater extent for maxillary sinus cancer than for other paranasal sites.[12] The reported incidence of lymph node metastasis at presentation varies from 10 to 15%, and nodal recurrence may occur in as many as 30% of patients.[13] The most common sites of involvement are the retropharyngeal and level II nodes. In patients who have SCC of the maxillary sinus, the risk of having lymph node metastasis on presentation correlates with extension of the primary tumor to the nasopharynx or oral cavity. The risk of developing regional metastasis after treatment correlates with local tumor recurrence.

Lymph node metastases signify more advanced disease and carry worse prognosis. When the primary disease can be addressed surgically and there is clinical evidence of nodal metastasis, a therapeutic nodal dissection should be performed. Management of the clinically N0 neck remains controversial, but elective nodal irradiation may be warranted in patients who have locally advanced disease.[12,14,15,16]

29.3.4 Distant Metastases

Although distant metastasis from cancer of the paranasal sinus does occur, failure to control the disease secondary to local recurrence is far more common. For SCC of the maxillary sinus, the rate of distant metastasis is approximately 10%, and it rarely occurs in the absence of local recurrence. Cancer of the ethmoid has a similar rate of distant metastasis, with adenocarcinoma having a slightly higher rate than squamous cell cancer (15–20% vs. 10%). In general, the most common sites for metastasis are the lung and bone.[12,16,17]

29.3.5 Staging

The most widely used staging system for sinonasal cancers is the American Joint Committee on Cancer (AJCC) tumor–node–metastasis system. There is a different staging system for cancer of the maxillary sinus than is used for ethmoid sinus and nasal cavity cancers. The nodal staging system for maxillary, ethmoid, and nasal cavity cancers is the same as for other sites in the head and neck and depends on the number, size, and laterality of involved lymph nodes. The classification from the most recent version, the 8th edition,[18] is shown in ▶ Table 29.1.

Table 29.1 Classification of sinonasal cancer according to the *AJCC Cancer Staging Manual*, 8th edition

Primary tumor (T-stage)		
Maxillary sinus	T1	Limited to the maxillary sinus mucosa, with no erosion or bone destruction
	T2	Bone erosion/destruction, including of hard palate or middle nasal meatus, except posterior wall of maxillary sinus and pterygoid plates
	T3	Invasion of bone of posterior wall of maxillary sinus, subcutaneous tissues, floor or medial wall of orbit, pterygoid fossa, or ethmoid sinuses
	T4a	Invasion of anterior orbital contents, skin of cheek, pterygoid plates, infratemporal fossa, cribriform plate, or sphenoid or frontal sinuses
	T4b	Invasion of orbital apex, dura, brain, middle cranial fossa, nasopharynx, clivus, or cranial nerves other than V_2
Nasal cavity and ethmoid sinus	T1	Limited to any one subsite, with or without bony invasion
	T2	Invasion into two subsites in a single region or extending to adjacent region in the nasoethmoidal complex, with or without bony invasion
	T3	Invasion of medial wall or floor of orbit, maxillary sinus, palate, or cribriform plate
	T4a	Invasion into anterior orbital contents or skin of nose or cheek; minimal extension into anterior cranial fossa, pterygoid plates, sphenoid or frontal sinuses
	T4b	Invasion into orbital apex, dura, brain, middle cranial fossa, nasopharynx, clivus, or cranial nerves other than V_2
Olfactory esthesioneuroblastoma	T1	Tumor isolated to nasal cavity and ethmoid sinuses
	T2	Tumor extends to sphenoid sinus or cribriform plate
	T3	Tumor extends to anterior cranial fossa or orbit, no dural invasion
	T4	Tumor invades dura or brain parenchyma
Regional lymph nodes (N-stage)[a]		
	N0	No regional lymph node metastasis
	N1	Metastasis in a single ipsilateral lymph node, ≤3 cm in greatest dimension
	N2a	Metastasis in a single ipsilateral lymph node, >3 cm and ≤6 cm
	N2b	Metastasis in multiple ipsilateral lymph nodes, none >6 cm
	N2c	Metastasis in bilateral or contralateral lymph nodes, none >6 cm
	N3	Metastasis in a lymph node >6 cm
Distant metastatic disease (M-stage)[b]		
	M0	No distant metastasis
	M1	Distant metastasis present

[a]Definitions apply to all subsites except olfactory esthesioneuroblastoma, which uses a N0 versus N1 system for positive and negative nodal metastases, respectively.
[b]Definitions apply to all subsites.

The majority of patients who have SNSCC (85%) present with advanced stage (T3–T4) cancer. Although the reported incidence of clinically evident lymph node metastasis presentation is around 10 to 15%, the overall risk of nodal involvement from SCC of the paranasal sinuses is closer to 30%.[15,16] Regional spread to the lymph nodes is uncommon in cancer confined within the sinus walls. After invasion into the overlying soft tissue and adjacent structures (e.g., the oral cavity), nodal involvement and even dissemination to distant sites are noted more frequently. Distant metastasis can be present in up to 10% of patients on initial diagnosis.[19]

29.4 Treatment

29.4.1 Surgery

Treatment of SNSCC depends on the stage and extent of disease. Early stage (T1–T2) tumors can be treated by single-modality therapy, more commonly surgery but in some selected cases radiation therapy. Patients who have localized disease showed 5-year survival rates of 86%, 80%, and 78% when receiving surgery, radiation and surgery, and radiation alone, respectively.[1] Endoscopic sinus surgery may be applied in selected cases, as discussed earlier, with relatively good outcomes comparable to those associated with open surgery.[20,21,22] The majority of patients who have more advanced and resectable disease are treated using surgery and postoperative radiation. Extension to the skull base is common, and craniofacial resection has enhanced our ability to resect locally advanced tumors successfully.[23,24,25]

Surgery followed by postoperative radiation therapy has been the accepted gold standard for most tumors of the sinonasal cavity. Hoppe et al published an 18-year experience at Memorial Sloane-Kettering Cancer Center in which 85 patients were treated for sinonasal cancers using surgical resection and postoperative radiation.[26] Most patients had SCC, T4 tumors, and tumors involving the maxillary sinus. Their 5-year estimates of local progression-free, disease-free, and overall survival rates were 62%, 55%, and 67%, respectively. The authors noted that squamous cell histology and cribriform plate involvement were independent predictors of local recurrence.

There is strong evidence that the use of combined surgery and adjuvant radiation therapy results in better tumor control and survival than radiation alone in patients who have cancer of the paranasal sinuses.[27] In 2009, Mendenhall et al reported the results of 109 patients who had sinonasal cancer treated between 1964 and 2005.[28] Within this group, 56 patients were treated using definitive radiation therapy, whereas 53 patients received surgery and postoperative radiation. Although the 5-year local control rate was 82% in patients who had T1 to T3 lesions, those patients who had T4 disease had a lower local control rate of 50%. Local control at 5 years was 43% after definitive radiation therapy versus 84% with primary surgery and adjuvant radiation therapy ($p < 0.0001$). Cause-specific survival rates were 81% and 54% for stage I to III and stage IV disease, respectively. This group concluded that the probability of local control and cause-specific survival is better after surgery and radiation therapy than after definitive radiation therapy. However, selection bias may have influenced the poor results of radiation therapy, considering that surgery was likely performed

only for patients who had resectable disease. Similarly, in 2009, Snyers et al reported a series of 168 patients treated between 1986 and 2006.[29] In all, 130 patients were treated with curative intent using surgery followed by postoperative radiotherapy, and 38 were considered inoperable and received radiotherapy alone ($n = 21$) or radiotherapy and chemotherapy ($n = 17$). For the entire population, the 5-year local control rate was 62% and regional control was 79%. Distant metastasis-free survival was 79%. Of the cases involving SCC or adenocarcinoma, patients who had stage I to III versus stage IV disease had local control rates at 5 years of 79% and 54%, respectively, comparable with the series reported by Mendenhall and colleagues.[28] Locally advanced disease that is not surgically resectable can be managed using radiation alone or using concurrent chemoradiation therapy. Radiation therapy alone in this setting yielded poor results, and more promising outcomes have been reported by the use of intensive regimens of chemotherapy followed by concurrent chemoradiation.[30]

The details of surgical management of sinonasal cancers are discussed in Chapter 16 of this book.

29.4.2 Management of the Neck

The incidence of lymph nodal metastasis at presentation ranges from 3 to 26%, and several authors have reported high rates of neck recurrences in untreated necks that can reach up to 30%.[13,14] Although the most frequently reported sites of lymphatic metastasis are level I and II, a significant part of the lymphatic drainage of the paranasal sinuses and the nasal cavity is directed to the retropharyngeal lymph nodes, which are inaccessible for palpation and are frequently overlooked. It is possible, then, that the true incidence of lymphatic spread of sinonasal malignancy is underestimated. The retropharyngeal lymph nodes are best evaluated using high-resolution imaging (CT or MRI) or PET-CT.

The overall risk of nodal metastasis either at diagnosis or as regional recurrence may depend on the histology and the stage and extent of the primary tumor. High-grade tumors such as SCC and sinonasal undifferentiated carcinoma have a relatively higher rate of nodal involvement, do advanced-stage (T3–T4) tumors.[16] Tumor extension into the oral cavity and nasopharynx is also associated with increased risk of nodal metastasis.[13,14]

Lymphatic metastasis to the cervical lymph nodes carries with it a poor prognosis in patients who have cancer of the sinonasal tract. In a study of 146 patients who had maxillary sinus cancer treated at MD Anderson Cancer Center,[16] patients presenting with node-negative versus node-positive disease had an estimated 5-year OS rate of 56% versus 44%, respectively ($p = 0.06$; ▶ Fig. 29.2).

Patients who have clinically positive lymph nodes require treatment of the neck, but prophylactic treatment of N0 patients remains controversial.[13] Because the risk of nodal metastasis is higher in patients who have high-grade and advanced-stage disease, it is generally recommended that the neck be electively treated in such patients. This policy of elective neck irradiation of patients who have advanced-stage and high-grade tumors was adopted at MD Anderson Cancer Center in 1991.[16] ▶ Fig. 29.3a shows the effect of elective neck radiation therapy (RT) on nodal control for node-negative (N0) patients who have squamous cell or undifferentiated carcinoma. Of the 36 patients in whom the ipsilateral neck was left untreated, 13 (36%) developed nodal recurrence versus only 3 (7%) of the 45 patients in whom elective neck irradiation was administered (p < 0.001). The use of elective neck treatment in these patients translated into a significant reduction in distant metastases (3% in treated vs. 20% in untreated at 5 years; p = 0.045) and an increase in recurrence-free survival (RFS) (67% in treated vs. 45% in untreated at 5 years; p = 0.025; ▶ Fig. 29.3b,c).

29.4.3 Radiation Therapy

Radiation therapy is frequently incorporated in the overall management of patients who have cancer of the nasal cavity and paranasal sinuses. Radiation therapy may be given with curative intent or as an adjuvant therapy before or after surgery. Radiation therapy may also be combined with chemotherapy, either as definitive treatment or as an adjunct to planned surgical resection. Radiation therapy may also be

used in the palliation of recurrent or unresectable tumors. Regardless of the treatment strategy, there is almost universal agreement that patients who have advanced-stage tumors are best treated using multimodal therapy, including surgery, radiation, and in some cases chemotherapy.[28,31]

External beam radiation or brachytherapy or both may be used as definitive local therapy in selected patients who have early-stage cancers of the nasal cavity.[32] Primary radiation therapy, however, has not been a well-accepted approach for definitive treatment of more advanced sinonasal cancers. This conclusion was partly based on the poor outcomes for patients who have advanced lesions and are concerned that radiation therapy does not adequately treat bony invasion, which is a frequent finding in patients who have sinonasal malignancies. In additions, several publications have reported increased incidence of radiation associated optic nerve injury and osteoradionecrosis when radiation therapy is administered as primary treatment.[28,29] Although some authors propose primary concurrent chemoradiation therapy for this site,[17,33] the majority of the published data on primary radiation therapy have been for tumors deemed not surgically resectable and have had a selection bias toward advanced disease.[28,29,34] In a study from Memorial Sloane-Kettering Cancer Center, the 5-year disease-free survival (DFS) and overall survival (OS) were 14%, and 15%, respectively, for 39 patients who had unresectable stage IVB paranasal sinus carcinomas treated with RT, with or without chemotherapy.[35] The majority of the recurrence (64%) was within the irradiated field. The investigators reported that the only significant factor for improved local progression-free survival and overall survival was a biologically equivalent dose of radiation of > 65 Gy and that treatment outcomes for patients who had unresectable sinonasal malignancies remained poor.

Delivering effective doses of radiation (60–70 Gy) for treatment of advanced sinonasal cancer using conventional radiotherapy is associated with serious morbidity, including blindness, brain necrosis, radiation-induced endocrinopathy attributed to hypothalamic–pituitary radiation damage, and osteoradionecrosis.[28,29] The use of three-dimensional conformal radiotherapy (3D-CRT) and intensity-modulated radiotherapy (IMRT) increases treatment accuracy by delivering tumoricidal doses to the tumor bed while

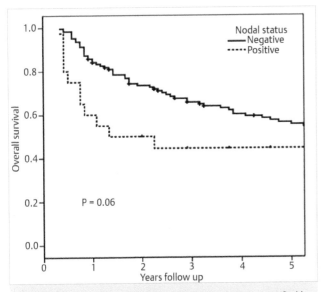

Fig. 29.2 Overall survival in patients with sinonasal cancer stratified by presenting T stage and nodal status.

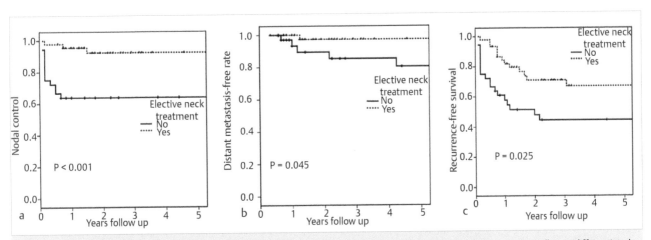

Fig. 29.3 Nodal control, distant metastasis-free survival, and recurrence-free survival rates for patients who had squamous cell or undifferentiated carcinoma treated using (n = 45) or without (n = 36) elective neck irradiation.

reducing radiation doses to nearby critical structures such as the optic nerves and the brain. Duprez et al examined the ocular complications of IMRT.[36] They reported on 130 patients treated using IMRT up to 70 Gy, of whom 101 patients were in the postoperative setting. The 5-year local control and overall survival were 59% and 52%, respectively. There was no radiation-induced blindness in 86 patients available for 6-month follow-up; 10 patients reported grade III tearing, and 1 patient had grade III visual impairment from ipsilateral retinopathy and neovascular glaucoma. Brain necrosis and osteoradionecrosis occurred in 6 patients and 1 patient, respectively. Chen et al analyzed 127 patients treated between 1960 and 2005.[37] The cohort was treated using conventional RT in 59 patients, 3D conformation in 45 patients, and IMRT in 23 patients. The 5-year OS, local control (LC), and DFS were not significantly different when analyzed by decade. However, the incidence of grade III to IV toxicity was 53%, 45%, 39%, 28%, and 16% for patients treated in the 1960s, 1970s, 1980s, 1990s, and 2000s. The authors concluded that improvements in therapeutic ratio were responsible for decreasing incidence of complications for patients treated throughout these decades.

More recently, charged particle radiation using beams of protons, carbon ions, helium ions, or other charged particles has held the promise of further enhancing high-dose delivery to tumor targets while limiting toxicity to normal tissue. The unique physical properties of charged particle therapy—with rapid falloff of dose beyond the Bragg peak (a sharp deposition of dose at a specific depth in tissue)—and its increased biological effectiveness compared with photon therapy might further augment treatment outcomes, not only by reducing the incidence and severity of complications but also by allowing an escalation in radiation dose to improve tumor control and survival, which cannot be achieved using photon therapy. A recent systematic review and meta-analysis compared the clinical outcomes of patients treated using charged particle therapy with those of individuals receiving photon therapy.[38] The study included 43 cohorts from 41 noncomparative observational studies, of which 30 cohorts were treated with photon therapy (1,186 patients) whereas 13 received charged particle therapy (286 patients). Median follow-up for the charged particle therapy group was 38 months (range 5–73), and that for the photon therapy group was 40 months (14–97). The pooled event rate of overall survival for charged particle therapy was significantly higher than that for photon therapy at the longest duration of follow-up (relative risk 1·27, 95% CI [confidence interval] 1·01–1·59; $p = 0.037$) and at 5 years (1·51, 1·14–1·99; $p = 0.0038$); see ▶ Table 29.2.

Locoregional control was also significantly better at the longest duration of follow-up for patients treated with charged particle therapy than for those receiving photon therapy (1·18, 1·01–1·37; $p = 0.031$), but not at 5 years (1·06, 0·68–1·67; $p = 0.79$). The pooled 5-year disease-free survival event rate was significantly higher for charged particle therapy than for photon therapy (1·93, 1·36–2·75; $p = 0.0003$), but not at longest follow-up (1·51, 1·00–2·30; $p = 0.052$). ▶ Table 29.3 shows the comparison of primary outcomes for cohorts receiving proton beam therapy versus those given IMRT. Disease-free survival at 5 years and locoregional control at longest follow-up were significantly higher in the proton beam therapy group. However, no other difference was noted between proton beam therapy and IMRT.

Table 29.2 Comparison of primary outcomes for charged particle therapy cohorts and photon therapy cohorts

	Cohorts (n)	Patients (n)	Event rate (95% CI)	I^2	Relative risk (95% CI)	p	NNT[a] (95% CI)
Overall survival[b]							
CPT	10	242	0.66 (0.56–0.79)	77.5%	1.27 (1.01–1.59)	0.037	7.09 (3.57–480.55)
Photon therapy	26	1,120	0.52 (0.46–0.60)	86.0%			
5-year overall survival							
CPT	6	146	0.72 (0.58–0.90)	80.1%	1.51 (1.14–1.99)	0.0038	4.12 (2.37–15.60)
Photon therapy	15	779	0.48 (0.40–0.57)	84.1%			
Disease-free survival[b]							
CPT	3	78	0.67 (0.48–0.95)	79.4%	1.51 (1.00–2.30)	0.052	
Photon therapy	8	411	0.44 (0.35–0.56)	76.5%			
5-year disease-free survival							
CPT	2	58	0.80 (0.67–0.95)	41.6%	1.93 (1.36–2.75)	0.0003	2.60 (1.74–5.15)
Photon therapy	6	341	0.41 (0.30–0.56)	80.9%			
Locoregional control[b]							
CPT	10	208	0.76 (0.68–0.86)	50.4%	1.18 (1.01–1.37)	0.031	8.55 (4.40–143.44)
Photon therapy	14	736	0.65 (0.59–0.71)	60.3%			
5-year locoregional control							
CPT	3	58	0.66 (0.43–1.02)	81.2%	1.06 (0.68–1.67)	0.79	
Photon therapy	8	546	0.62 (0.55–0.71)	73.0%			

Abbreviations: CI, confidence interval; CPT, charged particle therapy; NNT, number needed to treat.
Source: Reproduced with permission from Patel SH, Wang Z, Wong WW, et al, Charged particle therapy versus photon therapy for paranasal sinus and nasal cavity malignant diseases: a systematic review and meta-analysis, Lancet Oncol, 2014;15(9):1027–1038.
Note: $I^2 \geq 50\%$ suggests high heterogeneity across studies.
[a]Calculated when the difference between CPT and photon therapy was significant
[b]At longest duration of complete follow-up

Table 29.3 Comparison of primary outcomes for proton beam therapy cohorts and intensity-modulated radiation therapy cohorts

	Cohorts (n)	Patients (n)	Event rate (95% CI)	I^2	Relative risk (95% CI)	p
Overall survival[a]						
PBT	8	191	0.63 (0.53–0.76)	59.3%	1.02 (0.77–1.35)	0.89
IMRT	8	348	0.62 (0.50–0.77)	86.9%		
5-year overall survival						
PBT	5	124	0.66 (0.52–0.85)	69.7%	1.39 (0.99–1.94)	0.057
IMRT	4	212	0.48 (0.38–0.60)	45.1%		
Disease-free survival[a]						
PBT	2	56	0.49 (0.21–1.16)	83.6%	0.98 (0.40–2.42)	0.97
IMRT	3	187	0.50 (0.38–0.67)	69.3%		
5-year disease-free survival						
PBT	1	36	0.72 (0.59–0.89)		1.44 (1.01–2.05)	0.045
IMRT	3	187	0.50 (0.38–0.67)	69.3%		
Locoregional control[a]						
PBT	7	147	0.81 (0.71–0.92)	55.2%	1.44 (1.05–1.51)	0.011
IMRT	4	258	0.64 (0.57–0.72)	33.7%		
5-year locoregional control						
PBT	2	36	0.43 (0.09–2.10)	89.5%	0.73 (0.15–3.58)	0.70
IMRT	2	166	0.59 (0.52–0.67)	0.0%		

Abbreviations: CI, confidence interval; IMRT, intensity-modulated radiation therapy; PBT, proton beam therapy.
Source: Reproduced with permission from Patel SH, Wang Z, Wong WW, et al, Charged particle therapy versus photon therapy for paranasal sinus and nasal cavity malignant diseases: a systematic review and meta-analysis, Lancet Oncol, 2014;15(9):1027–1038.
Note: $I^2 \geq 50\%$ suggests high heterogeneity across studies.
[a]At longest duration of complete follow-up.

29.4.4 Chemotherapy

In an effort to improve local control and survival rates, chemotherapy is being increasingly incorporated in the management of patients who have cancer of the sinonasal tract and cranial base. Chemotherapy has been included in the treatment of squamous cell carcinoma (SCC), sinonasal undifferentiated carcinoma (SUNC), neuroendocrine carcinoma, esthesioneuroblastoma, and salivary gland carcinoma of the paranasal sinuses. Chemotherapy may be given as induction (neoadjuvant), adjuvant, maintenance, or palliative treatment. It may be combined with radiation in a sequential or concurrent fashion. Routes of administration include systemic (intravenous or oral), regional (intraarterial), and local (topical).

The incorporation of chemotherapy with radiation in a multimodality treatment approach seems to further enhance local control and perhaps disease-specific survival in patients who have advanced or high-grade cancer of the sinonasal tract. In the neoadjuvant setting, the most frequently used agents are platin-based, as a single agent or in combination with docetaxel, etoposide, ifosfamide, 5-fluorouracil, or cetuximab. (For pathology-specific regimens, please refer to the next section.) Potential benefits of induction chemotherapy are that it improves distant control, provides prognostic information, and can cytoreduce tumors and improve radiotherapy and surgical feasibility and tolerability.[30,39,40] Excellent long-term local control, overall survival, and disease-free survival were achieved in locoregionally advanced paranasal sinus cancer treated using induction chemotherapy, followed by surgery and postoperative concomitant chemoradiotherapy.[30] Induction chemotherapy achieved a clinical response in 87% of patients, and a complete

histologic response was documented at the time of surgery in half of these patients. The 10-year overall survival, disease-free survival, and local control rates were 56%, 73%, and 79%, respectively. These results are encouraging and may be superior to those achieved with surgery and radiation therapy. Further investigation of incorporating chemotherapy with radiation and surgery in a multimodal approach is warranted.[30]

More recently, Hanna et al reviewed the oncologic outcomes of patients who had advanced SCC of the paranasal sinuses treated with induction chemotherapy prior to definitive local therapy at MD Anderson Cancer Center.[39] All patients had T3 or T4 tumors, and 12 (26%) patients had clinical evidence of nodal metastasis, with an overall stage of III (20%) or IV (80%). More than two-thirds (67%) of the patients achieved at least a partial response to induction chemotherapy, 24% had progressive disease, and 9% had stable disease. Subsequent treatment after induction chemotherapy consisted of surgery usually followed by radiation or chemoradiation or by definitive radiation or chemoradiation with surgical salvage of any residual disease. Overall, surgical resection was performed in only 24 of 46 patients (52%) treated using induction chemotherapy. The 2-year survival for patients who had at least a partial response or stable disease after induction chemotherapy was 77%, in contrast with only 36% for patients who had progressive disease (▶ Fig. 29.4). The authors concluded that tumor response to induction chemotherapy in patients who have advanced SCC of the paranasal sinuses may be predictive of treatment outcome and prognosis. Favorable response to induction chemotherapy is associated with better survival and a reasonable chance of organ preservation.[39]

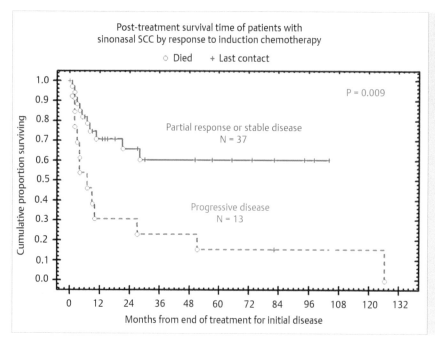

Fig. 29.4 Survival in patients who had sinonasal SCC by response to induction chemotherapy. (Reproduced with permission from Hanna EY, Cardenas AD, DeMonte F, et al, Induction chemotherapy for advanced squamous cell carcinoma of the paranasal sinuses, Arch Otolaryngol Head Neck Surg, 2011;137(1):78–81.)

Intra-arterial chemotherapy has been proposed with the intention of limiting radiation doses to critical structures and organ preservation. The University of Tennessee reported on 19 patients who had advanced stage tumors (84% with T4 disease) treated by intra-arterial high-dose cisplatin with concurrent radiation therapy followed by organ-sparing surgery.[33] The overall survival at 2 and 5 years was 68% and 53%, respectively. Ten patients developed grade III mucosal toxic effect, three patients developed hematologic toxic effect, and one patient developed confusion. One patient developed a treatment-limiting toxic effect (died of myocardial infarction). Homma et al reported similar favorable oncological results in 47 patients treated using intra-arterial cisplatin and conventional external-beam radiotherapy (65–70 Gy).[41] The 5-year overall survival rate was 69.3% for the cohort, with 74.5% experiencing grade III to IV toxicity. There were 25 late adverse reactions: osteonecrosis ($n = 7$), brain necrosis ($n = 2$), and ocular/visual problems ($n = 16$). The authors concluded that this regimen can cure the majority of patients who have advanced tumors and can facilitate organ preservation but that future studies should monitor late adverse reactions.

Topical chemotherapy has been reported to have favorable results in the treatment of sinonasal cancers. The regimen usually involves surgical debulking followed by a combination of repeated topical chemotherapy (5-fluorouracil) and necrotomy. The 5-year DFS has been reported in the range of 85%, comparable to surgery with postoperative radiation therapy.[42,43] Several reports from Japan have described the use of regional or local chemotherapy with radiation to reduce the extent of surgical resection of maxillary sinus cancer as demonstrating equal (and sometimes better) cure rates than conventional treatment consisting of radical surgery followed by radiation therapy. For example, a report described the outcome of 75 patients who had cancer of the maxillary sinus treated using surgery through a sublabial incision and tumor debridement, radiotherapy, and regional chemotherapy.[44] All 23 patients who had orbital involvement retained the orbital contents, and the majority demonstrated adequate ocular function. The authors concluded that combined therapy featuring conservative surgery, radiotherapy, and regional chemotherapy appears to be an effective method for local control and the preservation of ocular function.[44]

29.4.5 Outcome, Prognosis, and Tumor Biology

Several recent reviews report an improvement in 5-year overall survival of 30 to 60%.[1,19,20] The most significant predictor of survival remains disease stage, with 5-year overall survival for localized, regional, and distant disease being 83%, 41%, and 29%, respectively.[1] Recurrence after treatment occurs most frequently locally (36–69%), followed by regional (27–33%) and distant (15–35%).

To improve understandings of the biological features of SNSCC and to promote development of novel therapeutic strategies for this disease, identification of new molecular markers is essential. Because of the rarity of this tumor, however, few molecular studies have been conducted.[11] We have reported in 2014 that a comprehensive study of molecular markers in tumor specimens from 70 patients treated at MD Anderson Cancer Center for SNSCC, using tissue microarrays to explore new useful prognostic markers or novel therapeutic targets.[45] The markers we evaluated included high-risk human papillomavirus (HR-HPV) and its surrogate marker p16, the well-known cyclin-dependent kinase inhibitor p16 Ink4A; cyclin D1, a key factor for cell cycle G1/S transition; 3 receptor tyrosine kinases, epidermal growth factor receptor (EGFR), human epidermal growth factor receptor 2 (HER2), and c-Kit; tumor suppressor p53 and its downstream proapoptotic protein Bax; matrix metalloproteinases (MMP)-2 and MMP-9, which are known to be associated with tumor invasion and metastasis; vascular endothelial growth factor (VEGF), which stimulates vasculogenesis and angiogenesis; and DNA repair proteins Ku70 and

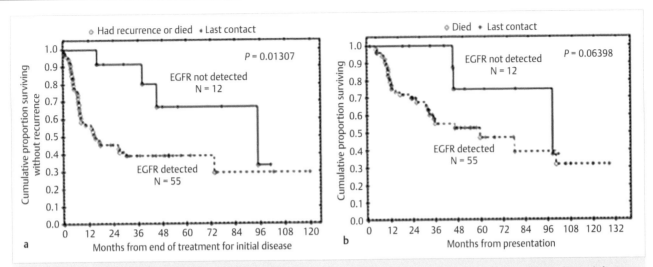

Fig. 29.5 Kaplan–Meier analyses of survival of patients who had sinonasal squamous cell carcinoma (SCC) according to epidermal growth factor receptor (EGFR) expression. (a) Patients who had an EGFR-positive tumor had significantly shorter disease-free survival than patients whose tumor did not express EGFR (p = 5.01307). (b) Patients who had an EGFR-positive tumor had a poorer overall survival rate than patients whose tumor did not express EGFR, but the difference was not statistically significant (p = 5.06398). (Reproduced with permission from Takahashi Y, Bell D, Agarwal G, et al, Comprehensive assessment of prognostic markers for sinonasal squamous cell carcinoma, Head & Neck 2014;36(8):1094–1102.)

excision repair cross-complementing 1 (ERCC1). EGFR, cyclin D1, MMP-2, MMP-9, Ku70, and ERCC1 were positive in more than half of the specimens. p16 Ink4A, VEGF, p53, and Bax were expressed in 10 to 40% of cases. For all the markers except HR-HPV, HER2, and c-Kit, differences in expression between normal and tumor tissues were significant by two-tailed Fisher exact test. The most significant finding in this study was that patients who had EGFR-positive SNSCC had a significantly poorer rate of DFS than patients who had EGFR-negative disease (p = .01307) (▶ Fig. 29.5a). Their OS rate was worse as well, but the difference was not statistically significant (p = .06398) (▶ Fig. 29.5b).

The rate of local recurrence was significantly worse for patients who had EGFR-positive disease (p = 0.0144). In summary, this study showed that EGFR protein expression may be a prognostic indicator for SNSCC. If this finding is confirmed by further studies, targeted inhibition of EGFR may be a new approach to treating patients who have SNSCC.[45]

References

[1] Sanghvi S, Khan MN, Patel NR, Yeldandi S, Baredes S, Eloy JA. Epidemiology of sinonasal squamous cell carcinoma: a comprehensive analysis of 4994 patients. Laryngoscope. 2014; 124(1):76–83

[2] Vazquez A, Khan MN, Blake DM, Patel TD, Baredes S, Eloy JA. Sinonasal squamous cell carcinoma and the prognostic implications of its histologic variants: a population-based study. Int Forum Allergy Rhinol. 2015; 5(1):85–91

[3] Nudell J, Chiosea S, Thompson LD. Carcinoma ex-Schneiderian papilloma (malignant transformation): a clinicopathologic and immunophenotypic study of 20 cases combined with a comprehensive review of the literature. Head Neck Pathol. 2014; 8(3):269–286

[4] Cheung FM, Lau TW, Cheung LK, Li AS, Chow SK, Lo AW. Schneiderian papillomas and carcinomas: a retrospective study with special reference to p53 and p16 tumor suppressor gene expression and association with HPV. Ear Nose Throat J. 2010; 89(10):E5–E12

[5] Lawson W, Schlecht NF, Brandwein-Gensler M. The role of the human papillomavirus in the pathogenesis of Schneiderian inverted papillomas: an analytic overview of the evidence. Head Neck Pathol. 2008; 2(2):49–59

[6] Vural E, Suen JY, Hanna E. Intracranial extension of inverted papilloma: an unusual and potentially fatal complication. Head Neck. 1999; 21(8):703–706

[7] Myers EN, Fernau JL, Johnson JT, Tabet JC, Barnes EL. Management of inverted papilloma. Laryngoscope. 1990; 100(5):481–490

[8] Vural E, Hutcheson J, Korourian S, Kechelava S, Hanna E, et al. Correlation of neural cell adhesion molecules with perineural spread of squamous cell carcinoma of the head and neck. Otolaryngology–Head and Neck Surgery. 2000; 122(5):717–720

[9] Hutcheson JA, Vural E, Korourian S, Hanna E. Neural cell adhesion molecule expression in adenoid cystic carcinoma of the head and neck. Laryngoscope. 2000; 110(6):946–948

[10] Hanna E, Vural E, Prokopakis E, Carrau R, Snyderman C, Weissman J. The sensitivity and specificity of high-resolution imaging in evaluating perineural spread of adenoid cystic carcinoma to the skull base. Arch Otolaryngol Head Neck Surg. 2007; 133(6):541–545

[11] Gil Z, Orr-Urtreger A, Voskoboinik N, et al. Cytogenetic analysis of sinonasal carcinomas. Otolaryngol Head Neck Surg. 2006; 134(4):654–660

[12] Cantù G, Bimbi G, Miceli R, et al. Lymph node metastases in malignant tumors of the paranasal sinuses: prognostic value and treatment. Arch Otolaryngol Head Neck Surg. 2008; 134(2):170–177

[13] Takes RP, Ferlito A, Silver CE, et al. The controversy in the management of the N0 neck for squamous cell carcinoma of the maxillary sinus. Eur Arch Otorhinolaryngol. 2014; 271(5):899–904

[14] Mirghani H, Hartl D, Mortuaire G, et al. Nodal recurrence of sinonasal cancer: does the risk of cervical relapse justify a prophylactic neck treatment? Oral Oncol. 2013; 49(4):374–380

[15] Guan X, Wang X, Liu Y, Hu C, Zhu G. Lymph node metastasis in sinonasal squamous cell carcinoma treated with IMRT/3D-CRT. Oral Oncol. 2013; 49(1): 60–65

[16] Bristol IJ, Ahamad A, Garden AS, et al. Postoperative radiotherapy for maxillary sinus cancer: long-term outcomes and toxicities of treatment. Int J Radiat Oncol Biol Phys. 2007; 68(3):719–730

[17] Robbins KT, Ferlito A, Silver CE, et al. Contemporary management of sinonasal cancer. Head Neck. 2011; 33(9):1352–1365

[18] Amin MB, Edge SB, Greene FL, et al. AJCC Cancer Staging Manual. 8th ed. New York: Springer; 2017

[19] Ansa B, Goodman M, Ward K, et al. Paranasal sinus squamous cell carcinoma incidence and survival based on Surveillance, Epidemiology, and End Results data, 1973 to 2009. Cancer. 2013; 119(14):2602–2610

[20] de Almeida JR, et al. Endonasal endoscopic surgery for squamous cell carcinoma of the sinonasal cavities and skull base: oncologic outcomes based on treatment strategy and tumor etiology. Head Neck. 2014

[21] Su SY, Kupferman ME, DeMonte F, Levine NB, Raza SM, Hanna EY. Endoscopic resection of sinonasal cancers. Curr Oncol Rep. 2014; 16(2):369

[22] Hanna E, DeMonte F, Ibrahim S, Roberts D, Levine N, Kupferman M. Endoscopic resection of sinonasal cancers with and without craniotomy: oncologic results. Arch Otolaryngol Head Neck Surg. 2009; 135(12):1219–1224

[23] Ganly I, Patel SG, Singh B, et al. Craniofacial resection for malignant paranasal sinus tumors: report of an international collaborative study. Head Neck. 2005; 27(7):575–584

[24] Gil Z, Fliss DM, Cavel O, Shah JP, Kraus DH. Improvement in survival during the past 4 decades among patients with anterior skull base cancer. Head Neck. 2012; 34(9):1212–1217

[25] Hentschel SJ, Vora Y, Suki D, Hanna EY, DeMonte F. Malignant tumors of the anterolateral skull base. Neurosurgery. 2010; 66(1):102–112, discussion 112

[26] Hoppe BS, Stegman LD, Zelefsky MJ, et al. Treatment of nasal cavity and paranasal sinus cancer with modern radiotherapy techniques in the postoperative setting—the MSKCC experience. Int J Radiat Oncol Biol Phys. 2007; 67(3):691–702

[27] Turner JH, Reh DD. Incidence and survival in patients with sinonasal cancer: a historical analysis of population-based data. Head Neck. 2012; 34(6):877–885

[28] Mendenhall WM, Amdur RJ, Morris CG, et al. Carcinoma of the nasal cavity and paranasal sinuses. Laryngoscope. 2009; 119(5):899–906

[29] Snyers A, Janssens GO, Twickler MB, et al. Malignant tumors of the nasal cavity and paranasal sinuses: long-term outcome and morbidity with emphasis on hypothalamic-pituitary deficiency. Int J Radiat Oncol Biol Phys. 2009; 73(5):1343–1351

[30] Lee MM, Vokes EE, Rosen A, Witt ME, Weichselbaum RR, Haraf DJ. Multimodality therapy in advanced paranasal sinus carcinoma: superior long-term results. Cancer J Sci Am. 1999; 5(4):219–223

[31] Guntinas-Lichius O, Kreppel MP, Stuetzer H, Semrau R, Eckel HE, Mueller RP. Single modality and multimodality treatment of nasal and paranasal sinuses cancer: a single institution experience of 229 patients. Eur J Surg Oncol. 2007; 33(2):222–228

[32] Allen MW, Schwartz DL, Rana V, et al. Long-term radiotherapy outcomes for nasal cavity and septal cancers. Int J Radiat Oncol Biol Phys. 2008; 71(2):401–406

[33] Samant S, Robbins KT, Vang M, Wan J, Robertson J. Intra-arterial cisplatin and concomitant radiation therapy followed by surgery for advanced paranasal sinus cancer. Arch Otolaryngol Head Neck Surg. 2004; 130(8):948–955

[34] Jansen EP, Keus RB, Hilgers FJ, Haas RL, Tan IB, Bartelink H. Does the combination of radiotherapy and debulking surgery favor survival in paranasal sinus carcinoma? Int J Radiat Oncol Biol Phys. 2000; 48(1):27–35

[35] Hoppe BS, Nelson CJ, Gomez DR, et al. Unresectable carcinoma of the paranasal sinuses: outcomes and toxicities. Int J Radiat Oncol Biol Phys. 2008; 72(3):763–769

[36] Duprez F, Madani I, Morbée L, et al. IMRT for sinonasal tumors minimizes severe late ocular toxicity and preserves disease control and survival. Int J Radiat Oncol Biol Phys. 2012; 83(1):252–259

[37] Chen AM, Daly ME, Bucci MK, et al. Carcinomas of the paranasal sinuses and nasal cavity treated with radiotherapy at a single institution over five decades: are we making improvement? Int J Radiat Oncol Biol Phys. 2007; 69(1):141–147

[38] Patel SH, Wang Z, Wong WW, et al. Charged particle therapy versus photon therapy for paranasal sinus and nasal cavity malignant diseases: a systematic review and meta-analysis. Lancet Oncol. 2014; 15(9):1027–1038

[39] Hanna EY, Cardenas AD, DeMonte F, et al. Induction chemotherapy for advanced squamous cell carcinoma of the paranasal sinuses. Arch Otolaryngol Head Neck Surg. 2011; 137(1):78–81

[40] Mak MP, Glisson BS. Is there still a role for induction chemotherapy in locally advanced head and neck cancer? Curr Opin Oncol. 2014; 26(3):247–251

[41] Homma A, Oridate N, Suzuki F, et al. Superselective high-dose cisplatin infusion with concomitant radiotherapy in patients with advanced cancer of the nasal cavity and paranasal sinuses: a single institution experience. Cancer. 2009; 115(20):4705–4714

[42] Knegt PP, Ah-See KW, vd Velden LA, Kerrebijn J. Adenocarcinoma of the ethmoidal sinus complex: surgical debulking and topical fluorouracil may be the optimal treatment. Arch Otolaryngol Head Neck Surg. 2001; 127(2):141–146

[43] Almeyda R, Capper J. Is surgical debridement and topical 5 fluorouracil the optimum treatment for woodworkers' adenocarcinoma of the ethmoid sinuses? A case-controlled study of a 20-year experience. Clin Otolaryngol. 2008; 33(5):435–441

[44] Nishino H, Miyata M, Morita M, Ishikawa K, Kanazawa T, Ichimura K. Combined therapy with conservative surgery, radiotherapy, and regional chemotherapy for maxillary sinus carcinoma. Cancer. 2000; 89(9):1925–1932

[45] Takahashi Y, Bell D, Agarwal G, et al. Comprehensive assessment of prognostic markers for sinonasal squamous cell carcinoma. Head Neck. 2014; 36(8):1094–1102

30 Nonsquamous Cell Carcinoma of the Nasal Cavity and Paranasal Sinuses

Paolo Castelnuovo, Mario Turri-Zanoni, Remo Accorona, Davide Mattavelli, Paolo Battaglia, and Piero Nicolai

Summary

Further to squamous cell carcinoma, which is the most frequent histology worldwide, other epithelial cancers may arise into the nasal cavity and paranasal sinuses, namely nonsquamous cell carcinomas, which originate with mucous membranes, minor salivary glands, and seromucinous glands. Essentially, these cancers are classified into the following subtypes: adenocarcinoma (intestinal and nonintestinal types), salivary gland carcinoma (adenoid cystic and non–adenoid cystic types), and poorly differentiated tumors such as sinonasal undifferentiated carcinoma (SNUC) and neuroendocrine carcinoma. A multidisciplinary approach is required for management of these diseases, because poorly differentiated tumors may benefit from nonsurgical treatments such as induction chemotherapy and/or exclusive radiochemotherapy, which should be tailored to the specific histology and stage of the tumor, taking also into account the age and general condition of the patient. Endoscopic endonasal surgery is emerging as a pivotal treatment for the surgical resection of these tumors, even if traditional craniofacial and transfacial approaches should be still considered in select cases of locally advanced diseases.

Keywords: anterior skull base, endoscopic endonasal surgery, ethmoid adenocarcinoma, paranasal sinus carcinoma, sinonasal cancer

30.1 Introduction

Nonsquamous cell carcinomas of the nasal cavity and paranasal sinuses originate from mucous membranes, minor salivary glands, and seromucinous glands and may be broadly classified into the following subtypes: adenocarcinoma (ADC; intestinal and nonintestinal types), salivary gland carcinoma (adenoid cystic and non–adenoid cystic types), and poorly differentiated tumors such as SNUC and neuroendocrine carcinoma.

Although squamous cell carcinoma of the nasal cavity and paranasal sinuses represents the most frequent histology worldwide, the incidence, site, and histological type of sinonasal cancers can vary in different geographical areas as a result of occupational, social, and genetic factors. In this regard, selected subtypes of nonsquamous cell carcinoma can represent the most frequent histology in specific areas, such as ADC in some European countries and undifferentiated carcinoma in Chinese endemic areas (e.g., Hong Kong).[1]

30.2 Adenocarcinoma

30.2.1 Incidence and Epidemiology

ADC represents the most common mucosal epithelial malignancy in Europe, although it comprises only the 20 to 30% of all sinonasal primary malignant tumors worldwide.[2] ADC usually presents in the fifth and sixth decades (mean age 58 years). It predominantly occurs in the ethmoid sinuses (85%) and olfactory region (13%), whereas a primary origin in the maxillary sinus is a rare event.[2,3] Because of their occupational exposure to wood and leather dusts, males are affected four times more frequently than women. Hard woods such as ebony, oak, and beech confer the highest risk of developing sinonasal ADCs, which is further increased by inhalation of formaldehyde or other substances normally used in the wood industry.[4] The strong correlation between intestinal-type ADC and exposure to wood and leather dusts makes this disease almost exclusive to carpenters and furniture makers. Accordingly, in many countries (Italy, Germany, Great Britain, Belgium, France, etc.), the tumor is considered an employment-related disease. Recent studies have shown that even short periods of exposure (< 5 years) can lead to an increased risk of ADC. In general, there is an average latency period of 40 years, although it can range between 20 and 70 years.[4] Despite this clear correlation, the molecular mechanisms leading to the development of sinonasal ADC are still unknown. Because wood dust does not have mutagenic properties, it is hypothesized that prolonged exposure to and irritation by wood dust particles stimulate cellular turnover by inflammatory pathways.[5]

30.2.2 Pathology

Sinonasal ADCs can be broadly divided into intestinal-type (ITAC) and non–intestinal-type (NITAC).

ITAC resembles ADC of the intestinal tract and shows a distinctive immunohistochemical phenotype, with all cases expressing CK20, CDX-2, and villin. These staining characteristics can also be found in precancerous lesions, as ITAC seems to be preceded by intestinal metaplasia of the respiratory mucosa, which is accompanied by a switch to an intestinal phenotype.[5]

Traditionally, two classifications of ITACs have been proposed. Barnes divided these tumors into five categories: papillary (18%), colonic (40%), solid (20%), mucinous (14%), and mixed (8%).[6] Kleinsasser and Schroeder divided ITACs into four categories: papillary tubular cylinder cell types I to III (I = well-differentiated, II = moderately differentiated, III = poorly differentiated), alveolar goblet type, signet-ring type, and transitional type.[7] Either classification is acceptable and related to prognosis, but because of its simplicity the Barnes classification is generally the most used.

NITACs are even rarer than ITACs and are merely divided into low- and high-grade subtypes, with the low grade presenting mostly in the ethmoid cells and the high grade in the maxillary sinus.[3] In this subset of ADC, occupational exposure has been rarely observed, and the grade of differentiation of tumor cells has been described as the most important prognostic factor.

30.2.3 Clinical Features

ADCs present with nasal obstruction, rhinorrhea, and epistaxis, which are often unilateral. Anosmia is generally the earliest symptom reported by patients but is generally underrated. Given the paucity of symptoms in early stages and the indolent growth of the tumor, diagnosis is usually late, with patients presenting for medical attention when they have advanced-stage tumors. Because the large majority of cases originate in the nasoethmoidal complex, the most frequent pattern of spread of disease follows the olfactory phyla toward the anterior cranial fossa.[8] Extension into the cranial cavity may result in neurological symptoms, such as headache. Extension may also occur into the pterygopalatine and infratemporal fossae with numbness or pain in the maxillary region. Cervical lymph node involvement at presentation can be seen in less than 6 to 8% of cases, with an added risk of neck recurrences that has been estimated to be around 4 to 6%.[9] Distant metastases are infrequent at presentation (1–3%) and generally involve the lung and liver. Notably, leptomeningeal metastasis has been described for advanced-stage ADC in a nonnegligible percentage of cases (5.4% of cases).[10] On endoscopic examination, ITAC commonly appears as an exophytic mass filling the olfactory cleft, usually at the level of the tail of the superior turbinate and bulging into the nasal cavity, often with a gray, necrotic, and friable appearance.

30.2.4 Treatment

Surgery is the mainstay for the treatment of sinonasal ADC. Endoscopic endonasal surgery is tailored to the extension of disease and may range from purely endonasal resection to an expanded resection including the ethmoidal roof and dura of the anterior skull base, from the posterior wall of the frontal sinus back to the planum sphenoidal (endoscopic resection with transnasal craniectomy).[8] Transnasal skull base reconstruction is performed using pedicled local flap such as naso-septal flap[11] and septal flip flap[12] whenever possible; however, in the large majority of cases, the nasal septum is involved by tumor and a multilayer skull base reconstruction using autologous materials such as fascia lata or iliotibial tract is recommended (▶ Fig. 30.1).[13] In cases of massive involvement of the

dura over the orbital roof or brain parenchyma infiltration, the endoscopic endonasal technique is combined with an external transcranial approach (cranioendoscopic resection).

In patients who have ITAC, in light of its association with occupational exposure, the entire ethmoid box has been traditionally considered to be at risk of harboring preneoplastic changes or developing metachronous lesions. Accordingly, a bilateral ethmoid labyrinth resection, including involved and uninvolved sides, has been generally suggested as prudent (▶ Fig. 30.2).[5] However, this policy has been recently challenged, with some Belgian authors having proposed unilateral surgical resection for unilateral extended ADCs, for which they have reported similar overall survival (OS) rates, with a slight increase in recurrence rate.[14,15] However, currently available data preclude any definitive conclusions, and additional studies of larger cohorts of patients, with longer follow-up, will be needed to adequately address this issue.

Endoscopic endonasal surgery is effective as a single treatment modality for early-stage (T1–T2) low-grade lesions that have been radically resected with negative margins.[16] In contrast, postoperative intensity-modulated radiotherapy (IMRT) improves survival rates for high-grade sinonasal ADCs (G3, signet-ring variant, solid type) regardless of the stage of disease at presentation. The role of adjuvant IMRT is also widely accepted for advanced-stage lesions (T3–T4) and in the presence of positive surgical margins.[10] Given the risk of leptomeningeal spread at diagnosis or late during follow-up, prophylactic brain irradiation can be considered in high-grade lesions with intracranial invasion.[10] Conversely, elective treatment of N0 neck lymph nodes is not recommended because of the low risk of regional metastases (6–8%) as reported in a large-scale review published in 2010.[1] Recently, proton therapy following surgical resection has shown promising results compared with conventional radiotherapy or IMRT, with superior local control rates for ADC (80 vs. 50–60%).[17]

Notably, in the presence of advanced-stage ITAC (T3–T4), a neoadjuvant chemotherapy regimen based on cisplatin, fluorouracil, and leucovorin followed by surgery and radiation has been proposed for tumors with wild-type or functional p53 protein that has been highly effective, showing promising results in terms of disease-free survival (DFS).[18] In addition, a

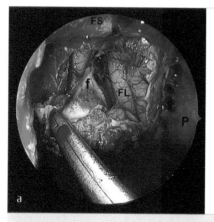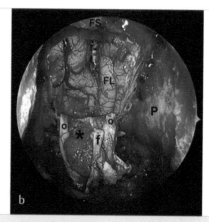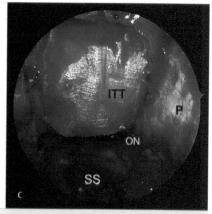

Fig. 30.1 Endoscopic resection with transnasal craniectomy (ERTC). **(a)** Anterior cranial fossa dura resection. **(b)** Removal of the intracranial part of the tumor (*black asterisk*). **(c)** Skull base reconstruction using the multilayer technique. f, falx cerebri; FL, frontal lobes; FS, frontal sinus; ITT, iliotibial tract; o, olfactory bulb and tract; ON, optic nerve; P, periorbit; SS, sphenoid sinus.

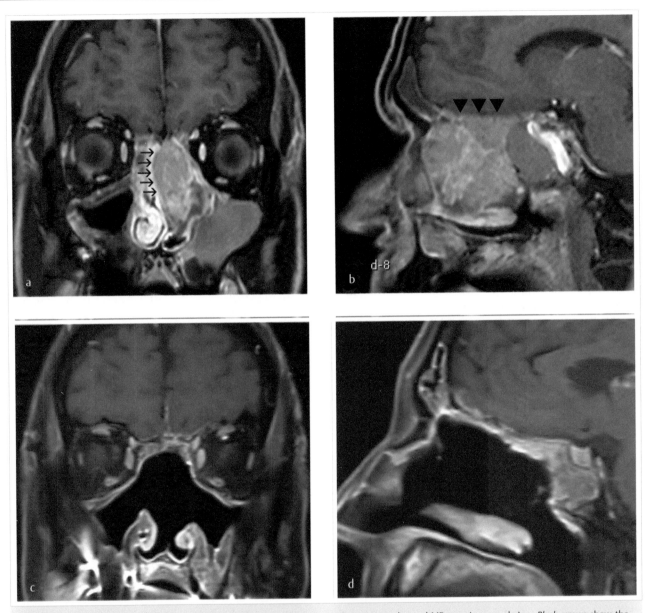

Fig. 30.2 Intestinal-type adenocarcinoma of the left ethmoid. **(a)** Preoperative contrast-enhanced MR scan in coronal view. *Black arrows* show the involvement of the nasal septum by the disease. **(b)** Preoperative MR scan in sagittal view. *Black arrowheads* point out the involvement of the anterior skull base. The patient has been submitted to endoscopic endonasal surgery with transnasal craniectomy followed by adjuvant irradiation (intensity-modulated radiotherapy, 62 Gy). The tumor was classified as pT4b for dural invasion. Contrast-enhanced MR scan in **(c)** coronal and **(d)** sagittal views showed no recurrence of disease after 5 years of follow-up.

subset of ITACs, mostly found in woodworkers, showed high expression of epithelial growth factor receptor (EGFR) on immunophenotyping, suggesting the possibility of using anti-EGFR therapy (**Video 30.1**).[19]

30.2.5 Outcome and Prognosis

The most important factors affecting survival in ADC are tumor stage and histological grade. A multicenter study from France analyzed a large cohort of 418 patients who had sinonasal ADC and found that stage of disease (T4), lymph node involvement, and intracranial extension were significantly associated with poorer outcomes.[20]

Recently, a large case series by Nicolai et al on 169 consecutive patients affected by ITAC reported DFS of 85.2%, 73.3%, and 71.7% at 1, 3, and 5 years, respectively, with OS of 93.0%, 80.5%, and 68.8% at 1, 3, and 5 years, respectively. OS and DFS were negatively affected by histological grade, advanced pT stage, dural and brain involvement, and positive surgical margins.[10] Recurrences were observed in 21.3% of cases: mainly local relapses (16%), leptomeningeal spread (5.4%), regional failure (1.8%), and distant metastases (6.5%). Comparable values of 5-year OS and recurrence rates were also reported by Camp et al (68% from a series of 123 patients)[21] and Vergez et al (62% from a series of 159 patients).[9] Overall, these data strongly support a definitive paradigm shift in the management of ITAC toward endoscopic surgery with or without adjuvant IMRT instead of external surgical techniques, which still play a role for only a small subset of patients.

Notably, in sinonasal ADC the follow-up period has a crucial impact on OS, in particular when unilateral resection was performed—as demonstrated by the Belgian experience, in which 5-year OS dropped from 83% on a midterm follow-up (median 42 months)[14] to 63% 3 years later (median follow-up 61 months).[15] This supports the need for strict postoperative endoscopic and radiological surveillance of patients, who should be regularly followed for at least 10 years to promptly detect late toxicities and local or distant recurrences.

30.3 Salivary Gland Carcinomas

30.3.1 Adenoid Cystic Carcinoma

Incidence and Epidemiology

Adenoid cystic carcinoma (AdCC) represents only 10% of salivary gland malignancies of any site, but it is the most frequent tumor arising in the minor salivary glands, accounting for about 60% of cases.[22,23,24,25,26,27] Consequently, it is by far the most frequent salivary tumor occurring in the nasal cavity and paranasal sinuses. The most involved subsites are the maxillary sinus (up to 45–50%), nasal cavity (20–30%), ethmoid (10%), and sphenoid sinus (4–5%).[23,27,28,29,30]

No etiologic factor has been recognized to date. The male: female ratio is variable in different series; the incidence in both genders is likely to be roughly equal, with a slight prevalence in women.[30] The peak age incidence is between the fifth and sixth decades of life. However, AdCC can arise at any age, and its occurrence in young adults is not rare.[23,28,29] It occurs mostly in Caucasians (over 70% of cases), followed by blacks, Asians, and Pacific Islanders (about 10% each).[30]

Pathology

AdCC has been classified into three different histologic subtypes: tubular, cribriform, and solid. Although several historical reports have stated that no correlation between histologic subtype and outcome is present,[31,32] Spiro et al and Batsakis et al suggested that the solid type is the most aggressive form and that its presence can negatively affect prognosis.[33,34] Accordingly, tumor grade has been correlated to evaluation of the prevalent histologic subtype. Two different scores are currently used:

- Spiro's score[33]:
  - Predominantly tubular, no solid
  - Mostly tubular, occasional solid
  - Mixed with substantial solid (> 50%)
- Szanto's score[35]:
  - Predominantly tubular, no solid
  - Predominantly cribriform, < 30% solid
  - Solid > 30%

Recently, van Weert et al retrospectively analyzed 81 patients surgically treated for head and neck AdCC to define the prognostic value of the two currently used grading systems and to propose a simplified scheme.[36] According to the authors, the presence of any solid component, irrespective of the proportion,

is a negative prognosticator and can effectively identify a subgroup of tumors with aggressive behavior and poor outcome.

This simplified score (presence vs. absence of solid form) is very promising due to its high interpathologist reliability, high reproducibility, and remarkable predictive value, comparable with traditional grading systems.[36]

The clinician should also be aware of a new pathologic entity called "high-grade transformation of AdCC." This rare and aggressive variant features dedifferentiated areas and a typical chromosomal translocation leading to MYB–NFIB fusion protein.[37]

Clinical Features

AdCC of the sinonasal tract is usually characterized by slow and indolent growth, with a distinctive tendency to spread along nerves (perineural and intraneural invasion) and along subperiosteal and submucosal planes (► Fig. 30.3).

Symptoms at presentation are usually scarce and subtle, and this feature is probably responsible for the high proportion of tumors diagnosed in the late stage (up to 76% of T3–T4 tumors

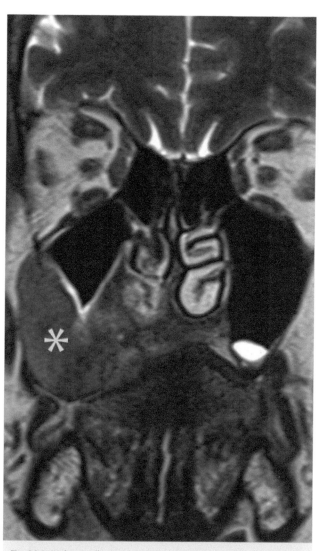

Fig. 30.3 Right maxillary adenoid cystic carcinoma: submucosal spread in the floor of the maxillary sinus and hard palate (*white asterisk*).

and up to 80% of tumors in stage IV).[23,28,38,39] The most frequent symptoms are nasal obstruction, facial pain, and epistaxis.[23] Other complaints specifically related to nerve infiltration have been reported, such as paraesthesia of the cheek or trigeminal neuralgia. Other signs (diplopia, epiphora, proptosis, dental instability, maxillary swelling, loss of visual acuity) are less common and suggest advanced disease.

Endoscopic examination usually shows a lobulated lesion covered by normal mucosa (▶ Fig. 30.4). Due to the almost omnipresent perineural spread of AdCC, clinical examination is often of little value to estimate tumor extension, and radiological studies such as MRI with contrast enhancement are essential.

Site-Specific Routes of Spread

The most critical means of spread of AdCC is along nerves, which can be regarded as the highway through which the tumor can overcome anatomical barriers and reach regions

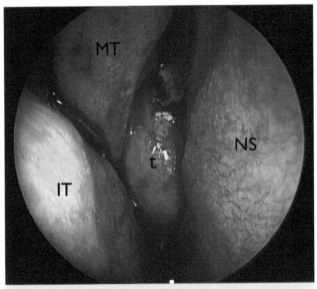

Fig. 30.4 Endoscopic appearance of nasoethmoidal adenoid cystic carcinoma. IT, inferior turbinate; MT, middle turbinate; NS, nasal septum; t, tumor.

distant from the site of origin. Herein, the most important patterns of spread are briefly summarized.

Maxillary Sinus

AdCC arising in the maxillary sinus can infiltrate the infraorbital nerve: by anterograde spread it can reach the premaxillary soft tissues, while by retrograde growth it can involve the maxillary nerve and Meckel's cave. Then, by anterograde route, the tumor can spread along any branch of the trigeminal nerve. For example, it can involve the supraorbital fissure and the orbit via the ophthalmic nerve, reaching other ocular nerves and/or the optic nerve; it can spread to the hard palate through the palatine nerves or reach the parotid region through the auriculotemporal nerve (branch of the mandibular nerve).

Another critical area is the pterygopalatine fossa (PPF), which can be involved either by direct tumor extension or by perineural spread. The PPF is a crossway of nerves (autonomic nerves arising from the pterygopalatine ganglion and anastomosing with branches of the trigeminal nerve) and vessels (branches of the maxillary artery, such as the infraorbital, posterosuperior alveolar, sphenopalatine, and vidian arteries, and so forth). Thus, from this fossa the tumor can reach infratemporal fossa and masticatory space, inferior orbital fissure and orbit, cavernous sinus and Meckel's cave, and middle cranial fossa (▶ Fig. 30.5).

Moreover, the tumor can extend along the carotid artery through the vidian nerve or by direct osseous permeation of the basisphenoid (▶ Fig. 30.6).

Finally, AdCC can also reach the facial nerve through either the aforementioned auriculotemporal nerve or the greater superficial petrosal nerve (which originates from the geniculate ganglion and gives origin to the vidian nerve by joining the deep petrosal nerve; ▶ Fig. 30.7).

Nasoethmoid

Nasoethmoid tumors can easily involve the anterior cranial fossa, either along olfactory nerves or by osseous permeation. Moreover, the orbit may be invaded via the ethmoidal vascular–nervous bundles. Finally, the tumor can reach the PPF via direct extension or vascular/neural spread and from there can spread to all the aforementioned structures.

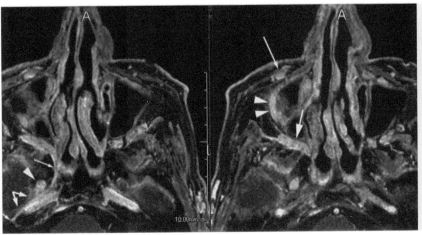

Fig. 30.5 Extensive perineural spread from right maxillary adenoid cystic carcinoma, involving pterygopalatine fossa (*short white arrow on the right*), vidian nerve (*white arrow on the left*), V_3 (*white arrowhead on the left*), greater petrosal nerve (*short coupled arrows on the left*), and infraorbital nerve (*white arrowheads on the right*); "resurfacing" nodule in the infraorbital soft tissues (*long white arrow on the right*).

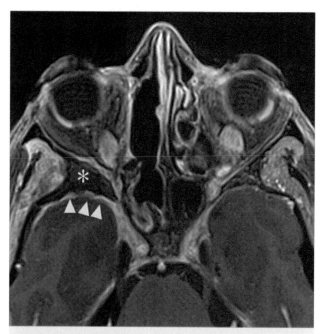

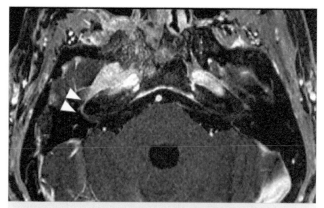

Fig. 30.7 Perineural spread from the pterygopalatine fossa to the geniculate ganglion and along the facial nerve (*white arrowheads*) via permeative invasion of the right basisphenoid and infiltration of the anterior foramen lacerum.

Fig. 30.6 Recurrent nasoethmoidal adenoid cystic carcinoma with permeative bone infiltration of the greater wing of the sphenoid (*asterisk*). Diffuse dural thickening (inflammatory reaction vs. infiltration) in the temporopolar region (*white arrowheads*).

Metastases

Lymph-node metastases are rare. In fact, AdCC per se displays little tendency toward lymphatic spread, and sinonasal tumors are usually at low risk of nodal metastasis owing to the scarcity of lymphatic vessels in this localization (with the exception of the hard palate and infratemporal fossa). The combination of these two aspects can explain the low incidence of nodal metastases (3.6–5.3%).[30,40]

Conversely, systemic spread is a frequent finding. Lungs are by far the most involved site, followed by liver, bone, and brain. Up to 5 to 7% of patients have metastases at presentation, whereas recurrence at distant sites can occur in about 40% of cases.[23,30]

Both local relapse and distant metastases may develop many years (up to 20) after primary treatment.[27,28]

Treatment

Surgery still plays a pivotal role in the treatment of sinonasal AdCC. The study of preoperative radiological imaging is of the utmost importance to estimating tumor extension, and surgical resection should be guided by meticulous examination of all possible avenues of spread of AdCC. All the named nerves adjacent to the tumor should be carefully inspected and perhaps also biopsied; if involved by tumor, they should be resected until clear margins are obtained. Critical areas, such as the PPF, should be always explored and possibly included in the resection. In addition, when the tumor is localized in proximity to bone, subperiosteal spread has to be ruled out by frozen section. Full-thickness resection of bone adjacent to the lesion is recommended in AdCC, not only when clear signs of permeation/erosion are detected, but also when the subperiosteal plane is invaded.[41]

In view of the insidious pattern of growth of AdCC and the complexity of sinonasal region, negative margins can be obtained in

only a minority of cases (about 40%) whatever the aggressiveness of the surgical plan.[23] A matter of debate is whether surgery is the ideal primary treatment when involvement of critical anatomical area (i.e., cavernous sinus) is clearly present. In view of the emerging role of new radiotherapies, as described later in this chapter, aggressive surgical resections should be balanced against their real effect on prognosis and morbidity, which can significantly worsen the patient's residual quality of life. In selected cases, a therapeutic plan combining surgical debulking with a minimal residual disease and subsequent radiotherapy can be considered to decrease overall morbidity. However, further clinical experience is needed to explore the validity of this paradigm. Treatment planning should always be discussed by an experienced multidisciplinary team.

Site-Specific Surgical Issues

Maxillary Sinus

Endoscopic medial maxillectomy is indicated only for tumors limited to the medial wall of the maxillary sinus. Otherwise, depending on the extension of the tumor, more aggressive surgical procedures such as subtotal, total, and radical extended maxillectomies are deemed necessary. Orbital clearance is indicated when the tumor transgresses the periorbita with macroscopic invasion of the orbital contents. If the tumor is in close contact with the anterior skull base, then the corresponding bony layer of the skull base should be removed. In case of involvement of olfactory phyla and/or (trans)dural invasion, resection of the dura and olfactory bulbs is mandatory.

Nasoethmoid

Whenever indicated, endoscopic endonasal surgery is the first choice for resection of nasoethmoid AdCC. In this setting, the advantages related to the endoscopic view (greater magnification of the surgical field, closer point of view, easier dissection of small anatomical structure) are particularly valuable to explore the possible pattern of spread of AdCC (submucosal/subperiosteal, invasion of PPF, etc.).

The main contraindications for a purely endoscopic approach are involvement of the anterior plate of the frontal sinus, massive involvement of the orbit, dural invasion over the orbit (lateral to the vertical line passing through the pupil), massive infiltration of the brain, massive involvement of the lacrimal pathway, and involvement of the hard palate or nasal bones. In these cases, combined cranioendoscopic approach or craniofacial resection are indicated.

Reconstruction

The goals of the reconstruction are to separate the sinonasal from the intracranial space and the oral cavity, allow dental prosthetic rehabilitation, and restore facial contour. Several options can be used to reconstruct maxillary defects: prosthesis (palatal obturator), pedicled flaps, and free flaps. According to Okay's classification,[42] for small defects (class Ia and Ib) an obturator or a fat pad pedicled flap can be adequate. For larger and more complex defects (class II and III z, f, zf), the use of osteomuscular/osteomuscular–fasciocutaneous free flaps (fibula, iliac crest, anterolateral thigh, and tip of the scapula) ensures better functional and aesthetic results.[43,44,45,46] In case of orbital exenteration, the reconstruction can be accomplished using an osteomuscolar/osteomuscolar–cutaneous free flap associated with orbital prosthesis; alternatively, a fasciocutaneous, myocutaneous, or fasciomyocutaneous free flap (rectus abdominis, anterolateral thigh) can be used to fill the orbital cavity.[44,46]

In case of dural resection, vascularized flaps (pericranial flap, nasoseptal flap) are the optimal choice for safer and faster healing. Multilayer reconstruction using autologous graft (i.e., iliotibial tract and fat) is an effective and safe alternative option when pedicled flaps are unavailable for oncological reasons or if their harvesting would result in unnecessary morbidity (i.e., harvesting of pericranial flap after pure endoscopic resections). Allogenic materials can be used when the reconstruction is completed by a vascularized flap. Finally, a free flap is almost never required to reconstruct an isolated anterior skull base defect.[8,47,48]

Nonsurgical Treatment

In view of the high frequency of positive microscopic margins, adjuvant radiotherapy is an essential treatment for locally advanced AdCC of the sinonasal tract.[41,49,50] Much as with surgery, fields of irradiation should be planned to take into account the possible pathways of spread of AdCC. For example, in case of perineural spread, all cranial nerves at risk should be irradiated up to their entry point in the skull base.

Promising data on the efficacy of heavy-ion therapy (carbon and proton) have been recently published, both as single-modality treatment for large inoperable AdCC and in an adjuvant setting.[51,52] Critical extensions of the tumor, predictable efficacy and morbidity of each treatment, expertise of the surgeon and radiation oncologist, and patient's willingness are all important factors to consider in treatment choice and planning.[41]

Chemotherapy is reserved for palliative treatment of metastatic disease; of note, the role of systemic therapies remains controversial, with no real benefit in primary, adjuvant, and palliative settings reported.[53]

Outcome and Prognosis

The natural history of AdCC is characterized by high risk of local relapse (▶ Fig. 30.8) and/or distant metastasis, typically many

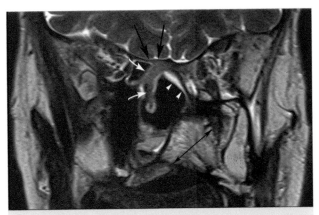

Fig. 30.8 Recurrence of left maxillary adenoid cystic carcinoma after left radical maxillectomy and reconstruction with osteomuscular-free flap (*black double-head arrow*). The submucosal–subperiosteal relapse (*white arrows*) in the residual ethmoid spreads to the vertical lamella of the right middle turbinate, while the overlying mucosa is intact and thickened (*arrowheads*). The periosteal layer of the skull base is still intact (*black arrows*).

years after primary treatment. Disease-specific survival (DSS) is quite high at 5 years (70%) but it drops at 10 years (40%) and further decreases at 20 years (15%).[23,30]

Recurrence rate is about 60% (range, 40–77%) with a slight prevalence of distant metastasis (40%) over local relapse (30%). Generally distant metastasis causes a remarkable decrease in survival rates (from about 65% to 20% at 5 years). Interestingly, lung and liver metastases are usually associated with a better prognosis (with a mortality rate of 50% at 4 years) than those of bone and brain (mortality rate ranging from 70% up to 100% at 1 year).[26,54,55,56,57,58] AdCC arising in the nasal cavity tends to have a better prognosis, whereas tumors originating in the sphenoid have the worst.

The most important negative prognostic factors are invasion of the skull base, pT4 classification, IV stage, solid subtype, and positive margins.[23,26,27,54,57] Perineural spread also has a negative effect on survival; in particular, intraneural invasion was a strong negative prognosticator in a large multicentric study on head and neck AdCC published in 2015.[58] The negative impact of the involvement of the orbit and infratemporal fossa is still unclear, as it did not reach statistical significance in the series from MD Anderson.[23]

Finally, it is worth remembering that the indolent and slow growth usually attributed to AdCC is typical of low- and intermediate-grade tumors. Conversely, high-grade variants (predominantly solid tumors, high-grade transformation of AdCC) can display a very aggressive biological behavior, resulting in advanced local disease and early regional and distant spread. Accordingly, the prognosis can be poor (5-year DSS ranging from 30 to 40%).[30]

30.3.2 Non–Adenoid Cystic Carcinoma Salivary Tumors

Non-AdCC salivary tumors (NAdCC) of the sinonasal tract are heterogeneous and very rare. Consequently, published evidence is confined to small case series and case reports. In general,

NAdCC are diagnosed at a relatively earlier stage than AdCC.[59] Because of the paucity of data, biological behavior, treatment strategy, and prognostic factors must be inferred by NAdCC of other subsites. Tumor grade is probably the most important parameter affecting biologic behavior and prognosis. Low- and intermediate-grade lesions display indolent growth, low tendency to spread along nerves and subperiosteal/perichondral planes, and favorable prognosis.[60,61,62,63,64] Generally, a less aggressive policy of surgical resection is advised in these cases, with adjuvant radiotherapy usually recommended only in locally advanced tumors.[41]

Conversely, high-grade tumors can display a more aggressive and rapid pattern of growth with perineural and lymphovascular spread. Accordingly, the surgical approach should be more aggressive and adjuvant radiotherapy is often required. Moreover, these tumors are associated with a high rate of distant metastasis. In fact, despite a reasonably good rate of local control, prognosis is still poor due to distant failure. The efficacy of chemotherapy is largely unsatisfactory; new regimens and target therapies are currently under investigation.[64]

30.4 Sinonasal Undifferentiated Carcinoma and Neuroendocrine Carcinoma

30.4.1 Incidence and Epidemiology

SNUC is a rare and very aggressive tumor that has a tendency to local invasion and distant spread. There is a male predominance (2–3:1). The age range is broad, usually ranging from the third to ninth decades, with median age at presentation the sixth decade.[1] There are no known etiologic agents. SNUCs are typically negative for Epstein–Barr virus. The anatomical sites mostly involved by the disease include the nasal cavity, ethmoid sinuses, and maxillary sinus, with a slight predominance for ethmoid sites (43% of cases).

Sinonasal neuroendocrine carcinomas (NECs) account for only 4% of all NECs, and very few cases have been reported. The majority of patients who have NEC are males. Although there seems to be an association with cigarette smoking, it is not as strong as for pulmonary NEC.[3] No specific risk factors for this tumor have been identified. Although the neoplasm has been described at any age between 16 and 77 years, the prevalent distribution is in the fifth and sixth decades. NEC most commonly arises in the superior or posterior nasal cavity (olfactory cleft) and often extends into the maxillary or ethmoid sinuses. Primary tumors of the maxillary or ethmoid sinuses without nasal involvement can be seen in approximately 45% of cases.[1]

30.4.2 Pathology

Several primary sinonasal cancers may present with an undifferentiated or poorly differentiated morphology characterized by small, medium, and large round or polygonal atypical cells. Differential diagnosis includes high-grade olfactory neuroblastoma, NEC, and SNUC. As a result, sinonasal poorly differentiated nonsquamous cell carcinomas pose significant diagnostic challenges for the pathologist, especially when specimens have limited volume. Su et al reported that up to 30% of sinonasal

malignancies referred to the Department of Pathology at the MD Anderson Cancer Center are given a different diagnosis on expert review.[65]

SNUC was originally described as a "high-grade epithelial neoplasm of the nasal cavity and paranasal sinuses of uncertain histogenesis without evidence of squamous or glandular differentiation."[66] This histopathologic entity was introduced only 30 years ago, so several cases previously included under another name (e.g., high-grade olfactory neuroblastoma [ONB], NEC, poorly differentiated nonkeratinizing squamous cell carcinoma [SCC]) should now be reclassified as SNUCs. Histologically, SNUC shows poorly defined nests, lobules, trabeculae, and sheets of tumor cells having no specific differentiation. The mitotic rate is very high, and tumor necrosis and apoptosis are often prominent. Lymphovascular and perineural invasion are common. The majority of SNUCs stain for simple cytokeratins (CK7, CK8, CK19) and show focal positivity for epithelial membrane antigen, neuron-specific enolase (NSE), and p53. Synaptophysin and chromogranin may show patchy, focal immunoreactivity. This finding supports the inclusion of SNUC within the spectrum of NEC,[65] although this is not universally accepted.

NECs can be classified into three main groups: well-differentiated neuroendocrine carcinoma (carcinoid tumor), moderately differentiated neuroendocrine carcinoma (atypical carcinoid tumor), and poorly differentiated NEC (small cell and large cell NEC).[3] This group of neoplasms should be characterized by some degree of epithelial differentiation as evidenced by the tumor's having arisen along a mucosal or epithelial site or its diffuse immunohistochemical expression of cytokeratins (CKAE1-AE3, CK8/18), and by immunohistochemical expression of neuroendocrine markers, such as CD56/N-CAM (widespread) together with synaptophysin, chromogranin (focal/variable), and NSE immunoreactivity.

Small cell NEC (also known as small cell carcinoma, oat cell carcinoma, and high-grade or poorly differentiated neuroendocrine carcinoma) is composed of small to intermediate-sized cells resembling those of small cell carcinoma of pulmonary or extrapulmonary origin.[67] Other microscopic hallmarks are the presence of necrosis, large numbers of apoptotic cells, and a high mitotic rate (10 mitoses per 10 high-power fields). The other variant of poorly differentiated NEC is the large cell type. This neoplasm has cells featuring moderate to abundant cytoplasm. The mitotic activity is the major histologic feature that distinguishes large cell neuroendocrine carcinoma from moderately differentiated neuroendocrine carcinoma (atypical carcinoid; > 10 mitoses per 10 high-power fields in large cell neuroendocrine carcinoma vs. 2–10 mitoses per 10 high-power fields in moderately differentiated neuroendocrine carcinoma).[68]

30.4.3 Clinical Features

Poorly differentiated nonsquamous cell carcinomas of the paranasal sinuses frequently originate from the ethmoid as a large, lobulated, or fungating mass with invasion of adjacent sinonasal structures as well as the orbit, skull base, or brain. Seventy to ninety percent of patients present with locally advanced disease (T4a–b), with orbital involvement reported in 50% of cases.[65] Patients are symptomatic, presenting with nasal obstruction, epistaxis, proptosis, cranial nerve palsies, visual disturbances, or pain. Symptoms are of relatively short duration (from weeks to months) compared with other sinonasal neoplasms, which frequently have a more gradual onset. In rare cases, sinonasal NEC may present with paraneoplastic syndromes characterized by elevated serum levels of adrenocorticotropic hormone and calcitonin.[1]

In contrast to the frequent presentation of locally advanced disease, only 5 to 13% of patients have nodal involvement of the neck at presentation. Conversely, the rates of distant metastasis are usually higher, ranging approximately between 25 and 30% and reaching a peak of 47.6% for small cell NEC.[69,70] Common sites of metastasis include lung, liver, and bone and bone marrow, particularly the vertebrae.

30.4.4 Treatment

The limited number of cases published, difficulties in diagnosis, and heterogeneous treatments used have limited establishment of ideal management in this subset of patients. Given the advanced stage of disease at presentation and the high incidence of distant failures, as well as their chemosensitivity, these tumors benefit from nonsurgical treatments as a first-line modality, leaving surgery as a salvage option. In this regard, aggressive trimodality treatment, including the integration of chemotherapy, radiotherapy, and surgery, has been reported to be an effective approach, although survival remains poor.[69,70] Since the early 2010, the role of induction chemotherapy has progressively emerged in the management of these aggressive cancers (► Fig. 30.9). The rate of response to induction chemotherapy could be used to stratify "responder" patients, who might be candidates for definitive chemoradiation, and "nonresponders," who may benefit from surgical resection followed by adjuvant radiotherapy or chemoradiotherapy.[2] Moreover, response to induction chemotherapy may also represent a strong prognostic factor that is able to predict OS rates. Chemotherapy regimens used in this neoadjuvant subset vary among institutions, but the most frequently adopted schemes include cisplatin and etoposide alternated with Doxorubicin and ifosfamide for NEC patients, whereas taxane and platinum-based agents or taxanes and 5-fluorouracil are frequently used for SNUC.[2]

At present, surgery is indicated when induction chemotherapy obtains poor results in tumor volume reduction and as a salvage procedure for persistence or local recurrence of disease after chemoradiation. Surgery should be performed provided that the patient is an acceptable surgical candidate and the tumor is resectable, using the less invasive technique possible and bearing in mind the goal of free-margin resection. Radiation therapy may be delivered using photons (e.g., IMRT) or heavy ion radiotherapy (carbon ion or proton beam). Elective irradiation of the neck and retropharyngeal nodes should be offered as a prudent procedure in such biologically aggressive cancers, especially when presenting in a locally advanced stage at diagnosis (**Video 30.2**).[69,70]

30.4.5 Outcome and Prognosis

Sinonasal Undifferentiated Carcinoma

Despite reports of very poor outcomes in the 1980s,[71] recent large series have shown 5-year OS ranging from 40 to 75%.[72] The MD Anderson Cancer Center reported an OS of 63% in a series of 18 patients, equally divided between neoadjuvant chemotherapy as the primary treatment modality in half of the cohort and surgery in the remainder.[73] Al-Mamgani et al published a series of 21 patients divided between chemoradiation therapy, neoadjuvant chemotherapy, and surgery as primary mode of treatment.[74] Patients who had resectable disease were selected for surgery with postoperative radiation or chemoradiation therapy. Those who had unresectable disease were offered either neoadjuvant chemotherapy or definitive chemoradiation therapy. Predictors of local control on multivariate analysis were T staging and treatment with three treatment modalities compared with two modalities.[74] Interestingly, this series reported the best survival outcomes ever published before (OS of 74%), suggesting that a tailored treatment approach is better than any single strategy.

The utility of neoadjuvant chemotherapy as a strategy for downstaging unresectable tumors before definitive surgery or radiation therapy has been described by Rischin et al in a series of 10 patients.[72] Four of seven patients treated using neoadjuvant cisplatin or carboplatin and 5-fluorouracil showed objective evidence of response, and two patients had stable disease with symptomatic improvement. One patient who had progressive disease died shortly after completing radiation therapy,

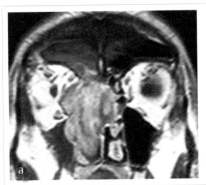 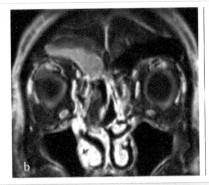 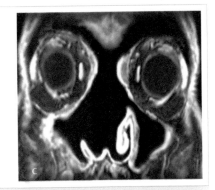

Fig. 30.9 Sinonasal undifferentiated carcinoma of the right ethmoid complex with orbital invasion. **(a)** Pretreatment MR scan in coronal view. **(b)** After three cycles of induction chemotherapy, a partial response was obtained with persistence of disease in the right ethmoid. A trimodality treatment with endoscopic surgery followed by adjuvant radiotherapy was planned. **(c)** Contrast-enhanced MR scan performed 2 years after treatment showed no recurrence of disease.

providing preliminary evidence that response to chemotherapy is a prognostic indicator and may be used to select patients for definitive treatment.[2] Moreover, Rischin et al supported the additional benefit of neoadjuvant chemotherapy in the reduction of systemic spread of disease, as demonstrated by their data: no patient who was treated with neoadjuvant chemotherapy followed by concurrent chemoradiation therapy developed distant metastasis, although both of the patients who were treated with surgery and radiation therapy did.[72]

Sinonasal Neuroendocrine Carcinoma

This is one of the most aggressive histologies, having a poor prognosis despite multimodality therapy. In a publication from MD Anderson on a series of 28 cases from 1990 to 2004, approximately 50% of the cohort received surgery as the primary treatment modality, whereas about a third received chemoradiotherapy.[70] The 5-year OS, DSS, and DFS rates were 66.9%, 78.5%, and 43.8%, respectively. The incidence of local, regional, and distant failure was 21%, 25%, and 18%, respectively—better than generally reported. Predictors of poor outcome were patients who had skull base or orbital involvement and tumors originating outside the nasal cavity. A complete response to neoadjuvant chemotherapy correlated with improved survival at 3 years. Moreover, patients who were treated with neoadjuvant chemotherapy presented regional and distant failure rates lower than expected (12.9% and 12.3%, respectively).

A systematic literature review by Rivero et al of patients who had small-cell NEC identified 80 patients, of whom 46.3% were alive after 30.8 months of mean follow-up and 49% had developed local, regional, or distant metastasis after a median time of 9 months.[67]

Only a few cases of large cell NEC have been reported in the sinonasal region. Outcome data are limited, but it is generally considered that they have the same poor prognosis as small cell NEC.[68]

30.5 Conclusion

Nonsquamous cell carcinoma of paranasal sinus represents a wide spectrum of histologies having different biological behaviors and different prognosis. Pathological diagnosis has a crucial role in determining optimal treatment strategies. Surgery still plays a pivotal role, although multimodality treatments and induction chemotherapy are essential, in selected settings, to improving survival. Multidisciplinary teams and a high level of expertise are mandatory in the management of such cancers.

References

[1] Lund VJ, Stammberger H, Nicolai P, et al. European Rhinologic Society Advisory Board on Endoscopic Techniques in the Management of Nose, Paranasal Sinus and Skull Base Tumours. European position paper on endoscopic management of tumours of the nose, paranasal sinuses and skull base. Rhinol Suppl. 2010; 22:1–143

[2] Castelnuovo P, Turri-Zanoni M, Battaglia P, Antognoni P, Bossi P, Locatelli D. Sinonasal malignancies of anterior skull base: histology-driven treatment strategies. Otolaryngol Clin North Am. 2016; 49(1):183–200

[3] El-Naggar AK, Chan JKC, Grandis JR, et al. WHO Classification of Head and Neck Tumours. WHO/IARC Classification of Tumours. 4th ed. Vol. 9, 2017

[4] Bonzini M, Battaglia P, Parassoni D, et al. Prevalence of occupational hazards in patients with different types of epithelial sinonasal cancers. Rhinology. 2013; 51(1):31–36

[5] Cantù G, Solero CL, Mariani L, et al. Intestinal type adenocarcinoma of the ethmoid sinus in wood and leather workers: a retrospective study of 153 cases. Head Neck. 2011; 33(4):535–542

[6] Barnes L. Intestinal-type adenocarcinoma of the nasal cavity and paranasal sinuses. Am J Surg Pathol. 1986; 10(3):192–202

[7] Kleinsasser O, Schroeder HG. Adenocarcinomas of the inner nose after exposure to wood dust. Morphological findings and relationships between histopathology and clinical behavior in 79 cases. Arch Otorhinolaryngol. 1988; 245(1):1–15

[8] Castelnuovo P, Battaglia P, Turri-Zanoni M, et al. Endoscopic endonasal surgery for malignancies of the anterior cranial base. World Neurosurg. 2014; 82(6) Suppl:S22–S31

[9] Vergez S, du Mayne MD, Coste A, et al. Multicenter study to assess endoscopic resection of 159 sinonasal adenocarcinomas. Ann Surg Oncol. 2014; 21(4):1384–1390

[10] Nicolai P, Schreiber A, Bolzoni Villaret A, et al. Intestinal type adenocarcinoma of the ethmoid: outcomes of a treatment regimen based on endoscopic surgery with or without radiotherapy. Head Neck. 2016; 38 Suppl 1:E996–E1003

[11] Hadad G, Bassagasteguy L, Carrau RL, et al. A novel reconstructive technique after endoscopic expanded endonasal approaches: vascular pedicle nasoseptal flap. Laryngoscope. 2006; 116(10):1882–1886

[12] Battaglia P, Turri-Zanoni M, De Bernardi F, et al. Septal flip flap for anterior skull base reconstruction after endoscopic resection of sinonasal cancers: preliminary outcomes. Acta Otorhinolaryngol Ital. 2016; 36(3):194–198

[13] Mattavelli D, Schreiber A, Ferrari M, et al. Three-layer reconstruction with iliotibial tract after endoscopic resection of sinonasal tumors: technical note. World Neurosurg. 2017; 101:486–492

[14] Bogaerts S, Vander Poorten V, Nuyts S, Van den Bogaert W, Jorissen M. Results of endoscopic resection followed by radiotherapy for primarily diagnosed adenocarcinomas of the paranasal sinuses. Head Neck. 2008; 30(6):728–736

[15] Van Gerven L, Jorissen M, Nuyts S, Hermans R, Vander Poorten V. Long-term follow-up of 44 patients with adenocarcinoma of the nasal cavity and sinuses primarily treated with endoscopic resection followed by radiotherapy. Head Neck. 2011; 33(6):898–904

[16] Turri-Zanoni M, Battaglia P, Lambertoni A, et al. Treatment strategies for primary early-stage sinonasal adenocarcinoma: A retrospective bi-institutional case-control study. J Surg Oncol. 2015; 112(5):561–567

[17] Dagan R, Bryant C, Li Z, et al. Outcomes of sinonasal cancer treated with proton therapy. Int J Radiat Oncol Biol Phys. 2016; 95(1):377–385

[18] Licitra L, Suardi S, Bossi P, et al. Prediction of TP53 status for primary cisplatin, fluorouracil, and leucovorin chemotherapy in ethmoid sinus intestinal-type adenocarcinoma. J Clin Oncol. 2004; 22(24):4901–4906

[19] Leivo I. Sinonasal adenocarcinoma: update on classification, immunophenotype and molecular features. Head Neck Pathol. 2016; 10(1):68–74

[20] Choussy O, Ferron C, Védrine PO, et al. GETTEC Study Group. Adenocarcinoma of ethmoid: a GETTEC retrospective multicenter study of 418 cases. Laryngoscope. 2008; 118(3):437–443

[21] Camp S, Van Gerven L, Poorten VV, et al. Long-term follow-up of 123 patients with adenocarcinoma of the sinonasal tract treated with endoscopic resection and postoperative radiation therapy. Head Neck. 2016; 38(2):294–300

[22] Kim KH, Sung MW, Chung PS, Rhee CS, Park CI, Kim WH. Adenoid cystic carcinoma of the head and neck. Arch Otolaryngol Head Neck Surg. 1994; 120(7):721–726

[23] Lupinetti AD, Roberts DB, Williams MD, et al. Sinonasal adenoid cystic carcinoma: the M. D. Anderson Cancer Center experience. Cancer. 2007; 110(12):2726–2731

[24] Sanghvi S, Patel NR, Patel CR, Kalyoussef E, Baredes S, Eloy JA. Sinonasal adenoid cystic carcinoma: comprehensive analysis of incidence and survival from 1973 to 2009. Laryngoscope. 2013; 123(7):1592–1597

[25] Li Q, Xu T, Gao JM, et al. Surgery alone provides long-term survival rates comparable to those of surgery plus postoperative radiotherapy for patients with adenoid cystic carcinoma of the palate. Oral Oncol. 2011; 47(3):170–173

[26] Marcinow A, Ozer E, Teknos T, et al. Clinicopathologic predictors of recurrence and overall survival in adenoid cystic carcinoma of the head and neck: a single institutional experience at a tertiary care center. Head Neck. 2014; 36(12):1705–1711

[27] Coca-Pelaz A, Rodrigo JP, Bradley PJ, et al. Adenoid cystic carcinoma of the head and neck—an update. Oral Oncol. 2015; 51(7):652–661

[28] Rhee CS, Won TB, Lee CH, et al. Adenoid cystic carcinoma of the sinonasal tract: treatment results. Laryngoscope. 2006; 116(6):982–986

[29] Ellington CL, Goodman M, Kono SA, et al. Adenoid cystic carcinoma of the head and neck: incidence and survival trends based on 1973–2007 Surveillance, Epidemiology, and End Results data. Cancer. 2012; 118(18):4444–4451

[30] Unsal AA, Chung SY, Zhou AH, Baredes S, Eloy JA. Sinonasal adenoid cystic carcinoma: a population-based analysis of 694 cases. Int Forum Allergy Rhinol. 2017; 7(3):312–320

[31] Matsuba HM, Spector GJ, Thawley SE, Simpson JR, Mauney M, Pikul FJ. Adenoid cystic salivary gland carcinoma: a histopathologic review of treatment failure patterns. Cancer. 1986; 57(3):519–524

[32] Pitman KT, Prokopakis EP, Aydogan B, et al. The role of skull base surgery for the treatment of adenoid cystic carcinoma of the sinonasal tract. Head Neck. 1999; 21(5):402–407

[33] Spiro RH, Huvos AG, Strong EW. Adenoid cystic carcinoma of salivary origin: a clinicopathologic study of 242 cases. Am J Surg. 1974; 128(4):512–520

[34] Batsakis JG, Luna MA, el-Naggar A. Histopathologic grading of salivary gland neoplasms: III. Adenoid cystic carcinomas. Ann Otol Rhinol Laryngol. 1990; 99(12):1007–1009

[35] Szanto PA, Luna MA, Tortoledo ME, White RA. Histologic grading of adenoid cystic carcinoma of the salivary glands. Cancer. 1984; 54(6):1062–1069

[36] van Weert S, van der Waal I, Witte BI, Leemans CR, Bloemena E. Histopathological grading of adenoid cystic carcinoma of the head and neck: analysis of currently used grading systems and proposal for a simplified grading scheme. Oral Oncol. 2015; 51(1):71–76

[37] Simpson RH, Skálová A, Di Palma S, Leivo I. Recent advances in the diagnostic pathology of salivary carcinomas. Virchows Arch. 2014; 465(4):371–384

[38] Amit M, Binenbaum Y, Sharma K, et al. Analysis of failure in patients with adenoid cystic carcinoma of the head and neck: an international collaborative study. Head Neck. 2014; 36(7):998–1004

[39] Seong SY, Hyun DW, Kim YS, et al. Treatment outcomes of sinonasal adenoid cystic carcinoma: 30 cases from a single institution. J Craniomaxillofac Surg. 2014; 42(5):e171–e175

[40] International Head and Neck Scientific Group. Cervical lymph node metastasis in adenoid cystic carcinoma of the sinonasal tract, nasopharynx, lacrimal glands and external auditory canal: a collective international review. J Laryngol Otol. 2016; 130(12):1093–1097

[41] Lombardi D, McGurk M, Vander Poorten V, et al. Surgical treatment of salivary malignant tumors. Oral Oncol. 2017; 65:102–113

[42] Okay DJ, Genden E, Buchbinder D, Urken M. Prosthodontic guidelines for surgical reconstruction of the maxilla: a classification system of defects. J Prosthet Dent. 2001; 86(4):352–363

[43] Genden EM, Wallace D, Buchbinder D, Okay D, Urken ML. Iliac crest internal oblique osteomusculocutaneous free flap reconstruction of the postablative palatomaxillary defect. Arch Otolaryngol Head Neck Surg. 2001; 127(7):854–861

[44] Piazza C, Paderno A, Taglietti V, Nicolai P. Evolution of complex palatomaxillary reconstructions: the scapular angle osteomuscular free flap. Curr Opin Otolaryngol Head Neck Surg. 2013; 21(2):95–103

[45] Fan S, Wang YY, Wu DH, et al. Intraoral lining with the fibular osteomyofascial flap without a skin paddle during maxillary and mandibular reconstruction. Head Neck. 2016; 38 Suppl 1:E832–E836

[46] Bianchi B, Bertolini F, Ferrari S, Sesenna E. Maxillary reconstruction using rectus abdominis free flap and bone grafts. Br J Oral Maxillofac Surg. 2006; 44(6):526–530

[47] Nicolai P, Battaglia P, Bignami M, et al. Endoscopic surgery for malignant tumors of the sinonasal tract and adjacent skull base: a 10-year experience. Am J Rhinol. 2008; 22(3):308–316

[48] Klatt-Cromwell CN, Thorp BD, Del Signore AG, Ebert CS, Ewend MG, Zanation AM. Reconstruction of skull base defects. Otolaryngol Clin North Am. 2016; 49(1):107–117

[49] Lloyd S, Yu JB, Wilson LD, Decker RH. Determinants and patterns of survival in adenoid cystic carcinoma of the head and neck, including an analysis of adjuvant radiation therapy. Am J Clin Oncol. 2011; 34(1):76–81

[50] Vander Poorten V, Hunt J, Bradley PJ, et al. Recent trends in the management of minor salivary gland carcinoma. Head Neck. 2014; 36(3):444–455

[51] Jensen AD, Poulakis M, Nikoghosyan AV, et al. Re-irradiation of adenoid cystic carcinoma: analysis and evaluation of outcome in 52 consecutive patients treated with raster-scanned carbon ion therapy. Radiother Oncol. 2015; 114(2):182–188

[52] Laurie SA, Licitra L. Systemic therapy in the palliative management of advanced salivary gland cancers. J Clin Oncol. 2006; 24(17):2673–2678

[53] Kokemueller H, Eckardt A, Brachvogel P, Hausamen JE. Adenoid cystic carcinoma of the head and neck—a 20 years experience. Int J Oral Maxillofac Surg. 2004; 33(1):25–31

[54] Oplatek A, Ozer E, Agrawal A, Bapna S, Schuller DE. Patterns of recurrence and survival of head and neck adenoid cystic carcinoma after definitive resection. Laryngoscope. 2010; 120(1):65–70

[55] Shen C, Xu T, Huang C, Hu C, He S. Treatment outcomes and prognostic features in adenoid cystic carcinoma originated from the head and neck. Oral Oncol. 2012; 48(5):445–449

[56] Amit M, Binenbaum Y, Sharma K, et al. Adenoid cystic carcinoma of the nasal cavity and paranasal sinuses: a meta-analysis. J Neurol Surg B Skull Base. 2013; 74(3):118–125

[57] van Weert S, Bloemena E, van der Waal I, et al. Adenoid cystic carcinoma of the head and neck: a single-center analysis of 105 consecutive cases over a 30-year period. Oral Oncol. 2013; 49(8):824–829

[58] Amit M, Binenbaum Y, Trejo-Leider L, et al. International collaborative validation of intraneural invasion as a prognostic marker in adenoid cystic carcinoma of the head and neck. Head Neck. 2015; 37(7):1038–1045

[59] Lopes MA, Santos GC, Kowalski LP. Multivariate survival analysis of 128 cases of oral cavity minor salivary gland carcinomas. Head Neck. 1998; 20(8):699–706

[60] McHugh CH, Roberts DB, El-Naggar AK, et al. Prognostic factors in mucoepidermoid carcinoma of the salivary glands. Cancer. 2012; 118(16):3928–3936

[61] Omlie JE, Koutlas IG. Acinic cell carcinoma of minor salivary glands: a clinicopathologic study of 21 cases. J Oral Maxillofac Surg. 2010; 68(9):2053–2057

[62] Ord RA, Salama AR. Is it necessary to resect bone for low-grade mucoepidermoid carcinoma of the palate? Br J Oral Maxillofac Surg. 2012; 50(8):712–714

[63] Patel TD, Vazquez A, Marchiano E, Park RC, Baredes S, Eloy JA. Polymorphous low-grade adenocarcinoma of the head and neck: a population-based study of 460 cases. Laryngoscope. 2015; 125(7):1644–1649

[64] Loh KS, Barker E, Bruch G, et al. Prognostic factors in malignancy of the minor salivary glands. Head Neck. 2009; 31(1):58–63

[65] Su SY, Bell D, Hanna EY. Esthesioneuroblastoma, neuroendocrine carcinoma, and sinonasal undifferentiated carcinoma: differentiation in diagnosis and treatment. Int Arch Otorhinolaryngol. 2014; 18 Suppl 2:S149–S156

[66] Frierson HF, Jr, Mills SE, Fechner RE, Taxy JB, Levine PA. Sinonasal undifferentiated carcinoma: an aggressive neoplasm derived from Schneiderian epithelium and distinct from olfactory neuroblastoma. Am J Surg Pathol. 1986; 10(11):771–779

[67] Rivero A, Liang J. Sinonasal small cell neuroendocrine carcinoma: a systematic review of 80 patients. Int Forum Allergy Rhinol. 2016; 6(7):744–751

[68] Kao HL, Chang WC, Li WY, Chia-Heng Li A, Fen-Yau Li A. Head and neck large cell neuroendocrine carcinoma should be separated from atypical carcinoid on the basis of different clinical features, overall survival, and pathogenesis. Am J Surg Pathol. 2012; 36(2):185–192

[69] Mourad WF, Hauerstock D, Shourbaji RA, et al. Trimodality management of sinonasal undifferentiated carcinoma and review of the literature. Am J Clin Oncol. 2013; 36(6):584–588

[70] Mitchell EH, Diaz A, Yilmaz T, et al. Multimodality treatment for sinonasal neuroendocrine carcinoma. Head Neck. 2012; 34(10):1372–1376

[71] Levine PA, Frierson HF, Jr, Stewart FM, Mills SE, Fechner RE, Cantrell RW. Sinonasal undifferentiated carcinoma: a distinctive and highly aggressive neoplasm. Laryngoscope. 1987; 97(8 Pt 1):905–908

[72] Rischin D, Porceddu S, Peters L, Martin J, Corry J, Weih L. Promising results with chemoradiation in patients with sinonasal undifferentiated carcinoma. Head Neck. 2004; 26(5):435–441

[73] Rosenthal DI, Barker JL, Jr, El-Naggar AK, et al. Sinonasal malignancies with neuroendocrine differentiation: patterns of failure according to histologic phenotype. Cancer. 2004; 101(11):2567–2573

[74] Al-Mamgani A, van Rooij P, Mehilal R, Tans L, Levendag PC. Combined-modality treatment improved outcome in sinonasal undifferentiated carcinoma: single-institutional experience of 21 patients and review of the literature. Eur Arch Otorhinolaryngol. 2013; 270(1):293–299

31 Esthesioneuroblastoma

Valerie J. Lund and David J. Howard

Summary

Esthesioneuroblastoma is a rare and unique tumor arising from olfactory epithelium, which prior to the advent of craniofacial surgery was associated with a poor prognosis. Conventional craniofacial resection doubled survival compared with previous treatments, and more recent advances in diagnosis and the combination of surgery and radiotherapy have further improved survival. The use of endoscopic surgery in selected cases has also reduced morbidity with similar outcomes. Genomic analysis of the tumor suggests new possibilities in targeted treatments in the future. However, lifelong follow-up is required irrespective of the treatment, because the natural history of this tumor extends over a lifetime.

Keywords: olfactory neuroblastoma, esthesioneuroblastoma, craniofacial resection, endoscopic surgery

31.1 Incidence and Epidemiology

In common with all tumors of the anterior skull base, esthesioneuroblastoma (ENB) is comparatively rare. This malignant neuroendocrine neoplasm classically arises from the olfactory mucosa and was first recognized by Berger et al in 1924, who coined the term *esthesioneuroepitheliome olfactif*.[1] However, a wide range of other terms has been used, including esthesioneurocytoma, esthesioneuroma, intranasal neuroblastoma, olfactory neuroepithelial tumor, and olfactory neuroblastoma. In 1966, Skolnik et al found only 97 cases reported in 42 papers in the English literature, with most authors having treated only two or three cases, and by 1989 O'Connor estimated that ≤ 300 cases had been published, which represented 1 to 5% of all malignant tumors of the nasal cavity.[2,3] However, this number had risen to 945 by 1997, not including a large series from the Armed Forces Institute of Pathology or another from the Institut Gustave-Roussy.[4,5,6] In 2000, the National Cancer Database included 664 cases from more than 500 U.S. hospitals over a 10-year period (1985–1995). In the last 40 years, this tumor is being described in increasing numbers, almost certainly due to increased awareness and improved histological techniques for diagnosis, and likely occurs in ~ 0.1/100,000 people/year. Even so, the difficulty of accruing large individual series compromises statistical analysis of outcomes. The authors, who work in a tertiary referral center, have managed 125 cases since 1970.

Hitherto, unlike for adenocarcinoma, occupational factors in the development of olfactory neuroblastoma have not been identified in men other than a single case report in a woodworker.[7] However, in rodents the administration of N-nitroso compounds has been reported to produce esthesioneuroepitheliomas when administered parenterally, orally, or topically, as has administration of bischloromethyl ether.[8,9,10,11]

There appears to be a slight male preponderance in the literature, and the tumor may occur over a wide age range (3–90 years), with a reported bimodal peak in the second/third decades and sixth/seventh decades.[3,12,13,14,15] In our own series, this male preponderance is more pronounced, with a 1.3:1 ratio, and the age range is 12 to 88 years (mean 48 years), though occurrence in children under 10 has occasionally been reported.[12,16]

Recent genomic analyses suggest that there may be some specific genetic variations that could predispose to the development of this tumor and that might provide therapeutic opportunities in the future.[17,18,19]

31.2 Pathology

Olfactory neuroblastoma generally arises in the nasal roof, corresponding to the anatomical distribution of the olfactory epithelium, which extends from the olfactory niche onto the upper nasal septum and superior turbinates on the lateral wall. Evidence for the origin of olfactory neuroblastoma from specialized olfactory epithelium, however, is somewhat circumstantial, though tumors occasionally found outside this distribution have been ascribed to ectopic olfactory epithelium.[5] Tumors arising in the cribriform niche can easily spread superiorly along olfactory fibers into the anterior cranial fossa to affect the olfactory bulb and tracts. The superior septum is often involved, and from thence the tumor may spread to the contralateral side and into the ethmoids and adjacent orbit. Earlier histological studies suggest that there is microscopic intracranial involvement in many patients even when not suggested by imaging and macroscopic appearance at surgery, but this has not been supported by more recent analysis.[20,21]

Macroscopically, the tumor is characteristically a polypoid reddish gray mass that bleeds readily. Microscopically, the tumor typically forms clusters of cells arranged in patterns, which vary from small nests surrounded by a fibrillary stroma to diffuse areas separated by fibrovascular septa. The cells may palisade around blood vessels, and occasionally true rosettes form. Hyam proposed a grading based on tumor differentiation, which is widely used.[5]

It had been suggested that ENB was part of the Ewing's sarcoma/peripheral neuroectodermal group of tumors, but this has not been supported by immunohistochemical studies.[22] However, it can present some difficulties in diagnosis, even when using modern techniques, and can be confused with a host of other small-cell tumors, such as lymphoma, malignant melanoma, peripheral neuroectodermal tumors, and sinonasal undifferentiated carcinoma, by those unfamiliar with sinonasal malignancy. This prompted Ogura and Schenck to describe ENB as the "great imposter."[23]

Immunohistochemistry using a broad panel of antibodies is usually employed to confirm the diagnosis. These include general neuroendocrine markers such as neuron-specific enolase (NSE), synaptophysin, chromogranin, and protein gene product–9.5 (PGP-9.5), which are usually positive.[24] S100 positivity can be demonstrated at the periphery of the tumor nests, and some tumors are also positive using MNF 116 and CAM 5.2, both of which are stains for certain cytokeratins. Conversely, LP

34, a high–molecular weight cytokeratin stain; epithelial membrane antigen (EMA); carcinoembryonic antigen (CEA); and glial fibrillary acidic protein (GFAP) are generally negative.

31.3 Staging

A number of staging systems have been proposed. Kadish et al's is a somewhat crude system that divides tumors into three stages[25]:

- Stage A: lesions confined to the nasal cavity
- Stage B: involvement of nasal cavity plus one or more of the paranasal sinuses
- Stage C: involvement beyond the nasal cavity, including the orbit, skull base, intracranial cavity, cervical lymph nodes, or systemic metastases

This can now be considerably refined by the use of modern imaging protocols validated by craniofacial resection.[26,27] However, neither the Kadish system nor subsequent modifications have proved entirely successful, largely owing to the late presentation of most patients and despite efforts to refine advanced disease by creating a stage D for metastases.[25,28] However, attempts to correlate both staging (Kadish/Morita) and histological grade (Hyam) have had variable success.[29,30] The staging system proposed by Dulgerov in 2001 is probably the most often used (▶ Table 31.1).[13]

31.4 Treatment

31.4.1 Clinical Features

The usual site of origin results in fairly innocuous symptoms initially, remarkable only for their sudden onset and unilaterality. As a consequence, there is often considerable delay in diagnosis, with some patients waiting for more than a year (24% of 40 cases reported by Schwabb et al).[6] There is little specific to this particular tumor, whose symptoms are common to all nasal cavity lesions: blockage, discharge, some epistaxis as a result of the tumor's vascularity, and hyposmia. In a series of 42 patients, unilateral obstruction occurred in 93%, epistaxis or serosanguineous discharge in 55%, and rhinorrhea in 30%.[15] Anosmia was

reported rarely (5%) in our patients, and invasion of the anterior cranial fossa is otherwise generally silent. As the tumor spreads to the orbit, patients may develop epiphora, displacement of the eye, diplopia, and eventually visual loss, though this last is usually a late phenomenon. Ocular symptoms occurred in 11% of our patients.[15] Curiously, in this series the left side was more often affected (62%) than the right (29%), with both sides affected at presentation in 9%. Occasionally involvement of the Eustachian orifice may result in otalgia and conductive hearing loss as a result of serous otitis media.

The incidence of cervical metastases varies considerably from report to report, compounded by the generally small numbers in each series. Rinaldo et al reported a lymph node metastatic frequency of 23.4% (range 5–100%), though only eight studies validated the diagnosis of ENB with immunohistochemistry.[14] A recent report by Nalavenkata et al found 7% at presentation and 9% during a mean follow-up of 41 months in 113 patients.[31]

Because ENB is a neuroendocrine tumor, it can be associated with paraneoplastic syndromes caused by inappropriate hormone production, such as antidiuretic hormone secretion (SIADH), first described by Bouche et al in 1967.[32] This has been estimated to occur in ~ 2% of cases, which has been our own experience, and may precede diagnosis of the tumor by some years (mean 3.5 years).[33] If suspected, immunohistochemical staining for arginine vasopressin confirms the diagnosis. Normalization of sodium and osmolality can be anticipated after tumor removal in most cases, and because disease recurrence can also manifest as SIADH, some authors consider sodium levels to be a form of tumor marker that could be monitored as part of routine follow-up.[33,34,35,36]

31.4.2 Imaging

Ideally, all patients are submitted to a preoperative imaging protocol, which employs a combination of high-resolution contrast-enhanced CT (coronal, axial, and sagittal planes) combined with multiplanar MRI enhanced with gadolinium diethylenetriamine penta-acetic acid (DTPA), which should include the neck. (▶ Fig. 31.1).[37] If available, ultrasound of the neck combined with fine-needle aspiration cytology is a useful screening technique having a high degree of accuracy.[38]

Many centers also undertake imaging for systemic metastases using PET-CT or MRI, although the incidence of systemic disease at presentation is extremely low.[39] Some clinicians have advocated 68Ga DOTATATE PET/CT because of its greater specificity for ENB.[40]

After surgery, all patients should also undergo a rigorous follow-up protocol of outpatient/office endonasal endoscopy together with MRI of the head and neck every 3 to 4 months for the first 2 years and then every 6 months thereafter.[26] Formal biopsy of any suspicious areas should be performed as required. Patients may develop recurrence many years after initial treatment (22 years from ostensibly curative treatment in one of our patients), which can occur anywhere in relation to the surgical field, orbit, or intracranial cavity, suggesting some local embolic phenomenon. Distant en plaque dural deposits are not uncommon, so the entire intracranial compartment should be visualized on MRI (▶ Fig. 31.2).

Initial imaging often suggests the diagnosis but also, more important, indicates extent.[37,41] No features are specific to ENB,

Table 31.1 Olfactory neuroblastoma: staging system after Dulguerov et al[13]

Stage	Characteristics
T1	Tumor involving the nasal cavity and/or paranasal sinuses (excluding the sphenoid sinus), sparing the most superior ethmoidal cells
T2	Tumor involving the nasal cavity and/or paranasal sinuses (including the sphenoid sinus), with extension to or erosion of the cribriform plate
T3	Tumor extending into the orbit or protruding into the anterior cranial fossa, without dural invasion
T4	Tumor involving the brain
N0	No cervical lymph node metastases
N1	Any form of cervical lymph node metastases
M0	No metastases
M1	Any distant metastases

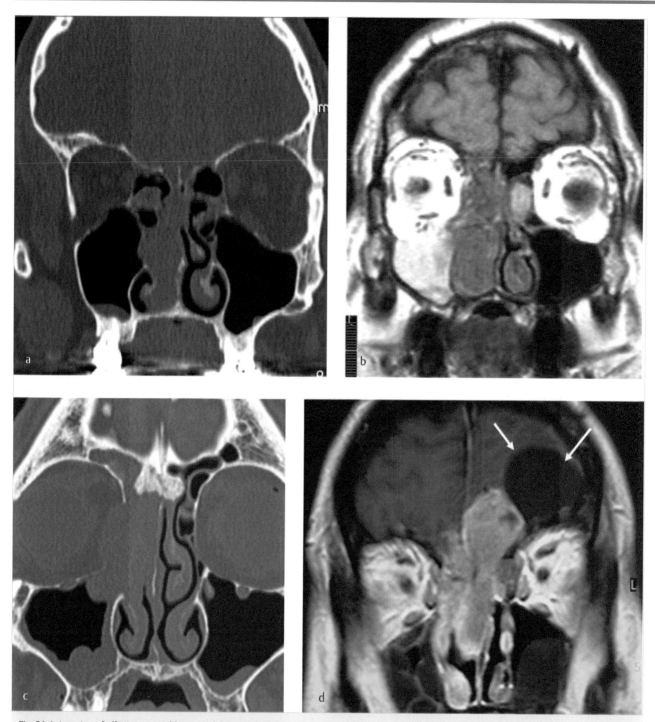

Fig. 31.1 Imaging of olfactory neuroblastoma. **(a)** Coronal CT showing a mass of olfactory neuroblastoma filling the right nasal cavity without obvious erosion of the skull base. **(b)** Coronal MRI (T1-weighted unenhanced) in the same patient, showing tumor confined to the nasal cavity and confirming suitability for an endoscopic resection. **(c)** Coronal CT in another patient showing olfactory neuroblastoma filling upper right nasal cavity and ethmoids with extension through the lamina papyracea and associated with new bone formation on the anterior skull base. **(d)** Coronal postgadolinium MRI scan in another patient showing olfactory neuroblastoma extending into anterior cranial cavity with an associated peritumoral cyst (*arrow*), requiring combined endoscopic and conventional craniofacial approach. ([a] and [b] reproduced with permission from Lund VJ, Howard DJ, Wei WI, Tumors of the Nose, Sinuses, and Nasopharynx, New York, NY: Thieme; 2012.)

but the position of the mass and associated bone erosion indicates a malignant nasal tumor and can be associated with intracranial peritumoral cysts. Coronal CT remains the most accurate method of demonstrating early anterior skull base erosion, whereas the addition of contrast enhancement and MRI shows extent of intracranial and orbital spread. Typical features are an intense signal on precontrast T2-weighted spin echo sequences and strong enhancement after gadolinium on T1-weighted sequences. However, even the most sophisticated imaging cannot be absolutely relied on to demonstrate involvement of the

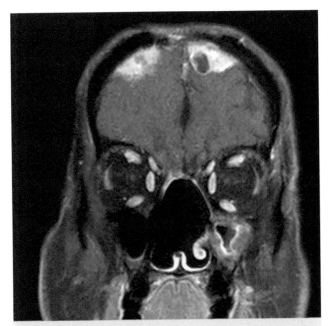

Fig. 31.2 Coronal MRI (T1 with gadolinium) showing dural deposits distant from the craniofacial cavity, found 11 years after treatment.

dura and orbital periosteum, which can be determined only by surgery with histological confirmation.

31.4.3 Treatment

The advent of craniofacial resection in the 1970s revolutionized the treatment of ENB, doubling survival figures, and rapidly became the "gold standard." In a 2001 meta-analysis, Dulgerov et al confirmed that this procedure, combined with radiotherapy, was the treatment of choice.[13]

31.4.4 Surgery

Craniofacial resection was introduced in the 1970s by Ketcham and others, providing the combination of an en bloc oncologic resection having low morbidity and excellent cosmesis.[42,43,44] By approaching the tumor from the nose and anterior cranial fossa, the operation directly addresses the origin and local spread of this tumor, allowing resection of dura and the olfactory system, including the olfactory epithelium, cribriform plate, olfactory bulb, and tracts. This directly deals with macro- and microscopic spread of disease, reducing local recurrence.[45,46]

There are many variations on the technique, but essentially all involve some form of craniotomy together with a nasal approach using various incisions and forms of repair. Use of a coronal incision in the scalp and a sublabial incision for a midfacial degloving can hide these scars, though the use of an extended lateral rhinotomy or a supraorbital spectacle incision heals well. The skull base repair may be effected using a pericranial flap or fascia lata and split skin. In our craniofacial series, which extended over 35 years, postoperative hospital stay has been, on average, 14 days, and major complications have been low.[46]

Prior to craniofacial resection, conventional wisdom dictated that the orbit should be sacrificed if tumor either was adjacent to or had transgressed the periosteum. However, it became clear that a significant proportion of these eyes could be salvaged without compromising survival. If the tumor has not penetrated the full thickness of orbital periosteum on frozen section, it is possible to resect it widely and skin graft the area. Nonetheless, the orbit should be cleared if there is full-thickness periosteal penetration or frank infiltration of orbital contents when cure would otherwise be possible.

In recent years, an endoscopic resection with curative intent has been used for selected cases, usually for those who are without significant intradural extension or who are a poor anesthetic risk. The endoscopic approach should not be regarded as a limited procedure, because it can encompass most of what was previously achieved by formal craniofacial approaches, including a wide-field resection of tissue, and also allows determination of the exact site of origin of the tumor.[21,26,47,48,49,50] Some authors have also suggested that olfactory function may be salvaged by preservation of one or both olfactory bulbs in selected cases.[51] If there is significant intradural or frontal lobe involvement, endoscopic and external craniotomy approaches can be combined.[52,53,54] Endoscopic surgery can also have a role in the management of localized recurrence.

There is insufficient evidence to support prophylactic treatment of the N0 neck, although a selective neck dissection is undertaken in the presence of disease.[55]

31.4.5 Radiotherapy

Radiation in this area must be carefully administered to deliver the maximum dose while preserving the adjacent brain and optic nerves. An external megavoltage beam and three-field technique has generally been used. An anterior port combined with wedged lateral fields delivers a dose of 60 to 70 Gy in 30 to 35 sessions over 6 to 7 weeks.[56]

Because of the proximity of the optic chiasm, intensity-modulated radiotherapy (IMRT) is preferred if available.[57] Generally, radiotherapy has been used as an adjunct to surgery, and postoperative delivery is preferred.[15,58]

Stereotactically guided radiotherapy has been used in combination with surgery, which may offer improved local control with minimal collateral damage, although numbers and follow-up preclude definitive evidence.[59] Similarly, the advantages of proton beam therapy remain to be determined owing to the present lack of numbers and follow-up.[56]

31.4.6 Chemotherapy

The use of concomitant chemotherapy has not been fully evaluated, though chemosensitivity has been found in retrospective series. ENB has been shown to respond to platinum-based regimes.[60,61,62,63,64] Cyclophosphamide, doxorubicin, docetaxel, irinotecan, and etoposide have also been used in more advanced disease.[65,66,67]

Since 1999 it has been our practice to give two courses of this adjunctive cisplatin at the beginning and halfway through the postoperative course of radiotherapy, based on data suggesting that doing so reduces recurrence.[64]

31.5 Outcome and Prognosis

Prior to the advent of conventional craniofacial resection (cCFR), the use of lateral rhinotomy and radiotherapy provided poor results of ≤ 40% at 5 years, largely due to its inability to deal with intracranial spread.[68,69,70] Craniofacial resection specifically addressed this area and allows removal of the olfactory bulbs and tracts, where microscopic disease might be residing undetected. As a result, when large series with long-term follow-up after craniofacial are considered, the 5-year overall survival is seen to have improved significantly or even to have doubled, as in our own series to 77%, or to 89% in that of Diaz et al.[15,71,72,73,74,75,76] However, there is continued loss over time, as well as local recurrence many years after treatment (range 12–144 months, mean 37 months, longest interval 22 years). In an earlier analysis of our cCFR series of 42 cases, disease-free survival dropped from 77% at 5 years to 53% at 10 years. In a further study of this cohort enlarged to 56 individuals, 15-year survival fell to 40%, underscoring the importance of long-term follow-up.[46]

The most frequent recurrence is local and occurred in 17% of our series, in keeping with other published series using craniofacial resection and radiotherapy. Local recurrence has been shown to be significantly decreased by the addition of radiotherapy (28% vs. 4%), but it does not seem to matter whether this is given before or after surgery, even when the therapeutic interval differs between pre- and postoperative administration.[15] This applies to both survival ($p = 0.52$) and complications ($p = 0.07$). Interestingly, previous treatment did not seem to affect 5-year actuarial survival, either, but in patients who developed local recurrence, 5-year survival after further salvage treatment was 54%. However, it should again be noted that the site of "local" recurrence can be anywhere and on either side of the nose, sinuses, orbit, or intracranial cavity, so follow-up must be especially vigilant if this disease is to be detected early.

A recent study of 95 of our ENB patients allowed comparison of 30 who underwent endoscopic sinus surgery (ESS), with 65 undergoing cCFR.[27] This showed significantly higher survival in those treated endoscopically (100% 5- and 97% 10-year overall survival), reflecting the selection of patients who have more limited disease but nonetheless confirming that this approach is at least as good as craniofacial resection, bringing much lower complication and morbidity rates (► Fig. 31.3).[27,77,78,79,80,81,82,83,84,85] As a consequence, our present approach for ENB treatment is as follows, as supported by a recent systematic review[86]:

- **T1, T2:** ESS plus radiotherapy, with or without adjuvant chemotherapy
- **T3:** ESS or ESS/conventional craniofacial resection (cCFR) plus radiotherapy, with or without adjuvant chemotherapy
- **T4:** cCFR plus radiotherapy, with or without adjuvant chemotherapy

A Cox regression analysis of the type of surgery, stage, orbital and/or brain involvement showed both orbital extension ($p = 0.002$) and intracranial involvement ($p = 0.022$) to be significant independent factors affecting outcome. Without orbital involvement, 5-year DFS was 88.3%, a figure that fell to 55.6% if periosteum was involved and to 25% with frank involvement of the globe (Mantel-Cox $p = 0.00$) (► Fig. 31.4). Similarly, disease-free survival (DFS) was significantly higher if there was no intracranial involvement (92.3% 5 years and 76.3% 10 years). If dura was involved, then 5-year survival was 68.9% and 10-year survival 56.8%, figures that fell to 41.7% and 10.4%, respectively, if there was intracerebral disease (Mantel-Cox $p = 0.000$; ► Fig. 31.5).

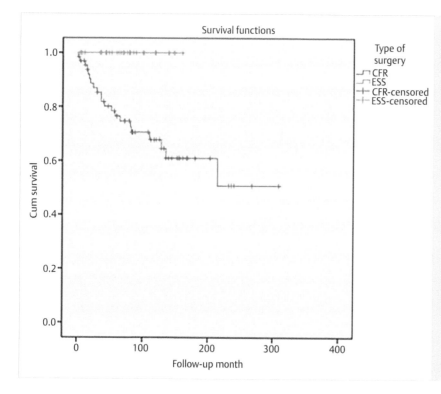

Survival functions

Fig. 31.3 Kaplan-Meier graph of overall survival comparing endoscopic sinus surgery (ESS) to cCFR. (Reproduced with permission from Lund VJ, Stammberger H, Nicolai P, et al, European position paper on endoscopic management of the nose, paranasal sinuses and skull base, Rhinology 2010; (Suppl 22), 105:86–100.)

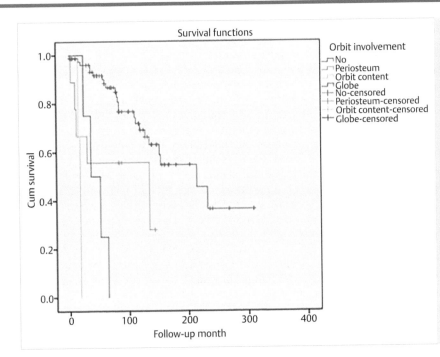

Fig. 31.4 Kaplan-Meier graph of disease-free survival according to orbital involvement. (Reproduced with permission from Lund VJ, Stammberger H, Nicolai P, et al, European position paper on endoscopic management of the nose, paranasal sinuses and skull base, Rhinology 2010; [Suppl 22], 105:86–100.)

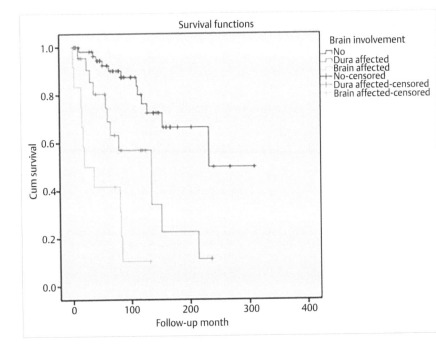

Fig. 31.5 Kaplan-Meier graph of disease-free survival according to intracranial involvement. (Reproduced with permission from Lund VJ, Stammberger H, Nicolai P, et al, European position paper on endoscopic management of the nose, paranasal sinuses and skull base, Rhinology 2010; [Suppl 22], 105:86–100.)

Cervical lymphadenopathy also constitutes an important prognostic factor. Koka et al showed a 29% survival with nodes versus 64% without nodes, which was supported by two subsequent meta-analyses.[13,14,87] Distant metastases with locoregional control are relatively rare (≤ 10%) and carry a poor prognosis.[15,62]

31.6 Conclusion

ENB is a rare nasal tumor that has a unique natural history. Its management requires experience in histopathology, radiology,

sinonasal surgery, and medical oncology. It is optimally treated by a combination of surgery and radiotherapy. Conventional craniofacial resection doubled survival compared with previous surgical treatments. However, endoscopic resection now offers an appropriate alternative in selected cases with minimal complications and morbidity. The role of chemotherapy remains to be determined, but genomic analysis may open up new avenues for treatment.[88] Lifelong follow-up is required irrespective of the treatment, for the natural history of this tumor extends over a lifetime.

References

[1] Berger L, Luc R, Richard D. L'estheioneuroepitheliome olfactif. Bull Assoc Fr Etud Cancer. 1924; 13:410–421

[2] Skolnik EM, Massari FS, Tenta LT. Olfactory neuroepithelioma: review of the world literature and presentation of two cases. Arch Otolaryngol. 1966; 84(6):644–653

[3] O'Connor TA, McLean P, Juillard GJ, Parker RG. Olfactory neuroblastoma. Cancer. 1989; 63(12):2426–2428

[4] Broich G, Pagliari A, Ottaviani F. Esthesioneuroblastoma: a general review of the cases published since the discovery of the tumour in 1924. Anticancer Res. 1997; 17 4A:2683–2706

[5] Hyams VJ. Olfactory neuroblastoma. In: Hyams VJ, Baksakis JG, Michaels L, eds. Tumours of the Upper Respiratory Tract and Ear. Washington, DC: Armed Forces Institute of Pathology; 1998:240–248

[6] Schwaab G, Micheau C, Le Guillou C, et al. Olfactory esthesioneuroma: a report of 40 cases. Laryngoscope. 1988; 98(8 Pt 1):872–876

[7] Magnavita N, Sacco A, Bevilacqua L, D'Alessandris T, Bosman C. Aesthesioneuroblastoma in a woodworker. Occup Med (Lond). 2003; 53(3):231–234

[8] Magee PN, Montesano R, Preussmann R. N-nitroso compounds and related carcinogens. In: Searle CE, ed. Chemical Carcinogens. Washington, DC: USA American Chemical Society; 1976:491–625

[9] Herrold KM. Induction of olfactory neuroepithelia tumours in Syrian hamsters by diethlynitrosamine. Cancer. 1964; 17:114–121

[10] Vollrath M, Altmannsberger M, Weber K, Osborn M. Chemically induced tumors of rat olfactory epithelium: a model for human esthesioneuroepithelioma. J Natl Cancer Inst. 1986; 76(6):1205–1216

[11] Leong BK, Kociba RJ, Jersey GC. A lifetime study of rats and mice exposed to vapors of bis(chloromethyl)ether. Toxicol Appl Pharmacol. 1981; 58(2):269–281

[12] Lund V, Howard D, Wei W. Tumors of the nose, sinuses and nasopharynx. New York: Thieme; 2014

[13] Dulguerov P, Allal AS, Calcaterra TC. Esthesioneuroblastoma: a meta-analysis and review. Lancet Oncol. 2001; 2(11):683–690

[14] Rinaldo A, Ferlito A, Shaha AR, Wei WI, Lund VJ. Esthesioneuroblastoma and cervical lymph node metastases: clinical and therapeutic implications. Acta Otolaryngol. 2002; 122(2):215–221

[15] Lund VJ, Howard D, Wei W, Spittle M. Olfactory neuroblastoma: past, present, and future? Laryngoscope. 2003; 113(3):502–507

[16] Kumar M, Fallon RJ, Hill JS, Davis MM. Esthesioneuroblastoma in children. J Pediatr Hematol Oncol. 2002; 24(6):482–487

[17] Valli R, De Bernardi F, Frattini A, et al. Comparative genomic hybridization on microarray (a-CGH) in olfactory neuroblastoma: analysis of ten cases and review of the literature. Genes Chromosomes Cancer. 2015; 54(12):771–775

[18] Czapiewski P, Kunc M, Haybaeck J. Genetic and molecular alterations in olfactory neuroblastoma: implications for pathogenesis, prognosis and treatment. Oncotarget. 2016; 7(32):52584–52596

[19] Capper D,. Engel N, Stichel D et al. A DNA methylation array-based re-definition of olfactory neuroblastoma. Acta Neuropathol. 2018; 136:255–271

[20] Harrison D. Surgical pathology of olfactory neuroblastoma. Head Neck Surg. 1984; 7(1):60–64

[21] Lund VJ, Wei WI. Endoscopic surgery for malignant sinonasal tumours: an eighteen year experience. Rhinology. 2015; 53(3):204–211

[22] Argani P, Perez-Ordoñez B, Xiao H, Caruana SM, Huvos AG, Ladanyi M. Olfactory neuroblastoma is not related to the Ewing family of tumors: absence of EWS/FLI1 gene fusion and MIC2 expression. Am J Surg Pathol. 1998; 22(4):391–398

[23] Ogura JH, Schenck NL. Unusual nasal tumors: problems in diagnosis and treatment. Otolaryngol Clin North Am. 1973; 6(3):813–837

[24] Lund VJ, Milroy C. Olfactory neuroblastoma: clinical and pathological aspects. Rhinology. 1993; 31(1):1–6

[25] Kadish S, Goodman M, Wang CC. Olfactory neuroblastoma: a clinical analysis of 17 cases. Cancer. 1976; 37(3):1571–1576

[26] Lund VJ, Stammberger H, Nicolai P, et al. European position paper on endoscopic management of tumours of the nose, paranasal sinuses and skull base. Rhinol Suppl. 2010;22:46–51

[27] Rimmer J, Lund VJ, Beale T, Wei WI, Howard D. Olfactory neuroblastoma: a 35-year experience and suggested follow-up protocol. Laryngoscope. 2014; 124(7):1542–1549

[28] Morita A, Ebersold MJ, Olsen KD, Foote RL, Lewis JE, Quast LM. Esthesioneuroblastoma: prognosis and management. Neurosurgery. 1993; 32(5):706–714, discussion 714–715

[29] Saade R, Roberts D, Ow Tj, et al. Prognosis and biology in esthesioneuroblastoma: staging versus grading dilemma—the MDACC experience. J Neurol Surg, Part B: Skull Base. Conference: 24th Annual Meeting North American Skull Base Society. Abstract 75, 2014

[30] Van Gompel JJ, Giannini C, Olsen KD, et al. Long-term outcome of esthesioneuroblastoma: Hyams grade predicts patient survival. J Neurol Surg B Skull Base. 2012; 73(5):331–336

[31] Nalavenkata SB, Sacks R, Adappa ND, et al. Olfactory neuroblastoma: Fate of the neck—a long-term multicenter retrospective study. Otolaryngol Head Neck Surg. 2016; 154(2):383–389

[32] Bouche J, Guiot G, Tessier P, Frèche C, Narcy P. [A further case of tumor of the olfactory placode]. Sem Hop. 1967; 43(9):587–591

[33] Gabbay U, Leider-Trejo L, Marshak G, Gabbay M, Fliss DM. A case and a series of published cases of esthesioneuroblastoma (ENB) in which long-standing paraneoplastic SIADH had preceded ENB diagnosis. Ear Nose Throat J. 2013; 92(10–11):E6

[34] Kunc M, Gabrych A, Czapiewski P, Sworczak K. Paraneoplastic syndromes in olfactory neuroblastoma. Contemp Oncol (Pozn). 2015;19(1):6–16

[35] Plasencia YL, Cortés MB, Arencibia DM, et al. Esthesioneuroblastoma recurrence presenting as a syndrome of inappropriate antidiuretic hormone secretion. Head Neck. 2006; 28(12):1142–1146

[36] Gray ST, Holbrook EH, Najm MH, Sadow PM, Curry WT, Lin DT. Syndrome of inappropriate antidiuretic hormone secretion in patients with olfactory neuroblastoma. Otolaryngol Head Neck Surg. 2012; 147(1):147–151

[37] Madani G, Beale T, Lund V. Imaging of sinonasal tumors. Seminars in Ultrasound. CT and MRI. 2009; 30(1):25–38

[38] Collins BT, Cramer HM, Hearn SA. Fine needle aspiration cytology of metastatic olfactory neuroblastoma. Acta Cytol. 1997; 41(3):802–810

[39] Broski SM, Hunt CH, Johnson GB, Subramaniam RM, Peller PJ. The added value of 18F-FDG PET/CT for evaluation of patients with esthesioneuroblastoma. J Nucl Med. 2012; 53(8):1200–1206

[40] Lapinska G, Jarzabski A, Dedecjus M. Esthesioneuroblastoma-evaluation of 68Ga-DOTATATE PET/CT imaging efficacy in diagnosing and treatment monitoring-initial experience. Eur J Nucl Med Mol Imaging. 2016; 43 Suppl 1:S323

[41] Pickuth D, Heywang-Köbrunner SH, Spielmann RP. Computed tomography and magnetic resonance imaging features of olfactory neuroblastoma: an analysis of 22 cases. Clin Otolaryngol Allied Sci. 1999; 24(5):457–461

[42] Ketcham AS, Van Buren JM. Tumors of the paranasal sinuses: a therapeutic challenge. Am J Surg. 1985; 150(4):406–413

[43] Clifford P. Transcranial approach for cancer of the antroethmoidal area. Clin Otolaryngol Allied Sci. 1977; 2(2):115–130

[44] Terz JJ, Young HF, Lawrence W, Jr. Combined craniofacial resection for locally advanced carcinoma of the head and neck I. Tumors of the skin and soft tissues. Am J Surg. 1980; 140(5):613–617

[45] Shah JP, Kraus DH, Bilsky MH, Gutin PH, Harrison LH, Strong EW. Craniofacial resection for malignant tumors involving the anterior skull base. Arch Otolaryngol Head Neck Surg. 1997; 123(12):1312–1317

[46] Howard DJ, Lund VJ, Wei WI. Craniofacial resection for tumors of the nasal cavity and paranasal sinuses: a 25-year experience. Head Neck 2006; 28(10):867–873

[47] Goffart Y, Jorissen M, Daele J, et al. Minimally invasive endoscopic management of malignant sinonasal tumours. Acta Otorhinolaryngol Belg. 2000; 54(2):221–232

[48] Walch C, Stammberger H, Anderhuber W, Unger F, Köle W, Feichtinger K. The minimally invasive approach to olfactory neuroblastoma: combined endoscopic and stereotactic treatment. Laryngoscope. 2000; 110(4):635–640

[49] Casiano RR, Numa WA, Falquez AM. Endoscopic resection of esthesioneuroblastoma. Am J Rhinol. 2001; 15(4):271–279

[50] Kassam A, Horowitz M, Welch W, et al. The role of endoscopic assisted microneurosurgery (image fusion technology) in the performance of neurosurgical procedures. Minim Invasive Neurosurg. 2005; 48(4):191–196

[51] Tajudeen BA, Adappa ND, Kuan EC, et al. Smell preservation following endoscopic unilateral resection of esthesioneuroblastoma: a multi-institutional experience. Int Forum Allergy Rhinol. 2016; 6(10):1047–1050

[52] Thaler ER, Kotapka M, Lanza DC, Kennedy DW. Endoscopically assisted anterior cranial skull base resection of sinonasal tumors. Am J Rhinol. 1999; 13(4):303–310

[53] Draf W, Schick B, Weber R, et al. Endoscopic micro-endoscopic surgery of nasal and paranasal sinus tumours. In: Stamm AC, Draf W, eds. Micro-Endoscopic Surgery of the Paranasal Sinuses and the Skull Base. Berlin, Germany: Springer; 2000:481–488

[54] Batra PS, Citardi MJ, Worley S, Lee J, Lanza DC. Resection of anterior skull base tumors: comparison of combined traditional and endoscopic techniques. Am J Rhinol. 2005; 19(5):521–528

[55] Zanation AM, Ferlito A, Rinaldo A, et al. When, how and why to treat the neck in patients with esthesioneuroblastoma: a review. Eur Arch Otorhinolaryngol. 2010; 267(11):1667–1671

[56] Lund VJ, Clarke PM, Swift AC, McGarry GW, Kerawala C, Carnell D. Nose and paranasal sinus tumours: United Kingdom National Multidisciplinary Guidelines. J Laryngol Otol. 2016; 130(S2) Suppl 2:S111–S118

[57] Dirix P, Vanstraelen B, Jorissen M, Vander Poorten V, Nuyts S. Intensity-modulated radiotherapy for sinonasal cancer: improved outcome compared to conventional radiotherapy. Int J Radiat Oncol Biol Phys. 2010; 78(4):998–1004

[58] Foote RL, Morita A, Ebersold MJ, et al. Esthesioneuroblastoma: the role of adjuvant radiation therapy. Int J Radiat Oncol Biol Phys. 1993; 27(4):835–842

[59] Unger F, Haselsberger K, Walch C, Stammberger H, Papaefthymiou G. Combined endoscopic surgery and radiosurgery as treatment modality for olfactory neuroblastoma (esthesioneuroblastoma). Acta Neurochir (Wien). 2005; 147(6):595–601, discussion 601–602

[60] Eden BV, Debo RF, Larner JM, et al. Esthesioneuroblastoma: long-term outcome and patterns of failure—the University of Virginia experience. Cancer. 1994; 73(10):2556–2562

[61] McElroy EA, Jr, Buckner JC, Lewis JE. Chemotherapy for advanced esthesioneuroblastoma: the Mayo Clinic experience. Neurosurgery. 1998; 42(5):1023–1027, discussion 1027–1028

[62] Levine PA, Gallagher R, Cantrell RW. Esthesioneuroblastoma: reflections of a 21-year experience. Laryngoscope. 1999; 109(10):1539–1543

[63] Kim DW, Jo YH, Kim JH, et al. Neoadjuvant etoposide, ifosfamide, and cisplatin for the treatment of olfactory neuroblastoma. Cancer. 2004; 101(10):2257–2260

[64] Nikapota A, Sevitt T, Lund VJ, et al. Outcomes of radical conformal radiotherapy and concomitant cisplatin chemotherapy for olfactory neuroblastoma—a review of a single centre experience. Abstr Am Soc Clin Oncol.. 2006; 24(18) Suppl:5555

[65] Loy AH, Reibel JF, Read PW, et al. Esthesioneuroblastoma: continued follow-up of a single institution's experience. Arch Otolaryngol Head Neck Surg. 2006; 132(2):134–138

[66] Mishima Y, Nagasaki E, Terui Y, et al. Combination chemotherapy (cyclophosphamide, doxorubicin, and vincristine with continuous-infusion cisplatin and etoposide) and radiotherapy with stem cell support can be beneficial for adolescents and adults with esthesioneuroblastoma. Cancer. 2004; 101(6):1437–1444

[67] Yoh K, Tahara M, Kawada K, et al. Chemotherapy in the treatment of advanced or recurrent olfactory neuroblastoma. Asia Pac J Clin Oncol. 2006; 2(4):180–184

[68] Shah JP, Feghali J. Esthesioneuroblastoma. Am J Surg. 1981; 142(4):456–458

[69] Appelblatt NH, McClatchey KD. Olfactory neuroblastoma: a retrospective clinicopathologic study. Head Neck Surg. 1982; 5(2):108–113

[70] Bailey BJ, Barton S. Olfactory neuroblastoma: management and prognosis. Arch Otolaryngol. 1975; 101(1):1–5

[71] Eriksen JG, Bastholt L, Krogdahl AS, Hansen O, Joergensen KE. Esthesioneuroblastoma—what is the optimal treatment? Acta Oncol. 2000; 39(2):231–235

[72] Resto VA, Eisele DW, Forastiere A, Zahurak M, Lee DJ, Westra WH. Esthesioneuroblastoma: the Johns Hopkins experience. Head Neck. 2000; 22(6):550–558

[73] Patel SG, Singh B, Polluri A, et al. Craniofacial surgery for malignant skull base tumors: report of an international collaborative study. Cancer. 2003; 98(6):1179–1187

[74] Constantinidis J, Steinhart H, Koch M, et al. Olfactory neuroblastoma: the University of Erlangen-Nuremberg experience 1975–2000. Otolaryngol Head Neck Surg. 2004; 130(5):567–574

[75] Diaz EM, Jr, Johnigan RH, III, Pero C, et al. Olfactory neuroblastoma: the 22-year experience at one comprehensive cancer center. Head Neck. 2005; 27(2):138–149

[76] Ow TJ, Hanna EY, Roberts DB, et al. Optimization of long-term outcomes for patients with esthesioneuroblastoma. Head Neck. 2014; 36(4):524–530

[77] Devaiah AK, Larsen C, Tawfik O, O'Boynick P, Hoover LA. Esthesioneuroblastoma: endoscopic nasal and anterior craniotomy resection. Laryngoscope. 2003; 113(12):2086–2090

[78] Nicolai P, Battaglia P, Bignami M, et al. Endoscopic surgery for malignant tumors of the sinonasal tract and adjacent skull base: a 10-year experience. Am J Rhinol. 2008; 22(3):308–316

[79] Snyderman CH, Carrau RL, Kassam AB, et al. Endoscopic skull base surgery: principles of endonasal oncological surgery. J Surg Oncol. 2008; 97(8):658–664

[80] Folbe A, Herzallah I, Duvvuri U, et al. Endoscopic endonasal resection of esthesioneuroblastoma: a multicenter study. Am J Rhinol Allergy. 2009; 23(1):91–94

[81] Castelnuovo P, Bignami M, Delù G, Battaglia P, Bignardi M, Dallan I. Endonasal endoscopic resection and radiotherapy in olfactory neuroblastoma: our experience. Head Neck. 2007; 29(9):845–850

[82] de Gabory L, Abdulkhaleq HM, Darrouzet V, Bébéar J-P, Stoll D. Long-term results of 28 esthesioneuroblastomas managed over 35 years. Head Neck. 2011; 33(1):82–86

[83] Song CM, Won T-B, Lee CH, Kim D-Y, Rhee C-S. Treatment modalities and outcomes of olfactory neuroblastoma. Laryngoscope. 2012; 122(11):2389–2395

[84] Komotar RJ, Starke RM, Raper DM, Anand VK, Schwartz TH. Endoscopic endonasal compared with anterior craniofacial and combined cranionasal resection of esthesioneuroblastomas. World Neurosurg. 2013; 80(1–2):148–159

[85] Ganly I, Patel SG, Singh B, et al. Complications of craniofacial resection for malignant tumors of the skull base: report of an International Collaborative Study. Head Neck. 2005; 27(6):445–451

[86] Fu TS, Monteiro E, Muhanna N, Goldstein DP, de Almeida JR. Comparison of outcomes for open versus endoscopic approaches for olfactory neuroblastoma: a systematic review and individual participant data meta-analysis. Head Neck. 2016; 38 Suppl 1:E2306–E2316

[87] Koka VN, Julieron M, Bourhis J, et al. Aesthesioneuroblastoma. J Laryngol Otol. 1998; 112(7):628–633

[88] Lechner M, Wells G, Steele C, et al. Clinical and mutation profiling of olfactory neuroblastoma, establishment of novel olfactory neuroblastoma cell culture model and results from drug screening ERS London 2018 Abstract

32 Melanoma of the Nasal Cavity and Paranasal Sinuses

Daniel P. McCormick and Dennis H. Kraus

Summary

Sinonasal melanoma is a rare and aggressive malignancy derived from melanocytes in the nasal cavity and paranasal sinuses. Symptoms vary by location, with paranasal sinus tumors often presenting at advanced stage because of their insidious growth. The staging system reflects their aggressive nature, with TNM staging beginning at T3. Optimal treatment is complete surgical resection. Postoperative radiation therapy is recommended for local control despite the absence of any proven benefit on overall survival (OS). Adjuvant chemotherapy or immunotherapy may incur an OS benefit. Recurrent, metastatic, or inoperable disease may be managed using primary radiation, chemotherapy, immunotherapy, and, more recently, checkpoint inhibitors. Despite these new therapies, estimated 10-year survival rate remains low, at 7%.

Keywords: mucosal melanoma, sinonasal, craniofacial, endoscopic resection, staging, immunotherapy, checkpoint inhibitors

32.1 Introduction

Melanoma is a malignancy of ectodermal origin that involves the skin in the vast majority of cases. The disease is classically divided according to the site of origin of the primary tumor: for example, cutaneous, noncutaneous, or unknown primary melanoma. Noncutaneous melanomas are infrequent and may be found in the retina, genitourinary tract, anus, and upper aerodigestive tract. The most frequent origin of noncutaneous melanoma is the eye (5.3%), followed by melanomas of unknown primary (2.2%) and mucosal melanomas (1.3%).[1] Mucosal melanomas of head and neck origin can arise in the oral cavity, oropharynx, nasal cavity, and paranasal sinuses.

Melanoma of the sinonasal cavity is a rare neoplasm that can involve various compartments of the respiratory mucosa. The first description of mucosal melanoma was by Weber in 1856.[2] Thirteen years later, Lucke reported the first resection of a nasal mucosal melanoma in a 52-year-old man who had "melanotic sarcoma."[3] One of the first reports of sinonasal melanoma is attributed to Viennois, who described the surgical extirpation of "polype melanique du nez" infiltrating the globe.[4] In 1885, Lincoln made the first report in the English literature of a "melanosarcoma" arising in the nasal antrum and treated with galvanocauterization.[5] Since then more than 1,950 cases of mucosal melanoma of the head and neck have been reported in the English literature, a third originating in the sinonasal area.[6] Significant progress has been made during the past decade in understanding the biology of melanomas, improved surgical technique, and its sensitivity to chemotherapy, radiotherapy, and immunotherapy.[7] However, because of the low prevalence of sinonasal melanoma, the pathophysiology of the disease, as well as the roles of radiotherapy and immunotherapy, remains controversial.

In this chapter, we review the current literature on paranasal and nasal mucosal melanomas, as well as the epidemiology, pathology, staging, and treatment of this disease.

32.2 Incidence and Epidemiology

The incidence of melanoma has been increasing 4 to 6% per year since 1973, a greater rate than for any other human cancer in the United States.[8] It is estimated that nearly 1 in 75 persons will develop melanoma during his or her lifetime.[9] The main factor believed to be involved in the significant rise in incidence of cutaneous melanoma is exposure to sunlight and ultraviolet radiation. Unlike melanoma of the skin, mucosal melanoma did not show any increase in incidence during this period, suggesting that a distinct pathophysiologic mechanism is associated with this tumor. However, a recent study by Marcus et al has shown an increase in sinonasal melanoma since 1989 and particularly in the decade from 1999 to 2009, although the researchers were unable to identify any causative factors.[10]

An analysis of the National Cancer Database performed over 9 years (1985–1994) showed that among 84,836 cases of malignant melanoma only 1,074 involved the mucosal membrane, half of which arose in the head and neck, with the sinonasal cavity being the most common site.[1] A more recent study pooling statistics from cancer registries across 27 states and 1 metropolitan area in the United States from 1996 to 2000 showed similar results, with only 1,806 cases of mucosal melanoma among 133,209 melanoma cases.[11] According to a report by the Armed Forces Institute of Pathology, sinonasal mucosal melanomas account for only 1% of all melanomas and for 0.6 to 4% of all tumors of the nasal cavity and paranasal sinuses.[12] Conley reported in his series that melanoma involved up to 6.7% of all sinonasal malignancies.[13] Ganly et al studied 1,307 patients who had malignant skull base tumors and found that 4% had sinonasal melanoma.[14] Lewis and Martin studied the incidence of malignant melanoma of the nasal cavity in Ugandan Africans and found that this disease accounted for 2.6% of all cases of melanoma.[15] In Denmark, melanoma of the upper aerodigestive tract accounts for 0.8% of all melanoma cases and for 8% of all head and neck melanomas.[16] Japanese have the highest rate of mucosal melanomas compared with Caucasians (4:1 relative rate), most commonly in the oral cavity.[17] Interestingly, the incidence of cutaneous melanoma among Japanese is lower than among Caucasians.

The mean age of presentation of sinonasal melanoma is 65, with a range of 50 to 80 years.[18,19,20] The gender distribution of sinonasal melanomas shows a slight male predominance.[21,22,23,24,25] Ganly et al have reported that of a total of 53 patients who had anterior skull base melanoma, 70% were males and 30% females.[14] Manolidis and Donald reviewed 172 cases of nasal melanomas and reported that 57% of the cases were males and 43% females.[26] Female patients who have cutaneous melanoma tend to have a better prognosis than men. However, similar outcomes occurred for males and females who had sinonasal melanoma in regard to long-term survival.[27,28,29]

The main factor involved in the development of cutaneous melanoma is exposure to sunlight and ultraviolet radiation, whereas the etiology of the ultraviolet light–protected mucosal melanoma remains unknown. Holmstrom and Lund have suggested that prolonged occupational exposure to formaldehyde may cause significant mucosal irritation, eventually causing paranasal malignant melanoma.[30] Similarly, Thompson et al reported formaldehyde exposure in 9 of 115 patients (7.8%) in whom a work history could be elicited.[12] The majority of these patients were painters, furniture makers, construction workers, and laundry workers. A joint Danish–Finnish–Swedish case-referent investigation initiated in 1977 studied the connection between nasal and sinonasal cancer and various occupational exposures. The authors found that formaldehyde was evenly distributed among cases involving different tumors of paranasal origin.[31]

The nasal cavity is the most common origin of head and neck mucosal melanomas (55–79%), followed by the oral cavity.[32,33,34,35] The lateral wall of the nasal cavity and the inferior turbinate are the most common origin of melanoma of the nasal mucosa. In the sinuses, the exact site of origin of melanoma is difficult to identify, because most tumors are diagnosed at advanced stage and frequently infiltrate multiple compartments. The most common site of origin for melanoma of the sinuses is the maxillary sinus, followed by the ethmoid and sphenoid sinuses.[26,29] Melanomas of the frontal sinus, as well as of the middle turbinate, superior turbinate, and cribriform plate, are very rare.[36] ▶ Table 32.1 shows the sites of origin of sinonasal melanomas among 563 patients reviewed in three different studies.[12,26,37]

Advanced-stage tumors most frequently involve multiple compartments. For example, in a recent multicenter study, Ganly et al reported that 50% of the patients who had skull base melanomas had tumors infiltrating the cribriform plate, 34% periorbital invasion, 26% orbital invasion, and 17% dural invasion.[14]

The majority of patients who have sinonasal melanomas present without regional or distant metastases at the time of diagnosis. Positive lymph nodes are found in 4 to 18% of patients at the time of diagnosis.[12,22,23,25] The incidence of lymph node involvement in patients who have mucosal melanoma of the oral cavity and oropharynx is 4.7 times higher than in patients who have sinonasal melanoma, owing to the dense lymphatic drainage of the oral cavity and oropharyngeal mucosa.[32] Distant metastases of sinonasal melanoma are rare at presentation. For example, Harrison et al reported that none of the 40 patients in their series had distant metastases at presentation.[22] In those patients who develop distant metastases, the most common sites are the lungs, bone, liver, brain, and skin.[32]

32.3 Pathology

The primary cell of origin of melanoma is the melanocyte, which can be found in the nasal and paranasal mucosa. These melanocytes have migrated as neuroectodermal derivatives and embedded in the endodermally derived respiratory mucosa.[38] It is estimated that the distribution of melanocytes in the respiratory mucosa is 1,500 cells per square millimeter—less than two-thirds the figure for those found in the skin.[39]

Mucosal melanosis is defined as a benign pigmented lesion characterized by pigmentation of basal keratinocytes with a normal or slightly increased number of melanocytes.[40] Association between mucosal melanosis and increased incidence of nasal or paranasal melanoma has been suggested by several authors.[15,41,42] Preexisting pigmentation of the sinonasal mucosa is seen in less than 10% of patients who have mucosal malignant melanoma.[43] Similarly, Thompson et al found preexisting melanosis in only 8% of the patients who had sinonasal melanoma.[12] The low rate of melanosis in patients who have mucosal melanoma indicates that most sinonasal melanomas arise de novo.

The majority of melanomas of the respiratory mucosa are large and polypoid and have a median thickness of 9 mm, significantly thicker than melanoma of the oral cavity.[44] Thompson et al reported a mean thickness of 7.2 mm (range 2–19 mm) and size of 24 mm (range 5–65 mm), and McLean et al had an average tumor depth > 10 mm for sinonasal melanoma, compared with 3.8 mm for oral.[12,45] Infrequently, mucosal melanoma in situ can be identified after biopsy of a suspected lesion (▶ Fig. 32.1). The authors found no correlation between survival and tumor thickness. Lee et al have found that depth of invasion > 7 mm is an independent factor for poor prognosis in patients who have mucosal melanomas of the head and neck.[46]

Melanoma has a notorious tendency to mimic other tumors, and in the sinonasal mucosa it can be easily confused with other tumors, which occur more commonly in this region. The challenge in making the diagnosis of sinonasal melanoma is more significant in cases of amelanotic melanoma and in the presence of ulceration. The Armed Forces Institute of Pathology study has previously shown that more than two-thirds of cases of sinonasal melanoma are misclassified as another neoplasm on initial pathologic evaluation.[12]

Histologically, mucosal melanoma cells may have different characteristics, such as small cells, spindle cells, epithelioid cells, and, rarely, pleomorphic cells.[24,47] Spindle cell melanoma appears sarcomatous and is composed of cells whose eosinophilic cytoplasm

Table 32.1 Site of origin of sinonasal melanomas[9,26,37]

Site	Manolidis and Donald Number (%)	Nandapalan et al Number (%)	Thompson et al[a] Number (%)
Nasal cavity			
Nasal NOS	159 (48)		34 (44)
Septum	44 (13)	61 (37)	20 (26)
Lateral wall	44 (13)	10 (6.7)	
Inferior turbinate	12 (3.7)	34 (6.1)	10 (13)
Middle turbinate	7 (2.1)	43 (26)	
Turbinate NOS	12 (3.7)		
Floor of nose	5 (1.5)	2 (1.2)	
Subtotal	283 (88)	150 (92)	64 (84)
Paranasal sinuses			
Maxillary sinus	32 (9.8)	5 (3)	3 (4)
Ethmoid sinus	8 (2.4)	8 (4.6)	
Frontal sinus	2 (0.6)		
Sinus NOS	21 (6.4)		9 (12.5)
Subtotal	63 (18.2)	13 (7.9)	12 (16)
Total	328 (100)	163 (100)	72 (100)

Abbreviation: NOS, not otherwise specific.
[a]In the other 39 patients, the specific compartment was not specified.

and nuclei may vary in shape and number. Epithelioid-type melanoma is characterized by large cells that have eosinophilic cytoplasm and acentric nucleus. Although melanomas display morphologic diversity, undifferentiated small round cells or polygonal cells are the most prominent cells found in sinonasal melanomas.[44,48] A pseudopapillary growth pattern is found in up to 25% of patients who have sinonasal melanomas, but not in melanoma of the oral cavity (▶ Fig. 32.2).[24,44]

The most significant factor in establishing the diagnosis of melanoma is melanin production and the appearance of junctional changes (▶ Fig. 32.3). Melanin pigment is found in two-thirds of cases of sinonasal melanoma and should be considered in a sinonasal myxoid tumor with melanin.[12] Such an example is melanoma botryoides, a polypoid tumor that contains small amounts of melanin with a botryoid or myxoid pattern.

Amelanotic tumors show similar biological behavior and prognosis as melanotic nasal melanomas but are more difficult

to diagnose than conventional melanomas.[49] A variant of melanoma, which does not contain melanin, is desmoplastic melanoma.[50] Rarely found in sinonasal melanoma, these cells are composed of amelanotic, poorly circumscribed fascicles and bundles of spindle cells with hyperchromatic nuclei.[51] Desmoplastic melanoma is a neurotrophic tumor, which frequently expresses aberrant p53 protein.[50] This variant of amelanotic malignant melanoma is difficult to differentiate from other soft tissue tumors of the nasal cavity, such as esthesioneuroblastoma, sarcoma, spindle cell carcinoma, and malignant peripheral nerve sheath tumors.[52]

Melanoma of the sinonasal mucosa often demonstrates deep invasion, necrosis, and vascular invasion. These characteristics are well-established predictors of reduced survival in cutaneous melanomas and melanomas of the head and neck.[44] Prasad et al have shown that 60% of paranasal melanomas are detected at an advanced stage, presenting with significant infiltration of skeletal muscles, cartilage, and bone at the time of surgery.[44]

Rarely nasal mucosal melanomas may show bone and osteoid formation.[12,53] Osteoid and metaplastic bone formation may be caused by repeated trauma, mesenchymal metaplasia, reparative reaction to bone invasion, and induction of bone formation of the surrounding tissues.[12]

Owing to the complicated differential diagnosis of this tumor, immunocytochemical staining is frequently required to establish the diagnosis of melanoma of the paranasal sinuses, particularly in cases of amelanotic variants. Melanoma stains positive for vimentin, HMB-45, and S100 protein. In contrast to cutaneous melanomas, paranasal melanoma is negatively stained for synaptophysin and actin leukocytic common antigen.[54,55] Interestingly, staining for P-97, which is frequently positive in melanoma of the esophageal mucosa, is not found in melanomas originating in the paranasal sinuses or nasal mucosa.[56,57] Other antigens, which are specifically stained in paranasal melanomas, are KC-2, SK-46, KBA-62 and PNL2.[58,59] Other melanoma-associated antigens found in the nasal cavity are tyrosinase (T311), D5, A103 (anti-melan-A/MART-1), and TRP-1.[42]

In a study of 44 sinonasal melanomas, Prasad et al found that all tumors were positive for tyrosinase, 98% for HMB-45, 95% for S100 protein, and 91% for D5.[60] They concluded that tyrosinase is the most sensitive marker for melanomas of nasal or

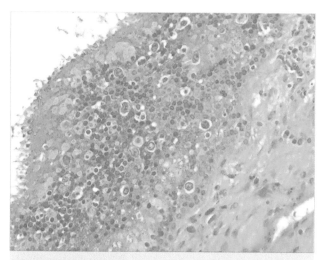

Fig. 32.1 Mucosal melanoma in situ. The photomicrograph shows mucosal melanoma confined to the sinonasal respiratory epithelium. The neoplastic melanocytes are three to four times larger than the benign surrounding cells. Convoluted nuclear membranes, as well as prominent nucleoli with increased nuclear to cytoplasmic ratio, can also be identified. 100 × H&E staining.

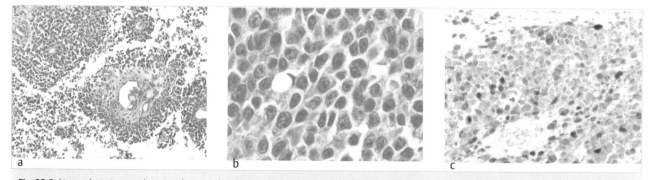

Fig. 32.2 Nonmelanotic nasopharyngeal mucosal melanoma. (a) Small round blue cells grow radially outward from central vessels, demonstrating the pseudopapillary architecture frequently seen in mucosal melanoma. (b) A photomicrograph of the specimen showing malignant cells arranged in a pavementlike sheet, with no evidence of pigmentation. Large cherry-red macronucleoli in the center of the cell nucleus are very characteristic but are not pathognomonic for melanoma. 600 × H&E staining. (c) Immunohistochemical staining for S100 in both the nucleus and the cytoplasm is indicative of malignant melanoma.

paranasal origin. Thompson et al studied 115 cases of sinonasal melanoma and found positive staining for S100 in 91% of the cases and HMB-45 in 76% of the cases.[12] Tyrosinase antigens were expressed in 77.7% of the cases. ▶ Table 32.2 shows the different antigens expressed in various tumors of the paranasal sinuses, including malignant melanoma.

Electron microscopy can be used as an adjunct for the diagnosis of melanoma in borderline cases and is very specific in identifying premelanosomes, a subcellular organelle present in melanomas. Wright and Heenan identified a subclass of premelanosomes with a high propensity to metastasize, but these premelanosomes are not found in all cases of mucosal melanoma.[22,61,62]

Because melanoma of the paranasal sinuses accounts for less than 7% of neoplasms involving this anatomical compartment, a proper differential diagnosis work-up is crucial for management of the disease. The microscopic differential diagnosis of sinonasal melanoma can be divided into three groups: small round blue cell tumors, pleomorphic cell tumors, and spindle cell tumors.[12] The first group includes tumors such as olfactory neuroblastoma, primitive neuroectodermal tumor, Ewing sarcoma, melanocytic neuroectodermal tumor of infancy, pituitary adenoma, lymphoma, plasmacytoma, small cell neuroendocrine carcinoma, and mesenchymal chondrosarcoma. The pleomorphic cells group includes sinonasal undifferentiated carcinoma, anaplastic large cell lymphoma, and rhabdomyosarcoma. The group of tumors characterized by spindle cells includes malignant peripheral nerve sheath tumor, fibrosarcoma, malignant fibrous histiocytoma, and synovial sarcoma.[12,48,63,64,65,66,67] Olfactory esthesioneuroblastoma can show similar morphology to melanoma; however, this tumor frequently shows neurofibrillary background, Homer-Wright rosettes, and focal sustentacular cell pattern even in high-grade tumors (Hyman grade II–IV). Furthermore, most esthesioneuroblastomas stain positive for neuron-specific enolase and chromogranin and negative for vimentin.

As described earlier, mucosal melanomas frequently lack melanin pigment and thus can be indistinguishable from other high-grade tumors, such as sinonasal undifferentiated carcinoma, undifferentiated nasopharyngeal carcinoma, poorly differentiated nonkeratinizing squamous cell carcinoma, small cell carcinoma, and anaplastic large cell lymphoma.[68] Fortunately, most epithelial tumors show strong cytokeratin immunostaining and fail to express S100 protein. Anaplastic large cell lymphoma does not stain for cytokeratin but expresses CD30 and anaplastic large cell lymphoma kinase proteins. Malignant peripheral nerve sheath tumors may also express S100 protein, complicating the pathologic diagnosis of melanoma. Malignant peripheral nerve sheath tumor does not express other antigens, such as HMB-45, which are frequently found in sinonasal melanoma.

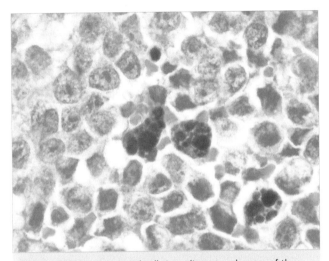

Fig. 32.3 Melanin pigmented cells in malignant melanoma of the sinonasal mucosa. The most important factor in establishing the diagnosis of melanoma is the appearance of malignant cells containing melanin. Unlike carcinoma, these cells have visible apparent spaces between their cytoplasmic borders.

Table 32.2 Histologic and antigenic characteristics of malignant melanoma and other undifferentiated tumors originating in the nasal and paranasal sinuses

	CK	NSE	CG	SYN	S100	HMB	LCA	CD56	CD99	VIM	DES	Myf4
SCC	+	–	–	–	–	–	–	–	–	–	–	–
SNUC	+	V	–	–	–	–	–	–	–	–	–	–
ONB	–	+	V	V	+[a]	–	–	–	–	–	–	–
SCUNC	+	+	+	+	+	–	–	–	–	–	–	–
MMM	–	–	–	–	+	+	–	–	–	+	–	–
T/NK ML	–	–	–	–	–	–	V	–	–	V	–	–
RMS	–	–	–	–	–	–	–	–	–	+	+	+
PNET/EWS	R +	V	–	V	V	–	–	–	+	+	–	–

Abbreviations: (+), positive; (–) negative; CD99, Ewing's marker; CG, chromogranin; CK, cytokeratin; DES, desmin; HMB, HMB 45 (as well as other melanocytic markers [melan A]); LCA,; MMM, mucosal malignant melanoma; NSE, neuron-specific enolase; ONB,; PNET/EWS, primitive (peripheral) neuroectodermal tumor/extraosseous Ewing's sarcoma; RMS, rhabdomyosarcoma; R +, rarely positive; SCC, squamous cell carcinoma; SCUNC, small-cell undifferentiated neuroendocrine carcinoma; SNUC, sinonasal undifferentiated carcinoma; SYN, synaptophysin; T/NK ML, nasal-type T/natural killer-cell lymphoma; VIM, vimentin; v, variably positive.
Source: Reproduced with permission from Brandwein MS, Rothstein A, Lawson W, et al, Sinonasal melanoma: a clinicopathologic study of 25 cases and literature meta-analysis, Arch Otolaryngol Head Neck Surg, 1997;123(3):290–296.
[a]Positive in the peripherally situated sustentacular cells.

32.4 Clinical Presentation and Findings

The clinical symptoms in patients who have paranasal sinus melanoma are frequently nonspecific and include pain, malaise, and weight loss. Other symptoms may be directly associated with the location of the primary tumor. Melanomas originating in the nasal septum may cause irritation and be visible to the patients.[69] This may explain why 75% of patients who have nasal mucosal melanoma are diagnosed early with a clinically localized disease, in comparison with those who have paranasal sinus melanoma. Most patients who have paranasal melanoma suffer from nasal discharge, recurrent epistaxis, or nasal obstruction (85–90% of cases). Thompson et al reported that 52 of 115 patients who had melanoma of the sinuses had epistaxis, 42 a visible mass, and 32 obstructive symptoms.[12] Pain (20%) and a visible facial mass (9%) occur in more advanced disease stages.[23] Signs representing orbital involvement are proptosis, ophthalmoplegia, decreased visual fields, and monocular blindness and are associated with poor prognosis.[14,46]

Most skin or oral cavity melanomas are more likely to be discovered by the patient or by the primary health care physician on routine examination, whereas sinonasal melanomas are inaccessible to self-examination and are routinely diagnosed at an advanced stage. The duration of the symptoms depends on the biological behavior of the disease. In cases of a slowly growing tumor of paranasal origin, airway obstruction may develop slowly, and the disease, which is obscured from the patient and the physician, may develop months or years before the diagnosis is established.[22] Most authors report mean symptom duration of 2 to 8 months.[16,23,34,46,70] Holdcraft and Gallagher have reported that 50% of their patients had suffered from symptoms for 1 to 4 months before diagnosis and that 30% had had symptoms for 6 to 24 months.[21] Thompson et al reported a mean duration of 8.2 months ranging from 2 weeks to 8 years.[12]

Evaluation of patients who have suspected sinonasal melanoma should include complete history and physical evaluation with emphasis on the head and neck. Fiberoptic evaluation of the paranasal sinuses and upper aerodigestive tract is indicated in all patients to evaluate the tumor extent and potential for resection (▶ Fig. 32.4). Radiologic evaluation should always include both CT and MRI of the head, neck, and paranasal sinuses for evaluation of bony and soft tissue involvement, respectively.[71] Patients should be evaluated for involvement of cranial nerve, orbit, skull base, dural, or brain infiltration using both CT and MRI.

Although perineural spread of disease occurs more commonly with squamous cell carcinoma and adenoid cystic carcinoma of the paranasal sinuses, malignant melanoma must also be included in this differential diagnosis, particularly if the patient's pathology is known to be desmoplastic melanoma. Imaging in patients who have malignant melanoma of the paranasal sinuses should focus on the likely potential for perineural spread. In a recent study of nine patients who had melanomas of the facial skin and paranasal sinuses (including five desmoplastic melanomas) with symptomatic cranial neuropathy, MR imaging demonstrated postgadolinium enhancement of the trigeminal nerve in all nine cases and of other cranial nerves in five cases.[72] Other findings included abnormal contrast

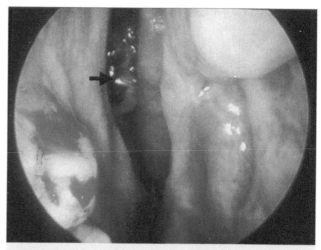

Fig. 32.4 Endoscopic photograph of a mucosal melanoma of the paranasal sinuses. Fiber-optic examination of the paranasal sinuses and upper aerodigestive tract is indicated in all patients prior to surgery so as to evaluate the tumor extent and the presence of a second primary. The photograph shows mucosal melanoma arising from the sinonasal mucosa (*arrow*).

enhancement and soft tissue thickening in the cavernous sinus, Meckel's cave, and/or the cisternal segment of the trigeminal nerve.

Suspicious neck metastases can be evaluated with CT, MRI, or ultrasound. Ultrasound-guided fine-needle biopsy can be used if indicated. Sentinel lymph node biopsy, which is frequently used for lymphatic mapping of cutaneous melanomas, is not a common practice for sinonasal disease.[73] Due to the high yield in staging metastatic disease, PET imaging now replaces staging techniques employing multiple imaging modalities (i.e., chest X-ray, neck and liver ultrasound, total body CT, and bone mapping).[74] Goerres et al have claimed that all mucosal melanomas of the head and neck can be visualized using FDG PET.[71] Large lesions that have a nodular growth are better demonstrated than lesions that have superficial mucosal spread. Similarly, lesions originating in the nasal vestibule are more challenging to identify than those in the posterior sinonasal complex owing to nonspecific uptake in the skin and muscles of the mouth.

Metastatic cutaneous melanoma to the paranasal sinuses is very rare and accounts for 1% of patients who have cutaneous melanoma.[48,75] Nevertheless, full work-up should be performed to exclude isolated metastasis of melanoma of the skin to the paranasal sinuses.

32.5 Staging

Prior to the 2009 release of the seventh edition of the American Joint Committee on Cancer's staging manual, there was no formal staging system for mucosal melanoma. This system (mmTNM) is still in the infancy of its general adoption, and several retrospective studies have assessed its validity in terms of the accuracy of predicted prognoses.

The current AJCC system for staging cutaneous melanoma has been in use since its major revision in 2003.[76] In this system, the prognosis of patients who have localized disease

(T1: tumors < 1.0 mm or T2: 1.0–2.0 mm in thickness) is good, whereas for patients who have melanomas > 2.0 mm in thickness, a worse survival rate is expected (T3, T4). Patients who have localized disease and no regional or distant metastases are classified as having stage I or II disease. In patients who have regional metastases (stage III), tumor burden is expressed as the number of positive nodes (N1 for a single node, N2 for 2–3 nodes, and N3 for ≥ 4 nodes). In patients who have distant metastatic disease (stage IV), the sites of metastases determine outcome, and M classification is graded from "a" to "c" accordingly (i.e., skin, lung, and visceral, respectively). As with cutaneous melanoma, the outcome of mucosal melanoma initially depends on the stage at presentation.[46] Unfortunately, because of the absence of histologic landmarks identifiable as a papillary and reticular dermis in the respiratory mucosa, the AJCC cutaneous classification system cannot be applied to this disease. Furthermore, sinonasal melanomas are frequently polypoid rather than deeply invasive, and tumor thickness cannot accurately predict the prognosis.[12]

The mmTNM system is similar to the cutaneous system, however, in that it is not location-based but rather emphasizes depth of invasion. In recognition of its aggressive behavior, the mmTNM staging system includes no early stages (T1/2). Any primary tumor involving epithelium or submucosa is automatically a T3, and those involving deep soft tissue, cartilage, or bone are T4a, whereas brain, dura, and skull base involvement is classified as T4b. Nodal disease is assessed simply for the absence (N0) or presence (N1) of regional metastases. Any distant metastasis qualifies as M1. The eighth edition of the AJCC staging manual no longer proposes prognostic stage grouping for mucosal melanoma (▶ Table 32.3).[77]

An alternative system for classification of sinonasal melanoma is the AJCC staging criteria for nasal and paranasal epithelial tumors (carTNM).[77] As described in detail in Chapter 29 of this book, this staging system considers the extent of the primary lesion (stage I–IV) and the presence of regional metastases (stage III–IV) or distant metastases (stage IV) as main prognostic indicators for survival. Notably, the AJCC TNM classification applies only to histologically confirmed carcinomas and was not validated for melanoma. Considering these limitations, few authors even prior to the introduction of the mmTNM had adopted the AJCC staging system for nasal and paranasal epithelial tumors in cases of sinonasal mucosal melanoma.[23,32,78]

The system most commonly used for staging mucosal melanoma of the head and neck was first suggested by Ballantyne.[79] In this classification, stage I disease represents tumors confined to the primary site, stage II the existence of positive regional lymph nodes, and stage III a distant metastatic disease. This system does not take into consideration the size and extent of the disease process, but it has been used repeatedly for classification of sinonasal melanomas and melanomas of the upper aerodigestive tract.[29,33,80] Because regional and metastatic disease is not common during initial diagnosis, most patients are characterized in the stage I group. Clearly, the main drawback of this staging system is its lack of ability to differentiate between patients who have localized disease and those who have advanced tumors and poor prognosis (i.e., orbital infiltration or intracranial extension).

Thompson et al studied a group of 115 patients who had sinonasal melanomas in an attempt to develop a validated staging

Table 32.3 AJCC TNM staging system for mucosal melanoma of the head and neck

T category	T criteria
T3	Tumors limited to the mucosa and immediately underlying soft tissue, regardless of thickness or greatest dimension—for example, polypoid nasal disease, pigmented or nonpigmented lesions of the oral cavity, pharynx, or larynx
T4	Moderately advanced or very advanced
T4a	Moderately advanced disease Tumor involving deep soft tissue, cartilage, bone, or overlying skin
T4b	Very advanced disease Tumor involving brain, dura, skull base, lower cranial nerves (IX, X, XI, XII), masticator space, carotid artery, prevertebral space, or mediastinal structures
N category	**N criteria**
NX	Regional lymph nodes cannot be assessed
N0	No regional lymph node metastases
N1	Regional lymph node metastases present
M category	**M criteria**
M0	No distant metastasis
M1	Distant metastasis present

Source: Adapted with permission from American Joint Committee on Cancer, Head and Neck Sites, 8th ed., Chicago, IL: Springer; 2017.

system by incorporating features of size, site, and regional and distant metastases into a single staging system.[12] The T classification of this staging system separates tumors localized to a single anatomical compartment (T1) and those involving more than one anatomical level (T2). The N classification accounts for the absence (N0) or presence (N1) of lymph node metastases (whether ipsilateral, bilateral, or contralateral). Patients who have T1 and T2 disease in the absence of regional or distant metastases are grouped into disease stages I and II, respectively. Stage III disease includes patients who have any T, N1, and M0, whereas patients who have distant metastases are classified as having stage IV disease. The TNM classification suggested by Thompson et al predicted patients' outcome based on the anatomical site of involvement and metastatic disease.

Prasad et al, at Memorial Sloan Kettering Cancer Center, suggested further microscopic classification of stage I (lymph node–negative) sinonasal melanoma.[81] Their microstaging system was performed according to disease invasion into three compartments: level I, melanoma in situ; level II, invasion into the lamina propria; and level III, invasion into deep tissue (i.e., skeletal muscles, bone, or cartilage). Kaplan-Meier analysis showed significant difference in 5-year disease-specific survival of patients who had level I (75%), level II (52%), and level III (23%).

Several studies have aimed to address the prognostic value of the various staging systems. Koivunen et al applied the mmTNM classification to 50 patients diagnosed with sinonasal malignant melanoma between 1990 and 2004 and found statistically significant survival differences in overall survival (OS) according to T stage.[82] Similarly, Kuauhyama et al directly compared the mmTNM with Ballantyne's staging system for 66 patients and found the mmTNM system superior in predicting prognosis.[83] However, when Michel et al compared all three systems in 32 patients (Ballantyne/Prasad, mmTNM and carTNM), they found that only the carTNM was significantly correlated with both OS and disease-free survival (DFS). The Ballantyne/Prasad and mmTNM systems correlated with survival only in patients who had metastatic disease in which OS was lower.[84] A further study at MD Anderson supported Michel et al's recommendations of using the carTNM system.[85]

32.6 Treatment

There is general consensus that surgery remains the treatment of choice for mucosal melanoma of sinonasal origin.[80] A recent report of the National Cancer Institute and the Centers for Disease Control and Prevention has demonstrated an absolute gain in OS of melanoma patients during the past decade.[86] The improvement in survival of cutaneous melanoma patients, despite the increase in incidence, is attributed to early detection and improvements in therapy. The mode of therapy for sinonasal melanoma awaits further evaluation owing to a lack of prospective studies and objective data for the benefit of adjuvant modalities such as postoperative radiotherapy, immunotherapy, and chemotherapy.

There has been some attempt to define the most appropriate treatment regimes using both meta-analysis and pooling from cancer databases, but owing to limitations with these studies, results are far from conclusive. The largest meta-analysis to date, by Gore et al, which pooled 39 case reports and 423 patients, came to the conclusion that there was no OS benefit for surgery with postoperative radiation therapy but that there might be a significant OS benefit with surgery and chemo-/immunotherapy because of its effect on distant metastatic disease. However, this was only level III evidence with a grade C recommendation.[87] In a retrospective study of 695 patients using the National Cancer Database, Konuthula et al analyzed treatment modalities and OS rates, but their only significant finding was that adjuvant radiation failed to confer an OS benefit. What's more, the database does not account for recurrences, and no data were available regarding its benefit for locoregional control.[88] These studies highlight the need for prospective, randomized controlled trials to guide future management.

32.6.1 Surgery

In the absence of distant metastases, complete tumor extirpation is the mainstay of treatment for malignant melanoma of the paranasal sinuses and nasal mucosa. Although negative margins after surgical resection are reported in more than 85% of patients, it is frequently not possible to achieve en bloc tumor resection, and 75% of patients will eventually develop local recurrence.[14] Two possible explanations for the high recurrence rate are (1) presence of multifocal disease and (2) submucosal lymphatic spread of melanoma cells in the respiratory mucosa, which is not clinically or radiographically apparent.[29] Freedman et al suggested multicentricity as a main factor predicting local recurrence after surgery.[23] Accordingly, wide surgical resection, without unnecessary compromise of function and cosmesis, is essential.

The route of spread for tumors originating in the anterior skull base and paranasal sinuses is determined by the complex anatomy of the craniofacial compartments. A tumor arising in the ethmoid sinus or paranasal cavity may invade laterally to the orbit, inferiorly to the maxillary antrum and palate, posteriorly to the nasopharynx and pterygopalatine fossa, and superiorly to the dura, brain, or cavernous sinus. The recent improvement of endoscopic technology now allows for the resection of benign neoplasms or early malignant neoplasms, with several studies, including a meta-analysis, having suggested comparable results.[89,90,91] However, for the majority of sinonasal melanoma, an open approach is more suitable for allowing extirpation of tumors in an en bloc fashion and with wide margins, in our opinion.

The type of surgery is planned according to the extent of the tumor. For small tumors involving the nasal septum, resection of the tumor along with the perichondrium and septal cartilage may be performed via lateral rhinotomy incision or endoscopically (▶ Fig. 32.5). However, these tumors also frequently infiltrate adjacent structures such as the hard palate, ethmoid sinuses, and medial maxillary walls. In such cases a unilateral or bilateral medial maxillectomy is performed via a lateral rhinotomy incision.

Conventional exposure of the infra- and suprastructure of the maxilla is achieved via a lateral rhinotomy with lip split or subciliary extension as indicated (▶ Fig. 32.6). Tumors infiltrating the cribriform plate and fovea ethmoidalis are safely accessed via the craniofacial or subcranial approach.[14] These approaches offer wide exposure of the tumor, allowing resection of the intracranial and extracranial extensions of the tumor.

Massive orbital involvement or orbital apex infiltration requires orbital exenteration. In this case, orbital exenteration is performed with radical maxillectomy or craniofacial resection as determined by the tumor's extension. Combinations of the craniofacial approach with transorbital and middle fossa approaches were described by Shah et al for malignant tumors of the anterior skull base and paranasal sinuses.[92] A combined facial translocation approach was also described and safely used by Hao et al for malignant tumors of the paranasal cavity.[93,94]

After resection of the primary tumor, the surgical margins should be evaluated for residual disease using multiple permanent sections at the periphery of resection, sampling bone, mucosa, soft tissue, and other tissue as indicated. Although complete tumor resection should be the goal of care for sinonasal melanoma, a recent analysis of 53 patients who had skull base melanoma showed no survival benefit of negative margins in this anatomical area.[14]

Dural and anterior skull base reconstruction is required after craniofacial resection. Dural reconstruction is performed principally using pericranial, galeal, temporalis fascia, or fascia lata grafts. Bovine pericardium can also be used for reconstruction. Fibrin glue is used to provide additional protection against cerebrospinal fluid leak. Reconstruction of the medial orbital walls is not typically performed. If indicated, a split calvarial bone graft, a fascia lata sling, or three-dimensional titanium mesh covered by pericranium are used for reconstruction of the orbital support. A temporalis muscle flap and a split-thickness skin graft to cover the orbital socket can be used after orbital exenteration. In cases of a radical maxillectomy with or without orbital exenteration, a lateral thigh free flap or a rectus abdominis musculocutaneous free flap may be used to obliterate this large defect and to support the obturator.

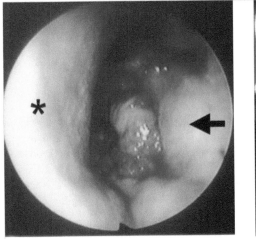
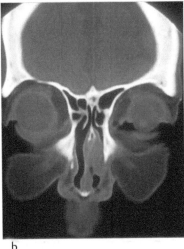
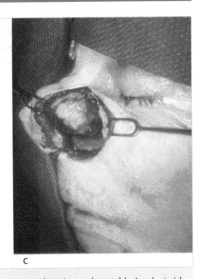

a   b   c

Fig. 32.5 Nonmelanotic melanoma of the nasal septum. **(a)** Endoscopic photograph of the lesion shows a nonmelanotic nasal septal lesion (*asterisk*, nasal septum; *arrow*, lateral nasal wall). **(b)** A preoperative coronal CT scan showing a left nasal septal lesion. **(c)** An intraoperative picture demonstrating exposure of the lesion. The type of surgery is planned according to the extent of the tumor. For small tumors involving the nasal septum, resection of the tumor along with the perichondrium and septal cartilage can be performed via lateral rhinotomy incision.

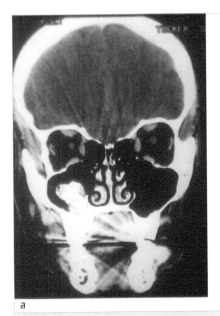
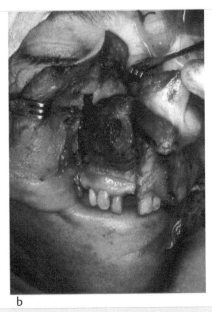
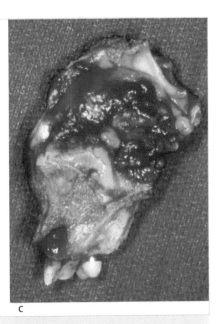

a   b   c

Fig. 32.6 Mucosal melanoma of the left maxillary sinus. **(a)** A preoperative coronal CT scan showing a hyperdense mass in the right maxillary antrum. **(b)** An intraoperative picture demonstrating exposure of the lesion. En bloc resection of the tumor along with a radical maxillectomy was achieved via the transfacial approach (lateral rhinotomy with lip split). **(c)** The excised specimen showing the melanotic lesion extending into the maxillary antrum.

Because neck lymph nodes are rarely encountered in cases of sinonasal melanoma, neck dissection should be performed only if regional metastases are identified, based on clinical or radiologic evaluation.

The postoperative complication rate after surgical resection of malignant skull base tumors is 36%.[14] Among patients treated with craniofacial resection for excision of sinonasal melanomas, postoperative mortality is 6% and major postoperative complications occur in 26% of the patients.

32.6.2 Radiation

The use of radiation therapy for treatment of melanoma is controversial. Despite the long-standing debate regarding the radio sensitivity of melanoma, there has been a significant increase in the use of adjuvant radiation therapy for the treatment of this disease.[1] Both clinical and basic science data indicate that melanoma cells have the ability to repair cellular damage, providing resistance to conventional fractionated radiation therapy.[95] It was therefore speculated that hypofractionation or high-dose-per-fractionation (HDPF) therapy would give more effective radiation treatment to these patients. Several nonrandomized, retrospective studies have reported improved locoregional control rates of patients who had high-risk cutaneous melanoma of the head and neck using conventional or hypofractionation adjuvant therapy compared with surgery alone.[96,97] Moreover, Raben et al reported 70% local control rate in 10 patients treated with the HDPF regimen after surgical resection of head and neck malignant melanoma, with minimal morbidity.[98] However, no change in OS was found in this study after hypofractionation adjuvant radiotherapy, owing to the development of disseminated disease. In patients who had mucosal melanoma, Patel et al reported no advantage of postoperative radiotherapy compared with surgery alone.[29]

In contrast, Ganly et al reported that postoperative radiation therapy was an independent positive predictor of overall, disease-specific, and recurrence-free survival on a multivariate analysis of patients who had skull base melanoma.[14] Patients treated with surgery and postoperative radiotherapy had 39% 3-year OS, compared with 18% in patients treated using surgery alone. Freedman et al reported no survival benefit for patients who had paranasal and nasal cavity melanoma treated using surgery and adjuvant radiotherapy, compared with those treated using surgery alone.[23] In the same study, it was reported that none of the 18 patients treated using radiation alone survived after 5 years.

Owens et al recently reported a retrospective evaluation of patients who had mucosal melanoma (23% with sinonasal disease) treated using surgery alone, surgery and adjuvant radiotherapy, or surgery and biochemotherapy, with or without adjuvant radiotherapy.[99] Radiation therapy was generally used as an adjuvant therapy for patients who had extensive disease. Patients who had sinonasal tumors received 6,000 cGy in 30 fractions, whereas those who had oral lesions received 3,000

cGy in 5 fractions. Biochemotherapy (cisplatin, vinblastine, and dacarbazine, with or without the addition of interferon alfa-2b and interleukin 2) was used almost exclusively in patients who had recurrent disease or distant metastases. The addition of radiotherapy tended to decrease the rate of local failure but did not prevent distant metastases or improve OS. Biochemotherapy regimens used for metastatic or recurrent disease had no significant impact on survival.

An evaluation of the impact of postoperative radiotherapy on local control and survival of patients who had head and neck mucosal melanoma was reported by Temam et al at the Institut Gustave-Roussy (Villejuif).[32] Sixty-nine patients who had local disease were managed by surgery without postoperative radiotherapy, two-thirds of whom had sinonasal disease. The study suggested that postoperative radiotherapy increased local control in patients who had small tumors but did not impact survival.

Most reports of definitive radiation therapy for mucosal melanomas involve small series of patients. Gilligan and Slevin reported one of the largest series of melanomas of the paranasal sinuses and nasal cavity treated using radiation alone.[25] Complete response was achieved in 79% of the 28 patients included in the study, with relatively low treatment morbidity. In this study, the overall 3- and 5-year survival rates were 49% and 18%, respectively (▶ Table 32.4).

Stern and Guillamondegui at MD Anderson Cancer Center reported two of five patients alive and disease-free 5 years after radiotherapy alone.[34] At Princess Margaret Hospital in Toronto, Canada, Harwood and Cummings reported 50% local control rate at 6 months to 4.2 years after primary radiotherapy (n = 10 patients).[100] Trotti and Peters reviewed a series of reports using radiotherapy alone for mucosal head and neck melanoma and concluded that 50 to 75% of the patients had documented complete response, with long-term control in 50 to 66%.[101] They concluded that in view of the poor results of radical surgery,

Table 32.4 Melanoma of the nasal and paranasal sinuses and survival

Study	Year	N	5-year survival	Impact of radiotherapy on survival
Holdcraft & Gallagher (18)	1968	39	10%	–
Freedman et al (20)	1973	56	30%	NS
Eneroth & Lundberg (91)	1975	24	17%	–
Harrison (19)	1976	40	27.5%	–
Trapp et al (16)	1987	17	25	–
Gilligan et al (22)[a]	1991	28	18%	–
Kingdom and Kaplan (15)	1995	17	20%	Prolonged
Harbo et al (92)	1997	25	24%	–
Brandwein et al (58)	1997	36	36%	–
Lund VJ et al (77)	1999	72	28%	NS
Owens et al (85)	2003	11	33%	NS
Thompson et al (9)	2003	115	42.6%	NS
Patel et al (26)	2002	35	47%	NS
Nakaya et al (93)	2004	16	31.8%	NS
Bridger et al (72)	2005	27	43%	–
Ganly et al (11)	2006	53	24%	>twofold increase

Abbreviation: NS, nonsignificant.
[a]Primary radiotherapy.

radiation should be seriously considered as the initial treatment of choice for primary mucosal melanomas of the head and neck. Albertsson et al reported the result of hyperfractionation radiation in combination with cisplatinum.[102] Three of four patients treated for local recurrence achieved local control. Radiation may also be appropriate as a primary treatment for patients who have unresectable disease, elderly patients, and patients who have high surgical risk or palliative intent.[103] External beam radiation may achieve local control, relieve pain, and decrease tumor compression on vital structures, including cranial nerves, the orbit, airway, and brain.

Radiation therapy has the potential for complications, especially if applied to the cranial base. Severe morbidity associated with radiation of the anterior skull base includes osteoradionecrosis, encephalomalacia, optic neuropathy, and retinopathy.[104] Radiation therapy has also been associated with a decreasing quality of life in patients with skull base malignancies.[105] Use of heavy particle radiation sources (i.e., proton or carbon ions), as well as accurate delivery using intensity-modulated radiation therapy, may be beneficial in enhancing therapeutic outcomes and reducing complication rates.

Fast neutron therapy was used to treat primary, recurrent, or metastatic cutaneous and mucosal melanoma in 48 patients, showing complete regression in 71%, with a 9% incidence of local recurrence.[106] The median survival was 14.5 months, and complications, including fibrosis and necrosis, occurred in 22% of patients. In another series, Linstadt et al reported local control in two of six patients treated with neon ions for melanoma located in a variety of sites, including paranasal sinus.[107] Promising results were found in a dose escalation study using carbon ions, reporting 100% 5-year local control rate in five patients who had mucosal melanoma.[108]

Currently, most centers are using radiation therapy in an adjuvant setting following surgical resection or in cases in which surgery in not possible or is refused by the patient both as an attempt at cure or for palliation.

32.6.3 Chemotherapy, Immunotherapy, and Checkpoint Inhibitors

There are no established adjuvant therapy regimes for mucosal melanoma, with treatment mostly regarded as palliative for recurrent, metastatic, or inoperable disease. A variety of chemotherapeutic agents, both as adjuvant or neoadjuvant therapy, have been used for treatment of distant disease based on extrapolation of data from treatment of patients who had cutaneous melanomas. These include cisplatinum, dacarbazine, vinca alkaloids and temozolomide. Unfortunately, most authors reported no advantage for chemotherapy in patients who had distant metastatic melanoma originating from a head and neck mucosal primary.[16,28,33,109]

Over the past decade, the mainstay of systemic therapy for treatment of metastatic disease has been immunotherapy or biological response modifiers with or without chemotherapy. The most frequently used biological response modifier is high-dose interferon alpha-2b (HDI/IFN alpha-2b), but interleukin-2 and bacillus Calmette-Guerin (BCG) vaccine have also been used. In 2002, the National Comprehensive Cancer Network recommended that high-risk patients who had localized cutaneous melanomas greater than 4.0 mm in thickness participate in adjuvant therapy clinical trials, including treatment using high-dose adjuvant IFN alpha-2b versus observation.[110] This recommendation was based on two studies performed by the Eastern Cooperative Oncology Group (trial 1684 and 1690); these were randomized controlled studies of IFN alpha-2b administered at maximum tolerated doses versus observation.[111] Another study showed a relapse-free survival advantage for high-dose interferon with no difference in OS.[112] Interestingly, although the trials did include a few mucosal melanoma patients, the efficacy in this subset was not specified.

Legha et al evaluated the use of concurrent biochemotherapy, including cisplatin, vinblastine, and dacarbazine, in combination with IFN-alpha and interleukin-2 in patients who had metastatic melanoma.[113] Among the 53 patients treated in this study, 21% achieved a complete response and 43% a partial response. The median survival was 11.8 months. The toxicities reported were severe myelosuppression, nausea, vomiting, and hypotension that required inpatient care and support. There were no treatment-related deaths. An anecdotal report that evaluated the utility of hormonal therapy with tamoxifen for palliative treatment of patients who had sinonasal melanoma reported good response in all three patients treated with the drug.[114]

With the increase in genetic profiling of mucosal melanomas identifying frequent oncogenes, including BRAF, NRAS and Kit, therapies aimed at targeting these mutations have been developed. The BRAF inhibitors vemurafenib and dabrafenib have shown increased survival in advanced stage BRAF-mutated metastatic mucosal melanoma.[115,116] However, unlike cutaneous melanoma, mucosal melanoma has much less frequent BRAF mutations.[117] Conversely, Kit mutations are frequent in mucosal melanoma but rarely reported in cutaneous melanoma. That said, c-Kit mutations are variable, with only selected alterations being oncogenic and thus a viable target for therapy.[118] When this is proven, c-Kit inhibitors such as imatinib have shown some benefit.[117,119,120]

There has also been recent work looking into immunomodulatory drugs or "checkpoint inhibitors," including CTLA-4 and PD-1/PD-L1 inhibitors. Ipilimumab is an anticytotoxic T-lymphocyte antigen 4 antibody that has been evaluated in two small studies of unresectable or metastatic mucosal melanoma. Although responses were observed, the rates were low, at 12% and 6%, respectively.[121,122] Programmed cell death-1 receptor (PD-1) and programmed cell death-ligand 1 receptor (PD-L1) have also been postulated as targeted therapy after the discovery that PD-L1 upregulation in metastatic melanoma might indicate a potential mechanism for immune response evasion.[123] Their clinical role requires further investigation.

Head-to-head trials comparing various therapies are lacking for adjuvant therapy after surgical excision. Recently Lian et al enrolled 189 patients at a single center who had AJCC stage II/III after surgical resection for surgery alone, adjuvant HDI (IFN-alpha2b), or adjuvant temozolomide plus cisplatin. They reported a statistically significant improvement in both recurrence-free survival (5.4, 9.4, and 20.8 months, respectively) and OS (21.2, 40.4, and 48.7 months, respectively) in those receiving temozolomide plus cisplatin versus observation or HDI.[124] However, this represents a single-institution study, and decisions regarding the use of adjuvant therapy for such patients should be made on an individual basis, extrapolating from available data from the cutaneous adjuvant trials and after discussion of anticipated results and morbidity with the patient.

32.7 Outcome and Prognosis

Of all patients who have mucosal melanomas of the head and neck, those who have disease involving the paranasal sinuses have the poorest outcome. Notably, tumors isolated to the nasal cavity are associated with the best prognosis of head and neck mucosal melanoma. Patients who have sinonasal melanomas have an interposed course of disease with multiple local or regional recurrences, followed by distant metastases and ultimately death from disseminated disease. Head and neck mucosal melanomas have a lower 5-year survival rate than cutaneous and ocular melanomas (32%, 75%, and 80%, respectively).[1] The estimated 10-year survival rate of these patients is 7%.[125] Despite the development of new surgical approaches and novel therapeutic agents, no significant increase in the OS of patients who have sinonasal and nasal cavity melanomas has been seen.

A recent study pooling data from the National Cancer Database for 695 patients showed a 5-year OS of 21.7% with a mean survival of 38.4 ± 1.7 months.[88] No statistically significant difference in OS was seen between patients receiving adjuvant radiation and those receiving surgery alone. These findings were similar to those of a previous cohort study performed by the Armed Forces Institute of Pathology that reported no influence of treatment modality on OS.[12] Among the 115 patients who participated in this study, no statistically significant difference was seen among patients managed by surgery alone, surgery with chemotherapy, surgery with radiotherapy, or surgery with combined therapy. After a mean follow-up of almost 14 years, 35% of the patients were alive or had died without evidence of disease. However, the aforementioned meta-analysis by Gore et al suggested a small statistically significant survival benefit for surgery with chemo-/immunotherapy.[87] Furthermore, in their series of 69 patients, Meng et al found a statistically significant benefit for both surgery plus radiation therapy and surgery plus chemoradiation therapy compared with surgery alone.[126]

Owens et al reported 14.3 months average interval to failure in patients who had sinonasal tumors (range 3–36 months), compared with 31.6 months in patients who had oral or oropharyngeal lesions (range 3–147 months).[99] For patients who had sinonasal disease, the OS rates at 3 and 5 years were 50% and 33%, respectively.

A large cohort of patients who had sinonasal melanoma who were undergoing craniofacial resection accumulated from multiple international institutions reported 3-year DFS and OS of 28% and 29%, respectively (▶ Fig. 32.7).[14] Orbital involvement was found to be an independent predictor of OS and disease-specific survival. For comparison, the overall 5-year survival of patients who had all malignant skull base tumors treated by the same group of surgeons was 54%, including for esthesioneuroblastoma (64%) and squamous cell carcinoma (50%).[127] Ganly et al demonstrated a threefold increase in OS and DFS after adjuvant conventional radiation therapy.[14] The risk of recurrence was fourfold in patients not receiving radiotherapy. As a result of incomplete data regarding precise staging, dose or delivery of radiation, and previous treatment, such retrospective studies must

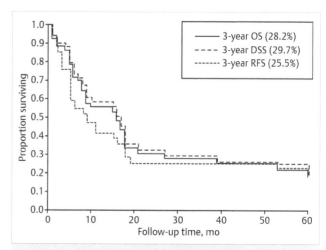

Fig. 32.7 Survival analysis of patients who had malignant melanoma of the paranasal sinuses. Three-year overall survival (OS), disease-specific survival (DSS), and recurrence-free survival (RFS) for craniofacial resection for malignant melanoma invading the skull base. (Reproduced with permission from Ganly I, Patel SG, Singh B, et al, Craniofacial resection for malignant melanoma of the skull base: report of an international collaborative study, Arch Otolaryngol Head Neck Surg, 2006;132(1):73–78.)

be interpreted with caution. Harrison et al reported 3-, 5-, and 10-year disease-specific survival of 47%, 28%, and 8%, respectively, with surgery alone.[22] Similar results were reported by Freedman and colleagues, who found 46% and 31% survival at 3 and 5 years among their group of patients treated using surgery and postoperative radiotherapy.[23] Once again, the discrepancies between the foregoing publications highlight the need for prospective randomized controlled trials in this area.

Local failure is a significant cause of mortality in patients who have sinonasal melanoma. Disease recurrence is common within the first 2 years of treatment, and late recurrence may be seen even after 5 years of follow-up. Freedman et al reported a series of 56 patients who had sinonasal melanoma, 34 of whom (60%) had recurrence in the primary site and 29% of whom underwent salvage resection of the tumor.[23] Patel et al reported local failure rate of 50%, nodal failure rate of 20%, and distant failure rate of 40% (▶ Fig. 32.8).[29] Only 6% of the patients in their study were eligible for salvage therapy.

Patients who have cutaneous melanoma and negative lymph nodes at presentation have a 5-year survival rate of 80% compared with 30% for those who have positive nodes. In contrast, patients who have mucosal melanoma of the head and neck have 27% and 19% 5-year survival for N0 and N + disease, respectively.[29,128] Similar results were found by Yii et al, who reported a 26% 5-year survival rate for patients who had localized disease, compared with a 0% 5-year survival rate for patients who had regional or distant metastases.[36] Temam et al reported that pathologic neck stage did not influence the OS of patients who had mucosal melanomas of the head and neck.[32]

In most patients, local recurrence is an ominous sign for ongoing distant disease. Although it is rare at presentation, 37% of patients will ultimately fail at distant sites, more than two-thirds of whom will also develop local or regional disease. Stern and Guillamondegui reported that 89% of patients who had local recurrence also developed disseminated disease.[34] The most

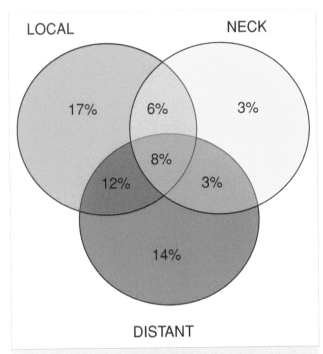

Fig. 32.8 Patterns of recurrence in sinonasal melanomas. No recurrence was found in 11 of the 35 patients (31.3%), isolated locoregional recurrence in 11 of 35 (31.3%), isolated distant failure in 4 of 35 (11.4%), and local and/or regional recurrence with distant failure in 9 of 35 patients (25.7%). (Reproduced with permission from Patel SG, Prasad ML, Escrig M, et al, Primary mucosal malignant melanoma of the head and neck, Head Neck, 2002;24(3):247–257.)

common sites of distant metastases are the lung and brain (33% and 14%, respectively). The median survival period from the time of detection of distant metastases to death is 7.1 months.[29]

Although there are reports of anecdotal cases in which the disease remained dormant for a long period, most patients who have sinonasal melanoma die of distant metastases, with or without local recurrence. The unpredictability of the clinical behavior of this tumor is commonly characterized by cases that have a prolonged clinical course despite repeated local recurrences and regional lymph node metastases.[122] Thus there is a lifelong risk of recurrence for all patients who have sinonasal mucosal melanoma. For this reason, lifelong surveillance of these patients is required. The value of salvage surgery for local recurrences and regional lymph node metastases cannot be predicted based on clinical and pathologic parameters alone. It is plausible that the course of disease is based on interactions between the primary tumor and the host's immune system, but the exact mechanism is not evident.

32.8 Conclusion

Melanoma of the nasal cavity and paranasal sinuses is an uncommon malignancy arising in the respiratory sinonasal mucosa. The majority of cases originate in the nasal cavity, followed by the paranasal sinuses. Whereas most head and neck melanomas are more likely to be discovered by the patient or during routine physical examination, sinonasal melanomas are not accessible to self-examination and are often diagnosed late,

resulting in poor survival. Melanoma tends to mimic other tumors pathologically, which can lead to misdiagnosis. Owing to the complicated differential diagnosis of this tumor, immunocytochemical staining is frequently required to establish the diagnosis of melanoma, particularly in cases of amelanotic variants. Surgery is considered the treatment of choice for primary mucosal melanoma of the sinonasal cavities. Because of the nature of this disease, complete tumor resection is challenging and the majority of those patients will eventually develop local recurrence. The high recurrence rate of sinonasal melanoma is secondary to a high incidence of multifocal disease and the presence of submucosal lymphatic spread of tumor cells. Thus all lesions require wide surgical resection, attempting to minimize unnecessary compromise of function and cosmesis. Of patients who have mucosal melanomas of the head and neck, those who have disease involving the paranasal sinuses have the poorest outcome, whereas tumors isolated to the nasal cavity are associated with a better prognosis. Local failure is a significant cause of mortality in these patients and is clearly associated with high rate of nodal recurrence and distant metastases. Most patients who have local recurrence are not amenable to curative salvage therapy.

The use of radiation therapy for treatment of melanoma is controversial. Recent studies have indicated that the addition of adjuvant radiotherapy tends to decrease the rate of local failure but has no significant impact on OS. Primary radiotherapy or chemotherapy is currently employed as palliative treatment of recurrent, inoperable, or metastatic disease or for patients who face unacceptable surgical risk. Unfortunately, most reports showed no survival advantage for chemotherapy in patients who had disseminated disease. The utility of other treatment modalities such as immunotherapy or biochemotherapy, as well as of heavy particle radiation sources and intensity-modulated radiation therapy, awaits further evaluation. Further studies are required for determination of the advantage of postoperative radiotherapy for treatment of patients who have sinonasal melanoma. Nevertheless, it is advisable to add hypofractionation radiotherapy after surgery—especially for treatment of sinonasal melanomas, which historically have been associated with a high incidence of local recurrence after surgery alone.

References

[1] Chang AE, Karnell LH, Menck HR, The American College of Surgeons Commission on Cancer and the American Cancer Society. The National Cancer Data Base report on cutaneous and noncutaneous melanoma: a summary of 84,836 cases from the past decade. Cancer. 1998; 83(8):1664–1678

[2] Weber CO. Chirurgische Ehrfahrungen und Untersuchungen, nebst zahlreichen Beobachtungen aus der chirurgischen Klinik und dem evangelischen Krahkenhause zu Bonn. Berlin: G. Reimer; 1859

[3] Lucke A. Die Lehre von den Geschwulsten in anatomischer und klinischer Beziehung in Handbuch d. allg. u. spec. chir. Erlangen; 1869:244

[4] Viennois L. Osteotomie du nez (Obs. II—Polype melanique du nez (melanosarcome) ayant detruit la paroi interne de l'orbite et refoulant le globe de l'oeil en avant: abaissement du nez comme operation preliminaire; ablation du polyp, pyohemie; mort huit jours apres). Lyon Med. 1872; 11:8–12

[5] Lincoln RP. A case of melano-sarcoma of the nose cured by galvanocauterization. N Y Med J. 1885; 42:406–407

[6] Lazarev S, Gupta V, Hu K, Harrison LB, Bakst R. Mucosal melanoma of the head and neck: a systematic review of the literature. Int J Radiat Oncol Biol Phys. 2014; 90(5):1108–1118

[7] Chin L. The genetics of malignant melanoma: lessons from mouse and man. Nat Rev Cancer. 2003; 3(8):559–570

[8] Wingo PA, Ries LA, Rosenberg HM, Miller DS, Edwards BK. Cancer incidence and mortality, 1973–1995: a report card for the U.S. Cancer. 1998; 82(6): 1197–1207

[9] Rigel DS. Malignant melanoma: incidence issues and their effect on diagnosis and treatment in the 1990s. Mayo Clin Proc. 1997; 72(4):367–371

[10] Marcus DM, Marcus RP, Prabhu RS, et al. Rising incidence of mucosal melanoma of the head and neck in the United States. J Skin Cancer. 2012; 2012: 231693

[11] McLaughlin CC, Wu XC, Jemal A, Martin HJ, Roche LM, Chen VW. Incidence of noncutaneous melanomas in the U.S. Cancer. 2005; 103(5):1000–1007

[12] Thompson LD, Wieneke JA, Miettinen M. Sinonasal tract and nasopharyngeal melanomas: a clinicopathologic study of 115 cases with a proposed staging system. Am J Surg Pathol. 2003; 27(5):594–611

[13] Conley JJ. Melanoma of the Head and Neck. 1st ed. New York, NY: Georg Thiem Verlag; 1990:154–178

[14] Ganly I, Patel SG, Singh B, et al. Craniofacial resection for malignant melanoma of the skull base: report of an international collaborative study. Arch Otolaryngol Head Neck Surg. 2006; 132(1):73–78

[15] Lewis MG, Martin JA. Malignant melanoma of the nasal cavity in Ugandan Africans: relationship of ectopic pigmentation. Cancer. 1967; 20(10): 1699–1705

[16] Andersen LJ, Berthelsen A, Hansen HS. Malignant melanoma of the upper respiratory tract and the oral cavity. J Otolaryngol. 1992; 21(3):180–185

[17] Takagi M, Ishikawa G, Mori W. Primary malignant melanoma of the oral cavity in Japan: with special reference to mucosal melanosis. Cancer. 1974; 34 (2):358–370

[18] Kingdom TT, Kaplan MJ. Mucosal melanoma of the nasal cavity and paranasal sinuses. Head Neck. 1995; 17(3):184–189

[19] Trapp TK, Fu YS, Calcaterra TC. Melanoma of the nasal and paranasal sinus mucosa. Arch Otolaryngol Head Neck Surg. 1987; 113(10):1086–1089

[20] Blatchford SJ, Koopmann CF, Jr, Coulthard SW. Mucosal melanoma of the head and neck. Laryngoscope. 1986; 96(9 Pt 1):929–934

[21] Holdcraft J, Gallagher JC. Malignant melanomas of the nasal and paranasal sinus mucosa. Ann Otol Rhinol Laryngol. 1969; 78(1):5–20

[22] Harrison DF. Malignant melanomata arising in the nasal mucous membrane. J Laryngol Otol. 1976; 90(11):993–1005

[23] Freedman HM, DeSanto LW, Devine KD, Weiland LH. Malignant melanoma of the nasal cavity and paranasal sinuses. Arch Otolaryngol. 1973; 97(4): 322–325

[24] Matias C, Corde J, Soares J. Primary malignant melanoma of the nasal cavity: a clinicopathologic study of nine cases. J Surg Oncol. 1988; 39(1):29–32

[25] Gilligan D, Slevin NJ. Radical radiotherapy for 28 cases of mucosal melanoma in the nasal cavity and sinuses. Br J Radiol. 1991; 64(768):1147–1150

[26] Manolidis S, Donald PJ. Malignant mucosal melanoma of the head and neck: review of the literature and report of 14 patients. Cancer. 1997; 80 (8):1373–1386

[27] Moore ES, Martin H. Melanoma of the upper respiratory tract and oral cavity. Cancer. 1955; 8(6):1167–1176

[28] Panje WR, Moran WJ. Melanoma of the upper aerodigestive tract: a review of 21 cases. Head Neck Surg. 1986; 8(4):309–312

[29] Patel SG, Prasad ML, Escrig M, et al. Primary mucosal malignant melanoma of the head and neck. Head Neck. 2002; 24(3):247–257

[30] Holmstrom M, Lund VJ. Malignant melanomas of the nasal cavity after occupational exposure to formaldehyde. Br J Ind Med. 1991; 48(1):9–11

[31] Hernberg S, Westerholm P, Schultz-Larsen K, et al. Nasal and sinonasal cancer: connection with occupational exposures in Denmark, Finland and Sweden. Scand J Work Environ Health. 1983; 9(4):315–326

[32] Temam S, Mamelle G, Marandas P, et al. Postoperative radiotherapy for primary mucosal melanoma of the head and neck. Cancer. 2005; 103(2):313–319

[33] Guzzo M, Grandi C, Licitra L, Podrecca S, Cascinelli N, Molinari R. Mucosal malignant melanoma of head and neck: forty-eight cases treated at Istituto Nazionale Tumori of Milan. Eur J Surg Oncol. 1993; 19(4):316–319

[34] Stern SJ, Guillamondegui OM. Mucosal melanoma of the head and neck. Head Neck. 1991; 13(1):22–27

[35] Yii NW, Eisen T, Nicolson M, et al. Mucosal malignant melanoma of the head and neck: the Marsden experience over half a century. Clin Oncol (R Coll Radiol). 2003; 15(4):199–204

[36] Ravid JM, Esteves JA. Malignant melanoma of the nose and paranasal sinuses and juvenile melanoma of the nose. Arch Otolaryngol. 1960; 72:431–444

[37] Nandapalan V, Roland NJ, Helliwell TR, Williams EM, Hamilton JW, Jones AS. Mucosal melanoma of the head and neck. Clin Otolaryngol Allied Sci. 1998; 23(2):107–116

[38] Zak FG, Lawson W. The presence of melanocytes in the nasal cavity. Ann Otol Rhinol Laryngol. 1974; 83(4):515–519

[39] Szabo G. The number of melanocytes in human epidermis. BMJ. 1954; 1 (4869):1016–1017

[40] Mannone F, De Giorgi V, Cattaneo A, Massi D, De Magnis A, Carli P. Dermoscopic features of mucosal melanosis. Dermatol Surg. 2004; 30(8): 1118–1123

[41] Cove H. Melanosis, melanocytic hyperplasia, and primary malignant melanoma of the nasal cavity. Cancer. 1979; 44(4):1424–1433

[42] Hofbauer GF, Böni R, Simmen D, et al. Histological, immunological and molecular features of a nasal mucosa primary melanoma associated with nasal melanosis. Melanoma Res. 2002; 12(1):77–82

[43] Bradley PJ. Primary malignant mucosal melanoma of the head and neck. Curr Opin Otolaryngol Head Neck Surg. 2006; 14(2):100–104

[44] Prasad ML, Busam KJ, Patel SG, Hoshaw-Woodard S, Shah JP, Huvos AG. Clinicopathologic differences in malignant melanoma arising in oral squamous and sinonasal respiratory mucosa of the upper aerodigestive tract. Arch Pathol Lab Med. 2003; 127(8):997–1002

[45] McLean N, Tighiouart M, Muller S. Primary mucosal melanoma of the head and neck: comparison of clinical presentation and histopathologic features of oral and sinonasal melanoma. Oral Oncol. 2008; 44(11):1039–1046

[46] Lee SP, Shimizu KT, Tran LM, Juillard G, Calcaterra TC. Mucosal melanoma of the head and neck: the impact of local control on survival. Laryngoscope. 1994; 104(2):121–126

[47] Crawford RI, Tron VA, Ma R, Rivers JK. Sinonasal malignant melanoma—a clinicopathologic analysis of 18 cases. Melanoma Res. 1995; 5(4):261–265

[48] Franquemont DW, Mills SE. Sinonasal malignant melanoma. A clinicopathologic and immunohistochemical study of 14 cases. Am J Clin Pathol. 1991; 96(6):689–697

[49] Chetty R, Slavin JL, Pitson GA, Dowling JP. Melanoma botryoides: a distinctive myxoid pattern of sino-nasal malignant melanoma. Histopathology. 1994; 24(4):377–379

[50] Prasad ML, Patel SG, Busam KJ. Primary mucosal desmoplastic melanoma of the head and neck. Head Neck. 2004; 26(4):373–377

[51] Batsakis JG, Regezi JA, Solomon AR, Rice DH. The pathology of head and neck tumors: mucosal melanomas, part 13. Head Neck Surg. 1982; 4(5):404–418

[52] Kilpatrick SE, White WL, Browne JD. Desmoplastic malignant melanoma of the oral mucosa. An underrecognized diagnostic pitfall. Cancer. 1996; 78(3): 383–389

[53] Hoorweg JJ, Loftus BM, Hilgers FJ. Osteoid and bone formation in a nasal mucosal melanoma and its metastasis. Histopathology. 1997; 31(5):465–468

[54] Ordóñez NG, Ji XL, Hickey RC. Comparison of HMB-45 monoclonal antibody and S-100 protein in the immunohistochemical diagnosis of melanoma. Am J Clin Pathol. 1988; 90(4):385–390

[55] Gown AM, Vogel AM, Hoak D, Gough F, McNutt MA. Monoclonal antibodies specific for melanocytic tumors distinguish subpopulations of melanocytes. Am J Pathol. 1986; 123(2):195–203

[56] Chello M, Marchese AR, Panza A, Mastroroberto P, Di Lello F. Primary malignant melanoma of the oesophagus with a left atrial metastasis. Thorax. 1993; 48(2):185–186

[57] Mohandas KM, Santhi Swaroop V, Dhir V, Vyas JJ. Primary malignant melanoma of the esophagus palliated with endoscopic laser therapy. Endoscopy. 1993; 25(8):551

[58] Uno Y, Saito R, Kanatani M, Hamaya K, Nose S. Malignant melanoma of the nasal cavity. Auris Nasus Larynx. 1994; 21(4):248–252

[59] Aung PP, Sarlomo-Rikala M, Lasota J, Lai JP, Wang ZF, Miettinen M. KBA62 and PNL2: 2 new melanoma markers—immunohistochemical analysis of 1563 tumors including metastatic, desmoplastic, and mucosal melanomas and their mimics. Am J Surg Pathol. 2012; 36(2):265–272

[60] Prasad ML, Jungbluth AA, Iversen K, Huvos AG, Busam KJ. Expression of melanocytic differentiation markers in malignant melanomas of the oral and sinonasal mucosa. Am J Surg Pathol. 2001; 25(6):782–787

[61] Wright JL, Heenan PJ. Electron microscopy findings in malignant melanoma of nose. ORL J Otorhinolaryngol Relat Spec. 1975; 37(4):233–236

[62] Henzen-Logmans SC, Meijer CJ, Ruiter DJ, Mullink H, Balm AJ, Snow GB. Diagnostic application of panels of antibodies in mucosal melanomas of the head and neck. Cancer. 1988; 61(4):702–711

[63] Brandwein MS, Rothstein A, Lawson W, Bodian C, Urken ML. Sinonasal melanoma: a clinicopathologic study of 25 cases and literature meta-analysis. Arch Otolaryngol Head Neck Surg. 1997; 123(3):290–296

[64] Lentsch EJ, Myers JN. Melanoma of the head and neck: current concepts in diagnosis and management. Laryngoscope. 2001; 111(7):1209–1222

[65] Mills SE, Fechner RE. "Undifferentiated" neoplasms of the sinonasal region: differential diagnosis based on clinical, light microscopic, immunohistochemical, and ultrastructural features. Semin Diagn Pathol. 1989; 6(4):316–328

[66] Nakhleh RE, Wick MR, Rocamora A, Swanson PE, Dehner LP. Morphologic diversity in malignant melanomas. Am J Clin Pathol. 1990; 93(6):731–740

[67] Wick MR, Stanley SJ, Swanson PE. Immunohistochemical diagnosis of sinonasal melanoma, carcinoma, and neuroblastoma with monoclonal antibodies HMB-45 and anti-synaptophysin. Arch Pathol Lab Med. 1988; 112(6): 616–620

[68] Ejaz A, Wenig BM. Sinonasal undifferentiated carcinoma: clinical and pathologic features and a discussion on classification, cellular differentiation, and differential diagnosis. Adv Anat Pathol. 2005; 12(3):134–143

[69] Kuwabara H, Takeda J. Malignant melanoma of the lacrimal sac with surrounding melanosis. Arch Pathol Lab Med. 1997; 121(5):517–519

[70] Hoyt DJ, Jordan T, Fisher SR. Mucosal melanoma of the head and neck. Arch Otolaryngol Head Neck Surg. 1989; 115(9):1096–1099

[71] Hammersmith SM, Terk MR, Jeffrey PB, Connolly SG, Colletti PM. Magnetic resonance imaging of nasopharyngeal and paranasal sinus melanoma. Magn Reson Imaging. 1990; 8(3):245–253

[72] Chang PC, Fischbein NJ, McCalmont TH, et al. Perineural spread of malignant melanoma of the head and neck: clinical and imaging features. AJNR Am J Neuroradiol. 2004; 25(1):5–11

[73] Civantos FJ, Moffat FL, Goodwin WJ. Lymphatic mapping and sentinel lymphadenectomy for 106 head and neck lesions: contrasts between oral cavity and cutaneous malignancy. Laryngoscope. 2006; 112(3)(Pt 2, Suppl 109):1–15

[74] Böni R, Böni RA, Steinert H, et al. Staging of metastatic melanoma by whole-body positron emission tomography using 2-fluorine-18-fluoro-2-deoxy-D-glucose. Br J Dermatol. 1995; 132(4):556–562

[75] Billings KR, Wang MB, Sercarz JA, Fu YS. Clinical and pathologic distinction between primary and metastatic mucosal melanoma of the head and neck. Otolaryngol Head Neck Surg. 1995; 112(6):700–706

[76] Balch CM, Buzaid AC, Soong SJ, et al. Final version of the American Joint Committee on Cancer staging system for cutaneous melanoma. J Clin Oncol. 2001; 19(16):3635–3648

[77] American Joint Committee on Cancer. Head and Neck Sites. 8th ed. Chicago, IL: Springer; 2017:55–184

[78] Bridger AG, Smee D, Baldwin MA, Kwok B, Bridger GP. Experience with mucosal melanoma of the nose and paranasal sinuses. ANZ J Surg. 2005; 75(4): 192–197

[79] Ballantyne AJ. Malignant melanoma of the skin of the head and neck: an analysis of 405 cases. Am J Surg. 1970; 120(4):425–431

[80] Mendenhall WM, Amdur RJ, Hinerman RW, Werning JW, Villaret DB, Mendenhall NP. Head and neck mucosal melanoma. Am J Clin Oncol. 2005; 28 (6):626–630

[81] Prasad ML, Patel SG, Huvos AG, Shah JP, Busam KJ. Primary mucosal melanoma of the head and neck: a proposal for microstaging localized, Stage I (lymph node-negative) tumors. Cancer. 2004; 100(8):1657–1664

[82] Koivunen P, Bäck L, Pukkila M, et al. Accuracy of the current TNM classification in predicting survival in patients with sinonasal mucosal melanoma. Laryngoscope. 2012; 122(8):1734–1738

[83] Luna-Ortiz K, Aguilar-Romero M, Villavicencio-Valencia V, et al. Comparative study between two different staging systems (AJCC TNM vs Ballantyne's) for mucosal melanomas of the Head & Neck. Med Oral Patol Oral Cir Bucal. 2016; 21(4):e425–e430

[84] Michel J, Perret-Court A, Fakhry N, et al. Sinonasal mucosal melanomas: the prognostic value of tumor classifications. Head Neck. 2014; 36(3): 311–316

[85] Moreno MA, Roberts DB, Kupferman ME, et al. Mucosal melanoma of the nose and paranasal sinuses, a contemporary experience from the M. D. Anderson Cancer Center. Cancer. 2010; 116(9):2215–2223

[86] Jemal A, Clegg LX, Ward E, et al. Annual report to the nation on the status of cancer, 1975-2001, with a special feature regarding survival. Cancer. 2004; 101(1):3–27

[87] Gore MR, Zanation AM. Survival in sinonasal melanoma: a meta-analysis. J Neurol Surg B Skull Base. 2012; 73(3):157–162

[88] Konuthula N, Khan MN, Parasher A, et al. The presentation and outcomes of mucosal melanoma in 695 patients. Int Forum Allergy Rhinol. 2017; 7(1): 99–105

[89] Lund VJ, Howard DJ, Harding L, Wei WI. Management options and survival in malignant melanoma of the sinonasal mucosa. Laryngoscope. 1999; 109 (2 Pt 1):208–211

[90] Rawal RB, Farzal Z, Federspiel JJ, Sreenath SB, Thorp BD, Zanation AM. Endoscopic resection of sinonasal malignancy: a systematic review and meta-analysis. Otolaryngol Head Neck Surg. 2016; 155(3):376–386

[91] Swegal W, Koyfman S, Scharpf J, et al. Endoscopic and open surgical approaches to locally advanced sinonasal melanoma: comparing the therapeutic benefits. JAMA Otolaryngol Head Neck Surg. 2014; 140(9):840–845

[92] Shah J. Nasal cavity and paranasal sinuses. In: Mosbey, ed. Head and Neck Surgery and Oncology. New York, NY: Elsevier; 2003:57–93

[93] Hao SP, Pan WL, Chang CN, Hsu YS. The use of the facial translocation technique in the management of tumors of the paranasal sinuses and skull base. Otolaryngol Head Neck Surg. 2003; 128(4):571–575

[94] Bilsky MH, Bentz B, Vitaz T, Shah J, Kraus D. Craniofacial resection for cranial base malignancies involving the infratemporal fossa. Neurosurgery. 2005; 57(4) Suppl:339–347

[95] Bentzen SM, Overgaard J, Thames HD, et al. Clinical radiobiology of malignant melanoma. Radiother Oncol. 1989; 16(3):169–182

[96] Ang KK, Byers RM, Peters LJ, et al. Regional radiotherapy as adjuvant treatment for head and neck malignant melanoma. Preliminary results. Arch Otolaryngol Head Neck Surg. 1990; 116(2):169–172

[97] Stevens G, Thompson JF, Firth I, O'Brien CJ, McCarthy WH, Quinn MJ. Locally advanced melanoma: results of postoperative hypofractionated radiation therapy. Cancer. 2000; 88(1):88–94

[98] Raben A, Zelefsky M, Harrison LB. High dose per fraction, short course irradiation for mucosal melanoma of the head and neck. Presented at the 4th International Head and Neck Society Meeting. Toronto, Canada, June 15, 1996

[99] Owens JM, Roberts DB, Myers JN. The role of postoperative adjuvant radiation therapy in the treatment of mucosal melanomas of the head and neck region. Arch Otolaryngol Head Neck Surg. 2003; 129(8):864–868

[100] Harwood AR, Cummings BJ. Radiotherapy for mucosal melanomas. Int J Radiat Oncol Biol Phys. 1982; 8(7):1121–1126

[101] Trotti A, Peters LJ. Role of radiotherapy in the primary management of mucosal melanoma of the head and neck. Semin Surg Oncol. 1993; 9(3): 246–250

[102] Albertsson M, Tennvall J, Andersson T, Biörklund A, Elner A, Johansson L. Malignant melanoma of the nasal cavity and nasopharynx treated with cisplatin and accelerated hyperfractionated radiation. Melanoma Res. 1992; 2 (2):101–104

[103] Wada H, Nemoto K, Ogawa Y, et al. A multi-institutional retrospective analysis of external radiotherapy for mucosal melanoma of the head and neck in Northern Japan. Int J Radiat Oncol Biol Phys. 2004; 59(2):495–500

[104] Garrott H, O'Day J. Optic neuropathy secondary to radiotherapy for nasal melanoma. Clin Exp Ophthalmol. 2004; 32(3):330–333

[105] Gil Z, Abergel A, Spektor S, et al. Quality of life following surgery for anterior skull base tumors. Arch Otolaryngol Head Neck Surg. 2003; 129(12): 1303–1309

[106] Blake PR, Catterall M, Errington RD. Treatment of malignant melanoma by fast neutrons. Br J Surg. 1985; 72(7):517–519

[107] Linstadt DE, Castro JR, Phillips TL. Neon ion radiotherapy: results of the phase I/II clinical trial. Int J Radiat Oncol Biol Phys. 1991; 20(4):761–769

[108] Mizoe JE, Tsujii H, Kamada T, et al. Organizing Committee for the Working Group for Head-and-Neck Cancer. Dose escalation study of carbon ion radiotherapy for locally advanced head-and-neck cancer. Int J Radiat Oncol Biol Phys. 2004; 60(2):358–364

[109] Jacquillat C, Khayat D, Banzet P, et al. Chemotherapy by fotemustine in cerebral metastases of disseminated malignant melanoma. Cancer Chemother Pharmacol. 1990; 25(4):263–266

[110] National Comprehensive Cancer Network, Inc Version 1.2005; 2005. www.nccn.org

[111] Kirkwood JM, Strawderman MH, Ernstoff MS, Smith TJ, Borden EC, Blum RH. Interferon alfa-2b adjuvant therapy of high-risk resected cutaneous melanoma: the Eastern Cooperative Oncology Group Trial EST 1684. J Clin Oncol. 1996; 14(1):7–17

[112] Kirkwood JM, Ibrahim JG, Sondak VK, et al. High- and low-dose interferon alfa-2b in high-risk melanoma: first analysis of intergroup trial E1690/ S9111/C9190. J Clin Oncol. 2000; 18(12):2444–2458

[113] Legha SS, Ring S, Eton O, et al. Development of a biochemotherapy regimen with concurrent administration of cisplatin, vinblastine, dacarbazine, interferon alfa, and interleukin-2 for patients with metastatic melanoma. J Clin Oncol. 1998; 16(5):1752–1759

[114] Seo W, Ogasawara H, Sakagami M. Chemohormonal therapy for malignant melanomas of the nasal and paranasal mucosa. Rhinology. 1997; 35 (1):19–21

[115] Chapman PB, Hauschild A, Robert C, et al. BRIM-3 Study Group. Improved survival with vemurafenib in melanoma with BRAF V600E mutation. N Engl J Med. 2011; 364(26):2507–2516

[116] Hauschild A, Grob JJ, Demidov LV, et al. Dabrafenib in BRAF-mutated metastatic melanoma: a multicentre, open-label, phase 3 randomised controlled trial. Lancet. 2012; 380(9839):358–365

[117] Chraybi M, Abd Alsamad I, Copie-Bergman C, et al. Oncogene abnormalities in a series of primary melanomas of the sinonasal tract: NRAS mutations and cyclin D1 amplification are more frequent than KIT or BRAF mutations. Hum Pathol. 2013; 44(9):1902–1911

[118] Wang X, Si L, Guo J. Treatment algorithm of metastatic mucosal melanoma. Linchuang Zhongliuxue Zazhi. 2014; 3(3):38

[119] Guo J, Si L, Kong Y, et al. Phase II, open-label, single-arm trial of imatinib mesylate in patients with metastatic melanoma harboring c-Kit mutation or amplification. J Clin Oncol. 2011; 29(21):2904–2909

[120] Carvajal RD, Antonescu CR, Wolchok JD, et al. KIT as a therapeutic target in metastatic melanoma. JAMA. 2011; 305(22):2327–2334

[121] Del Vecchio M, Di Guardo L, Ascierto PA, et al. Efficacy and safety of ipilimumab 3 mg/kg in patients with pretreated, metastatic, mucosal melanoma. Eur J Cancer. 2014; 50(1):121–127

[122] Postow MA, Luke JJ, Bluth MJ, et al. Ipilimumab for patients with advanced mucosal melanoma. Oncologist. 2013; 18(6):726–732

[123] Taube JM, Anders RA, Young GD, et al. Colocalization of inflammatory response with B7-h1 expression in human melanocytic lesions supports an adaptive resistance mechanism of immune escape. Sci Transl Med. 2012; 4 (127):127ra37

[124] Lian B, Si L, Cui C, et al. Phase II randomized trial comparing high-dose IFN-α2b with temozolomide plus cisplatin as systemic adjuvant therapy for resected mucosal melanoma. Clin Cancer Res. 2013; 19(16):4488–4498

[125] Eneroth CM, Lundberg C. Mucosal malignant melanomas of the head and neck with special reference to cases having a prolonged clinical course. Acta Otolaryngol. 1975; 80(5–6):452–458

[126] Meng XJ, Ao HF, Huang WT, et al. Impact of different surgical and postoperative adjuvant treatment modalities on survival of sinonasal malignant melanoma. BMC Cancer. 2014; 14:608

[127] Patel SG, Singh B, Polluri A, et al. Craniofacial surgery for malignant skull base tumors: report of an international collaborative study. Cancer. 2003; 98 (6):1179–1187

[128] Shah JP, Huvos AG, Strong EW. Mucosal melanomas of the head and neck. Am J Surg. 1977; 134(4):531–535

33 Sarcomas of the Skull Base

Ravin Ratan and Robert S. Benjamin

Summary

Sarcomas are a rare and diverse group of neoplasms, each having a distinct epidemiology and clinical behavior. Staging of sarcomas of the head and neck, and prognostication based on this staging, are currently being revised, as previous staging systems have proven inadequate. For most sarcomas of the head, including the skull base, complete surgical resection with pre- or postoperative radiation therapy is the standard of care. Chemotherapy can be applied in the neoadjuvant setting for patients who have tumors when complete resection may not be possible without tumor shrinkage or when the risk of local recurrence or systemic spread is high. Osteosarcoma, rhabdomyosarcoma, and hemangiopericytoma are among the sarcomas that may involve the base of skull and have distinct treatment considerations. Owing to the need for intensive coordination of multidisciplinary care, skull base sarcomas are best treated at high-volume specialty centers.

Keywords: soft tissue sarcoma, head and neck, sarcoma, osteosarcoma, skull base

33.1 Incidence and Epidemiology

Sarcomas are a group of more than 50 distinct neoplasms arising from mesenchymal tissue, each having a distinct natural history and biological behavior. Despite connective tissue's accounting for more than 75% of body weight, these tumors are rare: taken together, they account for less than 1% of cancers in adults and 15% of cancers in children. According to Surveillance, Epidemiology, and End Results Program (SEER) data, there were an estimated 3,300 new cases of bone sarcomas and 12,310 cases of soft tissue sarcoma in the United States in 2016, accounting for less than 1% of incident cancers in that year. An estimated 6,480 patients died from sarcoma during the same period.[1] Although sarcomas can occur anywhere in the body, the limbs, chest wall, and retroperitoneum are the most commonly encountered primary sites. Head and neck soft tissue sarcomas are less common, representing 4 to 10% of all soft tissue sarcomas and less than 1% of cancers occurring in the head and neck.[2] Bone sarcomas account for 20% of head and neck sarcomas and for 0.2% of cancers in the head and neck. In children, sarcomas are more common, with up to 35% of sarcomas originating in the head and neck.[3]

Although most sarcomas occur in the absence of a defined familial cancer syndrome, it is increasingly understood that monogenetic and polygenetic risk factors are present in nearly half of patients diagnosed with sarcoma.[4] Most clinically important are the rare but well-established cancer syndromes. Li-Fraumeni syndrome, caused by a mutation in *p53*, is the most commonly diagnosed hereditary genetic cancer syndrome in patients who have sarcoma. Patients who have Li-Fraumeni syndrome are at risk for a multitude of other rare and common cancers, including breast cancer, leukemias, and glioblastoma. Retinoblastoma, an uncommon cancer syndrome caused by a

null mutation of the *Rb1* gene, typically presents with bilateral retinoblastoma in childhood, though these patients are also at increased risk for osteosarcoma.[5] Both Li-Fraumeni and retinoblastoma syndrome patients are at increased risk for secondary malignancies when treated with radiation, so the use of radiation is (or, at least, should be) limited in the treatment of sarcomas in these patients.[6] Finally, patients who have neurofibromatosis type 1 have an approximately 10% lifetime risk of developing malignant peripheral nerve sheath tumors and are also at increased risk for development of rhabdomyosarcomas and gastrointestinal stromal tumors.[7,8,9]

Radiation-associated sarcomas are not limited to patients who have hereditary risk factors, though the prevalence is lower. It is estimated that the incidence of postirradiation sarcoma ranges from 0.03 to 0.3% of patients treated with radiation and is likely to be dose-dependent.[10]

Skull base sarcomas represent a comparatively rare subset of sarcomas in the head and neck, and most series that describe head and neck sarcomas include only a few of these patients. A diverse range of tumor subtypes occur in this area. In one large international collaborative series of patients who had anterior skull base sarcomas, 35.6% were low-grade sarcomas, 13% were osteosarcomas, 11.6% were rhabdomyosarcomas, and 9.6% were fibrosarcoma. The balance comprised an additional nine different sarcoma subtypes.[11] Sarcoma subtypes that affect the posterior skull base include chondrosarcoma and chordoma, both of which are addressed in other parts of this text.

33.2 Pathology

The fourth edition of the *WHO Classification of Tumours of Soft Tissue and Bone* recognizes more than 50 different sarcoma subtypes having distinct biologies and clinical behaviors. The most important distinction is whether the tumor originates in soft tissue or bone. For bone tumors, further classification into osteosarcoma, chondrosarcoma, or fibrosarcoma (or unclassified pleomorphic sarcoma) can be performed on the basis of the matrix present in the tumor (most commonly osteoid, chondroid, or not detectable).

Similarly, soft tissue tumors are classified according to their apparent lineage, with adipocytic, fibroblastic, smooth muscle, and vascular tumors accounting for the major categories.[12]

A particularly important aspect of sarcoma pathology is tumor grade. This is integrated into staging systems and, even more than traditional parameters such as tumor size and locoregional involvement, can be useful in predicting clinical behavior.[13] Two grading systems are used—one proposed by the National Cancer Institute and another by the Federation Nacionale des Centres de Lutte Contre le Cancer (FNCLCC); the latter is in more common use for its better ability to predict aggressive behavior.[14]

Considering the rarity of these tumors and the importance of an accurate diagnosis for treatment decisions, a correct diagnosis must be obtained whenever possible. In one series, expert review of histological diagnosis led to changing of the sarcoma subtype in 27% of cases, illustrating both the difficulties in diagnosing these rare tumors and the utility of expert review.[15]

33.3 Staging

Formal tumor, lymph node, metastasis (TNM) staging according to the criteria in the American Joint Committee on Cancer (AJCC) manual, seventh edition, has been of limited utility in predicting clinical behavior of sarcomas, particularly in the head and neck, where complex anatomy, frequent involvement of critical structures, and difficulty in performing adequate salvage surgery make local control particularly challenging. Consequently, these tumors are accompanied by a lower overall survival than similar tumors in other sites, a fact that has not historically been reflected in the staging system.[16] To address this, the AJCC Soft Tissue Sarcoma Expert Panel has proposed a separate TNM staging system for head and neck sarcomas in the eighth edition of the manual. The 5 cm cutoff that traditionally separates T1 and T2 tumors was not thought to be appropriate for tumors in this site, considering that approximately 70% of tumors in the head and neck are smaller than this. The eighth edition thus proposes a classification more in line with other head and neck malignancies, with T1 tumors being ≤2 cm, T2 being >2 to ≤4 cm, and T3 tumors being >4 cm. Notably, tumors with invasion of adjacent structures, including orbits and the skull base, are classified as T4. The prognostic significance of this system is as yet unknown—the AJCC's goal in proposing this classification was to enable prospective data collection with which to validate it. Accordingly, prognostic stage groups are not yet defined.[17]

Although local recurrence is an important route for treatment failure with base of skull tumors, in which resection with wide margins can be difficult, metastatic disease remains a driver of mortality, with major implications for management. All patients presenting with primary head and neck or base of skull sarcoma should undergo staging imaging of the primary tumor and CT imaging of the lungs to rule out metastatic disease. Patients who have osteosarcoma additionally require skeletal imaging as part of initial staging, including either PET-CT or bone scan, as these tumors can metastasize to other skeletal sites.

33.4 Treatment

33.4.1 Surgery

The surgical principles for management of skull base sarcomas are not materially different from other tumors that occur at these sites. The metastatic spread of sarcomas seldom involves lymph nodes, and extensive lymph node dissections that may be common for the treatment of carcinomas are not required during sarcoma resections in the absence of clinical lymph node involvement.[11] Wide local excision with microscopically negative margins is the standard of care for sarcomas of both soft tissue and bone, though the confines of the skull base can make this difficult to achieve.[18] In the International Collaborative Study Group series of anterior skull base sarcomas, involved sites included the orbit in 53% of patients and intracranial extension in 28% of patients.[11] Consequently, although adequate surgery alone does remain an acceptable standard of care in

those patients in whom it can be accomplished, multimodality therapy has an important role in the management of patients whose tumors are in proximity to or involving vital structures or who are otherwise not candidates for a wide excision.

33.4.2 Radiation

Multiple clinical reports have led to the routine use of adjuvant radiation therapy to aid in the local control of extremity soft tissue sarcomas. Two randomized prospective studies have demonstrated that administration of radiation in the adjuvant setting reduces the rate of local recurrence in extremity and or chest wall sarcomas, though neither demonstrated improvements in overall survival.[19,20]

There are fewer prospective data regarding the utility of radiation in patients who have head and neck sarcomas, though several retrospective studies support its use. Tran and colleagues at UCLA reported on 164 cases of head and neck sarcomas seen over a 33-year period. Patients receiving adjuvant radiation had a locoregional control rate of 90%, compared with 52% for those receiving surgery without radiation.[21] Also in support of adjuvant radiation therapy, a case series from the Princess Margaret Hospital suggested that head and neck sarcoma patients who had clear surgical margins had local relapse rates similar to those of patients with microscopically positive margins who received postoperative radiation therapy (26% versus 30%, respectively, at 5 years).[22] Data regarding radiation in skull base sarcomas is rare. In the series published by Prabhu and colleagues at MD Anderson Cancer Center, radiation was delivered postoperatively to 62%. The researchers were unable to identify a progression-free survival (PFS) or overall survival (OS) benefit, though admittedly the numbers involved in this study were small.[23]

The utility of preoperative rather than postoperative radiation has also been investigated. Possible advantages to preoperative treatment include lower required dose, smaller radiation field, and excision of treated tissues at the time of surgery. These considerations may allow sparing of radiosensitive structures near the tumor and minimization of late toxicities.[24,25] A prospective randomized study conducted by the National Cancer Institute of Canada Clinical Trials Group (NCIC CTG) in extremity sarcomas demonstrated a higher risk of wound healing complications in patients undergoing preoperative versus postoperative radiotherapy (35% vs. 17%) with similar disease outcomes.[24] Subsequent follow-up demonstrated that patients in the postoperative therapy cohort experienced greater fibrosis and trended to experience more edema and joint stiffness.[26]

A prospective series of patients receiving preoperative radiation in head and neck sarcoma and using the same criteria for definitions of wound complications from the NCIC CTG study was reported by the Princess Margaret Hospital. There the investigators documented a 20% rate of major wound complications, lower than that seen in extremity sarcoma studies. No patients had loss of vision, laryngeal function, or any neurological sequelae attributable to radiation therapy. The authors postulated that increased vascularity in the head and neck, and increased use of flaps for wound closure owing to cosmetic and functional considerations, might explain the lower-than-expected rate of wound complications.[27] Ultimately, the decision to favor preoperative versus postoperative radiation is a complex one that must take into account the expected sensitivity of the tumor to radiotherapy, the toxicity to adjacent tissues, expected margins, and the cosmetic and functional results of surgery. Additionally, many surgeons, including several at our own center, prefer to operate prior to radiation treatment. We suggest that the appropriate sequencing of therapies should be carefully considered for any patient who has base of skull sarcomas, ideally in a multidisciplinary conference setting at a specialty center.

33.4.3 Chemotherapy

The use of chemotherapy to treat unresectable or metastatic sarcoma has a history dating back to the 1960s. At that time, most sarcomas were treated with regimens that were most active against rhabdomyosarcomas and other pediatric sarcomas, with marginal activity in the subtypes that are more common in adults. Indeed, the employment of drugs such as vincristine, actinomycin, and cyclophosphamide in the treatment of pediatric rhabdomyosarcoma is as much a standard of care in 2017 as it was 50 years ago. For adult sarcomas, these drugs have limited activity, and the introduction of drugs such as doxorubicin and dacarbazine in the 1970s was the beginning of the divergence in treatment of adult sarcomas from pediatric tumors.

The choice of regimen is often impacted by goals of treatment. When given in the neoadjuvant setting, response rate (likelihood of a tumor shrinking) is considered of paramount importance in decreasing the likelihood of distant metastatic recurrence and facilitating an adequate resection. Whether this approach routinely succeeds in decreasing the extent of surgery is questionable. In one report of neoadjuvant chemotherapy for head and neck sarcomas, even with a response rate of 34%, the scope of surgery was lessened in only 13% of patients; 26% of patients had progression of disease on chemotherapy, and as a result 9% of patients had an increased scope of surgery.[28] This illustrates that the decision to employ neoadjuvant chemotherapy is one that should take into account the patient's risk of subsequently developing metastatic disease, the feasibility of resection prior to neoadjuvant treatment, and the patient's ability to tolerate intensive chemotherapy.

33.4.4 Doxorubicin

Doxorubicin has been used in the treatment of sarcoma for nearly half a century and, despite new drug approvals in 2012 and 2015 for the treatment of soft tissue sarcoma, remains the most efficacious agent in terms of response rate and impact on survival.[29] It has been noted that, unlike other tumors for which the drug is commonly used (including breast cancer, leukemias, and lymphomas), the administration of higher doses of doxorubicin to patients with sarcomas leads to higher response rates.[30] When used as a single agent, responses are low according to response evaluation criteria in solid tumors (RECIST)—in the range of 14% in a large study in 2014.[31] Consequently, the search for effective combinations has been of interest since the drug was introduced, starting with the alkylating agent dacarbazine.[29] Multiple trials have shown increased response rate to the combination of doxorubicin and dacarbazine over doxorubicin alone, but none of these has definitively shown an improvement in overall survival.[32,33,34]

A more modern combination, felt to be most active, is the combination of dose-intensive doxorubicin and ifosfamide, which was shown to have a response rate of 66% in the initial description and 26% by RECIST in a recent study, with a trend toward improvement in overall survival over doxorubicin alone.[31,35]

Whether doxorubicin and ifosfamide in combination improve overall survival over single-agent therapy remains controversial. The previously cited study, intended to settle this question, was powered to find a 10% improvement in overall survival. They found a 9% improvement, which missed the cutoff for statistical significance.[36] Additional evidence for combination chemotherapy can be found in the recently reported METASARC retrospective study conducted by the French Sarcoma Group, which looked at 2,165 patients treated in coordination with three sarcoma reference centers, with expert pathology review of all cases. In this study, patients who received combination chemotherapy in the front-line setting had improved overall survival over those who did not, to a statistically significant degree. Some of this effect might result from the selection of more fit patients for combination therapy—patients who might have done better regardless. Even so, this large and well-curated database provides the best available look at the natural history of patients treated for sarcoma and, in our opinion, is compelling evidence of the superiority of combination chemotherapy in appropriate patients. What is generally agreed on is that for patients who require tumor shrinkage to achieve palliation or to proceed to surgery, doxorubicin and ifosfamide in combination is the most active regimen. This has been incorporated into National Comprehensive Care Network (NCCN) guidelines.

The most recently examined doxorubicin-based combination uses a new anti-PDGFRα monoclonal antibody, olaratumab. The drug received accelerated approval from the FDA in 2016 for use in combination with doxorubicin on the basis of a 12-month improvement in overall survival over doxorubicin alone in a randomized phase II study. Interestingly, response rate was only modestly improved (18.2 vs. 11.9%), and the improvement in progression-free survival was also small (6.6 vs. 4.1 months).[37] A larger confirmatory phase III study has accrued but has not yet been reported. In view of its impressive overall survival benefits, this combination has gained widespread acceptance as front-line treatment for patients who have metastatic disease. For fit patients, we still favor doxorubicin and ifosfamide as front-line therapy considering the limited data available to support the survival benefit seen in the randomized doxorubicin and olaratumab phase II study.

33.4.5 Gemcitabine and Docetaxel

With the approval of gemcitabine for pancreas cancer and docetaxel for breast cancer in 1996, several phase II studies examined the activity of the drugs in sarcomas.[38,39,40,41,42,43,44] Gemcitabine clearly has single-agent activity, with response rates ranging from 3 to 18% in several phase II studies.[38,39,40,41] The response rate to single-agent docetaxel was more modest, ranging from 0 to 22%.[42,43,45] Considering the nonoverlapping toxicity, the combination of the two drugs was examined. Retrospective and early phase II studies suggested that the combination might result in synergistic activity, with response rates of 14 to 53%.[46,47] It was not clear whether this improved efficacy over gemcitabine alone was the result of optimal administration of the gemcitabine with use of a slower fixed-dose-rate infusion or of the addition of the marginally active docetaxel. To address this question, two randomized studies have been conducted. The first, conducted by the Sarcoma Alliance for Research Collaboration (SARC), enrolled patients who had a variety of soft tissue sarcomas. To minimize the number of patients required to get a statistically significant result, the trial employed Bayesian adaptive randomization to assign patients to treatment groups and determine when to stop the study. A total of 122 patients who had a variety of soft tissue sarcomas were assigned to receive either gemcitabine alone or gemcitabine and docetaxel. With the adaptive randomization, 73 patients received combination therapy and 49 received gemcitabine alone. Median progression-free survival was 6.2 months for the combination arm and 3.0 months for the single-agent arm. Overall survival was also improved, at 17.9 versus 11.5 months. Importantly, combination therapy was associated with more significant side effects and many more treatment discontinuations as a result of toxicity.[48]

In apparent conflict with these results is a second randomized study, conducted by the French Sarcoma Group, that randomized patients who had uterine and nonuterine leiomyosarcoma to gemcitabine and docetaxel versus gemcitabine alone. This study demonstrated no improvement in progression-free or overall survival with the addition of docetaxel to single-agent gemcitabine.[49] It should be noted, however, that the study was limited to patients who had leiomyosarcoma, whereas the patients who had the best results on the SARC study had unclassified pleomorphic sarcomas (called malignant fibrous histiocytoma at the time of the study). Furthermore, the French study used more gemcitabine in the control arm than the SARC study did.

Our approach has been to use gemcitabine and docetaxel in combination in fit patients, in most cases as a second-line treatment after doxorubicin-containing combination therapy. However, considering the mixed evidence regarding the importance of docetaxel in the combination, we are quick to dose reduce or eliminate the drug in patients of advanced age or marginal performance status or who have docetaxel-related toxicity.

33.4.6 Trabectedin

Approved in the United States in 2015 and in Europe in 2007, trabectedin has become an important treatment option, particularly for patients who have pretreated liposarcomas and leiomyosarcomas. It also has clear activity in several other sarcoma subtypes. The drug was initially isolated from a marine tunicate and is now produced synthetically. Its main mechanism of action appears to involve binding of the minor groove of DNA, though other mechanisms have also been implicated.[50] A number of phase II studies resulted in the approval of trabectedin for the treatment of soft tissue sarcomas in Europe in 2007.[51,52,53,54] Based on evidence of increased efficacy in leiomyosarcomas and liposarcomas, a phase III study was conducted that randomized patients who had those tumor types to treatment with trabectedin or dacarbazine. The study did not meet its primary endpoint of improved overall survival, but it did demonstrate significantly improved progression-free survival at 4.5 months for trabectedin and 1.5 months for the dacarbazine control.[55] Based on

these data, the FDA approved trabectedin in 2015 for patients who have liposarcomas and leiomyosarcomas previously treated with anthracycline based therapy.

Trabectedin has been of particular interest in patients who have chromosomal translocation-associated sarcomas, especially myxoid liposarcoma. A phase III study that randomized patients who had translocation-associated sarcomas to treatment with trabectedin versus doxorubicin has been conducted. Nearly half of the patients on the trial had myxoid liposarcoma. Ultimately, the study was not able to demonstrate a difference in PFS or OS, because too many of the patients received additional therapy prior to progression of disease and were subsequently censored. The study was ultimately underpowered, so definitive conclusions about relative efficacy of the two drugs in the front line cannot be drawn, although it is notable that 23.5% of patients in the trabectedin arm who were previously deemed unresectable proceeded to surgery.[56] Consequently, trabectedin is often used earlier than gemcitabine or other salvage therapies when treating myxoid liposarcoma, and to a lesser extent other translocation-associated tumors.

33.4.7 Eribulin

Approved for metastatic breast cancer in 2010, eribulin was approved for treatment of liposarcomas in 2015. The drug is an inhibitor of microtubule polymerization that is a derivative of a compound isolated from a marine sponge. An additional postulated mechanism of action is modulation of the tumor microenvironment and the metastatic potential of tumor cells.[57] Treatment using the agent is associated with increased number of microvessels and possible improved delivery of subsequent lines of therapy.[58]

A phase II study of eribulin conducted by the European Organization for Research and Treatment of Cancer (EORTC) demonstrated activity of the drug in patients who had synovial sarcoma, leiomyosarcoma, or adipocytic sarcoma. Based on a customary cutoff of 12 week PFS > 30% as the threshold for advancing a drug in development for sarcoma, patients who had liposarcoma or leiomyosarcoma were enrolled in a randomized phase III study of eribulin versus dacarbazine. The study demonstrated a 2-month improvement in overall survival in those treated with eribulin without a significantly improved progression-free survival or response rate. Interestingly, preplanned subgroup analysis suggested that liposarcomas had improved overall survival and that leiomyosarcomas had not.[59] Accordingly, the FDA approved eribulin in 2016 for the treatment of liposarcomas only rather than the entire studied population. Whether the lack of improvement in outcome for leiomyosarcomas was due to better-than-expected efficacy of dacarbazine in that group or poor efficacy of eribulin is unclear.

Subsequently presented data from the same phase III study showed that the survival benefit was significantly more pronounced (15.6 vs. 8.4 months) in liposarcomas alone than when leiomyosarcomas were included in the analysis. In contrast to the original study, this report demonstrated that in liposarcomas alone, PFS was modestly, though statistically significantly, improved after treatment with eribulin at 2.9 versus 1.7 months.[60]

33.4.8 Pazopanib

Pazopanib is a multitargeted tyrosine kinase inhibitor approved for the treatment of soft tissue sarcomas. The phase III PALETTE study, which led to the approval of pazopanib, excluded patients who had liposarcomas owing to lack of activity in an earlier study. The phase III trial demonstrated a 3-month improvement in progression-free survival with pazopanib over placebo (4.6 vs. 1.6 months), the primary endpoint of the study, but failed to demonstrate improved median overall survival. Six percent of patients in the pazopanib arm experienced a partial response, though a more substantial 67% of patients achieved stable disease (in contrast to 38% with placebo). Despite the modest response rate, the disease stabilization is of clinical interest. With limited options for patients who have metastatic or unresectable disease, pazopanib remains an important and commonly used palliative treatment option for patients who have progressed through other therapies.

33.5 Disease-Specific Considerations

33.5.1 Osteosarcoma

Although many varieties of soft tissue sarcoma can extend to involve the skull base, osteosarcomas are an exception in that they can arise from the skull base itself. This is a rare presentation, with head and neck osteosarcomas accounting for 10% of osteosarcoma cases. Of these, approximately 80 to 85% arise from the maxilla and mandible (jaw). The behavior of these tumors is distinct from the more common osteosarcoma of the long bones. The rate of distant metastatic disease is low, approximately 7 to 12% in two large single-institution reports. Local recurrence is more problematic, with rates of 18 to 34% in the same two case series.[61,62] Predictors of improved local control include tumors < 4 cm in size, fibrous histology, low histologic grade, and favorable response to chemotherapy. Positive margins are also intuitively associated with high risk for local relapse and are correlated with worsened overall survival. Retrospective data support the use of postoperative radiation therapy for patients who have positive margins at the time of surgery, demonstrating improved local control rates.[61]

Response to chemotherapy in head and neck sarcomas is also less robust than in more common limb osteosarcomas. In the Memorial Sloan Kettering series of patients receiving neoadjuvant chemotherapy, a relatively high 73% of patients had histologically poor responses to neoadjuvant treatment. Combined with lower metastatic potential, this apparently decreased chemosensitivity makes the routine use of neoadjuvant chemotherapy, which is standard for patients with osteosarcomas at other sites, less appealing for those who have jaw primaries.

Considering the lack of chemosensitivity and lower rates of distant metastatic disease, surgical resection without radiation or chemotherapy as up-front management of amenable tumors is an acceptable standard of care for jaw osteosarcomas. For tumors located in the mandible, where anatomy allows for relatively straightforward margin-negative resection, this is the most commonly applied treatment strategy. Tumors originating in the maxilla and other nonmandible skull sites, including the skull base, are often selected for neoadjuvant treatment on the basis of anticipated difficulty in obtaining negative margins. The data demonstrating improved outcomes treated in this fashion are limited, though Memorial Sloan Kettering demonstrated that patients who received neoadjuvant treatment had decreased rates of distant metastatic disease compared with historical controls.[62] Prognosis varies based on the case series, with 5-year overall survival rates ranging from 55 to 63% in several larger case series.[61,62,63]

The precise natural history of osteosarcomas arising in bones of the skull other than the mandible and maxilla is poorly characterized. We have seen metastatic disease from such tumors and thus treat osteosarcoma of the skull outside the jaw as if it were similar to that of other skeletal sites.

There is no universal agreement on optimal chemotherapy regimen for nongnathic osteosarcoma. Most regimens, including those used at our center, incorporate doxorubicin and cisplatin (AP). Many others also incorporate methotrexate into the treatment, resulting in the MAP regimen. Whether methotrexate improves outcomes when added to doxorubicin and cisplatin in adult patients is not clear, with two randomized studies having demonstrated no improvement in survival.[64,65] Nevertheless, based on the approach in the pediatric population, it is often employed in adult osteosarcoma patients. Typically, after a course of neoadjuvant therapy, the tumor is resected and additional adjuvant chemotherapy is administered. Here also, there is no clear standard of care, and many centers continue with MAP irrespective of the pathologic response seen at the time of surgery. They cite the EUROAMOS-1 trial, which demonstrated that intensification of adjuvant chemotherapy with ifosfamide and etoposide in addition to MAP in patients who had suboptimal (< 90%) necrosis did not improve outcomes over those who simply received additional MAP.[66]

The approach at our center has been to use doxorubicin and cisplatin in the neoadjuvant setting. Based on the level of tumor necrosis, we treat either with additional anthracycline-based therapy or, in poor responders, with high-dose ifosfamide followed by high-dose methotrexate. In our hands, this intensified approach in patients who have otherwise poorer prognoses results in similar outcomes irrespective of the level of necrosis.[67,68]

33.5.2 Rhabdomyosarcoma

Rhabdomyosarcoma is a rare tumor most commonly seen in children, in whom it constitutes more than 50% of soft tissue sarcomas—in contrast to adults, in whom the figure is closer to 3%. The childhood form of this disease carries a better prognosis, with cure rates as high as 70% when using multimodality treatment. In adults, the prognosis is poorer, with a 5-year OS of 45.7% in a large cohort of patients treated at the Istituto Nazionale Tumori in Milan, Italy. Of the 171 adult patients in this series, 53% had primary tumors in the head and neck. In this report, patients who received optimal chemotherapy (defined as a regimen containing an anthracycline along with cyclophosphamide or ifosfamide, given for at least eight cycles) and complete surgical resection, with radiation in the event that the tumor was incompletely resected, had a better outcome, with a 5-year OS of 61.5%. Illustrating the importance of appropriate chemotherapy in this disease, patients who did not receive chemotherapy had a 5-year relapse- and event-free survival of 39.4%, compared with 64.1% in the group that received optimal chemotherapy.[69] Thus, unlike other sarcomas of the head and neck, for which local therapy generally takes precedence, chemotherapy is a critical component of the treatment of this tumor type. Considering the apparent chemosensitivity, neoadjuvant treatment's likelihood of making surgery less extensive is likely to be higher than for other sarcomas.

Our approach to patients who have rhabdomyosarcoma is to use doxorubicin and ifosfamide at doses similar to other soft tissue sarcomas, with the addition of vincristine. Many other centers use vincristine, doxorubicin, and cyclophosphamide, often alternating with ifosfamide and etoposide. Actinomycin-D is more effective in these tumors than most adult sarcomas and can be used in place of doxorubicin, particularly when patients have received doxorubicin in the past. In the second line, topoisomerase inhibitors paired with alkylating agents are frequently used.

33.5.3 Solitary Fibrous Tumors

Solitary fibrous tumors (SFTs), previously called hemangiopericytomas, are rare tumors that historically were felt to arise from pericytes that can be found associated with capillaries throughout the body but that are now felt to be of fibroblastic origin.[70,71] As might be expected with a cell type so widely distributed throughout the body, SFTs can occur in a variety of locations. They often arise in the thoracic cavity as pleural-based lesions, though other common sites include the pelvic soft tissues, peritoneal cavity, and the dura.

Head and neck SFTs, including those of the dura, account for approximately 15 to 25% of these malignancies.[72,73] Clinical behavior can be difficult to predict based on pathologic features alone. These tumors can frequently be locally aggressive, and a minority of them have the ability to metastasize. The most common head and neck location is the dura.

Like other sarcomas, complete resection when possible is the favored treatment for these tumors, and the status of margins at the time of surgery is a predictor of the risk for local recurrence. In one case series published by Soyeur and colleagues at MD Anderson Cancer Center, patients undergoing gross total resection of dural SFT had a 5-year local control rate of 84%, with patients who underwent subtotal resection having a rate of 38%.[74]

The Soyeur study also attempted to look at the effect of radiation in the adjuvant setting, but too few patients received adjuvant radiation to be able to determine its efficacy. More convincingly in favor of adjuvant radiation treatment, a single-institution study of 17 patients who had intracranial SFT demonstrated a local recurrence rate of 12.5% in patients who received postoperative radiation, versus 88% in patients who did not.[75] For patients in whom resection is not an option, precision radiotherapy, including that using modalities such as fractioned stereotactic radiation therapy and Gamma Knife (Elekta), has been used in treating these tumors. In a series of 37 patients treated with precision radiotherapy for unresectable disease at the University of Heidelberg (including 25 patients who had tumors involving the skull base), PFS rate at 5 years was 79.5%. Most of these patients had undergone previous attempts at surgical excision.[76] Another series of 21 patients who had unresectable intracranial SFT treated using Gamma Knife radiotherapy was reported by investigators at the University of Virginia; 1-, 3-, and 5-year PFS rates were 90, 60.3, and 28.7%, with a 5-year survival after treatment of 81%.[77] These data suggest that radiosurgery may be a reasonable temporizing treatment, though with a high likelihood of eventual local recurrence.

Chemotherapy for SFT remains a somewhat poorly defined area. For patients who have unresectable or metastatic disease, systemic treatment is often the only option.

Park and colleagues at MD Anderson Cancer Center published a series of 14 patients treated with a combination of bevacizumab and temozolomide. The study demonstrated partial responses or stable disease, as assessed using the Choi criteria, in 13 of 14 patients. Median PFS was estimated at 9.7 months.[78] The regimen is reasonably well tolerated and remains our treatment of choice for patients who have SFT. Other agents that have broad activity against sarcoma subtypes, including doxorubicin, vincristine, cyclophosphamide, actinomycin, methotrexate, and dacarbazine, have been examined in this disease.[79,80,81] Older reports suggest several complete responses (CRs) and partial responses (PRs) with these agents, though our experience suggests that response rates are lower than might be expected based on these series.

33.6 Conclusion

Sarcomas represent a diverse family of distinct cancers that vary in their propensity for distant metastatic disease, predilection for local recurrence after resection, and responsiveness to medical and radiation therapy. The anatomical, functional, and cosmetic considerations involved in the local treatment of these tumors complicate their management, as do higher local recurrence rates than similar tumors at other body sites. Consequently, the ability to perform adequate surgery is a key determinant of overall prognosis. For localized cancers, chemotherapy and radiation can assist in providing adequate local control, though they are not curative modalities in the absence of surgery. For the patient who has metastatic disease, chemotherapy is the mainstay of treatment. Considering the rarity of these tumors and the need for intensive multidisciplinary coordination, consultation at specialty centers is critical to ensuring the best outcomes.[82]

References

[1] American Cancer Society. Cancer Facts and Figures 2016. Atlanta: American Cancer Society; 2016

[2] Stavrakas M, Nixon I, Andi K, et al. Head and neck sarcomas: clinical and histopathological presentation, treatment modalities, and outcomes. J Laryngol Otol. 2016; 130(9):850–859

[3] Sturgis EM, Potter BO. Sarcomas of the head and neck region. Curr Opin Oncol. 2003; 15(3):239–252

[4] Ballinger ML, Goode DL, Ray-Coquard I, et al. International Sarcoma Kindred Study. Monogenic and polygenic determinants of sarcoma risk: an international genetic study. Lancet Oncol. 2016; 17(9):1261–1271

[5] Hansen MF, Koufos A, Gallie BL, et al. Osteosarcoma and retinoblastoma: a shared chromosomal mechanism revealing recessive predisposition. Proc Natl Acad Sci U S A. 1985; 82(18):6216–6220

[6] Rodjan F, Graaf Pd, Brisse HJ, et al. Second cranio-facial malignancies in hereditary retinoblastoma survivors previously treated with radiation therapy: clinic and radiologic characteristics and survival outcomes. Eur J Cancer. 2013; 49(8):1939–1947

[7] Evans DG, Baser ME, McGaughran J, Sharif S, Howard E, Moran A. Malignant peripheral nerve sheath tumours in neurofibromatosis 1. J Med Genet. 2002; 39(5):311–314

[8] Ferrari A, Bisogno G, Macaluso A, et al. Soft-tissue sarcomas in children and adolescents with neurofibromatosis type 1. Cancer. 2007; 109(7): 1406–1412

[9] Miettinen M, Fetsch JF, Sobin LH, Lasota J. Gastrointestinal stromal tumors in patients with neurofibromatosis 1: a clinicopathologic and molecular genetic study of 45 cases. Am J Surg Pathol. 2006; 30(1):90–96

[10] Mark RJ, Bailet JW, Poen J, et al. Postirradiation sarcoma of the head and neck. Cancer. 1993; 72(3):887–893

[11] Gil Z, Patel SG, Singh B, et al. International Collaborative Study Group. Analysis of prognostic factors in 146 patients with anterior skull base sarcoma: an international collaborative study. Cancer. 2007; 110(5):1033–1041

[12] Fletcher CD, Bridge JA, Hogendoorn P, Mertens F, eds. WHO Classification of Tumours of Soft Tissue and Bone. 4th ed. Lyon: IARC; 2013

[13] Coindre JM, Terrier P, Bui NB, et al. Prognostic factors in adult patients with locally controlled soft tissue sarcoma. A study of 546 patients from the French Federation of Cancer Centers Sarcoma Group. J Clin Oncol. 1996; 14 (3):869–877

[14] Guillou L, Coindre JM, Bonichon F, et al. Comparative study of the National Cancer Institute and French Federation of Cancer Centers Sarcoma Group grading systems in a population of 410 adult patients with soft tissue sarcoma. J Clin Oncol. 1997; 15(1):350–362

[15] Presant CA, Russell WO, Alexander RW, Fu YS. Soft-tissue and bone sarcoma histopathology peer review: the frequency of disagreement in diagnosis and the need for second pathology opinions. The Southeastern Cancer Study Group experience. J Clin Oncol. 1986; 4(11):1658–1661

[16] Penel N, Mallet Y, Robin YM, et al. Prognostic factors for adult sarcomas of head and neck. Int J Oral Maxillofac Surg. 2008; 37(5):428–432

[17] O'Sullivan B, Maki RG, Agulnik M. AJCC Cancer Staging Manual. 8th ed. New York, NY: Springer Science + Business Media. 8th ed; 2017:499–505

[18] Balm AJ, Vom Coevorden F, Bos KE, et al. Report of a symposium on diagnosis and treatment of adult soft tissue sarcomas in the head and neck. Eur J Surg Oncol. 1995; 21(3):287–289

[19] Pisters PW, Harrison LB, Leung DH, Woodruff JM, Casper ES, Brennan MF. Long-term results of a prospective randomized trial of adjuvant brachytherapy in soft tissue sarcoma. J Clin Oncol. 1996; 14(3):859–868

[20] Yang JC, Chang AE, Baker AR, et al. Randomized prospective study of the benefit of adjuvant radiation therapy in the treatment of soft tissue sarcomas of the extremity. J Clin Oncol. 1998; 16(1):197–203

[21] Tran LM, Mark R, Meier R, Calcaterra TC, Parker RG. Sarcomas of the head and neck: prognostic factors and treatment strategies. Cancer. 1992; 70 (1):169–177

[22] Le Vay J, O'Sullivan B, Catton C, et al. An assessment of prognostic factors in soft-tissue sarcoma of the head and neck. Arch Otolaryngol Head Neck Surg. 1994; 120(9):981–986

[23] Prabhu SS, Diaz E, Sturgis EM, Myers JN, Suki D, Demonte F. Section on tumors: Mahaley Clinical Research Award: primary sarcomas of the skull base: an analysis of 63 cases. Clin Neurosurg. 2004; 51:340–342

[24] O'Sullivan B, Davis AM, Turcotte R, et al. Preoperative versus postoperative radiotherapy in soft-tissue sarcoma of the limbs: a randomised trial. Lancet. 2002; 359(9325):2235–2241

[25] Panwar U, Sankaye P. Preoperative versus postoperative radiotherapy in extremity soft tissue sarcoma: a changing trend towards preoperative radiotherapy in the UK. Clin Oncol (R Coll Radiol). 2015; 27(6):369–370

[26] Davis AM, O'Sullivan B, Turcotte R, et al. Canadian Sarcoma Group, NCI Canada Clinical Trial Group Randomized Trial. Late radiation morbidity following randomization to preoperative versus postoperative radiotherapy in extremity soft tissue sarcoma. Radiother Oncol. 2005; 75(1):48–53

[27] O'Sullivan B, Gullane P, Irish J, et al. Preoperative radiotherapy for adult head and neck soft tissue sarcoma: assessment of wound complication rates and cancer outcome in a prospective series. World J Surg. 2003; 27 (7):875–883

[28] DeMonte F. Soft tissue sarcomas of the skull base: time for a new paradigm. Cancer. 2007; 110(5):939–940

[29] Gottlieb JA, Baker LH, Quagliana JM, et al. Chemotherapy of sarcomas with a combination of Adriamycin and dimethyl triazeno imidazole carboxamide. Cancer. 1972; 30(6):1632–1638

[30] O'Bryan RM, Baker LH, Gottlieb JE, et al. Dose response evaluation of Adriamycin in human neoplasia. Cancer. 1977; 39(5):1940–1948

[31] Judson I, Verweij J, Gelderblom H, et al. European Organisation and Treatment of Cancer Soft Tissue and Bone Sarcoma Group. Doxorubicin alone versus intensified doxorubicin plus ifosfamide for first-line treatment of advanced or metastatic soft-tissue sarcoma: a randomised controlled phase 3 trial. Lancet Oncol. 2014; 15(4):415–423

[32] Omura GA, Major FJ, Blessing JA, et al. A randomized study of Adriamycin with and without dimethyl triazenoimidazole carboxamide in advanced uterine sarcomas. Cancer. 1983; 52(4):626–632

[33] Antman K, Crowley J, Balcerzak SP, et al. An intergroup phase III randomized study of doxorubicin and dacarbazine with or without ifosfamide and mesna in advanced soft tissue and bone sarcomas. J Clin Oncol. 1993; 11(7): 1276–1285

[34] Borden EC, Amato DA, Rosenbaum C, et al. Randomized comparison of three Adriamycin regimens for metastatic soft tissue sarcomas. J Clin Oncol. 1987; 5(6):840–850

[35] Patel SR, Vadhan-Raj S, Burgess MA, et al. Results of two consecutive trials of dose-intensive chemotherapy with doxorubicin and ifosfamide in patients with sarcomas. Am J Clin Oncol. 1998; 21(3):317–321

[36] Benjamin RS, Lee JJ. One step forward, two steps back. Lancet Oncol. 2014; 15 (4):366–367

[37] Tap WD, Jones RL, Van Tine BA, et al. Olaratumab and doxorubicin versus doxorubicin alone for treatment of soft-tissue sarcoma: an open-label phase 1b and randomised phase 2 trial [published correction appears in Lancet. 2016 Jul 30;388(10043):464]. Lancet. 2016;388(10043):488–497.

[38] Merimsky O, Meller I, Flusser G, et al. Gemcitabine in soft tissue or bone sarcoma resistant to standard chemotherapy: a phase II study. Cancer Chemother Pharmacol. 2000; 45(2):177–181

[39] Patel SR, Gandhi V, Jenkins J, et al. Phase II clinical investigation of gemcitabine in advanced soft tissue sarcomas and window evaluation of dose rate on gemcitabine triphosphate accumulation. J Clin Oncol. 2001; 19(15): 3483–3489

[40] Späth-Schwalbe E, Genvresse I, Koschuth A, Dietzmann A, Grunewald R, Possinger K. Phase II trial of gemcitabine in patients with pretreated advanced soft tissue sarcomas. Anticancer Drugs. 2000; 11(5):325–329

[41] Svancárová L, Blay JY, Judson IR, et al. Gemcitabine in advanced adult soft-tissue sarcomas: a phase II study of the EORTC Soft Tissue and Bone Sarcoma Group. Eur J Cancer. 2002; 38(4):556–559

[42] van Hoesel QG, Verweij J, Catimel G, et al. EORTC Soft Tissue and Bone Sarcoma Group. Phase II study with docetaxel (Taxotere) in advanced soft tissue sarcomas of the adult. Ann Oncol. 1994; 5(6):539–542

[43] Verweij J, Lee SM, Ruka W, et al. Randomized phase II study of docetaxel versus doxorubicin in first- and second-line chemotherapy for locally advanced or metastatic soft tissue sarcomas in adults: a study of the European Organization for Research and Treatment of Cancer Soft Tissue and Bone Sarcoma Group. J Clin Oncol. 2000; 18(10):2081–2086

[44] Edmonson JH, Ebbert LP, Nascimento AG, Jung SH, McGaw H, Gerstner JB. Phase II study of docetaxel in advanced soft tissue sarcomas. Am J Clin Oncol. 1996; 19(6):574–576

[45] Verweij J, Catimel G, Sulkes A, et al. EORTC Early Clinical Trials Group and the EORTC Soft Tissue and Bone Sarcoma Group. Phase II studies of docetaxel in the treatment of various solid tumours. Eur J Cancer. 1995; 31A Suppl 4:S21–S24

[46] Hensley ML, Maki R, Venkatraman E, et al. Gemcitabine and docetaxel in patients with unresectable leiomyosarcoma: results of a phase II trial. J Clin Oncol. 2002; 20(12):2824–2831

[47] Bay JO, Ray-Coquard I, Fayette J, et al. Groupe Sarcome Français. Docetaxel and gemcitabine combination in 133 advanced soft-tissue sarcomas: a retrospective analysis. Int J Cancer. 2006; 119(3):706–711

[48] Maki RG, Wathen JK, Patel SR, et al. Randomized phase II study of gemcitabine and docetaxel compared with gemcitabine alone in patients with metastatic soft tissue sarcomas: results of Sarcoma Alliance for Research through Collaboration study 002 [corrected]. J Clin Oncol. 2007; 25(19):2755–2763

[49] Pautier P, Floquet A, Penel N, et al. Randomized multicenter and stratified phase II study of gemcitabine alone versus gemcitabine and docetaxel in patients with metastatic or relapsed leiomyosarcomas: a Federation Nationale des Centres de Lutte Contre le Cancer (FNCLCC) French Sarcoma Group Study (TAXOGEM study). Oncologist. 2012; 17(9):1213–1220

[50] D'Incalci M, Galmarini CM. A review of trabectedin (ET-743): a unique mechanism of action. Mol Cancer Ther. 2010; 9(8):2157–2163

[51] Le Cesne A, Blay JY, Judson I, et al. Phase II study of ET-743 in advanced soft tissue sarcomas: a European Organisation for the Research and Treatment of Cancer (EORTC) soft tissue and bone sarcoma group trial. J Clin Oncol. 2005; 23(3):576–584

[52] Demetri GD, Chawla SP, von Mehren M, et al. Efficacy and safety of trabectedin in patients with advanced or metastatic liposarcoma or leiomyosarcoma after failure of prior anthracyclines and ifosfamide: results of a randomized phase II study of two different schedules. J Clin Oncol. 2009; 27(25):4188–4196

[53] Garcia-Carbonero R, Supko JG, Maki RG, et al. Ecteinascidin-743 (ET-743) for chemotherapy-naive patients with advanced soft tissue sarcomas: multicenter phase II and pharmacokinetic study. J Clin Oncol. 2005; 23(24):5484–5492

[54] Yovine A, Riofrio M, Blay JY, et al. Phase II study of ecteinascidin-743 in advanced pretreated soft tissue sarcoma patients. J Clin Oncol. 2004; 22(5):890–899

[55] Demetri GD, von Mehren M, Jones RL, et al. Efficacy and safety of trabectedin or dacarbazine for metastatic liposarcoma or leiomyosarcoma after failure of conventional chemotherapy: results of a phase III randomized multicenter clinical trial. J Clin Oncol. 2015

[56] Blay J-Y, Leahy MG, Nguyen BB, et al. Randomised phase III trial of trabectedin versus doxorubicin-based chemotherapy as first-line therapy in translocation-related sarcomas. Eur J Cancer. 2014; 50(6):1137–1147

[57] Dybdal-Hargreaves NF, Risinger AL, Mooberry SL. Eribulin mesylate: mechanism of action of a unique microtubule-targeting agent. Clin Cancer Res. 2015; 21(11):2445–2452

[58] Funahashi Y, Okamoto K, Adachi Y, et al. Eribulin mesylate reduces tumor microenvironment abnormality by vascular remodeling in preclinical human breast cancer models. Cancer Sci. 2014; 105(10):1334–1342

[59] Schöffski P, Chawla S, Maki RG, et al. Eribulin versus dacarbazine in previously treated patients with advanced liposarcoma or leiomyosarcoma: a randomised, open-label, multicentre, phase 3 trial. Lancet. 2016; 387(10028):1629–1637

[60] Chawla S, Schoffski P, Grignani G, et al. Subtype-specific activity in liposarcoma (LPS) patients (pts) from a phase 3, open-label, randomized study of erbulin (ERI) versus dacarbazine (DTIC) in pts with advanced LPS and leiomyosarcoma. J Clin Oncol. 2016:(suppl; abtr 11037)

[61] Guadagnolo BA, Zagars GK, Raymond AK, Benjamin RS, Sturgis EM. Osteosarcoma of the jaw/craniofacial region: outcomes after multimodality treatment. Cancer. 2009; 115(14):3262–3270

[62] Patel SG, Meyers P, Huvos AG, et al. Improved outcomes in patients with osteogenic sarcoma of the head and neck. Cancer. 2002; 95(7):1495–1503

[63] Ha PK, Eisele DW, Frassica FJ, Zahurak ML, McCarthy EF. Osteosarcoma of the head and neck: a review of the Johns Hopkins experience. Laryngoscope. 1999; 109(6):964–969

[64] Bramwell VH, Burgers MV, Souhami RL, et al. A randomized comparison of two short intensive chemotherapy regimens in children and young adults with osteosarcoma: results in patients with metastases: a study of the European Osteosarcoma Intergroup. Sarcoma. 1997; 1(3–4):155–160

[65] Souhami RL, Craft AW, Van der Eijken JW, et al. Randomised trial of two regimens of chemotherapy in operable osteosarcoma: a study of the European Osteosarcoma Intergroup. Lancet. 1997; 350(9082):911–917

[66] Marina NM, Smeland S, Bielack SS, et al. Comparison of MAPIE versus MAP in patients with a poor response to preoperative chemotherapy for newly diagnosed high-grade osteosarcoma (EURAMOS-1): an open-label, international, randomised controlled trial. Lancet Oncol. 2016; 17(10):1396–1408

[67] Wagner MJ, Livingston JA, Patel SR, Benjamin RS. Chemotherapy for bone sarcoma in adults. J Oncol Pract. 2016; 12(3):208–216

[68] Benjamin RS, Patel SR. Pediatric and adult osteosarcoma: comparisons and contrasts in presentation and therapy. Cancer Treat Res. 2009; 152:355–363

[69] Ferrari A, Dileo P, Casanova M, et al. Rhabdomyosarcoma in adults: a retrospective analysis of 171 patients treated at a single institution. Cancer. 2003; 98(3):571–580

[70] Stout AP, Murray MR. Hemangiopericytoma: a vascular tumor featuring Zimmermann's pericytes. Ann Surg. 1942; 116(1):26–33

[71] Stout AP. Hemangiopericytoma: a study of 25 cases. Cancer. 1949; 2(6):1027–1054

[72] Batsakis JG, Rice DH. The pathology of head and neck tumors: vasoformative tumors, part 9B. Head Neck Surg. 1981; 3(4):326–339

[73] McMaster MJ, Soule EH, Ivins JC. Hemangiopericytoma: a clinicopathologic study and long-term followup of 60 patients. Cancer. 1975; 36(6):2232–2244

[74] Soyuer S, Chang EL, Selek U, McCutcheon IE, Maor MH. Intracranial meningeal hemangiopericytoma: the role of radiotherapy: report of 29 cases and review of the literature. Cancer. 2004; 100(7):1491–1497

[75] Dufour H, Métellus P, Fuentes S, et al. Meningeal hemangiopericytoma: a retrospective study of 21 patients with special review of postoperative external radiotherapy. Neurosurgery. 2001; 48(4):756–762, discussion 762–763

[76] Combs SE, Thilmann C, Debus J, Schulz-Ertner D. Precision radiotherapy for hemangiopericytomas of the central nervous system. Cancer. 2005; 104(11):2457–2465

[77] Olson C, Yen CP, Schlesinger D, Sheehan J. Radiosurgery for intracranial hemangiopericytomas: outcomes after initial and repeat Gamma Knife surgery. J Neurosurg. 2010; 112(1):133–139

[78] Park MS, Patel SR, Ludwig JA, et al. Activity of temozolomide and bevacizumab in the treatment of locally advanced, recurrent, and metastatic hemangiopericytoma and malignant solitary fibrous tumor. Cancer. 2011; 117(21):4939–4947

[79] Beadle GF, Hillcoat BL. Treatment of advanced malignant hemangiopericytoma with combination Adriamycin and DTIC: a report of four cases. J Surg Oncol. 1983; 22(3):167–170

[80] Galanis E, Buckner JC, Scheithauer BW, Kimmel DW, Schomberg PJ, Piepgras DG. Management of recurrent meningeal hemangiopericytoma. Cancer. 1998; 82(10):1915–1920

[81] Wong PP, Yagoda A. Chemotherapy of malignant hemangiopericytoma. Cancer. 1978; 41(4):1256–1260

[82] Gutierrez JC, Perez EA, Moffat FL, Livingstone AS, Franceschi D, Koniaris LG. Should soft tissue sarcomas be treated at high-volume centers? An analysis of 4205 patients. Ann Surg. 2007; 245(6):952–958

34 Angiofibromas and Other Vascular Tumors of the Skull Base

Soma Subramaniam and Ricardo L. Carrau

Summary

Vascular tumors are a relatively rare entity in head and neck neoplasms. Angiofibromas account for most of these tumors. A summary of current staging systems is given. Management of angiofibroma is primarily endoscopic endonasal surgical resection, with preoperative embolization in most cases. The endonasal endoscopic transpterygoid approach is a useful technique in this scenario. The role of hormonal and targeted therapy is currently mainly adjuvant and requires further evaluation. A brief discussion of other vascular tumors is also provided.

Keywords: vascular tumor, angiofibroma, glomangiopericytoma, angiosarcoma, endonasal endoscopic transpterygoid approach, EETA, vascular endothelial growth factor, VEGF, mammalian target of rapamycin, mTOR, embolization

34.1 Introduction

Vascular tumors of the skull base, primarily angiofibromas, pose a significant surgical challenge because of their anatomical position, potential for expansion and bony destruction, and potential for significant perioperative bleeding. Methodical and systematic planning, exercising of sound surgical principles and technique, and provision of comprehensive perioperative care can help in surmounting these drawbacks. Angiofibroma is the most commonly encountered vascular tumor in this region. "Juvenile nasopharyngeal angiofibroma"[1] should be considered a misnomer, as it neither exclusively occurs in the juvenile age group nor truly arises from the nasopharynx.

The gross tumor specimen appearance can range from small and smooth to large and multilobulated, with color anywhere from light tan to reddish/purple. Erosions and ulcerations can be commonly seen on the surface of this tumor, if large. Histologically, it consists of two components: fibrous stroma and vascular spaces. The fibrous stroma is composed of spindle-shaped cells in a dense collagen matrix. Within this dense matrix is a vast network of irregular vascular channels of variable size. These endothelial-lined spaces lack the surrounding smooth muscle that is normally seen in blood vessels, which is the likely cause for the significant hemorrhage that occurs following manipulation.

The most common presentation of a sinonasal angiofibroma includes painless nasal obstruction, recurrent unilateral epistaxis, and a sinonasal or nasopharyngeal mass. The epicenter of the tumor origin is the lateral basisphenoid, between the sphenoid sinus and pterygopalatine fossa, in the region of the sphenopalatine foramen.[2,3] From its site of origin, it expands and erodes surrounding bone, taking the path of least resistance. It preferentially follows preformed pathways, medially to the nasal cavity, nasopharynx, and sphenoid sinus; laterally to the pterygopalatine fossa, gaining further access to the infratemporal fossa, as well as to the orbit via the inferior orbital fissure;

anteromedially into the maxillary and ethmoid sinus; and posteriorly/superiorly along the foramina of the vidian canal and foramen rotundum toward middle cranial fossa. Direct extension intracranially is also possible, eroding through the cribriform plate, fovea ethmoidalis, and planum sphenoidale.[4]

Other vascular tumors of the head and neck region include hemangioma, tufted angioma, glomangiopericytoma, angiosarcoma, and vascular polyps. Hemangioma, which usually presents in the infantile period, primarily affects the upper airway (subglottis of larynx), sinonasal tract, and nasal dorsum and has not been reported to originate in the skull base region. Similarly, tufted angioma and acquired lobular capillary hemangioma (pyogenic granuloma) affect primarily the cutaneous regions and anterior nasal cavity and do not generally originate in the skull base. Later in this chapter, we describe glomangiopericytoma (a distinct form of hemangiopericytoma) and angiosarcoma, two entities that have a predilection for the skull base.

34.2 Incidence and Epidemiology

Angiofibroma is a rare tumor, accounting for less than 0.5% of all head and neck neoplasms. A national study from Denmark noted an incidence per year of 3.7 cases per million males aged 10 to 24 years between 1981 and 2003.[5] It occurs mostly in adolescent males aged between 11 and young adulthood, although there have been reports of cases ranging from 6 years to 43 years, confirmed by histology.[6] In a recent systematic review, the mean age of presentation was 17.2 years.[7] There have been reports of this disease occurring in women, but these are rare instances and probably represent misreporting of other types of fibrovascular tumors rather than true angiofibromas. The data seem skewed toward larger case series from more populous countries, such as India and China, but the evidence does not suggest that angiofibroma exclusively involves any one ethnic group.[8]

34.3 Pathology

34.3.1 Angiofibroma

The pathological classification and etiology of angiofibromas have historically been points of disagreement and confusion among researchers owing to their relative rarity and unique morphology, as well as uncertainty about their etiology. Histologically, they consist of abundant fibroblastic stroma within which are embedded vascular channels of various sizes, ranging from capillaries to sinuses.[9] Clinically, angiofibromas exhibit locally aggressive characteristics. Angiofibroma has been variously described as hemangioma, vascular malformation,[10] hyperplastic lesion in response to inflammatory or allergic stimulus, excessive growth of paraganglionic tissue,[11] hamartoma,[12] and even extracolonic manifestation of familial adenomatous polyposis.[13] However, controversy remains over whether angiofibroma represents a hemangioma/vascular tumor or a vascular malformation.

As far back as 1982, Glowacki and Mulliken[14] published a histology-based classification of vascular lesions, essentially dividing this vast group of conditions into two groups—hemangiomas or vascular malformations. The key differentiating factor was histological evidence of increased mitotic activity and endothelial proliferation resulting in hyperplasia in the former, but no such proliferative activity, with normal mitotic activity, in the latter. In the modern era of immunohistochemical techniques for differentiating cell lines, the ability to detect proliferative markers with the aid of monoclonal antibodies has helped clarify this matter.

In vascular lesions, such as angiofibroma, markers for angiogenic stimulation would be the best indicators of vascular proliferation. These include VEGF (vascular endothelial growth factor), VEGFR or Flt-1/Flk-1 (vascular endothelial growth factor receptor), and CD34 antigen, as well as other associated proliferative indicators, such as FGF (fibroblast growth factor) and PCNA (proliferating cell nuclear antigen).[15] Multiple studies have confirmed that VEGF is the most prominent proangiogenic marker of this group.[16,17]

In 1994, Takahashi and colleagues found that FGF and VEGF protein levels were elevated in hemangiomas. By contrast, vascular malformations did not express bFGF and VEGF.[18] In 2006, Saylam and colleagues analyzed the VEGF immunoreactivity of 27 angiofibroma samples and concluded that Juvenile nasopharyngeal angiofibroma (JNA) was a vascular and proliferative tumor.[19] More recently, Zhang and colleagues[20] identified immunoreactivity of CD34 in both JNA and OCH (orbital cavernous hemangioma, also a misnomer, as histologically it has been better characterized as a vascular malformation). However, the CD34 immunostaining was significantly higher in JNA than in OCH. Such findings support the view that JNA has a characteristic of vasoproliferative activity, more consistent with a vascular tumor than with vascular malformation.

Another area of dispute is whether the neoplastic component of the tumor arises from the vascular component or from the fibroblastic stroma. Proponents of the vascular component theory suggest that incomplete regression of the first branchial arch artery results in the persistence of a residual vascular network in the region of the sphenopalatine foramen, which under the influence of hormonal surges in the periadolescent period results in tumor growth.[21] However, immunohistochemical studies have not consistently confirmed the relationship of positive hormone receptor status (e.g., androgen, estrogen, progesterone) within these tumors.[19,22,23] Conversely, increasing evidence suggests that the fibroblastic stroma is instead the focus of the neoplastic transformation. This is suggested by the immunohistochemical localization of beta-catenin only to the nuclei of stromal cells rather than to endothelial cells.[24]

Of interest, angiofibromas have been reported to occur up to 25 times more frequently among patients who have familial adenomatous polyposis. This finding suggests that alterations of the adenomatous polyposis coli (APC)/beta-catenin pathway may be involved in the pathogenesis of angiofibroma.[13,25]

34.3.2 Other Vascular Tumors

Glomangiopericytoma

Glomangiopericytoma (GPC), previously categorized as a sinonasal variant of hemangiopericytoma, is now considered a distinct tumor type under the 2005 World Health Organization classification of head and neck tumors.[26] The unencapsulated tumor is present beneath an intact respiratory epithelium, unless it has eroded through. The characteristic appearance is that of a "patternless" diffuse architecture, which may efface or surround normal tissue. The pattern of arrangement of the cells includes short fascicles, reticular pattern, or short palisades of closely packed cells. These cells are separated by a rich vasculature ranging from capillaries to large patulous spaces, giving the characteristic "staghorn" or "antlerlike" configuration. Other features include low mitotic activity (< 3/hpf), with absent to mild nuclear pleomorphism, mast cells, eosinophils, and extravasated erythrocytes. Necrosis and atypical mitoses are typically absent.[27]

The immunohistochemistry profile of GPCs includes reactivity with smooth muscle actin (SMA), nuclear b-catenin, cyclin-D, vimentin, and factor XIIIA (strong and diffuse reaction for the first of these three). It lacks expression of CD34, CD31, FVIII-R Ag, CD117, STAT6, bcl-2, AE1/AE3, CK7, EMA, desmin, S100 protein, GFAP, CD68, CD99, and NSE.

GPCs are a rare entity, accounting for less than 0.5% of all tumors in the sinonasal and skull region.[28] Several hundred cases have been reported in the literature, the majority of which have arisen within the nasal cavity and inferior/middle turbinates. The sinuses and skull base/intracranial extension have been involved less frequently. In an Armed Forces Institute of Pathology (AFIP) review of 104 GPC tumors, age at presentation was 5 to 86 years, with a mean of 62 years and approximate equal distribution of males/females.[28] Presenting symptoms include nasal obstruction and epistaxis, as well as rhinorrhea, facial pain, and infraorbital region numbness. Gross tumor appearance is polypoid, nontranslucent, beefy red to grayish pink, soft, edematous, and fleshy to friable in texture.

Treatment of GPCs is primarily surgery, even in the case of recurrences. Large case series have alluded to excellent 5-year survival of 90%[29,30] when complete surgical resection of the tumor has been achieved. Radiation treatment is generally reserved for unresectable disease.

Angiosarcoma

Angiosarcoma is a rare, high-grade malignant vascular tumor that accounts for less than 0.1% of all sinonasal malignancies and for 2% of all sarcoma.[31] In 10 cases of sinonasal tract angiosarcomas from AFIP, with age ranging from 13 to 81 years and almost equal male/female involvement, 8 arose from the nasal cavity and 2 from the maxillary sinus. The gross appearance of the tumor is vascular, generally purple to red, soft and friable, and it is often ulcerated with associated hemorrhage and necrosis. Microscopy reveals anastomosing vascular channels that appear tortuous and irregular, with small to large cavernous spaces. The endothelial cells are atypical, exhibiting pleomorphic nuclei with irregular nuclear contours and mitotic figures. Immunohistochemistry is characterized by immunoreactivity with Factor VIII-RA, CD34, CD31, and SMA but is nonreactive with keratin and S-100 protein. Ki67 is usually reactive (> 10%).[32]

Clinical presentation includes epistaxis, nasal obstruction, and nasal discharge. Treatment involves surgical resection, with possible adjuvant radiation and chemotherapy. Local recurrence following surgical resection occurs in more than 50% of cases and is the most common pattern of treatment failure. The majority of recurrences become apparent within 2 years of initial treatment. Regional metastases are less common, occurring in less than 20% of cases in most large series. Cervical lymph node metastases are more common in lesions arising from the scalp, and regional lymph node dissection is recommended in patients who have scalp lesions or palpable lymphadenopathy. Distant metastases occur in 30 to 50% of cases, with the lungs and liver most frequently involved. The overall 5-year survival for sinonasal angiosarcoma is generally poor, ranging from 12 to 33%.[33]

Traditional chemotherapy regimens have not been established but have included a combination of ifosfamide, paclitaxel, and doxorubicin for soft tissue sarcomas.[34] Bevacizumab, a humanized monoclonal antibody against VEGF, has shown some promise in helping to control inoperable cases of angiosarcomas of the head and neck in a few case reports.

34.4 Staging

For angiofibroma, imaging studies play a determining role in its diagnosis and staging. The anatomical detail that can be obtained from modern imaging has obviated the need to biopsy these lesions, thereby avoiding serious or catastrophic bleeding in the office. Biopsies are usually sent from the operating room after embolization. A combination of CT (provides bony anatomical detail) with MRI (provides good soft tissue detail, differentiates tumor from secretions, and is particularly useful for suspected orbital or intracranial extension) ascertains the extent of tumor spread.

Historically, several staging systems have been described for angiofibromas. The Andrews[35] and Radkowski[36] systems (largely based on the Sessions[37] system described 15 years earlier) have been the most widely used, as evidenced in a systematic review on this subject.[7] Other systems have been described, including the Fisch,[38] Chandler,[39] and Onerci[40] systems. Earlier systems did not consider the radiological features of modern imaging techniques and so have limited use. More recently, Snyderman and colleagues published the UPMC (University of Pittsburgh Medical Center) staging system.[41] This system considers the presence or absence of residual vascularity after embolization, indicating the possible recruitment of vessels beyond the internal maxillary artery, including the internal carotid artery or bilateral blood supply. In general, we prefer the Andrews and UPMC systems to stage angiofibroma. A summary of these staging systems is offered in ▶ Table 34.1.

Staging for angiosarcoma does not follow the American Joint Committee on Cancer (AJCC) system, which is applied to other soft tissue sarcomas. At present, there is no accepted staging for sinonasal angiosarcoma, although lymph node and distant metastasis is not common at initial presentation. Similarly, although a grading system of grades I through III is used in soft

Table 34.1 Angiofibroma staging systems

	Sessions 1981	Chandler 1984	Andrews 1989	Radkowski 1996	Onerci 2006	Snyderman 2010
Stage I	1a Limited to nose and NP 1b Extension into 1 or more sinuses	Limited to NP	Limited to NP, bone destruction negligible or limited to PPF	= Sessions	Nose, NP, ethmoid and sphenoid sinuses or minimal extension into PPF	Nasal cavity, medial PPF
Stage II	2a Minimal extension into PPF 2b Full occupation of PPF with or without erosion of orbit 2c ITF with or without cheek extension	Extension into nasal cavity or sphenoid sinus	Invading PPF or maxillary, ethmoid, or sphenoid sinus with bone destruction	= Sessions (IIC posterior to pterygoid plates)	Maxillary sinus, full occupation of PPF, extension to anterior cranial fossa, limited extension into ITF	Paranasal sinuses, lateral PPF; no residual vascularity
Stage III	IC extension	Tumor into antrum, ethmoid sinus, PPF, ITF, orbit, and/or cheek	**Invading ITF/orbit** IIIa No IC involvement IIIb With IC extradural (parasellar) involvement	Erosion of skull base: IIIa Minimal intracranial extension IIIb Extensive IC extension with/without cavernous sinus	Deep extension into cancellous bone at pterygoid base or body and GW sphenoid, significant lateral extension into ITF or pterygoid plates, orbital, cavernous sinus obliteration	Skull base erosion, orbit, ITF; no residual vascularity
Stage IV	N/A	IC extension	**Intracranial, intradural tumor** IVa Without cavernous sinus, pituitary, or optic chiasm infiltration IVb With cavernous sinus, pituitary, or optic chiasm infiltration	N/A	IC extension between pituitary gland and ICA, tumor localization lateral to ICA, middle fossa extension, and extensive IC extension	IV: Skull base erosion, orbit, ITF; **residual vascularity** V: IC extension, **residual vascularity** (M: medial extension, L: lateral extension)

Abbreviations: GW, greater wing; IC, intracranial; ITF, infratemporal fossa; NP, nasopharynx; PPF, pterygopalatine fossa.

tissue angiosarcoma, this system has not been applied to sino-nasal angiosarcoma. Grading has not yet been proven to have a clinical prognostic significance in sinonasal tract angiosarcomas, although further evaluation with a larger number of cases has been suggested.[42]

34.5 Treatment

34.5.1 Surgery

The mainstay treatment of angiofibromas and most other vascular tumors is surgery, but age, symptoms, and expected prognosis also influence the decision, especially for benign tumors. Surgical approaches for angiofibroma resection can be broadly classified into external and endonasal endoscopic approaches. External approaches may follow an anterior route, via midfacial degloving/endonasal, transantral, Denker's approach, or LeFort I or via Weber-Ferguson type incision, or a lateral route, via an infratemporal approach,[43] with or without a craniotomy (for cases of significant intracranial invasion). Inferior transpalatal approaches have also been described but have mostly fallen into disuse. Small tumors may be exposed and removed by removing the ipsilateral hard palate after raising the mucoperiosteum in a U-shaped fashion; however, these tumors are amenable to an endoscopic resection, which is associated with fewer sequelae and complications. Removal via transpalatal approaches that divide the soft palate were abandoned due to poor visualization of the tumor, association with significant blood loss, and negative effect on speech quality secondary to soft palate fibrosis and scarring. To determine the best surgical approach, one must consider multiple factors related to tumor (stage), patient, and surgeon/institution.

The endonasal endoscopic approach has become the preferred option to resect these tumors today in view of the better visualization, lower morbidity, lack of external scars, and lower level of blood loss. Nonetheless, although many of these tumors can in principle be resected via an endonasal endoscopic approach, whether they can be in practice depends on the level of expertise and resources available at a given institution. Most authors agree that patients whose tumors correspond with up to Andrews stage IIIa are candidates for an endoscopic endonasal approach. However, endoscopic approaches have also been described for resecting stage IIIb tumors (intracranial, extradural extension).[44] ▶ Table 34.2 summarizes the literature regarding endoscopic removal of angiofibromas over the past 15 years, analyzing the stage of tumor resected, rates of persistent/recurrent disease, and operative blood loss. Excluded from analysis were case series involving fewer than 10 patients, those in which tumor stage was not provided, and those involving inadequate or absent follow-up data.

The Endonasal Endoscopic Transpterygoid Approach

The endonasal endoscopic transpterygoid approach (EETA) is the initial surgical gateway that allows access to a variety of lateral and posterior surgical targets, including the infratemporal fossa (ITF), lateral nasopharynx (fossa of Rosenmuller), middle cranial fossa/Meckel's cave, cavernous sinus, petrous internal carotid artery (ICA), and foramen lacerum. We define the transpterygoid approach as one that requires either partial or complete resection of the pterygoid plates process. Its technical nuances have been previously described.[33] For a better understanding of its various modification and indications, the EETA (▶ Fig. 34.1)[45] has recently been classified into zones A–E, which match the extent of the transpterygoid dissection required by the surgical target (▶ Table 34.3).[46]

The most pertinent EETA types to this discussion are type D (partial or complete removal of the pterygoid plates and dissection of the petrous ICA), which is used for lesions requiring access to the infratemporal fossa and control of the petrous ICA, and type E (involving the removal of Eustachian tube in addition to the dissection involved in type D), which is used when access to the lateral nasopharynx is required.

Tumors that extend beyond Andrews stage IIIa (generally considered advanced-stage) may require staging the tumor resection. This may involve partial resection followed by a completion endonasal surgery at a later time or combination of an endonasal endoscopic approach with an external approach.

34.5.2 Radiation Therapy

Radiotherapy should not be considered as a first line of treatment for angiofibroma unless surgery is contraindicated. Secondary malignant transformation several decades post irradiation is a real and significant risk for young individuals.[47,48] In addition, radiation treatment can be associated with significant side effects or complications, which affect surrounding bone (osteoradionecrosis, growth impairment), brain (temporal lobe necrosis), and eyes (keratopathy and cataracts) as well as pituitary dysfunction (ranging from stunting of growth to panhypopituitarism).[49] In addition, radiation therapy rarely induces a complete tumor regression, but in other situations it may result in shrinkage of the tumor, which takes several years, with eventual tumor regrowth.[39] Historically, several groups reported on the use of primary radiotherapy as a single modality of treatment, largely seeking to avoid the risk of catastrophic bleeding during surgery.[50,51] However, with the availability of modern imaging and surgical tools and expertise, these risks have been minimized, making surgery the most viable and effective treatment option for many angiofibromas.

34.5.3 Medical Therapy

Chemotherapy

Evidence for the effectiveness chemotherapy is very limited and lacks results from randomized controlled trials. Attempts to treat angiofibroma using chemotherapy have been limited to a small series of patients who had advanced, recurrent, or inoperable tumors. In a study of five patients who had recurrent disease, use of combinations of doxorubicin, vincristine, dactinomycin, and cyclophosphamide produced a complete tumor response, with no further recurrence.[52] In another study, one patient who had advanced and unresectable disease underwent palliative treatment with Adriamycin and dacarbazine that yielded a partial response.[53]

Table 34.2 Endoscopic endonasal approach outcomes for sinonasal angiofibroma

Publication (year)	n	Staging system	Tumor stage	Mean follow-up (range, months)	Recurrent/residual disease	Cx	Blood loss (mean)
Jorrisen (2000)[a]	13	Radkowski/ Chandler/ Andrews/ Sessions	4 stage IA–IB 4 stage IIA–IIB 4 stage IIC 1 stage IIIA	35.3 (12–72)	1 for stage IIC after 6 mo (7.7%) 1 for stage IIIA after 4 mo (7.7%)	nil	NR
Roger (2002)[b]	20	Radkowski	4 stage I 7 stage II 9 stage IIIA	22	2 for stage IIIA (10%)	nil	350
Onerci (2003)[c]	12	Radkowski	8 stage IIC 4 stage III	6	2 for stage IIIA (16.7%)	nil	1,000
Nicolai (2003)[d]	15	Andrews	2 stage I 9 stage II 3 stage IIIA 1 stage IIIB	50 (24–93)	1 (6.7%)	nil	372
Hofmann (2005)[e]	21	Andrews	1 stage I 15 stage II 5 stage IIIa	51.7 (5–120)	3 (14.3%)	nil	225
Borghei (2006)[f]	23	Radkowski	14 stage IA–IB 9 stage IIA–IIB	33.1 (14–57)	1 for stage IIB (4.3%)	3 (synechiae)	450–1,600 (881)
Andrade (2007)[g]	12	Andrews	8 stage I 4 stage II	35 (12–60)	0	nil	200
Gupta (2008)[h]	28	Radkowski	6 stage I 20 stage IIA–IIB 2 stage IIC	(12–65)	1 (stage IIC)	1 intraop IMA bleed	168/360 (with/ without preop embolization)
Huang (2009)[i]	19	Radkowski	3 stage I 11 stage IIA–IIB 5 stage IIIA	34 (3–108)	0	nil	NR
Bleier (2009)[j]	10	Andrews	1 stage I 8 stage II 1 stage IIIA	24.4 (3.6–88.4)	0	nil	506
Midilli (2009)[k]	12	Radkowski	2 stage I 9 stage II 1 stage IIIA	92 (12–251)	0	NR	NR
Hackman (2009)[l]	15	Radkowski	4 stage I 6 stage II 5 stage IIIA–IIIB	480 (12–120)	0	1 retro-orbital bleed	280
Nicolai (2010)[m]	46	Onerci/ Andrews	5 stage I 24 stage II 17 stage III	73 (9–172)	4 (8.7%)	0	250–1,300 (580)
Ardehali (2010)[n]	47	Radkowski	21 stage IA–IIB 22 stage IIC 3 stage IIIA 1 stage IIIB	33.1 (8–74)	9	2 rupture of cavernous sinus, no mortality	770 (preop embolization) 1,402.6 (no preop embolization)
Frympas (2011)[o]	10	Radkowski	3 stage I 5 stage II 2 stage IIIA	23.7 (3–70)	1	1 (infraorbital nv hypoesthesia)	200–800 (444)
Lopez (2012)[p]	11	Andrews	1 stage I 10 stage II	96	0	nil	895
Martins (2013)[q]	17	Fisch	stage I & II	84	0	nil	300
El Sharkawy (2013)[r]	18	Radkowski	13 stage IA–IB 5 stage IIA	37.4 (14–72)	2	nil	342
Huang (2014)[s]	66	Radkowski	9 stage IA–IB 17 stage IIA–IIB 24 stage IIC 16 stage IIIA–IIIB	55 (6–182)	17 (28.3%) (all stage IIB or greater)	nil	800

Table 34.2 (Continued)

Publication (year)	n	Staging system	Tumor stage	Mean follow-up (range, months)	Recurrent/residual disease	Cx	Blood loss (mean)
Kopec (2014)[t]	10	Radkowski	8 stage IA–IB 2 stage IIA–IIB	42 (6–84)	1	nil	160
Janakiram (2016)[u]	15	Radkowski	15 stage IIA	12	3	nil	67.2

Abbreviations: Cx, complication; NR, not reported.

[a] Jorissen M, Eloy P, Rombaux P, Bachert C, Daele J. Endoscopic sinus surgery for juvenile nasopharyngeal angiofibroma. Acta Oto-rhino-laryngologica Belgica. 2000;54(2):201–219

[b] Roger G, Tran Ba Huy P, Froehlich P, et al. Exclusively Endoscopic Removal of Juvenile Nasopharyngeal Angiofibroma: Trends and Limits. Arch Otolaryngol Head Neck Surg. 2002;128(8):928–935.

[c] Onerci TM, Yücel OT, Oğretmenoğlu O. Endoscopic surgery in treatment of juvenile nasopharyngeal angiofibroma. Int J PediatrOtorhinolaryngol;67(2003):1219–1225

[d] Nicolai P, Berlucchi M, Tomenzoli D, et al. Endoscopic surgery for juvenile angiofibroma: when and how. The laryngoscope. 2003;113:775–782

[e] Hofmann T, Bernal-Sprekelsen M, Koele W, Reittner P, Klein E, Stammberger H. Endoscopic resection of juvenile angiofibromas—long term results. Rhinology. 2005;43:282–289

[f] Borghei P, Baradaranfar MH, Borghei SH, Sokhandon F. Transnasal endoscopic resection of juvenile nasopharyngeal angiofibroma without preoperative embolization. Ear, Nose & Throat Journal. 2006;85(11):740–746

[g] Andrade NA, Pinto JA, Nóbrega Mde O, Aguiar JE, Aguiar TF, Vinhaes ES. Exclusively endoscopic surgery for juvenile nasopharyngeal angiofibroma. Otolaryngol Head Neck Surg 2007;137: 492–496

[h] Gupta AK, Rajiniganth MG. Endoscopic approach to juvenile nasopharyngeal angiofibroma: our experience at a tertiary care centre. The Journal of laryngology and otology. 2008;122(11):1185–1189

[i] Huang J, Sacks R, Forer M Endoscopic resection of juvenile nasopharyngeal angiofibroma. Ann Otol Rhinol laryngo. 2009;118:764–768

[j] Bleier BS, Kennedy DW, Palmer JN, Chiu AG, Bloom JD, O'Malley BW. Current management of juvenile nasopharyngeal angiofibroma: a tertiary center experience 1999–2007. American Journal of Rhinology & Allergy 2007;23:328–330

[k] Midilli R, Karcı B, Akyildiz S. Juvenile nasopharyngeal angiofibroma: analysis of 42 cases and important aspects of endoscopic approach. International journal of pediatric otorhinolaryngology 2009;73(3):401–408

[l] Hackman T, Snyderman CH, Carrau R, Vescan A, Kassam A. Juvenile nasopharyngeal angiofibroma: The expanded endonasal approach. Am J Rhinol Allergy. 2009;23(1):95–99

[m] Nicolai P, Villaret AB, Farina D, et al. Endoscopic surgery for juvenile angiofibroma: a critical review of indications after 46 cases. Am J Rhinol Allergy. 2010;24(2):e67–e72

[n] Ardehali MM, Samimi Ardestani SH, Yazdani N, Goodarzi H, Bastaninejad S. Endoscopic approach for excision of juvenile nasopharyngeal angiofibroma: complications and outcomes. Am J Otolaryngol. 2010 Sep-Oct;31(5):343–349

[o] Fyrmpas G, Konstantinidis I, Constantinidis J. Endoscopic treatment of juvenile nasopharyngeal angiofibromas: our experience and review of the literature. Eur Arch Otorhinolaryngol. 2012;269(2):523–529

[p] López F, Suárez V, Costales M, Suárez C, Llorente JL. Treatment of juvenile angiofibromas: 18-year experience of a single tertiary centre in Spain. Rhinology 2012;50:95–103

[q] Martins MB, de Lima FV, Mendonça, de Jesus EP, Santos AC, Barreto VM, Santos RC Júnior. Nasopharyngeal angiofibroma: Our experience and literature review. Int Arch Otorhinolaryngol. 2013 Jan;17(1):14–19

[r] El Sharkawy AA. Endonasal endoscopic management of juvenile nasopharyngeal angiofibroma without angiographic embolization. Eur Arch Otorhinolaryngol. 2013 Jul;270(7):2051–2055

[s] Huang Y, Liu Z, Wang J, Sun X, Yang L, Wang D. Surgical management of juvenile nasopharyngeal angiofibroma: analysis of 162 cases from 1995 to 2012. Laryngoscope. 2014;124(8):1942–1946

[t] Kopeć T, Borucki Ł, Szyfter W (2014) fully endoscopic resection of juvenile nasopharyngeal angiofibroma own experience and clinical outcomes. Int J Pediatr Otorhinolaryngol 78: 1015–1018

[u] Janakiram TN, Sharma SB, Panicker VB. Endoscopic Excision of Non-embolized Juvenile Nasopharyngeal Angiofibroma: Our Technique. Indian J Otolaryngol Head Neck Surg. 2016 Sep;68(3):263–269

Antiandrogen Therapy and Other Hormonal Therapy

Considering that angiofibromas occur exclusively in adolescent males, there has been significant interest in understanding the hormonal role of testosterone and dihydrotesterone receptors in the pathogenesis of this disease. Immunohistochemical studies have demonstrated the presence of androgen receptors on angiofibroma specimens.[54] Following this rational, flutamide, a nonsteroidal androgen antagonist, has been studied by several groups. In some studies, flutamide produced a reduction in the volume of tumor size, but never a complete tumor regression. In one study, five male patients who had Fisch stage I to III lesions were treated preoperatively with 500 mg/day of flutamide for 6 weeks. CT post treatment showed reduction of tumor volume in four patients and increase in one, with an average volume reduction of 29%.[55] In another study involving 20 male patients who had Fisch stage II to IV lesions, a

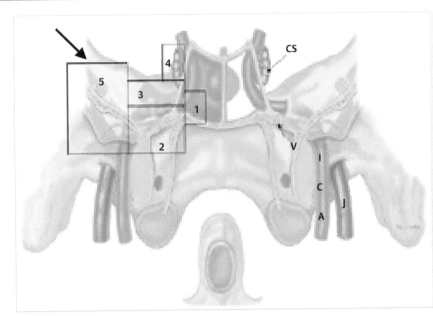

Fig. 34.1 The middle third of the clivus and petrous bone in the coronal plane. The five modular approaches are shown in the black boxes and relate to the course of the petrous ICA. The infrapetrous approaches consist of the medial petrous apex approach (Zone 1) and the petroclival approach (Zone 2). The suprapetrous approaches consist of the quadrangular space approach (Zone 3), superior cavernous sinus approach (Zone 4), and the transpterygoid/infratemporal approach (*black arrow*). The cavernous sinus (CS) is seen above, and the vidian canal (V) leading to the ICA is also demonstrated. Jugular vein (J). (Reproduced with permission from Kassam AB, Gardner P, Snyderman C, et al, Expanded endonasal approach: fully endoscopic, completely transnasal approach to the middle third of the clivus, petrous bone, middle cranial fossa, and infratemporal fossa, Neurosurgery Focus 2005;19:E6.)

Table 34.3 Endonasal endoscopic transpterygoid approaches

EETA	Region removed	Approach to
A	Partial removal (thinning) of pterygoid process	Pterygopalatine fossa (extended)
B	Anterior aspect of the base of the pterygoid process	Lateral recess of the sphenoid sinus
C	Base of the pterygoid process with dissection of vidian canal	Petrous apex/Meckel's cave
D	Partial or complete removal of the pterygoid plates with dissection of the petrous ICA	Extensive lesion requiring access to the infratemporal fossa and control of the petrous carotid artery
E	Partial or complete removal of the pterygoid plates with dissection of the petrous ICA and removal of the Eustachian tube	Nasopharyngeal malignancies, extensive tumors of the middle and posterior skull base (e.g., chordoma)

Abbreviations: ICA, internal carotid artery.
Source: Reproduced with permission from Kasemsiri P, Solares CA, Carrau RL, et al, Endoscopic endonasal transpterygoid approaches: anatomical landmarks for planning the surgical corridor, Laryngoscope 2013;123:811–815.

similar 6-week course of flutamide was completed and tumor volume was assessed by MRI. Prepubertal patients had a mean reduction of 2.3%, but two patients had significant increase in size. Conversely, postpubertal patients had a mean volume reduction of 16.5%, which was statistically significant. Three patients who had tumor recurrence showed reductions in tumor volume of 7%, 12%, and 18%.[56] These studies suggest that flutamide is not a curative treatment option but that it may have a role as an adjuvant treatment for control of tumor growth after surgical treatment or in nonoperable cases, particularly in postpubertal patients.

Antiestrogen tamoxifen has also been investigated, obtaining some tumor response. However, significant side effects are associated with its use that make it unsuitable for treatment of adolescent male patients.

Targeted Therapy, Beta-Blockers

As already described, most angiofibroma samples have been found to be VEGF-positive. Accordingly, VEGF inhibitors such as bevacizumab have the potential, in principle, to treat angiofibromas.

Another molecular target is the "mammalian target of rapamycin" (mTOR), which acts as the "master" switch that pri-

marily controls vascular growth via PI3 kinase and protein kinase B (PKB or AKT). The mTOR inhibitor sirolimus and its analogues have shown antiangiogenic activity in the treatment of kaposiform hemangioendotheliomas[57] and thus may have some effectiveness for treatment of angiofibroma.

Beta-blockers have been effectively used in the treatment of infantile hemangiomas, where it has been shown to reduce the expression of VEGF and induces apoptosis through the blockade of beta-1-adrenoceptors.[46] Its effect on angiofibroma control needs to be investigated.

34.6 Outcome and Prognosis

▶ Table 34.2 includes a list of major case series published since the year 2000, showing rates of complication and recurrence rates as well as other parameters. A direct comparison between the endonasal, endoscopic approach and the traditional external approaches is inherently flawed, being skewed as a result of a strong selection bias that entails choosing lower-stage tumors for the former but more advanced-stage lesions for the latter. However, when comparing series in which the endoscopic endonasal approach was performed for advanced-stage tumors with those using external approaches, the outcomes are at least comparable in terms of safety as well as rate of tumor recurrence. Accordingly, these findings and their added benefits of cosmesis preservation and better tumor visualization favor a shift toward use of the endonasal endoscopic approach for adequately selected patients.

34.7 Conclusion

Understandings of the genetics and etiology of JNA remain patchy and incomplete. Specific molecular targets for tumor growth will allow treatment of these vascular tumors more effectively while avoiding the morbidity associated with current treatments, including surgery. In the meantime, the endonasal endoscopic approach allows the resection of most tumors while avoiding facial incisions, offering improved visualization, decreased blood loss, shorter hospital stay, and superior cost-effectiveness.

References

[1] Chaveau C. Histoire des maladies du pharynx. Paris: Barriere; 1906

[2] Scholtz AW, Appenroth E, Kammen-Jolly K, Scholtz LU, Thumfart WF. Juvenile nasopharyngeal angiofibroma: management and therapy. Laryngoscope. 2001; 111(4 Pt 1):681–687

[3] Paris J, Guelfucci B, Moulin G, Zanaret M, Triglia JM. Diagnosis and treatment of juvenile nasopharyngeal angiofibroma. Eur Arch Otorhinolaryngol. 2001; 258(3):120–124

[4] Gupta AC, Murthy DP. Intracranial juvenile nasopharyngeal angiofibroma. Aust N Z J Surg. 1997; 67(7):477–482

[5] Glad H, Vainer B, Buchwald C, et al. Juvenile nasopharyngeal angiofibromas in Denmark 1981–2003: diagnosis, incidence, and treatment. Acta Otolaryngol. 2007; 127(3):292–299

[6] Lund V, Howard D, Wei W, et al. Chapter 9: Vasoform neoplasms and other lesions. In: Tumors of the Nose, Sinuses and the Nasopharynx. Thieme Book; 2014

[7] Boghani Z, Husain Q, Kanumuri VV, et al. Juvenile nasopharyngeal angiofibroma: a systematic review and comparison of endoscopic, endoscopic-assisted, and open resection in 1047 cases. Laryngoscope. 2013; 123(4):859–869

[8] Huang Y, Liu Z, Wang J, Sun X, Yang L, Wang D. Surgical management of juvenile nasopharyngeal angiofibroma: analysis of 162 cases from 1995 to 2012. Laryngoscope. 2014; 124(8):1942–1946

[9] Beham A, Fletcher CD, Kainz J, Schmid C, Humer U. Nasopharyngeal angiofibroma: an immunohistochemical study of 32 cases. Virchows Arch A Pathol Anat. 1993; 423:281–285

[10] Beham A, Beham-Schmid C, Regauer S, Auböck L, Stammberger H. Nasopharyngeal angiofibroma: true neoplasm or vascular malformation? Adv Anat Pathol. 2000; 7(1):36–46

[11] Girgis IH, Fahmy SA. Nasopharyngeal fibroma: its histo-pathological nature. J Laryngol Otol. 1973; 87(11):1107–1123

[12] Maurice M, Milad M. Pathogenesis of juvenile nasopharyngeal fibroma. (A new concept). J Laryngol Otol. 1981; 95(11):1121–1126

[13] Giardiello FM, Hamilton SR, Krush AJ, Offerhaus JA, Booker SV, Petersen GM. Nasopharyngeal angiofibroma in patients with familial adenomatous polyposis. Gastroenterology. 1993; 105(5):1550–1552

[14] Mulliken JB, Glowacki J. Hemangiomas and vascular malformations in infants and children: a classification based on endothelial characteristics. Plast Reconstr Surg. 1982; 69(3):412–422

[15] Roberts DM, Kearney JB, Johnson JH, Rosenberg MP, Kumar R, Bautch VL. The vascular endothelial growth factor (VEGF) receptor Flt-1 (VEGFR-1) modulates Flk-1 (VEGFR-2) signaling during blood vessel formation. Am J Pathol. 2004; 164(5):1531–1535

[16] Brieger J, Wierzbicka M, Sokolov M, Roth Y, Szyfter W, Mann WJ. Vessel density, proliferation, and immunolocalization of vascular endothelial growth factor in juvenile nasopharyngeal angiofibromas. Arch Otolaryngol Head Neck Surg. 2004; 130(6):727–731

[17] Ngan BY, Forte V, Campisi P. Molecular angiogenic signaling in angiofibromas after embolization: implications for therapy. Arch Otolaryngol Head Neck Surg. 2008; 134(11):1170–1176

[18] Takahashi K, Mulliken JB, Kozakewich HP, Rogers RA, Folkman J, Ezekowitz RA. Cellular markers that distinguish the phases of hemangioma during infancy and childhood. J Clin Invest. 1994; 93(6):2357–2364

[19] Saylam G, Yücel OT, Sungur A, Onerci M. Proliferation, angiogenesis and hormonal markers in juvenile nasopharyngeal angiofibroma. Int J Pediatr Otorhinolaryngol. 2006; 70(2):227–234

[20] Zhang M, Sun X, Yu H, Hu L, Wang D. Biological distinctions between juvenile nasopharyngeal angiofibroma and vascular malformation: an immunohistochemical study. Acta Histochem. 2011; 113(6):626–630

[21] Schick B, Plinkert PK, Prescher A. Aetiology of angiofibromas: reflection on their specific vascular component. Laryngorhinootologie. 2002; 81(4):280–284

[22] Montag AG, Tretiakova M, Richardson M. Steroid hormone receptor expression in nasopharyngeal angiofibromas: consistent expression of estrogen receptor beta. Am J Clin Pathol. 2006; 125(6):832–837

[23] Liu Z, Wang J, Wang H et al. Hormonal receptors and vascular endothelial growth factor in juvenile nasopharyngeal angiofibroma: immunohistochemical and tissue microarray analysis. Acta Otolaryngol. 2015 Jan;135(1):51–57

[24] Abraham SC, Montgomery EA, Giardiello FM, Wu TT. Frequent beta-catenin mutations in juvenile nasopharyngeal angiofibromas. Am J Pathol. 2001; 158 (3):1073–1078

[25] Ferouz AS, Mohr RM, Paul P. Juvenile nasopharyngeal angiofibroma and familial adenomatous polyposis: an association? Otolaryngol Head Neck Surg. 1995; 113(4):435–439

[26] Barnes L, Everson J, Reicchart P, Sidransky D. World Health Organization Classification of Tumors. Lyon: IARC Press; 2005

[27] Thompson LDR, Fanburg-Smith JC. Update on select benign mesenchymal and meningothelial sinonasal tract lesions. Head Neck Pathol. 2016; 10(1):95–108

[28] Thompson LD, Miettinen M, Wenig BM. Sinonasal-type hemangiopericytoma: a clinicopathologic and immunophenotypic analysis of 104 cases showing perivascular myoid differentiation. Am J Surg Pathol. 2003; 27(6):737–749

[29] Catalano PJ, Brandwein M, Shah DK, Urken ML, Lawson W, Biller HF. Sinonasal hemangiopericytomas: a clinicopathologic and immunohistochemical study of seven cases. Head Neck. 1996; 18(1):42–53

[30] Bignami M, Dallan I, Battaglia P, Lenzi R, Pistochini A, Castelnuovo P. Endoscopic, endonasal management of sinonasal haemangiopericytoma: 12-year experience. J Laryngol Otol. 2010; 124(11):1178–1182

[31] Aust MR, Olsen KD, Lewis JE, et al. Angiosarcomas of the head and neck: clinical and pathologic characteristics. Ann Otol Rhinol Laryngol. 1997; 106(11): 943–951

[32] Nelson BL, Thompson LD. Sinonasal tract angiosarcoma: a clinicopathologic and immunophenotypic study of 10 cases with a review of the literature. Head Neck Pathol. 2007; 1(1):1–12

[33] Sturgis EM, Potter BO. Sarcomas of the head and neck region. Curr Opin Oncol. 2003; 15(3):239–252

[34] Yang P, Zhu Q, Jiang F. Combination therapy for scalp angiosarcoma using bevacizumab and chemotherapy: a case report and review of literature. Chin J Cancer Res. 2013; 25(3):358–361

[35] Andrews JC, Fisch U, Valavanis A, Aeppli U, Makek MS. The surgical management of extensive nasopharyngeal angiofibromas with the infratemporal fossa approach. Laryngoscope. 1989; 99(4):429–437

[36] Radkowski D, McGill T, Healy GB, Ohlms L, Jones DT. Angiofibroma: changes in staging and treatment. Arch Otolaryngol Head Neck Surg. 1996; 122(2): 122–129

[37] Sessions RB, Bryan RN, Naclerio RM, Alford BR. Radiographic staging of juvenile angiofibroma. Head Neck Surg. 1981; 3(4):279–283

[38] Fisch U. The infratemporal fossa approach for nasopharyngeal tumors. Laryngoscope. 1983; 93(1):36–44

[39] Chandler JR, Goulding R, Moskowitz L, Quencer RM. Nasopharyngeal angiofibromas: staging and management. Ann Otol Rhinol Laryngol. 1984; 93(4 Pt 1):322–329

[40] Onerci TM, Yücel OT, Oğretmenoğlu O. Endoscopic surgery in treatment of juvenile nasopharyngeal angiofibroma. Int J Pediatr Otorhinolaryngol. 2003; 67 (11):1219–1225

[41] Snyderman CH, Pant H, Carrau RL, Gardner P. A new endoscopic staging system for angiofibromas. Arch Otolaryngol Head Neck Surg. 2010; 136(6): 588–594

[42] Weiss SW, Lasota J, Miettinen MM. Angiosarcoma of soft tissue. In: Fletcher CDM, Unni K, Mertens F, eds. Pathology and Genetics of Tumours of Soft Tissue and Bone, World Health Organization Classification of Tumours. Kleihues P, Sobin LH, series eds. Lyon, France: IARC Press; 2002:175–177

[43] Fisch U, Fagan P, Valavanis A. The infratemporal fossa approach for the lateral skull base. Otolaryngol Clin North Am. 1984; 17(3):513–552

[44] Langdon C, Herman P, Verillaud B, et al. Expanded endoscopic endonasal surgery for advanced stage juvenile angiofibromas: a retrospective multi-center study. Rhinology. 2016; 54(3):239–246

[45] Kassam AB, Gardner P, Snyderman C, Mintz A, Carrau R. Expanded endonasal approach: fully endoscopic, completely transnasal approach to the middle third of the clivus, petrous bone, middle cranial fossa, and infratemporal fossa. Neurosurg Focus. 2005; 19(1):E6

[46] Kasemsiri P, Solares CA, Carrau RL, et al. Endoscopic endonasal transpterygoid approaches: anatomical landmarks for planning the surgical corridor. Laryngoscope. 2013; 123(4):811–815

[47] Chen KT, Bauer FW. Sarcomatous transformation of nasopharyngeal angiofibroma. Cancer. 1982; 49(2):369–371

[48] Makek MS, Andrews JC, Fisch U. Malignant transformation of a nasopharyngeal angiofibroma. Laryngoscope. 1989; 99(10 Pt 1):1088–1092

[49] McAfee WJ, Morris CG, Amdur RJ, Werning JW, Mendenhall WM. Definitive radiotherapy for juvenile nasopharyngeal angiofibroma. Am J Clin Oncol. 2006; 29(2):168–170

[50] Lee JT, Chen P, Safa A, Juillard G, Calcaterra TC. The role of radiation in the treatment of advanced juvenile angiofibroma. Laryngoscope. 2002; 112(7 Pt 1):1213–1220

[51] Cummings BJ, Blend R, Keane T, et al. Primary radiation therapy for juvenile nasopharyngeal angiofibroma. Laryngoscope. 1984; 94(12 Pt 1): 1599–1605

[52] Goepfert H, Cangir A, Lee YY. Chemotherapy for aggressive juvenile nasopharyngeal angiofibroma. Arch Otolaryngol. 1985; 111(5):285–289

[53] Schick B, Kahle G, Hässler R, Draf W. [Chemotherapy of juvenile angiofibroma —an alternative?]. HNO. 1996; 44(3):148–152

[54] Hwang HC, Mills SE, Patterson K, Gown AM. Expression of androgen receptors in nasopharyngeal angiofibroma: an immunohistochemical study of 24 cases. Mod Pathol. 1998; 11(11):1122–1126

[55] Gates GA, Rice DH, Koopmann CF, Jr, Schuller DE. Flutamide-induced regression of angiofibroma. Laryngoscope. 1992; 102(6):641–644

[56] Thakar A, Gupta G, Bhalla AS, et al. Adjuvant therapy with flutamide for presurgical volume reduction in juvenile nasopharyngeal angiofibroma. Head Neck. 2011; 33(12):1747–1753

[57] Margolin JF, Soni HM, Pimpalwar S. Medical therapy for pediatric vascular anomalies. Semin Plast Surg. 2014; 28(2):79–86

35 Chordomas and Chondrosarcomas of the Skull Base

Joao Paulo Almeida, Franco DeMonte, Diana Bell, and Shaan M. Raza

Summary

This chapter discusses two rare tumors of the bony skull base: chordoma and chondrosarcoma. Although commonly discussed together, these are two distinct tumors, both pathologically and biologically. The epidemiology, pathology (histologic, immuno-histologic, and molecular), staging (when applicable), treatment (surgical, radiotherapeutic and chemotherapeutic), outcome, and prognosis for each tumor type are comprehensively discussed.

Keywords: chordoma, chondrosarcoma, brachyury, endonasal endoscopic resection, transcondylar approach, proton beam, spot-scanning, intensity-modulated radiation therapy, stereotactic radiosurgery, skull base tumor

35.1 Introduction

Chordomas and chondrosarcomas are rare tumors of the bony and cartilaginous skull base. Chordomas are difficult-to-treat invasive neoplasms that are thought to originate from remnants of the embryonic notochord. Chordoma arises primarily at the extremes of the axial skeleton, specifically the sacrococcygeal region and the clivus, and is associated with high rates of recurrence, morbidity, and mortality.[1] Unlike chordomas, skull base chondrosarcomas originate from areas of endochondral ossification, such as the petroclival, sphenopetrosal, spheno-occipital and petro-occipital synchondroses, and are usually associated with a better prognosis.[2]

Surgery is the primary treatment for both tumors. However, their invasiveness is associated with compression and encasement of cranial nerves and major vessels, which may limit the extent of surgical resection and contribute to high rates of recurrence. The comprehensive use of endoscopic and lateral skull base approaches has tremendously improved surgical outcomes in the modern era. Development of new radiation treatment modalities and better understanding of these tumors' behavior have contributed to modern treatment paradigms and improved prognosis. As in other skull base malignancies, current treatment of such tumors demands an integrated multidisciplinary approach involving neurosurgeons, ENT/head and neck surgeons, pathologists, radiation oncologists, and medical oncologists.

35.2 Epidemiology

Skull base chordomas and chondrosarcomas are rare tumors, having a combined incidence of 0.02/100,000 a year. They are more common in adults between the third and sixth decades but may occur at any age. Men tend to be slightly more affected then women.[1,3] Different ethnicities seem to be equally affected. Environmental risk factors have not been identified. Although patients who have chordomas and those who have chondrosarcomas have been grouped into a single population in previous studies, some differences between these tumors should be noted.

Chordomas represent 1 to 4% of all bone malignancies. They arise from the sacrum in approximately 50 to 60% of cases, from the skull base region (spheno-occipital/ nasal) in approximately 25 to 35%, from the cervical vertebrae in approximately 10%, and from the thoracolumbar vertebrae in approximately 5%.[4,5] They are more common in adulthood, but when present in the pediatric population they may be more aggressive and associated with a worse prognosis.[6]

Chondrosarcoma represents 4% of sarcomas reported in the literature and are the third most common bone malignancy, after multiple myeloma and osteosarcoma.[7] Chondrosarcomas involving the head and neck are rare tumors and account for only 1 to 12% of all chondrosarcomas.[3,7,8,9] Data from the National Cancer Database indicate that the median age at presentation for cranial chondrosarcoma is 51 years, with a slight male predominance (55%). Most cases (85%) occur in non-Hispanic white patients. Most cases present with low-grade conventional subtype, whereas mesenchymal and dedifferentiated subtypes represent 10 to 15% of chondrosarcomas of the skull base.[10,11]

35.3 Pathology

Chordomas and chondrosarcomas are bone and cartilaginous tumors, respectively, having different origins and histopathological and genetic characteristics. Although the literature has traditionally reported management paradigms and outcomes for these tumors collectively, they must be considered different entities. A pathologist who has expertise in bone and soft tissue sarcomas is imperative for the appropriate diagnosis and grading of these tumors. The development of immunohistochemical markers has facilitated their differentiation, especially with the recent observation of positive results for brachyury immunohistochemical staining in more than 95% of chordomas.[12]

35.3.1 Chordomas

Chordomas are locally aggressive bone neoplasms that arise from embryonic remnants of the notochord and show a dual epithelial–mesenchymal differentiation.[13] The classical chordoma (▶ Fig. 35.1) presents with physaliferous cells, which appear as clusters of large cells separated by fibrous septa into lobules and surrounded by basophilic extracellular matrix rich in mucin and glycogen.[14] Well-differentiated chordomas usually have solid sheets of adipocyte-like tumor cells, a myxoid matrix between tumor cells, and nuclei with atypia. Poorly differentiated chordomas shows proliferation of spindle-shaped tumor cells with pleomorphic nuclei, associated with occasional vacuolated tumor cells suggestive of notochordal differentiation.[15] Chondroid and dedifferentiated chordomas are rare subtypes that also affect the skull base. Chondroid chordomas have areas that resemble chondrosarcoma in addition to classic chordoma morphology. Dedifferentiated chordoma consists of two components: classic chordoma and a high-grade sarcomatous component that may resemble other high-grade sarcomas

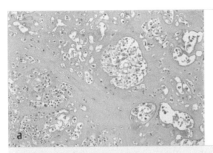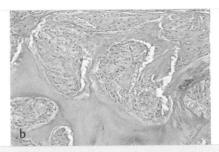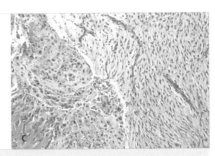

Fig. 35.1 Chordoma histological subtypes. **(a)** Chondroid type. **(b)** Conventional type. **(c)** Dedifferentiated type.

(e.g., osteosarcoma, fibrosarcomas). Prognosis of classical and chondroid subtypes is similar, but dedifferentiated chordomas have a much worse prognosis, dictated by the high-grade sarcoma component. Useful immunohistochemical markers for identification of chordomas include brachyury, epithelial markers, S100, and vimentin. Those are negative in chondrosarcomas and thus are useful for differentiation between those lesions.

The molecular pathways and genetic alterations present in chordomas are not completely understood, but some studies done in the last 10 years have added important contributions that may impact the future treatment of chordomas.[14,16] The PI3K/Akt/mTOR pathway is present in most chordomas and may play a crucial role in the pathogenesis of the tumor. The tuberous sclerosis complex (TSC) genes TSC 1 and 2 have also been associated with the development of these tumors.[15] In the last 5 years, transcriptome analysis studies demonstrated the upregulation of specific genes in skull base chordomas, including T (brachyury transcription factor), LMX1A, ZIC4, LHX4, and HOXA1.[14,16]

35.3.2 Chondrosarcomas

Chondrosarcomas are malignant tumors that produce cartilage matrix. In the skull base, they arise from regions of endochondral ossification, such as the petroclival region. These tumors are further categorized into four different histologic subtypes: conventional, mesenchymal, dedifferentiated, and clear cell. Most of these tumors (approximately 85%) are classified as conventional chondrosarcomas, but mesenchymal and dedifferentiated subtypes also affect the skull base (▶ Fig. 35.2).[17] The clear cell subtype has been reported only at other anatomical sites, not within the skull base.

Conventional chondrosarcomas are composed of multiple interconnecting lobules of varying size and chondroid or myxoid consistency, with a variable degree of cellularity, myxoid change, and calcification. The chondrocytes may have small or large hyperchromatic nuclei, with sporadic binucleation. These tumors are classified into three grades according to their nuclear size, hyperchromasia, cellularity, and mitotic activity.[18] Grade I chondrosarcomas represent most of these tumors. They are poorly cellular lesions, with chondrocytes that have a preponderance of small, densely straining nuclei, and retain a lacunar pattern. The intercellular background is usually chondroid, but there may be some myxoid components. Necrosis, nuclear atypia, and mitotic activity are not characteristics of this type of chondrosarcoma.

Grade II lesions present with areas of increased cellularity and enlarged, paler staining nuclei. A myxoid background is usually noted in areas having more cellularity. A low mitotic activity may be noted (fewer than 2 mitoses per 10 high-power fields [HPF]).

Grade III tumors characteristically display 2 or more mitoses per 10 HPF in the most cellular areas. There is usually a myxoid background associated with spindle or pleomorphic cells, and the lacunar pattern is predominantly lost. Foci of necrosis are usually seen.[17,18]

The mesenchymal subtype represents 2 to 13% of all chondrosarcomas. It is characterized by a bimorphic pattern with cellular zones of undifferentiated small or spindle cells and islands of hyaline cartilage. A hemangiopericytomatous vascular pattern and osteoclastic giant cells may be present. The cartilaginous area is positive for S100 protein, whereas the area with undifferentiated cells is consistently positive for CD99.[17] Dedifferentiated chondrosarcomas contain a well-differentiated component resembling a conventional subtype, as well as areas compatible with high-grade sarcoma, such as fibrosarcoma, osteosarcoma, or histiocytoma. The malignant area determines the prognosis and expected response to currently available chemotherapy protocols. Due to the presence of sarcomatous components, the prognosis of this subtype is significantly inferior to that presented by conventional chondrosarcomas. The clear cell subtype is extremely rare and represents about 1% of all chondrosarcomas. These low-grade malignant lesions consist of clear cells arranged in an indistinct lobular pattern, with round, large, centrally located nuclei having clear cytoplasm and distinct cytoplasmic membranes. They tend to have a better prognosis than the dedifferentiated and mesenchymal subtypes.

The molecular nature of chondrosarcomas has been less studied than that of chordoma. The hedgehog signaling pathway has been associated with chondrosarcomas. The induction of the parathyroid hormone-related protein (PTHLH) pathway (of the Indian hedgehog [IHH]/PTHLH pathway) and reactivation of bcl2 have been implicated in pathogenesis and progression of conventional chondrosarcomas, and bcl2 has been suggested as a reliable marker for the distinction between low-grade chondrosarcomas and enchondromas.[17,19]

35.4 Staging

There is no specific staging system for skull base chordomas and chondrosarcomas. The American Joint Committee on Cancer recommends a single tumor, node, metastasis, and histological grade classification (TNM+G) staging system for the

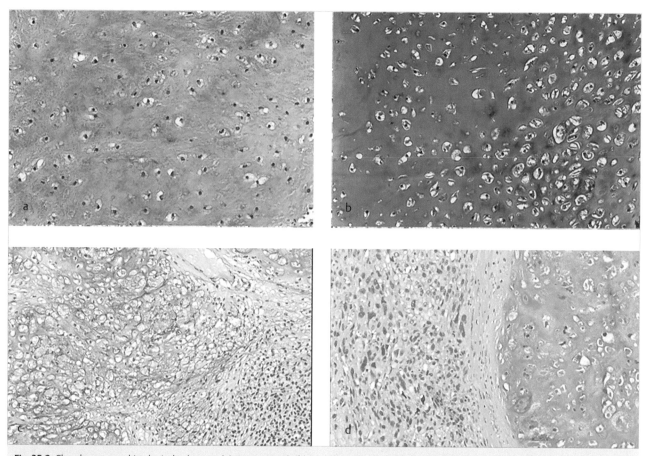

Fig. 35.2 Chondrosarcoma histological subtypes. **(a)** Conventional. **(b)** Dedifferentiated. **(c, d)** Mesenchymal.

different types of bone cancer, based on extension of the lesion, lymph node involvement, metastasis, and histological grade of the tumor. Additionally, it also describes a surgical staging system based on the stage, grade and site of the tumor. However, none of these staging systems has been correlated with outcomes in the skull base population.[20]

35.5 Treatment

Modern management of chordomas and chondrosarcomas of the skull base requires a multidisciplinary team of skull base surgeons, radiation oncologists, and clinical oncologists. Surgery remains crucial as a first line of treatment, but radiation has become increasingly important, especially when gross total resection is not possible and in cases having high-grade features.

35.5.1 Surgery

Surgical objectives are similar for both tumors: obtain tissue for diagnosis and achieve maximum safe resection and decompression of neurovascular structures for preservation and/or improvement of neurological function and quality of life. However, it is important to clearly delineate the expectations for an oncologic resection of a bony malignancy. Borrowing from concepts originating from spinal oncology, the Weinstein–Boriani–Biagini (WBB) classification for primary spinal column tumors delineates

the importance of addressing compartmental (vertebral body) and extracompartmental disease (i.e., tumor extension beyond the vertebral body) in an en bloc fashion. Although an en bloc resection is not feasible in the skull base, these concepts can be applied all the same. The bony skull base should be viewed as the originating compartment and any disease extension transdurally or into subcranial compartments (e.g., infratemporal fossa, longus capitis) viewed as extracompartmental extension. In general, an oncologic resection for any bony sarcoma should address compartmental and extracompartmental disease extensions.

The more aggressive behavior of chordomas demands an aggressive approach in order to maximize the chances of gross total resection and improve overall survival (OS) and progression-free survival (PFS). The first surgery, when planes for tumor dissection are preserved, is usually considered a unique opportunity to achieve maximal resection and long-term control of chordomas.[21] Surgical resection should thus be performed in centers that are expert in the management of chordomas, and a full discussion with the patient regarding the goals of surgery and potential complications should be undertaken prior to the surgical procedure. Different surgical approaches may be applied according to the goals of surgery (decompression vs. gross total resection) and the tumor's size, location, and relation with the dura mater, cranial nerves, and internal carotid artery (ICA). As a result, adequate case selection is mandatory. Skull base chordomas usually are midline tumors that affect the clivus and

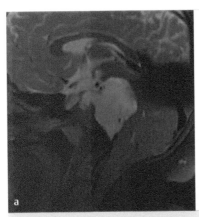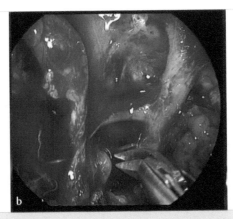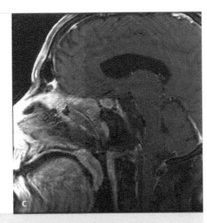

Fig. 35.3 Clival chordoma resected via expanded endonasal transclival approach. **(a)** Preoperative sagittal MRI T1-weighted with contrast demonstrating chordoma with extensive bony invasion and subdural disease extension with brainstem compression. **(b)** Intraoperative view of tumor dissection off vertebrobasilar system. **(c)** Postoperative imaging demonstrating resection.

in most cases do not invade the intradural space. Accordingly, these lesions often are medial to the ICA and cranial nerves, which favors resection through a midline, endoscopic endonasal approach (▶ Fig. 35.3).

An additional benefit of the endoscopic approach includes wide, less invasive exposure for drilling of potentially affected bone in the region. Though useful for a significant portion of clivus chordomas, this approach may be insufficient if the lesion is located lateral to the petrous and/or paraclival ICA or the cranial nerves or if large intradural components are present. In such cases, transcranial approaches should be considered, including posterior petrosectomy and far lateral/transcondylar or retrosigmoid approaches, for tumors having components in the posterior fossa, and an orbitozygomatic approach and its variations for lesions having lateral extensions into the cavernous sinus, middle fossa, and infratemporal fossa. Combination of endoscopic endonasal and transcranial approaches may be required in certain cases, especially in some chordomas, to achieve gross total resection.

Surgical results for chordomas have been mostly reported through retrospective single center observational studies. As an attempt to better evaluate the modern results of surgery, at least three meta-analysis have been recently published in the last 10 years.[22,23,24] As reported, gross total resection rates of endoscopic and transcranial approaches are 61 and 48%, respectively.[25] However, it is important to note that the extent of resection results is extremely variable in the literature, with rates of complete resection ranging from 0 to 73.7%.[23] Transcranial approaches seem to have been associated with higher rates of postoperative cranial nerve dysfunction and meningitis than endoscopic surgery; postoperative cerebrospinal fluid leak rates, however, were similar in open and endoscopic approaches and ranged from 5 to 10%.[23,25] It is important to emphasize the selection bias when discussing these results. Patients included in the open approaches cohort had a higher incidence of intradural invasion and larger tumors, whereas patients who underwent endoscopic endonasal surgery had smaller lesions with higher incidence of cavernous sinus invasion. The impact of extent of resection in the prognosis of chordomas has been demonstrated by multiple studies. In 2011 meta-analysis, Di Maio et al demonstrated that 5-year PFS was

87% in patients who had complete resection compared with 50% in patients with incomplete resection ($p < 0.0001$). The 5-year OS of patients who underwent complete and partial resection was 95% and 71%, ($p = 0.001$), respectively. Additionally, patients who underwent subtotal resection were 3.83 times more likely to experience a recurrence and 5.85 times more likely to die at 5 years than patients who underwent complete resection.[23]

Surgical management of recurrent chordomas is challenging and should consider the extent of recurrent disease and the modalities of treatment that were previously employed. The impact of surgery for management of recurrent chordomas was recently assessed by Raza et al.[21] The retrospective analysis of 29 patients with 55 recurrences treated at the MD Anderson Cancer Center demonstrated that reoperation of patients who had not received radiation therapy (RTX) was associated with improved median freedom from progression (FFP). However, if radiation had been used, the same benefit was not observed. For patients who have received only surgery, the presence of large recurrences may adversely impact the benefits to be gained through RTX. Reoperation may lead to further reduction of the tumor volume and decompression of the brainstem and cranial nerves, improving the results of radiation therapy.[26,27]

Understandings of the role of surgery in treating chondrosarcoma have been influenced by several reports published in the last 15 years. Surgery remains the first line of treatment, but goals of surgery depend on grade and subtype of chondrosarcoma. Grade I chondrosarcomas are slow-growing lesions that have low rates of recurrence, which do not seem to require gross total resection for improvement of survival rates.[2] In those cases, a less invasive approach may be useful, because the main objectives of the surgical procedure are removal of tumor for pathological analysis and decompression of cranial nerves and/or brainstem. In a recent study by the MD Anderson Cancer Center group, it was observed that gross total resection positively impacted PFS in conventional chondrosarcomas (111.8 vs. 42.9 months, $P = 0.201$), but statistical significance was not achieved.[2] Interestingly, surgery alone was effective for conventional grade I chondrosarcomas, even if postoperative residual tumor was present and no recurrence was noted in those cases

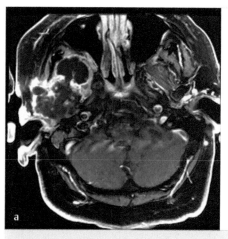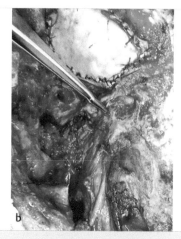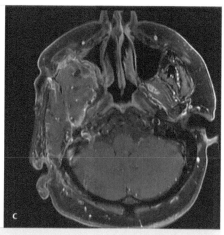

Fig. 35.4 Conventional grade III chondrosarcoma resected via subtemporal–infratemporal fossa approach. **(a)** Preoperative axial MRI T1-weighted with contrast demonstrating mass centered around right temporomandibular joint. **(b)** Intraoperative image after completion of skull base resection incorporating lateral temporal bone resection and mandibular condylectomy. **(c)** Postoperative imaging demonstrating gross total resection.

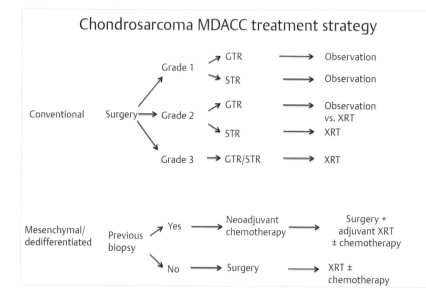

Fig. 35.5 Multimodality treatment algorithm for skull base chondrosarcomas employed at the University of Texas MD Anderson Cancer Center. (Reproduced with permission from Raza SM, Gidley PW, Meis JM, Grosshans DR, Bell D, DeMonte F, Multimodality treatment of skull base chondrosarcomas: the role of histology specific treatment protocols, Neurosurgery 2017;81:520–530.)

during a median follow-up of 67 months (range 13–248 months). Gross total resection seems to play a more important role in grade II and III chondrosarcomas, as suggested by 5-year PFS rates of 0% for subtotal resection and 67% for gross total resection. As discussed for chordomas, the surgical approach should be selected according to the location of the lesions and goals of surgery (▶ Fig. 35.4).

Chondrosarcomas are usually extradural parasellar lesions, centered in the petroclival region, with variable extensions into the cavernous sinus and/or cerebellopontine angle and jugular foramen regions. Depending on their growth pattern, chondrosarcomas may push the ICA and cranial nerves in the cavernous sinus laterally and create a relatively safe midline corridor that can be used for midline endoscopic approaches. Lesions located lateral to the cranial nerves in the posterior and middle fossa, as well as those having extensions into the temporal bone, mandible, and infratemporal fossa, should be considered for transcranial approaches and/or combined approaches.

Surgical treatment of mesenchymal and dedifferentiated subtypes is more challenging. The invasiveness of those lesions and the goals of surgery, which should attempt complete resection, may require more aggressive approaches. In this scenario, gross total resection is associated with significantly better PFS rates (58.2 vs. 1.0 month, $P < 0.05$).[2] A multidisciplinary approach is paramount in such cases (▶ Fig. 35.5). Infiltrative lesions previously diagnosed as mesenchymal or dedifferentiated chondrosarcomas subtypes may benefit from neoadjuvant chemotherapy for tumor reduction and improvement of extent of resection.

35.5.2 Radiation

Radiation treatment plays a major role in the management of chordomas. Adjuvant radiotherapy is recommended after surgical resection of skull base chordomas and is the main treatment modality for tumors deemed inoperable.[28] It is challenging and requires advanced planning, because it demands precise delivery of high doses of radiation to a relatively large field while avoiding damage to surrounding neural structures. Although most centers favor a strategy that maximizes radiation delivery to the tumor volume while respecting the tolerances of surrounding normal tissue, another school of thought favors sufficient irradiation, even at the cost of exceeding the dose threshold of surrounding normal tissue.[29] Conventional fractionated radiotherapy and proton therapy are the most common techniques, but stereotactic radiosurgery (SRS) and carbon ions have also been studied.[30,31] Hadrons have been gaining space in the treatment of chordomas and chondrosarcomas in the last 10 years. They can improve the radiobiological effect of radiation and minimize injury to surrounding neural tissue. These high-dose protons or charged particles include carbon ions, helium, and neon.[32,33]

Proton beam therapy is especially useful for treatment of skull base chordomas and chondrosarcomas. The initial results achieved in the 1980s and 1990s demonstrated the ability of this modality to deliver high doses of radiation (close to 70 Gy) while limiting the impact of radiation on the normal surrounding neurovascular structures, with 5-year control rates of 59 to 82%.[34,35,36] Proton beam radiotherapy has multiple favorable features for the management of chordomas.[28] Among the advantages of proton beam is the sudden dose decline beyond the target, which is related with the characteristic Bragg's peak effect of proton beam radiation. Another benefit is that protons or charged particles allow delivery of higher doses of radiation to the target volume, reducing the collateral radiation injury and improving radiobiological effect.[32] As a result, proton beam radiation therapy is able to deliver high radiation dosage more precisely than classic conventional fractionated therapy and may also be superior for tumor control and preservation of neurological function.[30,31,37]

For planning of RTX, the primary clinical target volume (CTV1) should include all volumes at risk for microscopic disease, including areas of preoperative tumor extension, and a second volume (CTV2) receiving a higher boost-dose of radiation should encompass any residual microscopic disease in the tumor bed after surgery. A third clinical target may be added to the treatment plan if gross residual lesions are present. Tumor seeding along the surgical corridor may occur in 5% of patients, and some groups suggest including the entire surgical corridor in the treatment plan.[37] Chordomas are radioresistant tumors and demand doses of at least 74 Gy, using conventional fractionation. This dose may lead to damage to brainstem, cranial nerves, and optic pathways around the lesion, so those structures should be contoured, and dosage constraint is recommended.

Hug et al reported the results of 58 patients (33 chordomas and 25 chondrosarcomas) treated with proton beam in a single center. The authors observed a 5-year local control rate of 59% for chordomas and 75% for chondrosarcomas.[38] Preradiation tumor volume > 25 mL and brainstem involvement were factors related to treatment failure. Grade III and IV toxicities were diagnosed in 4 (7%) of 58 patients and were symptomatic in 3 (5%). The failure of treatment was likely related to insufficient delivery of radiation to parts of the tumor, such as those in contact with the brainstem and cranial nerves. Austin et al analyzed 26 patients who had local tumor recurrence after

proton-based radiation therapy (proton RT) at Massachusetts General Hospital (MGH)/HCL and concluded, based on CT and MR review, that treatment in 75% of patients failed in regions receiving less than the prescribed dose because of normal tissue constraints.[39] The impact of tumor volume on the outcomes following RTX has also been demonstrated by Igati et al and McDonald et al.[26,40] In those studies, tumor volumes > 30 mL and > 20 mL, respectively, were associated with worse local control rates. Additionally, in the study by McDonald et al, it was observed that each additional 1 mL of tumor volume was linked with an increased risk of progression and brainstem compression, as well as that a radiation dose less than 74.5 Gy delivered to 1 mL of gross tumor volume (GTV) was predictive of treatment failure.[26] A meta-analysis by Matloob et al demonstrated that surgical resection followed by proton beam radiation was associated with 5-year disease control in 46 to 78% and 5-year survival rates of 66 to 87%.[32]

The most prevalent method for the delivery of proton radiotherapy is the passive scattering technique.[41] In 1980, Kanai proposed scanning a narrow pencil-beam in three dimensions through the target volume.[42] The flexibility of the spot scanning approach has been extended to deliver intensity-modulated proton therapy (IMPT), a direct equivalent to intensity-modulated radiotherapy (IMRT) with photons. Spot scanning provides greater control over the proximal aspects of the beam while improving conformity of the high-dose regions. A recent study from MD Anderson reported preliminary results with spot scanning proton therapy for chordomas and chondrosarcomas. The results demonstrated that compared with passive scanning, spot scanning plans provided improved high-dose conformity, sparing delivery to dose-limiting structures.[43] Ares et al reported a similar result using this technique, with 5-year local control rates of 81% for chordomas and 94% for chondrosarcomas and high-grade toxicity in 4 patients (6.25%).[41] No patient experienced brainstem toxicity.

Negative aspects related to proton beam therapy include the availability of fewer experienced facilities; dose distributions' being influenced to a greater degree by differences in density, so that air cavities and surgical hardware must be considered during the treatment planning process to a greater degree than is necessary for IMRT; and significantly higher cost.[31]

It is important to note that the evolution of photon-based linear accelerator therapy in the last 10 years has challenged the superiority of proton-based therapy for chordomas. The development of modern multileaf collimators (MLCs) allows for IMRT while onboard image-guidance (IG) systems permit near-real-time tracking during delivery, and robotic technology has been incorporated to ensure millimeter precision in dose delivery.[44] This has improved results, and several centers have adopted IG-IMRT for skull base chordoma and chondrosarcoma, delivering doses equivalent to those of proton therapy.[44,45,46] A recent study by Sahgal et al evaluated 24 patients who had skull base chordomas and who underwent surgery followed by IG-IMRT at the Princess Margaret Hospital/University of Toronto. The authors achieved a median total delivery dose of 76 Gy and obtained 5-year overall survival and local control rates of 85.6% and 65.3%, comparable to results reported after proton beam therapy. Emerging therapies, such as IMPT and in-room cone-beam CT, will likely impact the results of treatment of skull base chordomas.[44]

Like chordomas, chondrosarcomas require delivery of high radiation doses, > 60 Gy, usually delivered via IMRT/SRS or proton beam therapy. Similar limitations and side effects are present in the treatment of those tumors. The role of adjuvant radiotherapy for chondrosarcomas is not as clear as for chordomas.[2,47] Some centers recommend radiotherapy for all chondrosarcomas after surgery, whereas others select this treatment for tumors with aggressive features (conventional grade III or mesenchymal/dedifferentiated chondrosarcomas).[2,44] A recent study done by the MD Anderson group demonstrated that adjuvant radiotherapy significantly impacted PFS in conventional grade II and III chondrosarcomas (182 vs. 79 mo, $P < 0.05$) and had a positive trend for mesenchymal/dedifferentiated CSAs (43.5 vs. 22.0 mo).[2] Those results are similar to previously reported data that demonstrate 5-year overall survival and local control rates of 87.8% and 88.1%; they suggest that grade I skull base chondrosarcomas may have adjuvant radiation postponed but that other subtypes should receive postoperative radiotherapy (▶ Fig. 35.5).

Finally, it is important to note that the ideal technique for radiation delivery in both tumors is a matter of controversy. SRS is typically not useful as first-line adjuvant therapy, because chordomas require high dosing to cover the entire tumor bed. It is, however, a useful tool for the treatment of selected focal recurrences featuring small tumor volumes within or adjacent to previous radiation fields. As demonstrated in Raza et al in 2017, SRS may have an impact on the FFP of patients who have recurrent chordomas.[21] The largest SRS series to date, by the North American Gamma Knife Consortium, reports that optimal tumor control outcomes were achieved for tumor volumes less than 7 mL using a median marginal dose greater than 15 Gy.[46] Although previous radiation has not been demonstrated to negatively impact control after SRS, previous radiation fields can limit the marginal delivered dose. Adverse radiation events (ARE), as expected, may follow. In that same study, AREs occurred in 30% of patients having undergone previous radiation therapy and consisted of grade II/III events affecting the cranial nerves and pituitary gland.[46]

35.5.3 Chemotherapy

Chordomas have a risk for distant metastases regardless of histological subtype and a significant correlation with worsened outcomes.[21] Currently no drugs are specifically approved for the treatment of chordomas or chondrosarcomas. Classic chemotherapy agents have no significant effects on the treatment of those tumors except in the differentiated subtype, which has sarcomatous components. Currently, systemic therapy is used only in some patients who have advanced stages of disease, as an attempt to slow tumor progression.

Better understanding of the molecular pathways related to these tumors may change this scenario. Potentially relevant therapeutic targets have been identified in chordoma, including brachyury, mTOR, β-type platelet-derived growth factor receptor (PDGFRB), EGFR, and MET.[28] Imatinib mesylate, imatinib plus sirolimus or everolimus (mTOR inhibitors), sunitinib (tyrosine kinase inhibitor), EGFR inhibitors, and palbociclib (CDk4/6 inhibitor) have been tested in phase I and II trials with variable results.[48] Stacchiotti et al reported their experience with imatinib (RTK inhibitor) in 56 PDGFRB + patients.[49] With

overall tumor response at 6 months as the primary outcome defined by response evaluation criteria in solid tumors (RECIST) criteria (based on tumor size), the best response (partial response) was seen in 1.7% of the cohort; stable disease was seen in 70%.[50] Similar dismal results were also demonstrated with the use of lapatinib in a cohort of 18 EGFR + patients (overall response rate of 0.0%).[51] The most promising phase II study reported to date was by Bompas et al, assessing the role of sorafenib in 27 chordoma patients enrolled regardless of mutation status.[52] Employing similar RECIST defined outcomes, a partial response was seen in 3.7% of the cohort, whereas a majority of patients experienced stable disease with a 6-month PFS of 85.3%.

The brachyury overexpression in 95% of chordomas makes it a good target for immunotherapy treatment. A phase I study of yeast–brachyury GI-6301 vaccine and a larger phase II study comparing the results of radiotherapy alone versus radiotherapy plus the vaccine, are ongoing (NCT02383498).[53] Other potential targets are PD-L1 and PD-L2. Their overexpression has been previously demonstrated in preclinical studies and is the basis for the ongoing phase I trial NCT02989636, which evaluates the combination of SRS with concurrent and adjuvant PD-1 antibody, nivolumab, in patients who have recurrent or advanced chordomas.

Another factor relevant in the growing interest of targeted therapy for chordomas is that patients who have spinal chordomas have accounted for the majority of patients within the study cohorts. It is unclear, however, whether the pattern of genomic alterations is similar between skull base and spinal chordomas. Recent evidence, in fact, has identified significant genetic differences between skull base and spinal chordomas. Beyond potential biological differences between anatomical sites, the use of single agent targeted therapy is based on the assumption that a single pathway is more important than other pathways in tumor control. As further molecular information is gleaned and additional targeted therapies developed, multidrug therapy likely will have to be considered in order to simultaneously sequester different molecular drivers. For patients placed on targeted therapy based on mutations identified in preradiation surgical specimens, it is unclear whether the same targetable mutations exist in a radiated tumor. The impact of radiation in changing a tumor's genetic signature, and how this can impact targeted therapy, must be considered. Finally, considering the significant differences in survival and tumor control based on the pattern of distant metastasis (i.e., systemic vs. leptomeningeal disease (LMDD) likely resulting from differing biological mechanisms underscores the need for separate analyses.

Chemotherapy may be used as adjuvant treatment in mesenchymal and dedifferentiated chondrosarcomas. Mesenchymal chondrosarcomas and Ewing's sarcomas share some biological characteristics, so the same protocol, using anthracycline-based chemotherapy regimen, may be applied. This has been shown to have a positive impact on PFS ($P = 0.046$, hazard ratio (HR) = 0.482) and overall survival ($P = 0.004$, HR = 0.445). The positive benefits affected not only local disease recurrence but also incidence of systemic metastases.[54] Dedifferentiated chondrosarcoma treatment should be based on osteosarcoma treatment protocols, as recommended by the current National Comprehensive Cancer Network (NCCN) Bone Cancer Guidelines.

35.5.4 Outcome and Prognosis

As discussed, the prognoses of chordomas and chondrosarcomas differ significantly. Chordomas have a higher recurrence rate and lower PFS and OS rates. Classic factors that affect prognosis include subtype, extent of resection, and adjuvant radiotherapy. Patients who undergo gross total resection followed by radiotherapy have 5-year PFS and OS rates of 87% and 91%, respectively. Those who have dedifferentiated chordomas have a worse prognosis, dictated by the sarcomatous component of the tumor.

The prognosis of chondrosarcomas is significantly impacted by the grade and subtype of the lesion. Extent of resection and radiation play a lesser role in low-grade tumors. Conventional grade I tumors are slow-growing lesions that benefit from both gross total and subtotal resection. The low recurrence rates of these tumors justify postponing radiation, which can be used in cases of tumor regrowth. Conventional grade II/III tumors are more aggressive and demand adjuvant radiation for better OS and PFS rates. As observed in chordomas, dedifferentiated subtypes have significantly worse prognosis (median PFS of 24 months vs. 166 months for conventional subtype; $P < 0.05$).

35.6 Conclusion

Chordomas and chondrosarcomas are slow-growing tumors that affect the skull base and demand a combination of adequate diagnosis, surgery, and radiotherapy for optimal outcomes. Management of such rare tumors should be performed in centers that excel in skull base oncology, having ample experience with these tumors. The introduction of new techniques, such as endoscopic skull base surgery, proton beam therapy, and modern IG-IMRT, has positively impacted the prognosis of chordomas and chondrosarcomas. The development of new treatment modalities, such as immunotherapy and targeted therapy, may change the management of these tumors in the future and improve outcomes and patients' quality of life.

References

[1] Bohman LE, Koch M, Bailey RL, Alonso-Basanta M, Lee JY. Skull base chordoma and chondrosarcoma: influence of clinical and demographic factors on prognosis: a SEER analysis. World Neurosurg. 2014; 82(5):806–814

[2] Raza SM, Gidley PW, Meis JM, Grosshans DR, Bell D, DeMonte F. Multimodality treatment of skull base chondrosarcomas: the role of histology specific treatment protocols. Neurosurgery. 2017; 81(3):520–530

[3] Ellis MA, Gerry DR, Byrd JK. Head and neck chondrosarcomas: analysis of the Surveillance, Epidemiology, and End Results database. Head Neck. 2016; 38 (9):1359–1366

[4] Dasenbrock HH, Chiocca EA. Skull base chordomas and chondrosarcomas: a population-based analysis. World Neurosurg. 2015; 83(4):468–470

[5] McMaster ML, Goldstein AM, Bromley CM, Ishibe N, Parry DM. Chordoma: incidence and survival patterns in the United States, 1973–1995. Cancer Causes Control. 2001; 12(1):1–11

[6] Lau CS, Mahendraraj K, Ward A, Chamberlain RS. Pediatric chordomas: a population-based clinical outcome study involving 86 patients from the Surveillance, Epidemiology, and End Result (SEER) Database (1973–2011). Pediatr Neurosurg. 2016; 51(3):127–136

[7] Burningham Z, Hashibe M, Spector L, Schiffman JD. The epidemiology of sarcoma. Clin Sarcoma Res. 2012; 2(1):14

[8] Burkey BB, Hoffman HT, Baker SR, Thornton AF, McClatchey KD. Chondrosarcoma of the head and neck. Laryngoscope. 1990; 100(12):1301–1305

[9] Ruark DS, Schlehaider UK, Shah JP. Chondrosarcomas of the head and neck. World J Surg. 1992; 16(5):1010–1015, discussion 1015–1016

[10] Bloch O, Parsa AT. Skull base chondrosarcoma: evidence-based treatment paradigms. Neurosurg Clin N Am. 2013; 24(1):89–96

[11] Koch BB, Karnell LH, Hoffman HT, et al. National Cancer Database report on chondrosarcoma of the head and neck. Head Neck. 2000; 22(4):408–425

[12] Vujovic S, Henderson S, Presneau N, et al. Brachyury, a crucial regulator of notochordal development, is a novel biomarker for chordomas. J Pathol. 2006; 209(2):157–165

[13] Williams BJ, Raper DM, Godbout E, et al. Diagnosis and treatment of chordoma. J Natl Compr Canc Netw. 2013; 11(6):726–731

[14] Bell AH, DeMonte F, Raza SM, et al. Transcriptome comparison identifies potential biomarkers of spine and skull base chordomas. Virchows Arch. 2018; 472(3):489–497

[15] Yamaguchi T, Imada H, Iida S, Szuhai K. Notochordal tumors: an update on molecular pathology with therapeutic implications. Surg Pathol Clin. 2017; 10(3):637–656

[16] Bell D, Raza SM, Bell AH, Fuller GN, DeMonte F. Whole-transcriptome analysis of chordoma of the skull base. Virchows Arch. 2016; 469(4):439–449

[17] Kim MJ, Cho KJ, Ayala AG, Ro JY. Chondrosarcoma: with updates on molecular genetics. Sarcoma. 2011; 2011:405437

[18] Evans HL, Ayala AG, Romsdahl MM. Prognostic factors in chondrosarcoma of bone: a clinicopathologic analysis with emphasis on histologic grading. Cancer. 1977; 40(2):818–831

[19] Rozeman LB, Hameetman L, Cleton-Jansen AM, Taminiau AH, Hogendoorn PC, Bovée JV. Absence of IHH and retention of PTHrP signalling in enchondromas and central chondrosarcomas. J Pathol. 2005; 205(4):476–482

[20] Compton CC, American Joint Committee on Cancer. AJCC cancer staging atlas. New York, London: Springer; 2012

[21] Raza SM, Bell D, Freeman JL, Grosshans DR, Fuller GN, DeMonte F. Multimodality management of recurrent skull base chordomas: factors impacting tumor control and disease-specific survival. Oper Neurosurg (Hagerstown). 2018; 15(2):131–143

[22] Amit M, Na'ara S, Binenbaum Y, et al. Treatment and outcome of patients with skull base chordoma: a meta-analysis. J Neurol Surg B Skull Base. 2014; 75(6):383–390

[23] Di Maio S, Temkin N, Ramanathan D, Sekhar LN. Current comprehensive management of cranial base chordomas: 10-year meta-analysis of observational studies. J Neurosurg. 2011; 115(6):1094–1105

[24] Komotar RJ, Starke RM, Raper DM, Anand VK, Schwartz TH. The endoscope-assisted ventral approach compared with open microscope-assisted surgery for clival chordomas. World Neurosurg. 2011; 76(3–4):318–327, discussion 259–262

[25] Fraser JF, Nyquist GG, Moore N, Anand VK, Schwartz TH. Endoscopic endonasal transclival resection of chordomas: operative technique, clinical outcome, and review of the literature. J Neurosurg. 2010; 112(5):1061–1069

[26] McDonald MW, Linton OR, Moore MG, Ting JY, Cohen-Gadol AA, Shah MV. Influence of residual tumor volume and radiation dose coverage in outcomes for clival chordoma. Int J Radiat Oncol Biol Phys. 2016; 95(1):304–311

[27] Noël G, Feuvret L, Ferrand R, Boisserie G, Mazeron JJ, Habrand JL. Radiotherapeutic factors in the management of cervical-basal chordomas and chondrosarcomas. Neurosurgery. 2004; 55(6):1252–1260, discussion 1260–1262

[28] Stacchiotti S, Sommer J, Chordoma Global Consensus Group. Building a global consensus approach to chordoma: a position paper from the medical and patient community. Lancet Oncol. 2015; 16(2):e71–e83

[29] Catton C, O'Sullivan B, Bell R, et al. Chordoma: long-term follow-up after radical photon irradiation. Radiother Oncol. 1996; 41(1):67–72

[30] De Amorim Bernstein K, DeLaney T. Chordomas and chondrosarcomas: the role of radiation therapy. J Surg Oncol. 2016; 114(5):564–569

[31] Fernandez-Miranda JC, Gardner PA, Snyderman CH, et al. Clival chordomas: a pathological, surgical, and radiotherapeutic review. Head Neck. 2014; 36(6): 892–906

[32] Matloob SA, Nasir HA, Choi D. Proton beam therapy in the management of skull base chordomas: systematic review of indications, outcomes, and implications for neurosurgeons. Br J Neurosurg. 2016; 30(4):382–387

[33] Mohamad O, Sishc BJ, Saha J, et al. Carbon ion radiotherapy: a review of clinical experiences and preclinical research, with an emphasis on DNA damage/repair. Cancers (Basel). 2017; 9(6):9

[34] Austin-Seymour M, Munzenrider J, Goitein M, et al. Fractionated proton radiation therapy of chordoma and low-grade chondrosarcoma of the base of the skull. J Neurosurg. 1989; 70(1):13–17

[35] Saunders WM, Chen GT, Austin-Seymour M, et al. Precision, high dose radiotherapy. II. Helium ion treatment of tumors adjacent to critical central nervous system structures. Int J Radiat Oncol Biol Phys. 1985; 11(7): 1339–1347

[36] Suit HD, Goitein M, Munzenrider J, et al. Definitive radiation therapy for chordoma and chondrosarcoma of base of skull and cervical spine. J Neurosurg. 1982; 56(3):377–385

[37] Fagundes MA, Hug EB, Liebsch NJ, Daly W, Efird J, Munzenrider JE. Radiation therapy for chordomas of the base of skull and cervical spine: patterns of failure and outcome after relapse. Int J Radiat Oncol Biol Phys. 1995; 33(3): 579–584

[38] Hug EB, Loredo LN, Slater JD, et al. Proton radiation therapy for chordomas and chondrosarcomas of the skull base. J Neurosurg. 1999; 91(3):432–439

[39] Austin JP, Urie MM, Cardenosa G, Munzenrider JE. Probable causes of recurrence in patients with chordoma and chondrosarcoma of the base of skull and cervical spine. Int J Radiat Oncol Biol Phys. 1993; 25(3):439–444

[40] Igaki H, Tokuuye K, Okumura T, et al. Clinical results of proton beam therapy for skull base chordoma. Int J Radiat Oncol Biol Phys. 2004; 60(4):1120–1126

[41] Ares C, Hug EB, Lomax AJ, et al. Effectiveness and safety of spot scanning proton radiation therapy for chordomas and chondrosarcomas of the skull base: first long-term report. Int J Radiat Oncol Biol Phys. 2009; 75(4):1111–1118

[42] Kanai T, Kawachi K, Kumamoto Y, et al. Spot scanning system for proton radiotherapy. Med Phys. 1980; 7(4):365–369

[43] Grosshans DR, Zhu XR, Melancon A, et al. Spot scanning proton therapy for malignancies of the base of skull: treatment planning, acute toxicities, and preliminary clinical outcomes. Int J Radiat Oncol Biol Phys. 2014; 90(3): 540–546

[44] Sahgal A, Chan MW, Atenafu EG, et al. Image-guided, intensity-modulated radiation therapy (IG-IMRT) for skull base chordoma and chondrosarcoma: preliminary outcomes. Neuro-oncol. 2015; 17(6):889–894

[45] Hasegawa T, Ishii D, Kida Y, Yoshimoto M, Koike J, Iizuka H. Gamma Knife surgery for skull base chordomas and chondrosarcomas. J Neurosurg. 2007; 107 (4):752–757

[46] Kano H, Iqbal FO, Sheehan J, et al. Stereotactic radiosurgery for chordoma: a report from the North American Gamma Knife Consortium. Neurosurgery. 2011; 68(2):379–389

[47] Biermann JS, Chow W, Reed DR, et al. NCCN Guidelines insights: Bone Cancer, Version 2.2017. J Natl Compr Canc Netw. 2017; 15(2):155–167

[48] Colia V, Stacchiotti S. Medical treatment of advanced chordomas. Eur J Cancer. 2017; 83:220–228

[49] Stacchiotti S, Longhi A, Ferraresi V, et al. Phase II study of imatinib in advanced chordoma. J Clin Oncol. 2012; 30(9):914–920

[50] Eisenhauer EA, Therasse P, Bogaerts J, et al. New response evaluation criteria in solid tumours: revised RECIST guideline (version 1.1). Eur J Cancer. 2009; 45(2):228–247

[51] Stacchiotti S, Tamborini E, Lo Vullo S, et al. Phase II study on lapatinib in advanced EGFR-positive chordoma. Ann Oncol. 2013; 24(7):1931–1936

[52] Bompas E, Le Cesne A, Tresch-Bruneel E, et al. Sorafenib in patients with locally advanced and metastatic chordomas: a phase II trial of the French Sarcoma Group (GSF/GETO). Ann Oncol. 2015; 26(10):2168–2173

[53] Heery CR, Singh BH, Rauckhorst M, et al. Phase I trial of a yeast-based therapeutic cancer vaccine (GI-6301) targeting the transcription factor brachyury. Cancer Immunol Res. 2015; 3(11):1248–1256

[54] Frezza AM, Cesari M, Baumhoer D, et al. Mesenchymal chondrosarcoma: prognostic factors and outcome in 113 patients: a European Musculoskeletal Oncology Society study. Eur J Cancer. 2015; 51(3):374–381

36 Meningiomas

Jacob Freeman, Ashwin Viswanathan, and Franco DeMonte

Summary

Meningiomas are the most common intracranial tumors, and more than 40% of them occur at the skull base. Their epidemiology, etiology, pathology (histologic, immunohistologic, and molecular), clinical biology, observational management, treatment (surgical, radiotherapeutic and chemotherapeutic), outcome, and prognosis are comprehensively discussed.

Keywords: meningioma, atypical meningioma, anaplastic meningioma, Simpson grade, intensity-modulated radiation therapy, stereotactic radiosurgery, asymptomatic meningioma, skull base

36.1 Incidence/Epidemiology

Meningiomas account for 36.6% of all primary brain tumors and represent the most common nonmalignant central nervous system (CNS) neoplasm in adults.[1] According to data from the 2016 Central Brain Tumor Registry of the United States, which reflects reported cases of meningioma from 2009 to 2013, the incidence of meningioma nearly doubled, from 4.7 to 8.3 cases per 100,000 person-years, from 2004 to 2008.[1] This trend presumably reflects the use of MRI in the diagnosis of incidental meningioma, which occurs about 1% of the time according to a 2007 study of 2,000 adults aged 45 or older.[2] Women are diagnosed with meningioma at a ratio of 2.2:1 compared with men.[1] Between 2009 and 2013, the median age at diagnosis has risen from 63 to 66, and the incidence of meningioma continues to increase with increasing age.[1] Intracranial meningiomas outnumber spinal meningiomas by approximately 22:1. Although it is one of the most common intracranial tumors in adults, meningioma accounts for only 2.6% of all reported primary CNS tumors in children under 20. When stratified by age, adolescents aged 15 to 19 develop intracranial meningiomas more frequently (5%) than younger children (1.6%). The locations of most intracranial meningiomas are parasagittal, sphenoid ridge, or convexity. Forty percent of all meningiomas arise from the base of

the anterior, middle, or posterior fossa and are the most common skull base tumors. Sphenoid wing meningiomas make up about half of these; tuberculum sella and olfactory groove tumors the other half. Ectopic meningiomas have been described in the orbit, paranasal sinuses, skin, subcutaneous tissues, lung, mediastinum, and adrenal glands. ▶ Table 36.1 details the most common sites for meningiomas and their incidence.

36.2 Etiology

36.2.1 Trauma

Multiple case reports exist documenting intracranial dural-based,[3,4] intraosseus,[5] and extracranial cutaneous[6,7] meningiomas at the site of prior convexity or skull base injury. Likewise, several case–control studies have demonstrated an increased risk of meningioma genesis after head injury,[8,9,10,11,12] although these results have not been universally reproducible.[13,14] Recall bias has been suggested as a confounding factor limiting the effectiveness of case–control studies. Further epidemiological studies are necessary to validate and delineate a relationship.

36.2.2 Radiation

Exposure to ionizing radiation is a known etiological factor in the development of primary CNS tumors, with meningioma being the most common.[15] Of all radiation-induced tumors, the linear dose–response curve for development of meningioma is second only to that for sarcoma.[16] For a meningioma to be defined as radiation-induced, specific criteria have been proposed, including the following: (1) tumor was not present prior to irradiation, (2) tumor arose within the previously irradiated field, (3) a reasonable interval separated radiation therapy and detection of the second tumor, (4) tumor was confirmed histologically, (5) no family history is present of tumor predisposition syndrome such as phakomatosis, (6) histologic features differ from the primary tumor, and (7) tumor must not be recurrent or metastatic.[15,17,18] Compared with spontaneous meningiomas, radiation-induced meningiomas (RIMs) more commonly display higher World Health Organization (WHO) grade features and are more biologically aggressive tumors. For example, in two separate series of 10 RIMs, 50% were grade II or III (Galloway and Mack). Similarly, Al-Mefty et al reported a series of 16 RIMs, 38% of which were atypical or anaplastic tumors, with 100% of RIMs recurring at least once, 62% twice, and 17% thrice.[15] RIMs are more commonly multicentric rather than solitary[19,20] and demonstrate different cytogenetic changes, including less frequent NF-2 mutations and more frequent 1p and 6q mutations than their spontaneous counterparts.[15,21]

Examples of RIMs from both high- and low-dose exposure abound in the literature. High-dose exposure is loosely defined as therapeutic radiation used to treat another disease, and RIMs have been reported to develop after exposure to doses as low as 10 Gy[20,22] up to levels as high as 20 Gy[23] or 30 Gy. One of the first studies demonstrating the oncogenic potential of therapeutic

Table 36.1 Tumor location and incidence

Tumor location	Incidence
Parasagittal/falcine	25%
Convexity	19%
Sphenoid ridge	17%
Suprasellar (tuberculum)	9%
Posterior fossa	8%
Olfactory groove	8%
Middle fossa/Meckel's cave	4%
Tentorial	3%
Torcular	3%
Lateral ventricle	1–2%
Foramen magnum	1–2%
Orbit/optic nerve sheath	1–2%

radiation was published in 1974 by Modan and colleagues.[24] In this series, approximately 11,000 children who received high-dose radiation for treatment of tinea capitis, along with an age-matched cohort, were retrospectively followed for up to 23 years. Those exposed to the cranial radiation showed a relative risk of 9.5 for the development of meningioma. Similarly, children receiving high-dose prophylactic radiation to the neuroaxis for acute lymphoblastic leukemia have been shown to develop RIMs.[25]

RIMs developing after exposure to lower doses of radiation typically are from occupational, industrial, or environmental sources such as medical imaging (X-rays, CTs), nuclear power plants, or nuclear bombs, but the radiation dose from each of these is highly variable. For example, studies of atomic bomb survivors in Hiroshima and Nagasaki have shown a relative risk of 6.48 compared with non-exposed populations.[26,27] In the past few decades, the rising use of cellular telephones and the low-dose radiation levels to which they expose users prompted several large multinational studies evaluating the risk of brain tumor development.[28,29] The study results were congruent, demonstrating that cell phone use is not associated with an elevated risk of meningioma development. However, in the French CERENAT study, the heaviest cell phone users were found to have a 2.5-fold increased risk of meningioma development when considering lifelong radiation exposure.[28]

36.2.3 Infection

Viruses, and in particular polyomaviruses, have been studied as etiological agents of meningioma development. Simian virus 40 (SV40), a polyomavirus, is capable of transforming cells into those having a neoplastic phenotype.[30] The oncogenic and transforming properties of SV40 are related to expression of large tumor antigen (Tag), which is postulated to have a role in inactivating the tumor suppressor functions of p53, pRb, p107, and others.[31] Of 10 human meningioma samples analyzed, SV40 Tag was identified in 7 samples, the Tag-p53 complex in 3, and the Tag-pRb complex in 2.[32] In 2004, the first report linking SV40 exposure to meningioma was published.[33] The authors described a case of a scientist who had direct exposure to SV40 in the lab setting and who later developed an intracranial meningioma having identical SV40 DNA sequences. Although these data implicate SV40 in the pathogenesis of meningioma, other studies have not demonstrated the same results. In a study of 15 meningiomas, Rollison et al were unable to identify SV40 in any of the samples.[34] Similarly, in a larger series, Weggen et al found SV40 DNA in only 1 of 131 meningiomas sequenced.[35] Furthermore, Polymerase chain reaction (PCR) analysis for the Tag gene demonstrated a rate of 1 gene in every 250 tumor cells. Although the low frequency of SV40 and Tag DNA does not completely rule out a viral role in the pathogenesis of meningiomas, it appears to play a smaller role than was initially thought.

36.3 Genetics

36.3.1 Familial Meningioma Syndromes

The majority of meningiomas are sporadic tumors in patients having no history of brain tumors. However, familial meningiomas have been identified in a number of conditions, including

neurofibromatosis (NF) type 2 (NF2, 22q12.2), NF-1 (NF1, 17q11.2), Cowden's disease (PTEN, 10q23.31), Gorlin's or nevoid basal cell carcinoma syndrome (PTCH, 9q22.3), Li-Fraumeni syndrome (TP53, 17q11.2; CHEK2, 22q12.1), Gardner's syndrome (APC, 5q21–22), Rubinstein-Taybi syndrome (CREBBP, 16p13.3; EP300, 22q13), von Hippel-Lindau syndrome (VHL, 3p26–25; CCND1/cyclin D1, 11q13), Werner's syndrome (LMNA, 1q21.1; RECQL2, 8p12-p11.2), and multiple endocrine neoplasia Type 1 (MEN, 11q13), as well as melanoma/astrocytoma–brain tumor syndrome.[36,37]

36.3.2 Chromosomal Abnormalities

Meningiomas were one of the first solid tumors to be associated with a characteristic cytogenetic change—loss of heterozygosity (LOH) of chromosome 22. Forty to seventy percent of meningiomas exhibit LOH for markers from the chromosomal region 22q12.2, which encompasses the NF2 gene. NF2 encodes the protein merlin, which links membrane proteins to the cytoskeleton.[38] Biallelic inactivation of merlin results in loss of contact inhibition of cell proliferation and tumorigenesis.[39] Mutations in the NF2 gene have been reported in 30 to 60% of sporadic meningiomas. The frequency of NF2 mutations is similar among WHO grade I, II, and III meningiomas.[36,40] This finding suggests that NF2 gene inactivation may be an important initiation step in the formation of meningiomas but might not play a role in tumor progression.[37] Hansson et al used microarray-based comparative genomic hybridization to study 126 sporadic meningioma specimens.[41] They found the incidence of biallelic NF2 inactivation to be 52% in fibroblastic variants, compared with 18% in meningothelial histologies, suggesting that NF2 inactivation might not be a critical step in the formation of meningothelial meningiomas.[41] Instead, an alternate pathogenetic pathway could be deletion of the terminal segment of the long arm of chromosome 22 (22qter), as suggested by Yilmaz et al after the authors noted this specific genetic alteration in 26 of 36 patients (72%) who had meningothelial meningioma.[42]

Mutations on chromosome 1 represent the second most common genetic alteration in meningiomas.[41] Specific loss of the 1p36 locus has been associated with increased[43,44] and early[45] recurrence. In a large series of 247 grade I and II meningiomas, loss of 1p36 resulted in almost twice the number of recurrences as for patients who did not have 1p36 loss (33% vs. 18%).[43] Loss of chromosome 14q represents the third most common genetic abnormality after mutations in chromosomes 22 and 1.[46] As opposed to chromosome 22 loss, which occurs uniformly across all three grades of meningioma, 14q deletions occur in up to half of atypical meningiomas and the majority of anaplastic variants.[46] However, as with 1p loss, this genetic finding occurs at much lower rates in grade I meningiomas.[47] Not surprisingly, 14q deletions are associated with an increased risk of relapse and poorer prognosis.[48]

The increased recurrence rate of 14q deleted tumors was amply demonstrated in a 2017 meta-analysis of 742 patients who had meningioma, with an odds ratio for recurrence of 7.6 (95% CI: 4.3–13.6).[49] Similarly, 1q deletions were associated with an increased risk of recurrence (Overall Risk [OR] = 5.4; 95%CI: 3.6–8.1); however, chromosome 22 deleted tumors were far less likely to recur (OR = 1.6; 95%CI: 1.1–2.4).[49] With respect to meningioma, a specific locus of interest on chromosome 14q is the tumor suppressor gene maternally expressed gene 3 (MEG3), located at 14q32.[50] The antitumoral effect of MEG3 is mediated through activation of other tumor suppressor pathways, including p53 and Rb,[50,51] and through downregulation of MDM2, a gene encoding a protein responsible for p53 degradation.[51] MEG3 is overexpressed in normal arachnoidal cells but is not expressed in most meningiomas.[50] Among meningiomas, loss of MEG3 occurs more frequently in more aggressive recurrent tumors.[47,52] Work by Zhang et al in 2010 demonstrated that MEG3 is downregulated by epigenetic mechanisms such as CpG methylation within the promoter and the imprinting control region in meningiomas.[50] In addition, MEG3 suppression of DNA synthesis has been demonstrated via in vitro meningioma models, collectively demonstrating the tumor suppressor effect of MEG3.[50]

Chromosomal losses (1p, 6q, 10q, 14q, and 18q) and gains (1q, 9q, 12q, 15q, 17q, and 20q) have been associated with meningioma progression from low-grade to atypical.[53] Not infrequently, meningiomas express multiple genetic mutations, including LOH or co-deletion of 1p and 22q or 1p and 14q. These tumors demonstrate abnormal gene expression patterns on cDNA microarray analysis,[54] resulting in biologically more aggressive, higher-grade tumors[55] that have earlier recurrence rates.[45] Grade III or anaplastic tumors are associated with gains on 17q23 and losses on 9p. They may also demonstrate more frequent losses on 6q, 10, and 14q than are seen with atypical tumors.

36.3.3 Next-Generation Sequencing and NF2 Wild Type Mutations

Historically, meningioma has been considered a surgical disease: it most commonly exhibits slow growth with a low mitotic index, and surgical resection, if complete, is considered curative. Some low-grade tumors, however, behave more aggressively with early recurrence; others are in locations that prevent safe gross total resection; and still others are resistant to all available treatment methods, including surgery, radiation, and chemotherapy. Accordingly, a significant amount of genetic investigation has been undertaken to elucidate possible genetic targets for medical treatment in both nonresectable low-grade skull base meningiomas and recurrent high-grade tumors.[56,57,58] With the advent of next-generation sequencing, a rapid and relatively inexpensive whole genome sequencing technique, researchers have been able to identify specific mutation patterns among tumors of similar histologic grades. This has allowed the identification of subgroups of tumors that may be expected to recur earlier or more often, resulting in more specific behavior prediction. Furthermore, meningioma genotyping has identified specific molecular signatures of histologic phenotypes.[59] Taken together, next generation sequencing (NGS) is transforming the way meningiomas are categorized, from histologic subtype to specific genotype.[60]

Beginning in 2013, several oncogenic driver mutations were discovered in meningioma, including smoothened (SMO) and V-AKT murine thymoma viral oncogene homolog 1 (AKT1), both of which activate tumorigenic pathways in multiple cancers, including basal cell carcinoma, medulloblastoma, breast cancer, colorectal cancer, and lung cancer.[56,61] This was followed by the discovery of two additional oncogenic mutations: tumor necrosis factor receptor-associated factor 7 (TRAF7), which loses its normal apoptotic function when mutations occur in the WD40 binding domain, and Kruppel-like factor 4 (KLF4), which loses its normal regulatory role of cell differentiation due to a mutation in its zinc finger DNA binding site.[57,59] Several years later Abedalthagafi and colleagues discovered that phosphatidylinositol-4,5-bisphosphate 3-kinase catalytic subunit alpha (PIK3CA) mutations occur at a similar frequency as SMO, AKT1, TRAF7, and KLF4.[58] PIK3CA mutations exert a tumorigenic effect via activation of the AKT/mTOR pathway for cell growth and proliferation.[58]

With respect to mutation location and frequency, AKT1 and KLF4 are both frameshift mutations that occur at a single location—c.49G > A (p.E17K) and c.1225A > C (p.K409Q), respectively[40,56,57]—whereas SMO mutations most commonly involve p.L412F and p.W535 L changes. The most common mutation pattern in PIK3CA mutant tumors is p.H1047 R, which is found in a little less than half of tumors.[40] TRAF7 mutant tumors demonstrate variability in mutation locus, but 90% occur within the WD40 zinc finger DNA binding domain[40] and frequently co-occur with KLF4 and AKT1 mutations.

In general, these somatic mutations occur in about 5 to 10% of all meningiomas. They are mutually exclusive of NF2 mutant tumors, occurring only in NF2 wild type meningiomas[56,57,58,59] that are most commonly, but not always, low-grade. Interestingly, genotype seems to predict tumor location within the skull, where NF2 mutant meningiomas occur in the posterior fossa and tumors having TRAF7, AKT1, KLF4, SMO, and PIK3CA mutations most frequently occur in the anterior and middle fossa compartments along the midline.[56,58,59,60] In a retrospective review of 62 anterior skull base meningiomas by Strickland et al, 7 tumors demonstrated SMO mutations, of which 6 (82%) arose from the olfactory groove and 2 were grade II.[62] The authors concluded that olfactory groove meningiomas should be screened for SMO mutations.[62] Multiple recent meningioma sequencing studies have demonstrated that genotype predicts histologic phenotype.

In a 2013 study of 30 secretory meningiomas, Reuss et al found that all 30 tumors demonstrated the KLF4 K409Q mutation and that 29 exhibited the TRAF7 mutation within the WD40 binding domain.[59] The authors sequenced 267 other brain tumors, including other meningiomas, gliomas, metastases, glioneuronal tumors, and pituitary adenomas, along with 14 intraductal papillary mucinous neoplasms, 34 ductal adenocarcinoma, and 4 serous cystadenomas of the pancreas, without detecting the KLF4 mutation in any of the tumors; they detected TRAF7 in 8% of meningiomas. Taken together, these data support the conclusion that the KLF4/TRAF7 mutation defines the genetic signature of secretory meningioma. Similarly, germline loss of SMARCE1 has been demonstrated as a cause of both spinal and clear cell meningioma[63]; SMO mutations frequently result in meningothelial phenotype, and PIK3CA/AKT1 mutant tumors are most often of transitional or meningothelial histology.[56,58]

36.3.4 Gene Sequencing for Prognosis

Genetic sequencing experiments have demonstrated multiple prognostic implications of these NF2 WT mutations as well as other novel mutations that can help guide patient counseling and treatment and eventually inform the organization of a novel molecular grading system for meningioma. In a series of 79 olfactory groove meningiomas, those having SMO mutations occurred earlier and more than twice as often as AKT1 mutant tumors or wild type tumors, a finding that was independent of tumor grade.[64] In another series of 93 grade I and II skull base meningiomas, patients who had AKT1 mutant tumors had a shorter recurrence-free survival than their wild type counterparts.[65] Conversely, tumors that had the KLF4 K409Q mutation recur much later than KLF4 WT tumors and might represent a more benign subtype[65] TERT promoter mutational status has recently been identified as an extremely ominous genetic abnormality that can occur across all three histologic grades of meningioma and that results in shorter time to recurrence than anaplastic WT tumors.[66] In this study, the authors sequenced 267 tumors of grade I, II, and III histology, noting 16 tumors (6%) that had TERT promoter mutations: 2 grade I, 5 grade II, and 9 grade III. TERT promoter mutants demonstrated a significantly shorter recurrence-free survival (10 mo versus 179 mo, $p = 0.001$) than TERT WT tumors, regardless of grade. Furthermore, both grade I and 4/5 grade II mutant tumors demonstrated higher histologic grade features at recurrence. In view of the significance of this finding, the authors have suggested that TERT promoter mutational status be incorporated in the next meningioma grading system.[66]

Similarly, DNA methylation patterns identifying genetic groups at risk of earlier recurrence have been demonstrated.[67] BAP1 (BRCA1 associated protein-1) is a tumor suppressor gene that mediates its effects through chromatin modulation and transcription regulation. BAP1 germline mutations have been identified in a cancer predisposition syndrome that results in multiple tumors, including meningiomas, uveal melanoma, lung adenocarcinoma, and other cancers.[68] The frequency of BAP1 loss was studied in 57 rhabdoid meningiomas.[68] The authors identified 5 tumors (9%) with BAP1 loss, all of which were associated with a higher percentage of rhabdoid cells, higher grade (II or III), higher mitotic rate (> 5 mitoses/10 high-power fields [HPF]) and shorter time to recurrence than rhabdoid tumors with normal BAP1 expression.

Olar et al optimized a recurrence predictor using a training/validation approach and a support vector machine classification method with radial-basis smoothing kernel.[69] Three publicly available Affymetrix gene expression data sets (GSE9438, GSE16581, GSE43290) combining 127 newly diagnosed meningioma samples served as the training set. Unsupervised variable selection was used to identify an 18-gene gene expression profile (18-GEP) model that separated recurrences with a negligible root mean square error of 0.17. The characteristics of the training data set were as follows: WHO grade (I: 92 [73%], II: 32 [25%], III: 2 [2%]), median follow-up = 5.53 years (range: 0.05–25.42), recurrences = 18. This model was tested on 62 cases from their institution (validation data set [VD]) having similar demographics but enriched for cases featuring either long clinical follow-up or known recurrence. When applied to the VD, the 18-GEP separated recurrences with a misclassification error rate of 0.25 (log-rank $p = 0.0003$). 18-GEP was significantly predictive of tumor recurrence, independently ($p = 0.0008$, hazard ration [HR] = 4.61, 95%CI = 1.89–11.23]), and was predictive after adjustment for WHO grade, mitotic index, sex, tumor

location, and Simpson grade ($p = 0.0311$, HR = 9.28, 95% CI = [1.22–70.29]). The expression signature included genes encoding proteins involved in normal embryonic development, cell proliferation, tumor growth and invasion (FGF9, SEMA3C, EDNRA), angiogenesis (angiopoietin-2), cell cycle regulation (CDKN1A), membrane signaling (tetraspanin-7, caveolin-2), WNT-pathway inhibitors (DKK3), complement system (C1QA), and neurotransmitter regulation (SLC1A3, secretogranin-II).[69]

36.3.5 Genetic Underpinnings of Meningioma Development

Additionally, gene sequencing of meningiomas has begun to elucidate novel mechanisms of tumorigenesis. A 2017 meningioma sequencing experiment identified a subset of meningiomas with mutations in the RNA polymerase II gene POLR2A. RNA polymerase II is a key enzyme for transcription of protein coding genes in eukaryotes.[60] In this study, 775 tumors were sequenced and 23 tumors (3%) demonstrated the mutation. POLR2A mutants express elevated levels of WNT6 and significant downregulation of ZIC1/ZIC4, two proteins involved in meningeal cell differentiation. Specifically, WNT 6 is a protein secreted by nonneural ectoderm cells to cause the induction of neural crest cells, whereas ZIC1 is expressed by neural crest cells and results in meningeal cell differentiation. Thus the combination of elevated WNT6 and reduced ZIC1/ZIC4 would presumably result in higher numbers of dedifferentiated meningeal progenitor cells that could result in tumor formation.[60]

36.4 Tumor Biology

36.4.1 Growth Factors

Meningiomas express multiple growth factors and their receptors, including epidermal growth factor receptor (EGFR), basic fibroblast growth factor receptor (BFGFR), platelet-derived growth factor receptor (PDGFR), and vascular endothelial growth factor-A (VEGF-A). This suggests that autocrine growth factor secretion and autocrine loops may play a role in the growth of meningiomas.[70] This has been supported by experiments demonstrating meningioma cell growth and proliferation in the presence of growth factors.[71] An investigation by Smith et al demonstrated PDGFR-β expression in all 84 meningioma samples studied.[72] In addition, expression of BFGFR was found in 89% of benign meningiomas, whereas EGFR immunoreactivity was detected in 47% of benign meningiomas. In this study EGFR immunoreactivity was found to be a strong predictor of prolonged survival in patients who had atypical meningioma.[72] VEGF-A, which is also known as vascular permeability factor, is considered to be a key factor in angiogenesis and edema formation for meningiomas. Several studies have demonstrated VEGF-A levels in meningiomas to be associated with the extent of peritumoral edema,[73,74] and some smaller studies have postulated that VEGF-A mRNA expression may correlate with meningioma vascularity.[74,75] Furthermore, loss of the tumor suppressor gene MEG3, a finding commonly seen in meningiomas, has been correlated with increased levels of VEGF in MEG3 knockout mice, suggesting a possible underlying genetic role in the development of elevated vascularity seen in some meningiomas (Gordon). Other studies, however, have found no association between VEGF-A protein levels and microvessel density.[76] Multiple studies have assessed the effect of growth factor receptor inhibitors on meningioma growth. Unfortunately, the results from these studies have been largely underwhelming; the details are discussed in the chemotherapy treatment section of this chapter.

Transforming growth factor beta (TGF-β beta) 1, 2, and 3 along, with their receptors, are secreted and expressed by the leptomeninges and by meningioma tumor cells.[77] In vitro studies of WHO I meningiomas have demonstrated that tumor cell secretion of TGF-β reduces basal cell proliferation, thereby providing constant autocrine reduction and prevention of tumor growth.[78] In higher-grade meningiomas, however, TGF-β receptor levels are significantly reduced compared with grade I tumors, thereby compromising the inhibitory effect.[79]

36.4.2 Sex Steroid Receptors

The increased incidence of meningioma in women, along with the discovery of sex steroid receptors on meningioma tumor cells, has led to a significant amount of work examining whether endogenous or exogenous exposure to elevated levels of sex steroid increases risk of meningioma formation or tumor recurrence. Unfortunately, studies examining sex steroid sources, such as hormone replacement therapy and hormonal contraceptive use,[80,81,82,83,84,85] pregnancy,[86,87,88,89] age at menarche or menopause,[84] and breast cancer,[90,91] have been largely incongruous. Although the vast majority of grade I meningiomas express progesterone receptors (PRs), scarcely any are found on grade II or III tumors.[92,93,94,95] Most studies have found meningiomas to lack estrogen receptors (ERs), though some have found low concentrations of ERs in 5 to 33% of tumors.[96,97] Although some published data suggest that PR-positive tumors are less aggressive and are less likely to recur than those that exhibit ER-positivity, these studies are offset by data suggesting that there is no such relationship.[81,85,98]

Studies examining the risk of estrogen-only or estrogen/progesterone combination contraceptives on meningioma recurrence have demonstrated variable results.[99,100,101] Conversely, the few studies examining "ever-use" of exogenous, progesterone-only sources such as long-acting implantable and injectable contraceptives consistently demonstrated an elevated risk of meningioma genesis and recurrence.[81,85,102] In response to a rise in use of pure progesterone contraceptives, the risk of meningioma recurrence was reexamined in a recent 2017 study.[103] The authors studied 67 premenopausal women taking estrogen, estrogen/progesterone, or progesterone-only contraception who had surgically resected meningiomas and found that recurrence was higher in those taking pure progesterone than those taking estrogen only or a estrogen/progesterone combination (33% vs. 19%).[103] The progesterone-only group also demonstrated a significantly shorter time to recurrence (18 vs. 32 mo). These data suggest that progesterone-only contraception should be avoided in premenopausal women who have a known history of meningioma.

36.4.3 Somatostatin Receptors

Somatostatin receptors, and specifically somatostatin receptor subtype 2A (SSTR2A), are present at variable concentrations on most meningioma tumor cells.[104] Their presence can be confirmed in the clinical preoperative setting using octreotide nuclear scintigraphy, or postoperatively in the laboratory via immunohistochemistry.[105] The SSTR2A mediates the antiproliferative effects of somatostatin on meningioma tumor cells.[106] This was demonstrated in an in vitro study of 80 SSTR2A-positive meningiomas, in which a somatostatin analog significantly decreased cell proliferation in 88% of the tumors but no cell death was observed.[107]

36.4.4 Growth Hormone Receptors

Growth hormone receptors are present on meningioma tumor cells. Activation of the growth hormone/insulin-like growth factor 1 (GH/IGF-1) axis significantly increases the growth rate of meningiomas and has sparked investigation into inhibitors as treatment options.[108]

36.5 Pathology

Meningiomas arise from the arachnoidal cap cells of the arachnoid villi/granulations.[109] The WHO 2016 classification divides meningiomas into three grades: benign (grade I), atypical (grade II), and anaplastic or malignant (grade III).[110] Approximately 80% of meningiomas are WHO grade I and possess a low risk of recurrence or aggressive growth. Grade II meningiomas account for 15 to 20% of all meningiomas, whereas grade III tumors constitute only 1 to 3% meningiomas.[48] Grade II and grade III meningiomas are characterized by a greater likelihood of recurrence or of aggressive growth. The WHO 2016 retained the same classification system for meningioma, based on the number of mitotic figures (MFs) per 10 HPF in the area of highest mitotic activity. The only change for meningioma grading in the WHO 2016 is that the presence of tumor brain invasion in an otherwise grade I tumor now requires reclassification as a grade II tumor (▶ Table 36.2).

Meningiomas of any grade may exhibit invasion of brain parenchyma, which is characterized by fingerlike projections of tumor cells without an intervening layer of leptomeninges. The presence of brain invasion confers a greater risk for recurrence, similar to that seen for atypical meningiomas. Proliferative indices were not included in the grading criteria for meningiomas owing to significant differences in technique and interpretation

Table 36.2 2016 WHO classification of meningiomas

WHO I (<4 mitoses/10 HPF)	WHO II (4–20 mitoses/ 10 HPF)	WHO III (4–20 mitoses/ 10 HPF)
Meningothelial	Atypical	Anaplastic
Fibrous (fibroblastic)	Grade I with brain invasion	Papillary
Transitional (mixed)	Chordoid	
Psammomatous	Clear cell	
Secretory		
Angiomatous		
Microcystic		
Lymphoplasmacyte-rich		
Metaplastic		

between laboratories.[111] Likewise, nuclear atypia and invasion into bone or soft tissue does not affect grade.

36.5.1 WHO Grade I

Meningothelial, fibrous, and transitional meningiomas are the three most common histological variants of grade I meningiomas. Less common subtypes include psammomatous, angiomatous, microcystic, lymphoplasmacyte-rich, and secretory meningiomas (▶ Fig. 36.1). Chordoid, clear cell, papillary, and rhabdoid variants of meningiomas are often associated with more aggressive tumor behavior and are consequently not classified as grade I tumors. Benign grade I meningiomas may also invade surrounding structures, including the skull, dural sinuses, orbit, and soft tissues.

Meningothelial meningioma is a common variant in which tumor cells form lobules surrounded by thin collagenous septae. Tumor cells are uniform, resembling normal arachnoid cap cells, and may show central clearing. Rounded eosinophilic cytoplasmic protrusions into the nucleus, termed pseudoinclusions, are also seen. Whorls and psammoma bodies, when present, are less well defined than those seen in fibrous, psammomatous, or transitional meningiomas. Fibrous meningiomas are formed by spindle-shaped cells that resemble fibroblasts. These spindle-shaped cells form intersecting fascicles and are embedded in a collagen-rich and reticulin-rich matrix. Transitional or mixed meningioma is a common histological subtype that contains features of both meningothelial and fibrous meningiomas. Both the lobular arrangement of meningothelial meningiomas and the fascicular pattern of fibrous variants may be seen next to one another. They usually demonstrate extensive whorl formation in which the tumor cells form concentric cell layers by wrapping around each other. When the whorl formations hyalinize and calcify, they form structures known as psammoma bodies. Secretory meningiomas are rare grade I meningiomas with secretory globules (pseudopsammomas) that result in extensive peritumoral edema,[112] which appears very aggressive on imaging. Although the extent of edema does not correlate with the proliferation index, it is associated with immunohistochemical presence of carcinoembryonic antigen and cytokeratin.[113,114,115]

36.5.2 WHO Grade II

According to the WHO 2016 criteria, a meningioma is classified as atypical if it demonstrates brain invasion, has ≥ 4 mitoses per 10 HPF, or meets three of the five following criteria: increased cellularity, high nuclear to cytoplasmic ratio (small cells), prominent nucleoli, uninterrupted patternless or sheetlike growth, or foci of spontaneous (not induced by embolism) necrosis.[110] Two meningioma variants, clear-cell and chordoid, have been found to have higher recurrence rates even in the absence of the foregoing criteria, leading to their classification as atypical meningiomas (▶ Fig. 36.2).

Clear cell meningioma is a rare meningioma variant composed of sheets of polygonal cells whose clear, glycogen-rich cytoplasm is positive for periodic acid Schiff. They also demonstrate dense perivascular and interstitial collagen deposition. Clear cell tumors are more commonly found in the cauda equina or the cerebellopontine angle and tend to affect younger patients. Chordoid meningiomas are typically supratentorial tumors and have regions that are histologically similar to

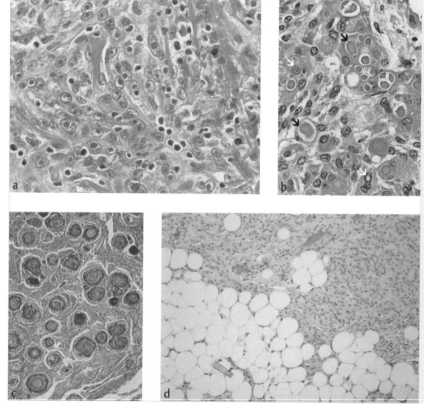

Fig. 36.1 (a–d) World Health Organization grade I meningioma subtypes: collage of the microscopic appearance of all the different grade I subtypes.

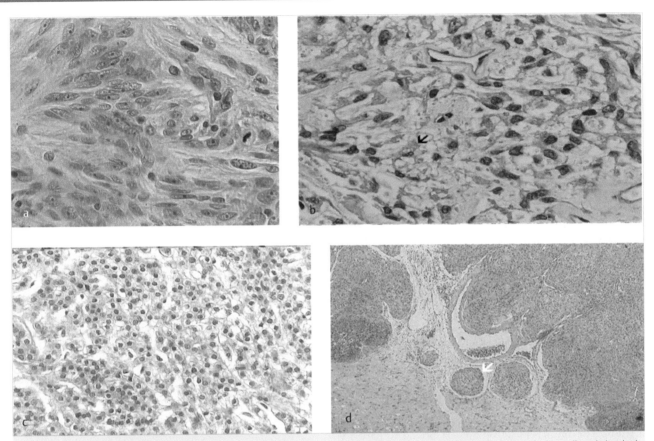

Fig. 36.2 (a–d) World Health Organization grade II meningioma subtypes: collage of the microscopic appearance of atypical, clear cell, and chordoid meningioma as well as a picture of brain invasion.

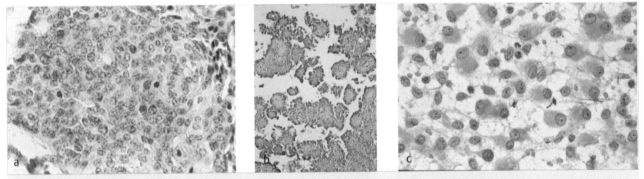

Fig. 36.3 (a–c) World Health Organization grade III meningioma subtypes: collage of the microscopic appearance of anaplastic, papillary, and rhabdoid meningioma.

chordoma. They may have cords of small epithelioid tumor cells that contain eosinophilic cytoplasm residing in a basophilic, mucin-rich matrix.[53]

36.5.3 WHO Grade III

Malignant meningiomas are characterized by a highly elevated mitotic index of > 20 mitoses per 10 HPF and can pathologically resemble sarcoma, carcinoma, or melanoma. In addition, large areas of necrosis can usually be seen. Papillary and rhabdoid meningiomas are consistently associated with malignant behavior and are therefore classified as WHO grade III tumors

(▶ Fig. 36.3).[116] Papillary meningioma has a propensity to affect younger patients, commonly exhibits brain invasion, and may show distant metastases. The rhabdoid variant is a rare tumor that contains sheets of large rhabdoid cells whose eosinophilic cytoplasm contains whorled intermediate filaments and eccentric nuclei (Perry 1998). The median survival is less than 2 years, and the recurrence rate is 50 to 80% after surgical resection.[117]

36.5.4 Immunohistochemistry

Epithelial membrane antigen (EMA) is the most commonly used marker in pathological analysis of meningiomas, and most tumors show at least scattered positivity for this antigen.[118] All meningiomas also strongly express vimentin.[119] Tissue micro-array immunohistochemistry (TMA-IHC) has proven to be an efficient and reliable method for analyzing biomarkers in meningioma. Using TMA-IHC, Lusis et al found EMA reactivity in 100% of meningiomas regardless of grade and E-cadherin immunoreactivity in 91% of all meningiomas and 90% of anaplastic meningiomas.[92] These markers, however, are not specific for meningiomas.

Immunohistochemistry has also proved useful in quantifying the proliferative index for meningiomas with the antibody MIB-1, which targets the proliferation marker Ki-67. Elevated proliferative indices as measured by MIB-1 labeling have been associated with an increased risk of recurrence.[120] Mean MIB-1 labeling indices are 0.7 to 2.2% for grade I meningiomas, 2.1 to 9.3% for grade II meningiomas, and 11 to 16.3% for grade III meningiomas.[121] MIB-1 labeling indices of greater than 5% suggest a greater likelihood of recurrence.

Similarly, an antibody that specifically recognizes the phosphorylated histone H3 (PHH3) has been effectively used as an aid in grading meningiomas.[122] During mitosis, phosphorylation of the Ser-10 residue of histone H3 reaches a maximum. Consequently, immunostaining with anti-PHH3 allows the observer to rapidly focus on the most mitotically active areas of the tumor. In 2015, Olar et al evaluated the mitotic index (number of mitoses per 1,000 tumor cells) in 363 meningiomas using PHH3 IHC.[123] In multivariate analysis, mitotic index was significantly associated with recurrence free survival ($P < 0.01$) after adjustment for Simpson grade, WHO grade, and MIB-1 index.

36.6 Treatment

36.6.1 Surgery

Complete surgical excision is the treatment of choice for meningiomas. In 1957, Simpson published a landmark paper examining the effect of degree of meningioma resection on recurrence rates following surgery.[124] Tumor resections were divided into five categories:

- I: macroscopically complete resection of tumor, bone, and dura
- II: macroscopically complete resection of tumor with dural coagulation
- III: complete tumor resection without dural coagulation
- IV: subtotal resection
- V: simple decompression

Kinjo et al further suggested a grade 0 resection in which an additional 2 cm margin of dura is excised as a means for further reducing the rate of recurrence.[125] A direct relationship between Simpson grade and 10-year symptomatic recurrence rate was demonstrated as follows: grade I (9%), grade II (19%), grade III (29%), grade IV (44%), grade V (100%). As a result, this scale has been adopted by neurosurgeons as a means of quantifying degree of meningioma resection. However, most attempts to re-create Simpson's results have failed to demonstrate a significant difference in recurrence rate among grades I, II, and III.[126, 127,128,129]

The extent of resection has since been strongly confirmed as the primary factor influencing meningioma recurrence rate.

The 10-year progression-free survival data range from 61 to 80% for a gross total resection and from 37 to 45% for a subtotal resection.[130,131] Nanda et al reported 20-year follow-up data for 112 WHO grade I meningiomas, noting a significant difference in tumor recurrence rate between grades 0 and I and grades II and IV (2.9% vs. 31%, $p = 0.0001$), a finding that was statistically similar when evaluating degree of resection using the Shinsu resection grading scale.[132]

The ability to achieve a safe, complete resection is influenced by invasion into eloquent cortex, tumor involvement of dural sinuses, growth into cranial nerves such as is commonly seen in cavernous sinus meningiomas, association with vascular structures, tumor location and size, and previous surgery or radiation.[109] The vast majority of meningiomas are surrounded by a layer of arachnoid that separates the tumor from the brain, cranial nerves, and blood vessels. By accessing this arachnoidal plane, the surgeon is able to minimize the chance of injury to neurovascular structures. Fortunately, an arachnoid plane can frequently be visualized on MRI T2 fluid-attenuated inversion recovery (FLAIR) images and when present has been correlated with improved surgical outcomes.[133] Internal debulking of the tumor facilitates the delineation of the arachnoid plane by allowing the edge of the tumor to collapse inward. Meningiomas may attach to or surround cerebral arteries diminishing the diameter of the vessel, but only very rarely do they invade the arterial walls.

Convexity Meningiomas

Convexity meningiomas comprise approximately 15% of all meningiomas, although there are more atypical or anaplastic tumors in the convexity than in the skull base,[134] they possess the greatest potential for cure. By definition, convexity meningiomas do not arise from the skull base and do not involve the dural sinuses; hence they allow for excision of a wide dural margin. Recurrent and/or aggressive meningiomas might not have the normal arachnoidal layer separating them from the cerebrum, and they require careful sharp dissection under the operating microscope to minimize cortical injury. Once the tumor and a wide dural margin have been resected, the dural defect may be repaired using a variety of autograft, allograft, xenograft, or synthetic options, including pericranium, fascia lata, temporalis fascia, cadaveric dura, bovine pericardium, and synthetic collagen matrix. In 2010, Sanai et al evaluated a series of 141 supratentorial meningiomas for perioperative risk. As expected, the risk profile was quite low, with no intraoperative complications, and had a postoperative neurosurgical and medical complication rate of 10%.[135] Surgical complications included hematoma requiring evacuation, cerebrospinal fluid (CSF) leak, and operative site infection. Seventy-five percent of tumors were WHO grade I; the remaining 25% were grade II. Simpson grade 0 or I resection was achieved in 122 patients (87%) and at median radiographic follow-up of 3.7 years (range 1–10 years), six patients (4%) had radiographic evidence of tumor recurrence.[135]

Parasagittal/Parafalcine Meningiomas

Cushing and Eisenhardt defined the parasagittal meningioma as one that fills the parasagittal angle, with no brain tissue between the tumor and the superior sagittal sinus (SSS).[136] Parasagittal meningiomas account for 17 to 32% of meningiomas, and the primary consideration in their removal is management of the SSS and the cerebral veins that drain into it. A variety of classification systems have been created based on the degree of meningioma invasion into the cerebral venous sinus. The classification described by Sindou et al stratified these tumors from those that only attached to the outer surface of the sinus wall to those associated with complete sinus occlusion, with or without preservation of one free wall.[137] Surgical approaches and management included simple dissection of the meningioma off the lateral wall of the sinus (for type I invasion), sagittal sinus reconstruction (type II–IV invasion), and excision or bypass of the sinus in the case of a totally occluded sinus (type V and VI invasion).[137] In a 2011 series of 61 parasagittal/falcine meningiomas with superior sagittal invasion, 33 of 55 tumors with partial occlusion were resected. Grade I tumors with gross total resection were compared with those that had subtotal resection wherein a small piece was left within the lumen of the sinus. Over an average of 7.6 years of follow-up, there was no difference in tumor control rate. The authors thus recommend consideration of radiation for growing residual tumor in the middle or posterior third of the SSS in view of the risk for venous infarction.[138] Given the advancements in neurosurgical instrumentation, coupled with the benign nature of the tumor residual in the SSS, the authors advocate for consideration of a modern approach using conformal radiation as a surgical adjuvant treatment for recurrent tumors.

Olfactory Groove/Planum Sphenoidale and Tuberculum Sellae Meningiomas

Olfactory groove planum sphenoidale and tuberculum sellae tumors comprise approximately 10% of meningiomas apiece.[139] These tumors are generally midline with similar blood supply (ethmoidal branches of the ophthalmic arteries, the anterior branch of the middle meningeal artery, and the meningeal branches of the ICA). Pre- and intraoperative measures for control of tumor blood supply include embolization and extracranial ligation,[140] although correct selection of an approach allowing for early control of these vessels often negates the need for other preoperative interventions. For surgical planning, many factors must be considered, including the location of the optic nerves relative to the tumor, with OGMs/planum meningiomas displacing the optic nerve inferiorly but tuberculum sellae meningiomas growing from below and pushing the optic nerve superiorly.[139]

In the modern neurosurgical era, surgical approach via an open craniotomy versus endoscopic endonasal approach (EEA) is a frequently discussed and debated topic. Open approaches include variations of a bifrontal craniotomy with or without removal of the orbital bandeau[139,141] and modified versions of the pterional approach with or without removal of the orbital roof.[142] Although the EEA is used for meningiomas involving all three fossae, those involving the anterior skull base have been met with the greatest success and lowest side effect profile. Nevertheless, despite the use of lumbar drains and modern reconstruction techniques, CSF leak remains a significant complication of the EEA, even in the anterior skull base. This possible complication must be considered when selecting an approach. For OGMs, the EEA should be reserved for anosmic patients who had small to medium-sized tumors (3–4 cm) without lateral extension beyond the orbits and without extension into the frontal sinus, where gross total resection (GTR) and reconstruction are much more difficult.[143,144] Preservation of olfaction has been historically considered impossible with the EEA, but reports of unilateral endonasal approaches with meticulous attention paid to the nasoseptal flap and olfactory epithelium suggest that it may be spared in some cases and in others may be negatively impacted but not lost.[145,146,147]

Sphenoid Wing Meningiomas

Sphenoid wing meningiomas are the second most common type of meningiomas, after the parasagittal type. These meningiomas are classified according to their point of origin along the sphenoid ridge and include spheno-orbital meningiomas involving the sphenoid wing and orbit that are characterized by hyperostosis of the sphenoid bone, progressive painless proptosis, vision loss, abnormal ocular motility, and occasional trigeminal neuropathies secondary to foraminal encroachment. Considering their frequent involvement of the superior orbital fissure, optic canal and cavernous sinus complete resection is impossible without significant morbidity. Accordingly, modern series are beginning to adapt a more conservative approach with subtotal resection for reversal of proptosis and preservation of vision, followed by stereotactic radiation for progression or recurrence.[148,149]

The internal carotid, the middle and anterior cerebral arteries and their branches, and the optic, oculomotor, and olfactory nerves are the neurovascular structures at greatest risk during the surgical removal of sphenoid wing meningiomas. The importance of the relationship between these tumors and the nearby vasculature was evaluated in a recent review of surgically resected sphenoid wing meningiomas.[150] In this study the authors demonstrate that degree of vascular encasement by the tumor predicted postoperative ischemic outcome, prompting consideration of subtotal resection in cases of complete encasement. The presence of the arachnoidal layer allows for meningiomas to be microsurgically separated from these structures even though there may be a marked distortion of the normal anatomy of the region.

Posterior Fossa Meningiomas

Posterior fossa meningiomas account for 10% of all intracranial meningiomas. Almost half these meningiomas are located in the cerebellopontine angle, whereas 40% are tentorial or cerebellar convexity tumors, 9% are petroclival, and 6% involve the foramen magnum. A standard retrosigmoid craniotomy allows sufficient exposure for the removal of most meningiomas of the cerebellopontine angle, whereas the supra- and infratentorial and presigmoid approaches may be necessary for petroclival meningiomas. Foramen magnum meningiomas may require a far lateral or transoccipital condylar approach for optimal access. Following tumor debulking and devascularization, the tumor is dissected from the brainstem; the basilar, vertebral, and cerebellar arteries; and the trochlear, trigeminal, abducens, facial, vestibulocochlear, and lower cranial nerves. Meningiomas involving the tentorium and cerebellar convexity have the transverse sinus as their main area of concern. Postoperative sequela of iatrogenic transverse/sigmoid narrowing or thrombosis following posterior fossa approaches for these tumors is relatively benign, with very few complications reported.[151]

36.6.2 Radiation

External Beam Radiation Therapy

Though complete surgical resection is the ultimate goal in treating patients who have meningioma, this is not always possible with an acceptable level of morbidity. When subtotal resection is chosen to minimize morbidity, or in cases of higher-grade tumor recurrence, radiation therapy has been shown to be an effective adjuvant treatment option.[130,152] Fractionated external beam radiation therapy (EBRT) is often selected for large skull base tumors that exceed the size limits of stereotactic radiosurgery (SRS). Recommended doses generally range from 50 to 55 Gy in fractions of 1.8 to 2.0 Gy, typically administered five times per week. The planning target volume can include only the gross tumor volume or the gross tumor volume, plus a margin depending on the grade of the meningioma (2 cm margin recommended for anaplastic meningioma). Targeting the dural tail of meningiomas remains a subject of controversy.[153]

Radiation therapy is an integral part of the treatment of meningiomas. In patients who have undergone a subtotal resection followed by adjuvant EBRT, 5-year progression-free survival has been 77 to 91%.[152,154,155,156,157] In a retrospective analysis of 140 patients treated using subtotal resection followed by EBRT, Goldsmith et al reported a 5-year progression-free survival rate of 85% for benign meningiomas and 58% for malignant tumors.[152] Soyeur et al more recently compared gross total resection, subtotal resection plus adjuvant EBRT, and subtotal resection followed by radiotherapy at tumor progression.[154] Over a mean follow-up of 7.7 years, the 5-year progression-free survival for gross total resection was 77%, whereas that for subtotal resection alone was 38%. Patients who underwent subtotal resection and adjuvant radiotherapy had a 5-year progression-free survival rate of 91%. The overall survival for the three groups was not statistically different and was no different than for the age-match general population.

In another series by Mendenhall et al, 101 patients who had benign skull base meningioma were treated either primarily or after subtotal resection with radiation therapy and demonstrated 92% local control and cause-specific survival rates at 15 years.[158] In addition, EBRT has become an integral part of the management of optic nerve sheath meningiomas. In their evaluation of 64 patients with long-term follow-up, Turbin et al concluded that EBRT led to more favorable outcomes than surgical resection, observation, or surgical resection plus EBRT.[159] Several other studies have produced similar results.[153,160]

Current methods of treatment planning and delivery have led to decreased toxicity profiles associated with EBRT compared with the 38% rate reported in earlier literature.[161] The complication rate for radiation therapy is 2.2 to 3.6% and includes cognitive decline, pituitary insufficiency, and radiation-induced neoplasms.[152,161,162]

Stereotactic Radiosurgery and Radiotherapy

Stereotactic radiation techniques have emerged as an important alternative to conventional EBRT allowing for highly conformal,

single-dose, or hypofractionated treatment schedules for complex skull base meningioma targets. Three modalities exist for SRS: linear accelerator (LINAC), including the Cyberknife (mobile LINAC); Gamma Knife (Elekta); and particle beam (proton or carbon ion). Tumors most appropriate for SRS are smaller than 3.5 cm, with little surrounding edema, in locations where dose constraints for critical structures, including the optic apparatus, cochlea, and brainstem, can be respected.[163] The radiobiologic differences between radiation methods are beyond the scope of this chapter, but it is important to understand that for meningiomas, single high-dose SRS does not rely as heavily on cells' being in a mitotic, dividing state to achieve a cell kill effect and thus may be a more effective treatment option when feasible.[164]

To compare optimal imaging for SRS treatment of meningiomas, Khoo et al compared clinical target volumes using CT and MRI for patients with skull base meningiomas undergoing radiation therapy. They found that MR- and CT-based target volumes provided complementary data regarding tumor involvement in soft tissue and bony regions, respectively.[165] Consequently, MR and CT fusion images are optimal for treatment planning of smaller meningiomas. For larger meningiomas, CT-based planning is usually adequate.

Fractionated stereotactic radiotherapy (SRT) allows for precise stereotactic targeting and steep dose gradients, whereas the fractionated schedule adds the benefit of allowing normal tissues to heal between treatments. LINAC, a photon-based radiation therapy, is the primary modality used for SRT and is used with a relocatable frame. Gamma Knife radiosurgery, using a cobalt-60 source, emits highly focused gamma rays to a specific target. Although accuracy and dose to healthy surrounding tissues are frequently debated, Gamma Knife is generally felt to be more precise than the frameless Cyberknife alternative. Gamma Knife radiosurgery, however, is limited to radiation of the cranial and subcranial compartment, whereas LINAC options can be used to treat other areas of the body as well. Particle beam (proton and carbon ion) treatment as boost therapy to standard photon irradiation, as well as standalone treatment, has been investigated in low-grade skull base meningiomas as well as higher grade II and III tumors, with promising results.[166] In an early study of seven patients who had grade I–III meningiomas treated using particle therapy, including proton therapy for low-grade cavernous tumors or standard photon radiation (50 Gy) with carbon boost 18 GyE for grade II/III tumors, a small shrinkage effect was noted at the first scan, and no recurrence was noted at last follow-up.[166]

SRS and SRT have shown promising results as both primary and adjuvant therapies for meningioma. Numerous retrospective studies since the 1990s have demonstrated 5-year local control rates with SRS of 86 to 99%, tumor regression rates of 28 to 70%, and symptom improvement in 8 to 65% of patients.[163] In their experience treating patients who had benign meningiomas less than 3.5 cm in average diameter, Pollock et al found that radiosurgery yielded results comparable to those seen with a Simpson's grade I surgical resection.[167] However, compared with a population who underwent a Simpson's grade II, III, or IV resection, SRS yielded a higher rate of progression-free survival.[167] The 3- and 7-year rates of progression-free survival for SRS were 100% and 95%, respectively, whereas those seen for Simpson's grade I was 100% and 96%, for Simpson's grade II were 91% and 82%, and for Simpson's grade III and IV were 68% and 34%, respectively.

More recently, Kollova et al reported their experience treating 325 benign meningiomas using either primary or adjuvant SRS.[168] Patients had a mean tumor volume of 4.4 mL, and the authors achieved a tumor control rate of 97.9% at 5 years. Improvement in neurological symptoms such as imbalance, oculomotor palsy, trigeminal symptoms, hemiparesis, and vertigo occurred in 61.9% of patients. The permanent toxicity rate was 5.7%, a figure that included seizures, trigeminal symptoms, hemiparesis, and others. Toxicity after radiosurgery is usually the result of either symptomatic edema or cranial neuropathies. In particular, the special sensory nerves (optic and vestibulocochlear) appear the most sensitive.[169] Vascular occlusion after SRS is a rare complication but is estimated to occur in 1 to 2% of cases.[170] The pathogenesis is thought to involve luminal narrowing after radiation-induced endothelial damage. Although SRS is often used as an adjuvant treatment option for recurrent high-grade meningioma, its effect on tumor control decreases as grade increases.[171,172]

As with SRS, SRT has shown high rates of progression-free survival of 98 to 100% over a mean follow-up of 21 to 68 months.[173,174] Studies have also shown average reductions in tumor volume of 33% at 24 months and 36% at 36 months with SRT.[175] Acute toxicities of SRT are generally mild and can include alopecia, skin erythema, and fatigue. The rate of late toxicity ranges from 2 and 13%. Late complications include hypopituitarism, visual deterioration, cognitive impairment, and tinnitus.[163]

Timing of adjuvant therapy for patients who have benign meningioma and who have undergone total or subtotal resection is still a matter of controversy. Although retrospective data lend credence to the use of adjuvant radiation therapy after gross total resection of atypical meningioma,[176] there are no prospective, randomized data to support this practice. Fortunately, however, the ROAM/EORTC-1308 trial examining radiation versus observation following resection of grade II meningiomas is under way and should help clarify this issue.[177]

36.6.3 Chemotherapy

Use of chemotherapy for treatment-resistant meningioma has been investigated extensively over the years. Unfortunately, the multitude of trials exploring most classes of standard chemotherapeutic agents have been met with largely disappointing results. Of all the chemotherapy drug trials conducted for meningioma, one of the best results came from a prospective study of 14 patients who had progressive malignant meningioma, who were given cyclophosphamide, Adriamycin, and vincristine (3 cycles for GTR and 6 cycles for STR) after surgery and radiation.[178] The authors reported a median time to progression of 4.6 years and median overall survival of 5.3 years—a finding significantly better than that associated with surgery alone. Hydroxyurea is an oral ribonucleotide reductase inhibitor that arrests meningioma cell division in the S phase of the cell cycle and induces apoptosis.[179] Though this agent has been effective in in vitro and in vivo studies, treatment of patients who have recurrent or unresectable meningiomas has shown little benefit, with the best results being no more than 1 year of progression-free survival.[180,181,182]

Temozolomide, an alkylating agent that has been used for treatment of malignant gliomas, showed no benefit for treating refractory meningiomas in a phase II trial[183]; however, in vitro trials of high-mobility group nucleosome-binding protein-5 (HMGN5) inhibition that demonstrated temozolomide sensitization deserve further investigation.[184] Irinotecan (CPT-11), a topoisomerase-1 inhibitor, has been shown to inhibit in vitro cultures of human meningioma cell lines and in vivo studies using a subcutaneous tumor model.[185] However, a phase II study evaluating CPT-11 in patients who had recurrent meningioma was stopped prematurely when all patients demonstrated tumor progression within 6 months.[186]

36.6.4 Hormone Therapy

The presence of hormone receptors on meningioma tumor cells sparked a plethora of trials investigating the clinical efficacy of using inhibitors of these receptors in treatment of recurrent meningioma. Mifepristone (RU486) is a progesterone blocker that has been shown to inhibit the growth of cultured human meningioma tissue and meningioma in animal models.[187] In a 2015 double blind, prospective phase III trial, 164 patients who had unresectable meningioma were given either mifepristone or placebo for 2 years.[188] At follow-up there were no differences between the two groups in failure-free survival or overall survival. Similarly, a phase II trial of tamoxifen, an ER antagonist, for treatment resistant meningioma was largely ineffective, with tumor progression noted in 10 patients within 6 weeks of treatment.[189] Somatostatin receptors are present on meningioma cells, and in vitro studies examining somatostatin analogs have demonstrated an inhibitory effect on growth of meningioma cells. Unfortunately, degree of receptor expression does not correlate with clinical response,[190] and thus far, somatostatin analogs have not proven effective for recurrent receptor-positive meningioma in the clinical setting. Specifically, one pilot study and two phase II prospective trials evaluating a total of 39 patients demonstrated 5 partial radiographic responses and a median time to progression of 4 to 5 months.[190,191,192] Although somatostatin analog therapy has been mostly unsuccessful, somatostatin receptor-targeted radionuclide therapy with[90]Y-DOTATOC may be another option, a few trials having shown promise.[193,194] Yttrium-90 is a radioactive isotope that is combined with DOTATOC, a tetraazocyclo-dodecanetetraacetic acid–modified somatostatin analog. In a trial of 15 patients who had recurrence, receptor positive meningioma stable disease was achieved in 13 patients at 24-month follow-up.[194]

Similarly, in a phase II clinical trial of somatostatin-based radiopeptide therapy, DOTATOC was radiolabeled with 90Y and 177Lu and administered to 34 patients who had progressive meningioma.[194] In this study, stable disease was achieved in 23 patients (65.6%) with a mean overall survival (OS) of 8.6 years from recruitment. As with other forms of hormone antagonist therapy for meningioma, growth hormone receptor antagonist showed promise in the lab but does not appear to have a significant clinical effect, although the latter has not been studied in prospective controlled fashion. In 2001, McCutcheon et al demonstrated reduction of tumor growth in mice that had been xenografted with human meningioma tumors after administration of pegvisomant, a growth hormone receptor inhibitor.[195] Unfortunately, a 2005 case report of a woman who had acromegaly and a skull base meningioma treated with pegvisomant demonstrated no appreciable inhibitory effect on the tumor. Rather, over a period of 5 years of surveillance, the tumor grew in volume to nine times its original size.[196]

36.6.5 Growth Factor Receptor Inhibitors

Meningiomas express high levels of growth factor receptors.[197,198] Unfortunately, trials testing EGFR inhibitors such as erlotinib and gefitinib[199] as well as imatinib, a PDGFR inhibitor,[200] have failed to demonstrate significant growth inhibition of recurrent meningioma. Antiangiogenic drugs, including sunitinib[201,202] and bevacizumab,[203,204,205] have been explored as well in case reports, retrospective series, and a few phase II trials, suggesting a possible antitumoral effect in receptor positive tumors, although randomized clinical trials await.

36.6.6 Immunotherapy

Interferon-α is cytokine that has been used as an effective treatment for multiple cancers, including hairy cell leukemia,[206] chronic myelogenous leukemia,[207] renal cell carcinoma,[208] and melanoma.[209] Initial lab studies examining the effect of interferon-α on meningiomas demonstrated an inhibitory growth[210] and antiangiogenic effect,[211] prompting a few clinical studies, including of combination interferon-α and 5-fluorouracil[212] and of interferon-α as a solo treatment.[213] Although these series demonstrated effective prolongation of time to recurrence in a small group of patients who had aggressive, recurrent meningioma, interferon-α frequently induces a flulike state that is very poorly tolerated.

Immune checkpoint inhibitors that boost the immune response to tumors have received a lot of attention for their successful use in melanoma and other tumors. Early work in this area has demonstrated an elevated number of programmed death ligand 1 (PD-L1) tumor cells in higher-grade meningiomas, suggesting a possible role for immune checkpoint inhibitors in these tumors.[214] Accordingly, clinical studies evaluating PD-L1 inhibitors pembrolizumab and nivolumab are under way.

36.6.7 Targeted Molecular Therapy

In addition to immunotherapy, therapeutics that target specific genetic mutations may hold promise as a medical alternative for recurrent, aggressive meningioma. Select mutations, including SMO and AKT1, provide targetable sites for medical treatments that already exist. Accordingly, research is under way to test the efficacy of these medications in mutation-positive meningiomas. At present, a single case report exists demonstrating a positive antitumoral effect from targeted treatment of a patient with a multifocal, skull base, recurrent AKT1-mutant tumor treated using surgery, radiation, and two chemotherapeutic agents: somatostatin and sorafenib.[215] After the fourth recurrence, the histology was upgraded to III and pulmonary metastases were identified. Genetic screening identified the AKT1 mutation, and the patient was started on an AKT1 inhibitor. At 2-year follow-up, imaging demonstrated

a slight reduction in the volume of intracranial disease and stability of pulmonary disease.

36.6.8 Viral Oncolytic Therapy

Viral oncolytic therapy has been tested in the lab with herpes simplex virus, demonstrating a tumor-killing effect in xenografted mice that had meningioma[216] and high-dose adenovirus, producing an oncolytic effect on meningioma cells in culture.[217]

36.7 Asymptomatic Meningioma

One-third to two-fifths of all meningiomas are asymptomatic at diagnosis.[109,218] Several studies have assessed the growth rate of these incidentally identified meningiomas.[218,219,220] Olivero et al found that 10 of 45 patients who had asymptomatic meningiomas exhibited tumor growth. Over an average imaging follow-up of 47 months, the average tumor growth in these 10 patients was 2.4 mm/year.[220] Yano et al found that only 37% of asymptomatic meningiomas showed tumor growth and that only 6% of patients became symptomatic over a mean follow-up of 3.9 years.[218] Patients who had tumors larger than 3 cm at diagnosis or who had T2-hyperintense tumors were more likely to become symptomatic over time, whereas patients who had calcified tumors were less likely to.[218] In the subgroup of patients 70 years and older the surgical morbidity associated with asymptomatic tumors was 9.4%, compared with 4.4% in patients younger than 70 years. Furthermore, the surgical morbidity in this group exceeded the morbidity in the observation-alone cohort (6%). Hence, for asymptomatic meningiomas, Yano et al recommended serial neuroimaging and close clinical monitoring.[218] Careful observation, with another imaging study 3 months after the first, is recommended to identify atypical or anaplastic growth patterns, with another scan 6 months later to detect any growth, and then yearly scans thereafter, representing a reasonable method of managing patients who have asymptomatic tumors.

References

[1] Ostrom QT, Gittleman H, Xu J, et al. CBTRUS statistical report: primary brain and other central nervous system tumors diagnosed in the United States in 2009–2013. Neuro-oncol. 2016; 18 suppl_5:v1–v75

[2] Vernooij MW, Ikram MA, Tanghe HL, et al. Incidental findings on brain MRI in the general population. N Engl J Med. 2007; 357(18):1821–1828

[3] Caroli E, Salvati M, Rocchi G, Frati A, Cimatti M, Raco A. Post-traumatic intracranial meningiomas. Tumori. 2003; 89(1):6–8

[4] François P, N'dri D, Bergemer-Fouquet AM, et al. Post-traumatic meningioma: three case reports of this rare condition and a review of the literature. Acta Neurochir (Wien). 2010; 152(10):1755–1760

[5] Kotzen RM, Swanson RM, Milhorat TH, Boockvar JA. Post-traumatic meningioma: case report and historical perspective. J Neurol Neurosurg Psychiatry. 1999; 66(6):796–798, 798

[6] Borggreven PA, de Graaf FH, van der Valk P, Leemans CR. Post-traumatic cutaneous meningioma. J Laryngol Otol. 2004; 118(3):228–230

[7] Pacheco Compaña FJ, Midón Míguez J, Avellaneda Oviedo EM, Busto Lodeiro E. Post-traumatic cutaneous meningioma. Arch Plast Surg. 2016; 43(4):381–384

[8] Monteiro GT, Pereira RA, Koifman RJ, Koifman S. Head injury and brain tumours in adults: a case-control study in Rio de Janeiro, Brazil. Eur J Cancer. 2006; 42(7):917–921

[9] Preston-Martin S, Paganini-Hill A, Henderson BE, Pike MC, Wood C. Case-control study of intracranial meningiomas in women in Los Angeles County, California. J Natl Cancer Inst. 1980; 65(1):67–73

[10] Preston-Martin S, Pogoda JM, Schlehofer B, et al. An international case-control study of adult glioma and meningioma: the role of head trauma. Int J Epidemiol. 1998; 27(4):579–586

[11] Preston-Martin S, Yu MC, Henderson BE, Roberts C. Risk factors for meningiomas in men in Los Angeles County. J Natl Cancer Inst. 1983; 70(5):863–866

[12] Phillips LE, Koepsell TD, van Belle G, Kukull WA, Gehrels JA, Longstreth WT, Jr. History of head trauma and risk of intracranial meningioma: population-based case-control study. Neurology. 2002; 58(12):1849–1852

[13] Annegers JF, Laws ER, Jr, Kurland LT, Grabow JD. Head trauma and subsequent brain tumors. Neurosurgery. 1979; 4(3):203–206

[14] Inskip PD, Mellemkjaer L, Gridley G, Olsen JH. Incidence of intracranial tumors following hospitalization for head injuries (Denmark). Cancer Causes Control. 1998; 9(1):109–116

[15] Al-Mefty O, Topsakal C, Pravdenkova S, Sawyer JR, Harrison MJ. Radiation-induced meningiomas: clinical, pathological, cytokinetic, and cytogenetic characteristics. J Neurosurg. 2004; 100(6):1002–1013

[16] Inskip PD, Sigurdson AJ, Veiga L, et al. Radiation-related new primary solid cancers in the childhood cancer survivor study: comparative radiation dose response and modification of treatment effects. Int J Radiat Oncol Biol Phys. 2016; 94(4):800–807

[17] Cahan WG, Woodard HQ, Higinbotham NL, et al. Sarcoma arising in irradiated bone; report of 11 cases. Cancer. 1948; 1(1):3–29

[18] Umansky F, Shoshan Y, Rosenthal G, Fraifeld S, Spektor S. Radiation-induced meningioma. Neurosurg Focus. 2008; 24(5):E7

[19] Sadetzki S, Flint-Richter P, Ben-Tal T, Nass D. Radiation-induced meningioma: a descriptive study of 253 cases. J Neurosurg. 2002; 97(5):1078–1082

[20] Musa BS, Pople IK, Cummins BH. Intracranial meningiomas following irradiation—a growing problem? Br J Neurosurg. 1995; 9(5):629–637

[21] Shoshan Y, Chernova O, Juen SS, et al. Radiation-induced meningioma: a distinct molecular genetic pattern? J Neuropathol Exp Neurol. 2000; 59(7):614–620

[22] Strojan P, Popović M, Jereb B. Secondary intracranial meningiomas after high-dose cranial irradiation: report of five cases and review of the literature. Int J Radiat Oncol Biol Phys. 2000; 48(1):65–73

[23] Harrison MJ, Wolfe DE, Lau TS, Mitnick RJ, Sachdev VP. Radiation-induced meningiomas: experience at the Mount Sinai Hospital and review of the literature. J Neurosurg. 1991; 75(4):564–574

[24] Modan B, Baidatz D, Mart H, Steinitz R, Levin SG. Radiation-induced head and neck tumours. Lancet. 1974; 1(7852):277–279

[25] Salvati M, Cervoni L, Puzzilli F, Bristot R, Delfini R, Gagliardi FM. High-dose radiation-induced meningiomas. Surg Neurol. 1997; 47(5):435–441, discussion 441–442

[26] Shintani T, Hayakawa N, Hoshi M, et al. High incidence of meningioma among Hiroshima atomic bomb survivors. J Radiat Res (Tokyo). 1999; 40(1):49–57

[27] Sadamori N, Shibata S, Mine M, et al. Incidence of intracranial meningiomas in Nagasaki atomic-bomb survivors. Int J Cancer. 1996; 67(3):318–322

[28] Coureau G, Bouvier G, Lebailly P, et al. Mobile phone use and brain tumours in the CERENAT case-control study. Occup Environ Med. 2014; 71(7):514–522

[29] Cardis E, Armstrong BK, Bowman JD, et al. Risk of brain tumours in relation to estimated RF dose from mobile phones: results from five Interphone countries. Occup Environ Med. 2011; 68(9):631–640

[30] Topp WC, Lane D, Pollack R. Transformation by SV40 and polyomavirus. In: Tooze J, ed. DNA Tumor Viruses. New York, NY: Cold Spring Harbor Laboratory Press, Inc.; 1981:200–301

[31] Fanning E. Simian virus 40 large T antigen: the puzzle, the pieces, and the emerging picture. J Virol. 1992; 66(3):1289–1293

[32] Zhen HN, Zhang X, Bu XY, et al. Expression of the simian virus 40 large tumor antigen (Tag) and formation of Tag-p53 and Tag-pRb complexes in human brain tumors. Cancer. 1999; 86(10):2124–2132

[33] Arrington AS, Moore MS, Butel JS. SV40-positive brain tumor in scientist with risk of laboratory exposure to the virus. Oncogene. 2004; 23(12):2231–2235

[34] Rollison DE, Utaipat U, Ryschkewitsch C, et al. Investigation of human brain tumors for the presence of polyomavirus genome sequences by two independent laboratories. Int J Cancer. 2005; 113(5):769–774

[35] Weggen S, Bayer TA, von Deimling A, et al. Low frequency of SV40, JC and BK polyomavirus sequences in human medulloblastomas, meningiomas and ependymomas. Brain Pathol. 2000; 10(1):85–92

[36] Wellenreuther R, Kraus JA, Lenartz D, et al. Analysis of the neurofibromatosis 2 gene reveals molecular variants of meningioma. Am J Pathol. 1995; 146(4):827–832

[37] Simon M, Boström JP, Hartmann C. Molecular genetics of meningiomas: from basic research to potential clinical applications. Neurosurgery. 2007; 60(5):787–798

[38] Pečina-Šlaus N. Merlin, the NF2 gene product. Pathol Oncol Res. 2013; 19(3):365–373

[39] Morrison H, Sherman LS, Legg J, et al. The NF2 tumor suppressor gene product, merlin, mediates contact inhibition of growth through interactions with CD44. Genes Dev. 2001; 15(8):968–980

[40] Yuzawa S, Nishihara H, Tanaka S. Genetic landscape of meningioma. Brain Tumor Pathol. 2016; 33(4):237–247

[41] Hansson CM, Buckley PG, Grigelioniene G, et al. Comprehensive genetic and epigenetic analysis of sporadic meningioma for macro-mutations on 22q and micro-mutations within the NF2 locus. BMC Genomics. 2007; 8:16

[42] Yilmaz Z, Sahin FI, Atalay B, et al. Chromosome 1p36 and 22qter deletions in paraffin block sections of intracranial meningiomas. Pathol Oncol Res. 2005; 11(4):224–228

[43] Ruiz J, Martínez A, Hernández S, et al. Clinicopathological variables, immunophenotype, chromosome 1p36 loss and tumour recurrence of 247 meningiomas grade I and II. Histol Histopathol. 2010; 25(3):341–349

[44] Hamilton BO, Sy JS, Megyesi JF, Ang LC. Her2neu amplification associates with co-deletion 1p/14q in recurrent meningiomas. Can J Neurol Sci. 2013; 40(3):361–365

[45] Maillo A, Orfao A, Espinosa AB, et al. Early recurrences in histologically benign/grade I meningiomas are associated with large tumors and coexistence of monosomy 14 and del(1p36) in the ancestral tumor cell clone. Neuro-oncol. 2007; 9(4):438–446

[46] Bi WL, Abedalthagafi M, Horowitz P, et al. Genomic landscape of intracranial meningiomas. J Neurosurg. 2016; 125(3):525–535

[47] Menon AG, Rutter JL, von Sattel JP, et al. Frequent loss of chromosome 14 in atypical and malignant meningioma: identification of a putative "tumor progression" locus. Oncogene. 1997; 14(5):611–616

[48] Lamszus K. Meningioma pathology, genetics, and biology. J Neuropathol Exp Neurol. 2004; 63(4):275–286

[49] Och W, Szmuda T, Sikorska B, et al. Recurrence-associated chromosomal anomalies in meningiomas: single-institution study and a systematic review with meta-analysis. Neurol Neurochir Pol. 2016; 50(6):439–448

[50] Zhang X, Gejman R, Mahta A, et al. Maternally expressed gene 3, an imprinted noncoding RNA gene, is associated with meningioma pathogenesis and progression. Cancer Res. 2010; 70(6):2350–2358

[51] Zhou Y, Zhong Y, Wang Y, et al. Activation of p53 by MEG3 non-coding RNA. J Biol Chem. 2007; 282(34):24731–24742

[52] Balik V, Srovnal J, Sulla I, et al. MEG3: a novel long noncoding potentially tumour-suppressing RNA in meningiomas. J Neurooncol. 2013; 112(1):1–8

[53] Riemenschneider MJ, Perry A, Reifenberger G. Histological classification and molecular genetics of meningiomas. Lancet Neurol. 2006; 5(12):1045–1054

[54] Martínez-Glez V, Alvarez L, Franco-Hernández C, et al. Genomic deletions at 1p and 14q are associated with an abnormal cDNA microarray gene expression pattern in meningiomas but not in schwannomas. Cancer Genet Cytogenet. 2010; 196(1):1–6

[55] Kumar S, Kakkar A, Suri V, et al. Evaluation of 1p and 14q status, MIB-1 labeling index and progesterone receptor immunoexpression in meningiomas: adjuncts to histopathological grading and predictors of aggressive behavior. Neurol India. 2014; 62(4):376–382

[56] Brastianos PK, Horowitz PM, Santagata S, et al. Genomic sequencing of meningiomas identifies oncogenic SMO and AKT1 mutations. Nat Genet. 2013; 45(3):285–289

[57] Clark VE, Erson-Omay EZ, Serin A, et al. Genomic analysis of non-NF2 meningiomas reveals mutations in TRAF7, KLF4, AKT1, and SMO. Science. 2013; 339(6123):1077–1080

[58] Abedalthagafi M, Bi WL, Aizer AA, et al. Oncogenic PI3K mutations are as common as AKT1 and SMO mutations in meningioma. Neuro-oncol. 2016; 18(5):649–655

[59] Reuss DE, Piro RM, Jones DT, et al. Secretory meningiomas are defined by combined KLF4 K409Q and TRAF7 mutations. Acta Neuropathol. 2013; 125(3):351–358

[60] Clark VE, Harmancı AS, Bai H, et al. Recurrent somatic mutations in POLR2A define a distinct subset of meningiomas. Nat Genet. 2016; 48(10):1253–1259

[61] Domingues P, González-Tablas M, Otero Á, et al. Genetic/molecular alterations of meningiomas and the signaling pathways targeted. Oncotarget. 2015; 6(13):10671–10688

[62] Strickland MR, Gill CM, Nayyar N, et al. Targeted sequencing of SMO and AKT1 in anterior skull base meningiomas. J Neurosurg. 2017; 127(2): 438–444

[63] Smith MJ, Wallace AJ, Bennett C, et al. Germline SMARCE1 mutations predispose to both spinal and cranial clear cell meningiomas. J Pathol. 2014; 234 (4):436–440

[64] Boetto J, Bielle F, Sanson M, Peyre M, Kalamarides M. SMO mutation status defines a distinct and frequent molecular subgroup in olfactory groove meningiomas. Neuro-oncol. 2017; 19(3):345–351

[65] Yesilöz Ü, Kirches E, Hartmann C, et al. Frequent AKT1E17K mutations in skull base meningiomas are associated with mTOR and ERK1/2 activation and reduced time to tumor recurrence. Neuro-oncol. 2017; 19(8): 1088–1096

[66] Sahm F, Schrimpf D, Olar A, et al. TERT promoter mutations and risk of recurrence in meningioma. J Natl Cancer Inst. 2015; 108(5)

[67] Olar A, Wani KM, Wilson CD, et al. Global epigenetic profiling identifies methylation subgroups associated with recurrence-free survival in meningioma. Acta Neuropathol. 2017; 133(3):431–444

[68] Abdel-Rahman MH, Pilarski R, Cebulla CM, et al. Germline BAP1 mutation predisposes to uveal melanoma, lung adenocarcinoma, meningioma, and other cancers. J Med Genet. 2011; 48(12):856–859

[69] Olar A, Goodman LD, Wani KM, et al. A gene expression signature predicts recurrence-free survival in meningioma. Oncotarget. 2018; 9(22):16087–16098

[70] Todo T, Adams EF, Fahlbusch R, Dingermann T, Werner H. Autocrine growth stimulation of human meningioma cells by platelet-derived growth factor. J Neurosurg. 1996; 84(5):852–858, discussion 858–859

[71] Peyre M, Salaud C, Clermont-Taranchon E, et al. PDGF activation in PGDS-positive arachnoid cells induces meningioma formation in mice promoting tumor progression in combination with Nf2 and Cdkn2ab loss. Oncotarget. 2015; 6(32):32713–32722

[72] Smith JS, Lal A, Harmon-Smith M, Bollen AW, McDermott MW. Association between absence of epidermal growth factor receptor immunoreactivity and poor prognosis in patients with atypical meningioma. J Neurosurg. 2007; 106(6):1034–1040

[73] Goldman CK, Bharara S, Palmer CA, et al. Brain edema in meningiomas is associated with increased vascular endothelial growth factor expression. Neurosurgery. 1997; 40(6):1269–1277

[74] Provias J, Claffey K, delAguila L, Lau N, Feldkamp M, Guha A. Meningiomas: role of vascular endothelial growth factor/vascular permeability factor in angiogenesis and peritumoral edema. Neurosurgery. 1997; 40(5):1016–1026

[75] Samoto K, Ikezaki K, Ono M, et al. Expression of vascular endothelial growth factor and its possible relation with neovascularization in human brain tumors. Cancer Res. 1995; 55(5):1189–1193

[76] Lamszus K, Lengler U, Schmidt NO, Stavrou D, Ergün S, Westphal M. Vascular endothelial growth factor, hepatocyte growth factor/scatter factor, basic fibroblast growth factor, and placenta growth factor in human meningiomas and their relation to angiogenesis and malignancy. Neurosurgery. 2000; 46 (4):938–947, discussion 947–948

[77] Johnson MD, Federspiel CF, Gold LI, Moses HL. Transforming growth factor-β and transforming growth factor β-receptor expression in human meningioma cells. Am J Pathol. 1992; 141(3):633–642

[78] Johnson MD, Okediji E, Woodard A. Transforming growth factor-β effects on meningioma cell proliferation and signal transduction pathways. J Neurooncol. 2004; 66(1–2):9–16

[79] Johnson MD, Shaw AK, O'Connell MJ, Sim FJ, Moses HL. Analysis of transforming growth factor β receptor expression and signaling in higher grade meningiomas. J Neurooncol. 2011; 103(2):277–285

[80] Benson VS, Kirichek O, Beral V, Green J. Menopausal hormone therapy and central nervous system tumor risk: large UK prospective study and meta-analysis. Int J Cancer. 2015; 136(10):2369–2377

[81] Korhonen K, Raitanen J, Isola J, Haapasalo H, Salminen T, Auvinen A. Exogenous sex hormone use and risk of meningioma: a population-based case-control study in Finland. Cancer Causes Control. 2010; 21(12):2149–2156

[82] Qi ZY, Shao C, Huang YL, Hui GZ, Zhou YX, Wang Z. Reproductive and exogenous hormone factors in relation to risk of meningioma in women: a meta-analysis. PLoS One. 2013; 8(12):e83261

[83] Johnson DR, Olson JE, Vierkant RA, et al. Risk factors for meningioma in postmenopausal women: results from the Iowa Women's Health Study. Neuro-oncol. 2011; 13(9):1011–1019

[84] Lee E, Grutsch J, Persky V, Glick R, Mendes J, Davis F. Association of meningioma with reproductive factors. Int J Cancer. 2006; 119(5):1152–1157

[85] Wigertz A, Lönn S, Mathiesen T, Ahlbom A, Hall P, Feychting M, Swedish Interphone Study Group. Risk of brain tumors associated with exposure to exogenous female sex hormones. Am J Epidemiol. 2006; 164(7):629–636

[86] Hatiboglu MA, Cosar M, Iplikcioglu AC, Ozcan D. Sex steroid and epidermal growth factor profile of giant meningiomas associated with pregnancy. Surg Neurol. 2008; 69(4):356–362, discussion 362–363

[87] Roelvink NC, Kamphorst W, van Alphen HA, Rao BR. Pregnancy-related primary brain and spinal tumors. Arch Neurol. 1987; 44(2):209–215

[88] Goldberg M, Rappaport ZH. Neurosurgical, obstetric and endocrine aspects of meningioma during pregnancy. Isr J Med Sci. 1987; 23(7):825–828

[89] Bickerstaff ER, Small JM, Guest IA. The relapsing course of certain meningiomas in relation to pregnancy and menstruation. J Neurol Neurosurg Psychiatry. 1958; 21(2):89–91

[90] Custer BS, Koepsell TD, Mueller BA. The association between breast carcinoma and meningioma in women. Cancer. 2002; 94(6):1626–1635

[91] Mehta D, Khatib R, Patel S. Carcinoma of the breast and meningioma: association and management. Cancer. 1983; 51(10):1937–1940

[92] Lusis EA, Chicoine MR, Perry A. High throughput screening of meningioma biomarkers using a tissue microarray. J Neurooncol. 2005; 73(3):219–223

[93] Brandis A, Mirzai S, Tatagiba M, Walter GF, Samii M, Ostertag H. Immunohistochemical detection of female sex hormone receptors in meningiomas: correlation with clinical and histological features. Neurosurgery. 1993; 33(2): 212–217, discussion 217–218

[94] Gabos S, Berkel J. Meta-analysis of progestin and estrogen receptors in human meningiomas. Neuroepidemiology. 1992; 11(4–6):255–260

[95] Strik HM, Strobelt I, Pietsch-Breitfeld B, Iglesias-Rozas JR, Will B, Meyermann R. The impact of progesterone receptor expression on relapse in the long-term clinical course of 93 benign meningiomas. In Vivo. 2002; 16(4): 265–270

[96] Hsu DW, Efird JT, Hedley-Whyte ET. Progesterone and estrogen receptors in meningiomas: prognostic considerations. J Neurosurg. 1997; 86(1):113–120

[97] Rubinstein AB, Loven D, Geier A, Reichenthal E, Gadoth N. Hormone receptors in initially excised versus recurrent intracranial meningiomas. J Neurosurg. 1994; 81(2):184–187

[98] Pravdenkova S, Al-Mefty O, Sawyer J, Husain M. Progesterone and estrogen receptors: opposing prognostic indicators in meningiomas. J Neurosurg. 2006; 105(2):163–173

[99] Claus EB, Black PM, Bondy ML, et al. Exogenous hormone use and meningioma risk: what do we tell our patients? Cancer. 2007; 110(3):471–476

[100] Michaud DS, Gallo V, Schlehofer B, et al. Reproductive factors and exogenous hormone use in relation to risk of glioma and meningioma in a large European cohort study. Cancer Epidemiol Biomarkers Prev. 2010; 19(10): 2562–2569

[101] Jhawar BS, Fuchs CS, Colditz GA, Stampfer MJ. Sex steroid hormone exposures and risk for meningioma. J Neurosurg. 2003; 99(5):848–853

[102] Piper JG, Follett KA, Fantin A. Sphenoid wing meningioma progression after placement of a subcutaneous progesterone agonist contraceptive implant. Neurosurgery. 1994; 34(4):723–725, discussion 725

[103] Harland TA, Freeman JL, Davern M, et al. Progesterone-only contraception is associated with a shorter progression-free survival in premenopausal women with WHO Grade I meningioma. J Neurooncol. 2017:[Epub ahead of print]

[104] Dutour A, Kumar U, Panetta R, et al. Expression of somatostatin receptor subtypes in human brain tumors. Int J Cancer. 1998; 76(5):620–627

[105] Schulz S, Pauli SU, Schulz S, et al. Immunohistochemical determination of five somatostatin receptors in meningioma reveals frequent overexpression of somatostatin receptor subtype sst2A. Clin Cancer Res. 2000; 6(5): 1865–1874

[106] He Y, Yuan XM, Lei P, et al. The antiproliferative effects of somatostatin receptor subtype 2 in breast cancer cells. Acta Pharmacol Sin. 2009; 30(7): 1053–1059

[107] Graillon T, Romano D, Defilles C, et al. Octreotide therapy in meningiomas: in vitro study, clinical correlation, and literature review. J Neurosurg. 2016; •••:1–10

[108] Friend KE, Radinsky R, McCutcheon IE. Growth hormone receptor expression and function in meningiomas: effect of a specific receptor antagonist. J Neurosurg. 1999; 91(1):93–99

[109] Drummond KJ, Zhu JJ, Black PM. Meningiomas: updating basic science, management, and outcome. Neurologist. 2004; 10(3):113–130

[110] Louis DN, Ohgaki H, Wiestler OD, et al. World Health Organization Histological Classification of Tumours of the Central Nervous System. France: International Agency for Research on Cancer; 2016

[111] Perry A, Louis DN, Scheithauer BW, et al. Meningiomas. In: Kleihues P, Cavanee WK, eds. Pathology and Genetics of Tumors of the Nervous System: World Health Organization Classification of Tumors Lyon, France: IARC Press; 2007

[112] Alguacil-Garcia A, Pettigrew NM, Sima AA. Secretory meningioma. A distinct subtype of meningioma. Am J Surg Pathol. 1986; 10(2):102–111

[113] Colakoğlu N, Demirtaş E, Oktar N, Yüntem N, Islekel S, Ozdamar N. Secretory meningiomas. J Neurooncol. 2003; 62(3):233–241

[114] Probst-Cousin S, Villagran-Lillo R, Lahl R, Bergmann M, Schmid KW, Gullotta F. Secretory meningioma: clinical, histologic, and immunohistochemical findings in 31 cases. Cancer. 1997; 79(10):2003–2015

[115] Buhl R, Hugo HH, Mihajlovic Z, Mehdorn HM. Secretory meningiomas: clinical and immunohistochemical observations. Neurosurgery. 2001; 48(2):297–301, discussion 301–302

[116] Perry A, Scheithauer BW, Stafford SL, Abell-Aleff PC, Meyer FB. "Rhabdoid" meningioma: an aggressive variant. Am J Surg Pathol. 1998; 22(12):1482–1490

[117] Perry A, Scheithauer BW, Stafford SL, Lohse CM, Wollan PC. "Malignancy" in meningiomas: a clinicopathologic study of 116 patients, with grading implications. Cancer. 1999; 85(9):2046–2056

[118] Schnitt SJ, Vogel H. Meningiomas: diagnostic value of immunoperoxidase staining for epithelial membrane antigen. Am J Surg Pathol. 1986; 10(9):640–649

[119] Artlich A, Schmidt D. Immunohistochemical profile of meningiomas and their histological subtypes. Hum Pathol. 1990; 21(8):843–849

[120] Bruna J, Brell M, Ferrer I, Gimenez-Bonafe P, Tortosa A. Ki-67 proliferative index predicts clinical outcome in patients with atypical or anaplastic meningioma. Neuropathology. 2007; 27(2):114–120

[121] Matsuno A, Nakaguchi H, Nagashima T, Fujimaki T, Yoshiyuki Osamura R. Histopathological analyses and proliferative potentials of intracranial meningiomas using bromodeoxyuridine and MIB-1 immunohistochemistry. Acta Histochem Cytochem. 2005; 38:9–15

[122] Ribalta T, McCutcheon IE, Aldape KD, Bruner JM, Fuller GN. The mitosis-specific antibody anti-phosphohistone-H3 (PHH3) facilitates rapid reliable grading of meningiomas according to WHO 2000 criteria. Am J Surg Pathol. 2004; 28(11):1532–1536

[123] Olar A, Wani KM, Sulman EP, et al. Mitotic index is an independent predictor of recurrence-free survival in meningioma. Brain Pathol. 2015; 25(3):266–275

[124] Simpson D. The recurrence of intracranial meningiomas after surgical treatment. J Neurol Neurosurg Psychiatry. 1957; 20(1):22–39

[125] Kinjo T, al-Mefty O, Kanaan I. Grade zero removal of supratentorial convexity meningiomas. Neurosurgery. 1993; 33(3):394–399, discussion 399

[126] Naumann M, Meixensberger J. Factors influencing meningioma recurrence rate. Acta Neurochir (Wien). 1990; 107(3–4):108–111

[127] Adegbite AB, Khan MI, Paine KW, Tan LK. The recurrence of intracranial meningiomas after surgical treatment. J Neurosurg. 1983; 58(1):51–56

[128] Oya S, Kim SH, Sade B, Lee JH. The natural history of intracranial meningiomas. J Neurosurg. 2011; 114(5):1250–1256

[129] Heald JB, Carroll TA, Mair RJ. Simpson grade: an opportunity to reassess the need for complete resection of meningiomas. Acta Neurochir (Wien). 2014; 156(2):383–388

[130] Condra KS, Buatti JM, Mendenhall WM, Friedman WA, Marcus RB, Jr, Rhoton AL. Benign meningiomas: primary treatment selection affects survival. Int J Radiat Oncol Biol Phys. 1997; 39(2):427–436

[131] Mirimanoff RO, Dosoretz DE, Linggood RM, Ojemann RG, Martuza RL. Meningioma: analysis of recurrence and progression following neurosurgical resection. J Neurosurg. 1985; 62(1):18–24

[132] Nanda A, Bir SC, Konar S, Maiti TK, Bollam P. World Health Organization Grade I convexity meningiomas: study on outcomes, complications and recurrence rates. World Neurosurg. 2016; 89:620–627.e2

[133] Thenier-Villa JL, Alejandro Galárraga Campoverde R, Ramón DE LA Lama Zaragoza A, Conde Alonso C. Predictors of morbidity and cleavage plane in surgical resection of pure convexity meningiomas using cerebrospinal fluid sensitive image subtraction magnetic resonance imaging. Neurol Med Chir (Tokyo). 2017; 57(1):35–43

[134] Kane AJ, Sughrue ME, Rutkowski MJ, et al. Anatomic location is a risk factor for atypical and malignant meningiomas. Cancer. 2011; 117(6):1272–1278

[135] Sanai N, Sughrue ME, Shangari G, Chung K, Berger MS, McDermott MW. Risk profile associated with convexity meningioma resection in the modern neurosurgical era. J Neurosurg. 2010; 112(5):913–919

[136] Cushing H, Eisenhardt L. Meningiomas: Their Classification, Regional Behaviour, Life History, and Surgical End Results. Springfield, IL: Charles C Thomas; 1938

[137] Sindou MP, Alvernia JE. Results of attempted radical tumor removal and venous repair in 100 consecutive meningiomas involving the major dural sinuses. J Neurosurg. 2006; 105(4):514–525

[138] Sughrue ME, Rutkowski MJ, Shangari G, Parsa AT, Berger MS, McDermott MW. Results with judicious modern neurosurgical management of parasagittal and falcine meningiomas: clinical article. J Neurosurg. 2011; 114(3):731–737

[139] Hentschel SJ, DeMonte F. Olfactory groove meningiomas. Neurosurg Focus. 2003; 14(6):e4

[140] Manjila S, Cox EM, Smith GA, et al. Extracranial ligation of ethmoidal arteries before resection of giant olfactory groove or planum sphenoidale meningiomas: 3 illustrative cases with a review of the literature on surgical techniques. Neurosurg Focus. 2013; 35(6):E13

[141] González-Darder JM, Pesudo-Martínez JV, Bordes-García V, et al. [Olfactory groove meningiomas. Radical microsurgical treatment through the bifrontal approach]. Neurocirugia (Astur). 2011; 22(2):133–139

[142] Downes AE, Freeman JL, Ormond DR, Lillehei KO, Youssef AS. Unilateral tailored fronto-orbital approach for giant olfactory groove meningiomas: technical nuances. World Neurosurg. 2015; 84(4):1166–1173

[143] Koutourousiou M, Fernandez-Miranda JC, Wang EW, Snyderman CH, Gardner PA. Endoscopic endonasal surgery for olfactory groove meningiomas: outcomes and limitations in 50 patients. Neurosurg Focus. 2014; 37(4):E8

[144] Schwartz TH. Should endoscopic endonasal surgery be used in the treatment of olfactory groove meningiomas? Neurosurg Focus. 2014; 37(4):E9

[145] Youssef AS, Sampath R, Freeman JL, Mattingly JK, Ramakrishnan VR. Unilateral endonasal transcribriform approach with septal transposition for olfactory groove meningioma: can olfaction be preserved? Acta Neurochir (Wien). 2016; 158(10):1965–1972

[146] Tajudeen BA, Adappa ND, Kuan EC, et al. Smell preservation following endoscopic unilateral resection of esthesioneuroblastoma: a multi-institutional experience. Int Forum Allergy Rhinol. 2016; 6(10):1047–1050

[147] Upadhyay S, Buohliqah L, Dolci RLL, Otto BA, Prevedello DM, Carrau RL. Periodic olfactory assessment in patients undergoing skull base surgery with preservation of the olfactory strip. Laryngoscope. 2017; 127(9):1970–1975

[148] Freeman JL, Davern MS, Oushy S, et al. Spheno-orbital meningiomas: a 16-year surgical experience. World Neurosurg. 2017; 99:369–380

[149] Bowers CA, Sorour M, Patel BC, Couldwell WT. Outcomes after surgical treatment of meningioma-associated proptosis. J Neurosurg. 2016; 125(3):544–550

[150] McCracken DJ, Higginbotham RA, Boulter JH, et al. Degree of vascular encasement in sphenoid wing meningiomas predicts postoperative ischemic complications. Neurosurgery. 2017; 80(6):957–966

[151] Jean WC, Felbaum DR, Stemer AB, Hoa M, Kim HJ. Venous sinus compromise after pre-sigmoid, transpetrosal approach for skull base tumors: a study on the asymptomatic incidence and report of a rare dural arteriovenous fistula as symptomatic manifestation. J Clin Neurosci. 2017; 39:114–117

[152] Goldsmith BJ, Wara WM, Wilson CB, Larson DA. Postoperative irradiation for subtotally resected meningiomas: a retrospective analysis of 140 patients treated from 1967 to 1990. J Neurosurg. 1994; 80(2):195–201

[153] Rogers L, Mehta M. Role of radiation therapy in treating intracranial meningiomas. Neurosurg Focus. 2007; 23(4):E4

[154] Soyuer S, Chang EL, Selek U, Shi W, Maor MH, DeMonte F. Radiotherapy after surgery for benign cerebral meningioma. Radiother Oncol. 2004; 71(1):85–90

[155] Barbaro NM, Gutin PH, Wilson CB, Sheline GE, Boldrey EB, Wara WM. Radiation therapy in the treatment of partially resected meningiomas. Neurosurgery. 1987; 20(4):525–528

[156] Miralbell R, Linggood RM, de la Monte S, Convery K, Munzenrider JE, Mirimanoff RO. The role of radiotherapy in the treatment of subtotally resected benign meningiomas. J Neurooncol. 1992; 13(2):157–164

[157] Taylor BW, Jr, Marcus RB, Jr, Friedman WA, Ballinger WE, Jr, Million RR. The meningioma controversy: postoperative radiation therapy. Int J Radiat Oncol Biol Phys. 1988; 15(2):299–304

[158] Mendenhall WM, Morris CG, Amdur RJ, Foote KD, Friedman WA. Radiotherapy alone or after subtotal resection for benign skull base meningiomas. Cancer. 2003; 98(7):1473–1482

[159] Turbin RE, Thompson CR, Kennerdell JS, Cockerham KP, Kupersmith MJ. A long-term visual outcome comparison in patients with optic nerve sheath meningioma managed with observation, surgery, radiotherapy, or surgery and radiotherapy. Ophthalmology. 2002; 109(5):890–899, discussion 899–900

[160] Brower JV, Amdur RJ, Kirwan J, Mendenhall WM, Friedman W. Radiation therapy for optic nerve sheath meningioma. Pract Radiat Oncol. 2013; 3(3):223–228

[161] al-Mefty O, Kersh JE, Routh A, Smith RR. The long-term side effects of radiation therapy for benign brain tumors in adults. J Neurosurg. 1990; 73(4): 502–512

[162] Glaholm J, Bloom HJG, Crow JH. The role of radiotherapy in the management of intracranial meningiomas: the Royal Marsden Hospital experience with 186 patients. Int J Radiat Oncol Biol Phys. 1990; 18(4):755–761

[163] Elia AE, Shih HA, Loeffler JS. Stereotactic radiation treatment for benign meningiomas. Neurosurg Focus. 2007; 23(4):E5

[164] Amichetti M, Amelio D, Minniti G. Radiosurgery with photons or protons for benign and malignant tumours of the skull base: a review. Radiat Oncol. 2012; 7:210

[165] Khoo VS, Adams EJ, Saran F, et al. A Comparison of clinical target volumes determined by CT and MRI for the radiotherapy planning of base of skull meningiomas. Int J Radiat Oncol Biol Phys. 2000; 46(5):1309–1317

[166] Rieken S, Habermehl D, Haberer T, Jaekel O, Debus J, Combs SE. Proton and carbon ion radiotherapy for primary brain tumors delivered with active raster scanning at the Heidelberg Ion Therapy Center (HIT): early treatment results and study concepts. Radiat Oncol. 2012; 7:41

[167] Pollock BE, Stafford SL, Utter A, Giannini C, Schreiner SA. Stereotactic radiosurgery provides equivalent tumor control to Simpson Grade 1 resection for patients with small- to medium-size meningiomas. Int J Radiat Oncol Biol Phys. 2003; 55(4):1000–1005

[168] Kollová A, Liscák R, Novotný J, Jr, Vladyka V, Simonová G, Janousková L. Gamma Knife surgery for benign meningiomas. J Neurosurg. 2007; 107(2):325–336

[169] Tishler RB, Loeffler JS, Lunsford LD, et al. Tolerance of cranial nerves of the cavernous sinus to radiosurgery. Int J Radiat Oncol Biol Phys. 1993; 27(2): 215–221

[170] Barami K, Grow A, Brem S, Dagnew E, Sloan AE. Vascular complications after radiosurgery for meningiomas. Neurosurg Focus. 2007; 22(3):E9

[171] Wojcieszynski AP, Ohri N, Andrews DW, Evans JJ, Dicker AP, Werner-Wasik M. Reirradiation of recurrent meningioma. J Clin Neurosci. 2012; 19(9): 1261–1264

[172] Friedman WA, Murad GJ, Bradshaw P, et al. Linear accelerator surgery for meningiomas. J Neurosurg. 2005; 103(2):206–209

[173] Debus J, Wuendrich M, Pirzkall A, et al. High efficacy of fractionated stereotactic radiotherapy of large base-of-skull meningiomas: long-term results. J Clin Oncol. 2001; 19(15):3547–3553

[174] Jalali R, Loughrey C, Baumert B, et al. High precision focused irradiation in the form of fractionated stereotactic conformal radiotherapy (SCRT) for benign meningiomas predominantly in the skull base location. Clin Oncol (R Coll Radiol). 2002; 14(2):103–109

[175] Henzel M, Gross MW, Hamm K, et al. Significant tumor volume reduction of meningiomas after stereotactic radiotherapy: results of a prospective multicenter study. Neurosurgery. 2006; 59(6):1188–1194, discussion 1194

[176] Rydzewski NR, Lesniak MS, Chandler JP, et al. Gross total resection and adjuvant radiotherapy most significant predictors of improved survival in patients with atypical meningioma. Cancer. 2017:[Epub ahead of print]

[177] Jenkinson MD, Javadpour M, Haylock BJ, et al. The ROAM/EORTC-1308 trial: radiation versus observation following surgical resection of atypical meningioma: study protocol for a randomised controlled trial. Trials. 2015; 16:519

[178] Chamberlain MC. Adjuvant combined modality therapy for malignant meningiomas. J Neurosurg. 1996; 84(5):733–736

[179] Schrell UM, Rittig MG, Anders M, et al. Hydroxyurea for treatment of unresectable and recurrent meningiomas. I. Inhibition of primary human meningioma cells in culture and in meningioma transplants by induction of the apoptotic pathway. J Neurosurg. 1997; 86(5):845–852

[180] Loven D, Hardoff R, Sever ZB, et al. Non-resectable slow-growing meningiomas treated by hydroxyurea. J Neurooncol. 2004; 67(1–2):221–226

[181] Newton HB, Slivka MA, Stevens C. Hydroxyurea chemotherapy for unresectable or residual meningioma. J Neurooncol. 2000; 49(2):165–170

[182] Ragel BT, Gillespie DL, Kushnir V, Polevaya N, Kelly D, Jensen RL. Calcium channel antagonists augment hydroxyurea- and ru486-induced inhibition of meningioma growth in vivo and in vitro. Neurosurgery. 2006; 59(5):1109–1120, discussion 1120–1121

[183] Chamberlain MC, Tsao-Wei DD, Groshen S. Temozolomide for treatment-resistant recurrent meningioma. Neurology. 2004; 62(7):1210–1212

[184] He J, Liu C, Wang B, Li N, Zuo G, Gao D. HMGN5 blockade by siRNA enhances apoptosis, suppresses invasion and increases chemosensitivity to temozolomide in meningiomas. Int J Oncol. 2015; 47(4):1503–1511

[185] Gupta V, Su YS, Samuelson CG, et al. Irinotecan: a potential new chemotherapeutic agent for atypical or malignant meningiomas. J Neurosurg. 2007; 106(3):455–462

[186] Chamberlain MC, Tsao-Wei DD, Groshen S. Salvage chemotherapy with CPT-11 for recurrent meningioma. J Neurooncol. 2006; 78(3):271–276

[187] Matsuda Y, Kawamoto K, Kiya K, Kurisu K, Sugiyama K, Uozumi T. Antitumor effects of antiprogesterones on human meningioma cells in vitro and in vivo. J Neurosurg. 1994; 80(3):527–534

[188] Ji Y, Rankin C, Grunberg S, et al. Double-blind phase III randomized trial of the antiprogestin agent mifepristone in the treatment of unresectable meningioma: SWOG S9005. J Clin Oncol. 2015; 33(34):4093–4098

[189] Goodwin JW, Crowley J, Eyre HJ, Stafford B, Jaeckle KA, Townsend JJ. A phase II evaluation of tamoxifen in unresectable or refractory meningiomas: a Southwest Oncology Group study. J Neurooncol. 1993; 15(1):75–77

[190] Johnson DR, Kimmel DW, Burch PA, et al. Phase II study of subcutaneous octreotide in adults with recurrent or progressive meningioma and meningeal hemangiopericytoma. Neuro-oncol. 2011; 13(5):530–535

[191] Chamberlain MC, Glantz MJ, Fadul CE. Recurrent meningioma: salvage therapy with long-acting somatostatin analogue. Neurology. 2007; 69(10): 969–973

[192] Norden AD, Ligon KL, Hammond SN, et al. Phase II study of monthly pasireotide LAR (SOM230C) for recurrent or progressive meningioma. Neurology. 2015; 84(3):280–286

[193] Gerster-Gilliéron K, Forrer F, Maecke H, Mueller-Brand J, Merlo A, Cordier D. 90Y-DOTATOC as a therapeutic option for complex recurrent or progressive meningiomas. J Nucl Med. 2015; 56(11):1748–1751

[194] Marincek N, Radojewski P, Dumont RA, et al. Somatostatin receptor-targeted radiopeptide therapy with 90Y-DOTATOC and 177Lu-DOTATOC in progressive meningioma: long-term results of a phase II clinical trial. J Nucl Med. 2015; 56(2):171–176

[195] McCutcheon IE, Flyvbjerg A, Hill H, et al. Antitumor activity of the growth hormone receptor antagonist pegvisomant against human meningiomas in nude mice. J Neurosurg. 2001; 94(3):487–492

[196] Drake WM, Grossman AB, Hutson RK. Effect of treatment with pegvisomant on meningioma growth in vivo. Eur J Endocrinol. 2005; 152(1):161–162

[197] Arnli MB, Backer-Grøndahl T, Ytterhus B, et al. Expression and clinical value of EGFR in human meningiomas. PeerJ. 2017; 5:e3140

[198] Yang SY, Xu GM. Expression of PDGF and its receptor as well as their relationship to proliferating activity and apoptosis of meningiomas in human meningiomas. J Clin Neurosci. 2001; 8 Suppl 1:49–53

[199] Norden AD, Raizer JJ, Abrey LE, et al. Phase II trials of erlotinib or gefitinib in patients with recurrent meningioma. J Neurooncol. 2010; 96(2):211–217

[200] Wen PY, Yung WK, Lamborn KR, et al. Phase II study of imatinib mesylate for recurrent meningiomas (North American Brain Tumor Consortium study 01–08). Neuro-oncol. 2009; 11(6):853–860

[201] Kaley TJ, Wen P, Schiff D, et al. Phase II trial of sunitinib for recurrent and progressive atypical and anaplastic meningioma. Neuro-oncol. 2015; 17(1): 116–121

[202] Raheja A, Colman H, Palmer CA, Couldwell WT. Dramatic radiographic response resulting in cerebrospinal fluid rhinorrhea associated with sunitinib therapy in recurrent atypical meningioma: case report. J Neurosurg. 2017; 127(5):965–970

[203] Shih KC, Chowdhary S, Rosenblatt P, et al. A phase II trial of bevacizumab and everolimus as treatment for patients with refractory, progressive intracranial meningioma. J Neurooncol. 2016; 129(2):281–288

[204] Nayak L, Iwamoto FM, Rudnick JD, et al. Atypical and anaplastic meningiomas treated with bevacizumab. J Neurooncol. 2012; 109(1):187–193

[205] Lou E, Sumrall AL, Turner S, et al. Bevacizumab therapy for adults with recurrent/progressive meningioma: a retrospective series. J Neurooncol. 2012; 109(1):63–70

[206] Golomb HM, Jacobs A, Fefer A, et al. Alpha-2 interferon therapy of hairy-cell leukemia: a multicenter study of 64 patients. J Clin Oncol. 1986; 4(6):900–905

[207] Niederle N, Moritz T, Kloke O, et al. Interferon alfa-2b in acute- and chronic-phase chronic myelogenous leukaemia: initial response and long-term results in 54 patients. Eur J Cancer. 1991; 27 Suppl 4:S7–S14

[208] Neidhart JA. Interferon therapy for the treatment of renal cancer. Cancer. 1986; 57(8) Suppl:1696–1699

[209] Creagan ET, Ahmann DL, Frytak S, Long HJ, Itri LM. Recombinant leukocyte A interferon (rIFN-alpha A) in the treatment of disseminated malignant melanoma: analysis of complete and long-term responding patients. Cancer. 1986; 58(12):2576–2578

[210] Koper JW, Zwarthoff EC, Hagemeijer A, et al. Inhibition of the growth of cultured human meningioma cells by recombinant interferon-alpha. Eur J Cancer. 1991; 27(4):416–419

[211] Folkman J, Ingber D. Inhibition of angiogenesis. Semin Cancer Biol. 1992; 3 (2):89–96

[212] Zhang ZJ, Wang JL, Muhr C, Smits A. Synergistic inhibitory effects of interferon-alpha and 5-fluorouracil in meningioma cells in vitro. Cancer Lett. 1996; 100(1–2):99–105

[213] Kaba SE, DeMonte F, Bruner JM, et al. The treatment of recurrent unresectable and malignant meningiomas with interferon alpha-2B. Neurosurgery. 1997; 40(2):271–275

[214] Han SJ, Reis G, Kohanbash G, et al. Expression and prognostic impact of immune modulatory molecule PD-L1 in meningioma. J Neurooncol. 2016; 130 (3):543–552

[215] Weller M, Roth P, Sahm F, et al. Durable control of metastatic AKT1-mutant WHO grade 1 meningothelial meningioma by the AKT inhibitor, AZD5363. J Natl Cancer Inst. 2017; 109(3):1–4

[216] Nigim F, Esaki S, Hood M, et al. A new patient-derived orthotopic malignant meningioma model treated with oncolytic herpes simplex virus. Neuro-oncol. 2016; 18(9):1278–1287

[217] Grill J, Lamfers ML, van Beusechem VW, et al. Oncolytic virotherapy of meningiomas in vitro with replication-competent adenovirus. Neurosurgery. 2005; 56(1):146–153, discussion 153–154

[218] Yano S, Kuratsu J, Kumamoto Brain Tumor Research Group. Indications for surgery in patients with asymptomatic meningiomas based on an extensive experience. J Neurosurg. 2006; 105(4):538–543

[219] Nakamura M, Roser F, Michel J, Jacobs C, Samii M. The natural history of incidental meningiomas. Neurosurgery. 2003; 53(1):62–70, discussion 70–71

[220] Olivero WC, Lister JR, Elwood PW. The natural history and growth rate of asymptomatic meningiomas: a review of 60 patients. J Neurosurg. 1995; 83 (2):222–224

37 Schwannomas of the Skull Base

Michael Gleeson

Summary

The incidence, natural history, presentation and management of cranial nerve schwannomas are discussed in relation to their site according to evidence mainly acquired and published over the last 20 years.

Keywords: vestibular schwannoma, trigeminal schwannoma, facial schwannoma, jugular foramen schwannoma, hypoglossal schwannoma, surgical treatment, stereotactic radiotherapy

37.1 Introduction

Cranial nerve schwannomas form the backbone of any skull base surgeon's clinical practice. Vestibular schwannomas are by far the most common, but schwannomas can develop on any of the cranial and spinal nerves. Although usually solitary, generally slow-growing, and benign, a very small number either are malignant or become malignant over time. Their growth rate varies and is certainly not uniform, and a few eventually undergo spontaneous involution. Bilateral vestibular schwannomas (VSs) develop in patients who have NF2 along with multiple schwannomas on the other cranial nerves. Schwannomas are next most commonly found on the trigeminal, facial, vagal, glossopharyngeal, and hypoglossal cranial nerves, in that order of frequency.

With the introduction of MRI, the true incidence and natural history of intracranial schwannomas has become apparent. In the light of this knowledge, the management of these tumors has changed considerably. Relatively small tumors that might previously have been resected are now subject to a period of observation first, with serial MR scans to determine their growth pattern before deciding on treatment. Only those found to be enlarging or causing brainstem compression are considered to be in need of treatment by either stereotactic radiosurgery or resection as appropriate. Despite the benign nature of these tumors, their management can have a very significant impact on quality of life, even in uncomplicated cases. Furthermore, the presence of multiple tumors puts a completely different complexion on how these patients should be managed.

37.2 Incidence and Epidemiology

Vestibular schwannomas (VSs) are traditionally thought to account for 8 to 10% of primary intracranial, extra-axial tumors and for 85% of tumors found in the cerebellopontine angle. These data have been acquired from postmortem autopsy material that likely missed countless intrameatal tumors and from archived operative registers at major institutions. The true incidence of cranial nerve schwannomas has almost certainly yet to be determined accurately, for improvements in imaging over time have continued to reveal smaller and smaller tumors, as first highlighted by a study undertaken by Tos, Charabi, and Thomsen,[1] who were in the unique position of having access to the entire medical records of Denmark with respect to VS. Over

three consecutive time periods they observed a steady increase in newly diagnosed tumors. They attributed this to increased awareness among otolaryngologists of the diagnosis of VS and better access to CT and later MRI. By 1995, their observed incidence had risen from 7.8 tumors per million population per year in 1983 to 12.4 tumors per million. This increase was largely due to the earlier detection of small intracanalicular tumors. In a later study, it was estimated that eventually as many as 1 per 1000 individuals would be diagnosed with a VS in their lifetime.[2]

The peak incidence of solitary intracranial schwannomas is between the sixth and seventh decades of life regardless of the site of the tumor. In a recent study of 23,739 patients who had VSs diagnosed between 2004 and 2010 in the United States, there was no overall difference in incidence between males and females. When comparing age and gender, incidence was slightly higher in females between 35 and 54 years of age and higher in males between 65 and 84 years. Asian Pacific Islanders had the highest incidence, followed by whites, Alaskan natives, and American Indians. Incidence was significantly lower in Hispanics.[3] Similar racial differences have been recorded elsewhere in the world. Although this might be due to genetic or environmental factors, it could equally well be influenced by differences in diagnostic practices and health care provision.

The data for the incidence of other cranial nerve schwannomas are far more vague. Trigeminal schwannomas, the next most common, are said to account for 0.07 to 0.36% of all intracranial tumors and anywhere from 0.8 to 8% of intracranial schwannomas, based on data first quoted by Cushing, then propagated and embellished through subsequent generations.[4] The best that can be said of facial and jugular foramen schwannomas are that they are uncommon and that hypoglossal schwannomas are extremely rare, based on single institutional experiences and small series case reports.[5] The same can be said for schwannomas that develop on the other cranial nerves.

Cranial nerve schwannomas are extremely common in patients who have neurofibromatosis type 2 (NF2), and indeed presence of multiple intracranial schwannomas is among the diagnostic criteria for the condition (▶ Table 37.1).[6] In a study of the distribution of non–vestibular cranial nerve schwannomas in 83 patients who had NF2, oculomotor and trigeminal schwannomas were those most commonly present at the time of first radiological evaluation (▶ Table 37.2).[7] The birth incidence of patients who have NF2 is 1/33,206 population per year, with a prevalence of 1/56,161 of the population. The median age at diagnosis of de novo case is 23 years (range 4–48 years) and is significantly earlier in patients who have first-degree relatives who also have NF2: median age 20 years (range 3–39 years).

37.3 Pathology

Schwannomas are benign nerve sheath tumors in the vast majority of cases. In very large series, 0.2% have been reported to be malignant.[3] Mutations are found throughout the coding

Table 37.1 Diagnostic criteria for NF2

Primary finding	Added features required for diagnosis
Bilateral VS	None
First-degree relative with NF2	Unilateral VS or: Any 2 other NF2-associated lesions: meningioma, schwannoma, glioma, cataracts
Unilateral VS	Any 2 other NF2-associated lesions: meningioma, schwannoma, glioma, cataracts
Multiple meningiomas	Unilateral VS or: Any 2 other NF2-associated lesions: meningioma, schwannoma, glioma, cataracts

Abbreviations: NF2, neurofibromatosis type 2; VS, vestibular schwannoma.
Source: Data from Ardern-Holmes S, Fisher G, North K, Neurofibromatosis type 2: presentation, major complications, and management with a focus on the paediatric age group, Journal of Child Neurology 2017;32:9–22.

Table 37.2 Location and size of nonvestibular schwannomas at first evaluation

Volume (mL)	Mean	Standard deviation	N (%)
III: Oculomotor	0.23	0.26	10 (15.6)
IV: Trochlear	0.08	–	1 (1.5)
V: Trigeminal	0.56	1.58	46 (76)
VI: Abducens	0.03	–	1 (1.5)
IX: Glossopharyngeal	3.35	–	1 (1.5)
X: Vagus	0.51	0.62	3 (4.7)
XI: Accessory	0.08	–	1 (1.5)
XII: Hypoglossal	0.04	–	1 (1.5)
Total	0.52	1.40	64

Source: Data from Fisher LM, Doherty JK, Lev MH, Slattery WH, Distribution of non-vestibular cranial nerve schwannomas in neurofibromatosis 2, Otology & Neurotology 2007;28:1083–1090.

sequence on chromosome 22q8. They are formed by Schwann cells that show a loss of the NF2 gene product Merlin (moesinerzin-radixin–like protein), also known as schwannomin.

Macroscopically, schwannomas form round masses that are usually encapsulated. They grow expansively and often contain thinly spread nerve bundles on the surface. Degenerative changes caused by infarctlike necrosis are often seen. Microscopic appearances are of a variable pattern of neoplastic Schwann cells. Zones of compact cells with nuclear palisading are referred to as Antoni A areas or Verucay bodies, whereas paucicellular zones where the cells have indistinct processes are termed Antoni B areas. All schwannomas show a pericellular reticulin pattern formed by basement membranes. Their vasculature is often thickened and hyalinized, and the tumors can contain lipidized cells and haemosiderin. Occasionally schwannomas contain significant amounts of melanin, in which case they are called melanotic schwannomas. Other morphological variants include ancient schwannomas that have bizarre cellular forms and occasional mitotic figures but that are not malignant.

Schwannomas express S100 and Sox10 and may focally express GFAP (glial fibrillary acidic protein). Tumor cells have a basement membrane that can be visualized using a reticulin silver stain or immunostaining for collagen type IV. Displaced axons on the surface of the tumor, usually within the capsule, can be visualized using neurofilament immunostaining (▶ Fig. 37.1).

37.3.1 Neurofibromatosis Type 2

Historically, NF2 has been subgrouped by the severity of its symptoms, initially into the Gardner (mild) and Wishart (severe) subtypes. In 1995 a genotype–phenotype was described that has since been further confirmed and clarified.[8,9,10] Mutations of the NF2 gene can cause a loss of the gene product, merlin; a reduction in protein function; or a gain of protein function. Those leading to the production of a truncated protein, such as nonsense or frameshift mutations, tend to be linked to more severe disease than those caused by large deletions, missense mutations, and in-frame deletions.[11] Patients who have mutations that result in truncated protein rather than loss of protein expression tend to present and be diagnosed at a much younger age than others and have a higher prevalence/proportion of meningiomas, spinal tumors, and other cranial nerve schwannomas (not VS). Their VSs become symptomatic earlier in terms of hearing loss and tinnitus. They also develop paraesthesia, wasting, weakness, and headaches at an early stage.[10]

In contrast to solitary schwannomas, those associated with NF2 tend to be multinodular in appearance, suggesting a multifocal origin.

37.3.2 Mosaicism

More than 50% of people who have NF2 have no family history of the disease and develop the mutation in a de novo manner. De novo mutations may happen at either the prezygotic or the postzygotic stage. Prezygotic mutations take place in the germline cells of either parent, whereas postzygotic mutations take place in any cell after fertilization and cell division. Patients whose mutation takes place in the postzygotic stage may develop mosaicism, in which only a proportion of their total body cells contain the mutation. In this way, the individual may develop severe, mild, or incomplete disease phenotypes depending on the type and proportion of their tissues affected. In short, patients' tumors may be limited to a specific anatomical area.

37.3.3 Schwannomatosis

Schwannomatosis is a clinically related disease entity characterized by benign schwannomas distributed throughout the nervous system. It is often difficult to distinguish from NF2, particularly the mosaic form. Although bilateral VSs are pathognomonic of NF2, even unilateral VSs are very uncommon in patients who have schwannomatosis. Both conditions are associated with meningioma, albeit at a much higher incidence in patients who have NF2 than those who have schwannomatosis. Germline mutations of the NF2 gene are not present in patients who have schwannomatosis, but somatically acquired

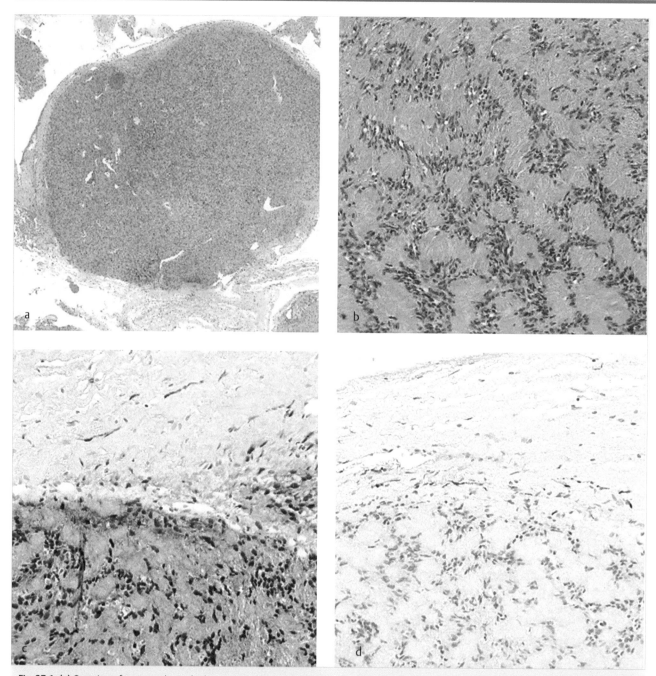

Fig. 37.1 **(a)** Overview of a resected spinal schwannoma showing the well-demarcated, encapsulated tumor. **(b)** Detail showing the palisading growth of tumor cells with incipient formation of so-called Verocay bodies. **(c)** S100 immunostaining. The lower part shows the positive nuclei and cytoplasm of the tumor. The upper part shows the fibrous capsule. Note the nerve fibers within the peritumoral capsule. (The Schwann cells are S100-positive.) **(d)** Immunostaining for neurofilament, which specifically labels subcapsular nerve fibers. Scale bar: **(a)** 2 mm, **(b)** 200 μm, **(c, d)** 100 μm. (Courtesy of Professor Sebastian Brandner.)

mutations are present in the tumors. Mutations of the chromatin remodeling gene on chromosome 22, SMARCB1 (SWI/SNF-related matrix-associated actin-dependent regulator of chromatin subfamily B member 1), are responsible for 20% of patients who have schwannomatosis, and there is a much higher detection rate of approximately 50% in patients who have familial disease. Patients who have an additional mutation of the LZTR1 (leucine-zipper–like transcription regulator 1 gene) confers an increased risk of developing a VS.[12,13]

37.4 Staging and Presentation

The functions of a staging system are twofold: First, to define criterion points in tumor growth and symptomatology that are associated with a significant change in outcome prognosis, so that patients can be given properly informed consent. Second, to guide the clinician in treatment selection and the surgeon in assessing optimal approach and likely complications.

37.4.1 Vestibular Schwannoma

Most VSs present with a progressive, unilateral hearing loss associated with tinnitus and a disturbance of balance that is often misdiagnosed and that precedes the hearing loss by months or even years. Some may cause a sudden sensorineural hearing loss and symptoms referable to the facial nerve, such as facial twitching, disturbances of taste, and, less commonly, facial palsy. As the tumor increases in size, molds, and begins to compress the brainstem, a trigeminal deficit develops and some patients present with neuralgia. In the latter stages, further compression of the brainstem causes obstructive hydrocephalus; by that time vagal and glossopharyngeal deficits may be interfering with swallowing.[14]

In the first instance, most surgeons simply classify tumors on a 5-point scale based on MRI appearance and maximal axial measurements. Thus a VS may be intrameatal, either filling the internal auditory canal (IAC) or only partially filling it. Small tumors would have a maximal extrameatal diameter of 1.9 cm, medium tumors 2.0 to 3.4 cm, large tumors 3.5 to 4.4 cm, and giant tumors 4.5 cm or larger. The Hanover radiological VS classification scheme is favored by many and is of some utility, being more detailed (▶ Table 37.3). Improvements to this scheme might be to record whether cerebrospinal fluid (CSF) was present between the lateral end of the internal auditory meatus and the medial end of the tumor, which would indicate the possibility of a better prognosis if hearing preservation surgery were anticipated. Similarly, there is no category for intralabyrinthine tumors or those spreading from the lateral end of the IAC into the labyrinth, for which there is no hope for hearing using surgical means (▶ Fig. 37.2).

For some national databases, specific measurements are now required. Three measurements taken at 90° to a plane passing through the internal auditory meatus along the posterior wall of the temporal bone are recorded: maximal axial diameter, maximal anteroposterior diameter, and maximal craniocaudal dimension. Until reliable, reproducible, and accurate volume measurements are a standard part of the software supplied with MR scanners, these measurements and the Hannover classification scale should be used. Even then, it is likely that volume measurements will merely contribute more information to the radiation oncologists who quote their stereotactic fields in cubic centimeters.

37.4.2 Trigeminal Schwannoma

Most trigeminal schwannomas remain asymptomatic until they have attained significant size. Some will have been diagnosed simply because they are part of the tumor load in a newly diagnosed patient who has NF2. Those that are symptomatic present with a progressive sensory deficit in one of the divisions of the cranial nerve, pain, or neuralgia. A few will press on adjacent cranial nerves, such as the abducens, trochlear, or oculomotor nerves, and be discovered during investigation of diplopia.

Jefferson described a classification in 1953 that others have since modified in various ways. Trigeminal schwannomas can develop anywhere along the course of the nerve, although the majority arise at the entry site of the trigeminal root into Meckel's cave. The most recent classification, a modification of that described by Samii,[4] recognized six distinct groups based on their origin and extension (▶ Table 37.4).[15,16] Most large surgical series group their cases similarly, even if not using a standardized notation, while recommending suitable approaches for each group (▶ Fig. 37.3).

37.4.3 Facial Schwannoma

There are no staging systems for facial nerve schwannomas—merely a recognition that schwannomas can develop on any segment of the nerve from the cerebello-pontine angle (CPA) and internal auditory canal, through the fallopian canal in the temporal bone to its course in the retromandibular fossa and parotid gland (▶ Fig. 37.4).

More attention has been focused on the predilection or origin in the perigeniculate region and on optimal time and methods of management.[17,18] Most present with a very slowly progressive facial weakness that may take many months to become noticeable. Those who have tumor in the retromandibular fossa are more concerned about the visible mass in their neck and, even though tumor extends into their temporal bones, have no facial weakness. Some such tumors are misdiagnosed as salivary

Table 37.3 Hannover radiological vestibular schwannoma classification

Tumor radiological grade	Extension
T1	Purely intrameatal
T2	Intra- and limited extrameatal extension
T3A	Filling the CPA but not reaching the brainstem
T3B	Filling the CPA and touching the brainstem
T4A	Compressing the brainstem
T4B	Hydrocephalus secondary to compression of the fourth ventricle

Abbreviation: CPA, cerebello-pontine angle.

Table 37.4 Modified Samii classification of trigeminal schwannomas

Type	Extension	Approach
A	Extracranial tumor with small extension into the middle fossa	V3: ITF type D + EMFA V2: Endoscopic TM
B	Middle fossa tumor with extracranial extension	IMF + ITF type D or endoscopic TM
C	Middle fossa tumor	Intra- or extradural MFA
D	Posterior fossa tumor	RS
E	Dumbbell-shaped tumor in middle and posterior fossa	Staged RS & MFA
F	Tumor with extracranial and middle and posterior fossa extensions	Staged approaches

Abbreviations: EMFA, extradural middle fossa approach; IMF, intradural middle fossa; ITF, infratemporal fossa. infratemporal fossa approach; MFA, middle fossa approach; RS, retrosigmoid; TM, transmaxillary approach.

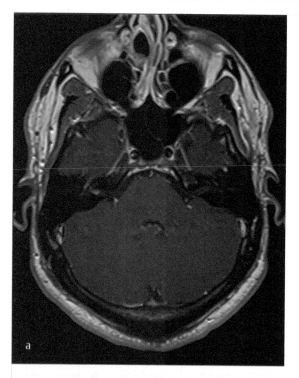
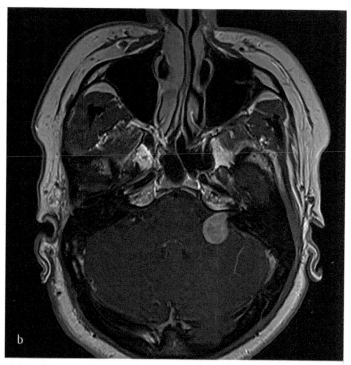
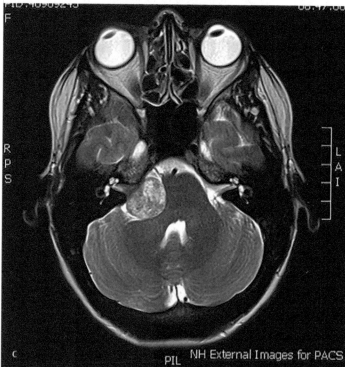
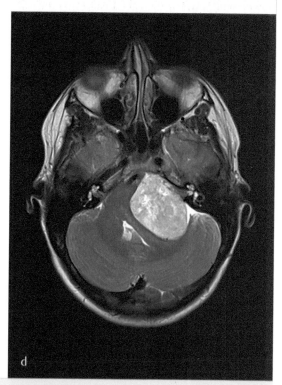

Fig. 37.2 **(a)** T1 right VS; **(b)** T3b left VS; **(c)** T4a right VS; **(d)** T4b left VS. VS, vestibular schwannoma.

gland tumors with disastrous results. Tumor spread into the middle ear causes a conductive hearing loss, whereas those extending into the labyrinthine segment of the fallopian canal or IAC produce a sensorineural loss. Destruction of the roof of the IAC is typical of tumors that arise in the labyrinthine segment of the nerve.

37.4.4 Jugular Foramen Schwannoma

Few surgeons have personal clinical experience of significant size, and the largest reported series of 204 patients was acquired by a meta-analysis of case reports published over a 23-year period.[19] These tumors tend to present relatively late,

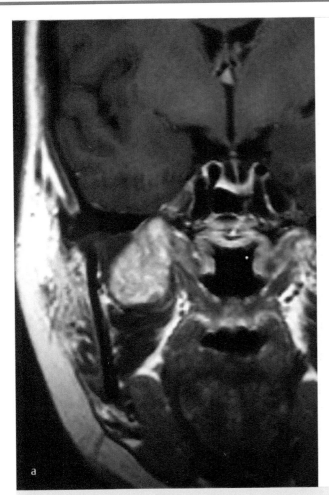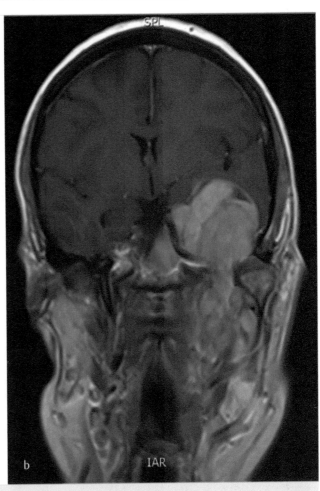

Fig. 37.3 (a) Type A tumor just entering the foramen ovale. (b) Type B tumor with significant components in both the middle fossa and extracranially.

because they grow very slowly and are not suspected until a neural deficit is acquired, by which time it is difficult to know from which lower cranial nerve the tumor arose—although the vagus and glossopharyngeal nerves are most often implicated. Many are found coincidentally on scans undertaken for other purposes and before the tumor has caused any neural deficit at all. The most common presenting symptoms are a husky voice, dysphagia, ataxia, hearing loss, and tinnitus, which may be pulsatile, for the tumors tend to obstruct or impede the venous outflow through the jugular bulb. Very rarely, jugular foramen schwannomas may present with glossopharyngeal neuralgia syncope syndrome. Sudden onset pharyngeal neuralgic pain, sometimes precipitated by turning the neck to one side, is followed by profound bradycardia, hypotension, and impaired consciousness.[20]

The simple scheme devised by Kaye[19] and modified by Pellet[21] has been adopted for most reported cases. Samii et al[22] made a significant modification to this scheme to emphasize that the grade should also help define the most appropriate surgical approach, particularly for patients who have intraosseous tumor (▶ Table 37.5; ▶ Fig. 37.5).

Table 37.5 Classification of jugular foramen schwannomas

Class	Definition	Surgical approach
A	Tumor confined to cisternal part of the nerves; no significant extension into the JF	RS
B1	Intraosseous tumor inside the JF	EA-RS infralabyrinthine approach
B2	Intraosseous tumor with significant extension into the cisternal space	EA-RS infralabyrinthine approach
B3	Intraosseous tumor with significant extension into the infratemporal fossa	EA transcervical approach
C	Tumor arising from the extracranial part of the nerve	Transcervical approach
D	Dumbbell-shaped tumor with intracranial, intraosseous, and extracranial parts	Combined transcervical, EA-RS, and infralabyrinthine approach

Abbreviations: EA-RS, endoscopic-assisted retrosigmoid; JF, jugular foramen; RS, retrosigmoid.

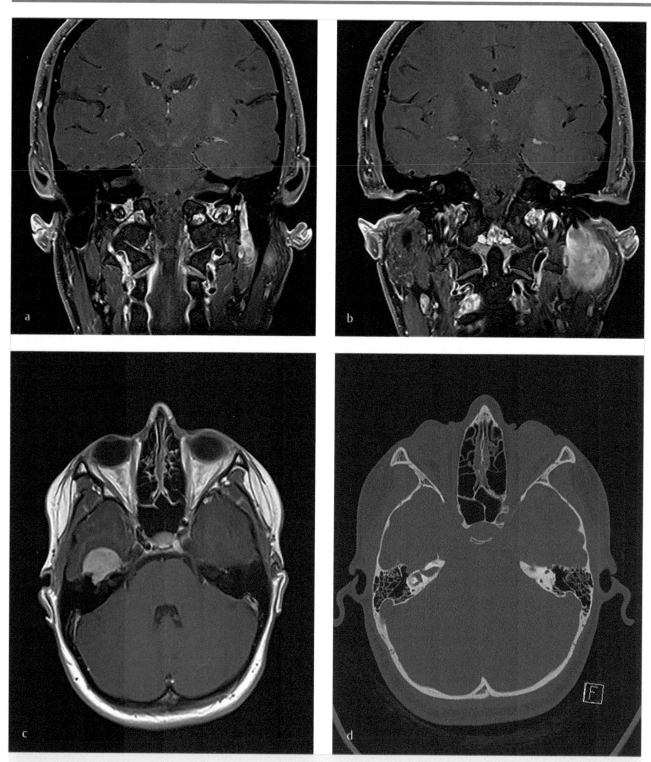

Fig. 37.4 (a,b) The facial schwannoma extends from the retromandibular region in the parotid, through the entire length of the fallopian canal, to the lateral end of the IAC and has broken through the floor of the middle cranial fossa in the perigeniculate region. **(c,d)** The facial schwannoma has eroded the roof of the IAC and extends in to the middle cranial fossa. IAC, internal auditory canal.

37.4.5 Hypoglossal Schwannoma

Hypoglossal schwannomas are extremely rare and may be completely intracranial, intracranial and extracranial, or completely extracranial. Most patients present with a slowly progressive wasting of the tongue. Suboccipital headache exacerbated by neck movements is said to be an early sign of intracranial tumors. Large tumors may present with cerebellar and brainstem signs or even jugular foramen syndrome.[5]

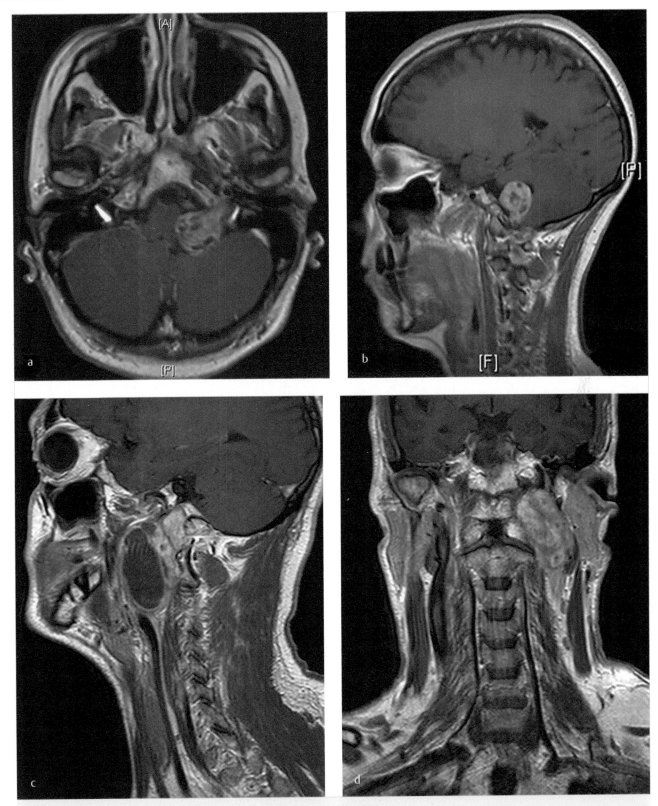

Fig. 37.5 (a,b) Type B2 jugular foramen schwannoma. **(c,d)** Type C vagal schwannoma.

37.5 Treatment and Outcomes

As already stated, clinical data collected over the last 20 years has increased our knowledge of intracranial schwannomas and their natural history and growth patterns. It has changed views on their best management. Advances in both surgical and radiation techniques have made some more easily and successfully managed. Even more recently, over the last 10 years, drugs have been developed and trialed that have a part to play in the treatment of patients who have NF2. Nevertheless there remain some tumors, regardless of their site of origin, that pose a significant threat to the patient's life as well as to the quality of the patient's life if surgery is part of the management plan.

37.5.1 Vestibular Schwannoma Management

Clinical Observation: "Wait and Scan"

A very large percentage of skull base schwannomas are now detected when they are extremely small. This is particularly the case with VSs, for which increased awareness of the significance of unilateral auditory and vestibular symptoms, together with increased access to MR scanners, has increased the frequency of their diagnosis. There is no urgency to treat these tumors, especially if they are not touching or compressing the brainstem. Patients lose little by a period of clinical observation with interval scans, for at least 30% might never need any further intervention. There is a potential loss of candidacy for hearing preservation surgery while waiting and observing in up to 50%, whereas less than 10% lose their candidacy for stereotactic radiotherapy. In an extensive review of the literature, Portier et al[23] found estimates of successful hearing preservation by surgery of up to 60%, but the average was much less—just 31%. This huge range can be explained by a lack of consistency in how hearing results are reported. So although about 50% lose their candidacy for hearing preservation surgery by observation, in reality the figure is 15%—that being the percentage of those in whom it could have been successful. Whether that percentage might have been greater had their tumors not grown, or had those patients lost their hearing without further growth, is simply not known.

Surgery

Assuming that the patient is fit for surgery, microsurgical resection is the time-honored gold-standard treatment option for all VSs that are shown to be growing or simply to be too large to observe or treat by other means. Current consensus is to reserve microsurgical resection for tumors that have an axial diameter within the angle greater than 2.5 cm. Patient choice has largely driven this management protocol. Those patients who have smaller tumors tend to choose stereotactic radiotherapy regardless of their age, although most surgeons prefer to treat patients under 30 years using microsurgery. Other indications for surgery include those patients who have severe vertigo, which is not usually helped or abolished by radiosurgery, and those whose radiosurgery has failed to stop tumor growth.

The retrosigmoid and translabyrinthine are the most commonly used approaches, and both are suitable for any size of tumor. The retrosigmoid approach is relatively quick and offers the advantage of possible hearing preservation. The translabyrinthine approach destroys any residual hearing and cannot be employed in the presence of middle ear or mastoid sepsis. Certain anatomical features, such as a very high jugular bulb, anteriorly placed sigmoid sinus, or hypoplastic temporal bone,

might also suggest that a retrosigmoid approach would be preferable. The middle fossa approach is suitable for small tumors largely restricted to the IAC, in which hearing preservation is the aim.

Outcome and prognosis after surgical resection are dependent on the size of the tumor. Similarly, complications develop more frequently when resecting large tumors than smaller ones. Death; stroke; cerebellar contusion; venous sinus injury; CSF leak; and trigeminal, abducens, and lower cranial nerve palsies more often complicate the resection of large and giant tumors. A total resection is nearly always the aim but is sometimes not possible without inflicting loss of facial nerve function. A case can be made for near total removal, particularly in very large or giant tumors, followed by interval scans and radiosurgery if the residual disease continues to grow. In this way, facial nerve function is optimized and preserved longer. The most frequent outcome measure quoted in large series is anatomical preservation of the facial nerve. However, anatomical preservation does not guarantee functional integrity, and functional results are rarely scored by an independent third party. It is fair to say that good facial nerve outcomes, House-Brackmann grade I to II, are achieved in about 90% of cases for small tumors but rarely in more than 25% for large and giant tumors. Recurrence rates are not often quoted, but recurrence is certainly encountered.

Radiation

The efficacy of stereotactic radiosurgery is now well established, and it is preferred as the first-line therapy for smaller VSs. It certainly preserves hearing for longer in most, although some patients' hearing may continue to deteriorate over time. It has radically changed the management of vestibular tumors worldwide over the past 20 years.[24] Failure to control growth rate is associated with radiosurgery, just as with microsurgery, and cannot be predicted or ignored. The marginal dose has been reduced so that radiation-induced complications are avoided while maintaining equivalent tumor control. Some radiation oncologists are now treating 3 cm tumors. Currently 5- and 10-year tumor control rates in excess of 90% are achieved and additional microsurgery avoided in over 97% of cases. In a large proportion of those in whom tumor growth is not controlled, additional radiosurgery is well tolerated and is successful.[25] Surgical resection after stereotactic radiosurgery is more complicated, for the arachnoid becomes condensed around the tumor and the facial nerve becomes more difficult to dissect free from it without destroying function. For the majority in which salvage surgery is required, a subtotal or near total resection is the only way to preserve facial nerve function as well as that of the trigeminal nerve.

37.5.2 Management of Vestibular Schwannoma in NF2

It is universally accepted that maintaining good quality of life must be the overriding aim of management for these patients. Most are destined to become profoundly deaf over time, and it is our duty to retain as much normal hearing as possible while minimizing collateral damage for as long as possible.

Surgery

Microsurgical resection of VSs in NF2 is much more difficult than in sporadic tumors. The tumors are often nodular and multifocal within the eighth nerve complex, and frequently the VS is in collision with another schwannoma that has developed on the facial nerve. The tumors are also less vascular than their sporadic counterparts.[26] These factors alone make hearing preservation surgery almost impossible even if the tumor is small enough to otherwise allow consideration. Furthermore, facial nerve outcomes are far worse than in sporadic cases—and most NF2 VSs are too large from the outset. Finally, in very small tumors with normal hearing, there is no way to predict which VS will inflict a complete hearing loss first. A complete bilateral hearing loss is a huge handicap for the patient that cochlear implants and auditory brainstem implants help to some extent, but it should never be precipitated unless surgery is required to save life. Some consider that this protocol stifles the development of microsurgical techniques for this group of patients, and it must be recognized that a few surgeons are extremely skilled in hearing preservation techniques. For them, it is reasonable to weigh up the potential advantages for the patient of removing a very small tumor from a hearing ear and preserving at least the cochlear nerve, if not hearing. If the patient and the patient's parents are properly and accurately consented, an ethical case can be made for this type of intervention. However, it must be remembered that the fundamental biological fault that has caused this condition cannot be cured by surgery and that other tumors in the same vicinity are likely to arise subsequently.

Stereotactic Radiotherapy

Despite early reports of radiation therapy's having induced malignant change,[27] this appears to be far less common than originally thought. Stereotactic radiotherapy should certainly be considered in NF2 and the normal boundaries in terms of tumor volume stretched slightly to give the patient the best chance of avoiding surgery. Significant case series estimate tumor control in 60 to 80% at 5 years, with hearing preservation in 73% at 1 year, diminishing to 48% at 5 years, with low risk of injury to the facial and trigeminal nerves.[28,29]

Chemotherapy

Bevacizumab (Avastin) is the most widely studied targeted therapy for NF2. This IgG1 monoclonal antibody, which binds biologically active vascular endothelial growth factor (VEGF), has been used in a large number of patients who have NF2. It has been shown to produce a significant reduction in tumor volume (< 20%) and improvement in hearing function in a number of these patients.[30,31] Tumor shrinkage has been sustained with continuous use of the drug but tends to regress when the drug is discontinued. The toxicity profile of bevacizumab is relatively well known, and it appears to be well tolerated. It does have a negative effect on wound healing, so surgery is not advised while the drug is being used.[32] Phase II studies are also under way on a number of drugs, including lapatinib, sorafenib, nilotinib, and PTC299, an inhibitor of VEGF synthesis.

37.5.3 Management of Trigeminal Schwannoma

Cushing stated "that is possible of course that a method may someday be evolved whereby a Gasserian neuroma or meningioma, even after it has crossed the ridge, may be safely removed. Should this come to pass, it will be another conquest for neurosurgery." The management of trigeminal schwannomas has moved on a bit since then, if only to recognize that very significant morbidity can be inflicted by over-enthusiastic surgery.

A period of observation with serial scans to document growth rate before devising a management plan applies to trigeminal schwannomas as much as, if not more than, it does to all other cranial base schwannomas, particularly those arising in patients who have NF2. Some might never require active intervention. Potential complications resulting from collateral damage to adjacent cranial nerves are very significant.

Surgery

Surgery remains the mainstay of treatment for most who require resection or radical debulking. Complete tumor removal may not be possible or wise, particularly for tumors that invade the cavernous sinus. The best approach will be determined by the site of origin and spread of the tumor, as indicated in Table 37-4. Total or near total resection is achieved in only about 70% of cases, following which a period of clinical observation with interval scans is wise before considering adjunctive radiosurgery.

Stereotactic Radiosurgery

Stereotactic radiosurgery (SRS) using either Gamma Knife or CyberKnife has come to challenge the place of surgery as the first-line treatment for trigeminal schwannomas. Significantly sized series comparable to those published for microsurgery have been published with medium-length periods of follow-up, making a good case for combination therapy after surgical debulking or for recurrent disease.[33,34]

37.5.4 Management of Facial Schwannomas

The major management dilemma for a patient who has a facial schwannoma is when and not how to treat it. Historically, surgical resection was the only treatment modality employed, and with it came complete loss of facial function. Restoration of facial symmetry and acceptable facial movement relied on various grafting techniques that were not always as satisfactory as either the patient or the surgeon would have liked. Operating only when facial palsy was well established meant that a large proportion of the muscle motor end plates had probably been lost and with them the chance for a better functional outcome. Operating too soon probably denied the patient many months or years of acceptable facial function. The advent of stereotactic radiosurgery has encouraged some to use it in selected cases.[35] The author's experience using it for the patient in ▶ Fig. 37.4 resulted in a complete resolution of facial nerve function and no further loss of hearing acuity. We are entering a new era and must learn which facial schwannomas are suitable for stereotactic radiosurgery.

37.5.5 Management of Jugular Foramen Schwanommas

Some schwannomas have probably completed their growth when first detected and will lie dormant for decades. Unless there is a substantial amount of tumor molding or compression of the brainstem, an expectant approach is best for most patients, with interval scans. The previously held view that the treatment of choice for these tumors was surgical no longer holds.

Surgery

Surgical resection should be advised only for large schwannomas and for patients who persist in requesting surgery despite adequate consent. The choice of approach is dictated by the site of origin and stage of the tumor. Intracranial tumor is best removed using a retrosigmoid approach combined with an infralabyrinthine exposure of the jugular foramen. Those tumors largely restricted to the parapharyngeal space can be managed by a transcervical approach combined with an infralabyrinthine exposure to removed disease in the jugular fossa and foramen.

Stereotactic Radiosurgery

Stereotactic radiosurgery should be considered if a schwannoma is growing and of an appropriate size, especially if it has not produced a palsy. Similarly, if a small vagal schwannoma has already produced a palsy, stereotactic radiosurgery should be considered or at least discussed first. A multi-institutional retrospective study of Gamma Knife radiosurgery for 117 patients who had jugular foramen schwannomas reported 3- and 5-year progression-free survival rates of 91% and 89%, respectively.[36]

37.5.6 Management of Hypoglossal Schwannomas

These tumors are so rare, and so many present with large intracranial extension, that surgical resection or debulking is appropriate. More recently, stereotactic radiosurgery has been employed either up front or to manage residual tumor in an attempt to limit cranial nerve damage.[5]

References

[1] Tos M, Charabi S, Thomsen J. Incidence of vestibular schwannomas. Laryngoscope. 1999; 109(5):736–740

[2] Evans DGR, Moran A, King A, Saeed S, Gurusinghe N, Ramsden R. Incidence of vestibular schwannoma and neurofibromatosis 2 in the North West of England over a 10-year period: higher incidence than previously thought. Otol Neurotol. 2005; 26(1):93–97

[3] Kshettry VR, Hsieh JK, Ostrom QT, Kruchko C, Barnholtz-Sloan JS. Incidence of vestibular schwannomas in the United States. J Neurooncol. 2015; 124(2):223–228

[4] Samii M, Migliori MM, Tatagiba M, Babu R. Surgical treatment of trigeminal schwannomas. J Neurosurg. 1995; 82(5):711–718

[5] Suri A, Bansal S, Sharma BS, et al. Management of hypoglossal schwannomas: single institutional experience of 14 cases. J Neurol Surg B Skull Base. 2014; 75(3):159–164

[6] Ardern-Holmes S, Fisher G, North K. Neurofibromatosis type 2: presentation, major complications, and management with a focus on the paediatric age group. J Child Neurol. 2017; 32(1):9–22

[7] Fisher LM, Doherty JK, Lev MH, Slattery WH, III. Distribution of nonvestibular cranial nerve schwannomas in neurofibromatosis 2. Otol Neurotol. 2007; 28(8):1083–1090

[8] Seizinger BR, Martuza RL, Gusella JF. Loss of genes on chromosome 22 in tumorigenesis of human acoustic neuroma. Nature. 1986; 322(6080):644–647

[9] Mérel P, Hoang-Xuan K, Sanson M, et al. Screening for germ-line mutations in the NF2 gene. Genes Chromosomes Cancer. 1995; 12(2):117–127

[10] Selvanathan SK, Shenton A, Ferner R, et al. Further genotype–phenotype correlations in neurofibromatosis 2. Clin Genet. 2010; 77(2):163–170

[11] Evans DGR, Trueman L, Wallace A, Collins S, Strachan T. Genotype/phenotype correlations in type 2 neurofibromatosis (NF2): evidence for more severe disease associated with truncating mutations. J Med Genet. 1998a; 35(6):450–455

[12] Piotrowski A, Xie J, Liu YF, et al. Germline loss-of-function mutations in LZTR1 predispose to an inherited disorder of multiple schwannomas. Nat Genet. 2014; 46(2):182–187

[13] Smith MJ, Isidor B, Beetz C, et al. Mutations in LZTR1 add to the complex heterogeneity of schwannomatosis. Neurology. 2015; 84(2):141–147

[14] Matthies C, Samii M. Management of 1000 vestibular schwannomas (acoustic neuromas): clinical presentation. Neurosurgery. 1997; 40(1):1–9, discussion 9–10

[15] Guthikonda B, Theodosopoulos PV, van Loveren H, Tew JM, Jr, Pensak ML. Evolution in the assessment and management of trigeminal schwannoma. Laryngoscope. 2008; 118(2):195–203

[16] Ramina R, Mattei TA, Sória MG, et al. Surgical management of trigeminal schwannomas. Neurosurg Focus. 2008; 25(6):E6

[17] McMonagle B, Al-Sanosi A, Croxson G, Fagan P. Facial schwannoma: results of a large case series and review. J Laryngol Otol. 2008; 122(11):1139–1150

[18] Wilkinson EP, Hoa M, Slattery WH, III, et al. Evolution in the management of facial nerve schwannoma. Laryngoscope. 2011; 121(10):2065–2074

[19] Kaye AH, Hahn JF, Kinney SE, Hardy RW, Jr, Bay JW. Jugular foramen schwannomas. J Neurosurg. 1984; 60(5):1045–1053

[20] Saman Y, Whitehead D, Gleeson M. Jugular foramen schwannoma presenting with glossopharyngeal neuralgia syncope syndrome. J Laryngol Otol. 2010; 124(12):1305–1308

[21] Pellet W, Cannoni M, Pech A. The widened transcochlear approach to jugular foramen tumors. J Neurosurg. 1988; 69(6):887–894

[22] Samii M, Babu RP, Tatagiba M, Sepehrnia A. Surgical treatment of jugular foramen schwannomas. J Neurosurg. 1995; 82(6):924–932

[23] Portier F, Lot G, Herman P, Salvan D, George B, Tran Ba Huy P. [Hearing preservation in vestibular schwannoma surgery: indications, techniques and results in the literature since 1990]. Neurochirurgie. 2000; 46(4):358–368, discussion 368–369

[24] Mackeith SA, Kerr RS, Milford CA. Trends in acoustic neuroma management: a 20-year review of the Oxford Skull Base Clinic. J Neurol Surg B Skull Base. 2013; 74(4):194–200

[25] Klijn S, Verheul JB, Beute GN, et al. Gamma Knife radiosurgery for vestibular schwannomas: evaluation of tumor control and its predictors in a large patient cohort in the Netherlands. J Neurosurg. 2016; 124(6):1619–1626

[26] Sobel RA. Vestibular (acoustic) schwannomas: histologic features in neurofibromatosis 2 and in unilateral cases. J Neuropathol Exp Neurol. 1993; 52(2):106–113

[27] Shin M, Ueki K, Kurita H, Kirino T. Malignant transformation of a vestibular schwannoma after Gamma Knife radiosurgery. Lancet. 2002; 360(9329):309–310

[28] Mathieu D, Kondziolka D, Flickinger JC, et al. Stereotactic radiosurgery for vestibular schwannomas in patients with neurofibromatosis type 2: an analysis of tumor control, complications, and hearing preservation rates. Neurosurgery. 2007; 60(3):460–468, discussion 468–470

[29] Rowe JG, Radatz MW, Walton L, Soanes T, Rodgers J, Kemeny AA. Clinical experience with Gamma Knife stereotactic radiosurgery in the management of vestibular schwannomas secondary to type 2 neurofibromatosis. J Neurol Neurosurg Psychiatry. 2003; 74(9):1288–1293

[30] Plotkin SR, Stemmer-Rachamimov AO, Barker FG, II, et al. Hearing improvement after bevacizumab in patients with neurofibromatosis type 2. N Engl J Med. 2009; 361(4):358–367

[31] Mautner VF, Nguyen R, Kutta H, et al. Bevacizumab induces regression of vestibular schwannomas in patients with neurofibromatosis type 2. Neuro-oncol. 2010; 12(1):14–18

[32] Blakeley JO, Evans DG, Adler J, et al. Consensus recommendations for current treatments and accelerating clinical trials for patients with neurofibromatosis type 2. Am J Med Genet A. 2012; 158A(1):24–41

[33] Yianni J, Dinca EB, Rowe J, Radatz M, Kemeny AA. Stereotactic radiosurgery for trigeminal schwannomas. Acta Neurochir (Wien). 2012; 154(2):277–283

[34] Champ CE, Mishra MV, Shi W, et al. Stereotactic radiotherapy for trigeminal schwannomas. Neurosurgery. 2012; 71(2):270–277

[35] Fezeu F, Lee CC, Dodson BK, et al. Stereotactic radiosurgery for facial nerve schwannomas: a preliminary assessment and review of the literature. Br J Neurosurg. 2015; 29(2):213–218

[36] Hasegawa T, Kato T, Kida Y, et al. Gamma Knife surgery for patients with jugular foramen schwannomas: a multiinstitutional retrospective study in Japan. J Neurosurg. 2016; 125(4):822–831

38 Paragangliomas of the Head and Neck

Matthew Mifsud and Patrick J. Gullane

Summary

Paragangliomas of the head and neck are a unique collection of rare neoplasms. Their neuroendocrine origin necessitates a unique management approach, requiring comprehensive genetic and biochemical assessment in addition to a more standard tumor work-up. A variety of surgical and radiotherapeutic strategies can be employed to manage appropriately selected cases. However, many of these tumors exhibit an indolent natural history, progressing slowly over a patient's lifetime. Consequently, a conservative observational strategy is often efficacious, limiting treatment-associated morbidity and helping optimize patient quality of life.

Keywords: head and neck paraganglioma, head and neck neuroendocrine tumor, glomus tumor, jugulotympanic tumor, carotid body tumor

38.1 Introduction

The human paraganglionic system comprises a highly specialized neurosecretory epithelium (composed of chromaffin cells) found within the adrenal medulla and along neuronal/vascular adventitia within extra-adrenal paraganglia.[1,2,3] All elements of this system share a common neural crest origin and are characterized by catecholamine production and storage.[4] A clear link exists to the autonomic nervous system, with sympathetic paraganglia generally found in the abdomen and thorax, whereas those of parasympathetic origin cluster exclusively within the neck and skull base.[5] The most well-known head and neck sites are the carotid bifurcation (carotid body), jugular foramen, and tympanic plexus. However, paraganglionic tissue may also be found along the course of the vagus and glossopharyngeal nerves, including within the larynx, nasal cavity, orbits, and trachea.[1,3,6]

Extra-adrenal paragangliomas are rare neuroendocrine neoplasms, which comprise only 10% of all chromaffin cell tumors (with pheochromocytomas encompassing the other 90%); only about 3% of these lesions occur in the head and neck.[2,7] Although catecholamine hypersecretion is a unique concern with paragangliomas, this is an uncommon concern within the head and neck (only 3–4% of cases) because of their parasympathetic origin.[8] As a consequence, they most commonly present as benign, slow-growing, and hypervascular tumors with potential symptomatology linked to anatomical site of origin.[7,8] Although surgical resection has been the historic treatment of choice for all paragangliomas, the association with key neurovascular structures is associated with significant morbidity (e.g., speech/swallowing disorder, severe blood loss, not insignificant stroke risk) and has led to an ever more complex treatment algorithm that increasingly emphasizes the potential role of observation.[6,7]

38.2 Incidence and Epidemiology

The rarity of head and neck paragangliomas (HNPGs) makes the true disease incidence rate somewhat difficult to ascertain.

Most estimates suggest an incidence that ranges from 1 in 30,000 to 100,000 within the general population.[8,9,10,11,12] They are generally most common in the fourth to sixth decades of life and show a strong female preponderance (roughly 2/3:1).[3,7,13] Familial and sporadic variants exist. Multicentric lesions (occurring either synchronous or metachronous with the primary presenting tumor) occur in 10 to 20% of patients, but this phenomenon is far more common in those who have documented hereditary disorders.[6,14,15] Because all HNPGs are derived from the same neural crest–derived cellular line, they share a unified pathologic appearance.[3,14,16] Accordingly, they are classified on the basis of anatomical site of origin, with carotid body (CBP), jugulotympanic (JTP), and vagal (VP) paragangliomas the most common (▶ Table 38.1).[2,7,9,17]

Several genetic mechanisms are known to play a key role in tumorigenesis and are discussed hereafter. Although some of these mechanisms may play a contributory role even in sporadic (nonfamilial) HNPGs, the underlying pathophysiologic basis for HNPGs remains poorly defined. There is however a key association, between chronic hypoxic states and tumor development (specifically at the carotid body).[1,18,19] This was first noted in the 1960s and 1970s among Peruvians, who live at high altitudes in the Andes Mountains (2,105–4,350 meters above sea level).[9,20,21] Reduced atmospheric oxygen seems to provoke carotid body hyperplasia; particularly large and heavy carotid bodies are thus common in this population. The prevalence of

Table 38.1 Basic features of common head and neck paragangliomas

	Carotid body	Jugulotympanic	Vagal
Origin	Carotid body	Paraganglion of jugular bulb and the tympanic plexus	Usually the ganglion nodosum
Location	At the carotid bifurcation	The middle ear and surrounding lateral skull base	The parapharyngeal space, above the carotid bifurcation
Frequency[a]	57%	30%	13%
Clinical features	Most often these present as an asymptomatic and slowly enlarging mass at the angle of the mandible. They are known to splay the external and internal carotid arteries on imaging (the "lyre sign").	Symptoms related to middle ear localization: • Conductive hearing loss • Otalgia • Bleeding from ear • Tinnitus • Facial palsy Examination will most often reveal a violaceous middle ear mass behind an intact tympanic membrane.	Often present as slowly enlarging neck masses. At least one lower cranial nerve deficit, particularly unilateral vocal fold palsy, occurs in 35–65% of patients at presentation. On imaging, typically displaces both the external/internal carotid arteries anteromedially.

[a]The relative frequency across series of all head and neck paragangliomas.

paragangliomas is correspondingly elevated, being roughly 10 times more frequent than among those living at sea level.[9,19] Although the mechanism underlying chronic hypoxic stimulation is not clearly understood, this effect has been confirmed for other medical conditions, including cystic fibrosis, cyanotic heart disease, and central alveolar hypoventilation, in which the prevalence of HNPG is also increased.[9]

38.2.1 Genetics of Head and Neck Paragangliomas

Advances in molecular genetics over the past thirty years, have identified some genetic driver event as a cause of more than 50% of pheochromocytomas and paragangliomas (▶ Table 38.2).[22] Inherited paraganglioma syndromes, for example, are now known to be associated with germline mutations in one of at least 12 different genes. More recently, somatic mutations have been identified in related genetic elements within sporadic paraganglioma cases.[10,13,22,23] How these nonheritable mutations are acquired, and their association with the pathogenesis of sporadic paragangliomas, is a particularly intriguing new area of study.[4,23]

Hereditary paragangliomas, can be broadly grouped into two clusters on the bases of gene expression profiles.[22,24] The first cluster includes mutations in the von Hippel-Lindau (VHL), succinate dehydrogenase (SDH) subunits, and hypoxia-inducible factor 2A (HIF2A) genes.[22] These genetic elements are involved in the hypoxia–angiogenesis pathway, acting to modulate a transcription factor known as HIF, which is typically upregulated within oxygen-sensitive tissue in response to hypoxia. Mutations in VHL, SDH, or HIF2A thus seemingly create a state

of pseudohypoxemia, inducing a persistent angiogenesis (and thus tumorigenesis), a condition that can be presumed to be similar to that experienced by individuals living at high altitude.[9,19,22,24] The second genetic cluster is more heterogeneous and is rarely associated with HNPGs. It includes genes associated with specific protein signaling [neurofibromin 1 (NF1), RET], mitogenesis [MYC-associated factor X (MAX)], and protein trafficking (TMEM127) pathways.[4]

Mutations mapped to the succinate dehydrogenase gene family (SDHA, SDHB, SDHC, SDHD, and SDHAF2) are the cause of a group of familial paraganglioma syndromes (known as PGL1–5), most specifically associated with HNPGs.[7,10,25,26,27] These genes encode subunits of mitochondrial complex II, which is involved in the aerobic electron transport chain and Krebs cycle. The inheritance pattern of SDH mutations is somewhat unique. Although an autosomal dominant pattern is exhibited, there is both age-dependent penetrance and almost 100% maternal imprinting.[10,28,29] Accordingly, phenotypic expression of the disease state is dependent on patient age, with the average presentation in the third decade of life.[28,30] Maternal imprinting is an epigenetic phenomenon in which alleles inherited from the mother become inactivated. Consequently, an affected father has a roughly 50% chance of disease transmission, whereas affected mothers can only transmit inactivated genes, which could be reactivated in the next generation.[10,28,29]

Contrary to the previously dogmatic 10% rule, current evidence suggests that roughly 30% of all paragangliomas possess a familial germline mutation.[4,23,24,28,29,30] The PGLs in particular are generally characterized by five key features: (1) a positive family history, (2) young age (≤ 45), (3) preceding or simultaneous pheochromocytoma, (4) multiple paragangliomas, and (5) male gender.[13,30] It is interesting to note this male predominance, which is contrary to the female predominance observed with sporadic tumors. The precise disease phenotype is, however, dependent on the exact succinate dehydrogenase defect present. SDHD mutations (the leading cause of familial HNPGs), for example, are associated with multifocality. SDHB mutations, by contrast, are associated with a particularly high rate of malignant paraganglioma (> 30% risk).[2,7,13,24]

Because the price of genomic screening costs from $1,000 to $2,000, a targeted genetic screening approach has generally been advocated based on the five key clinical predictors outlined in the preceding paragraph.[25,30] More recent advances in molecular testing have led others to advocate for universal genetic testing (targeting SDHB, SDHC, SDHD, and VHL) given a > 10% likelihood of heritable mutations in otherwise presumed sporadic cases.[23,25,26,30] Another important consideration is the rapidly growing list of associated somatic and germline mutations now linked to these tumors, with potential clinically relevant consequences for patient and family members alike. Genetic counseling should at the very least be advocated in the majority of cases to help guide this process.[25]

Table 38.2 Paraganglioma associated genetic mutations

Syndrome	Genes	Related conditions
Hereditary paraganglioma[a]	SDHA SDHAF2 SDHB SDHC SDHD	Multiple paragangliomas + pheochromocytoma, and • Gastrointestinal stromal tumors • Renal cell carcinoma • Pituitary adenomas
Von Hippel–Lindau Syndrome	VHL	CNS hemangioblastoma Pheochromocytoma Renal cell carcinoma Renal/pancreatic cysts Endolymphatic sac tumors
Neurofibromatosis type I	NF1	Cutaneous neurofibromas Malignant peripheral nerve sheath tumors Optic gliomas
Multiple endocrine neoplasia (2A and 2B)	RET	Medullary thyroid carcinoma Pheochromocytoma Marfanoid habitus Mucosal neuromas
Others	HIF2	Polycythemia Somatostatinomas
	MAX	None known

Abbreviations: CNS, central nervous system; HIF2, hypoxia, inducible factor 2; MAX, MYC-associated factor.
[a]Hereditary paragangliomas are associated with succinate dehydrogenase gene (SDH) mutations.

38.2.2 Malignant Paraganglioma

Malignant paragangliomas are a rare entity responsible for 3 to 5% of these lesions within the head and neck.[13] Interestingly, the likelihood of malignancy is dependent on tumor anatomical localization, being particularly likely for vagal (16–19%) lesions.[6,31] Diagnosis is generally made on the basis of metastatic disease considering the difficulty distinguishing from benign lesions on histopathology.[6,13,31,32] However, the presence of significant invasion of local structures is considered to represent malignant disease by certain authors.[33] Although isolated regional cervical lymph node spread is most common (55–70% of cases), distant disease dissemination (when occurring) is most common to bone, lung, and liver.[13,32] Interestingly regional spread is particularly common for malignant carotid body tumors (94% of cases), whereas distant metastasis is more common for malignancies at other sites.[31,32] Overall survival for patients receiving treatment (surgery ± adjuvant radiotherapy [XRT]) for disease isolated to the head and neck is high—roughly 80 to 90% at 5 years.[31,32] Treatment results become disappointing, however, in cases involving distant metastatic spread.[13,31,32]

38.3 Pathology

Paragangliomas and pheochromocytomas are highly vascular neuroendocrine tumors that share a uniform histopathologic appearance.[1,3,14] They are generally surrounded by a pseudocapsule that may show evidence of capsular penetration/vascular invasion, but these findings are not diagnostic of malignancy.[14] Architecturally, a classic "Zellballen" pattern is described, with tumor cells arranged in round oval nests that vary in size (▶ Fig. 38.1). Two cell types are present the predominant chief cells (type I epithelioid cells) and sustentacular cells (type II supporting cells).[1,3,14]

The chief cells are of neuroendocrine lineage and thus possess catecholamine-containing granules. They are often characterized by nuclear enlargement and a varying cytoplasmic component that ranges from granular eosinophilic to deeply basophilic.[14] These cells stain positive for neuroendocrine histochemical markers such as chromogranin, synaptophysin,

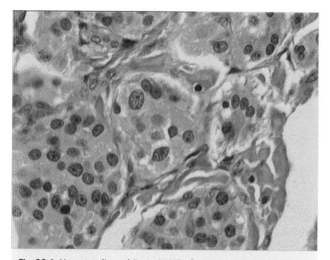

Fig. 38.1 Hematoxylin and Eosin (H&E) of a paraganglioma showing the classic "Zellballen" pattern. This is characterized by the presence of uniform clusters of round to polygonal cells (chief cells) surrounded by a rich fibrovascular network that includes supporting sustentacular cells.

NSE, and CD56. The sustentacular cells are a group of stromal cells that act like neural glia in creating a supportive/vascular network around chief cell nests.[14] These cells have a unique immunohistochemical pattern and are uniformly s100 protein-positive.

Catecholamine synthesis is an important hallmark of the paraganglionic system. This biosynthetic pathway uses a series of enzymatic catalysts to convert precursor substrates (phenylalanine and tyrosine) into functional catecholamines (dopamine, norepinephrine, and epinephrine).[4] Catecholamine catabolism also uniquely occurs within paraganglionic tissue (including tumors) through the action of catecholamine-O-methyl transferase, producing a group of metabolites known as metanephrines.[4,34] HNPGs rarely cause symptomatic catecholamine secretion (< 4%), because the parasympathetic derived tissue lacks the downstream enzymatic mechanism needed to produce epinephrine.[4,6,13,14,35] These tumors do, however, tend to produce dopamine, so the associated metanephrine methoxytyramine may be detectable even in clinically silent tumors.[34] Despite the rarity of hypersecretory HNPGs, the potential life-threatening nature of functional tumors and risk of multicentricity lead most authors to recommend biochemical screening by measurement of 24-hour urinary or plasma metanephrines.[4,33,34]

38.4 Staging

Because most HNPGs are benign, traditional staging systems are not applicable. Site-specific disease classifications have, however, been devised, particularly as a means of guiding surgical resection (▶ Table 38.3). Since 1971, carotid body tumors have been stratified based on the Shamblin system.[6,7,13] Shamblin class I tumors simply splay (but do not invade the carotid vessels), whereas Class III tumors completely encase both the internal and external carotid artery (▶ Fig. 38.2). Higher-class lesions thus require more extensive resection (and potentially carotid artery reconstruction), leading to an increasingly higher risk of treatment-related morbidity. For JTPs, two separate staging systems are commonly referenced: Fisch-Mattox and Glasscock-Jackson.[13,36] The Fisch-Mattox system incorporates all these lesions into a single continuum, whereas Glasscock-Jackson denotes tympanic and jugular bulb tumors separately. No specific staging system is in use for VPs.

38.5 Treatment

The obvious challenge posed by HNPGs is that of balancing the potential treatment associated with tumor-specific morbidity in a population of patients who most often present with benign asymptomatic disease. The concern is, of course, unrestrained growth and local invasiveness, which may lead to both progressive cranial nerve and neurovascular deficits.[6,7] Similar morbidities are, however, caused by curative treatment protocols, with a > 10% likelihood of potentially serious adverse outcomes reported in most series.[6,7,37] Unfortunately, a uniformly accepted treatment algorithm does not exist. A detailed pretreatment clinical work-up, knowledge of patient-specific comorbidities/risk tolerance, and an understanding of disease natural history are thus essential to guide management decision making.

Table 38.3 Site-specific head and neck paraganglioma classification systems

Carotid body paragangliomas		
	I	Splaying the carotid bifurcation with little attachment to carotid vessels
Shamblin classification	II	Partial surrounding of internal and external carotid artery
	III	Complete encasement of internal and external carotid arteries

Jugulotympanic paraganglioma		
	A	Tumor entirely within middle ear space
	B	Tumor only within middle ear and mastoid
Fisch-Mattox classification	C	Tumor within the infralabyrinthine temporal bone or petrous apex
	D1	Tumor with < 2 cm of intracranial extension
	D2	Tumor with ≥ 2 cm of intracranial extension

Glasscock-Jackson classification	Tympanic	Jugular
I	Small mass limited to promontory	Small tumor involving jugular bulb, middle ear, and mastoid
II	Tumor completely filling middle ear space	Tumor extends under IAC, may have intracranial extension
III	Tumor filling middle ear and extending into mastoid	Tumor extends to petrous apex, may have intracranial extension
IV	Tumor filling middle ear and extending into mastoid or through tympanic membrane to fill EAC; may involve anterior ICA	Tumor extends beyond petrous apex into clivus or infratemporal fossa; may have intracranial extension

Abbreviations: EAC, external auditory canal; IAC, internal auditory canal; ICA, internal carotid artery.

During the initial clinical encounter, disease symptomatology particularly related to the function of potentially at-risk cranial nerves (VII–XII), must be assessed. In most situations, anatomical (and potentially functional imaging) can be used for accurate tumor categorization, with biopsy only rarely indicated.[6,38,39,40] Contrast-enhanced MRI is particularly useful, as these tumors exhibit an almost pathognomonic "salt-and-pepper" appearance on T2-weighted imaging, characterized by a high degree of contrast enhancement and vascular flow voids (▶ Fig. 38.3).[6,40] In cases being considered for surgical management, the addition of MR/CT angiography is advocated to better map the association between the tumor and surrounding vascular anatomy. The use of functional imaging techniques (e.g., ^{123}I/^{131}I-metaiodobenzyl-guanidine scintigraphy,[111] In-DTPA pentetreotide scans, SPECT/CT) are also proposed, both as a means of defining the individual tumor natural history and as a screen for metachronous paragangliomas.[39,40] However, the optimal role of these various techniques remains under investigation.[24,39,40]

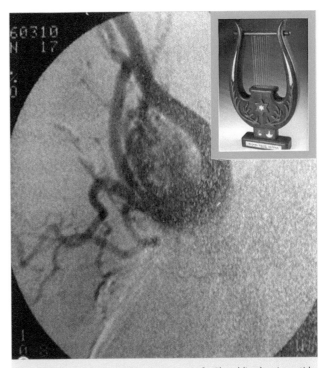

Fig. 38.2 Classic angiographic appearance of a Shamblin class I carotid body tumor. Note the presence of a vascular blush found to splay the external and internal carotid arteries. This is referred to as the "lyres sign," mimicking the appearance of the stringed instrument used during antiquity.

38.5.1 Observation

The concept of applying a noninterventional approach to HNPGLs is based on a presumed indolent natural history. This was first outlined by van der May et al from Leiden University, in the Netherlands. They reviewed 52 cases of JTPs with prolonged follow-up (mean 13.5-year follow up); although most were treated surgically (radical vs. subtotal resection), 13 cases were observed.[41] None of the patients died from tumor or developed distant metastasis, but the likelihood of cranial nerve deficits was two times higher in the surgical cohort.[41,42] A more recent update by this group reviewed 48 HNPGs (in 26 patients, as a result of familial disease variants), managed initially with observation. Further reinforcing the indolent nature of these tumors (at least in the Dutch population), they calculated a slow tumor growth rate (0.83 mm/y) with a median time to tumor doubling of 10.2 years.[43] However, the growth rate was incredibly variable, with doubling time ranging from 0.6 to 21.5 years.[43] Rapid growth was most common in intermediate-sized tumors (0.8 to 4.5 mL), indicating size as a potential prognostic factor of disease progression. They propose a volume increase of ≥ 20% (a criterion reached by 60% of tumors) to be a clear sign of tumor enlargement and potential threshold for intervention.[43]

A collection of studies has further elaborated on the potential utility of observation for jugular paragangliomas in particular.[42,44] A combined 39 patients (Fisch type C and D) have been managed using this approach, with only 3 eventually requiring treatment. During the period of follow-up, tumor

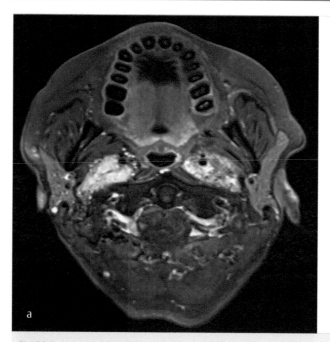
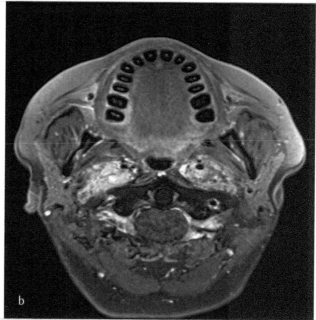

Fig. 38.3 Contrast-enhanced axial T2-weighted MR imaging of a 47-year-old female patient who had bilateral carotid body tumors. Observation was selected in this case, with no appreciable change in tumor size from **(a)** 2010 to **(b)** 2013. Note the classic "salt-and-pepper" appearance of both tumors.

growth occurred in only 30 to 40% of cases, with a slow tumor growth rate (< 1 mm/y) reported in most patients. However, this cohort, by and large, included older patients (> 65) with generally < 10 years of follow-up, limiting the potential applicability to younger individuals.[42,44]

The Vanderbilt university group has also reported a series of 47 cervical paragangliomas (in 43 patients), managed without intervention. Similar to the other series, an indolent natural history was noted, with tumor growth in only 38% of cases and a mean growth rate of 0.2 cm/year.[45] None of these cases required aggressive management, and no new cranial nerve deficits arose during the observation period—which, again, was relatively short-term (mean 5 y).[45]

38.5.2 Surgery

Surgical resection is to some extent still considered the gold standard of treatment for HNPGs, for gross total resection (GTR) is the only true curative option. Technical nuances are addressed in other sections within this book, so we instead outline the logical framework underlying surgical management of these neoplasms. The overall likelihood of achieving a GTR is roughly 90% in most surgical series. When achieved, there is a high likelihood of long-term disease control (> 90%).[8,11,13,37,46,47] The potential limitation of radical treatment is, however, the likelihood of significant acute complications (e.g., wound infection, cerebrovascular accident, cerebrospinal fluid leak) and chronic treatment-specific morbidity (e.g., hearing loss, dysphonia, dysphagia/aspiration, facial weakness) as a result of cranial nerve deficits.[7,8,37,46,47]

A combination of both patient- and tumor-specific variables, including anatomical site of origin, tumor size, patient comorbidities, and established staging systems, can be used to help risk-stratify the likelihood of severe postoperative complications. Tympanic paragangliomas, for example, are most often contained by the temporal bone.[42,48] Because these cases generally present with pulsatile tinnitus, aural fullness, and conductive hearing loss, surgery is particularly advantageous given the potential for symptom improvement. Regardless of tumor extent, resection (either GTR or subtotal if tumor is adherent to critical structures) also has a low (< 2%) risk of cranial neuropathy or vascular injury.[48]

CBPs are somewhat more challenging considering the need for major vessel manipulation intraoperatively. However, isolated tumors in young patients without evidence of atherosclerotic disease, small size (< 5 cm), and low Shamblin classification can be readily managed with low likelihood of neurovascular complications and reasonably low rate (< 20%) of chronic cranial nerve deficits (▶ Fig. 38.4; ▶ Fig. 38.5).[7,49,50]

Advanced carotid body tumors, conversely, require complex surgical approaches that may necessitate carotid artery reconstruction and that are associated with as high as a 40% rate of permanent neurologic deficit. Radical intervention in these cases must thus be considered with greater caution.[13,49] Bilateral carotid body tumors pose a particularly unique challenge considering the potential for baroreceptor failure and severe resistant hypertension. If surgery is to be considered, the smaller tumor (having the lower likelihood of complications) is often addressed first, allowing various treatment options (surgery, observation, or XRT) to be considered for the contralateral side.[6,7]

Surgery for jugular and VPs are particularly likely to be associated with adverse complications.[37,44,46,47] VPs, for example, effectively require vagal sacrifice to allow tumor extirpation with a postoperative deficit in > 90% of cases. The majority of patients will require extensive rehabilitation (e.g., prolonged swallowing therapy, feeding tube use and medialization laryngoplasty) to achieve reasonable upper airway function.[37,46,47,51] For larger tumors, presence of additional acute lower cranial nerve deficits can prevent appropriate adaptation to the vagal sacrifice, leading to prolonged functional morbidity. The lateral skull base localization of jugular paragangliomas are particularly technically challenging. This equates to a lower rate of tumor control, a relatively high rate of cranial nerve sacrifice, and the greatest risk (about 10%) of acute life-threatening complications (e.g., cerebrospinal fluid leak, severe aspiration, meningitis, and stroke).[37,46] Nonsurgical treatment options are thus particularly attractive for the majority of these jugular and VPs.

There are a few situations in which surgical management of HNPGs should be strongly considered. First, as discussed, low-risk tympanic and carotid body tumors are ideal candidates,

considering the high likelihood of tumor control with low morbidity. Catecholamine-secreting tumors (though rare) should be resected owing to the life-threatening nature of hypersecretory episodes and the potential for XRT to worsen this symptomatology.[7,24] Finally, malignant paragangliomas with disease isolated to the neck should be managed surgically when feasible (± adjuvant XRT) to optimize the likelihood of cure and locoregional disease control.[31,32,52]

38.5.3 Radiotherapy

Because our understanding of the potential morbidity of surgery has increased, so has the role of XRT. Although it has been traditionally thought of as a palliative option, a large body of literature has suggested comparative effectiveness with radical surgical resection.[6] It is important to realize that "cure" is defined differently in patients who are managed with XRT. The optimal posttreatment outcome is the presence of an asymptomatic mass without disease progression.[17] Both conventional and stereotactic XRT have been used for HNPGs. For conventional fractionated XRT, a dose of 45 Gy is advocated regardless of tumor size and location.[17,53,54] There is no evidence that more radical XRT has any advantage for local control, and the low doses used for these tumors promotes a favorable side effect profile. Hypofractionated stereotactic XRT is generally given in one or several (3–5) settings to a dose around the tumor margins of 12 to 25 Gy.[55,56]

Long-term tumor control rates for XRT (both conventional and stereotactic) are reported as > 90 to 95% by multiple authors.[6,17,37,53,54,55,56] For example, a University of Florida group reported a 10-year 96% local control rate in 156 HNPGs managed using XRT alone at a median follow-up of 8.7 years (ranging from 1 to > 30).[17] Of the five recurrent cases, all were identified within 10 years of treatment completion. The literature for stereotactic radiosurgery is less robust but suggests similarly high control rates in systematic reviews of small single-institution series.[55]

XRT (particularly in series of low-dose XRT) is generally well tolerated, with serious adverse events reported in < 10% of

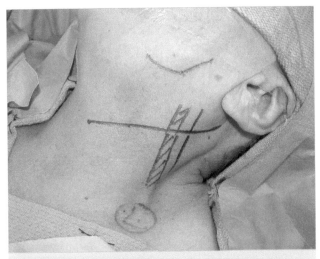

Fig. 38.4 A standard submandibular approach for cervical paragangliomas. This can be used for most tumors now considered for upfront resection (e.g., Shamblin class I carotid body tumors), affording appropriate exposure of the tumor and key surrounding neurovascular structures.

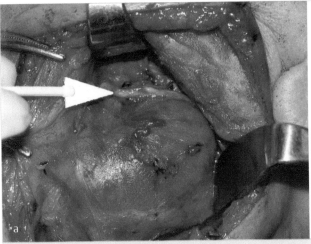
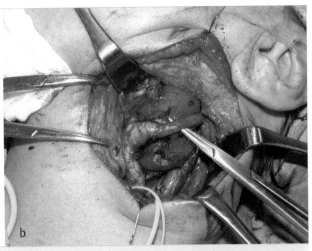

Fig. 38.5 Intraoperative photographs showing resection of Shamblin class I carotid body tumor. **(a)** Note proximity of hypoglossal nerve (labeled with surgical sponge) along the superior aspect of the tumor. This is distracted into a more superficial position by the bulk of the tumor. **(b)** Dissection of both internal and external carotid arteries circumferentially is needed, even in relatively small carotid body tumors, to ensure complete resection.

cases.[17,37,54] Potential complications include xerostomia, osteonecrosis, brain necrosis, and sensorineural hearing loss. One potential concern is the theoretical acceleration of carotid stenosis after XRT, as has been noted in the treatment of head and neck squamous cell carcinoma. However, no definitive case of late stroke has been identified in a radiated paraganglioma patient, indicating that the impact of low-dose XRT on carotid atherosclerosis is likely negligible.[17,53] The potential advantage of stereotactic radiosurgery is the highly conformal nature of treatment, which potentially spares dose to surrounding tissue. This may limit complications for skull base tumors but, interestingly, comes at the price of higher rates of sensorineural hearing loss, because cranial nerve VIII is particularly sensitive to hypofractionated therapy.[55]

38.6 Outcome and Prognosis

The overall prognosis for the majority of patients who have paragangliomas of the head and neck is excellent, with an expected normal life span. These neoplasms' impact (if any) on quality of life is dependent on a variety of clinical variables, including the underlying genetic background (with potential for multicentric vs. malignant disease), the individual tumor's natural history, and the treatment approach selected. A conservative multidisciplinary management plan should be advocated in all cases. A traditional primary surgical approach should be reserved for selected cases of small/favorable tumors (localized to the tympanic and carotid body paraganglia) considering the high likelihood of curative resection with limited risk of long-term morbidity. The majority of benign nonfunctional tumors should, by contrast, receive an observational approach. Intervention (most often XRT) can then be customized to a tumor's individualized biology, reserved for cases with clear evidence of progression. Lifelong clinical assessment is an obvious necessity in this population, particularly for those who have hereditary paraganglioma syndromes, considering the continuing risk of secondary paragangliomas or pheochromocytomas.

Outcomes for the rare population of patients who have malignant HNPGs is more limited. Five-year relative survival rates are 59.5% for all patients but range from 77% for those who have regional disease to only 12% for those have distant metastasis at presentation. Surgery (± adjuvant XRT) remains the ideal choice for those who have regional disease failure; options for those who have disease dissemination are limited.

38.7 Conclusion

Paragangliomas of the head and neck are a unique collection of rare neoplasms. The neuroendocrine origin of these tumors poses a unique set of challenges, with comprehensive genetic and biochemical assessment essential to appropriate clinical care. The indolent natural history characteristic of the majority of cases should guide treatment planning. A variety of surgical and radiotherapeutic strategies is available in appropriately selected cases. A conservative observational strategy, however, is often efficacious, limiting treatment-associated morbidity and helping optimize patient quality of life.

References

[1] Barnes L, Tse LL, Hunt JL, Micahels L. Tumours of the paraganglionic system. In: Barnes L, Eveson JW, Reichart P, Sidransky D. World Health Organization Classification of Tumors: Pathology & Genetics of Head and Neck Tumours. Lyon: IARC Press; 2005:361–370

[2] Kim Y, Goldenberg D. Anatomy, physiology, and genetics of paragangliomas. Oper Tech Otolaryngol–Head Neck Surg. 2016; 27:2–6

[3] Wang B, Zagzag D, Nonaka D. Tumors of the nervous system. In: Barnes L, ed. Surgical Pathology of the Head and Neck. Vol. 2. 3rd ed. New York. Informa Healthcare; 2009:669–773

[4] Tischler AS, Pacak K, Eisenhofer G. The adrenal medulla and extra-adrenal paraganglia: then and now. Endocr Pathol. 2014; 25(1):49–58

[5] Lee JA, Duh QY. Sporadic paraganglioma. World J Surg. 2008; 32(5):683–687

[6] Hu K, Persky MS. Treatment of head and neck paragangliomas. Cancer Contr. 2016; 23(3):228–241

[7] Moore MG, Netterville JL, Mendenhall WM, Isaacson B, Nussenbaum B. Head and neck paragangliomas: an update on evaluation and management. Otolaryngol Head Neck Surg. 2016; 154(4):597–605

[8] Anttila T, Häyry V, Nicoli T, et al. A two-decade experience of head and neck paragangliomas in a whole population-based single centre cohort. Eur Arch Otorhinolaryngol. 2015; 272(8):2045–2053

[9] Baysal BE, Myers EN. Etiopathogenesis and clinical presentation of carotid body tumors. Microsc Res Tech. 2002; 59(3):256–261

[10] Badenhop RF, Jansen JC, Fagan PA, et al. The prevalence of SDHB, SDHC, and SDHD mutations in patients with head and neck paraganglioma and association of mutations with clinical features. J Med Genet. 2004; 41(7):e99

[11] Obholzer RJ, Hornigold R, Connor S, Gleeson MJ. Classification and management of cervical paragangliomas. Ann R Coll Surg Engl. 2011; 93(8):596–602

[12] Kollert M, Minovi AA, Draf W, Bockmühl U. Cervical paragangliomas—tumor control and long-term functional results after surgery. Skull Base. 2006; 16(4):185–191

[13] Hunt JL. Chapter 28: Diseases of the paraganglia system. In: Thompson LDR, Goldblum JR. Head and Neck Pathology. 2nd ed. Philadelphia, PA: Elsevier Inc; 2013:668–678

[14] Capatina C, Ntali G, Karavitaki N, Grossman AB. The management of head-and-neck paragangliomas. Endocr Relat Cancer. 2013; 20(5):R291–R305

[15] Szymańska A, Szymański M, Czekajska-Chehab E, Gołąbek W, Szczerbo-Trojanowska M. Diagnosis and management of multiple paragangliomas of the head and neck. Eur Arch Otorhinolaryngol. 2015; 272(8):1991–1999

[16] Unsicker K, Huber K, Schütz G, Kalcheim C. The chromaffin cell and its development. Neurochem Res. 2005; 30(6–7):921–925

[17] Gilbo P, Morris CG, Amdur RJ, et al. Radiotherapy for benign head and neck paragangliomas: a 45-year experience. Cancer. 2014; 120(23):3738–3743

[18] Baysal BE. A phenotypic perspective on mammalian oxygen sensor candidates. Ann N Y Acad Sci. 2006; 1073:221–233

[19] Favier J, Gimenez-Roqueplo AP. Pheochromocytomas: the (pseudo)-hypoxia hypothesis. Best Pract Res Clin Endocrinol Metab. 2010; 24(6):957–968

[20] Saldana MJ, Salem LE, Travezan R. High altitude hypoxia and chemodectomas. Hum Pathol. 1973; 4(2):251–263

[21] Arias-Stella J, Valcarcel J. Chief cell hyperplasia in the human carotid body at high altitudes; physiologic and pathologic significance. Hum Pathol. 1976; 7(4):361–373

[22] Dahia PLM. Pheochromocytoma and paraganglioma pathogenesis: learning from genetic heterogeneity. Nat Rev Cancer. 2014; 14(2):108–119

[23] Currás-Freixes M, Inglada-Pérez L, Mancikova V, et al. Recommendations for somatic and germline genetic testing of single pheochromocytoma and paraganglioma based on findings from a series of 329 patients. J Med Genet. 2015; 52(10):647–656

[24] Corssmit EP, Romijn JA. Clinical management of paragangliomas. Eur J Endocrinol. 2014; 171(6):R231–R243

[25] Brito JP, Asi N, Bancos I, et al. Testing for germline mutations in sporadic pheochromocytoma/paraganglioma: a systematic review. Clin Endocrinol (Oxf). 2015; 82(3):338–345

[26] Mannelli M, Castellano M, Schiavi F, et al. Italian Pheochromocytoma/Paraganglioma Network. Clinically guided genetic screening in a large cohort of Italian patients with pheochromocytomas and/or functional or nonfunctional paragangliomas. J Clin Endocrinol Metab. 2009; 94(5):1541–1547

[27] Iacobone M, Schiavi F, Bottussi M, et al. Is genetic screening indicated in apparently sporadic pheochromocytomas and paragangliomas? Surgery. 2011; 150(6):1194–1201

[28] Drovdlic CM, Myers EN, Peters JA, et al. Proportion of heritable paraganglioma cases and associated clinical characteristics. Laryngoscope. 2001; 111 (10):1822–1827

[29] van der Mey AGL, Maaswinkel-Mooy PD, Cornelisse CJ, Schmidt PH, van de Kamp JJP. Genomic imprinting in hereditary glomus tumours: evidence for new genetic theory. Lancet. 1989; 2(8675):1291–1294

[30] Neumann HPH, Erlic Z, Boedeker CC, et al. Clinical predictors for germline mutations in head and neck paraganglioma patients: cost reduction strategy in genetic diagnostic process as fall-out. Cancer Res. 2009; 69(8):3650–3656

[31] Sethi RV, Sethi RK, Herr MW, Deschler DG. Malignant head and neck paragangliomas: treatment efficacy and prognostic indicators. Am J Otolaryngol–Head Neck Med Surg. 2013; 34(5):431–438

[32] Lee JH, Barich F, Karnell LH, et al. American College of Surgeons Commission on Cancer, American Cancer Society. National Cancer Data Base report on malignant paragangliomas of the head and neck. Cancer. 2002; 94(3):730–737

[33] Chen H, Sippel R, Pacak K. The NANETS consensus guideline for the diagnosis and management of neuroendocrine tumors: pheochromocytoma, paraganglioma & medullary thyroid cancer. Pancreas. 2010; 39(6):775–783

[34] Eisenhofer G, Peitzsch M. Laboratory evaluation of pheochromocytoma and paraganglioma. Clin Chem. 2014; 60(12):1486–1499

[35] Osinga TE, Korpershoek E, de Krijger RR, et al. Catecholamine-synthesizing enzymes are expressed in parasympathetic head and neck paraganglioma tissue. Neuroendocrinology. 2015; 101(4):289–295

[36] Sweeney AD, Carlson ML, Wanna GB, Bennett ML. Glomus tympanicum tumors. Otolaryngol Clin North Am. 2015; 48(2):293–304

[37] Suárez C, Rodrigo JP, Bödeker CC, et al. Jugular and vagal paragangliomas: systematic study of management with surgery and radiotherapy. Head Neck. 2013; 35(8):1195–1204

[38] Adams MS, Bronner-Fraser M, Badenhop RF, et al. Paragangliomas of head and neck: a surgical challenge. Cancer. 2014; 1(3):659–664

[39] Gimenez-Roqueplo AP, Caumont-Prim A, Houzard C, et al. EVA Investigators. Imaging work-up for screening of paraganglioma and pheochromocytoma in SDHx mutation carriers: a multicenter prospective study from the PGL. J Clin Endocrinol Metab. 2013; 98(1):E162–E173

[40] Taïeb D, Varoquaux A, Chen CC, Pacak K. Current and future trends in the anatomical and functional imaging of head and neck paragangliomas. Semin Nucl Med. 2013; 43(6):462–473

[41] van der Mey AGL, Frijns JHM, Cornelisse CJ, et al. Does intervention improve the natural course of glomus tumors? A series of 108 patients seen in a 32-year period. Ann Otol Rhinol Laryngol. 1992; 101(8):635–642

[42] Carlson ML, Sweeney AD, Wanna GB, Netterville JL, Haynes DS. Natural history of glomus jugulare: a review of 16 tumors managed with primary observation. Otolaryngol Head Neck Surg. 2015; 152(1):98–105

[43] Jansen JC, van den Berg R, Kuiper A, van der Mey AG, Zwinderman AH, Cornelisse CJ. Estimation of growth rate in patients with head and neck paragangliomas influences the treatment proposal. Cancer. 2000; 88(12):2811–2816

[44] Prasad SC, Mimoune HA, D'Orazio F, et al. The role of wait-and-scan and the efficacy of radiotherapy in the treatment of temporal bone paragangliomas. Otol Neurotol. 2014; 35(5):922–931

[45] Langerman A, Athavale SM, Rangarajan SV, Sinard RJ, Netterville JL. Natural history of cervical paragangliomas: outcomes of observation of 43 patients. Arch Otolaryngol Head Neck Surg. 2012; 138(4):341–345

[46] Neskey DM, Hatoum G, Modh R, et al. Outcomes after surgical resection of head and neck paragangliomas: a review of 61 patients. Skull Base. 2011; 21 (3):171–176

[47] Netterville JL, Jackson CG, Miller FR, Wanamaker JR, Glasscock ME. Vagal paraganglioma: a review of 46 patients treated during a 20-year period. Arch Otolaryngol Head Neck Surg. 1998; 124(10):1133–1140

[48] Carlson ML, Sweeney AD, Pelosi S, Wanna GB, Glasscock ME, III, Haynes DS. Glomus tympanicum: a review of 115 cases over 4 decades. Otolaryngol Head Neck Surg. 2015; 152(1):136–142

[49] Luna-Ortiz K, Rascon-Ortiz M, Villavicencio-Valencia V, Herrera-Gomez A. Does Shamblin's classification predict postoperative morbidity in carotid body tumors? A proposal to modify Shamblin's classification. Eur Arch Otorhinolaryngol. 2006; 263(2):171–175

[50] Papaspyrou K, Mewes T, Rossmann H, et al. Head and neck paragangliomas: Report of 175 patients (1989–2010). Head Neck. 2012; 34(5):632–637

[51] Bradshaw JW, Jansen JC. Management of vagal paraganglioma: is operative resection really the best option? Surgery. 2005; 137(2):225–228

[52] Moskovic DJ, Smolarz JR, Stanley D, et al. Malignant head and neck paragangliomas: Is there an optimal treatment strategy? Head Neck Oncol. 2010; 2:23

[53] Suárez C, Rodrigo JP, Mendenhall WM, et al. Carotid body paragangliomas: a systematic study on management with surgery and radiotherapy. Eur Arch Otorhinolaryngol. 2014; 271(1):23–34

[54] Dupin C, Lang P, Dessard-Diana B, et al. Treatment of head and neck paragangliomas with external beam radiation therapy. Int J Radiat Oncol Biol Phys. 2014; 89(2):353–359

[55] Marchetti M, Pinzi V, Tramacere I, Bianchi LC, Ghielmetti F, Fariselli L. Radiosurgery for paragangliomas of the head and neck: another step for the validation of a treatment paradigm. World Neurosurg. 2017; 98:281–287

[56] Lieberson RE, Adler JR, Soltys SG, Choi C, Gibbs IC, Chang SD. Stereotactic radiosurgery as the primary treatment for new and recurrent paragangliomas: is open surgical resection still the treatment of choice? World Neurosurg. 2012; 77(5–6):745–761

39 Pituitary Adenomas

Amol Raheja and William T. Couldwell

Summary

Pituitary adenomas are among the most common intracranial neoplasms, and they account for 10 to 15% of all intracranial tumors. The vast majority of pituitary adenomas (PAs) are benign and present incidentally or with hypopituitarism, hormonal hypersecretion, and local mass effect. Significant advances, including availability of more sensitive diagnostic hormonal assays, improvement in neuroimaging modalities, refinement in surgical techniques, and innovation of novel adjuvant therapeutic options, have contributed to the contemporary management of PAs. Comprehensive management of PAs includes a multidisciplinary approach involving a team of neurosurgeons, neuroradiologists, neuropathologists, medical and radiation oncologists, and endocrinologists. In this chapter, we discuss the epidemiology, pathology, classification, clinical presentation, diagnostic work-up, therapeutic options, and outcomes of PAs in the modern era of medicine.

Keywords: pituitary adenoma, epidemiology, classification, diagnostic work-up, therapeutic options, treatment outcomes

39.1 Introduction

Pituitary adenomas (PAs) are predominantly benign tumors that are commonly encountered in neurosurgical practice. They represent one of the most common intracranial tumor, being diagnosed in almost one in five patients.[1] Understandings of the pathogenesis and clinical manifestations of PAs continue to evolve. Significant advances, including availability of more sensitive diagnostic hormonal assays, improvement in neuroimaging modalities, refinement in surgical techniques, and innovation of novel adjuvant therapeutic options, have contributed to the contemporary management of PAs. Comprehensive management of PAs includes a multidisciplinary approach involving a team of neurosurgeons, neuroradiologists, neuropathologists, medical and radiation oncologists, and endocrinologists. In this chapter, we discuss the epidemiology, pathology, classification, clinical presentation, diagnostic work-up, therapeutic options, and outcomes of PAs in the modern era of medicine.

39.2 Prevalence, Incidence, and Epidemiology

PAs are among the most common intracranial neoplasms, accounting for 10 to 15% of all intracranial tumors.[2] It is estimated from autopsy studies that approximately 15 to 25% of the general population harbors undiagnosed PA; most however, go unnoticed throughout life.[1,3,4,5] The prevalence and incidence of PA are estimated at 80 to 90 per 100,000 population and 0.5 to 8.2 per 100,000 population, respectively.[2,3] The incidence of PA appears to vary according to age, sex, and ethnicity.[3] It is reported to be higher in blacks, in whom PAs

account for more than 20% of tumors originating in the central nervous system.[3]

The majority of PAs are smaller than 5 mm in diameter and lack clinical significance. The clinically relevant tumors are generally either nonfunctional macroadenomas (>1 cm) or functional tumors. Nonfunctional PAs (NFPAs) account for approximately 14 to 28% of all clinically relevant PAs and about 50% of all macroadenomas.[6] The remaining clinically relevant PAs are functional tumors and commonly microadenomas (≤1 cm) (▶ Fig. 39.1). Among functional tumors, 50 to 60% secrete prolactin (Prl), 30% secrete growth hormone (GH), 15 to 25% secrete adrenocorticotrophic hormone (ACTH), and 0.5 to 3% secrete thyroid-stimulating hormone (TSH), leading to the development of Forbes-Albright syndrome, acromegaly, Cushing's disease, and secondary hyperthyroidism, respectively.[3]

Overall, prolactinomas and NFPAs are the two most commonly encountered PAs in clinical practice.[3] The most common subtype diagnosed in adolescents is Prl-secreting tumor. The vast majority of microadenomas are observed in women in their second or third decade of life. Men generally present later, in their fourth or fifth decade, almost always with macroadenomas.[3] Some series report a higher rate of PA diagnosis in females of reproductive age, probably because the gonadal axis is affected in the early part of the natural history of the disease, leading to infertility and bringing the patients to clinical attention. Pituitary carcinomas (PCs) are very rare, having a mean age at presentation of 44 years and developing with equal frequency in both sexes.[2]

Acromegaly is characterized by GH hypersecretion, caused in more than 95% of cases by pituitary somatotroph adenoma. The annual incidence of acromegaly in the United States is approximately 3 to 4 cases per million, with a prevalence of 40 to 60 per million people. It is estimated that worldwide burden of acromegaly patients is about 40 to 130 million cases.[7] Because of its insidious development and the slow progression of clinical symptoms, acromegaly frequently remains undiagnosed for many years and is commonly diagnosed in the third to fifth decade of life. Accordingly, at the time of diagnosis, the majority of GH-secreting tumors are macroadenomas. Prompt initiation of treatment for acromegalic patients is of paramount importance, because there is a two to four times greater a risk of mortality from uncontrolled disease than in the general population.[7]

The incidence of Cushing's disease is 1.2 to 2.4 per million, and its prevalence is about 40 per million population.[8,9] Cushing's disease accounts for 75 to 80% of cases of ACTH-dependent Cushing's syndrome. It is most commonly diagnosed in the third to fourth decade of life and is eight times more common in women than men.[8,9] ACTH-secreting pituitary tumors are also the most common PA encountered in prepubertal children. Overall, there is a 4.8-fold higher mortality rate in patients who have Cushing's disease than in the general population, especially from cardiovascular and cerebrovascular events.[8,9]

The incidence of thyrotropinoma has ranged from 0.05 to 0.32 per million per year, and the reporting of cases has increased, probably because of the increase in awareness among treating physicians.[10,11] Most of the patients are diagnosed in

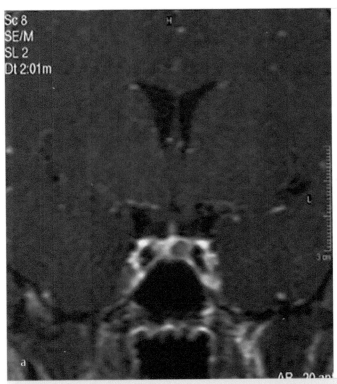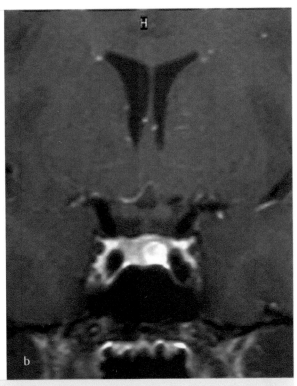

Fig. 39.1 Pituitary functional microadenoma. This patient is a 35-year-old woman who has hyperprolactinemia (120 ng/mL). **(a)** A small tumor is visualized during dynamic T1-weighted MR imaging. Note that after very early contrast administration, the tumor appears hypointense and is readily visible, because the normal gland avidly demonstrates contrast enhancement. **(b)** More delayed images demonstrate a reversal of enhancement pattern, with the dye washing out of the gland and the tumor demonstrating delayed enhancement.

their fifth or sixth decade of life, and there does not seem to be a sex predilection.[10,11] Prolactinomas constitute about 40% of PAs and 50 to 60% of all functional pituitary tumors. Most of these tumors are small, intrasellar, and slow-growing, and they are found predominantly in premenopausal women.[12,13,14] Larger prolactinomas do occur, but more frequently in men and younger women. Giant prolactinomas (>4 cm) constitute only 2 to 3% of all prolactinomas.[12,13,14] Most NFPAs express gonadotropins or their subunits (α and β), whereas approximately 15% of NFPAs are silent adenomas that can express, but not secrete, other pituitary hormones (Prl, GH, ACTH, and TSH). Approximately 30% of NFPAs are null cell adenomas—that is, they do not express or secrete any hormone.[6] Although the vast majority of PAs are benign, a subset of these tumors can exhibit a more aggressive clinical course, with higher recurrence rates and resistance to conventional therapies. Approximately 25 to 55% of PAs demonstrate invasion of dura, bone, the cavernous sinuses, and surrounding anatomical structures, with macroadenomas having a greater tendency to invade than microadenoma.[2]

39.3 Pathology

39.3.1 Classification

PAs can be classified according to multiple criteria, including radiological, histopathological, immunohistochemical, clinical, functional, and tumor dimensions.[15,16,17] One of the earliest classification systems for PA was proposed by Hardy[18]; it was based primarily on sellar enlargement with or without bony destruction and on the pattern/symmetricity of tumor extension. Subsequently, Kovacs and Horvath[19] presented another classification based on the ultrastructural details of the tumor as highlighted on electron microscopy. The more recent Knosp classification[20] is based on the radiological extent of cavernous invasion by the tumor and its precise relationship to the cavernous carotid artery. These classification schemes do not take into account subtyping based on hormonal expression by tumor cells. Advancements have enabled the evolution of pathological classification of PA from a histochemical classification (i.e., acidophilic, basophilic, and chromophobic PA) to an immunohistochemical-based one (i.e., lactotrophic, somatotrophic, corticotrophic, gonadotrophic, thyrotrophic, and null cell adenomas).[15] Electron microscopy has further helped delineate additional subtypes based on the arrangement of ubiquitous cytoplasmic constituents and appearance of specific morphology.

Besides the enzymatic immunohistochemistry (IHC) assay, the functional status of the tumor is defined primarily by the clinical symptoms produced by hormonal hypersecretion. Clinically, a PA can be classified as either functional (hormone-secreting) or nonfunctional (non–hormone-secreting). Functional tumors can manifest clinically as acromegaly (GH excess), Cushing's disease/Nelson's syndrome (ACTH excess), Forbes-Albright syndrome (prolactinoma, Prl excess), or secondary hyperthyroidism (TSH excess). PA can be classified on the basis of the tumor dimensions into microadenoma (≤1 cm) and macroadenoma (>1 cm).[3] Some authors have labeled macroadenomas that are larger than 4 cm in any dimension as giant PAs.

39.3.2 World Health Organization Grading

The currently valid 2016 World Health Organization (WHO) classification system employs the use of modern sensitive enzymatic assays to ascertain the hormonal expression in PA apart from the histopathological ultrastructural details identified on electron microscopy.[21] This classification differentiates PA into three histopathological grades that also correspond to their associated biological behavior: typical benign adenomas, atypical adenomas, and PCs.[16] Classical or typical PA is the most commonly observed variant and has the lowest growth potential. Atypical adenomas, accounting for approximately 2.7 to 15% of PA, represent an intermediate-grade tumor exhibiting more aggressive biological behavior, an increased growth potential, and a higher likelihood of tumor recurrence. They are characterized by a Ki-67 labeling index > 3%, excessive p53 immunoreactivity, and an increased rate of mitosis. In addition, invasiveness of the tumor is another essential criterion for the diagnosis of atypical adenoma.[2,15,22] PC is the most aggressive variant, demonstrating malignant behavior with evidence of cerebrospinal or systemic metastases. It is a rare entity, accounting for < 1% of symptomatic pituitary tumors. Although de novo development of PC cannot be excluded, in most cases PC arises from a preexisting macroadenoma exhibiting invasive and proliferative features. The usual latency period for the development of PC from its benign variant is 7 years, although it varies depending on the tumor subtype.[2,15,22]

Limitations of Current WHO Grading: Invasion and Proliferation

One of the major caveats to the currently valid WHO grading system is the linkage of proliferation parameters to tumor invasiveness when defining atypical adenomas.[15,16,23,24] This creates two specific groups of tumors within the classification

of typical PA, one having proliferative-only characteristics and other invasive-only. Both these tumor groups will be classified as WHO grade I benign PA, but their biological behavior, natural history of progression, and tumor recurrence rates are quite different from typical PA, being neither invasive nor proliferative. Accordingly, based on the French collaborative study on prognostic factors for PA, Trouillas et al[24] proposed a new five-grade classification scheme for PA, attempting to reclassify invasive tumors and segregate them from proliferative ones so as to better predict the long-term functional outcome within each tumor grade. Besides uncoupling the invasiveness and proliferation, they also precisely defined the diagnostic prerequisites for invasiveness and proliferative tumors. Invasion is defined as histological and/or radiological (MRI) signs of cavernous sinus (▶ Fig. 39.2) or sphenoid sinus invasion (▶ Fig. 39.3). Proliferation is defined as the presence of at least two of three criteria: Ki-67 labeling index > 1% (Bouin-Hollande fixative) or > 3% (formalin fixative); mitoses, $n > 2/10$ per high-powered field; and p53 positive (> 10 strongly positive nuclei).[24] Similarly, Saeger et al[16] have also proposed another modification to the currently valid WHO grading that highlights the importance of segregating invasiveness and proliferation as prognostic markers.

39.3.3 Pathogenesis and Biomarkers of Tumor Aggressiveness

Although the precise molecular mechanisms involved in the pathogenesis of PA are unknown, it is now accepted that PA onset is related to proto-oncogene mutations, overexpression of activating genes, or loss of tumor suppressor genes.[4] The initiating events lead to proliferative gain of function in a single monoclonal pituitary cell population, subsequently leading to clonal expansion by tumor-promoting molecules.[4] Recent evidence points toward a pivotal role for epigenetic modifications,

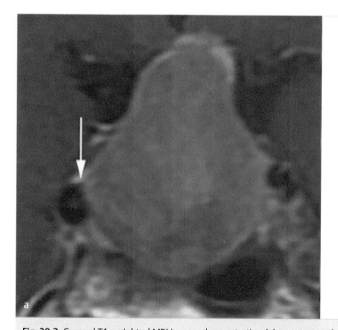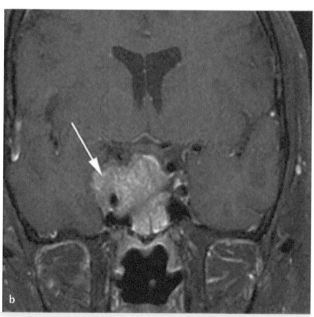

Fig. 39.2 Coronal T1-weighted MRI images demonstrating **(a)** tumor growth adjacent to and compressing the cavernous sinus and **(b)** true invasion of the cavernous sinus, where the carotid is demonstrated being encased by tumor.

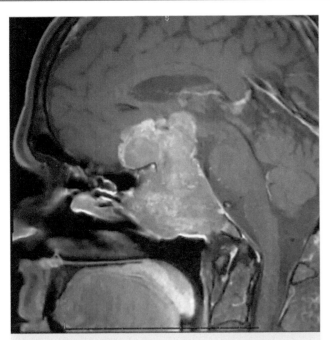

Fig. 39.3 Sagittal MRI with contrast enhancement demonstrating invasive pituitary macroadenoma. The tumor is invading and filling the sphenoid sinus, and the clivus is eroded.

microRNAs, and long noncoding RNAs in the pathogenesis of PAs.[4] One of the most important prognostic factors for PAs is the accurate classification of tumor based on hormone content and subtyping with reference to ultrastructural details. Biomarkers of aggressiveness primarily include histological subtype, Ki-67 labeling index, p53 expression, and markers of invasion and proliferation.[6,15,22] PA variants often associated with aggressive natural history include densely granulated lactotroph adenomas, acidophil stem cell adenomas, sparsely granulated somatotroph adenomas, thyrotroph adenomas, Crooke's cell adenomas, sparsely granulated corticotroph adenomas, null cell adenomas, and silent subtype 3 adenomas.[6,15,22] Other novel markers potentially acting as surrogates for aggressive biological behavior include genomic imbalance (11q allelic loss), DNA aneuploidy, germline mutations associated with MEN1 (multiple endocrine neoplasia-1), MEN 4, Carney's complex, familial isolated PA and succinate dehydrogenase syndrome, micro-RNAs, p27, senescence markers (p16, p21, β-galactosidase), growth factors (epidermal growth factor, vascular endothelial growth factor) and their receptors (EGFR, VEGFR), matrix metalloproteinase, neural cell adhesion molecule, and Galectin-3.[6,15,22] Apart from these syndromes, familial clustering of pituitary tumors has also been reported in the Utah population.[25]

39.4 Clinical Presentation, Diagnostic Work-up, and Remission Criteria

Most PAs still present with either signs or symptoms of hormonal hypersecretion, hypopituitarism, or mass effect.[3] Hypersecretion may manifest as acromegaly, Cushing's disease, amenorrhea–galactorrhea syndrome, or secondary hyperthyroidism.

Conversely, hypopituitarism may present as generalized fatigue, weakness, or reduced libido from gonadal dysfunction; cold intolerance and weight gain from hypothyroidism; nausea, vomiting, and hemodynamic instability from adrenal insufficiency; or stunted growth and failure to thrive from somatotroph deficiency.[3] Finally, the clinical manifestations of direct mass effect include visual field defects (most commonly bitemporal hemianopia) along with diminution of visual acuity from optic apparatus compression; ptosis, miosis, trigeminal neuralgia, and diplopia from cavernous sinus involvement; headache from dural and diaphragma sellar stretching; eating, behavior, and vigilance disturbances from hypothalamic dysfunction; and complex partial seizures from temporal lobe compression. Presenting symptoms in children are primarily the result of endocrine dysfunction, for visual field deficits are reported in only 5% of cases.[3]

Diagnostic work-up includes radiological imaging, endocrinological work-up, and ophthalmological evaluation to classify a tumor and assess the preoperative status of the patient. A fat-saturated, thin-slice, gadolinium-enhanced MRI of the brain (pituitary protocol) is the standard imaging of choice. Dynamic gadolinium-enhanced MRI of the brain is the diagnostic imaging of choice for pituitary microadenomas. The dynamic scan displays the time course of contrast enhancement rather than just the final postcontrast images, thereby improving the sensitivity of picking up small microadenomas not otherwise visualized on standard imaging methods. Microadenomas appear as areas of delayed contrast enhancement compared with the surrounding normal pituitary tissue on early postcontrast images.

Endocrinological work-up includes fasting 8 a.m. serum Prl, T3, T4, TSH, GH, insulinotropic growth factor (IGF-1), cortisol, ACTH, luteinizing hormone (LH), follicle-stimulating hormone (FSH), and estrogen (for women) or testosterone (for men). Ophthalmological examination includes the assessment of visual acuity, visual field charting, funduscopy, and oculomotor function assessment. Disease-specific symptoms, diagnostic tests, and remission criteria are described hereafter.

39.4.1 Pituitary Incidentaloma and Nonfunctional Pituitary Adenoma

With the advent and widespread availability of better neuroimaging modalities and more frequent cranial screening performed for unrelated causes, an increasing number of PAs are being diagnosed incidentally.[26] These "incidentalomas" are not necessarily asymptomatic, although they are almost always nonfunctional in nature.[27] They are associated with pituitary dysfunction in about 15% of patients and with visual deficits in about 5% of patients. Although the majority of these tumors are microincidentalomas, approximately a third are macroincidentalomas, which may demonstrate significant increase in size over time and will require some intervention. On the contrary, nonfunctioning microincidentalomas smaller than 5 mm usually do not grow much and rarely require active intervention other than radiological surveillance. Only 5% of microincidentalomas exceed 10 mm size in their natural course of disease.[27]

Nonfunctioning pituitary macroadenomas generally lead to compression of the pituitary gland and some degree of pituitary dysfunction. GH deficiency is the most frequent abnormality, followed by gonadotropin (LH, FSH), ACTH, and TSH deficiencies.[6,28] Marginal elevation of serum Prl levels (usually up to 100 ng/mL, occasionally more) can be seen with nonfunctioning macroadenomas because of the loss of the inhibitory effect of dopamine from the hypothalamus on Prl secretion, a phenomenon known as "stalk effect."[6,28] The risk of apoplexy is minimal (1%, and 10% at 5 years) but is greater in macroadenomas adjacent to optic apparatus, and especially in those requiring anticoagulation therapy.[6,28] Direct mass effect may lead to visual decline and is the most common presenting complaint of adults who have nonfunctioning macroadenomas.

39.4.2 Acromegaly

Clinical manifestations of acromegaly include coarsening of facial features, malocclusion of teeth, prognathism, and enlargement of forehead, tongue, hands and feet. Onset of GH excess from tumor secretion prior to fusion of the bony epiphysis will result in gigantism (▶ Fig. 39.4). Complications linked to GH and IGF-1 excess in acromegaly include premature atherosclerosis, hypertrophic cardiomyopathy, diabetes mellitus, arthritis, polyps of the colon, carpel tunnel syndrome, and obstructive sleep apnea syndrome.[29,30] Serum GH and IGF-1 levels screen for acromegaly, and an oral glucose tolerance test confirms the diagnosis.[29,30,31,32] Current consensus guidelines published in 2010[31] unanimously accept the biochemical remission criteria as normalization of age-adjusted IGF-1 levels plus either a random GH < 1 µg/L in patients treated medically or glucose-suppressed GH < 0.4 µg/L in patients treated using other modalities, except pegvisomant (GH receptor antagonist), for which only IGF-1 levels are used.

39.4.3 Cushing's Disease

Cushing's disease is characterized by excessive ACTH secretion by PA, leading to surplus cortisol secretion by the adrenal glands and ultimately resulting in diabetes mellitus, hypertension, cardiovascular disease, hypercoagulability, weight gain, central obesity, moon facies, abdominal purple striae, easy bruisability, increased facial and body hair, osteoporosis, proximal muscle weakness, and neurocognitive and psychiatric disturbances.[8,33] Although rare, Cushing's disease is associated with significant clinical, social, economic, and quality-of-life burdens. Frequently, the diagnosis is delayed because of the gradual presentation of the constellation of heterogeneous clinical signs and symptomatology, which present over a period of a couple years.[8,33] Per Endocrine Society Clinical Practice Guidelines,[34,35] screening tests to diagnose Cushing's disease include 24-hour urinary free cortisol excretion test, midnight salivary cortisol assay, and 1-mg dexamethasone suppression test. To distinguish ectopic ACTH secretion from Cushing's disease, bilateral inferior petrosal sinus sampling with corticotropin-releasing hormone (CRH) stimulation is the gold-standard test. It has a sensitivity of 80 to 100% and a specificity of more than 95%.[34,35,36]

Because baseline central–peripheral gradients have suboptimal accuracy, CRH/desmopressin stimulation must be performed for optimal results. However, this test has a limited role in lateralizing the tumor.[34,35,36] The false-negative results in this test can occur because of unilateral or bilateral anatomical variants in the petrosal venous system. Jugular venous sampling is another less invasive alternative for this test[34,35,36]; however,

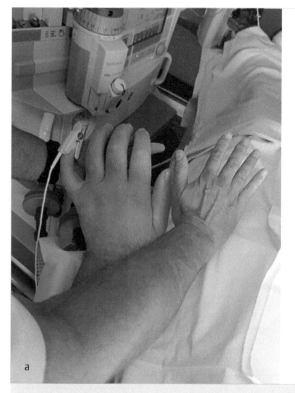
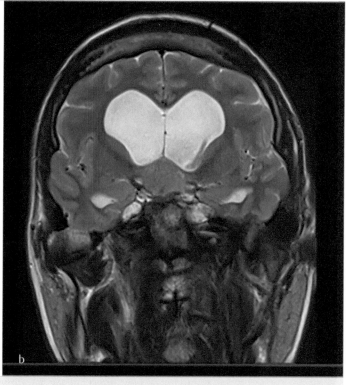

Fig. 39.4 Acromegaly with gigantism. **(a)** Note the size of the left hand of the patient in comparison with the hand of the senior author. The patient in this picture exceeded 8 feet in height. **(b)** MRI study demonstrates tumor extending superiorly to fill the third ventricle.

the high-dose dexamethasone suppression test is much more readily available, less invasive, and dynamic. A screening MRI/CT scan of the chest and abdomen is recommended when looking for a primary malignancy with ectopic ACTH production.[34,35,36]

Criteria for biochemical remission for Cushing's disease after surgery are affected by perioperative use of injectable steroids and the use of adjuvant medical therapy in the form of metyrapone, ketoconazole, and mifepristone, which has resulted in the lack of a universal definition for endocrine remission.[8,33] To streamline the criteria, the Endocrine Society clinical practice guideline published in 2008[33] advised withholding perioperative or postoperative glucocorticoids until testing for biochemical remission is complete. They recommended that a postoperative day 1 morning serum cortisol < 2 µg/dL is an indication of remission.[33] In addition, close monitoring for any signs of hypoadrenalism should be performed during the immediate postoperative period, and a maintenance dose glucocorticoid replacement should be instituted as soon as biochemical remission is proven. This replacement may need to be continued for approximately 6 to 18 months.[33]

Patients who have serum cortisol levels between 2 and 5 µg/dL are also considered to be in possible remission, because their tumor recurrence rates are similar to those in patients who have cortisol levels < 2 µg/dL (estimated at approximately 10% at 10 years postoperatively).[33] Nevertheless, this subset of patients is referred to as having subclinical Cushing's disease. They are advised to undergo repeat serum cortisol testing more frequently than those who have definite remission criteria. Patients who have serum cortisol levels persistently exceeding 5 µg/dL up to 6 weeks after surgery are considered to have persistent disease and should be considered for repeat surgery, adjuvant radiation, or medical-based therapies.[33] Besides other supplementary diagnostic tests (such as 24-h urinary free cortisol levels), midnight salivary cortisol levels, serum ACTH levels, and low-dose dexamethasone suppression tests can also be performed to confirm the endocrine remission.[8,33] Apart from these static biochemical tests, further dynamic biochemical tests such as CRH stimulation test, desmopressin stimulation test, and metyrapone stimulation tests can also be performed, although these tests have no specific advantage over the more traditional static tests.[8,33,37]

39.4.4 Prolactinoma

Prolactinomas are associated with endocrine dysfunction, which affects gonadal function, and neurological deficits caused by mass effect. Their clinical manifestation includes Forbes-Albright syndrome, including amenorrhea, galactorrhea, and infertility in women. In men, it presents as decreased libido, sexual dysfunction, erectile dysfunction, infertility, and occasionally gynecomastia.[12,13,14] In addition, hypoestrogenism and hypoandrogenism associated with hyperprolactinemia can lead to osteoporosis in both sexes. Serum Prl levels can rise because of any pituitary tumor causing compression on the posterior pituitary gland ("stalk effect").[12,13,14] However, serum Prl levels > 100 ng/mL are suggestive of prolactinoma, and serum levels > 200 ng/mL are highly suggestive of Prl-secreting tumor. Serum Prl levels of 100 to 250 ng/mL suggest the presence of a microprolactinoma, and levels > 250 ng/mL typically indicate macroprolactinoma.[12,13,14] At times even a giant invasive prolactinoma

may reveal a serum prolactin level within normal range. This phenomenon, known as the "hook effect," occurs because of oversaturation of a prolactin-detecting antibody assay. Accordingly, to appropriately judge prolactin levels, serial dilution assay should also be performed.[12,13,14] Other common causes of elevation of serum Prl levels also need to be ruled out; these include pregnancy, primary hypothyroidism, chronic renal failure, liver cirrhosis, drug-induced hyperprolactinemia, pseudoprolactinomas from stalk effect, macroprolactinemia, and physiological elevations.[12,13,14] Hence the initial laboratory tests in a case of suspected prolactinoma should include biochemical testing to rule out renal and liver insufficiencies, TSH levels, and a pregnancy test for women. Postoperative day 1 serum Prl level of < 10 ng/mL are associated with nearly 100% cure rates in microprolactinoma patients.

39.4.5 Thyrotropinoma

Thyrotropinomas are rare pituitary tumors that present with the same symptoms as primary hyperthyroidism: palpitations, heat intolerance, increased sweating, restlessness, weight loss, and goiter. They may present with mass effect symptoms and hypopituitarism.[10,11] They are often diagnosed late and are usually macroadenomas at the time of presentation. In most of the earlier studies, 70 to 90% of TSH-producing tumors were macroadenomas, with a latency period between onset of symptoms and diagnosis of approximately 4.5 to 9 years.[10,11] More recent studies report an increasing proportion of microadenomas at the time of diagnosis. The severity of clinical symptomatology is disproportionately low considering the amount of serum TSH and T4 elevation in thyrotropinomas when compared with corresponding patients who have untreated primary hyperthyroidism. These patients have an increased propensity to develop thyroid cancer because of the uninhibited TSH stimulation of thyroid cells.[10,11] Hence periodic screening for thyroid nodules using high-resolution ultrasound is recommended to detect the possible development of thyroid cancer. This diagnosis is usually considered when the TSH levels are inappropriately elevated or normal in a hyperthyroid individual who has increased serum T4 levels, regardless of presence of visible tumor on imaging.[10,11]

The differential diagnosis includes early phase of destructive thyroiditis, inconsistent thyroid replacement of hypothyroidism, recurrence of primary hypothyroidism, assay interference with heterophilic antibodies, acute psychiatric disease, use of amiodarone medication, and genetic causes, including resistance to thyroid hormone (RTH α and β), elevated serum thyroid hormone-binding proteins, and familial dysalbuminemic hyperthyroxinemia.[10,11] Undetectable TSH levels 7 days after surgery are highly predictive of successful outcome.

39.4.6 Pituitary Apoplexy

Pituitary apoplexy is a rare but sometimes life-threatening condition caused by infarcts or bleeds within the pituitary tumor, leading to both acute hypopituitarism and rapidly expanding intracranial mass, which may cause permanent visual loss if not treated immediately.[38,39,40,41] Pituitary apoplexy has an estimated prevalence of 6.2 cases per 100,000 persons and an incidence of 0.17 episodes per 100,000 person-years.[38,39,40] It occurs in 0.6 to 10% of all cases of PA, has a discrete predominance in males, and frequently occurs in the fifth or sixth decade of life.[38,39,40] It is typically characterized by sudden severe headache, visual loss, ophthalmoplegia, and altered mental status. Anterior pituitary hormone dysfunction is present in about 80% of patients at initial presentation.[38,39,40] The most critical deficiency is ACTH, observed in about 70% of cases, which may manifest with hypotension and hyponatremia. An acute hemorrhagic component can be visualized on CT scan (▶ Fig. 39.5), whereas MRI is most beneficial for subacute and chronic stages of apoplexy. Interestingly, mucosal thickening is often seen within the sphenoid sinus adjacent to the apoplectic tumor. Peripheral enhancement is typically seen in most cases; rarely, an empty sella may be present. Factors predisposing toward the development of pituitary apoplexy include vascular flux alterations during surgery, radiotherapy, and postspinal anesthesia; acute increase in blood flow during physical activity and systemic hypertension; dynamic stimulatory tests of pituitary

gland during provocative tests; hypoglycemia with insulin administration; coagulation disturbances with the use of anticoagulation and presence of thrombocytopenia; pregnancy; sickle cell anemia; estrogen replacement; lymphocytic leukemia; head trauma; and cessation of dopamine agonist therapy.[38,39,40] Occasionally, pituitary apoplexy may occur in microadenomas.[42]

39.5 Treatment

The goal of treatment for asymptomatic incidentalomas is primarily conservative, employing a "wait-and-watch" policy. Conversely, the management goals of symptomatic PA treatment include removing the tumor or reducing the tumor burden to alleviate the mass effect, preventing tumor recurrence, normalizing hormonal secretion (for functional tumors), and preserving normal pituitary function. In particular, the reversal of hormonal excess aims to reduce associated morbidity and mortality risks to the patient. At each stage of management, potential

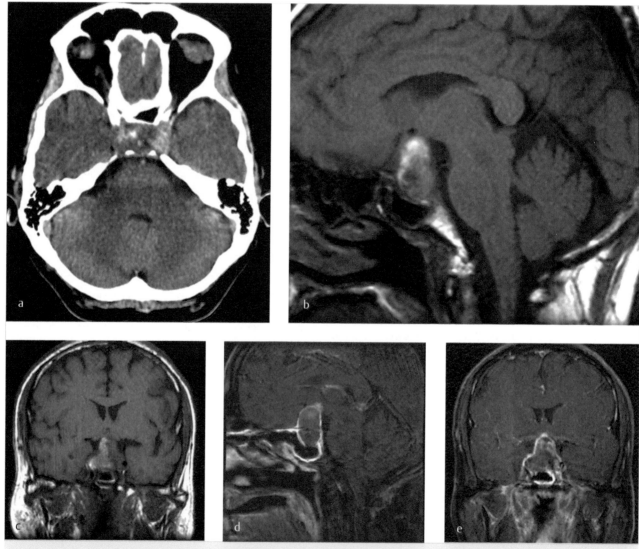

Fig. 39.5 Pituitary apoplexy. The patient presented with headache, nausea, and visual loss. (a) Note the high density within the sellar region on the axial noncontrast CT scan, indicating blood. On (b) sagittal and (c) coronal MRI precontrast images, high-intensity signal is noted. After contrast, the lesion is noted in (d) sagittal and (e) coronal images to have a variegated enhancement pattern, with mucosal thickening and enhancement adjacent to the apoplectic pituitary tumor.

iatrogenic morbidity needs to be weighed against the frequently benign nature of PA, a balance that must be considered on a case-by-case basis. Although surgery is at the forefront of the treatment paradigm, there is still a significant role for expectant management, medical therapies, adjuvant stereotactic radiosurgery (SRS)/fractionated stereotactic radiotherapy (FSRT), and chemotherapeutic agents in patients who have PA.

39.5.1 Conservative Management

Because microincidentalomas grow much more slowly than macroincidentalomas do, microincidentalomas are usually monitored using repeat imaging to ascertain the growth rate of the lesion. Nonfunctional microincidentalomas of < 5 mm size require no surveillance, and those ≥ 5 mm do not require surgical resection but rather require close radiological surveillance at 6 months and subsequently at 2 years.[27] Conversely, macroincidentalomas demonstrate tumor progression in 20 to 24% and 34 to 40% of patients at 4- and 8-year follow-up, respectively; thus they are followed more cautiously and the threshold for active intervention is lower.[27] Nonfunctioning macroincidentalomas situated remote from the optic apparatus are monitored with MRI along with complete hormonal profile (to look for anterior pituitary dysfunction) every year, then every 2 years.[27] When the macroincidentaloma is in proximity to the optic apparatus and is managed conservatively using surveillance rather than surgery, MRI is recommended at 6 months with hormonal profile and ophthalmological evaluation. Subsequently, annual MRI is advised along with hormonal and visual assessment every 6 months.[27]

If there is a tumor remnant after initial surgical decompression of a symptomatic NFPA, two options are available: simple surveillance or adjuvant therapy. The appropriate treatment decision has to be made in agreement with the patient and involves a multidisciplinary approach. The factors weighed in the decision-making process are the clinical profile of the patient, including age, comorbid status, and ability to undergo prolonged surveillance; tumor morphology, including size, pattern of extension, relation to the optic apparatus, and evidence of cavernous sinus invasion; pathological findings, including WHO grading, IHC, Ki-67 labeling index, and p53 expression; remnant progression; presence or absence of hypopituitarism; and availability of, and experience with, adjuvant therapeutic options in the treating center. Often in such cases, unless an elevated growth potential is reflected by the tumor, postponing radiotherapy is usually recommended until radiological progression is manifested, because the efficacy is comparable regardless of whether treatment is immediate or postponed.[28]

39.5.2 Surgery

The surgical success rate is dependent on patient age; tumor size, pattern of extension, WHO grade and precise ultrastructural morphology, degree of invasiveness, and proliferation potential; the magnitude of hormonal hypersecretion (for functional tumors); and the experience level of the surgeon.[7]

Microscopic vs. Endoscopic Transsphenoidal Surgery

Surgical approaches to pituitary tumors have evolved dramatically since the early times of Schloffer and Cushing. Transsphenoidal surgery fell out of favor until the 1960s, when Dott, Guiot, and Hardy repopularized the procedure.[43,44] A major driving force behind the evolution of the current surgical techniques has been the improvement in surgical optics and instrumentation, which have fueled the trend toward progressive minimalism. A microscopic transsphenoidal approach has been the gold-standard procedure of choice for treatment of the majority of PAs. Subsequently, Carrau and Jho and Cappabianca et al conceived and developed endoscope-guided transsphenoidal surgery, which has been accepted as a valid alternative to the traditional microscopic transsphenoidal approach.[43,44] Advocates of the endoscopic approach report better visualization with the panoramic view, as well as reduced patient discomfort and improved quality of life, whereas the proponents of the microscopic approach report better tactile sense with three-dimensional visualization and greater familiarity with using the microscope.[43,44,45,46] Much conflicting evidence exists in the literature regarding the relative pros and cons of each technique. A definite advantage of endoscopic approach is in extended skull base surgeries and when tackling giant PAs[43,44,45,46]; however, these extensive skull base approaches are commonly associated with large skull base defects requiring multilayered reconstructions. Despite adequate measures, cerebrospinal fluid (CSF) leak rates are substantial in such cases when compared with transcranial approaches.[43,44,45,46]

In the largest meta-analysis to date comparing the short-term outcome of endoscopic (24 data sets, 3,518 patients) versus microscopic (22 data sets, 2,125 patients) PA surgery, Ammirati et al[45] found significantly higher incidence of vascular complications in endoscopic group than in the microscopic group ($p < 0.0001$). No other statistically significant differences were noted between the two techniques for any other variable. They inferred that endoscopy does not offer any significant advantage over the gold-standard microscopic transsphenoidal approach, although they recommended a prospective multicentric randomized controlled trial to demonstrate any superiority of one procedure over another.

Transsphenoidal Surgery: Indications

Transsphenoidal surgery is the first-line treatment for all symptomatic PAs except prolactinomas. It can also be a second-line treatment for Prl-secreting tumors that are resistant to medical management. Considering the primarily benign nature of disease, radiation treatment is usually not considered prior to surgical decompression of the tumor.[46] Surgery is also indicated as an emergency measure in patients presenting with pituitary apoplexy and compressive symptoms, irrespective of the tumor subtype.[38] Surgery for incidentalomas is reserved primarily for any tumor demonstrating progression, cases of tumor-related hypopituitarism, tumors causing compression of the optic chiasm, patients who have possible malignancy, patients who desire to become pregnant in the short term, noncompliant patients, or cases involving elevated risk of pituitary apoplexy.[27,46] Surgery for prolactinomas is indicated for women who have macroprolactinomas who are also contemplating pregnancy; patients who have resistance to or intolerance of dopamine agonists; patients who have large cystic tumors for which medical management is unlikely to be beneficial; patients who have CSF leakage post tumor shrinkage; patients who are dependent on antipsychotic medications, because dopamine agonist therapy may precipitate psychotic episodes; patients who have acute visual loss; and patients who have prolactinomas presenting with pituitary apoplexy and symptoms of local mass effect, as well as in cases requiring reduction of tumor bulk to increase sensitivity to pharmacological therapy.[14,46]

In addition, an analysis of cost efficacy by Jethwa et al[47] demonstrated that transsphenoidal surgical resection of microprolactinomas, either microscopic or endoscopic, appears to be more cost-effective than lifelong medical therapy in young patients who have a life expectancy of more than 10 years. Repeat surgery is indicated for NFPAs if complete resection of the recurrence is feasible, for symptomatic optic chiasm compression (to create a safety margin between the tumor and optic apparatus ahead of adjuvant radiotherapy), and in cases of postradiotherapy progression.[6,28] Transient or permanent levothyroxine supplementation may be required after resection of thyrotropinomas, because postoperative TSH usually becomes undetectable after complete tumor resection and may remain low for many months to follow.[11]

Transcranial Surgery: Indications

Indications for transcranial approaches have traditionally included a small sella turcica that has a large extrasellar component, tumors that have large parasellar and subfrontal extensions, very large tumors (▶ Fig. 39.6), nonpneumatized or unfavorable sphenoid sinus anatomy, coexisting internal carotid artery or anterior cerebral artery aneurysm, presence of "kissing" carotids, and the presence of firm or fibrous PAs (identified during prior surgical procedure).[48]

Alternative Surgical Procedures

Bilateral adrenalectomy should be considered in the comprehensive treatment algorithm for patients who have persistent Cushing's disease after failed pituitary surgery, especially for those who have severe sequelae of hypercortisolism or who desire pregnancy.[49] This procedure has demonstrated remarkable improvement in clinical signs and symptoms of Cushing's disease, but it also has some serious long-term complications, including adrenal crisis and Nelson's syndrome associated with hyperpigmentation and aggressive pituitary tumor growth. In a select subset of patients, total thyroidectomy is required for recurrent tumors refractory to conventional treatment or in patients who are at risk of thyroid storm.[11]

39.5.3 Medical Therapy

Acromegaly

The available medical therapies for GH-secreting PAs include somatostatin receptor ligands (SRLs, such as octreotide and lanreotide), dopamine agonists (e.g., cabergoline), and GH receptor antagonists (e.g., pegvisomant); they are recommended when surgical success is not technically feasible, after subtotal resection of secretory adenomas, and immediately subsequent to radiotherapy during the latency period prior to reduction in GH levels.[29,30,32,50] Pharmacological treatment of acromegaly helps improve left ventricular hypertrophy, cardiac dysfunction, hypertension, and obstructive sleep apnea, but its effect on joints and soft tissue tumors may be irreversible. These

SRLs are usually considered the mainstay of medical therapy when used as either adjuvant or primary medical therapy.[29,30,32,50] Theoretically, preoperative medical management with SRLs improves acromegaly-related symptoms, decreases arterial stiffness and improves endothelial function; reduces soft tissue swelling, especially in the upper respiratory tract; and induces better blood pressure control, thus potentially reducing the risks associated with anesthesia and surgery. However, the precise role of preoperative treatment with SRLs is still uncertain because of the heterogeneity of methodology, low overall surgical cure rates, variable study designs, and conflicting results in the current literature.

It seems that SRL treatment 3 months prior to surgery may improve short-term surgical remission rates, but this apparent benefit does not translate into higher long-term remission rates.[29,30,32,50] One possible explanation for this observation could be the fact that carry-over effects from SRLs could last for a few months after surgery, leading to a false impression of better remission rates in the short term. In addition, the potential role of SRLs in reducing perioperative risk from acromegaly-associated cardiopulmonary complications also needs to be evaluated more extensively before SRLs can be included in the mainstream preoperative treatment regime for acromegalic patients.

Developing novel pharmacological approaches to patients who have acromegaly include pasireotide (somatostatin receptor 5 binding profile); oral octreotide with transient permeability enhancer to enable gut absorption; use of antisense oligonucleotide of 20 bases that binds to the GH receptor mRNA and inhibits translation of receptor protein; and a targeted secretion inhibitor, combining botulinum toxin and a GH-releasing hormone chimera molecule that binds to adenoma cells expressing GHRH receptor, leading to internalization of botulinum toxin and inhibition of GH secretion. However, some of these approaches are still in experimental phases.[29,30,32,50]

Cushing's Disease

The available medical management options include the end-tissue directed/glucocorticoid receptor antagonist, mifepristone; drugs directly blocking adrenal gland function (steroidogenesis inhibitors), including ketoconazole, metyrapone, and mitotane; and drugs targeting the corticotroph tumors at the pituitary level, including SRL to somatostatin (SST) receptor 5, pasireotide; cabergoline (dopamine D2 receptor agonist, DA); peroxisome proliferator-activated receptor gamma (PPARγ) agonists, including rosiglitazone and pioglitazone; and retinoic acid acting on retinoic acid receptors.[8,34,51] Pasireotide is a novel multireceptor ligand somatostatin analog with a high binding affinity to SST receptor 5, the predominant receptor in human corticotroph adenoma cells.[34] Its primary indications are for treatment of recurrent hypercortisolism after surgery and for patients who are not appropriate candidates for primary surgical resection. Primary side effects of pasireotide are similar to those of octreotide and include nausea, diarrhea, gallstones, and hyperglycemia.[34] Steroidogenesis inhibitors may achieve normocortisolemia and are often used as bridge therapy until definitive reduction of ACTH is achieved by surgery or radiation. Their effectiveness can be increased by combination therapies. Accumulating evidence suggests that epidermal

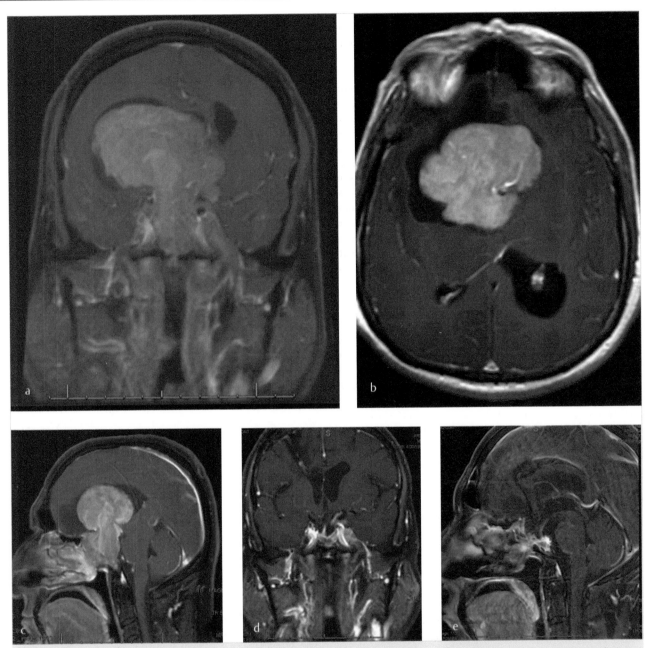

Fig. 39.6 Massive pituitary tumor with intracranial extension. This 45-year-old man presented with cognitive decline and visual loss. Preoperative MRI images with contrast demonstrate tumor with a large mass invading the frontal lobes: **(a)** coronal, **(b)** axial, and **(c)** sagittal T1-weighted images with contrast enhancement. He underwent a transcortical excision of the tumor with gross total resection, including the sellar component, as shown in **(d)** coronal and **(e)** sagittal views.

growth factor receptor (EGFR) and cyclin E-CDK2, which are the key regulators of Rb-mediated G1/S checkpoint in the cell cycle, may be promising targets for treating ACTHomas.[51]

Prolactinoma

Medical management with bromocriptine and cabergoline is the first line of management of prolactin secreting PAs according to the 2011 Endocrine Society guidelines.[12,13,14] Because of the lower side-effect profile, cabergoline is associated with higher drug compliance. However, cabergoline is more costly than bromocriptine, so from a financial perspective, bromocriptine is

a reasonable option. The long-term side effect profile of dopamine agonists includes gastrointestinal disturbances, valvular heart disease, and postural hypotension. Dopamine agonist therapy withdrawal may be contemplated for patients whose Prl levels have normalized, with no tumor on MRI or reduction of tumor size by at least 50% and no invasion of critical structures for a minimum of 2 years.[12,13,14] Gradual drug withdrawal while carefully titrating serum Prl levels may be attempted after about 4 years of dopamine agonist therapy. Recurrences are usually observed during the first 6 months to 1 year of drug withdrawal. As a result, regular follow-ups are necessary at 3-month intervals for the first year, then annually for 5 years post withdrawal, to monitor serum Prl levels and tumor recurrence. However, treatment often needs to be continued for life, because hyperprolactinemia tends to recur in a significant proportion of patients (~ 80%) after the medication is discontinued.[12,13,14]

Resistance to dopamine agonist therapy is defined as inability to normalize serum Prl levels and failure to decrease macroprolactinoma size by ≥ 50% at the maximal conventional doses.[12,13,14] Failure of medical management occurs in approximately 25 to 33% of patients with bromocriptine therapy and 10 to 15% of patients with cabergoline therapy. The possible underlying mechanisms for dopamine agonist therapy resistance in prolactinomas can be reduction in D2 dopamine receptor density, decrease in the number of nerve growth factor receptors, dysregulation of cell proliferation, and differentiation and alterations in intracellular signal transduction pathways. Treatment approaches for patients who have drug resistance to dopamine agonists include switching over to other drugs, increasing the dose beyond the conventional dosages, transsphenoidal surgery, and radiation therapy. Reduction of endogenous estrogen, use of selective estrogen receptor modulators, and aromatase inhibitors are potential experimental approaches.[12,13,14]

Thyrotropinoma

Cosecretion of GH and Prl may be seen in about 16% and 10% patients who have thyrotropinoma, respectively. Most thyrotroph cells express a variable number of somatostatin receptors, particularly the SSTR2 and SSTR5 receptors, as well as dopamine receptors.[11] The presence of somatostatin and dopamine receptors on thyrotroph cells has provided the therapeutic rationale for using SRL and dopamine agonists in the treatment of thyrotropinomas. As an alternative adjuvant therapeutic option to radiation therapy for residual or recurrent thyrotropinoma, SRL therapy has demonstrated reasonable biochemical, remission, and tumor shrinkage rates.[11] The high cost of treatment is the primary limiting factor for SRL therapy. Conversely, the treatment response with DA therapy is variable, with the best results obtained for tumors with cosecretion of TSH and Prl hormones.[11]

39.5.4 Radiation Therapy

Stereotactic Radiosurgery vs. Fractionated Stereotactic Radiotherapy

The two available modalities for adjuvant radiation therapy in the treatment algorithm of PA are SRS and FSRT.[52,53] With advances in high-resolution imaging, image guidance, dosage planning, and radiation dose-shielding options, both SRS and FSRT have been demonstrated to be relatively well tolerated while having excellent accuracy and safety profiles. Both have been used as an effective second-/third-line treatment for patients who have either functional or nonfunctional PA who are not cured after surgery and who do not respond to, or who wish to avoid, long-term medical therapy. They can also be offered as a first-line treatment for NFPA patients who are at extremely high surgical risk. SRS has some specific advantages over FSRT when it comes to PA treatment. With dose escalation and reduction in number of fractions comes a greater biological effect on late-responding tissues, such as PA cells, than with early-responding tissues.[52,53]

For functioning adenomas, SRS appears to provide a more rapid rate of endocrine remission. In addition, the convenience of single-session treatment with SRS versus multiple sessions for FSRT skews the clinician's and patient's judgment in favor of SRS more often. However, patients who have large tumor volume, irregular residual tumor shape, or close proximity of tumor to radiosensitive structures such as visual apparatus and brainstem are not suitable candidates for SRS and thus should opt for FSRT to limit the risk of delayed toxicities. The efficacy rate for FSRT is slightly lower than SRS and is again dependent on tumor subtype and functional status.[52,53]

Photon vs. Proton Beam Therapy

SRS uses multiple low-energy radiation beams designated to converge on a precise stereotactic target, resulting in high-dose radiation to a specific target with a sharp fall-off in radiation exposure outside the target. It may be delivered as photons (Leksell Gamma Knife [Elekta] and CyberKnife [Accuray]) or as charged particles such as proton beam therapy. Charged particles have the advantage of more steep radiation dose fall-off after delivering energy to the intended target and thus are conceptually superior to photon beam therapy. Because of the limited availability and higher costs associated with proton beam therapy, it is not commonly used for pituitary tumors.

In general, NFPAs are more radiosensitive than their functional counterparts. The mean marginal radiation dosages to the 50% isodose line for NFPA and functional pituitary adenoma (FPA) are 12 to 18 Gy and 18 to 30 Gy, respectively. There seems to be a differential radiosensitivity between specific subtypes of secretory PAs as well, the explanation for which is yet obscure. Overall, Cushing's disease demonstrates the highest rates of biochemical remission, followed by acromegaly and prolactinoma.[52,53] Possible factors responsible could include patient selection, tumor volume, radiation dose, use of suppressive medications, and duration of follow-up. Antisecretory medical therapies are generally withheld around the radiation treatment time so as to boost the efficacy of SRS, especially for acromegaly and prolactinomas—possibly because there is reduction in radiosensitivity of adenoma cells secondary to decreased cell division when exposed to SRL and dopamine agonist therapies. Additionally, SRLs may act as free radical scavengers, thereby reducing the DNA damage after ionizing radiation in GH-secreting tumor cells.[14,32]

Complications of Radiation Therapy

Delayed hypopituitarism is the most common complication after SRS or FSRT for PA patients. The risk of SRS-induced delayed hypopituitarism, which is reported to be ~ 28 to 42%, can be reduced by performing a pituitary transposition (hypophysopexy) using a spacer in the form of autologous fat graft placed between normal pituitary gland and residual tumor in the cavernous sinus.[14,52,53] This helps increase the effective distance between the radiosurgical target and normal functioning gland, thereby reducing the effective biological dose to the normal gland. Known risk factors predisposing towards SRS-induced hypopituitarism include target volume > 4 mL, residual tumor proximity to the pituitary gland and stalk, maximum dose received by the pituitary gland > 15 Gy and by the distal infundibulum > 17 Gy, no healthy pituitary gland seen on MRI, preexisting partial hypopituitarism, and history of prior radiotherapy. Steeper dose fall-off, improved conformality in radiation planning, and adequate shielding may help minimize the risk of other neurological deficits arising after SRS. Rare toxicities of SRS include radiation necrosis of adjacent parenchyma, internal carotid artery stenosis/occlusion, and radiation-induced secondary malignancy.[14,52,53]

39.5.5 Chemotherapy

Temozolomide (TMZ) is an oral chemotherapeutic alkylating agent; it has a favorable side-effect profile and has demonstrated activity against Pas.[5,54] Its nonoverlapping toxicity and ability to induce rapid tumor regression make it a potentially important adjunctive treatment option. It has been tried for heavily pretreated PAs and carcinomas resistant or refractory to conventional therapeutic options. Besides TMZ, other chemotherapeutic options such as lomustine, 5-flurouracil, cisplatin, carboplatin, and etoposide have also been tried.[5,54] TMZ has been the most consistently reported agent, with the most favorable efficacy and side effect profile for pituitary tumors. The treatment response can be as high as 55% for aggressive PAs and as high as 58% for PCs. Although the association of O^6-methylguanine-DA methyltransferase (MGMT) with the treatment responsiveness of TMZ is not as well validated in pituitary tumors as with glioma therapy, several studies have suggested its importance in selectively choosing appropriate pituitary tumor patients for predicting the therapeutic benefit of TMZ.[5,54]

The degree of MGMT expression appears to be inversely related to TMZ therapy response, although the literature is divided on this. Recent evidence suggests that mutations in mismatch repair proteins such as MSH6 could render pituitary tumors resistant to TMZ.[5,54] Immediate toxicity of TMZ primarily includes hematological suppression, which is often short-lived and can be easily managed with dose reduction. The other common side effects include nausea, constipation, and fatigue. The delayed and permanent toxicities can include development of iatrogenic myelodysplastic syndrome and acute myeloid leukemia. These permanent complications are quite rare, however, with an estimated incidence of < 0.1%.[5,54]

39.6 Pituitary Adenoma in Pregnancy

Among prolactinoma patients during pregnancy, tumor growth causing significant symptoms and requiring intervention has been reported to occur in 2.4% of those who have microadenomas, 21% of those who have macroadenomas without prior radiation or surgery, and 4.7% of those who have macroadenomas with prior surgery or irradiation.[55,56] Both the dopamine agonist cabergoline and bromocriptine have been found to be safe for consumption during pregnancy (FDA category B), but the number of studies citing the safety data for bromocriptine in pregnancy is about sevenfold that of cabergoline. Thus it is generally advisable to withhold cabergoline therapy as soon as pregnancy is confirmed. If it is necessary to continue medical therapy during pregnancy, as in cases of aggressive macroadenoma or adenoma close to optic apparatus, the decision must be made only after detailed discussion with the patient's family.

In many cases, medical therapy is completely withheld and radiological surveillance using plain MRI is done every trimester. Surgery, when indicated, must be performed during the second trimester of gestation.[55,56]

For acromegalic women who become pregnant while on medical management with SRLs, GH receptor antagonists, or dopamine agonists, cessation of medical therapy is advised, primarily on the basis of lack of a body of data demonstrating the safety of their use in pregnant acromegalic patients. ACTH-secreting adenomas should be resected using a transsphenoidal approach in the second trimester of pregnancy.[55,56] Pregnancies in women harboring TSHomas are exceedingly rare, with only a few case reports available in the literature. Accordingly, an individualistic approach and informed decision should be used for such cases.

39.7 Outcome and Prognosis

Diabetes insipidus (DI) is a common complication after pituitary surgery, and its effects can be transient or permanent. Neurogenic DI occurs subsequent to injury to magnocellular neurons in the hypothalamus, which produces and transports arginine vasopressin and forms the hypothalamo–hypophyseal tract. DI leads to dilute high-volume urine output and increased serum osmolality. Factors affecting DI rates include pituitary tumor size, adherence to surrounding structures, surgical approach, and tumor histopathology.[57] The overall rate of visual field improvement with transsphenoidal surgical tumor decompression is ~ 80%. Early visual improvement after surgical decompression is attributed to restoration of axoplasmic flow, whereas delayed recovery is because of optic nerve remyelination and remodeling. More specific visual testing via optic coherence tomography, visual evoked potential, and pattern electroretinogram may further help prognosticate the long-term visual outcome.[58] PCs are often radioresistant and are associated with poor prognosis, and approximately 80% of these patients die within 8 years.[22]

39.7.1 Acromegaly

Prognosis in acromegaly is determined by the pattern and extent of organ system involvement. Untreated acromegaly reduces life expectancy by ~ 10 years, and mortality commonly occurs due to cardiovascular, cerebrovascular, metabolic, and respiratory comorbidities. Specifically, lung and bowel cancers account for ~ 70% of all acromegaly-related neoplasms, and cancer mortality is 4.6-fold higher in acromegalic men than in the normal male population. Using a comparative effectiveness research analysis integrating efficacy, cost, and quality of life for available treatment strategies to tackle GH-secreting pituitary microadenoma, Marko et al concluded that choice of management therapy must be individualized for each patient who has acromegaly.[7] On the basis of their analysis, they listed treatment strategies in decreasing order of efficacy as transsphenoidal surgery, pegvisomant therapy, SRL treatment, and SRS. Among these, one-time surgery and SRS were more cost-effective than lifelong medical therapy. Similarly, quality-of-life data analysis demonstrated that curative surgery is the best available option, followed by pegvisomant therapy, SRL treatment, and SRS.

The efficacy of surgery in acromegalic patients is estimated to be 72 to 95% for intrasellar microadenomas and 40 to 68% for noninvasive macroadenomas.[7] In the hands of experienced neurosurgeons, overall complication rates for transsphenoidal pituitary surgery are < 5%. The most common complications include hyponatremia as a result of syndrome of inappropriate antidiuretic hormone hypersecretion, CSF leak, oculomotor nerve paresis, visual deterioration, carotid artery injury, epistaxis, infection, and DI. The average rate of permanent hypopituitarism after transsphenoidal surgery is estimated to be ~ 2 to 3%.[7] The surgical mortality is estimated to be around 0.1%. The reporting for recurrence rates is not consistent and is quite variable across different studies, although it averages ~ 6% for all completely resected pituitary tumors treated via transsphenoidal surgery.[7] The mean remission rate for reoperations in such cases is 37% (range 8–59%).[50] The mean endocrine remission rate of SRS for acromegalic patients is 43.6% (range 0–82%) with an average latency period of 2 years.[53] Neurological deficits and hypopituitarism occur in 1.8% (range 0–11%) and 15.3% (range 0–40%) of cases, respectively. Factors associated with postradiosurgical endocrine remission include higher prescribed radiation dose, lower pretreatment GH and IGF-1 levels, and withholding of hormone-suppressive medications prior to SRS therapy.[7,30,53]

The efficacy of SRLs to attain biochemical remission is 40 to 85%, again varying according to remission criteria used in various studies. Overall, the remission rates are quite similar when comparing their use as a primary or adjuvant therapy.[7,29,30,32,50] Tumor volume reduction is commonly observed with SRL therapy concordant to the reduction in GH secretion, and it normally occurs within 3 months of therapy initiation. SRL therapy use, however, is limited by the high cost of treatment and the side-effect profile, which includes the risks of cholelithiasis, abdominal pain, and transient diarrhea. Frequent monitoring of blood glucose and HbA1C levels is necessary, because SRLs have a negative influence on glucose metabolism. Pegvisomant is a genetically modified GH analog that acts as a competitive inhibitor at the receptor level to block the action of native GH. It acts at peripheral sites as a GH receptor antagonist and is indicated to normalize uncontrolled IGF-1 levels following maximum therapy with other modalities. Using its maximal dosage, IGF-1 normalization rates of 82% have been achieved.[7,29,30,32,50]

The treatment effect is maximized in patients after surgery. Initial apprehension toward paradoxical increase in tumor size limited its widespread use, but most recent literature has suggested otherwise, demonstrating a reduction in tumor volume in ~ 12 to 19% of treated patients and tumor growth in < 2% of treated patients. Side effects of pegvisomant include elevation of liver enzymes, especially when used in conjunction with SRLs, for which the reported risk is 27 to 34%. Other side effects include injection site lipodystrophy, fatigue, dizziness, headaches, perspiration, and abdominal bloating. In contrast to SRLs, pegvisomant has beneficial effects on glucose metabolism.[7,29,30,32,50]

Bromocriptine tends to normalize IGF-1 with only very high doses, which are not well tolerated by ~ 10% of patients.[7,29,30,32,50] High-dose cabergoline therapy is better tolerated and has shown better efficacy than bromocriptine for patients who have modest elevations of serum IGF-1 levels to approximately two times the upper limit of normal; however, its efficacy is still lower (~ 40%)

than that of other contemporary therapeutic options. It works better for tumors demonstrating cosecretion of Prl hormone. The side-effect profile of cabergoline includes nausea, vomiting, headaches, nasal congestion, and dizziness. Bromocriptine causes much more severe gastrointestinal symptoms. The long-term use of higher doses of cabergoline may be limited by the development of cardiac valvular disease, necessitating regular cardiac checkups with echocardiography.[7,29,30,32,50]

39.7.2 Cushing's Disease

Transsphenoidal surgery is the mainstay of therapy, which leads to remission rates ranging from 65 to 93%, with a median time to relapse ranging from 20 to 84 months.[59] The recurrence rates remain relatively high at 20 to 25% on long-term follow-up. Better remission rates can be attained if meticulous dissection using the pseudocapsule of the adenoma is performed to ensure complete tumor resection. If there is residual tumor after first surgery, it may be worthwhile to explore the whole gland again. Repeat transsphenoidal surgery is effective in obtaining remission in 61 to 73% of patients who have disease relapse, but if the residual tumor is still not found, partial or total hypophysectomy should be contemplated. Disease remission occurs in ~ 60 to 75% in this subset of patients.[59] Rates of endocrine remission with SRS are 16.7 to 87%, with an average latency period of 1 year.[53] Risk of new onset or worsening of existing neurological deficits was 3.4% on average. The incidence of hypopituitarism after radiosurgery is slightly higher, at an average of 24.9%, than that of NFPA, probably because of the higher dose of radiation received by normal pituitary gland and pituitary stalk. Pasireotide efficacy in normalizing urinary free cortisol levels has been reported in up to 28% of patients, which can be further increased to 50% or more by adding cabergoline and ketoconazole therapies to the treatment regime.[8,34] Cabergoline is generally effective in achieving normal urinary free cortisol (UFC) levels in ~ 40% of Cushing's disease patients.[8,34]

39.7.3 Prolactinoma

Dopamine agonist therapy is the first-line therapy for prolactinomas in normalizing serum Prl levels, reducing tumor volume, and reversing gonadal dysfunction. They can restore gonadal function in ~ 80 to 90% of patients who have microprolactinomas.[12,13,14] Similarly, normalization of Prl levels can be achieved in up to 85% of patients who have previously untreated macroprolactinoma, with tumor shrinkage of at least 25% seen in ~ 80% of patients. Serum Prl should be monitored annually while on medical treatment. Normalization of Prl after surgery can be achieved in 80 to 90% for microadenomas and in 40% for macroadenomas.[12,13,14] For prolactinomas, endocrine remission rates after SRS average ~ 29.4% (range 0–83%).[53] In general, biochemical remission rates for prolactinomas after SRS tend to be worse than those with Cushing's disease and acromegaly, even when taking into account preradiosurgical patient and tumor attributes.[53] As with acromegaly, the rates of endocrine remission rates seem to improve by taking patients off dopamine agonist therapy while they undergo SRS therapy. Iatrogenic neurological deficits and delayed hypopituitarism occur, on average, in 3.6% of cases (range 0–14%) and 15.7% of cases (range 0–45%), respectively. Because hypopituitarism has independently been associated with reduced life expectancy, patients need regular endocrine testing and treatment of any identified hormonal deficiencies. Although quite rare, side effects of SRS other than neurological deficits and hypopituitarism include trigeminal neuralgia, temporal lobe epilepsy with seizures, radiation necrosis, and carotid artery stenosis.

39.7.4 Thyrotropinoma

Transsphenoidal surgery is the treatment of choice for thyrotropinoma; up to 85.5% of cases have complete radiological remission, and 71.4 to 100% of patients develop biochemical remission after surgery.[11] The overall recurrence rate after remission from surgery is ~ 31%. SRLs are also known to suppress TSH levels by acting on the SSTR2 and 5 receptors present on thyrotroph cells, and they can reduce TSHoma tumor volume by > 20% in up to 50% of cases.[11] Overall, SRLs may lead to normalization of thyroid function tests in up to 73 to 100% of cases and a reduction in tumor volume in 20 to 70%. The latency period for the normalization of thyroid function after starting SRLs has been between 10 days and 20 months. Radiation therapy, when used as an adjuvant therapy, helps in achieving biochemical remission in ~ 36.3 to 100% of cases over the long term.[53] Ensuring at least a 3-mm gap between the optic apparatus and tumor can reduce the incidence of visual decline after SRS therapy. If the tumor closely abuts the optic apparatus, hypofractionated SRS or FSRT may be used to optimize visual outcome. In addition, using the shielding technique and ensuring radiation dose of < 8 to 10 Gy to the optic apparatus can also prevent long-term visual loss.

39.7.5 Pituitary Apoplexy and Nonfunctional Pituitary Adenoma

Prompt treatment with fluids and injectable hydrocortisone is the mainstay of medical management for pituitary apoplexy. In the event of pituitary apoplexy, early surgical decompression of the tumor (preferably within 1 wk) has been associated with good outcomes.[38] When giving long-term hormone supplementation, glucocorticoids and testosterone are generally required in ~ 60 to 80% of patients, thyroxine in ~ 60%, and desmopressin in ~ 10 to 15%.[38] Gross total resection rates in the recent literature have approached ~ 80% for NFPA.[6,28] The morbidity of early postoperative adrenal insufficiency ranges from 0.96 to 12.90%, with an overall morbidity of 5.55%.[60] The risk for adrenal insufficiency is not governed by the perioperative steroid supplementation. Morning serum cortisol of < 60 nmol/L at 3 days after surgery is highly specific and highly sensitive for adrenal insufficiency, whereas > 270 nmol/L is highly specific and highly sensitive for adrenal sufficiency. The intermediate range (60–270 nmol/L) morning serum cortisol needs further evaluation to better ascertain the requirement for steroid supplementation in perioperative period.[60]

In patients in whom apparently complete tumor resection is achieved (based on postoperative imaging), the recurrence risk is around 10 to 20% at 5 years and 30% at 10 years. In cases of postoperative tumor residual, recurrence risk ranges from 25 to 40% at 5 years and exceeds 50% at 10 years.[6,28] Recovery of visual loss correlates with duration and severity of visual field defect, and ~ 80 to 90% of patients show some improvement

through almost 1 year after surgery. The chance of recovery of hypopituitarism is ~ 30% after surgery, and there is a 5 to 10% risk of aggravating or inducing hypopituitarism.[6,28] Overall, the risk of new-onset DI is < 5%. For NFPA, tumor control rates with SRS range from 83 to 100% and neurological deficits are uncommon, at an average of 2.1% (range 0–7.1%).[53] Delayed hypopituitarism is reported in approximately 12% of patients (range 0–39%). Tumor volume < 4 to 5 mL appears to have the optimal response to SRS.

39.7.6 Follow-up Surveillance Protocol

In addition to standard postoperative care, serum electrolytes and osmolality must be regularly checked along with strict intake/output charting. In addition to urine-specific gravity, central venous pressure and daily weight must be assessed to optimize fluid and electrolyte balance.[61] The radiological assessment after surgery is generally deferred until at least 3 months to avoid misinterpreting postoperative inflammation and edema as tumor remnants. If there is a tumor remnant or suspicious imaging findings with ill-defined enhancement, follow-up MRI is repeated annually for 5 years and then every 2 to 3 years in the absence of tumor progression. Finally, the imaging schedule is tailored according to each case scenario and clinical judgment based on the remnant tumor dimensions, distance between tumor and optic apparatus, and presence of doubt about remnant progression. If there was preexisting visual compromise, repeat ophthalmological checkup is recommended at 3 months after surgery and includes visual acuity testing, visual field charting, funduscopy, and oculomotor examination. This must be repeated every 6 months until maximal improvement is achieved.

A comprehensive endocrinological evaluation should be performed at 4 to 6 weeks postoperatively. If there is no postoperative deficiency, further exploration is unnecessary unless there is progression of a tumor remnant or a new recurrence. In the case of postoperative hormonal deficiency, monthly monitoring for 6 to 12 months is required to tailor replacement therapy. Preoperative thyrotroph deficiency should be reassessed postoperatively after interruption of thyroxine therapy for at least 1 month. Considering the long biological half-life of IGF-1, accurate assessment of IGF-1 levels after surgery requires a period of 3 to 4 months for the level to stabilize. By contrast, GH has a very short half-life, so its role in the assessment of biochemical remission during the immediate postoperative period is paramount. The incidence of recurrence in acromegalic patients appears to peak around 1 to 5 years after surgery, although recurrences have been observed more than 10 years after initial cure,[50] requiring continuation of surveillance imaging and hormonal assays until at least 10 years after surgery. It can subsequently be tailored to the individual patient's requirements.

39.8 Conclusion

The vast majority of PAs are benign and present incidentally or with hypopituitarism, hormonal hypersecretion, and local mass effect. As the tumor grows beyond the confines of sella, it may impinge on the visual apparatus, leading to visual decline. Effective medical therapy is available for prolactinomas, whereas surgery remains the mainstay for most of the other pituitary tumors. Radiation treatment is often the second or third line of management, commonly reserved for nonresectable lesions and those refractory to first-line treatments. Novel medical therapies and chemotherapeutic agents may help optimize the long-term functional outcomes. Comprehensive management of PA requires a multidisciplinary collaboration among a team of neurosurgeons, neuroradiologists, neuropathologists, medical and radiation oncologists, and endocrinologists.

References

[1] Ezzat S, Asa SL, Couldwell WT, et al. The prevalence of pituitary adenomas: a systematic review. Cancer. 2004; 101(3):613–619

[2] Chatzellis E, Alexandraki KI, Androulakis II, Kaltsas G. Aggressive pituitary tumors. Neuroendocrinology. 2015; 101(2):87–104

[3] Jane J, Jr, Laws E, Jr. Surgical Treatment of Pituitary Adenomas. Endotext [Internet]. South Dartmouth, MA: MDText.com, Inc.; 2000

[4] Grizzi F, Borroni EM, Vacchini A, et al. Pituitary adenoma and the chemokine network: a systemic view. Front Endocrinol (Lausanne). 2015; 6:141

[5] Lin AL, Sum MW, DeAngelis LM. Is there a role for early chemotherapy in the management of pituitary adenomas? Neuro-oncol. 2016; 18(10):1350–1356

[6] Cámara Gómez R. Non-functioning pituitary tumors: 2012 update. Endocrinol Nutr. 2014; 61(3):160–170

[7] Marko NF, LaSota E, Hamrahian AH, Weil RJ. Comparative effectiveness review of treatment options for pituitary microadenomas in acromegaly. J Neurosurg. 2012; 117(3):522–538

[8] Rutkowski MJ, Breshears JD, Kunwar S, Aghi MK, Blevins LS. Approach to the postoperative patient with Cushing's disease. Pituitary. 2015; 18(2):232–237

[9] Sharma ST, Nieman LK, Feelders RA. Comorbidities in Cushing's disease. Pituitary. 2015; 18(2):188–194

[10] Beck-Peccoz P, Persani L, Lania A. Thyrotropin-secreting pituitary adenomas. In: De Groot LJ, Chrousos G, Dungan K, Feingold KR, Grossman A, Hershman JM, et al., eds. Endotext [Internet]. South Dartmouth, MA: MDText.com, Inc.; 2015

[11] Amlashi FG, Tritos NA. Thyrotropin-secreting pituitary adenomas: epidemiology, diagnosis, and management. Endocrine. 2016; 52(3):427–440

[12] Molitch ME. Management of medically refractory prolactinoma. J Neurooncol. 2014; 117(3):421–428

[13] Wong A, Eloy JA, Couldwell WT, Liu JK. Update on prolactinomas. Part 1: Clinical manifestations and diagnostic challenges. J Clin Neurosci. 2015; 22(10):1562–1567

[14] Wong A, Eloy JA, Couldwell WT, Liu JK. Update on prolactinomas. Part 2: Treatment and management strategies. J Clin Neurosci. 2015; 22(10):1568–1574

[15] Raverot G, Vasiljevic A, Jouanneau E, Trouillas J. A prognostic clinicopathologic classification of pituitary endocrine tumors. Endocrinol Metab Clin North Am. 2015; 44(1):11–18

[16] Saeger W, Honegger J, Theodoropoulou M, et al. Clinical impact of the current WHO classification of pituitary adenomas. Endocr Pathol. 2016; 27(2):104–114

[17] Lloyd R, Kovacs K, Young W Jr, et al. Pituitary tumors: introduction. In: DeLellis R, Lloyd R, Heitz P, Eng C, eds. WHO Classification of Tumors of the Endocrine Organs: Pathology and Genetics of Endocrine Organs. Lyon, France: IARC Press; 2004:10–13

[18] Hardy J. Transsphenoidal surgery of hypersecreting pituitary tumors. In: Kohler PO, Ross GT, eds. Diagnosis and treatment of pituitary tumors: proceedings of a conference sponsored jointly by the National Institute of Child Health and Human Development and the National Cancer Institute, January 15–17, 1973, Bethesda, Md. Amsterdam: Excerpta medica, 1973;179–198

[19] Kovacs K, Horvath E. Tumors of the pituitary gland. Washington, DC: Armed Forces Institute of Pathology; 1986

[20] Knosp E, Steiner E, Kitz K, Matula C. Pituitary adenomas with invasion of the cavernous sinus space: a magnetic resonance imaging classification compared with surgical findings. Neurosurgery. 1993; 33(4):610–617, discussion 617–618

[21] Louis D, Ohgaki H, Wiestler O, Cavenee W. World Health Organization histological classification of tumours of the central nervous system. Lyon, France: International Agency for Research on Cancer; 2016

[22] Sav A, Rotondo F, Syro LV, Di Ieva A, Cusimano MD, Kovacs K. Invasive, atypical and aggressive pituitary adenomas and carcinomas. Endocrinol Metab Clin North Am. 2015; 44(1):99–104

[23] Saeger W, Petersenn S, Schöfl C, et al. Emerging histopathological and genetic parameters of pituitary adenomas: clinical impact and recommendation for future WHO classification. Endocr Pathol. 2016; 27(2):115–122

[24] Trouillas J, Roy P, Sturm N, et al. members of HYPOPRONOS. A new prognostic clinicopathological classification of pituitary adenomas: a multicentric case-control study of 410 patients with 8 years post-operative follow-up. Acta Neuropathol. 2013; 126(1):123–135

[25] Couldwell WT, Cannon-Albright L. A heritable predisposition to pituitary tumors. Pituitary. 2010; 13(2):130–137

[26] Sivakumar W, Chamoun R, Nguyen V, Couldwell WT. Incidental pituitary adenomas. Neurosurg Focus. 2011; 31(6):E18

[27] Galland F, Vantyghem MC, Cazabat L, et al. Management of nonfunctioning pituitary incidentaloma. Ann Endocrinol (Paris). 2015; 76(3):191–200

[28] Chanson P, Raverot G, Castinetti F, Cortet-Rudelli C, Galland F, Salenave S, French Endocrinology Society non-functioning pituitary adenoma workgroup. Management of clinically non-functioning pituitary adenoma. Ann Endocrinol (Paris). 2015; 76(3):239–247

[29] Fleseriu M, Hoffman AR, Katznelson L, on behalf of the AACE Neuroendocrine and Pituitary Scientific Committee. American Association of Clinical Endocrinologists and American College of Endocrinology disease state clinical review: management of acromegaly patients: what is the role of pre-operative medical therapy? Endocr Pract. 2015; 21(6):668–673

[30] Melmed S, Colao A, Barkan A, et al. Acromegaly Consensus Group. Guidelines for acromegaly management: an update. J Clin Endocrinol Metab. 2009; 94(5):1509–1517

[31] Giustina A, Chanson P, Bronstein MD, et al. Acromegaly Consensus Group. A consensus on criteria for cure of acromegaly. J Clin Endocrinol Metab. 2010; 95(7):3141–3148

[32] Giustina A, Chanson P, Kleinberg D, et al. Acromegaly Consensus Group. Expert consensus document: a consensus on the medical treatment of acromegaly. Nat Rev Endocrinol. 2014; 10(4):243–248

[33] Biller BM, Grossman AB, Stewart PM, et al. Treatment of adrenocorticotropin-dependent Cushing's syndrome: a consensus statement. J Clin Endocrinol Metab. 2008; 93(7):2454–2462

[34] Ceccato F, Scaroni C, Boscaro M. Clinical use of pasireotide for Cushing's disease in adults. Ther Clin Risk Manag. 2015; 11:425–434

[35] Nieman LK, Biller BM, Findling JW, et al. The diagnosis of Cushing's syndrome: an Endocrine Society Clinical Practice Guideline. J Clin Endocrinol Metab. 2008; 93(5):1526–1540

[36] Pecori Giraldi F, Cavallo LM, Tortora F, et al. Altogether to Beat Cushing's Syndrome Group. The role of inferior petrosal sinus sampling in ACTH-dependent Cushing's syndrome: review and joint opinion statement by members of the Italian Society for Endocrinology, Italian Society for Neurosurgery, and Italian Society for Neuroradiology. Neurosurg Focus. 2015; 38(2):E5

[37] Pendharkar AV, Sussman ES, Ho AL, Hayden Gephart MG, Katznelson L. Cushing's disease: predicting long-term remission after surgical treatment. Neurosurg Focus. 2015; 38(2):E13

[38] Glezer A, Bronstein MD. Pituitary apoplexy: pathophysiology, diagnosis and management. Arch Endocrinol Metab. 2015; 59(3):259–264

[39] Johnston PC, Hamrahian AH, Weil RJ, Kennedy L. Pituitary tumor apoplexy. J Clin Neurosci. 2015; 22(6):939–944

[40] Oldfield EH, Merrill MJ. Apoplexy of pituitary adenomas: the perfect storm. J Neurosurg. 2015; 122(6):1444–1449

[41] Liu JK, Couldwell WT. Pituitary apoplexy in the magnetic resonance imaging era: clinical significance of sphenoid sinus mucosal thickening. J Neurosurg. 2006; 104(6):892–898

[42] Randall BR, Couldwell WT. Apoplexy in pituitary microadenomas. Acta Neurochir (Wien). 2010; 152(10):1737–1740

[43] Berker M, Hazer DB, Yücel T, et al. Complications of endoscopic surgery of the pituitary adenomas: analysis of 570 patients and review of the literature. Pituitary. 2012; 15(3):288–300

[44] Raheja A, Couldwell WT. Microsurgical resection of skull base meningioma—expanding the operative corridor. J Neurooncol. 2016; 130(2):263–267

[45] Ammirati M, Wei L, Ciric I. Short-term outcome of endoscopic versus microscopic pituitary adenoma surgery: a systematic review and meta-analysis. J Neurol Neurosurg Psychiatry. 2013; 84(8):843–849

[46] Miller BA, Ioachimescu AG, Oyesiku NM. Contemporary indications for transsphenoidal pituitary surgery. World Neurosurg. 2014; 82(6) Suppl:S147–S151

[47] Jethwa PR, Patel TD, Hajart AF, Eloy JA, Couldwell WT, Liu JK. Cost-effectiveness analysis of microscopic and endoscopic transsphenoidal surgery versus medical therapy in the management of microprolactinoma in the United States. World Neurosurg. 2016; 87:65–76

[48] Marquez Y, Tuchman A, Zada G. Surgery and radiosurgery for acromegaly: a review of indications, operative techniques, outcomes, and complications. Int J Endocrinol. 2012; 2012:386401

[49] Katznelson L. Bilateral adrenalectomy for Cushing's disease. Pituitary. 2015; 18(2):269–273

[50] Mathioudakis N, Salvatori R. Management options for persistent postoperative acromegaly. Neurosurg Clin N Am. 2012; 23(4):621–638

[51] Fukuoka H. New potential targets for treatment of Cushing's disease: epithelial growth factor receptor and cyclin-dependent kinases. Pituitary. 2015; 18(2):274–278

[52] Chen Y, Li ZF, Zhang FX, et al. Gamma Knife surgery for patients with volumetric classification of nonfunctioning pituitary adenomas: a systematic review and meta-analysis. Eur J Endocrinol. 2013; 169(4):487–495

[53] Sheehan JP, Xu Z, Lobo MJ. External beam radiation therapy and stereotactic radiosurgery for pituitary adenomas. Neurosurg Clin N Am. 2012; 23(4):571–586

[54] Liu JK, Patel J, Eloy JA. The role of temozolomide in the treatment of aggressive pituitary tumors. J Clin Neurosci. 2015; 22(6):923–929

[55] Araujo PB, Vieira Neto L, Gadelha MR. Pituitary tumor management in pregnancy. Endocrinol Metab Clin North Am. 2015; 44(1):181–197

[56] Molitch ME. Endocrinology in pregnancy: management of the pregnant patient with a prolactinoma. Eur J Endocrinol. 2015; 172(5):R205–R213

[57] Schreckinger M, Szerlip N, Mittal S. Diabetes insipidus following resection of pituitary tumors. Clin Neurol Neurosurg. 2013; 115(2):121–126

[58] Fraser CL, Biousse V, Newman NJ. Visual outcomes after treatment of pituitary adenomas. Neurosurg Clin N Am. 2012; 23(4):607–619

[59] Dallapiazza RF, Oldfield EH, Jane JA, Jr. Surgical management of Cushing's disease. Pituitary. 2015; 18(2):211–216

[60] Tohti M, Li J, Zhou Y, Hu Y, Yu Z, Ma C. Is peri-operative steroid replacement therapy necessary for the pituitary adenomas treated with surgery? A systematic review and meta analysis. PLoS One. 2015; 10(3):e0119621

[61] Edate S, Albanese A. Management of electrolyte and fluid disorders after brain surgery for pituitary/suprasellar tumours. Horm Res Paediatr. 2015; 83(5):293–301

40 Craniopharyngiomas

Alan Siu, Sanjeet Rangarajan, Christopher J. Farrell, Marc Rosen, and James J. Evans

Summary

Craniopharyngiomas are histologically benign but clinically aggressive tumors that primarily involve the sellar/suprasellar region. The clinical management can be quite complex owing to the adjacent anatomical structures, so a greater understanding of the anatomy and clinical course is critical to optimizing the treatment of these lesions. Additional insights have also resulted from genetic studies. Clinical management involves a multidisciplinary approach that includes neurosurgery, endocrinology, ophthalmology, and possibly oncology. Surgical management remains the mainstay of treatment. Newer, less invasive therapies continue to be developed that can aid in the more comprehensive management of these tumors.

Keywords: craniopharyngioma, adamantinomatous, papillary, Rathke's pouch

40.1 Introduction

Craniopharyngiomas are particularly difficult intracranial neoplasms to remove and are associated with high recurrence rates. These tumors are theorized to originate from degeneration of the epithelial remnants of Rathke's pouch and the craniopharyngeal duct. As a result, craniopharyngiomas can involve the length of the craniopharyngeal duct from the sella, parasellar, and suprasellar areas. These locations along the cranial base, coupled with the propensity of the tumor to adhere to critical structures such as the hypothalamus, optic chiasm, and neurovasculature, necessitates a well-planned and well-executed surgical resection to minimize complications. Overall gross total resection rates have benefited greatly from the introduction of minimally invasive skull base techniques that use an endoscopic endonasal approach to enrich the viewing angles, facilitating more maximal resection while minimizing complications. Despite this operative advancement, the overall treatment of craniopharyngiomas still requires a multidisciplinary team that includes neurosurgery, otolaryngology, endocrinology, neuro-oncology, and radiation oncology.

40.2 Incidence and Epidemiology

Craniopharyngiomas are benign World Health Organization (WHO) grade I intracranial tumors that originate from the remnants of Rathke's pouch. Although craniopharyngiomas constitute less than 1% of all primary central nervous system tumors, they are the most common nonglial tumor in children.[1] The incidence of craniopharyngiomas is estimated at 0.13 per 100,000 person-years, with a bimodal age distribution between 5 to 14 years and 65 to 74 years and a higher prevalence in childhood.[2] There is no gender or race predilection.

Two pathological types of craniopharyngiomas have been described. The adamantinomatous subtype is more common in children, accounting for 5 to 10% of pediatric intracranial malignancies, whereas the papillary form occurs almost exclusively in adults.

Craniopharyngiomas are most commonly found in the suprasellar region but can extend along the entire length of the craniopharyngeal duct into the sella and parasellar regions. Pan et al described five growth patterns of craniopharyngiomas based on their relationship to the arachnoid sleeve that surrounds the pituitary stalk.[3] Three basic growth patterns have been observed—infradiaphragmatic (sellar), subarachnoid extraventricular, and subpial intraventricular (third ventricle)—based on their origin from infrasellar, infradiaphragmatic, transinfundibular, suprasellar, subarachnoid, or subpial ventricular locations.

40.3 Pathology

Craniopharyngiomas are epithelial neoplasms believed to form from the squamous epithelial rests or the remnants of the primitive craniopharyngeal duct, most commonly found at the level of the infundibulum. Traditionally, two histological types of craniopharyngiomas are described: adamantinomatous and papillary. Adamantinomatous craniopharyngiomas may develop from remnants of Rathke's pouch. These tumors are grossly characterized as a spongy mass with cystic components that contain dark fluid with lipid and polarized cholesterol crystals. Histologically, adamantinomatous craniopharyngiomas are defined by the presence of nests and trabeculae of epithelium within a loose fibrous stroma. They also contain areas of wet keratin, calcifications, and cholesterol clefts. Papillary craniopharyngiomas are characterized as a solid tumor consisting of well-differentiated, monomorphic squamous epithelial cells that form distinct papillae within a fibrovascular core. This subtype can easily be differentiated from its counterpart by the lack of cystic spaces filled with "motor oil" fluid, wet keratin, calcifications, or xanthogranulomatous change.

Genetic studies for craniopharyngiomas have shown promise in developing targeted therapies. Comparative genetic studies have indicated an overexpression of CTNNB1 and BRAF V600E mutations in more than 90% of adamantinomatous and papillary craniopharyngiomas, respectively.[4,5,6] BRAF V600E mutations are known to cause other cancers via the constitutive activation of MAPK signaling pathway, which promotes cell proliferation. A phase II clinical trial is under way to determine the utility of BRAF inhibitors in the treatment of papillary craniopharyngiomas. CTNNB1 mutations are also associated with other cancers, because accumulation of nuclear B-catenin leads to activation of the Wnt signaling pathway and cellular proliferation.[7] Overactivation of the Wnt/B-catenin pathway has been demonstrated to induce craniopharyngioma formation in the mouse model.[7] Further characterization of the Wnt/B-catenin pathway and its role in the progression of adamantinomatous craniopharyngiomas may prove critical to the development of additional targeted therapies.[8]

Immunohistochemistry has traditionally been of limited utility owing to the poor understanding of the genetic alterations associated with craniopharyngiomas. In general, craniopharyngiomas stain positive for cytokeratins, epithelial membrane antigen, and carcinoembryonic antigen. Adamantinomatous craniopharyngiomas are also positive for beta-catenin. However, in light of recent findings of the high incidence of genetic mutations for CTNNB1 and BRAF V600E, immunohistochemistry will most likely play an increasingly significant role in diagnosis and treatment. In 2015, BRAF mutation status was used to successfully differentiate papillary craniopharyngioma from Rathke's cleft cyst.[9] The presence of B-catenin can also be used to differentiate between the adamantinomatous and papillary subtypes.

Recent genomic and transcriptomic studies have yielded additional insights into the molecular drivers.[10] In addition to the Wnt/B-catenin pathway, adamantinomatous craniopharyngiomas were found to also have dysregulation of the epidermal growth factor receptor (EGFR) and sonic hedgehog (SHH) signaling pathways. These studies point to a multifactorial involvement driving tumor progression and necessitate further studies to develop effective targeted therapies.

40.4 Staging

The decision to intervene is largely dependent on a combination of clinical and radiographic factors. Despite advancements in the nonoperative treatment of craniopharyngiomas, surgical resection remains the mainstay of intervention, with radiation and chemotherapy serving adjuvant roles.[11] The extent of surgical resection and overall prognosis are largely a function of the tumor growth pattern as it relates to the adjoining critical neurovascular structures. Several studies have offered topographical classification schemes based on the tumor location and its association to surrounding structures, such as the diaphragma sella, optic chiasm, pituitary stalk, and third ventricle. These schemes can aid in operative planning, including surgical approach and expected morbidity.

Surgical intervention in the case of a newly diagnosed craniopharyngioma is dependent on symptoms, tumor size, and evidence of growth with serial imaging. Although asymptomatic patients who have large suprasellar lesions may be observed, many surgeons advocate for early surgical resection to optimize complete removal at the outset, the better to prevent a limited removal in the future.[12] Regardless, a multisystem neurologic, ophthalmologic, and endocrinologic comprehensive assessment is necessary to determine the sequelae of this tumor.

40.5 Preoperative Assessment

40.5.1 Clinical Assessment

The initial work-up includes a comprehensive neurologic, endocrinologic, and visual assessment. Additionally, consultation with otolaryngology should be pursued for preoperative planning if an endoscopic endonasal approach is considered. In general, the clinical sequelae of craniopharyngiomas can be divided into five categories:

- **Endocrine:** Hypopituitarism occurs in up to 82% of patients who have craniopharyngiomas, secondary to compression of the pituitary gland, infundibulum, or hypothalamus.[12,13,14] Growth hormone deficiency is the most common hormonal deficit, the clinical manifestations of which can vary depending on age.[15] In the prepubescent population, short stature and delayed sexual development are common. Hypocortisolemia occurs in up to 62% of patients and can be potentially fatal.[12,13,16] Additional manifestations may include infertility, amenorrhea, and galactorrhea as a result of hyperprolactinemia due to stalk effect, occurring in up to 55% of patients. Diabetes insipidus is much less common preoperatively. A complete pituitary serologic panel should be obtained, including luteinizing hormone, follicle-stimulating hormone, estrogen, testosterone, thyroid-stimulating hormone, free thyroxine, adrenocorticotrophic hormone, cortisol, growth hormone, insulin growth factor-1, and prolactin levels. About 82% of patients will have evidence of endocrine deficiency in one or more axes.[15,17]

- **Ophthalmologic:** Deficits in visual acuity and visual fields, most often bitemporal hemianopia, are common manifestations resultant from direct compression of the optic nerves and chiasm by craniopharyngiomas, occurring in up to 84% of patients.[18,19,20] Objective findings of optic nerve atrophy and papilledema may result either from direct compression or, secondarily, from hydrocephalus. Comprehensive testing by an ophthalmologist or optometrist is necessary preoperatively. Visual deficits can often stabilize or recover from surgical decompression, with the likelihood of visual recovery dependent on the duration and severity of the visual deficit.[14]

- **Hypothalamic:** Manifestations of hypothalamic dysfunction are mainly in the form of hyperphagia and obesity but can also include daytime sleepiness, behavioral changes, and imbalances in homeostasis (blood pressure, temperature, heart rate, thirst). Preoperative weight gain is quite common.[21,22,23] There is no current effective treatment for hypothalamic obesity, but careful nutrition and exercise may help. Hyperphagia and obesity may also occur postoperatively as a result of hypothalamic injury.[24]

- **Hydrocephalus:** Obstructive hydrocephalus occurs in up to 30% of patients and commonly indicates tumor extension into the third ventricle with obstruction of the foramen of Monro.[25] A retrochiasmatic origin is often implicated.[1] Symptoms may include nausea/vomiting and papilledema, but headaches are by far the most common complaint.[12] The presence of symptomatic hydrocephalus may necessitate preoperative spinal fluid diversion in the form of an external ventricular drain or ventriculoperitoneal shunt.

- **Frontotemporal effects:** Large craniopharyngiomas can result in mass effect and edema in the frontal and temporal lobes, which can cause behavioral changes and altered mentation.[18,19] In extreme cases, apathy, urinary incontinence, and hypersomnia can also be present.

40.5.2 Radiographic Assessment

Preoperative CT and MRI studies provide important insights for preoperative planning. The CT is optimal for bony anatomy and can yield critical insights with which to guide the surgical approach when endonasal techniques are used, such as septal deviations, concha bullosa, sphenoethmoidal air cells, and the location of sphenoid septations as they relate to the carotid artery. Craniopharyngiomas are also known to contain calcifications, which also can be best appreciated on CT scan. MRI is critical for preoperative planning and is excellent for characterization of the degree of tumor extension, including by identifying encasement of surrounding neurovascular structures, such as the optic nerves/chiasm, internal carotid arteries, anterior cerebral arteries, pituitary gland, and infundibulum. It may also be useful for predicting the degree of involvement of the hypothalamus as evidenced by fluid-attenuated inversion recovery (FLAIR) hyperintensity. These considerations can often guide the surgical approach, because an open transcranial approach is traditionally favored for tumors with a large degree of lateral extension, a postfixed chiasm, or a small intercarotid distance. Aside from these exceptions, the extended endoscopic approach is a robust procedure that has provided excellent outcomes in our experience.[26,27]

A thorough understanding of skull base anatomy is critical for operative success. Several classification schemes have been described to guide the choice of operative approach. The earliest classification scheme included the Hoffman classification, which described the location of the craniopharyngioma relative to the optic chiasm.[28] Yasargil et al further differentiated the tumor location relative to the diaphragma sella, whereas Samii et al described a classification scheme based on the vertical projection of the tumor.[29,30] In the era of endoscopic approaches, Kassam et al developed a classification scheme centered on the location of the infundibulum.[31]

More recently, a comprehensive anatomical classification system was developed to guide aggressive surgical resection.[32] This scheme classified craniopharyngiomas based on tumor origin into four possible groups: intrasellar, prechiasmatic, retrochiasmatic, and intraventricular types (▶ Fig. 40.1).

Consistent with the previous classification scheme by Kassam et al, lesions that have significant extension into the third ventricle were considered suboptimal for an endoscopic approach and alternative transcranial approaches such as the interhemispheric or translamina terminalis approach were recommended.[31] Ideal

locations for endonasal craniopharyngioma resection include the intrasellar and prechiasmatic types without lateral extension. The orbitozygomatic and transpetrosal approaches were advocated for prechiasmatic tumors with lateral extension and the retrochiasmatic craniopharyngiomas, respectively. Although technically more difficult, in our experience and others, retrochiasmatic lesions can be approached endoscopically with great success once a learning curve is overcome.[27,33,34,35,36,37]

Preoperative characterization of tumor adherence and attachment to surrounding structures, specifically the hypothalamus, are gaining greater attention.[38] The determination of hypothalamic involvement preoperatively is critical both in determining the limits of resection and counseling of the patient regarding postoperative risk for hypothalamic dysfunction (hyperphagia, obesity, behavioral dysfunction), which can be a debilitating consequence and result in significant reduction in quality of life.[39] Van Gompel et al identified T2 signal change and irregular contrast enhancement as predictors of hypothalamic involvement.[40] Puget et al developed a grading scheme centered on hypothalamic preservation at the cost of gross total resection for tumors that clearly involved the hypothalamus. They were able to achieve good functional outcomes and tumor control using adjuvant radiotherapy.[39] These scoring systems were recently externally validated in a separate cohort and point to the importance of examining the preoperative MRI for prognostication.[41]

40.6 Postoperative Considerations

It is of critical importance to discuss with the patient the possible postoperative complications that can be life-changing. The

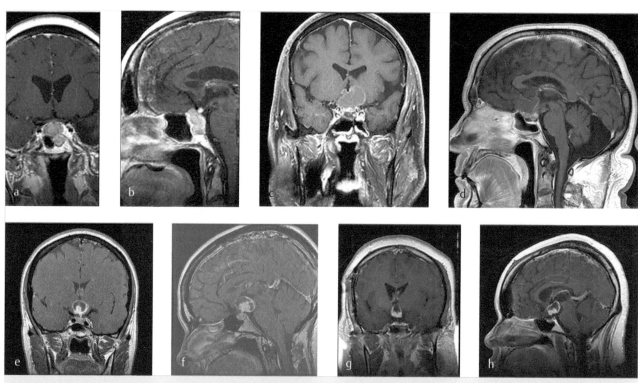

Fig. 40.1 (a, b) Intrasellar, **(c, d)** prechiasmatic, **(e, f)** retrochiasmatic, and **(g, h)** intraventricular types.

patient should be counseled on the potential for hypothalamic dysfunction with symptoms of obesity and hyperphagia and endocrine dysfunction, including diabetes insipidus and panhypopituitarism. The outcome of these preoperative conversations can guide intraoperative management decisions.

40.7 Treatment

The current treatment paradigm for craniopharyngiomas is multidisciplinary, with surgery remaining the cornerstone of treatment. Surgical intervention can be extremely challenging due to the infiltration and adherence of the tumor to surrounding critical structures such as the hypothalamus, vasculature, and cranial nerves.[38] The ideal treatment goal is gross total surgical resection resulting in disease cure with functional preservation, but the involvement of neurovascular structures often necessitates subtotal resection and subsequent adjuvant therapies to maintain function and quality of life. The following six factors should be taken into consideration when intervention is necessary.

40.7.1 Management of Hydrocephalus

Hydrocephalus is present in up to 30% of patients at diagnosis. The initial triage step involves differentiation of acute versus chronic hydrocephalus and determination of the severity of symptoms. In the setting of acute hydrocephalus with severe symptoms, immediate cerebral spinal fluid diversion is necessary using either a perioperative external ventricular drain or a staged surgical procedure with initial placement of an ventriculoperitoneal shunt. In the setting of chronic hydrocephalus or absence of acute symptoms, surgical resection of the tumor alone will typically result in the resolution of hydrocephalus.

40.7.2 Perioperative Endocrine Management

Preoperative hypocortisolemia is uncommon but if present will necessitate preoperative stress dosing with hydrocortisone or dexamethasone, which can also aid in control of vasogenic edema and aseptic meningitis. Perioperative fluid balance should be maintained, as a small proportion of patients experience diabetes insipidus preoperatively. In patients who have volume depletion, mannitol or other diuretic agents should not be administered. Patients should otherwise be maintained on their outpatient endocrine replacement medications as scheduled.

40.7.3 Management of Tumor-Related Cysts

Not infrequently, craniopharyngiomas may exist primarily in a cystic form or be composed of both solid and cystic elements. Significant tumor extension superiorly into the lateral ventricle or laterally toward the sylvian fissure may necessitate a transcranial approach for adequate access. This is especially true for the cystic component, with lateral extension limiting complete removal endoscopically. Adjuvant procedures to address a residual or recurrent cyst may include stereotactic needle aspiration or Ommaya reservoir placement. The placement of the reservoir can facilitate future aspirations as needed, as well as possible intratumoral administration of colloidal radioisotopes or chemotherapeutic agents.[42]

40.7.4 Presence of Calcifications

Calcifications are observed in 45 to 57% of craniopharyngiomas.[15] The location of calcifications relative to surrounding neurovascular structures is an important consideration for preventing iatrogenic injury when resecting the calcifications intraoperatively. This may also limit the ability to achieve a gross total resection.

40.7.5 Relationship to Surrounding Structures

Third Ventricle

The degree of infiltration into the third ventricle can dictate the surgical approach. A tumor that is entirely isolated within the body of the third ventricle or the optic recess with an intact floor of the third ventricle is suboptimal for the endoscopic endonasal route, so a craniotomy route would be recommended.[31]

Hypothalamus

An appreciation of the degree of tumor invasion of the hypothalamus is critical to minimize postoperative morbidity. Muller et al differentiated the anterior and posterior hypothalamus using the mammillary bodies as the landmark.[43] The presence of a clear cerebrospinal fluid (CSF) cleft signifies absence of hypothalamic invasion but is an infrequent finding. Other determinants of hypothalamic invasion, including T2 or FLAIR hyperintensity, may be associated with a difficult surgical dissection plane along the walls of the hypothalamus.[40] However, intraoperative assessment remains the gold standard, necessitating careful and limited dissection in this area to minimize irreversible complications.

Optic Pathways

The optic nerves and chiasm can be displaced and compressed by the tumor. It is important to appreciate the location of these structures on preoperative imaging and as early as possible during the operation in order to minimize iatrogenic injury. Preservation of the vasculature supplying the optic chiasm and nerves is critical during tumor dissection. Several classification schemes already mentioned underscore the importance of considering the location of the tumor relative to the chiasm as prechiasmatic or retrochiasmatic.[28,32]

Pituitary Stalk

The location of the infundibulum is a very important consideration in guiding the surgical approach and counseling the patient regarding potential postoperative development of diabetes insipidus and endocrinopathy. Retroinfundibular lesions are suboptimal for an endoscopic approach if preservation of the infundibulum is of primary importance, but stalk preservation may be accomplished through greater bony removal of the sellar floor.[31,33,34] Oftentimes, craniopharyngiomas invade or originate from the pituitary stalk. In these settings, radical resection requires sacrifice of the infundibulum and often results in permanent diabetes insipidus and hypopituitarism.

Cerebrovasculature

It is important to appreciate the location of the internal carotid arteries and their branches, including the anterior cerebral arteries and posterior communicating arteries, preoperatively. Dense adherence of craniopharyngiomas to the large arteries of the skull base is a common reason for subtotal resection. However, with careful dissection, an arachnoid plane can often be identified and developed, facilitating separation of these vessels from the capsule of the tumor.

40.7.6 Degree of Lateral Extension

Significant extension of the tumor lateral to the internal carotid artery or optic nerve can prohibit effective resection via an endonasal approach, and tumors exhibiting these significant lateral extensions are more suitable for a transcranial approach.

Surgical success is contingent on detailed preoperative planning and recognition of possible anatomical limitations intraoperatively. If necessary to avoid injury to critical neurovascular structures, subtotal resection should be performed with a plan for adjuvant therapy. The extent of surgical resection necessary for long-term control is highly debatable. Some surgeons advocate for aggressive surgical resection to minimize recurrence, cyst formation, and improve overall survival, whereas others report that subtotal removal and adjuvant radiation provides similar long-term tumor control to that possible through gross total resection, with less surgical risk.[44,45]

40.8 Surgical Approaches

The options for the surgical approach for resection of craniopharyngiomas can be broadly divided into transcranial and endoscopic endonasal techniques (▶ Fig. 40.2). The specific surgical approach is governed by the location of the pathology in combination with the surgeon's experience.

40.8.1 Transcranial Approaches

Subfrontal Approach

This approach is used primarily for suprasellar lesions. The addition of a transbasal translamina terminalis extension provides greater exposure to the anterior third ventricle.[46,47] A recent retrospective study highlighted the strength of the subfrontal approach in providing exposure along the vertical axis from the sella to the third ventricle, with gross total resection achieved in 91% of cases.[48]

Frontotemporal Approach

This is the workhorse approach and as such is familiar to nearly all neurosurgeons. This approach provides access to the sellar/parasellar region through the opticocarotid and oculomotor-carotid triangles. The assumption is that the tumor will have increased the spaces within these triangles, which are otherwise narrow. The advantages with this approach are its ability to provide direct access to the lateral portion of the tumor and to facilitate direct optic nerve decompression via an anterior

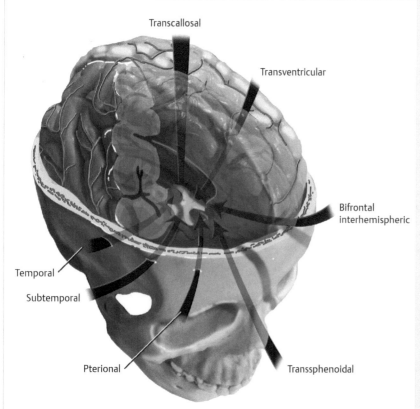

Fig. 40.2 Approaches to resection of a craniopharyngioma.

clinoidectomy and unroofing of the optic canal. In addition, injuries to major vascular structures are better managed by this approach. A key extension is an orbital osteotomy to improve basal visualization. Additional variants are the supraorbital and minipterional approaches, which have not been extensively studied.[49]

Interhemispheric Approach

This approach is used for craniopharyngiomas that exhibit significant extension within the third ventricle or through the foramen of Monro to the lateral ventricles.

Transpetrosal Approach

This lateral approach is typically used for retrochiasmatic tumors that have extension into the third ventricle and interpeduncular fossa. It allows for excellent visualization of the hypothalamus and pituitary stalk. The major disadvantages are retraction on the temporal lobe and the need to traverse neurovascular structures and cranial nerves during the dissection.

Intracavitary Therapy/Cyst Aspiration

This approach is typically considered in the setting of large predominantly cystic tumors with the goals of decreasing mass effect and improving endocrinopathy. As expected, simple cyst drainage is associated with higher rates of recurrence than other surgical interventions are.[42] As an important adjunct, or alternative, to surgical resection in select cystic cases, the catheter can be placed in the cyst and used for injection of radioisotopes or chemotherapeutic agents.

40.8.2 Endoscopic Approach

Endoscopic Endonasal Transtuberculum/Transplanum Approach

This approach is largely indicated for midline lesions between the carotid arteries and medial to the optic nerves with limited lateral extension. Intrasellar, preinfundibular, and prechiasmatic lesions are optimal but not required. Relative contraindications include tumors located exclusively in the third ventricle, but even these lesions can be approached with sufficient experience.[22]

The expanded endoscopic endonasal approach carries many advantages over traditional transcranial approaches. The approach accesses natural corridors to provide direct visualization to the tumor without the need for brain retraction. There is, however, a steep learning curve that requires a unique skill set. Although reliable repair of skull base defects had traditionally plagued the success of endoscopic approaches, contemporary techniques using multilayered closures have dramatically reduced the incidence of CSF leaks to less than 5% at experienced centers.

40.9 Adjuvant Therapies

Various options are available for the treatment of residual or recurrent craniopharyngiomas.

40.9.1 Radiation

Stereotactic radiation is a commonly employed therapy for craniopharyngiomas and may be delivered as radiotherapy or radiosurgery.

Radiotherapy

Radiotherapy is delivered through various methodologies, such as photon stereotactic radiotherapy and proton beam therapy. There is currently no class I data to suggest superiority of any modality for the treatment of craniopharyngiomas, but each method has its theoretical advantage. The advantage of stereotactic radiotherapy is that it is delivered in multiple fractions, which reduces the impact of the radiation on radiosensitive normal structures such as the optic apparatus. This is an especially important feature in the context of craniopharyngiomas due to the proximity to the chiasm. Intensity-modulated radiation therapy provides the capability to conform treatment plans to irregular shapes or volumes by modulating the intensity of the individual beams, thereby limiting radiation exposure to critical structures and providing improved dose homogeneity. Proton beam therapy can deliver large doses of radiation with limited exit dose to surrounding tissues, which is advantageous when near critical structures. Some complications of radiotherapy include endocrinopathy, vasculitis, neurobehavioral changes, and visual deficits.

Stereotactic Radiosurgery

Stereotactic radiosurgery is defined by the delivery of a single high-dose fraction of conformal radiation to the target. Accordingly, its application is limited by the target's proximity to critical structures, with the radiation delivery dose to the optic chiasm ideally limited to less than 8 to 10 Gy. Leskell Gamma Knife (Elekta) and linear accelerators are the most common devices for this type of photon delivery. This technique is optimal for smaller targets with sufficient distance between the tumor and critical radiation-sensitive structures. A major disadvantage with radiosurgery is the observation that treatment can result in an increase in the size of the cystic component, which can require subsequent interventions for cyst decompression.[50,51,52] As with all radiation therapies, radiosurgery may result in delayed development of endocrinopathy, vasculitis, neurobehavioral changes, and visual deficits.

40.9.2 Intracavitary Radiation

Stereotactic delivery of a colloidal radioisotope into the cystic component of craniopharyngiomas has been extensively reported without a general consensus on the optimal therapeutic agent.[53,54,55,56,57] The two most commonly used radioisotopes are yttrium-90 and phosphorus-32, which are beta-emitting isotopes. These two radioisotopes have similarly limited penetrance to surrounding tissues.

40.9.3 Chemotherapy

Systemic Chemotherapy

Systemic chemotherapy has not been studied extensively and is considered a last-line therapy for aggressive craniopharyngiomas refractory to alternative therapies. Various regimens of chemotherapy have been reported but have not been extensively studied.[58,59] Systemic administration of interferon-α for the treatment of craniopharyngiomas has also been reported.

Intracavitary Chemotherapy

Intracavitary chemotherapy is an accepted alternative for the treatment of the cystic component of craniopharyngiomas. The two most common agents are bleomycin and interferon-α.

40.9.4 Targeted Therapies

Recent studies into the genetic underpinnings of craniopharyngiomas have yielded promising avenues for targeted treatments. The papillary type of craniopharyngioma is strongly associated with BRAF V600E mutations. Targeted therapies for this specific mutation have previously been successful for other types of cancers.[6] A recent case report identified a successful response using BRAF and MEK inhibitors for a patient who had recurrent papillary-type craniopharyngioma.[60] This study points to a promising treatment modality for papillary-type craniopharyngiomas with BRAF inhibitors such as vemurafenib and dabrafenib. As of 2019, a phase II clinical trial is in process to evaluate the benefit of BRAF inhibitors for papillary craniopharyngiomas. Targeted therapies for the Wnt pathway are currently in development. A recent in vitro study did find an impact of inhibition of the EGFR pathway in sensitizing adamantinomatous craniopharyngiomas to radiation.[61]

40.10 Outcomes and Prognosis

Surgical intervention remains the cornerstone of treatment for craniopharyngiomas and offers the best opportunity for a cure. Successful surgical resection is largely dependent on tumor consistency, presence of arachnoid dissection planes, and degree of adherence to surrounding critical neurovascular structures, including hypothalamus. A multitude of surgical approaches are available to achieve the goal of maximal resection, yet class I and II data assessing comparative outcomes using these approaches are lacking. However, a large body of comparative literature does exist in the form of retrospective reviews and meta-analyses that has yielded some insight as it relates to outcomes. A major confounder of these studies is the divergence in the goals of surgery. Some have advocated for a radical surgical resection, even at the risk of increasing morbidity, to improve progression-free survival, whereas others have promoted a more conservative resection complemented by adjuvant therapies to preserve quality of life.[32,62,63,64]

40.10.1 Comparison of Surgical Approaches

Patient selection is a critical step to achieving successful surgical resection. Certain craniopharyngiomas are suboptimal for an endoscopic endonasal approach—namely, those with lateral extension beyond the internal carotid artery, complete vascular encasement, and isolated location in the third ventricle. These lesions are often best approached via a transcranial route. Given

these exceptions, a multitude of studies have compared the traditional transcranial to endoscopic approaches. The advent of the endoscopic endonasal approaches has greatly facilitated the resection of properly selected craniopharyngiomas with decreased morbidity and at least equivalent tumor-control rates compared with transcranial approaches, but the learning curve to successfully employing endoscopic approaches can be steep.[27,65] The primary advantage of the endoscopic approach is the direct line of sight provided along the long axis of the tumor without the need for brain retraction. The inferior optic chiasm and retrochiasmatic regions are also well visualized, which minimizes potential blind spots and allows for early decompression of these structures. The greatest disadvantage of the endoscopic approaches has been postoperative CSF leakage, although CSF leak rates have dramatically improved with the advent of multilayered closures and use of the nasoseptal flap. In contrast, transcranial approaches are versatile, with a multitude of options to attack complex lesions. The disadvantages with the traditional transcranial approaches are brain injury from retraction and small operative corridors between critical neurovascular structures that can increase the risk of visual deficits and vascular injury.[65] A blind spot underneath the optic chiasm can also increase the likelihood of residual tumor.

In 2012, Komotar et al performed a large systematic review of the literature comparing endoscopic endonasal approaches with both transsphenoidal microscopic and transcranial approaches.[65] The endoscopic approaches resulted in higher rates of gross total resection (67% vs. 43%) and postoperative improvement in vision compared with the transcranial cohort. However, the CSF leak rate was also higher in the endoscopic cohort (18.4%) than in the transsphenoidal microscopic (9.0%) and transcranial (2.6%) groups. Jeswani et al found in their institutional experience equivocal outcomes comparing endoscopic with transcranial approaches.[66]

More recently, Wannemuehler et al published their single-institution comparison of transcranial approaches with the extended endoscopic approach, which found similar resection rates (gross total resection rate [GTR] about 55%) but associated significantly improved visual outcomes with the endoscopic approach.[67] Additional morbidities, including diabetes insipidus and endocrinopathy, were similar between the groups, at about 50%. Although postoperative CSF leakage was observed only in the endonasal group, this result did not meet statistical significance. For craniopharyngiomas that can be treated using either approach, the endoscopic approach was more likely to result in gross total resection (90% vs. 40%), visual recovery, and overall fewer complications than with the transcranial approaches.[36] Prospective randomized comparisons are needed to determine the definitive advantage of one surgical approach over the other, but the data at least indicate the noninferiority of endoscopic approaches to transcranial approaches.

40.10.2 Overall Survival

Contemporary multimodality treatment strategies for craniopharyngiomas have resulted in improved overall survival rates, estimated to be up to 94% at 10 years.[44,68,69] Gross total resection improves survival, with 10-year survival rates up to 100%, compared with 86% for partial removal. The addition of radiation to partial removal can increase survival up to 100% at 10 years.[44,68,70] However, definitive class I data comparing the treatment strategies of aggressive surgical resection with subtotal resection complemented by adjuvant radiation are lacking.

40.10.3 Morbidities Associated with Surgical Intervention

The most common postoperative morbidities are endocrinologic, ophthalmologic, and hypothalamic dysfunction. Endocrinopathies are seen in almost all patients postoperatively, the most common of which are growth hormone, gonadotrophins, ACTH, TSH, and ADH.[17,63] A meta-analysis by Sughrue et al found that the development of an endocrinopathy was more frequently associated with gross total resection than with subtotal resection plus radiation.[71] Postoperative visual deficits are reported to occur in upward of 48% of patients and most commonly affect patients who have preexisting deficits.[17,44] Hypothalamic obesity is estimated to affect up to 61% of patients.[17] Cognitive dysfunction is estimated to affect 40% of patients at 10 years.[67,68]

40.10.4 Overall Risk of Recurrence

The extent of resection is critical to progression-free survival. Rates of recurrence for a gross total resection can be as high as 50% after 10 years, which is significantly lower than partial or subtotal resection.[72] Mortini et al found that recurrence most frequently occurred within the first 3 years, with overall progression-free survival of 76.2% and 64.8% at 5 and 10 years, respectively.[68] Predictors of recurrence were residual tumor, which decreased progression-free survival rates from 84.9% to 48.3% at 5 years. Age, tumor size, tumor subtype, tumor location, Ki-67, and the presence of calcifications have been inconsistent predictors of recurrence.[72] Adjuvant therapies have a reported benefit in controlling disease progression.[69,73,74] Randomized trials would be necessary to determine the effectiveness of radiation in reducing the risk of recurrence.

40.10.5 Adjuvant Therapy

A thorough multimodal treatment plan is necessary to treat residual and recurrent disease. In a systematic review performed by Gopalan et al, Gamma Knife radiosurgery dosage of up to 16.4 Gy resulted in 75% overall tumor control, with the greatest occurring for solid tumors (90%) and the worst for mixed solid-cystic tumors (59%).[75] Morbidity and mortality were estimated to be 4 to 5% overall, but an increase in the cystic component can occur in up to 20% of cases.[50,51,52] Fractionated stereotactic radiotherapy also resulted in good long-term local control rates of 92% and 88% at 10 and 20 years, respectively.[76] Thus radiation is an effective complement to surgical resection, resulting in excellent overall survival.

Intracavitary irradiation can improve the cystic component in 71 to 88% of cases, with about a 10% risk of increasing its size.[15] Intracavitary phosphorus-32 was successful in controlling cyst growth in 82% of cases, but overall progression-free survival at 5 years was 52%, owing largely to tumor growth outside the field.[55] Brachytherapy is optimal for monocystic tumors. Potential complications include toxicity to surrounding tissues resulting in damage to the hypothalamus, optic apparatus, stroke, and parenchymal edema.

40.10.6 Management of Recurrence

Recurrence can occur in up to 62% of patient at 10 years despite initial gross total resection.[15,44,68] Most recurrences are evident within the first 3 years.[68] Residual tumor was the strongest predictor of progression. The data for management of recurrent craniopharyngiomas are sparse. Treatment options include reoperation, radiation, chemotherapy, and observation. Turel et al recently described their single-center experience, in which 20% were successfully observed.[77] Of those needing intervention, 86% achieved gross total resection of their recurrent tumor. The presence of a recurrence does not preclude reoperation, which can often improve patient outcomes.[62] The extended endonasal approach has been advocated as an effective treatment for achieving good resection rates, particularly when the previous surgery was transcranial.[77,78] In the case of a cyst recurrence, stereotactic aspiration with a needle or Ommaya reservoir placement are potential options. Although the data are quite limited, preliminary studies support observation, followed by reoperation if needed.

40.11 Conclusion

Harvey Cushing described craniopharyngiomas as the "most forbidding of the intracranial tumors."[79] The intimate relationship of these tumors with the hypothalamus, optic apparatus, internal carotid arteries, and surrounding perforators necessitates a comprehensive evaluation and perioperative plan for management, which often includes multimodal treatment strategies. The expanded endoscopic endonasal approach has been shown to be a promising option for resection of midline craniopharyngiomas with minimal lateral extension. Adjuvant therapies, specifically stereotactic radiation, are effective adjuncts in controlling residual/recurrent disease. Novel gene-based therapies show promise and will likely change the treatment paradigm for craniopharyngiomas.

References

[1] Hoffman HJ. Surgical management of craniopharyngioma. Pediatr Neurosurg. 1994; 21 Suppl 1:44–49

[2] Bunin GR, Surawicz TS, Witman PA, Preston-Martin S, Davis F, Bruner JM. The descriptive epidemiology of craniopharyngioma. Neurosurg Focus. 1997; 3 (6):e1

[3] Pan J, Qi S, Liu Y, et al. Growth patterns of craniopharyngiomas: clinical analysis of 226 patients. J Neurosurg Pediatr. 2016; 17(4):418–433

[4] Brastianos PK, Taylor-Weiner A, Manley PE, et al. Exome sequencing identifies BRAF mutations in papillary craniopharyngiomas. Nat Genet. 2014; 46(2): 161–165

[5] Larkin SJ, Ansorge O. Pathology and pathogenesis of craniopharyngiomas. Pituitary. 2013; 16(1):9–17

[6] Martinez-Gutierrez JC, D'Andrea MR, Cahill DP, Santagata S, Barker FG, II, Brastianos PK. Diagnosis and management of craniopharyngiomas in the era of genomics and targeted therapy. Neurosurg Focus. 2016; 41(6):E2

[7] Martinez-Barbera JP. Molecular and cellular pathogenesis of adamantinomatous craniopharyngioma. Neuropathol Appl Neurobiol. 2015; 41(6):721–732

[8] Apps JR, Martinez-Barbera JP. Molecular pathology of adamantinomatous craniopharyngioma: review and opportunities for practice. Neurosurg Focus. 2016; 41(6):E4

[9] Schweizer L, Capper D, Hölsken A, et al. BRAF V600E analysis for the differentiation of papillary craniopharyngiomas and Rathke's cleft cysts. Neuropathol Appl Neurobiol. 2015; 41(6):733–742

[10] Robinson LC, Santagata S, Hankinson TC. Potential evolution of neurosurgical treatment paradigms for craniopharyngioma based on genomic and transcriptomic characteristics. Neurosurg Focus. 2016; 41(6):E3

[11] Sainte-Rose C, Puget S, Wray A, et al. Craniopharyngioma: the pendulum of surgical management. Childs Nerv Syst. 2005; 21(8–9):691–695

[12] Halac I, Zimmerman D. Endocrine manifestations of craniopharyngioma. Childs Nerv Syst. 2005; 21(8–)(9):640–648

[13] Hopper N, Albanese A, Ghirardello S, Maghnie M. The pre-operative endocrine assessment of craniopharyngiomas. J Pediatr Endocrinol Metab. 2006; 19 Suppl 1:325–327

[14] Campbell PG, McGettigan B, Luginbuhl A, Yadla S, Rosen M, Evans JJ. Endocrinological and ophthalmological consequences of an initial endonasal endoscopic approach for resection of craniopharyngiomas. Neurosurg Focus. 2010; 28(4):E8

[15] Karavitaki N, Cudlip S, Adams CB, Wass JA. Craniopharyngiomas. Endocr Rev. 2006; 27(4):371–397

[16] Di Battista E, Naselli A, Queirolo S, et al. Endocrine and growth features in childhood craniopharyngioma: a mono-institutional study. J Pediatr Endocrinol Metab. 2006; 19 Suppl 1:431–437

[17] Van Effenterre R, Boch AL. Craniopharyngioma in adults and children: a study of 122 surgical cases. J Neurosurg. 2002; 97(1):3–11

[18] Carmel PW, Antunes JL, Chang CH. Craniopharyngiomas in children. Neurosurgery. 1982; 11(3):382–389

[19] Banna M. Craniopharyngioma in adults. Surg Neurol. 1973; 1(4):202–204

[20] Banna M, Hoare RD, Stanley P, Till K. Craniopharyngioma in children. J Pediatr. 1973; 83(5):781–785

[21] Hoffmann A, Boekhoff S, Gebhardt U, et al. History before diagnosis in childhood craniopharyngioma: associations with initial presentation and long-term prognosis. Eur J Endocrinol. 2015; 173(6):853–862

[22] Nishioka H, Fukuhara N, Yamaguchi-Okada M, Yamada S. Endoscopic endonasal surgery for purely intrathird ventricle craniopharyngioma. World Neurosurg. 2016; 91:266–271

[23] Müller HL, Emser A, Faldum A, et al. Longitudinal study on growth and body mass index before and after diagnosis of childhood craniopharyngioma. J Clin Endocrinol Metab. 2004; 89(7):3298–3305

[24] Müller HL. Craniopharyngioma and hypothalamic injury: latest insights into consequent eating disorders and obesity. Curr Opin Endocrinol Diabetes Obes. 2016; 23(1):81–89

[25] Zuccaro G. Radical resection of craniopharyngioma. Childs Nerv Syst. 2005; 21(8–9):679–690

[26] Kenning TJ, Beahm DD, Farrell CJ, Schaberg MR, Rosen MR, Evans JJ. Endoscopic endonasal craniopharyngioma resection. J Neurosurg. 2012; 32 Suppl:E5

[27] Kshettry VR, Do H, Elshazly K, et al. The learning curve in endoscopic endonasal resection of craniopharyngiomas. Neurosurg Focus. 2016; 41(6):E9

[28] Hoffman HJ, De Silva M, Humphreys RP, Drake JM, Smith ML, Blaser SI. Aggressive surgical management of craniopharyngiomas in children. J Neurosurg. 1992; 76(1):47–52

[29] Yaşargil MG, Curcic M, Kis M, Siegenthaler G, Teddy PJ, Roth P. Total removal of craniopharyngiomas: approaches and long-term results in 144 patients. J Neurosurg. 1990; 73(1):3–11

[30] Samii M, Tatagiba M. Surgical management of craniopharyngiomas: a review. Neurol Med Chir (Tokyo). 1997; 37(2):141–149

[31] Kassam AB, Gardner PA, Snyderman CH, Carrau RL, Mintz AH, Prevedello DM. Expanded endonasal approach, a fully endoscopic transnasal approach for the resection of midline suprasellar craniopharyngiomas: a new classification based on the infundibulum. J Neurosurg. 2008; 108(4):715–728

[32] Morisako H, Goto T, Goto H, Bohoun CA, Tamrakar S, Ohata K. Aggressive surgery based on an anatomical subclassification of craniopharyngiomas. Neurosurg Focus. 2016; 41(6):E10

[33] Liu JK, Christiano LD, Patel SK, Eloy JA. Surgical nuances for removal of retrochiasmatic craniopharyngioma via the endoscopic endonasal extended transsphenoidal transplanum transtuberculum approach. Neurosurg Focus. 2011; 30(4):E14

[34] Sankhla SK, Jayashankar N, Khan GM. Extended endoscopic endonasal transsphenoidal approach for retrochiasmatic craniopharyngioma: surgical technique and results. J Pediatr Neurosci. 2015; 10(4):308–316

[35] Zacharia BE, Amine M, Anand V, Schwartz TH. Endoscopic endonasal management of craniopharyngioma. Otolaryngol Clin North Am. 2016; 49(1):201–212

[36] Moussazadeh N, Prabhu V, Bander ED, et al. Endoscopic endonasal versus open transcranial resection of craniopharyngiomas: a case-matched single-institution analysis. Neurosurg Focus. 2016; 41(6):E7

[37] Dehdashti AR, Ganna A, Witterick I, Gentili F. Expanded endoscopic endonasal approach for anterior cranial base and suprasellar lesions: indications and limitations. Neurosurgery. 2009; 64(4):677–687, discussion 687–689

[38] Prieto R, Pascual JM, Rosdolsky M, et al. Craniopharyngioma adherence: a comprehensive topographical categorization and outcome-related risk stratification model based on the methodical examination of 500 tumors. Neurosurg Focus. 2016; 41(6):E13

[39] Puget S, Garnett M, Wray A, et al. Pediatric craniopharyngiomas: classification and treatment according to the degree of hypothalamic involvement. J Neurosurg. 2007; 106(1) Suppl:3–12

[40] Van Gompel JJ, Nippoldt TB, Higgins DM, Meyer FB. Magnetic resonance imaging-graded hypothalamic compression in surgically treated adult craniopharyngiomas determining postoperative obesity. Neurosurg Focus. 2010; 28(4):E3

[41] Mortini P, Gagliardi F, Bailo M, et al. Magnetic resonance imaging as predictor of functional outcome in craniopharyngiomas. Endocrine. 2016; 51(1):148–162

[42] Rachinger W, et al. Cystic craniopharyngiomas: microsurgical or stereotactic treatment? Neurosurgery. 2017;80(5):733–743

[43] Müller HL, Gebhardt U, Teske C, et al. Study Committee of KRANIOPHARYNGEOM 2000. Post-operative hypothalamic lesions and obesity in childhood craniopharyngioma: results of the multinational prospective trial KRANIOPHARYNGEOM 2000 after 3-year follow-up. Eur J Endocrinol. 2011; 165(1):17–24

[44] Karavitaki N, Brufani C, Warner JT, et al. Craniopharyngiomas in children and adults: systematic analysis of 121 cases with long-term follow-up. Clin Endocrinol (Oxf). 2005; 62(4):397–409

[45] Masson-Cote L, Masucci GL, Atenafu EG, et al. Long-term outcomes for adult craniopharyngioma following radiation therapy. Acta Oncol. 2013; 52(1):153–158

[46] Liu JK. Modified one-piece extended transbasal approach for translamina terminalis resection of retrochiasmatic third ventricular craniopharyngioma. Neurosurg Focus. 2013; 34(1 Suppl):Video 1

[47] Liu JK, Christiano LD, Gupta G, Carmel PW. Surgical nuances for removal of retrochiasmatic craniopharyngiomas via the transbasal subfrontal translamina terminalis approach. Neurosurg Focus. 2010; 28(4):E6

[48] Du C, Feng CY, Yuan XR, et al. Microsurgical management of craniopharyngiomas via a unilateral subfrontal approach: a retrospective study of 177 continuous cases. World Neurosurg. 2016; 90:454–468

[49] Wilson DA, Duong H, Teo C, Kelly DF. The supraorbital endoscopic approach for tumors. World Neurosurg. 2014; 82(6) Suppl:S72–S80

[50] Chung WY, Pan DH, Shiau CY, Guo WY, Wang LW. Gamma Knife radiosurgery for craniopharyngiomas. J Neurosurg. 2000; 93 Suppl 3:47–56

[51] Lee CC, Yang HC, Chen CJ, et al. Gamma Knife surgery for craniopharyngioma: report on a 20-year experience. J Neurosurg. 2014; 121 Suppl:167–178

[52] Lamiman K, Wong KK, Tamrazi B, et al. A quantitative analysis of craniopharyngioma cyst expansion during and after radiation therapy and surgical implications. Neurosurg Focus. 2016; 41(6):E15

[53] Voges J, Sturm V, Lehrke R, Treuer H, Gauss C, Berthold F. Cystic craniopharyngioma: long-term results after intracavitary irradiation with stereotactically applied colloidal beta-emitting radioactive sources. Neurosurgery. 1997; 40(2):263–269, discussion 269–270

[54] Van den Berge JH, Blaauw G, Breeman WA, Rahmy A, Wijngaarde R. Intracavitary brachytherapy of cystic craniopharyngiomas. J Neurosurg. 1992; 77(4):545–550

[55] Maarouf M, El Majdoub F, Fuetsch M, et al. Stereotactic intracavitary brachytherapy with P-32 for cystic craniopharyngiomas in children. Strahlenther Onkol. 2016; 192(3):157–165

[56] Kickingereder P, Maarouf M, El Majdoub F, et al. Intracavitary brachytherapy using stereotactically applied phosphorus-32 colloid for treatment of cystic craniopharyngiomas in 53 patients. J Neurooncol. 2012; 109(2):365–374

[57] Hasegawa T, Kondziolka D, Hadjipanayis CG, Lunsford LD. Management of cystic craniopharyngiomas with phosphorus-32 intracavitary irradiation. Neurosurgery. 2004; 54(4):813–820, discussion 820–822

[58] Bremer AM, Nguyen TQ, Balsys R. Therapeutic benefits of combination chemotherapy with vincristine, BCNU, and procarbazine on recurrent cystic craniopharyngioma: a case report. J Neurooncol. 1984; 2(1):47–51

[59] Lippens RJ, Rotteveel JJ, Otten BJ, Merx H. Chemotherapy with Adriamycin (doxorubicin) and CCNU (lomustine) in four children with recurrent craniopharyngioma. Eur J Paediatr Neurol. 1998; 2(5):263–268

[60] Brastianos PK, Shankar GM, Gill CM, et al. Dramatic response of BRAF V600E mutant papillary craniopharyngioma to targeted therapy. J Natl Cancer Inst. 2015; 108(2):djv310

[61] Stache C, Bils C, Fahlbusch R, et al. Drug priming enhances radiosensitivity of adamantinomatous craniopharyngioma via downregulation of survivin. Neurosurg Focus. 2016; 41(6):E14

[62] Elliott RE, Hsieh K, Hochm T, Belitskaya-Levy I, Wisoff J, Wisoff JH. Efficacy and safety of radical resection of primary and recurrent craniopharyngiomas in 86 children. J Neurosurg Pediatr. 2010; 5(1):30–48

[63] Yang I, Sughrue ME, Rutkowski MJ, et al. Craniopharyngioma: a comparison of tumor control with various treatment strategies. Neurosurg Focus. 2010; 28(4):E5

[64] Schoenfeld A, Pekmezci M, Barnes MJ, et al. The superiority of conservative resection and adjuvant radiation for craniopharyngiomas. J Neurooncol. 2012; 108(1):133–139

[65] Komotar RJ, Starke RM, Raper DM, Anand VK, Schwartz TH. Endoscopic endonasal compared with microscopic transsphenoidal and open transcranial resection of craniopharyngiomas. World Neurosurg. 2012; 77(2):329–341

[66] Jeswani S, Nuño M, Wu A, et al. Comparative analysis of outcomes following craniotomy and expanded endoscopic endonasal transsphenoidal resection of craniopharyngioma and related tumors: a single-institution study. J Neurosurg. 2016; 124(3):627–638

[67] Wannemuehler TJ, Rubel KE, Hendricks BK, et al. Outcomes in transcranial microsurgery versus extended endoscopic endonasal approach for primary resection of adult craniopharyngiomas. Neurosurg Focus. 2016; 41(6):E6

[68] Mortini P, Losa M, Pozzobon G, et al. Neurosurgical treatment of craniopharyngioma in adults and children: early and long-term results in a large case series. J Neurosurg. 2011; 114(5):1350–1359

[69] Rajan B, Ashley S, Gorman C, et al. Craniopharyngioma—a long-term results following limited surgery and radiotherapy. Radiother Oncol. 1993; 26(1):1–10

[70] Minniti G, Saran F, Traish D, et al. Fractionated stereotactic conformal radiotherapy following conservative surgery in the control of craniopharyngiomas. Radiother Oncol. 2007; 82(1):90–95

[71] Sughrue ME, Yang I, Kane AJ, et al. Endocrinologic, neurologic, and visual morbidity after treatment for craniopharyngioma. J Neurooncol. 2011; 101 (3):463–476

[72] Mortini P, Gagliardi F, Boari N, Losa M. Surgical strategies and modern therapeutic options in the treatment of craniopharyngiomas. Crit Rev Oncol Hematol. 2013; 88(3):514–529

[73] Zhang YQ, Ma ZY, Wu ZB, Luo SQ, Wang ZC. Radical resection of 202 pediatric craniopharyngiomas with special reference to the surgical approaches and hypothalamic protection. Pediatr Neurosurg. 2008; 44(6):435–443

[74] Stripp DC, Maity A, Janss AJ, et al. Surgery with or without radiation therapy in the management of craniopharyngiomas in children and young adults. Int J Radiat Oncol Biol Phys. 2004; 58(3):714–720

[75] Gopalan R, Dassoulas K, Rainey J, Sherman JH, Sheehan JP. Evaluation of the role of Gamma Knife surgery in the treatment of craniopharyngiomas. Neurosurg Focus. 2008; 24(5):E5

[76] Harrabi SB, Adeberg S, Welzel T, et al. Long term results after fractionated stereotactic radiotherapy (FSRT) in patients with craniopharyngioma: maximal tumor control with minimal side effects. Radiat Oncol. 2014; 9: 203

[77] Cavallo LM, Prevedello DM, Solari D, et al. Extended endoscopic endonasal transsphenoidal approach for residual or recurrent craniopharyngiomas. J Neurosurg. 2009; 111(3):578–589

[78] Dhandapani S, et al. Endonasal endoscopic reoperation for residual or recurrent craniopharyngiomas. J Neurosurg. 2017;126(2):418–430

[79] Cushing H. The Craniopharyngiomas: Intracranial Tumors: Notes upon a Series of Two Thousand Verified Cases with Surgical Mortality Percentages Pertaining Thereto. Springfield: Thomas; 1932

41 Epidermoids, Dermoids, and Other Cysts of the Skull Base

Samuel P. Gubbels, Bruce J. Gantz, Paul W. Gidley, and Franco DeMonte

Summary

This chapter discusses several histopathologically distinct lesions that only rarely affect the skull base. These lesions are primarily developmental in nature, although cholesterol granulomas are likely secondary to alterations in air cells occasionally present in the petrous apex. The epidemiology, etiology, embryology, pathophysiology, clinical biology, treatment, outcome, and prognosis are comprehensively discussed.

Keywords: epidermoid, dermoid, cholesterol granuloma, arachnoid cyst, endonasal endoscopic fenestration, infralabyrinthine/infracochlear approach, skull base lesion

41.1 Introduction

Cystic lesions of the skull base, in general, represent growth of normally occurring tissues in abnormal or aberrant locations rather than true neoplasia. Though skull base cysts are uncommon lesions, the difficulty in obtaining their complete removal and the potential morbidity incurred in their treatment make patients who have them quite memorable to the neurotologist and/or neurosurgeon involved in their care. This chapter reviews the clinical and pathological findings of the most common cysts affecting the skull base and discusses the diagnosis and treatment of these lesions.

41.2 Epidermoids

41.2.1 Incidence and Epidemiology

In 1829, the French pathologist Cruveilhier was the first to offer a systematic description of a series of epidermoids, which he termed "pearly tumors."[1] Cruveilhier reported the incidental finding at autopsy of a large epidermoid tumor in a man who had died of a head injury. In describing this case, along with two cases previously reported by Dumeril and Le Prestre, Cruveilhier commented on the notable size and extent that epidermoid tumors may attain without producing symptoms.[1,2] These lesions were known as "Cruveilhier's pearly tumors" until Muller in 1838 first used the term *cholesteatoma* to describe them after noting the presence of cholesterol crystals within the matrix of the lesions.[3] The prolific German pathologist Rudolf Virchow in 1855 concluded that *pearly tumor* was the more correct term to be used in the description of these lesions, for he found presence of cholesterol crystals to be inconsistent.[4] Bostroem in 1897 coined the term *epidermoids* to describe these lesions, and this term is the most commonly used today.[5]

Epidermoids represent 0.2 to 1.5% of all intracranial tumors and 6 to 14% of all tumors of the cerebellopontine angle (CPA), where they are the third most common lesion, after only schwannomas and meningiomas.[6,7,8] Approximately 30 to 60% of all epidermoids occur in the CPA, followed, in decreasing order of frequency, by the parasellar region, paraclival area, lateral recess of fourth ventricle, and petrous apex.[6,9,10,11,12,13] In addition to the intracranial locations already listed, epidermoids can occur in the diploë of the calvarium (intraosseous), where they can present as a painless swelling with an associated calvarial defect.[14] Intraosseous epidermoids represent up to 25% of cases in two larger series and are to be differentiated from the intracranial type of these lesions.[15,16]

The age of incidence of intracranial epidermoids is from birth to 80 years, with the majority identified by the third or fourth decades of life.[6,17] A male preponderance has been reported, with a male:female ratio of 5:4.[9,18,19] Multiple epidermoid tumors almost never occur, and no familial predisposition to the development of these lesions has been reported. In 2005, intracranial epidermoid cysts have been reported in three patients who had craniovertebral junction anomalies—the first known association of these lesions with other congenital malformations.[20]

41.2.2 Embryology

In 1854, Von Remak proposed that epidermoids occurred due to an error in embryological development leading to entrapment of keratinizing ectodermal elements, with subsequent growth of the aberrantly located tissue. The timing of this embryological event is postulated to have occurred at the time of closure of the neural groove, between the third and fifth week of development.[21,22,23,24] Von Remak's theory continues to be the most widely accepted theory for the formation of these lesions, though the timing of the embryological error and subtype (neuro vs. cutaneous ectoderm) of the entrapped tissue has been the source of debate through the decades.[25,26,27] Other theories regarding the origin of epidermoids have been proposed, including Virchow's theory of squamous metaplasia and Fleming and Botterel's multipotential embryonic cell rest theory.[4,28] More recent publications have proposed a modification of Fleming and Botterel's theory whereby multipotential cells are carried from a medial to lateral position along with migrating otic capsular elements during embryogenesis.[29,30,31] Kountakis demonstrated migratory properties of CPA epidermoid cells in vitro similar to those of acquired cholesteatomas and, because these properties are unique to epithelium of the first branchial groove, concluded that epidermoids originate from the first branchial groove.[32] Though this theory does not rule out theories such as Virchow's or Fleming and Botterel's, it does indirectly support the concept that entrapment of would-be first branchial cleft epithelium during embryogenesis ultimately leads to epidermoid formation.

41.2.3 Pathology

Epidermoids' characteristic appearance makes them easily recognized on gross inspection. The external surface is silky with a white-gold, mother-of-pearl appearance and sheen, often with multiple delicate vessels evident on the surface. The capsule can be lobulated or smooth and tears easily with application of a shearing force. The tumor is malleable and compresses easily owing to the caseous core of squamous debris. Section of the cyst reveals a capsule consisting of a thin layer of stratified, keratinizing squamous epithelium, often with multiple foci of calcification, surrounded by a thin layer of fibrous soft tissue. The cyst is filled with desquamated keratin debris and cholesterol crystals having a soft, waxy texture. The keratin debris within the core has a lamellar or onion-skin gross appearance and is essentially avascular (▶ Fig. 41.1).[6,9,33]

Some epidermoids have a high triglyceride content in addition to the presence of cholesterol crystals. The growth rate of epidermoids is linear and to be differentiated from the exponential pattern seen with a neoplasm, either benign or malignant.[24] It is only the basal layers of an epidermoid that undergo cell division, followed by progressive maturation and ultimately death of the overlying layers of the epithelium, which eventually slough into the central core of the lesion. With time the central, nonviable core represents the bulk of the epidermoid, with the viable cells displaced circumferentially toward the periphery of the lesion. Because of this growth pattern and the slow rate of expansion, epidermoids characteristically envelop surrounding nerves, vessels, and other critical structures rather than displacing them like most benign neoplasms. After filling the intracranial subarachnoid space from which it originated, the epidermoid then extends to adjacent spaces, eroding bone in the process.[31] The capsule of the cyst typically insinuates itself into surrounding structures as it erodes the bone in the area, conforming to anatomical features in the area as it expands. In addition to engulfing cranial nerves and vessels in the area, epidermoids can cause atrophy, ischemic injury, and paresis due to the interaction with the cerebral and cerebellar parenchyma.[35] This pattern of growth, combined with the relative friability of the epithelial layer, makes complete extirpation of these lesions difficult and, not infrequently, impossible without the sacrifice of the involved vessels and nerves, which is to be avoided.

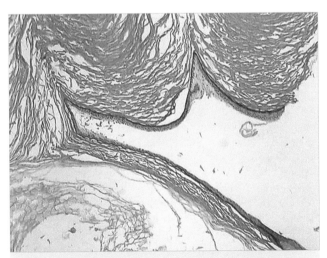

Fig. 41.1 Photomicrograph of a resected posterior fossa epidermoid cyst. A layer of simple squamous epithelium lines the cyst, which contains lamellae of keratin debris.

41.2.4 Clinical Manifestations

Because of their slow rate and pattern of growth, epidermoids can be asymptomatic, found incidentally on imaging performed for other reasons. More commonly epidermoids will present with a long, protracted course of sometimes mild and vague clinical manifestations. Early series of patients who had epidermoids reported some who had duration of symptoms attributable to the lesion of as long as 53 years.[34] Modern imaging has enabled earlier identification of these lesions, with some reports of duration of symptoms similar to those reported in series of acoustic neuromas.[11,16,36,37,38] Even so, some modern series report delays in diagnosis of 20 years or longer.[11,13,30,36]

Epidermoids present with a spectrum of symptoms similar to those seen with an acoustic neuroma or other expansile lesion of the CPA—namely, cranial nerve deficits, which occur in 80 to 90% of patients.[30,31] Cranial nerve VIII is most commonly involved (40–93%) in most series of intracranial epidermoids and may manifest as hearing loss, vertigo, tinnitus, disequilibrium, or gait disturbance.[16,30,31,36,38,39,40,41] Some have found the facial nerve to be more frequently affected on presentation.[35] In contrast to the stretch injury to the facial nerve that can occur in cases of acoustic neuroma, epidermoids are thought to engulf the facial nerve and cause axonotmesis or neurotmesis due to the resulting ischemic injury, generally manifesting as facial weakness or hemifacial spasm.[42] Trigeminal nerve involvement, producing symptoms of facial pain, numbness, corneal reflex abnormalities, and masticator muscle weakness, is more common on presentation (25–52%) in epidermoids than acoustic neuromas.[13,16,30,31,36,38,40] The facial pain seen in cases of epidermoid tumors is atypical for trigeminal neuralgia in that it is longer in duration and may not be accompanied by sensory or motor dysfunction of cranial nerve V.[43]

Three mechanisms have been proposed to account for the trigeminal neuralgia seen with epidermoids: direct compression of the nerve root, indirect compression of the nerve due to vessel displacement from the enlarging cyst and toxic neuritis as a result of cyst content leakage.[6,36,44] Larger epidermoids may involve cranial nerves III, IV, VI, IX, X, and XI, producing visual deficits, diplopia, hoarseness, and dysphagia. Headache occurs frequently with epidermoids and may be due to the expansile nature of the lesion (which may also produce papilledema secondary to increased intracranial pressure) or to a toxic effect from leakage of the cyst contents.[30,31,35,36] Seizures due to epidermoids have been described but are an uncommon manifestation of the disease.[45]

41.2.5 Radiology

Please refer to Chapter 4 of this book for a detailed discussion of the imaging characteristics of epidermoid cysts of the skull base. ▶ Fig. 41.2 shows representative imaging of a right-sided CPA epidermoid.

41.2.6 Treatment

Epidermoids of the skull base are best treated using surgical excision. Chemotherapy has no role in the treatment of these lesions, for they are not true neoplasms. The use of external

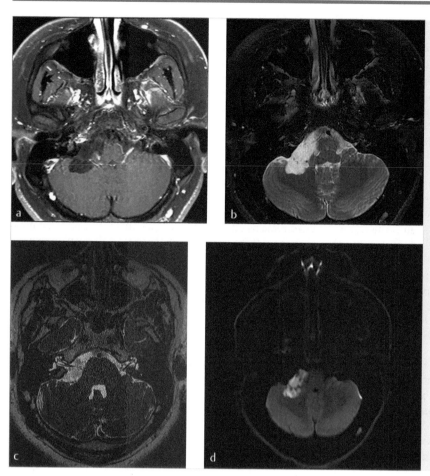

Fig. 41.2 **(a)** Axial T1-weighted MRI reveals an epidermoid cyst in the cerebellopontine angle, exerting mass effect on the lateral cerebellum. The lesion is hypointense and without enhancement. **(b)** Axial T2-weighted MRI reveals this lesion to be hyperintense on T2 sequences. **(c)** Axial constructive interference in steady state (CISS) images clearly identify the vestibulocochlear and facial nerves traversing the lesion. **(d)** Axial diffusion-weighted imaging reveals restricted diffusion within the cyst.

beam radiation therapy has been reported in one case of a recurrent epidermoid but should be reserved for symptomatic treatment of patients who are not surgical candidates, if any.[46] In general, complete cyst removal should be pursued in all cases but, because of the infiltrative nature of these lesions, may not be possible without incurring significant morbidity and even mortality. Epidermoids engulf and become intimately involved with surrounding neurovascular structures, making complete excision difficult if not impossible without risking potentially devastating consequences from sacrifice of cranial nerves, vascular injury, or damage to the cerebellum, brainstem, or temporal lobe. Incomplete excision, leaving cyst matrix on cranial nerves and vasculature intimately involved with the lesion, is an acceptable alternative in some cases, for "recurrence may occur slowly and reoperation may not be required for many years."[7,36,43] The rates of total cyst excision vary considerably in published series, with rates as low as 0% and as high as 80 to 97%.[11,30,31,35] Second operations are required in up to a third of patients, generally many years after initial resection.[43]

Multiple approaches have been employed to access and excise these lesions, including suboccipital, translabyrinthine, transotic, transcochlear, subtemporal, and petrosal routes.[31,35,36,47,48] These approaches are beyond the scope of this chapter, but detailed descriptions of these approaches can be found in Chapter 18 (suboccipital), Chapters 18, 21, and 26 (translabyrinthine, transotic, transcochlear), Chapter 19 (subtemporal), and Chapters 18, 24, and 26 (petrosal).

41.2.7 Outcome and Prognosis

The rates of total cyst removal vary from 0 to 97% in modern published series, with rates of recurrence requiring a second operation ranging from 0 to 36%. Overall published recurrence rates range from 0 to 55% of patients, and the reported time to recurrence of epidermoids ranges from 36 to 264 months, highlighting the importance of long-term follow-up with periodic MRI surveillance in all patients who have epidermoids, regardless of whether total excision was achieved at the initial surgery.[43] Mortality rates in modern series range from 0 to 16%, a significant improvement from the premicrosurgical era.[43]

Complications of surgery for epidermoids of the skull base are similar to those seen in the treatment of other CPA neoplasms, including cerebrospinal fluid (CSF) leak, cranial nerve injury, infection, aseptic meningitis, hydrocephalus, pulmonary embolus, headache, seizures, and aspiration.[31,36,48] Cranial nerve VIII is the most frequently injured during excision of these lesions, though many series employ a translabyrinthine, possibly transcochlear approach to address these lesions, which may skew the interpretation of the rates of postoperative cranial nerve VIII dysfunction. It is difficult to assess the rates of such dysfunction postoperatively from published series owing to variability in the reporting of preexisting dysfunction, lack of mention of whether hearing preservation was attempted, and absence of clear descriptions of the nature of the postoperative dysfunction (vestibular vs. auditory, conductive vs. sensorineural hearing loss, means of auditory assessment). Nevertheless, reported rates of hearing preservation (as loosely defined) when attempted range from 15 to 72%.[17,31,36,48] Similarly, interpretation of the rates of cranial nerve VII dysfunction postoperatively is difficult owing to variability in reporting but ranges from an 8 to 50% incidence of some level of facial nerve dysfunction.[17,31,36,38] It is important to note that most series include patients who had some degree of preoperative facial nerve dysfunction or who had the facial nerve mobilized to enable complete cyst removal, both of which would clearly bias the reported rates of postoperative dysfunction.

In general, the rates of postoperative cranial nerve dysfunction after removal of intracranial epidermoids are highly variable and potentially subject to a number of factors, including age, coexistent medical problems, level of preoperative dysfunction, extent of nerve involvement by the epidermoid, meticulousness of cyst dissection and tissue handling, level of scrutiny in the evaluation of postoperative dysfunction, and administration of corticosteroids. Furthermore, the risk of injury to the facial and other involved cranial nerves is higher than for acoustic tumors of similar size because of epidermoids' tendency to encircle the nerves.[45] Intraoperative neurophysiological monitoring of involved cranial nerves, especially the facial nerve, is recommended.[49]

When assessing the outcomes of surgical interventions for epidermoids of the skull base, it is important to appreciate the natural history of these lesions with their associated morbidity and mortality. Reported complications associated with untreated intracranial epidermoids include hearing loss, facial weakness, facial numbness, lower cranial neuropathies, diplopia, blindness, headaches, cerebellar dysfunction, encephalitis, seizures, hydrocephalus, and death.[31,35,45] Recurrent aseptic meningitis occurring spontaneously in the setting of an epidermoid has been described in a number of reports—in some as the initial presentation of the lesion.[43] In addition, aseptic meningitis occurring after excision of epidermoid tumors has been reported in many series, thought to be secondary to a toxic effect of spilled keratin debris within the subarachnoid space.[30,31,35,36] Evaluation and management of patients who have epidermoid cysts requires vigilance for the development of aseptic meningitis and initiation of treatment using corticosteroids, and possibly antibiotics, if suspected.

A rare but feared complication of intracranial epidermoids is the development of squamous cell carcinoma, whether a de novo lesion discovered at the first operation for epidermoid, incidentally at autopsy, or, more frequently, in the setting of an incompletely resected lesion.[31,50,51,52,53,54,55,56,57,58,59] Most reports describe a delay of 3 months to 33 years before discovery of carcinoma in the setting of an incompletely excised lesion.[22,52,60,61,62,63,64,65,66] There appeared to be a male predominance, and patients typically had rapidly progressive and more severe symptoms than seen in benign epidermoids. Some patients had an episode of aseptic meningitis prior to the development of carcinoma within the epidermoid, supporting the concept that chronic inflammation of the cyst matrix ultimately leads to malignant transformation, analogous to the pattern seen when carcinoma develops within a burn scar or area of chronic ulceration. Enhancement of a portion of an incompletely resected epidermoid tumor on CT or MRI, especially in the presence of atypical or severe symptoms, should signal the possibility of carcinoma.[31,67] Improved clinical

outcomes have been described with the use of adjuvant treatment with radiation.[51,52,53,54,56,63,64,68,69,70,71] Asahi described an improvement in mean survival from 4 months to 15 months with the addition of external beam radiation therapy to surgical resection of carcinoma arising within an intracranial epidermoid.[60] Tamura reviewed the use of stereotactic radiotherapy in the setting of carcinoma arising within an intracranial epidermoid and found median survival times of 1, 18, and 44 months with the use of surgery alone, surgery plus external beam radiation, and surgery plus stereotactic radiotherapy, respectively—differences that the authors found to be statistically significant.[72] Murase stressed the importance of combination chemotherapy and radiation in the treatment of these lesions, though the benefit of adding chemotherapy in these cases remains unproven.[60,68] Despite these measures, the prognosis overall for carcinoma in the setting of an epidermoid of the skull base remains poor.[31,45,60]

41.3 Dermoids

41.3.1 Incidence and Epidemiology

Dermoids, like epidermoids, are cysts lined by stratified, keratinizing squamous epithelium but differ from epidermoids in that they also contain mesodermal elements such as hair, sebaceous glands, sweat glands or, rarely, teeth, bone, or cartilage.[43,73,74] Dermoids are to be differentiated from teratomas, which are true neoplasms that originate from a misplaced rest of embryonic germ cells which progress to form a tumor composed of well-differentiated tissue derivatives of all three germ layer in an organlike pattern.[75] Like epidermoids, dermoids grow through the division of the outer lining of the cyst with progressive expansion of the core of the cyst as cellular debris accumulates. The growth pattern again is linear, not exponential as with a true neoplasm.[30]

Verratus in 1745 was the first to identify a dermoid on autopsy of a 40-year-old woman who died from a febrile illness.[76] Masses of hair, in addition to abundant squamous debris, were found in pathological examination of the lesion. In 1860 Lannelogue and Achard reported the first posterior fossa dermoid occurring in a child.[77] Six years later, Toynbee and Hinton described cystic lesions with "masses of hair" within the mastoid and middle ear space.[78,79] The first reported attempt at surgical removal of an intracranial dermoid was by Horrax in 1922, but not until 1934 was a dermoid successfully removed from the posterior fossa, by Tytus and Pennybacker.[80,81] Intracranial dermoids are rare lesions, accounting for 0.04 to 0.7% of all intracranial neoplasms, with incidence a quarter to half that of intracranial epidermoids.[33,75,82,83,84,85,86,87] Dermoids can occur in many intracranial locations both intra- and extradurally and are thought to typically occur in more midline locations than epidermoids do.[88] Above the tentorium, dermoids occur most frequently in the frontobasal, suprasellar, parasellar, cavernous sinus, and temporal regions.[84,89,90,91] Infratentorial locations for dermoids include the occiput, CPA, and prepontine areas. Dermoids have also been reported within the temporal bone in the mastoid complex, tympanum, and petrous apex.[92,93,94] Dermoids can occur in all age groups but are found more frequently in children than epidermoids are, especially when considering dermoids of the posterior fossa.[95] In reviewing multiple case reports of posterior fossa dermoids, one study found a median age of 2 years (range 6 months to 27 years), with relatively equal sex distribution.[88] Dermoids of the posterior fossa have been associated with Klippel-Feil syndrome in a number of reports.[96,97,98,99,100,101,102,103] There are three case reports in the literature of dermoids in children who had Goldenhar syndrome, though this association is less clear.[104,105,106] No familial predilection to the development of intracranial dermoids has been reported.

41.3.2 Embryology

Similar embryological events are thought to lead to the formation of dermoids and epidermoids (see previously). Some have postulated that dermoids form as a result of the aberrant adherence of primitive mesodermal cells to developing intracranial veins.[107] The predilection of dermoids for a midline position has been theorized to occur when cutaneous ectoderm is drawn intracranially as the falx cerebri or tentorium are forming from the fusion of two leaflets of dura.[88]

41.3.3 Pathology

Dermoid cysts are similar in appearance to epidermoids but have a variable number of hairs or dermal appendages (sebaceous or sweat glands) present. Fat is often present within dermoid cysts in addition to desquamated debris. Teeth, bone, cartilage, salivary glands, nerves, and lymph nodes have been reported in dermoids but are rare.[75,108] Dermoids have a variable growth rate and size on presentation, with some reports of large posterior fossa masses in children and others of small, limited tympanic lesions in adults.[95,109] Dermoids, especially those occurring in the posterior fossa, can have an associated dermal sinus that can be complete or incomplete in its connection. In 1952, Logue and Till proposed a classification based on the position of the cyst relative to the dura and connection to an associated occipital dermal sinus: (1) extradural cyst with complete dermal sinus, (2) intradural cyst without an associated sinus, (3) intradural cyst with an incomplete dermal sinus, and (4) intradural dermoid cyst with a complete dermal sinus.[110] In addition, dermoids may be either extra axial or intra axial in location, the most common intra-axial sites being the fourth ventricle or cerebellar vermis.[88] Lunardi found that the mean age of children who had dermoid cyst of the posterior fossa with an associated dermal sinus was 2.4 years, whereas dermoids without a dermal sinus tended to be discovered in older children (age 9 on average), indicating that the presence of a dermal sinus will often lead to an earlier diagnosis of the intracranial component.[95] In addition to intradural and extradural locations, dermoids have been classified as interdural when they are located between dural layers within the cavernous sinus, an uncommon location generally presenting with an oculomotor palsy.[89,111,112]

Rupture of dermoid and, less commonly, epidermoid cysts occurring spontaneously or during surgical removal, is a well-documented complication that can result in significant morbidity. The mechanism of spontaneous rupture of dermoid cysts is unclear, though Stendel hypothesized that glandular secretion under age-dependent hormonal changes leads to rapid enlargement with subsequent rupture and spillage of fatty contents in the subarachnoid space and ventricular system.[75] Rupture of dermoid

cysts after head trauma and during surgery have also been described.[113,114] Aseptic meningitis is the most frequent complication that can result from rupture of an intracranial dermoid and may lead to cranial nerve fibrosis or obstructive hydrocephalus due to occlusion of the ventricular outlets.[21,22,114,115,116,117,118] Rupture of intracranial dermoids can also cause an acute or delayed cerebral vasospasm with resultant ischemia, though the pathophysiology of this process is unclear.[21,119,120,121,122] The presence of fat within the subarachnoid space and ventricular system following rupture of dermoids has been well described and has been known to persist for years (▶ Fig. 41.3).[21,117,123,124]

41.3.4 Clinical Manifestations

Intracranial dermoids cause a spectrum of symptoms similar to those seen with epidermoids (see previously). Dermoids located in the cavernous sinus can cause paresis of cranial nerves III, IV, VI, V1, and V2. Ruptured intracranial dermoids most commonly present with headaches, seizures, and, when ischemia has occurred, sensory or motor defects.[21] However, rupture of an intracranial epidermoid may occur without symptoms.[74,123] Martinez-Lage and colleagues suggest that, at least in the case of dermoids of the posterior fossa, tumors reach a "critical size" of 3 cm at which most patients develop symptoms and because of this recommend removal prior to the lesion reaching this point.

41.3.5 Radiology

Please refer to Chapter 4 for a discussion of the imaging characteristics of dermoid cysts of the skull base. ▶ Fig. 41.3 shows representative imaging of a left middle and posterior fossa dermoid with evidence of rupture.

41.3.6 Treatment

Intracranial dermoid cysts are optimally treated with complete surgical removal, including the total removal of any associated dermal sinus, if present. Given the difficult anatomical relationships often encountered with these lesions, complete removal is sometimes impossible. When rupture of an intracranial dermoid has occurred, thorough irrigation of the subarachnoid space is recommended.[21,75] The use of a corticosteroid containing solution to irrigate the operative field has been advocated as a way to prevent the development of aseptic meningitis when rupture of a dermoid or epidermoid cyst has occurred.[31,38,39,40,114]

41.3.7 Outcome and Prognosis

Published reports with follow-up of 6 to 22 years have shown freedom from recurrence following removal of dermoid cysts, including subtotal resection in one patient.[81,95,125] Recurrence of incompletely resected dermoids has been reported three times in the literature, in contrast to subtotally resected epidermoids.[16,33,44,84,88,126] Whether this reflects a lower propensity for recurrence with dermoids rather than simply a lower incidence of the disease is unclear. Periodic monitoring with contrast-enhanced MRI scanning after removal of dermoids is recommended.

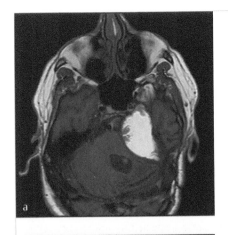
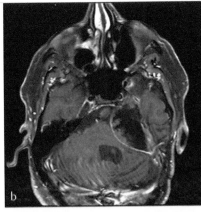
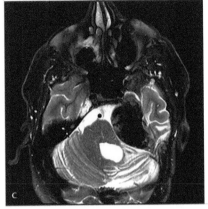
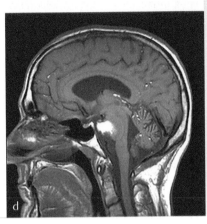

Fig. 41.3 (a) Axial T1-weighted MRI reveals a dermoid cyst spanning the left middle and posterior skull base. The mass is of high signal intensity on T1-weighted imaging. (b) Axial T1-weighted, fat-suppressed MRI reveals suppression of the predominately fatty content of this dermoid cyst. (c) Axial T2-weighted MRI reveals that this lesion is hypointense of T2 imaging. (d) Sagittal T1-weighted MRI reveals scattered T1-hyperintense droplets of fatty dermoid cyst content indicative of prior cyst rupture.

41.4 Cholesterol Granulomas

41.4.1 Incidence and Epidemiology

Cholesterol granulomas, though the most common cystic lesion of the petrous apex, are rare, affecting approximately 0.6 per million people in the general population.[127,128]

41.4.2 Pathophysiology

Their etiology is debated, with two alternative theories of formation.[127,128,129] One theory invokes the obstruction of the air cells of the petrous apex as the inciting event. This leads to resorption of the air and the creation of a vacuum into which blood is drawn and trapped. A second theory proposes that extensive pneumatization of the petrous apex leads to the exposure of bone marrow–filled spaces, which bleed into and obstruct the outflow tract. Although the etiology is debated, the crucial event is bleeding into the air cells and a reactive inflammatory response.

41.4.3 Pathology

The cyst has a fibrous capsule and contents that are viscous and motor oil–like and that contain cholesterol crystals. There is also evidence of chronic granulomatous inflammation with giant cell reaction.

41.4.4 Clinical Manifestations

Headache and dizziness are common symptoms, but many are incidentally identified on cranial imaging. Occasionally specific symptoms of facial paresthesia and/or pain, hearing loss, and facial weakness occur.

41.4.5 Radiology

CT scans reveal a non-enhancing cyst with smooth-edged erosion of bone and loss of internal bony structure. Cholesterol granulomas are typically hyperintense on both T1- and T2-weighted sequences. Their hypointensity on diffusion-weighted sequences further differentiates them from epidermoids (▶ Fig. 41.4).

41.4.6 Treatment

The two management options that currently exist for cholesterol granuloma are observation and surgical drainage. Many incidentally identified cholesterol granulomas do not become symptomatic or grow. In a collaborative natural history study from Vanderbilt University and the Mayo Clinic-Rochester, 85.7% of patients had no reported symptom progression or radiographic growth over a median follow-up of 27.8 months (range 6.4–221.5 months). Of the 10 patients (14.3%) who experienced symptom progression or radiographic growth, 3 went on to surgical drainage and 7 continued with observation. In this study, patients who had large lesions (average 3 cm diameter) and multiple symptoms were more likely to be managed with surgery rather than observation.[129]

The goal of surgical management is to create an avenue of persistent drainage from the cyst into an air-containing region

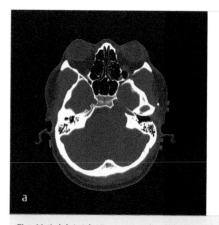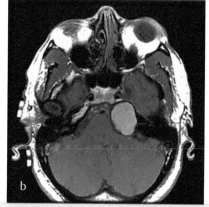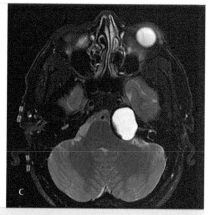

Fig. 41.4 (a) Axial CT scan reveals smooth erosion of the left petrous apex in this patient who has a cholesterol granuloma. (b) Axial T1-weighted MRI identifies the T1-hyperintense nature typical of cholesterol granuloma. (c) Axial T2-weighted MRI similarly reveals the lesion to be T2-hyperintense.

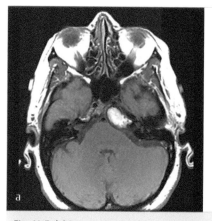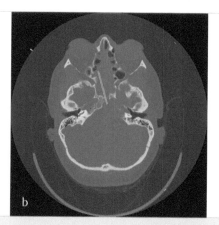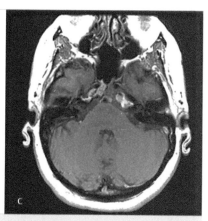

Fig. 41.5 (a) Preoperative axial T1-weighted MRI of a left petrous apex cholesterol granuloma presenting to the posterior aspect of the sphenoid sinus. The patient, a 37-year-old woman, presented with subjective left facial numbness initially in the mandibular nerve distribution but then progressing to all three trigeminal nerve divisions. (b) Postoperative axial CT scan reveals the surgical fenestration of the cyst into the sphenoid sinus and the placement of a Silastic stent. (c) Postoperative axial T1-weighted MRI reveals significant resolution of the cyst. There was complete resolution of the patient's preoperative symptom complex.

of the head. The most common procedures are an endonasal endoscopic drainage into the sphenoid sinus, or a transtemporal infralabyrinthine/infracochlear approach.[129,130,131]

The choice of approach requires a careful assessment of the availability of an adequate and safe surgical corridor for drainage. For endonasal approaches there must be space between the medial wall of the cyst and the lateral wall of the paraclival internal carotid artery; see case example 1 in ▶ Fig. 41.5. Lesions behind the internal carotid artery are best approached via the infralabyrinthine/infracochlear route; see case example 2 in ▶ Fig. 41.6.

41.4.7 Outcome and Prognosis

In well-selected patients the surgical outcomes are similar between approaches. Symptom improvement can be expected in 90% of patients. Cyst recurrence has an incidence of 7 to 13%. The need for stents to maintain the drainage pathway is an unresolved issue.

41.5 Arachnoid Cysts

41.5.1 Incidence and Epidemiology

The first report of an intracranial arachnoid cyst was by Bright in 1831, describing them as "serous cysts forming in connection with the arachnoid."[132] Maunsell in 1899 first described an arachnoid cyst in the posterior fossa, but not until 1932 did Mullin report the first one such lesion in the CPA, followed by Aubry in 1937.[133,134,135] Since then there have been many reports of arachnoid cysts in the posterior fossa.[136,137,138,139,140,141,142,143,144,145,146,147]

Arachnoid cysts represent 1% of all intracranial lesions and occur most commonly in the middle fossa at the sylvian fissure.[148,149] The CPA is the second most common site for the development of arachnoid cysts. Temporal bone involvement with arachnoid cysts, though well described, is rare.[144,147,148,150,151,152,153,154,155,156] There appears to be a male preponderance with arachnoid cysts, at least with regard to those involving the

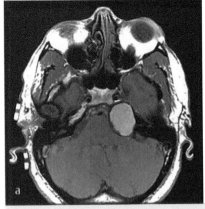
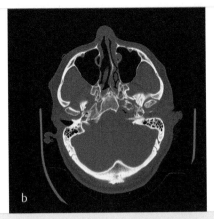
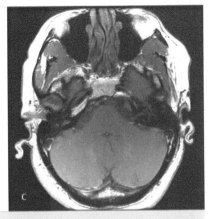

Fig. 41.6 **(a)** Preoperative axial T1-weighted MRI reveals the endoscopically unfavorable location of this cholesterol granuloma posterolateral to the internal carotid artery. The patient, a 33-year-old man, had headache and left-sided tinnitus. **(b)** Postoperative axial CT details the trajectory of the infralabyrinthine/infracochlear approach for drainage of the cyst. A Silastic catheter is in place. **(c)** Postoperative axial T1-weighted MRI reveals near-complete cyst resolution. His headaches resolved, although he still has intermittent tinnitus.

middle fossa.[145,149,157] The mean age at surgery for arachnoid cysts in one review was 31 years, although 70% of patients who have arachnoid cysts become symptomatic in childhood and 60 to 90% of reported patients are children.[144,145,158,159,160] This discrepancy is most likely a reflection of the vague symptoms that typify these lesions and the consequent delay in diagnosis and/ or treatment that results from the often nonspecific symptoms. Sinha and colleagues have reported a left-sided predominance for arachnoid cysts.

Arachnoid cysts have been associated with congenital anomalies such as polycystic kidney disease as well as with developmental syndromes such as Kabuki, Goldenhar, Chudley-McCullough, trisomy-12, and Criduchat.[161,162,163,164,165,166] In addition, bilateral temporal arachnoid cysts have been well documented in association with glutaric aciduria type I patients, in whom the increased catabolism associated with surgical interventions may produce devastating worsening of neurological status.[167,168,169,170,171] Familial arachnoid cysts have been described by multiple groups, but the pattern of inheritance remains unclear.[149,164,169,172,173,174]

41.5.2 Embryology and Pathophysiology

Primary (or "true") arachnoid cysts are congenital malformations thought to form at gestational week 15 when the roof of the fourth ventricle opens through the foramina of Luschka and Magendie into the cisterna magna.[147,152,154] Secondary arachnoid cysts can result from trauma, neoplasia, infection, radiation, or hemorrhage and are thought to develop due to an adhesive arachnoiditis potentially caused by any of these insults.[45,155,175] With regard to primary lesions, Starkman hypothesized that as the fourth ventricle opens into the cisterna, aberrant flow of CSF causes a splitting or duplication of the arachnoid membrane that, with further filling, results in the formation of an arachnoid cyst.[176] Petrous apex arachnoid cysts are thought to arise from CSF pulsations through arachnoid granulations in areas of weakened dura overlying congenital bony dehiscences or irregularities in the petroclival fissure. With arachnoid cyst formation and

continued, chronic pulsation further bone erosion of the petrous apex occurs, creating a smooth, scalloped defect.[146,152,155]

A similar but distinct entity is a CSF cephalocele of the petrous apex, which is a diverticulum of all of the layers of the meninges creating a similar bony defect (▶ Fig. 41.7).[177] Isaacson and colleagues hypothesized that a CSF cephalocele may result from increased intracranial pressure transmitting into Meckel's cave via a patent porus trigeminus.[147] In their series, three of four patients who had a CSF cephalocele were found to have an empty sella, a finding that others have associated with increased intracranial pressure.[178,179,180]

Three mechanisms have been proposed to explain the expansion of arachnoid cysts. One theory is that intracystic hemorrhage results in the establishment of an osmotic gradient, causing subsequent enlargement of the cyst due to fluid shifts. Another mechanism implicates active secretion of fluid by the internal lining of the cyst as the cause of expansion, a theory supported by the finding of Na$^+$/K$^+$-ATPase pumps in the cells lining the cyst.[181] Further support for this theory was provided by the finding of ectopic choroid plexus within some arachnoid cysts.[182] The most widely accepted theory regarding the expansion of arachnoid cysts describes a ball valve mechanism of CSF trapping within the cyst, driven by intermittent increases in intracranial pressure.[150,183]

41.5.3 Pathology

Histologically arachnoid cysts are CSF spaces surrounded by a thin membrane a few cell layers thick. The cyst lining resembles normal arachnoid tissue that has been split at its membrane and encloses the fluid cavity.[175] The lining consists of pseudostratified epithelial cells with surface microvilli evident on electron microscopy. Rengachary and Watanabe described four histological findings to differentiate the wall of an arachnoid cyst from normal arachnoid: (1) splitting of the arachnoid membrane at the margin of the cyst, (2) a very thick layer of collagen in the cyst wall, (3) the absence of traversing trabecular processes within the cyst, and (4) the presence of hyperplastic arachnoid cells in the cyst wall, which presumably participate in collagen synthesis.[184]

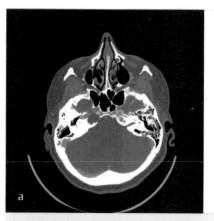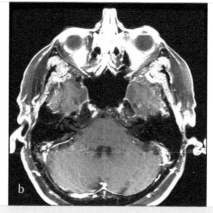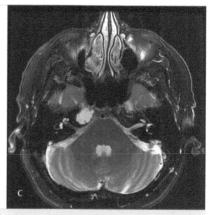

Fig. 41.7 **(a)** Axial CT reveals a very well circumscribed nonsclerotic lesion of the right petrous apex, consistent with meningocele. **(b)** Axial T1-weighted MRI reveals the lesion to be T1-hypointense, consistent with CSF. **(c)** Axial T2-weighted MRI clearly identifies this petrous apex "cephalocele."

41.5.4 Classification

Vaquero proposed a classification system for arachnoid cysts of the posterior fossa on anatomical location as follows: laterocerebellar, supracerebellar, retrocerebellar, clival, and mixed.[185] Laterocerebellar cysts occupy the CPA and petrous apex and are generally smaller than those seen in other locations. Differentiation of arachnoid cysts in this area from epidermoids requires MRI scanning with fluid-attenuated inversion recovery (FLAIR) and diffusion-weighted image (DWI) sequences. Retrocerebellar cysts occupy the midline posterior to the cerebellum and can be quite large, with significant compression of the cerebellar parenchyma. Supracerebellar arachnoid cysts originate from the quadrigeminal cistern and extend posteriorly along the tentorium with a tendency to cause hydrocephalus. Clival cysts displace the brainstem posteriorly, can extend laterally to the CPA, and are rare.

41.5.5 Clinical Manifestations

Arachnoid cysts are highly variable in the spectrum and severity of the symptoms they cause, much like epidermoids and dermoids. Incidental, asymptomatic arachnoid cysts have been encountered commonly since the advent and widespread use of MRI and CT scanning in the setting of head trauma and as part of the work-up of other neurological complaints.[186,187] The most frequent presentations of an arachnoid cyst are headache (sometimes associated with nausea and vomiting) and signs of cerebellar dysfunction, including dysmetria and gait disturbance.[144] Arachnoid cysts can cause both communicating and noncommunicating hydrocephalus through compression of the ventricular system or blockage of CSF outflow, causing the typical spectrum of associated symptoms seen in hydrocephalus from other causes. Cysts in the CPA or petrous apex typically present with tinnitus, hearing loss, vertigo, and dizziness.[147,150,188,189,190] Facial paralysis due to an arachnoid cyst has been described but is uncommon.[156,191,192,193] Other unusual presentations include hemifacial spasm, trigeminal neuralgia, narcolepsy, seizures, visual loss, otalgia, meningitis, and otorrhea.[147,150,159,194,195,196,199] A review by Jallo found that the time of onset of symptoms to diagnosis varied from 4 weeks to 12 months, reflecting the vague symptomatology on presentation of these lesions.[147]

41.5.6 Radiology

Please refer to Chapter 4 for a discussion of the imaging characteristics of arachnoid cysts of the skull base. ▶ Fig. 41.8 shows representative imaging of a right posterior fossa arachnoid cyst.

41.5.7 Treatment

In general, asymptomatic patients who have an arachnoid cyst do not require treatment and can be followed clinically and through periodic radiological examinations to monitor for growth or the development of symptoms.[144,147,197,198] However, some authors argue that in the case of a large, asymptomatic lesion, the potential for rapid deterioration and even death from intracystic hemorrhage after minor head trauma is significant enough to justify operative intervention.[199,200,201] Indications for surgery to treat arachnoid cysts include demonstrated growth, neural compression, hydrocephalus, and refractory symptoms referable to the lesion.[144,148] Surgical treatment options include shunting (cystoperitoneal or ventriculoperitoneal for associated hydrocephalus), fenestration (either open or endoscopic), and microsurgical resection or marsupialization. Cystoperitoneal shunting has the advantage of low morbidity and mortality but leads to shunt dependency. Even so, many authors feel that cystoperitoneal shunting should be the initial surgical procedure for most arachnoid cysts, especially if hydrocephalus is present.[138,158,185,202,203,204,205] Ventriculoperitoneal shunting is recommended in cases of communicating hydrocephalus due to an arachnoid cyst but is not used as the sole treatment modality in the case of posterior fossa lesions, owing to the risk of upward tentorial herniation with progressive enlargement of the primary lesion.[149,204,205,206]

Open surgical interventions for arachnoid cysts include fenestration, marsupialization, and/or resection. Fenestration has been advocated by many surgeons, for it avoids shunt dependency, allows direct inspection and biopsy of the cyst, and seems to provide long-term results with few reported failures.[144,158,160,185,203,207] However, some authors have reported that cyst fenestration alone does not reliably treat associated hydrocephalus, if present—presumably because there is blockage of the CSF flow in the subarachnoid space, perhaps because of the presence of blood and cellular debris. Accordingly, many patients

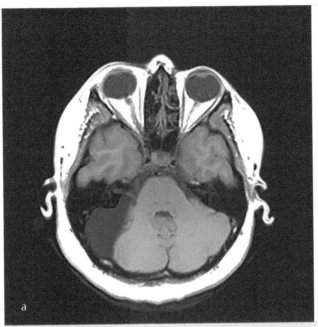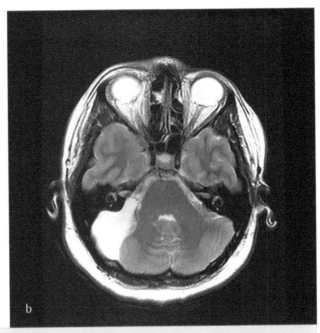

Fig. 41.8 **(a)** Axial noncontrast T1-weighted MRI. A right posterior fossa arachnoid cyst is visualized. Note the scalloping to the posterior petrous surface of the temporal bone. **(b)** Axial T2-weighted MRI. The cyst contains T2 hyperintense fluid consistent with CSF.

who have had cyst fenestration still require ventriculoperitoneal (or lumboperitoneal) shunting to treat continued ventriculomegaly.[207,208] In the treatment of CPA epidermoid cysts, some authors advocate resection of the medial, lateral, and posterior walls of the cyst with fenestration of the remaining portion. Advantages to this approach are that it provides optimal treatment by preventing subarachnoid blood and debris from causing future arachnoiditis and obstruction.[144,147,206] With this approach, any cyst membrane that may be adherent to brainstem, cerebellum, major vessels, or cranial nerves is left in place. Arachnoid cysts of the petrous apex can be approached through retrosigmoid, middle fossa, or infracochlear approaches. The infracochlear approach provides decompression of petrous apex cysts only. In contrast, an extradural middle fossa approach has been advocated by many groups, because it allows for removal of cyst lining and obliteration of the defect to prevent future infection or CSF leakage in cases of both arachnoid cysts and CSF cephaloceles.[147,177,209,210]

41.5.8 Outcome and Prognosis

Ciricillo and colleagues reported on a series of 40 pediatric patients who had arachnoid cysts over a 10-year period.[204] Five patients did not require intervention, but 15 underwent cyst fenestration, of whom 12 required shunting for improvement after a median follow-up of 8 years. The remaining 20 patients underwent shunting procedures, and 6 of them required subsequent shunt revision. Based on these results, the authors recommended shunting as the initial procedure for children who have arachnoid cysts. Levy reported on 39 patients who had middle fossa arachnoid cysts and who underwent cyst fenestration. Fifteen patients had either hydrocephalus or macrocephaly and required ventriculoperitoneal shunting in addition to fenestration.[208] Raffel presented a series of 29 arachnoid cysts

in children in the middle and posterior fossae. Fenestration alone was successful in 22, but 7 needed additional cystoperitoneal shunting.

Samii and colleagues reported a series of 12 patients who had CPA arachnoid cysts treated using cyst resection or maximal fenestration through a suboccipital approach. One patient had palsies of cranial nerves VII and VIII, but all 12 patients improved symptomatically with this approach, with no mortality by 3-year follow-up.[206] Jallo used a similar approach in five pediatric patients who had CPA arachnoid cysts, including one who had failed previous cystoperitoneal shunting. All five patients were successfully treated using this approach, with a mean follow-up of 5 years, leading the authors to recommend microsurgical treatment for CPA arachnoid cysts as the optimal initial treatment.[144]

References

[1] Cruveilhier J. Anatomie physiologique du corps humain, vol. II. Paris, France: Balliere; 1829

[2] Bailey P. Cruveilhier's "tumeur perlee.". Surg Gynecol Obstet. 1920; 31: 390–401

[3] Muller J. Uber den feineren Bau und die Formen der krankhaften Geschwulste. Vol. 1. Berlin, Germany: G Reimer; 1838

[4] Virchow R. Uber Perlgeschwultse. Virchows Arch A Pathol Anat Histopathol. 1855; 8:371–418

[5] Bostroem E. Ueber die pialen epidermoide, dermoide und dermalen dermoide. Zbl Pathol. 1897; 8:1–98

[6] Nager GT. Epidermoids involving the temporal bone: clinical, radiological and pathological aspects. Laryngoscope. 1975; 85(12 Pt 2) Suppl 2:1–21

[7] Lalwani AK. Meningiomas, epidermoids, and other nonacoustic tumors of the cerebellopontine angle. Otolaryngol Clin North Am. 1992; 25(3): 707–728

[8] Findeisen L. WT. Uber intracranielle Epidermoide. Zentralbl Neurochir. 1937; 2:301–315

[9] Zulch K. Brain Tumors: Their Biology and Pathology. 3rd ed. Berlin, Germany: Springer-Verlag; 1986

[10] Schiffer D. Brain Tumors: Biology, Pathology and Clinical References. 2nd ed. Berlin, Germany: Springer-Verlag; 1997

[11] Berger MS, Wilson CB. Epidermoid cysts of the posterior fossa. J Neurosurg. 1985; 62(2):214–219

[12] Netsky MG. Epidermoid tumors. Review of the literature. Surg Neurol. 1988; 29(6):477–483

[13] Talacchi A, Sala F, Alessandrini F, Turazzi S, Bricolo A. Assessment and surgical management of posterior fossa epidermoid tumors: report of 28 cases. Neurosurgery. 1998; 42(2):242–251, discussion 251–252

[14] Kuzeyli K, Duru S, Cakir E, Baykal S, Ceylan S, Aktürk F. Epidermoid tumor of the occipital bone. Neurosurg Rev. 1996; 19(2):109–112

[15] Obrador S, Lopez-Zafra JJ. Clinical features of the epidermoids of the basal cisterns of the brain. J Neurol Neurosurg Psychiatry. 1969; 32(5):450–454

[16] Yamakawa K, Shitara N, Genka S, Manaka S, Takakura K. Clinical course and surgical prognosis of 33 cases of intracranial epidermoid tumors. Neurosurgery. 1989; 24(4):568–573

[17] Grey PL, Moffat DA, Hardy DG. Surgical results in unusual cerebellopontine angle tumours. Clin Otolaryngol Allied Sci. 1996; 21(3):237–243

[18] Bartlett J. Tumors of the lateral ventricle. Except choroid plexus tumors. In: Vinken PJ, Bruyn GW, ed. Handbook of Clinical Neurology, Vol. II. Amsterdam, The Netherlands: North Holland Publishing; 1974:596–609

[19] Lakhdar A, Sami A, Naja A, et al. [Epidermoid cyst of the cerebellopontine angle. A surgical series of 10 cases and review of the literature]. Neurochirurgie. 2003; 49(1):13–24

[20] Chandra PS, Gupta A, Mishra NK, Mehta VS. Association of craniovertebral and upper cervical anomalies with dermoid and epidermoid cysts: report of four cases. Neurosurgery. 2005; 56(5):E1155

[21] El-Bahy K, Kotb A, Galal A, El-Hakim A. Ruptured intracranial dermoid cysts. Acta Neurochir (Wien). 2006; 148(4):457–462

[22] Abramson RC, Morawetz RB, Schlitt M. Multiple complications from an intracranial epidermoid cyst: case report and literature review. Neurosurgery. 1989; 24(4):574–578

[23] Schijman E, Monges J, Cragnaz R. Congenital dermal sinuses, dermoid and epidermoid cysts of the posterior fossa. Childs Nerv Syst. 1986; 2(2):83–89

[24] Alvord EC, Jr. Growth rates of epidermoid tumors. Ann Neurol. 1977; 2(5):367–370

[25] Boestroem E. Uber die pialen Epidermoide, Dermoide und Lipome und duralen Dermoide. Centralbl Allg Path Anat. 1897; 8:1–98

[26] Scholtz E. Einige Bemerkungen uber das meningaele Cholesteatom in Anschluss an einenFall von Cholesteatom des III Ventrikels. Virchow's Arch Path Anat. 1906; 184:225–273

[27] Baumann CH, Bucy PC. Paratrigeminal epidermoid tumors. J Neurosurg. 1956; 13(5):455–468

[28] Fleming JF, Botterell EH. Cranial dermoid and epidermoid tumors. Surg Gynecol Obstet. 1959; 109:403–411

[29] Sano K. Intracranial dysembryogenetic tumors: pathogenesis and their order of malignancy. Neurosurg Rev. 2001; 24(4):162–167, discussion 168–170

[30] Yaşargil MG, Abernathey CD, Sarioglu AC. Microneurosurgical treatment of intracranial dermoid and epidermoid tumors. Neurosurgery. 1989; 24(4):561–567

[31] Kaylie DM, Warren FM, III, Haynes DS, Jackson CG. Neurotologic management of intracranial epidermoid tumors. Laryngoscope. 2005; 115(6):1082–1086

[32] Kountakis SE, Chang CY, Gormley WB, Cabral FR. Migration of intradural epidermoid matrix: embryologic implications. Otolaryngol Head Neck Surg. 2000; 123(3):170–173

[33] Love JG, Kernohan JM. Dermoid and epidermoid tumors (cholesteatomas) of the central nervous system. JAMA. 1936; 107:1876–1883

[34] Ulrich J. Intracranial Epidermoids. A study on their distribution and spread. J Neurosurg. 1964; 21:1051–1058

[35] de Souza CE, Sperling NM, da Costa SS, Yoon TH, Abdel Hamid M, de Souza RA. Congenital cholesteatomas of the cerebellopontine angle. Am J Otol. 1989; 10(5):358–363

[36] Samii M, Tatagiba M, Piquer J, Carvalho GA. Surgical treatment of epidermoid cysts of the cerebellopontine angle. J Neurosurg. 1996; 84(1):14–19

[37] Vinchon M, Pertuzon B, Lejeune JP, Assaker R, Pruvo JP, Christiaens JL. Intradural epidermoid cysts of the cerebellopontine angle: diagnosis and surgery. Neurosurgery. 1995; 36(1):52–56, discussion 56–57

[38] Mohanty A, Venkatrama SK, Rao BR, Chandramouli BA, Jayakumar PN, Das BS. Experience with cerebellopontine angle epidermoids. Neurosurgery. 1997; 40(1):24–29, discussion 29–30

[39] Sabin HI, Bordi LT, Symon L. Epidermoid cysts and cholesterol granulomas centered on the posterior fossa: twenty years of diagnosis and management. Neurosurgery. 1987; 21(6):798–805

[40] Altschuler EM, Jungreis CA, Sekhar LN, Jannetta PJ, Sheptak PE. Operative treatment of intracranial epidermoid cysts and cholesterol granulomas: report of 21 cases. Neurosurgery. 1990; 26(4):606–613, discussion 614

[41] De Micheli E, Bricolo A. The long history of a cerebello-pontine angle epidermoid tumour—a case report and lessons learned. Acta Neurochir (Wien). 1996; 138(3):350–354

[42] Antoli-Candela F, Jr, Stewart TJ. The pathophysiology of otologic facial paralysis. Otolaryngol Clin North Am. 1974; 7(2):309–330

[43] Antonio SM. DK, Della Cruz A. Epidermoid cysts of the cerebellopontine angle. In: Jackler RK, ed. Neurotology. Philadelphia, PA: Elsevier/Mosby; 2005:841–849

[44] Jamjoom AB, Jamjoom ZA, al-Fehaily M, el-Watidy S, al-Moallem M, Nain-Ur-Rahman. Trigeminal neuralgia related to cerebellopontine angle tumors. Neurosurg Rev. 1996; 19(4):237–241

[45] Eisenman DVE, Selesnick SH. Unusual tumors of the internal auditory canal and cerebellopontine angle. In: Jackler RK, Driscoll C, eds. Tumors of the Ear and Temporal bone. Philadelphia, PA: Lippincott, Williams & Wilkins; 2000:236–275

[46] Parikh S, Milosevic M, Wong CS, Laperriere N. Recurrent intracranial epidermoid cyst treated with radiotherapy. J Neurooncol. 1995; 24(3):293–297

[47] Lunardi P, Fortuna A, Cantore G, Missori P. Long-term evaluation of asymptomatic patients operated on for intracranial epidermoid cysts: comparison of the diagnostic value of magnetic resonance imaging and computer-assisted cisternography for detection of cholesterin fragments. Acta Neurochir (Wien). 1994; 128(1–4):122–125

[48] Moffat DA, Quaranta N, Baguley DM, Hardy DG, Chang P. Staging and management of primary cerebellopontine cholesteatoma. J Laryngol Otol. 2002; 116(5):340–345

[49] Conley F. Epidermoid and dermoid tumors: clinical features and surgical management. In: Wilkins RH, ed. Neurosurgery. New York: McGraw-Hill; 1985:668–673

[50] Kveton JF, Glasscock ME, III, Christiansen SG. Malignant degeneration of an epidermoid of the temporal bone. Otolaryngol Head Neck Surg. 1986; 94(5):633–636

[51] Nishio S, Takeshita I, Morioka T, Fukui M. Primary intracranial squamous cell carcinomas: report of two cases. Neurosurgery. 1995; 37(2):329–332

[52] Dubois PJ, Sage M, Luther JS, Burger PC, Heinz ER, Drayer BP. Case report: malignant change in an intracranial epidermoid cyst. J Comput Assist Tomogr. 1981; 5(3):433–435

[53] Gi H, Yoshizumi H, Nagao S, Nishioka T, Uno J, Fujita Y. [C-P angle epidermoid carcinoma: a case report]. No Shinkei Geka. 1990; 18(11):1041–1045

[54] Giangaspero F, Manetto V, Ferracini R, Piazza G. Squamous cell carcinoma of the brain with sarcoma-like stroma. Virchows Arch A Pathol Anat Histopathol. 1984; 402(4):459–464

[55] Lewis AJ, Cooper PW, Kassel EE, Schwartz ML. Squamous cell carcinoma arising in a suprasellar epidermoid cyst: case report. J Neurosurg. 1983; 59(3):538–541

[56] Mori Y, Suzuki Y, Tanasawa T, Yoshida J, Wakabayashi T, Kobayashi T. [A case report of epidermoid carcinoma in the cerebello-pontine angle]. No Shinkei Geka. 1995; 23(10):905–909

[57] Bondeson L, Fält K. Primary intracranial epidermoid carcinoma. Acta Cytol. 1984; 28(4):487–489

[58] Landers JW, Danielski JJ. Malignant intracranial epidermoid cyst: report of a case with leptomeningeal spread. Arch Pathol. 1960; 70:419–423

[59] Yamanaka A, Hinohara S, Hashimoto T. Primary diffuse carcinomatosis of the spinal meninges accompanied with a cancerous epidermal cyst of the base of the brain; report of a case of autopsy. Gan. 1955; 46(2–3):274–276

[60] Asahi T, Kurimoto M, Endo S, Monma F, Ohi M, Takami M. Malignant transformation of cerebello-pontine angle epidermoid. J Clin Neurosci. 2001; 8(6):572–574

[61] Ogata N, Jochum W, Aguzzi A, Fournier JY, Yonekawa Y. Total removal of a primary intracranial squamous cell carcinoma invading the brain stem. Surg Neurol. 1996; 46(5):477–480

[62] Fox H, South EA. Squamous cell carcinoma developing in an intracranial epidermoid cyst (cholesteatoma). J Neurol Neurosurg Psychiatry. 1965; 28:276–281

[63] Knorr JR, Ragland RL, Smith TW, Davidson RI, Keller JD. Squamous carcinoma arising in a cerebellopontine angle epidermoid: CT and MR findings. AJNR Am J Neuroradiol. 1991; 12(6):1182–1184

[64] Matsuno A, Shibui S, Ochiai C, Inoya H, Takakura K. [Primary intracranial epidermoid carcinoma accompanied with epidermoid cyst in the cerebellopontine angle—a case report]. No Shinkei Geka. 1987; 15(8):851–858

[65] Nishiura I, Koyama T, Handa J, Amano S. Primary intracranial epidermoid carcinoma—case report. Neurol Med Chir (Tokyo). 1989; 29(7):600–605

[66] Toglia JU, Netsky MG, Alexander E, Jr. Epithelial (epidermoid) tumors of the cranium: their common nature and pathogenesis. J Neurosurg. 1965; 23(4):384–393

[67] Lo WWMS-BL. Tumors of the temporal bone and cerebellopontine angle. In: Som P, CH, eds. Head and Neck Imaging. St. Louis: Mosby; 1996:1449–1534

[68] Murase S, Yamakawa H, Ohkuma A, et al. Primary intracranial squamous cell carcinoma—case report. Neurol Med Chir (Tokyo). 1999; 39(1):49–54

[69] Garcia CA, McGarry PA, Rodriguez F. Primary intracranial squamous cell carcinoma of the right cerebellopontine angle. J Neurosurg. 1981; 54(6):824–828

[70] Goldman SA, Gandy SE. Squamous cell carcinoma as a late complication of intracerebroventricular epidermoid cyst. Case report. J Neurosurg. 1987; 66(4):618–620

[71] Salazar J, Vaquero J, Saucedo G, Bravo G. Posterior fossa epidermoid cysts. Acta Neurochir (Wien). 1987; 85(1–2):34–39

[72] Tamura K, Aoyagi M, Wakimoto H, et al. Malignant transformation eight years after removal of a benign epidermoid cyst: a case report. J Neurooncol. 2006; 79(1):67–72

[73] Smith AS. Myth of the mesoderm. AJNR Am J Neuroradiol. 1989; 10(2):449

[74] Smith AS, Benson JE, Blaser SI, Mizushima A, Tarr RW, Bellon EM. Diagnosis of ruptured intracranial dermoid cyst: value MR over CT. AJNR Am J Neuroradiol. 1991; 12(1):175–180

[75] Stendel R, Pietilä TA, Lehmann K, Kurth R, Suess O, Brock M. Ruptured intracranial dermoid cysts. Surg Neurol. 2002; 57(6):391–398, discussion 398

[76] Verratus. De Bononiensi scientiarum et atrium instituto atque academia comentarii. Bononiae. 1745; 2(1):1–184

[77] Lannelongue EA. Traite des Kystes congenitaux. Paris: 1886

[78] Toynbee J. Hairs in the mastoid cells. Trans Pathol Soc London. 1866; 17:274

[79] Hinton J. Sebaceous tumors and hairs in the tympanum of a boy. Trans Pathol Soc London. 1866; 17:275

[80] Horrax G. A consideration of the dermal versus the epidermal cholesteatomas having their attachment in the cerebral envelopes. Arch Neurol Psychiatry. 1922; 8:265–285

[81] Pennybacker J, Tytus JS. Pearly tumours in relation to the central nervous system. J Neurol Neurosurg Psychiatry. 1956; 19(4):241–259

[82] Leutner C, Keller E, Pauleit D, et al. [An epidermoid of the sphenoid bone and a ruptured intracranial dermoid—a case report]. RoFo Fortschr Geb Rontgenstr Nuklearmed. 1998; 168(2):202–204

[83] Rubin G, Scienza R, Pasqualin A, Rosta L, Da Pian R. Craniocerebral epidermoids and dermoids: a review of 44 cases. Acta Neurochir (Wien). 1989; 97(1–2):1–16

[84] Arseni C, Dănăilă L, Constantinescu AI, Carp N, Decu P. Cerebral dermoid tumours. Neurochirurgia (Stuttg). 1976; 19(3):104–114

[85] Guidetti B, Gagliardi FM. Epidermoid and dermoid cysts. Clinical evaluation and late surgical results. J Neurosurg. 1977; 47(1):12–18

[86] MacCarty CS, Leavens ME, Love JG, Kernohan JW. Dermoid and epidermoid tumors in the central nervous system of adults. Surg Gynecol Obstet. 1959; 108(2):191–198

[87] Manlapaz JS. Ruptured intracranial dermoid; report of a case and survey of previously reported cases. Am J Surg. 1960; 100:723–730

[88] Martínez-Lage JF, Ramos J, Puche A, Poza M. Extradural dermoid tumours of the posterior fossa. Arch Dis Child. 1997; 77(5):427–430

[89] Akdemir G, Dağlioğlu E, Ergüngör MF. Dermoid lesion of the cavernous sinus: case report and review of the literature. Neurosurg Rev. 2004; 27(4):294–298

[90] Hamer J. Diagnosis by computerized tomography of intradural dermoid with spontaneous rupture of the cyst. Acta Neurochir (Wien). 1980; 51(3–4):219–226

[91] Caldarelli M, Colosimo C, Di Rocco C. Intra-axial dermoid/epidermoid tumors of the brainstem in children. Surg Neurol. 2001; 56(2):97–105

[92] Fried MP, Vernick DM. Dermoid cyst of the middle ear and mastoid. Otolaryngol Head Neck Surg. 1984; 92(5):594–596

[93] Vrabec JT, Schwaber MK. Dermoid tumor of the middle ear: case report and literature review. Am J Otol. 1992; 13(6):580–581

[94] Behnke EE, Schindler RA. Dermoid of the petrous apex. Laryngoscope. 1984; 94(6):779–783

[95] Lunardi P, Missori P, Gagliardi FM, Fortuna A. Dermoid cysts of the posterior cranial fossa in children. Report of nine cases and review of the literature. Surg Neurol. 1990; 34(1):39–42

[96] Roberts AP. A case of intracranial dermoid cyst associated with the Klippel-Feil deformity and recurrent meningitis. Arch Dis Child. 1958; 33(169):222–225

[97] Whittle IR, Besser M. Congenital neural abnormalities presenting with mirror movements in a patient with Klippel-Feil syndrome: case report. J Neurosurg. 1983; 59(5):891–894

[98] Diekmann-Guiroy B, Huang PS. Klippel-Feil syndrome in association with a craniocervical dermoid cyst presenting as aseptic meningitis in an adult: case report. Neurosurgery. 1989; 25(4):652–655

[99] Dickey W, Hawkins SA, Kirkpatrick DH, McKinstry CS, Gray WJ. Posterior fossa dermoid cysts and the Klippel-Feil syndrome. J Neurol Neurosurg Psychiatry. 1991; 54(11):1016–1017

[100] Kuribayashi K, Nakasu S, Matsumura K, Matsuda M, Handa J. [Dermoid cyst in the fourth ventricle associated with Klippel-Feil syndrome]. No To Shinkei. 1993; 45(8):747–751

[101] Kennedy PT, McAuley DJ. Association of posterior fossa dermoid cyst and Klippel-Feil syndrome. AJNR Am J Neuroradiol. 1998; 19(1):195–, discussion 196

[102] Hinojosa M, Tatagiba M, Harada K, Samii M. Dermoid cyst in the posterior fossa accompanied by Klippel-Feil syndrome. Childs Nerv Syst. 2001; 17(1–2):97–100

[103] Sharma MS, Sharma BS, Yadav A, Khosla VK. Posterior fossa dermoid in association with Klippel-Feil syndrome—a short report. Neurol India. 2001; 49(2):210–212

[104] Murphy MJ, Risk WS, VanGilder JC. Intracranial dermoid cyst in Goldenhar's syndrome: case report. J Neurosurg. 1980; 53(3):408–410

[105] Shirakuni T, Yamasaki S, Sato H. [An infant case of Goldenhar syndrome associated with intracranial lesions]. No To Hattatsu. 1985; 17(3):251–255

[106] Wilson GN. Cranial defects in the Goldenhar syndrome. Am J Med Genet. 1983; 14(3):435–443

[107] Lunardi P, Missori P, Rizzo A, Gagliardi FM. Chemical meningitis in ruptured intracranial dermoid. Case report and review of the literature. Surg Neurol. 1989; 32(6):449–452

[108] Hyams V, Batsakis J, Michaels L. Tumors of the Upper Respiratory Tract and Ear, vol. 25. Washington, D.C.: Armed Forces Institute of Pathology; 1988:201–206

[109] Howie TO. A case of dermoid or developmental cyst of the middle-ear cavity. J Laryngol Otol. 1962; 76:62–66

[110] Logue V, Till K. Posterior fossa dermoid cysts with special reference to intracranial infection. J Neurol Neurosurg Psychiatry. 1952; 15(1):1–12

[111] Nakagawa K, Ohno K, Nojiri T, Hirakawa K. [Interdural dermoid cyst of the cavernous sinus presenting with oculomotor palsy: case report]. No Shinkei Geka. 1997; 25(9):847–851

[112] North KN, Antony JH, Johnston IH. Dermoid of cavernous sinus resulting in isolated oculomotor nerve palsy. Pediatr Neurol. 1993; 9(3):221–223

[113] Phillips WE, II, Martinez CR, Cahill DW. Ruptured intracranial dermoid tumor secondary to closed head trauma: computed tomography and magnetic resonance imaging. J Neuroimaging. 1994; 4(3):169–170

[114] Carvalho GA, Cervio A, Matthies C, Samii M. Subarachnoid fat dissemination after resection of a cerebellopontine angle dysontogenic cyst: case report and review of the literature. Neurosurgery. 2000; 47(3):760–763, discussion 763–764

[115] Cavazzani P, Ruelle A, Michelozzi G, Andrioli G. Spinal dermoid cysts originating intracranial fat drops causing obstructive hydrocephalus: case reports. Surg Neurol. 1995; 43(5):466–469, discussion 469–470

[116] Karabulut N, Oguzkurt L. Tetraventricular hydrocephalus due to ruptured intracranial dermoid cyst. Eur Radiol. 2000; 10(11):1810–1811

[117] Larsson EM, Brandt L, Holtås S. Persisting intraventricular fat-fluid levels following surgery on a ruptured dermoid cyst of the posterior fossa. Acta Radiol. 1987; 28(4):489–490

[118] Martin R, Knone A, Schuknecht B, Kuhn W. Rapid development of occlusion hydrocephalus by intraventricular fat possibly derived from a ruptured dermoid cyst. J Neurol Neurosurg Psychiatry. 1989; 52(1):134–135

[119] Ahmad I, Tominaga T, Ogawa A, Yoshimoto T. Ruptured suprasellar dermoid associated with middle cerebral artery aneurysm: case report. Surg Neurol. 1992; 38(5):341–346

[120] Ford K, Drayer B, Osborne D, Dubois P. Case report: transient cerebral ischemia as a manifestation of ruptured intracranial dermoid cyst. J Comput Assist Tomogr. 1981; 5(6):895–897

[121] Mikhael MA. Transient spasm of carotid siphon complicating ruptured cranial dermoid cyst. Radiology. 1982; 144(4):824

[122] Ecker RD, Atkinson JL, Nichols DA. Delayed ischemic deficit after resection of a large intracranial dermoid: case report and review of the literature. Neurosurgery. 2003; 52(3):706–710

[123] Messori A, Polonara G, Serio A, Gambelli E, Salvolini U. Expanding experience with spontaneous dermoid rupture in the MRI era: diagnosis and follow-up. Eur J Radiol. 2002; 43(1):19–27

[124] Oursin C, Wetzel SG, Lyrer P, Bächli H, Stock KW. Ruptured intracranial dermoid cyst. J Neurosurg Sci. 1999; 43(3):217–220, discussion 220–221

[125] Lepintre J, Labrune M. [Congenital dermal fistulae communicating with the central nervous system. 21 operated cases in children]. Neurochirurgie. 1970; 16(4):335–348

[126] Hamel E, Frowein RA, Karimi-Nejad A. Intracranial intradural epidermoids and dermoids: surgical results of 38 cases. Neurosurg Rev. 1980; 3 (4):215–219

[127] Sweeney AD, Osetinsky LM, Carlson ML, et al. The natural history and management of petrous apex cholesterol granulomas. Otol Neurotol. 2015; 36(10):1714–1719

[128] Raghavan D, Lee TC, Curtin HD. Cholesterol granuloma of the petrous apex: a 5-year review of radiology reports with follow-up of progression and treatment. J Neurol Surg B Skull Base. 2015; 76(4):266–271

[129] Eytan DF, Kshettry VR, Sindwani R, Woodard TD, Recinos PF. Surgical outcomes after endoscopic management of cholesterol granulomas of the petrous apex: a systematic review. Neurosurg Focus. 2014; 37(4):E14

[130] Cömert E, Cömert A, Çay N, Tunçel Ü, Tekdemir İ. Surgical anatomy of the infralabyrinthine approach. Otolaryngol Head Neck Surg. 2014; 151(2):301–307

[131] Scopel TF, Fernandez-Miranda JC, Pinheiro-Neto CD, et al. Petrous apex cholesterol granulomas: endonasal versus infracochlear approach. Laryngoscope. 2012; 122(4):751–761

[132] Bright R. Diseases of the Brain and Nervous System, Part I. London: Longman, Resse, Orme, Brown and Green; 1831:437–439

[133] Maunsell H. Subtentorial hydatid tumor removed by trephining: recovery. N Z Med J. 1889; 2:151–156

[134] Mullin W. Circumscribed arachnoid cyst giving symptoms of an acoustic neuroma. Trans Am Otol Soc. 1932; 22:72–101

[135] Aubry M, Ombredanne M. Etude Oto-Neurologique et Chirurgicale du Vertige. Indications et Resultats De la Chirurgie Intracranienne Du Nerf Auditif. Paris: Masson and Cie; 1937:100–122

[136] Lehman RA, Fieger HG, Jr. Arachnoid cyst producing recurrent neurological disturbances. Surg Neurol. 1978; 10(2):134–136

[137] Alker GJ, Jr, Glasauer FE, Leslie EV. Radiology of a large cisterna magna cyst: a case report. Arch Neurol. 1979; 36(6):376–379

[138] di Rocco C, Caldarelli M, di Trapani G. Infratentorial arachnoid cysts in children. Childs Brain. 1981; 8(2):119–133

[139] Handa J, Nakano Y, Aii H. CT cisternography with intracranial arachnoidal cysts. Surg Neurol. 1977; 8(6):451–454

[140] McDonald JV, Colgan J. Arachnoidal cysts of posterior fossa: their pneumoencephalographic appearance. Neurology. 1964; 14:643–646

[141] Williams B. Subarachnoid pouches of the posterior fossa with syringomyelia. Acta Neurochir (Wien). 1979; 47(3–4):187–217

[142] Pappas DG, Brackmann DE. Arachnoid cysts of the posterior fossa. Otolaryngol Head Neck Surg. 1981; 89(2):328–332

[143] Gomez MR, Yanagihara T, MacCarty CS. Arachnoid cyst of the cerebellopontine angle and infantile spastic hemiplegia: case report. J Neurosurg. 1968; 29(1):87–90

[144] Jallo GI, Woo HH, Meshki C, Epstein FJ, Wisoff JH. Arachnoid cysts of the cerebellopontine angle: diagnosis and surgery. Neurosurgery. 1997; 40(1):31–37, discussion 37–38

[145] Buongiorno G, Ricca G. Supratentorial arachnoid cyst mimicking a Ménière's disease attack. J Laryngol Otol. 2003; 117(9):728–730

[146] Thijssen HO, Marres EH, Slooff JL. Arachnoid cyst simulating intrameatal acoustic neuroma. Neuroradiology. 1976; 11(4):205–207

[147] Isaacson B, Coker NJ, Vrabec JT, Yoshor D, Oghalai JS. Invasive cerebrospinal fluid cysts and cephaloceles of the petrous apex. Otol Neurotol. 2006; 27(8):1131–1141

[148] Kandenwein JA, Richter HP, Börm W. Surgical therapy of symptomatic arachnoid cysts—an outcome analysis. Acta Neurochir (Wien). 2004; 146(12):1317–1322

[149] Sinha S, Brown JI. Familial posterior fossa arachnoid cyst. Childs Nerv Syst. 2004; 20(2):100–103

[150] Bohrer PS, Chole RA. Unusual lesions of the internal auditory canal. Am J Otol. 1996; 17(1):143–149

[151] Cheung SW, Broberg TG, Jackler RK. Petrous apex arachnoid cyst: radiographic confusion with primary cholesteatoma. Am J Otol. 1995; 16(5):690–694

[152] Batra A, Tripathi RP, Singh AK, Tatke M. Petrous apex arachnoid cyst extending into Meckel's cave. Australas Radiol. 2002; 46(3):295–298

[153] Schuknecht HF, Gao YZ. Arachnoid cyst in the internal auditory canal. Ann Otol Rhinol Laryngol. 1983; 92 6 Pt 1:535–541

[154] Abbott R. The endoscopic management of arachnoidal cysts. Neurosurg Clin N Am. 2004; 15(1):9–17

[155] Falcioni M, Caruso A, Taibah A, et al. Arachnoid cysts of the petrous apex in a patient with vestibular schwannoma. Otolaryngol Head Neck Surg. 2000; 123(5):657–658

[156] Kacker A, Bent JP, Abbott R. Non-communicating arachnoid cyst of the temporal bone presenting as facial nerve paralysis in an infant. Int J Pediatr Otorhinolaryngol. 1999; 49(2):151–154

[157] Wester K. Peculiarities of intracranial arachnoid cysts: location, sidedness, and sex distribution in 126 consecutive patients. Neurosurgery. 1999; 45(4):775–779

[158] Galassi E, Tognetti F, Frank F, Fagioli L, Nasi MT, Gaist G. Infratentorial arachnoid cysts. J Neurosurg. 1985; 63(2):210–217

[159] Higashi S, Yamashita J, Yamamoto Y, Izumi K. Hemifacial spasm associated with a cerebellopontine angle arachnoid cyst in a young adult. Surg Neurol. 1992; 37(4):289–292

[160] Hoffman HJ, Hendrick EB, Humphreys RP, Armstrong EA. Investigation and management of suprasellar arachnoid cysts. J Neurosurg. 1982; 57(5):597–602

[161] Allen A, Wiegmann TB, MacDougall ML. Arachnoid cyst in a patient with autosomal-dominant polycystic kidney disease. Am J Kidney Dis. 1986; 8(2):128–130

[162] Kara B, Kayserili H, Imer M, Calişkan M, Ozmen M. Quadrigeminal cistern arachnoid cyst in a patient with Kabuki syndrome. Pediatr Neurol. 2006; 34 (6):478–480

[163] Hajje MJ, Nachanakian A, Haddad J. [Goldenhar syndrome and arachnoid cyst]. Arch Pediatr. 2003; 10(4):353–354

[164] Welch KO, Tekin M, Nance WE, Blanton SH, Arnos KS, Pandya A. Chudley-McCullough syndrome: expanded phenotype and review of the literature. Am J Med Genet A. 2003; 119A(1):71–76

[165] Masuno M, Fukushima Y, Sugio Y, Kuroki Y. Partial distal 12q trisomy with arachnoid cyst. Jinrui Idengaku Zasshi. 1987; 32(1):39–43

[166] Balci S, Oguz KK. Cri-du-chat syndrome associated with arachnoid cyst causing triventricular hydrocephalus. Clin Dysmorphol. 2001; 10(4):289–290

[167] Hald JK, Nakstad PH, Skjeldal OH, Strømme P. Bilateral arachnoid cysts of the temporal fossa in four children with glutaric aciduria type I. AJNR Am J Neuroradiol. 1991; 12(3):407–409

[168] Martínez-Lage JF, Casas C, Fernández MA, Puche A, Rodriguez Costa T, Poza M. Macrocephaly, dystonia, and bilateral temporal arachnoid cysts: glutaric aciduria type 1. Childs Nerv Syst. 1994; 10(3):198–203

[169] Jamjoom ZA, Okamoto E, Jamjoom AH, al-Hajery O, Abu-Melha A. Bilateral arachnoid cysts of the sylvian region in female siblings with glutaric aciduria type I: report of two cases. J Neurosurg. 1995; 82(6):1078–1081

[170] Renner C, Razeghi S, Uberall MA, Hartmann P, Lehnert W. Clinically asymptomatic glutaric aciduria type I in a 4 5/12-year-old girl with bilateral temporal arachnoid cysts. J Inherit Metab Dis. 1997; 20(6):840–841

[171] Lütcherath V, Waaler PE, Jellum E, Wester K. Children with bilateral temporal arachnoid cysts may have glutaric aciduria type 1 (GAT1); operation without knowing that may be harmful. Acta Neurochir (Wien). 2000; 142 (9):1025–1030

[172] Handa J, Okamoto K, Sato M. Arachnoid cyst of the middle cranial fossa: report of bilateral cysts in siblings. Surg Neurol. 1981; 16(2):127–130

[173] Pomeranz S, Constantini S, Lubetzki-Korn I, Amir N. Familial intracranial arachnoid cysts. Childs Nerv Syst. 1991; 7(2):100–102

[174] Tolmie JL, Day R, Fredericks B, Galea P, Moffett AW. Dominantly inherited cerebral dysplasia: arachnoid cyst associated with mild mental handicap in a mother and her son. J Med Genet. 1997; 34(12):1018–1020

[175] Nager G. Epidermoids (congenital cholesteatomas). In: Nager G, ed. Pathology of the Ear and Temporal Bone, vol. I. Baltimore, MD: Williams & Wilkins; 1993:710–742

[176] Starkman SP, Brown TC, Linell EA. Cerebral arachnoid cysts. J Neuropathol Exp Neurol. 1958; 17(3):484–500

[177] Moore KR, Fischbein NJ, Harnsberger HR, et al. Petrous apex cephaloceles. AJNR Am J Neuroradiol. 2001; 22(10):1867–1871

[178] Prichard CN, Isaacson B, Oghalai JS, Coker NJ, Vrabec JT. Adult spontaneous CSF otorrhea: correlation with radiographic empty sella. Otolaryngol Head Neck Surg. 2006; 134(5):767–771

[179] Foley KM, Posner JB. Does pseudotumor cerebri cause the empty sella syndrome? Neurology. 1975; 25(6):565–569

[180] Weisberg LA. Housepian EM, Saur DP. Empty sella syndrome as complication of benign intracranial hypertension. J Neurosurg. 1975; 43(2):177–180

[181] Go KG, Houthoff HJ, Blaauw EH, Havinga P, Hartsuiker J. Arachnoid cysts of the sylvian fissure. Evidence of fluid secretion. J Neurosurg. 1984; 60(4):803–813

[182] Schuhmann MU, Tatagiba M, Hader C, Brandis A, Samii M. Ectopic choroid plexus within a juvenile arachnoid cyst of the cerebellopontine angle: cause of cyst formation or reason of cyst growth. Pediatr Neurosurg. 2000; 32(2):73–76

[183] Tirakotai W, Schulte DM, Bauer BL, Bertalanffy H, Hellwig D. Neuroendoscopic surgery of intracranial cysts in adults. Childs Nerv Syst. 2004; 20(11–12):842–851

[184] Rengachary SS, Watanabe I. Ultrastructure and pathogenesis of intracranial arachnoid cysts. J Neuropathol Exp Neurol. 1981; 40(1):61–83

[185] Vaquero J, Carrillo R, Cabezudo JM, Nombela L, Bravo G. Arachnoid cysts of the posterior fossa. Surg Neurol. 1981; 16(2):117–121

[186] Garcia-Bach M, Isamat F, Vila F. Intracranial arachnoid cysts in adults. Acta Neurochir Suppl (Wien). 1988; 42:205–209

[187] Eskandary H, Sabba M, Khajehpour F, Eskandari M. Incidental findings in brain computed tomography scans of 3000 head trauma patients. Surg Neurol. 2005; 63(6):550–553

[188] Hadley MN, Grahm TW, Daspit CP, Spetzler RF. Otolaryngologic manifestations of posterior fossa arachnoid cysts. Laryngoscope. 1985; 95(6):678–681

[189] Haberkamp TJ, Monsell EM, House WF, Levine SC, Piazza L. Diagnosis and treatment of arachnoid cysts of the posterior fossa. Otolaryngol Head Neck Surg. 1990; 103(4):610–614

[190] Pollice PA, Bhatti NI, Niparko JK. Imaging quiz case 1: posterior fossa arachnoid cyst. Arch Otolaryngol Head Neck Surg. 1997; 123(7):762–, 764–765

[191] Sumner TE. Benton C, Marshak G. Arachnoid cyst of the internal auditory canal producing facial paralysis in a three-year-old child. Radiology. 1975; 114(2):425–426

[192] Bonora G, Manzoni D, Frattini D, Gruppioni A, De la Pierre L. [Facial paralysis secondary to arachnoid cysts: description of a case in a girl with precocious puberty]. Pediatr Med Chir. 1989; 11(3):343–345

[193] Diwan AG, Agarwal SI, Lakade SM, Krishna KK. Facial paralysis due to arachnoid cyst. J Assoc Physicians India. 2005; 53:544

[194] Babu R, Murali R. Arachnoid cyst of the cerebellopontine angle manifesting as contralateral trigeminal neuralgia: case report. Neurosurgery. 1991; 28(6):886–887

[195] Nakano H, Ogashiwa M. Complete remission of narcolepsy after surgical treatment of an arachnoid cyst in the cerebellopontine angle. J Neurol Neurosurg Psychiatry. 1995; 58(2):264

[196] Gelabert-González M. [Intracranial arachnoid cysts]. Rev Neurol. 2004; 39(12):1161–1166

[197] Becker T, Wagner M, Hofmann E, Warmuth-Metz M, Nadjmi M. Do arachnoid cysts grow? A retrospective CT volumetric study. Neuroradiology. 1991; 33(4):341–345

[198] Punzo A, Conforti R, Martiniello D, Scuotto A, Bernini FP, Cioffi FA. Surgical indications for intracranial arachnoid cysts. Neurochirurgia (Stuttg). 1992; 35(2):35–42

[199] Ehrensberger J, Gysler R, Illi OE, et al. Congenital intracranial cysts: clinical findings, diagnosis, treatment and follow-up. A multicenter, retrospective long-term evaluation of 72 children. Eur J Pediatr Surg. 1993; 3(6):323–334

[200] McCullough DC, Harbert JC, Manz HJ. Large arachnoid cysts at the cranial base. Neurosurgery. 1980; 6(1):76–81

[201] Chao TK. Middle cranial fossa arachnoid cysts causing sensorineural hearing loss. Eur Arch Otorhinolaryngol. 2005; 262(11):925–927

[202] Mason TB, II, Chiriboga CA, Feldstein NA, Kartha K, Khandji AG. Massive intracranial arachnoid cyst in a developmentally normal infant: case report and literature review. Pediatr Neurol. 1997; 16(1):59–62

[203] Anderson FM, Segall HD, Caton WL. Use of computerized tomography scanning in supratentorial arachnoid cysts: a report on 20 children and four adults. J Neurosurg. 1979; 50(3):333–338

[204] Ciricillo SF, Cogen PH, Harsh GR, Edwards MS. Intracranial arachnoid cysts in children: a comparison of the effects of fenestration and shunting. J Neurosurg. 1991; 74(2):230–235

[205] Harsh GRT, IV, Edwards MS, Wilson CB. Intracranial arachnoid cysts in children. J Neurosurg. 1986; 64(6):835–842

[206] Samii M, Carvalho GA, Schuhmann MU, Matthies C. Arachnoid cysts of the posterior fossa. Surg Neurol. 1999; 51(4):376–382

[207] Raffel C, McComb JG. To shunt or to fenestrate: which is the best surgical treatment for arachnoid cysts in pediatric patients? Neurosurgery. 1988; 23(3):338–342

[208] Levy ML, Meltzer HS, Hughes S, Aryan HE, Yoo K, Amar AP. Hydrocephalus in children with middle fossa arachnoid cysts. J Neurosurg. 2004; 101(1) Suppl:25–31

[209] Schick B, Draf W, Kahle G, Weber R, Wallenfang T. Occult malformations of the skull base. Arch Otolaryngol Head Neck Surg. 1997; 123(1):77–80

[210] Mulcahy MM, McMenomey SO, Talbot JM, Delashaw JB, Jr. Congenital encephalocele of the medial skull base. Laryngoscope. 1997; 107(7):910–914

42 Fibro-Osseous Lesions of the Skull Base

Panagiotis Kerezoudis, Kyle D. Perry, Colin L. W. Driscoll, and Michael J. Link

Summary

Fibrous dysplasia is a degenerative bone disorder characterized by the replacement of normal bone with abnormal fibrous tissue. This challenging condition often necessitates a multidisciplinary approach for optimal screening and management of the affected individuals. In the absence of comorbidities, such as growth hormone (GH) excess or secondary bone disorders, these lesions are typically slow-growing, without any significant functional consequences. For patients who have enlarging bony mass and associated cosmetic problems, it is recommended that surgical management be postponed until after skeletal maturity is achieved, when lesions typically are quiescent and progress more slowly. Surgical resection or contouring of the abnormal bone with immediate skull reconstruction might be warranted when new symptoms appear or rapid lesion growth is observed; in such cases the patient should be informed of the risk of regrowth. Medical management is primarily used for the management of refractory pain at the lesion site, which these patients commonly experience. Biphosphonates are one of the most frequently prescribed and effective medications. In the absence of symptomatic cranial nerve involvement, such as optic nerve compression, or external auditory canal narrowing, conservative management is preferred. Evidence of rapid lesion growth, new onset of pain or paresthesias, or visual or hearing changes may require immediate surgical referral and evaluation. Considering the unpredictable course and recurrent nature of the disease, meticulous long-term follow-up of this patient population is of paramount importance.

Keywords: fibrous dysplasia, skull base, surgery, adults, pediatrics

42.1 Introduction

Fibrous dysplasia (FD) is a benign genetic bone disorder that is characterized by the replacement of normal bone with abnormal fibrous tissue proliferation.[1,2] The first report in the literature is credited to Dr. von Recklinghausen (1891), who more than a century ago described, patients who had a pathologic condition of the bone that was characterized by deformity and fibrotic changes, which he called osteitis fibrosa generalisata.[3] The term *fibrous dysplasia* was introduced by Lichtenstein in 1938.[4] Finally, in 1937, McCune, Albright, and colleagues recognized the entity of osteodystrophia fibrosa disseminata, defined by endocrinopathies, cutaneous hyperpigmentation, and precocious puberty in females associated with polyostotic FD.[5,6] The differential diagnosis often includes Paget's disease, intraosseous meningioma, or metastasis (▶ Table 42.1).

42.2 Illustrative Case

A 20-year-old right-handed man with a past medical history of severe FD involving the left skull base presented with enlarging

Table 42.1 Differential diagnosis of skull base fibrous dysplasia in children and adults

Differential diagnosis	How to differentiate
Paget's disease	Predilection for cranial vault Spares facial bones Affects older people
Cemento-ossifying fibroma	Usually more well-defined Smooth margins Tumorlike concentric expansion
Intraosseous meningioma	Presence of intracranial compartment Dural tail sign
Metastases	Typically associated with little expansion and avid contrast enhancement

occipital mass and progressive left-sided hearing loss. He had prior surgical history of left external auditory canaloplasty for his hearing loss. For a short period his hearing had improved, but serial imaging suggested progression of the FD with restenosis of the left external auditory canal (EAC). He also complained of constant tinnitus and suffered with repeated cerumen impaction. Additionally, he reported a long history of headaches, occipital in nature, that started at age 15, usually lasting 15 minutes to 48 hours. Review of symptoms and clinical examination did not reveal any signs or symptoms of cranial nerve compression. Audiogram was consistent with conductive hearing loss. Brain CT imaging revealed progressive enlargement of his temporo-occipital mass, with scattered areas of cystic degeneration as well as significant narrowing of the EAC (▶ Fig. 42.1; ▶ Fig. 42.2).

MRI showed only mild evidence of brain parenchyma compression and no radiographic findings of secondary Chiari's malformation (▶ Fig. 42.3). Digital subtraction angiography was notable for narrowing of the left sigmoid sinus (▶ Fig. 42.4).

Out of concern for possible malignant transformation of the lesion—considering the prominent cystic degeneration, the nondurable canaloplasty, and the worsening hearing loss—an operation was offered to resect a large portion of the occipital bone FD and to more thoroughly decompress the stenotic EAC. Accordingly, the patient underwent bioccipital craniectomy, resection of the dysplastic bone, left mastoidectomy and partial petrosectomy, decompression of the sigmoid sinus, and revision canaloplasty of the left EAC. At 7-year follow-up, the residual FD remained radiographically stable in size and the EAC was still patent.

42.3 Incidence and Epidemiology

FD is a relatively rare disease, accounting for approximately 7% of benign bone lesions.[7] The true incidence is unknown, as many cases are asymptomatic. It can be divided into three forms. Monostotic, involving only one bone, is the mildest and most common form, representing about 70% of all cases.[1] It is typically diagnosed during the second or third decade of life,

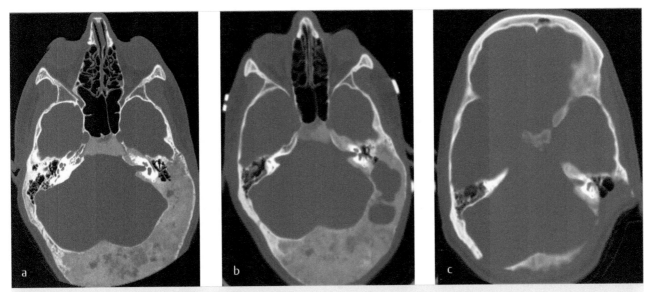

Fig. 42.1 (a) Axial CT scan of the head shows changes consistent with fibrous dysplasia involving the occipital and temporal bones. (b) Follow-up CT after 5 years, on the date of surgery, reveals significant cystic degenerative change. (c) Four-month postoperative CT shows good decompression contour to the patient.

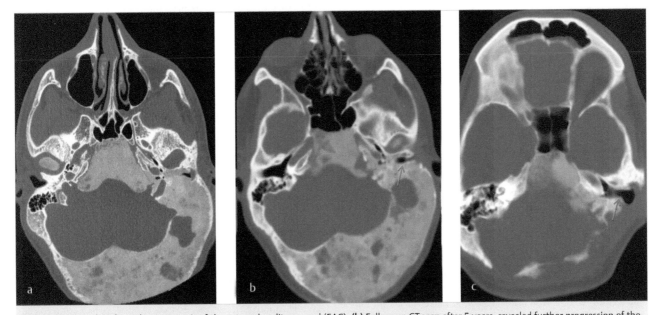

Fig. 42.2 (a) Axial CT from shows stenosis of the external auditory canal (EAC). (b) Follow-up CT scan after 5 years, revealed further progression of the fibrous dysplasia, and the patient was experiencing increasing difficulty with hearing and cerumen impaction. (c) Axial CT 4 months after EAC decompression showing a widely patent intact EAC (*red arrow*).

primarily involving the femur, the ribs, and the craniofacial bones.[8,9,10] The polyostotic form (approximately 30%) has an earlier onset, most often in childhood, with extensive and severe skeletal and craniofacial involvement. The last and most serious form of the disorder, McCune-Albright syndrome (MAS; less than 3% of cases), is associated with short stature secondary to premature closure of the epiphyses as well as endocrine abnormalities and pigmented cutaneous lesions.[5,6] Other syndromes within the spectrum of polyostotic FD are Jaffe-Lichtenstein syndrome, which is characterized by cafe-au-lait skin lesions, and

Mazabraud syndrome, which is defined by the presence of intramuscular myxomas.[7,11]

The incidence of craniofacial involvement in FD has been reported to be 10 to 25% in the monostotic form and 50 to 90% in the polyostotic form.[12,13,14] Lesions in FD are typically slow-growing and are often identified incidentally, particularly in the monostotic forms, or when facial asymmetry and gradual swelling become apparent. Also, FD may be discovered when cranial imaging with CT or MRI is performed for nonspecific symptoms such as headache.

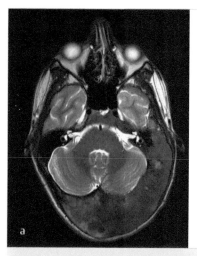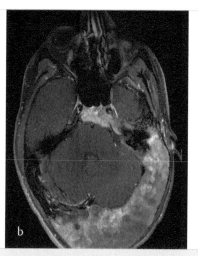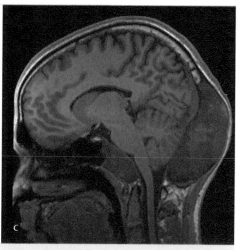

Fig. 42.3 Head MRIs, February 2008. **(a)** Axial T2 showing the dysplastic occipital and temporal bone with scattered areas of cystic degeneration. **(b)** Axial T1 postgadolinium reveals heterogeneous contrast enhancement. **(c)** Sagittal T1 shows a prominent bony mass rising from the patient's occiput. There is no evidence of compression of the adjacent brain parenchyma or secondary Chiari's malformation.

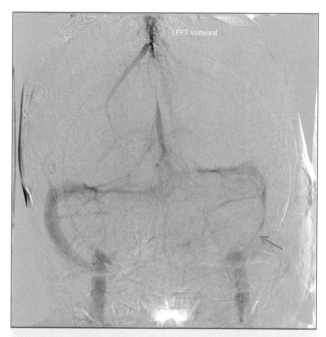

Fig. 42.4 Digital subtraction angiography. The left sigmoid sinus is markedly narrowed (*red arrow*) but appears still patent.

42.4 Pathology

42.4.1 Gene Mutation

FD is a genetic disease caused by somatic mutations (i.e., after fertilization in somatic cells) in the *GNAS1* gene, which is located on chromosome 20q and encodes the alpha subunit of a stimulatory G protein.[15,16] The mutation results in formation of excess cyclic adenosine monophosphate (cAMP) in mutated cells, which in turn is thought to prevent the differentiation of cells within the osteoblastic lineage.[17] This excess of cAMP also contributes to the overexpression of interleukin (IL)-6 by

mutated osteoblastic cells, activating the surrounding osteoclasts and causing the bony lesions to expand.[14,16,17]

Variability in disease severity and progression is related to the stage at which the postzygotic mutation occurred.[14,15,18] Severe disease is typically associated with an early mutational event such that all three germ cell layers (endoderm, mesoderm, and ectoderm) are affected with a more widespread distribution of mutant cells, such as that seen in MAS. It is also postulated that somatic mutations that occur later in life result in a limited distribution of the mutant cells and that the resulting phenotype is less severe, as seen in monostotic FD.[14,15,18] This hypothesis might also provide a biological rationale for monostotic FD's not converting to polyostotic disease over time.

42.4.2 Histologic Findings

FD lesions are characterized by the gradual replacement of normal bone with firm and rubbery fibrous tissue. They are microscopically identifiable by the irregular trabeculae of woven bone intermixed with a connective tissue stroma (▶ Fig. 42.5).[2] Skull lesions tend generally to have a firmer consistency than those in the long bones, which have greater proportion of bony spicules.[19] Furthermore, as lesions expand, they become cystic and can occasionally be vascular. Overall, lesions may vary in bone density as well as in the cellularity and vascularity of the fibrous stroma.[2]

42.4.3 Associated Endocrinopathies

In children, the most commonly encountered endocrinopathy in MAS is precocious puberty, predominantly in girls. In adults, hyperthyroidism, acromegaly, and renal phosphate wasting are the most common endocrine complications of MAS.[18,20] GH excess occurs in approximately 20% of patients who have MAS and has been associated with an increase in the relative risk (RR) for complete encasement of the optic nerve (RR = 4.1) and optic neuropathy (RR = 3.8).[21]

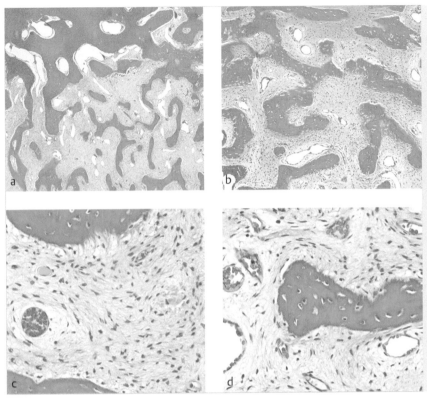

Fig. 42.5 (a) Fibrous dysplasia encapsulated by a well-defined border of sclerotic bone (100 × H&E). (b) Curvilinear bone trabeculae of fibrous dysplasia. The bone lacks the peripheral osteoblasts seen in other entities (200 × H&E). (c) The stroma of fibrous dysplasia is typically composed of bland-appearing fibroblast-like cells with delicate collagen fibers (400 × H&E). (d) High-power examination of the bone in fibrous dysplasia. The trabeculae are often composed of immature woven bone (400 × H&E).

42.4.4 Pain Pathophysiology

Pain is a common manifestation in FD and is often the presenting symptom of the disease.[22,23,24] Although not yet fully elucidated, proposed mechanisms suggest ectopic sprouting and formation of neuroma-like structures by sensory and sympathetic nerve fibers within the dysplastic skeleton.[23] Endogenous stromal cells as well as inflammatory and immune cells accumulate in the area of the lesion and secrete nerve growth factor (NGF), which binds to the TrkA receptor on the nerve fibers, promoting their pathological reorganization and providing an anatomical substrate that promotes skeletal pain.[23,25,26]

42.5 Nonsurgical Management

Currently, no medical treatment option is available to cure or arrest the progression of FD. Conservative management is typically employed in cases of asymptomatic, nondisfiguring lesions, and it primarily aims to control pain symptoms, which are present in up to 67% of patients.[23] Interestingly, pain intensity does not seem to correlate with disease burden. In a study of 78 patients (34 children and 44 adults), adults were more likely to report worse pain scores than children, suggesting an age-related increase in the prevalence of pain in FD.[23]

Pain is commonly undertreated; patients often need multiple analgesic medications, including nonsteroidal anti-inflammatory drugs (NSAIDs) with or without opioids. Biphosphonates, such as alendronate, pamidronate, or zoledronic acid constitute a class of drugs prescribed to patients who have FD for management of pain and reduction of the lesion growth rate.[27,28,29] Clinical studies have demonstrated mixed results with regard to the efficacy of bisphosphonates and FD-related pain, featuring limited

sample sizes and with most studies examining all skeletal regions, not just the craniofacial sites.

In a study by Chapurlat and colleagues, approximately 20% of patients were treated with bisphosphonates, and 75% reported pain relief or improvement from this class of drugs compared with 50% for NSAIDs.[23] Plotkin and colleagues examined 18 children and adolescents who had polyostotic FD or MAS treated using IV pamidronate therapy and noticed a decrease in reported pain, serum alkaline phosphatase, and urinary N-telopeptides.[30] However, they did not notice radiographic or histomorphometric improvement of the FD lesions.[30]

In another report of 13 patients who had MAS and who were treated with pamidronate for 2 to 6 years, a decrease in long bone pain, fracture rate, and bone turnover markers was found, with the most encouraging results in adults.[29] Chan and colleagues followed three children younger than 5 years old who had MAS treated with pamidronate and noted a decrease in long bone pain and fracture rate. The facial lesions remained stable, whereas the lesions located in the long bones continued to expand.[31] Considering this variation in response between children and adults who have FD, and the dubious safety of prolonged bisphosphonate use in children, further studies are needed to provide insight into the effectiveness of biphosphonates for slowing the progression of the lesion and addressing intractable FD pain. Apart from biphosphonates, NSAIDs, and opioids, potential future therapeutic strategies include monoclonal antibodies that block the osteoclast-induced bone remodeling (e.g., denosumab,[32] tocilizumab[33]), as well as blockers of peripheral sensitization (e.g., NGF/TrkA inhibitors). Pregabalin is also considered, having been shown to attenuate neuropathic pain and ectopic reorganization of nerve fibers.[23]

Underlying endocrinopathies, and particularly growth hormone (GH) excess, might accelerate the growth of the lesion. Accordingly, there must be concomitant control and management of the underlying endocrinopathy. Finally, it is worth mentioning that radiotherapy represents a historical treatment option for the management of FD. However, its effectiveness is limited, and it has been shown to be associated with malignant transformation of the lesions.[34]

42.6 Surgical Management

Surgery remains the primary treatment modality for the management of patients who have FD. In general, surgical treatment is generally avoided in young patients; because revision surgery is often necessary, it makes most sense to defer treatment as long as possible in an attempt to reduce the total number of procedures that any single patient might have to endure. It is worth emphasizing, however, that there is always some risk of regrowth, even when surgery is performed after puberty.[14] Kusano and colleagues found in their long-term follow-up of 11 patients that the growth of monostotic FD was arrested in adolescence, but polyostotic FD was less predictable.[35] In cases that warrant surgical intervention, a variety of techniques can be employed, ranging from endoscopic decompression of the orbital walls to contouring or complete orbitofrontal craniotomy with resection of the lesion and immediate reconstruction of the bony defect, such as in patients who have a monostotic or aggressive lesion.[36,37,38]

42.6.1 Restoration of Facial Aesthetics

Surgical intervention for the restoration of facial aesthetics can be performed at any age. The risk of regrowth is greater in younger patients.[39] Accordingly, the literature suggests waiting until patients are beyond puberty and are skeletally mature, with their lesions stable in growth.[40] The selection of excisional surgery over contouring depends on a constellation of factors, including patient age, type of FD, lesion location and growth rate, associated symptoms, aesthetic disturbance, and patient preference. Evidence from the 2000s suggests that a radical approach followed by surgical reconstruction is associated with higher rates of successful elimination of the underlying diseased bone and prevention of relapse.[41] This can be achieved using synthetic materials or using free fibula or autologous rib bone grafts, with good functional and aesthetic results.

42.6.2 Optic Canal Involvement

FD involving the skull base usually affects frontal, ethmoid, sphenoid, and temporal bone.[2,42] Common findings include eye proptosis, hypertelorism, and dystopia, as well as visual loss. Other reported findings include nasolacrimal duct obstruction, lid closure difficulty, trigeminal neuralgia, and extraocular muscle palsy. The optimal management of FD in the region of the optic nerve is a matter of contention among surgeons. Owing to the paucity of large scale studies and long-term follow-up, guidelines on the optimal management of patients who have FD are limited. Overall, patients can be categorized into those who have no evidence of optic neuropathy, who have gradual optic neuropathy, and who have acute visual disturbance.[14]

No Evidence of Optic Neuropathy

Several studies have shown that close observation is an acceptable practice for asymptomatic cases, because optic neuropathy and vision loss are not necessarily the natural progression in encased optic nerves.[8,13,21,38,43,44] Cutler and colleagues reported that 88% of their series (87 patients) had no evidence of optic neuropathy despite complete encasement of the optic nerve by the dysplastic bone.[21] Interestingly, no relationship between patient age and degree of involvement of the optic canal has been established, suggesting that optic canal encasement is not simply an inevitable consequence of increasing age. Lee and colleagues conducted a case–control study of patients who had extensive cranial base FD and concluded that observation with regular ophthalmologic examinations in patients who have asymptomatic encasement is a reasonable treatment option that obviates the need for optic nerve decompression despite significant narrowing of the optic canal.[13]

Surgical intervention should also be avoided in the absence of vision loss or optic neuropathy for fear of potential surgical complications, most notably severe damage to the optic nerve secondary to nerve traction, thermal damage, postoperative edema, or hemorrhage as the main suspected causes. Although steroids have been proposed as well, benefits are based on limited evidence and are transient.[1,45]

Gradual Optic Neuropathy

Optic neuropathy is difficult to evaluate and follow, because the changes may be gradual and subtle, without evidence of papilledema or visual compromise. Clinical observation has shown that a patient's vision decreases in very advanced cases in which the optic canal is severely encased and the optic nerve greatly compressed.[8,13,21,38,43,44] As previously mentioned, GH excess increases the risk of optic neuropathy. Accordingly, referral to an endocrinologist for prompt evaluation of GH excess and hormone suppression is also imperative to disease control. During optic nerve decompression, the surgeon needs to carefully remove the bone surrounding the optic canal using a high-speed drill, with constant irrigation for cooling.[46] Attention should also be paid during endoscopic removal of the optic canal floor, as it might likewise lead to unintentional damage to the optic nerve.[46] Postoperative recovery of visual loss is unfortunately unpredictable and largely depends on the severity and the duration of the preoperative visual loss. In the largest surgical series to date, Chen and colleagues have proposed that visual loss of more than 1 month's duration is not reversible by decompression.[47] The same author team also preserved effective vision in 67% of the patients who were experiencing visual compromise.[47] Similarly, Henderson estimated that 50% of the patients will salvage their vision.[1,48] However, there are reported cases of postoperative blindness following orbital decompression,[1,49] which might be attributed to postoperative edema or occlusion of the ophthalmic artery secondary to thrombosis, hemorrhage, or spasm.[1,49,50,51,52]

Acute Visual Disturbance

Acute visual changes usually develop due to secondary disorders, such as mucocele and aneurysmal bone cyst (ABC).[13,53] Most commonly, acute visual deterioration is thought to occur due to intralesional hemorrhage associated with ABC and subsequent compression of the optic nerve.[37,54] Accordingly, patients who have a documented cystic lesion near the optic canal or who have increased GH require vigilant observation. In cases of acute vision loss, management of increased pressure using acetazolamide with or without steroids and urgent surgical decompression might be indicated.

Temporal Bone Involvement

The temporal bone is commonly affected (> 70%) in patients who have craniofacial polyostotic FD or MAS[55]; nevertheless patients remain asymptomatic in the majority of the cases.[56,57] DeKlotz and colleagues found that nearly 85% of patients had normal or near normal hearing in spite of the high incidence of temporal bone involvement in the polyostotic cases.[55] Ten percent of the patients had conductive hearing loss, and approximately 4% had sensorineural or mixed hearing loss. Furthermore, the degree of hearing loss was mild in most instances (77%) and did not correlate to the amount of disease involvement of the temporal bone.

Hearing loss is attributed to EAC narrowing as a result of the expansile surrounding FD or fixation of the ossicles from adjacent involved bone. The narrowing of the EAC can result in cerumen impaction, external otitis, or cholesteatoma.[55,58] Involvement of the middle ear or Eustachian tube may lead to chronic otitis media and cholesteatoma. Although rare, some case reports have suggested that the contouring and excision of the surrounding dysplastic lesion can lead to exacerbation or regrowth of the lesion in polyostotic forms or in MAS. In more advanced cases, sensorineural hearing loss may occur secondary to impingement of the vestibulocochlear nerve within the internal auditory canal (IAC). Consistent with this, there have been cases of reversal of hearing loss after decompression of the IAC.[59] However, in most cases of sudden or gradual loss, decompression does not result in hearing improvement. Because hearing is fragile and can deteriorate suddenly, some surgeons advocate prophylactic decompression when there is significant and progressive stenosis, hoping thereby to preserve hearing. Evidence of hearing changes on audiometric testing, including auditory brainstem response testing, may help in distinguishing patients who are at higher risk. Interestingly, extensive and progressive disease involving the IAC does not predictably result in sensorineural hearing or vestibular or facial nerve deficits.

In light of these concerns, after the temporal bone is discovered to be involved, a comprehensive audiology examination and periodic exams by an otolaryngologist are recommended. Unless symptoms are severe or progress rapidly, watchful waiting is generally advisable until the growth has slowed or the patient passes puberty. Surgery for the EAC is typically reserved for cases of recurrent otitis externa, canal cholesteatoma, or near total ear canal stenosis. In such cases, canaloplasty with some skin grafting to reline the expanded bony canal is the treatment option. Chance of recurrence is high, however, with almost half of all patients requiring two or more operations.[2] The wider the ear canal is made, the longer another surgery can be avoided, but there may be a less favorable cosmetic outcome.

Finally, another rare finding secondary to temporal bone involvement is facial weakness or paralysis resulting from compression of the facial nerve in the petrous temporal bone.[60,61] Unfortunately, the precise location of the symptomatic compression may be impossible to determine, necessitating extensive surgery through both a middle fossa and a transmastoid approach. In contrast to a sudden sensorineural hearing loss resulting from nerve compression in the IAC, it is more likely that the facial nerve will recover after decompression. Accordingly, a prophylactic decompression of a "threatened" facial nerve is not indicated.

42.6.3 Control of Secondary Lesions

Several types of additional lesions might develop in the setting of the primary FD lesion: benign, such as mucocoele and ABC, and malignant, most often osteosarcoma. These lesions might be responsible for rapid growth and symptom exacerbation. Furthermore, complications such as sinus obstruction or nasal stenosis may require surgical treatment. Treatment in these situations is dictated by the nature of the secondary disorder and requires a multidisciplinary approach.

42.7 Outcomes and Prognosis

The natural history of FD is generally difficult to predict; a study conducted at the National Institutes of Health consisting of 109 patients over 32 years showed that 90% of craniofacial lesions present by the age of 3 to 4 years.[14] According to one study, the average duration of disease progression was 9.8 years and the mean age at arrest of progression 19.2 years.[62,63] Progression of disease is also more rapid with the polyostotic type. Interestingly, it appears that monostotic FD does not progress to polyostotic FD or MAS.[64]

Some studies have suggested that biochemical markers of bone turnover, including serum osteocalcin, bone-specific alkaline phosphatase, and C-terminal type I collagen crosslinks, can be used to monitor disease activity and response to treatment.[18,65]

42.8 Secondary Disorders

Malignant transformation of FD lesions is very rare; it has been estimated to range between 0.5 and 4%, with a mean interval of 15 years from the time of diagnosis.[66,67] The craniofacial region is the most common site of involvement, followed by the femur, tibia, and pelvis.[68] The most frequently reported malignancy is osteosarcoma (68%), followed by various other histologic types, including fibrosarcoma, chondrosarcoma, and malignant fibrohistiocytoma.[66,68,69] Diagnosis might be challenging, particularly in cases of low-grade osteosarcoma.[70,71] In such cases, immunohistochemical analysis of resected specimens with MDM2 and CDK4 may assist in distinguishing FD from a malignancy, for malignancies will often express MDM2 or CDK4.[70,71] Features suggestive of malignant transformation include rapid increase of the lesion size, new onset of pain or tenderness, and changes in imaging characteristics.[68] In such cases, extensive resection with adequate margins is imperative to successful treatment of the lesion.

ABC is another type of lesion that might develop in the setting of a primary FD lesion.[70] This is an uncommon, reactive bone lesion consisting of an arteriovenous malformation. Very few cases of ABCs affecting the cranial bones with FD have been reported.[71]

42.9 Conclusion

In summary, FD is a challenging bone disorder that requires a multidisciplinary approach for optimal screening and management of affected individuals. In the absence of comorbidities, such as GH excess or secondary disorders, these lesions are typically slow-growing, without any functional consequences. To avoid enlarging bony mass and cosmetic problems, it is recommended that surgical management be postponed until after skeletal maturity is achieved, when lesions typically are quiescent and progress more slowly. If new symptoms or rapid lesion growth are observed, then surgical resection or contouring of the abnormal bone with immediate skull reconstruction might be warranted; in such cases the patient should be informed of the risk of regrowth. Medical management is primarily used for management of refractory pain at the lesion site from which these patients commonly suffer. Biphosphonates are one of the most frequently prescribed and effective medications. In the absence of symptomatic cranial nerve involvement, such as optic nerve compression, or EAC narrowing, conservative management is preferred. Evidence of rapid lesion growth, new onset of pain or paresthesias, or visual or hearing changes warrants immediate surgical referral and evaluation. Considering the unpredictable course of the disease, meticulous long-term follow-up of this patient population is of paramount importance.

References

[1] Ricalde P, Horswell BB. Craniofacial fibrous dysplasia of the fronto-orbital region: a case series and literature review. J Oral Maxillofac Surg. 2001; 59(2): 157–167, discussion 167–168

[2] Lustig LR, Holliday MJ, McCarthy EF, Nager GT. Fibrous dysplasia involving the skull base and temporal bone. Arch Otolaryngol Head Neck Surg. 2001; 127 (10):1239–1247

[3] von Recklinghausen FD, Reimer G. Die Fibröse Oder Deformirende Ostitis, Die Osteomalacie Und Die Osteoplastische Carcinose in Ihren Gegenseitigen Beziehungen. Berlin: Georg Reimer; 1891

[4] Lichtenstein L. Polyostotic fibrous dysplasia. Arch Surg. 1938; 36(5):874–898

[5] Albright F, Butler AM, Hampton AO, Smith P. Syndrome characterized by osteitis fibrosa disseminata, areas of pigmentation and endocrine dysfunction, with precocious puberty in females: report of five cases. N Engl J Med. 1937; 216(17):727–746

[6] McCune DJ, Bruch H. Osteodystrophia fibrosa: report of a case in which the condition was combined with precocious puberty, pathologic pigmentation of the skin and hyperthyroidism, with a review of the literature. Am J Dis Child. 1937; 54(4):806–848

[7] Parekh SG, Donthineni-Rao R, Ricchetti E, Lackman RD. Fibrous dysplasia. J Am Acad Orthop Surg. 2004; 12(5):305–313

[8] Lee JS, FitzGibbon EJ, Chen YR, et al. Clinical guidelines for the management of craniofacial fibrous dysplasia. Orphanet J Rare Dis. 2012; 7 Suppl 1:S2

[9] Ippolito E, Bray EW, Corsi A, et al. European Pediatric Orthopaedic Society. Natural history and treatment of fibrous dysplasia of bone: a multicenter clinicopathologic study promoted by the European Pediatric Orthopaedic Society. J Pediatr Orthop B. 2003; 12(3):155–177

[10] Lisle DA, Monsour PAJ, Maskiell CD. Imaging of craniofacial fibrous dysplasia. J Med Imaging Radiat Oncol. 2008; 52(4):325–332

[11] Biagini R, Ruggieri P, Boriani S, Picci P. The Mazabraud syndrome: case report and review of the literature. Ital J Orthop Traumatol. 1987; 13(1):105–111

[12] Rahman AMA, Madge SN, Billing K, et al. Craniofacial fibrous dysplasia: clinical characteristics and long-term outcomes. Eye (Lond). 2009; 23(12): 2175–2181

[13] Lee JS, FitzGibbon E, Butman JA, et al. Normal vision despite narrowing of the optic canal in fibrous dysplasia. N Engl J Med. 2002; 347(21):1670–1676

[14] Ricalde P, Magliocca KR, Lee JS. Craniofacial fibrous dysplasia. Oral Maxillofac Surg Clin North Am. 2012; 24(3):427–441

[15] DiCaprio MR, Enneking WF. Fibrous dysplasia: pathophysiology, evaluation, and treatment. J Bone Joint Surg Am. 2005; 87(8):1848–1864

[16] Riminucci M, Liu B, Corsi A, et al. The histopathology of fibrous dysplasia of bone in patients with activating mutations of the Gs α gene: site-specific patterns and recurrent histological hallmarks. J Pathol. 1999; 187 (2):249–258

[17] Bianco P, Riminucci M, Majolagbe A, et al. Mutations of the GNAS1 gene, stromal cell dysfunction, and osteomalacic changes in non-McCune-Albright fibrous dysplasia of bone. J Bone Miner Res. 2000; 15(1):120–128

[18] Chapurlat RD, Orcel P. Fibrous dysplasia of bone and McCune–Albright syndrome. Best Pract Res Clin Rheumatol. 2008; 22(1):55–69

[19] Nager GT, Kennedy DW, Kopstein E. Fibrous dysplasia: a review of the disease and its manifestations in the temporal bone. Ann Otol Rhinol Laryngol Suppl. 1982; 92:1–52

[20] Collins MT, Chebli C, Jones J, et al. Renal phosphate wasting in fibrous dysplasia of bone is part of a generalized renal tubular dysfunction similar to that seen in tumor-induced osteomalacia. J Bone Miner Res. 2001; 16(5): 806–813

[21] Cutler CM, Lee JS, Butman JA, et al. Long-term outcome of optic nerve encasement and optic nerve decompression in patients with fibrous dysplasia: risk factors for blindness and safety of observation. Neurosurgery. 2006; 59(5): 1011–1017, discussion 1017–1018

[22] Kelly MH, Brillante B, Collins MT. Pain in fibrous dysplasia of bone: age-related changes and the anatomical distribution of skeletal lesions. Osteoporos Int. 2008; 19(1):57–63

[23] Chapurlat RD, Gensburger D, Jimenez-Andrade JM, Ghilardi JR, Kelly M, Mantyh P. Pathophysiology and medical treatment of pain in fibrous dysplasia of bone. Orphanet J Rare Dis. 2012; 7 Suppl 1:S3

[24] Chapurlat RD, Delmas PD, Liens D, Meunier PJ. Long-term effects of intravenous pamidronate in fibrous dysplasia of bone. J Bone Miner Res. 1997; 12 (10):1746–1752

[25] Skaper SD, Pollock M, Facci L. Mast cells differentially express and release active high molecular weight neurotrophins. Brain Res Mol Brain Res. 2001; 97 (2):177–185

[26] Ehrhard PB, Erb P, Graumann U, Otten U. Expression of nerve growth factor and nerve growth factor receptor tyrosine kinase Trk in activated CD4-positive T-cell clones. Proc Natl Acad Sci U S A. 1993; 90(23):10984–10988

[27] Liens D, Delmas PD, Meunier PJ. Long-term effects of intravenous pamidronate in fibrous dysplasia of bone. Lancet. 1994; 343(8903):953–954

[28] Chao K, Katznelson L. Use of high-dose oral bisphosphonate therapy for symptomatic fibrous dysplasia of the skull. J Neurosurg. 2008; 109(5): 889–892

[29] Matarazzo P, Lala R, Masi G, Andreo M, Altare F, de Sanctis C. Pamidronate treatment in bone fibrous dysplasia in children and adolescents with McCune-Albright syndrome. J Pediatr Endocrinol Metab. 2002; 15 Suppl 3: 929–937

[30] Plotkin H, Rauch F, Zeitlin L, Munns C, Travers R, Glorieux FH. Effect of pamidronate treatment in children with polyostotic fibrous dysplasia of bone. J Clin Endocrinol Metab. 2003; 88(10):4569–4575

[31] Chan B, Zacharin M. Pamidronate treatment of polyostotic fibrous dysplasia: failure to prevent expansion of dysplastic lesions during childhood. J Pediatr Endocrinol Metab. 2006; 19(1):75–80

[32] Boyce AM, Chong WH, Yao J, et al. Denosumab treatment for fibrous dysplasia. J Bone Miner Res. 2012; 27(7):1462–1470

[33] Tocilizumab in fibrous dysplasia of bone, ClinicalTrials.gov. https://clinicaltrials.gov/ct2/show/NCT01791842. Accessed April 1, 2017

[34] Edgerton MT, Persing JA, Jane JA. The surgical treatment of fibrous dysplasia: with emphasis on recent contributions from cranio-maxillo-facial surgery. Ann Surg. 1985; 202(4):459–479

[35] Kusano T, Hirabayashi S, Eguchi T, Sugawara Y. Treatment strategies for fibrous dysplasia. J Craniofac Surg. 2009; 20(3):768–770

[36] Pletcher SD, Metson R. Endoscopic optic nerve decompression for nontraumatic optic neuropathy. Arch Otolaryngol Head Neck Surg. 2007; 133(8): 780–783

[37] Amit M, Fliss DM, Gil Z. Fibrous dysplasia of the sphenoid and skull base. Otolaryngol Clin North Am. 2011; 44(4):891–902, vii–viii

[38] Tan Y-C, Yu C-C, Chang C-N, Ma L, Chen Y-R. Optic nerve compression in craniofacial fibrous dysplasia: the role and indications for decompression. Plast Reconstr Surg. 2007; 120(7):1957–1962

[39] Nowinski D, Messo E, Hedlund A, Hirsch J-M. Computer-navigated contouring of craniofacial fibrous dysplasia involving the orbit. J Craniofac Surg. 2011; 22 (2):469–472

[40] Choi JW, Lee SW, Koh KS. Correction of proptosis and zygomaticomaxillary asymmetry using orbital wall decompression and zygoma reduction in craniofacial fibrous dysplasia. J Craniofac Surg. 2009; 20(2):326–330

[41] Valentini V, Cassoni A, Marianetti TM, Terenzi V, Fadda MT, Iannetti G. Craniomaxillofacial fibrous dysplasia: conservative treatment or radical surgery? A retrospective study on 68 patients. Plast Reconstr Surg. 2009; 123 (2):653–660

[42] Van Tilburg W. Fibrous dysplasia. Handb Clin Neurol. 1972; 14:163–212

[43] Chen Y-R, Chang C-N, Tan Y-C. Craniofacial fibrous dysplasia: an update. Chang Gung Med J. 2006; 29(6):543–549

[44] Amit M, Collins MT, FitzGibbon EJ, Butman JA, Fliss DM, Gil Z. Surgery versus watchful waiting in patients with craniofacial fibrous dysplasia—a meta-analysis. PLoS One. 2011; 6(9):e25179

[45] Lei P, Bai H, Wang Y, Liu Q. Surgical treatment of skull fibrous dysplasia. Surg Neurol. 2009; 72 Suppl 1:S17–S20

[46] Chen YR, Breidahl A, Chang CN. Optic nerve decompression in fibrous dysplasia: indications, efficacy, and safety. Plast Reconstr Surg. 1997; 99(1):22–30, discussion 31–33

[47] Henderson JW. Fibro-osseous, osseous, and cartilaginous tumors of orbital bone. Orbital Tumors. 3rd ed. New York, NY: Raven Press, 1994;155–161

[48] Edelstein C, Goldberg RA, Rubino G. Unilateral blindness after ipsilateral prophylactic transcranial optic canal decompression for fibrous dysplasia. Am J Ophthalmol. 1998; 126(3):469–471

[49] Sofferman RA. Harris P. Mosher Award thesis. The recovery potential of the optic nerve. Laryngoscope. 1995; 105(7 Pt 3 Suppl 72):1–38

[50] Leong LTY, Ming BJCC. Craniofacial fibrous dysplasia involving the orbit: a case report and literature review. Asia Pac J Ophthalmol (Phila). 2015; 4(3):151–154

[51] Michael CB, Lee AG, Patrinely JR, Stal S, Blacklock JB. Visual loss associated with fibrous dysplasia of the anterior skull base: case report and review of the literature. J Neurosurg. 2000; 92(2):350–354

[52] Collins MT. Spectrum and natural history of fibrous dysplasia of bone. J Bone Miner Res. 2006; 21 Suppl 2:99–P104

[53] DeKlotz T. Audio-otologic phenotypes of polyostotic fibrous dysplasia. In: Meeting of the American Academy of Otolaryngology San Francisco, CA; 2011

[54] Sataloff RT, Graham MD, Roberts BR. Middle ear surgery in fibrous dysplasia of the temporal bone. Am J Otol. 1985; 6(2):153–156

[55] Megerian CA, Sofferman RA, McKenna MJ, Eavey RD, Nadol JB, Jr. Fibrous dysplasia of the temporal bone: ten new cases demonstrating the spectrum of otologic sequelae. Am J Otol. 1995; 16(4):408–419

[56] Lambert PR, Brackmann DE. Fibrous dysplasia of the temporal bone: the use of computerized tomography. Otolaryngol Head Neck Surg. 1984; 92(4):461–467

[57] Morrissey DD, Michael Talbot J. Fibrous Dysplasia of the Temporal Bone: Reversal of Sensorineural Hearing Loss after Decompression of the Internal Auditory Canall. Laryngoscope. 1997;107(10):1336–1340.

[58] Zaytoun GM, Dagher WI, Rameh CE. Recurrent facial nerve paralysis: an unusual presentation of fibrous dysplasia of the temporal bone. Eur Arch Otorhinolaryngol. 2008; 265(2):255–259

[59] Wang Y-C, Chen Y-A. Fibrous dysplasia of the temporal bone presenting as an external auditory canal mass. Otolaryngol Head Neck Surg. 2009; 141(5):655–656

[60] Maher CO, Friedman JA, Meyer FB, Lynch JJ, Unni K, Raffel C. Surgical treatment of fibrous dysplasia of the skull in children. Pediatr Neurosurg. 2002; 37 (2):87–92

[61] St. Clair EG, McCutcheon IE. Skull tumors. In: Winn H, ed. Youmans Neurological Surgery. Elsevier; 2011:1666–1691

[62] Hart ES, Kelly MH, Brillante B, et al. Onset, progression, and plateau of skeletal lesions in fibrous dysplasia and the relationship to functional outcome. J Bone Miner Res. 2007; 22(9):1468–1474

[63] Chapurlat RD. Medical therapy in adults with fibrous dysplasia of bone. J Bone Miner Res. 2006; 21 Suppl 2:114–119

[64] Reis C, Genden EM, Bederson JB, Som PM. A rare spontaneous osteosarcoma of the calvarium in a patient with long-standing fibrous dysplasia: CT and MR findings. Br J Radiol. 2008; 81(962):e31–e34

[65] Ameli NO, Rahmat H, Abbassioun K. Monostotic fibrous dysplasia of the cranial bones. Neurosurg Rev. 1981; 4(2):71–77

[66] Ruggieri P, Sim FH, Bond JR, Unni KK. Malignancies in fibrous dysplasia. Cancer. 1994; 73(5):1411–1424

[67] Yabut SM, Jr, Kenan S, Sissons HA, Lewis MM. Malignant transformation of fibrous dysplasia: a case report and review of the literature. Clin Orthop Relat Res. 1988(228):281–289

[68] Nishio J, Iwasaki H, Takagi S, et al. Low-grade central osteosarcoma of the metatarsal bone: a clinicopathological, immunohistochemical, cytogenetic and molecular cytogenetic analysis. Anticancer Res. 2012; 32(12):5429–5435

[69] Yoshida A, Ushiku T, Motoi T, et al. Immunohistochemical analysis of MDM2 and CDK4 distinguishes low-grade osteosarcoma from benign mimics. Mod Pathol. 2010; 23(9):1279–1288

[70] Diah E, Morris DE, Lo L-J, Chen Y-R. Cyst degeneration in craniofacial fibrous dysplasia: clinical presentation and management. J Neurosurg. 2007; 107(3):504–508

[71] Itshayek E, Spector S, Gomori M, Segal R. Fibrous dysplasia in combination with aneurysmal bone cyst of the occipital bone and the clivus: case report and review of the literature. Neurosurgery. 2002; 51(3):815–817, discussion 817–818

Index

Note: Page numbers set **bold** or *italic* indicate headings or figures, respectively.

Index